Clinical Veterinary Microbiology

Clinical Veterinary Microbiology

Edited by **Andrea Santoro**

SYRAWOOD
PUBLISHING HOUSE
New York

Published by Syrawood Publishing House,
750 Third Avenue, 9th Floor,
New York, NY 10017, USA
www.syrawoodpublishinghouse.com

Clinical Veterinary Microbiology
Edited by Andrea Santoro

International Standard Book Number: 978-1-68286-065-6 (Hardback)

Printed in the United States of America.

Contents

Preface

Veterinary microbiology focuses on the diseases caused by microbes such as bacteria, etc. primarily among livestock, dairy animals and other domesticated animals. It also covers zoonoses amongst wild animals. This book provides a comprehensive overview of veterinary microbiology. It encompasses relevant research from different parts of the world highlighting microbial genetics, different types of diseases, their management, epidemiology, etc. This book will be beneficial for veterinarians, pharmaceutical research personnel, students, and public health professionals.

Various studies have approached the subject by analyzing it with a single perspective, but the present book provides diverse methodologies and techniques to address this field. This book contains theories and applications needed for understanding the subject from different perspectives. The aim is to keep the readers informed about the progress in the field; therefore, the contributions were carefully examined to compile novel researches by specialists from across the globe.

Indeed, the job of the editor is the most crucial and challenging in compiling all chapters into a single book. In the end, I would extend my sincere thanks to the chapter authors for their profound work. I am also thankful for the support provided by my family and colleagues during the compilation of this book.

Editor

1

Plant-based solutions for veterinary immunotherapeutics and prophylactics

Igor Kolotilin[1], Ed Topp[2†], Eric Cox[3†], Bert Devriendt[3†], Udo Conrad[4†], Jussi Joensuu[5†], Eva Stöger[6†], Heribert Warzecha[7†], Tim McAllister[8†], Andrew Potter[9,10†], Michael D McLean[11†], J Christopher Hall[12†] and Rima Menassa[1,2*]

Abstract

An alarming increase in emergence of antibiotic resistance among pathogens worldwide has become a serious threat to our ability to treat infectious diseases according to the World Health Organization. Extensive use of antibiotics by livestock producers promotes the spread of new resistant strains, some of zoonotic concern, which increases food-borne illness in humans and causes significant economic burden on healthcare systems. Furthermore, consumer preferences for meat/poultry/fish produced without the use of antibiotics shape today's market demand. So, it is viewed as inevitable by the One Health Initiative that humans need to reduce the use of antibiotics and turn to alternative, improved means to control disease: vaccination and prophylactics. Besides the intense research focused on novel therapeutic molecules, both these strategies rely heavily on the availability of cost-effective, efficient and scalable production platforms which will allow large-volume manufacturing for vaccines, antibodies and other biopharmaceuticals. Within this context, plant-based platforms for production of recombinant therapeutic proteins offer significant advantages over conventional expression systems, including lack of animal pathogens, low production costs, fast turnaround and response times and rapid, nearly-unlimited scalability. Also, because dried leaves and seeds can be stored at room temperature for lengthy periods without loss of recombinant proteins, plant expression systems have the potential to offer lucrative benefits from the development of edible vaccines and prophylactics, as these would not require "cold chain" storage and transportation, and could be administered in mass volumes with minimal processing. Several biotechnology companies currently have developed and adopted plant-based platforms for commercial production of recombinant protein therapeutics. In this manuscript, we outline the challenges in the process of livestock immunization as well as the current plant biotechnology developments aimed to address these challenges.

Table of contents

* Correspondence: rima.menassa@agr.gc.ca
†Equal contributors
[1]Department of Biology, University of Western Ontario, 1151 Richmond St, London, ON, Canada
[2]AAFC, Southern Crop Protection and Food Research Centre, 1391 Sandford St, London, ON, Canada
Full list of author information is available at the end of the article

1. Introduction

The health and well-being of food-bearing animals is a major preoccupation for any livestock, poultry or fish producer. Endemic disease or epidemic outbreaks represent a very significant financial risk to the producer due to loss of animals, production of animals that are not marketable, and reduction in feed conversion efficiency. The potential risk to consumers from contaminated food is an important public health concern, and very significant investments are made by the agri-food industry to ensure safe food products. Nevertheless, an estimated 9.4 million cases of illness due to consumption of food contaminated with known pathogens occurs annually in the United States [1]. Thus, it is critically important that primary producers ensure the health of their livestock for public health, animal welfare and business profitability reasons.

The key to minimizing animal morbidity and mortality is the employment of good production practices. Best practices will vary according to the production system, but land-based agriculture will typically include provision of uncontaminated feed and water, adequate ventilation and air quality, biosecurity, robust surveillance of animal health, and the judicious use of antimicrobial agents and parasiticides for disease prevention and treatment, when warranted. Prominent in the animal health toolbox are antibiotics. It can be reasonable to assume that the availability of antibiotics will become increasingly constrained as legitimate public alarm over the looming spectre of catastrophic antibiotic resistance in human medicine is translated into action at the farm level. Furthermore, the development of antibiotic resistance will progressively reduce antibiotic therapy options available to veterinarians. More restricted use of veterinary antibiotics will result from market-driven forces, as consumers increasingly demand antibiotic-free food, and through the policies of governments and codes of practice of veterinary practitioners that promote judicious use [2]. Within this evolving environment, newly developed vaccines and immunotherapeutic agents offer the potential to lessen the need for antibiotics for disease control, and offer veterinary practitioners much needed tools [3].

The global market for animal vaccines is estimated to be currently worth $5.8 billion, and is anticipated to grow with a compound annual growth rate of 8.1% to a value of $8.6 billion by 2018 [4]. The efficacy of a vaccine, the ease with which it can be employed, and the overall benefit in terms of increased productivity must be competitive with other disease management options. Recent advances in immunology and in biotechnology, specifically the development of methods to produce potent vaccines very cost-effectively using plant-based bioreactors have the potential to make vaccines an even more attractive proposition. Furthermore, in cases where vaccination cannot be used to prevent disease, the production of antibodies in plants for passive immunotherapy and infectious disease control holds great promise.

This review paper will cover animal immunization essentials and will present the latest developments in plant biotechnology for the production of veterinary therapeutics. Specific aspects discussed will include high-level recombinant protein production in plant-based systems, the ability to use unpurified material for treatment, the possibility of oral rather than parenteral delivery, low cost of protein/vaccine production, very short turnaround time from conception to large-scale manufacturing, and the ability to "stack" genes encoding antigens and adjuvants to create potent multi-target vaccines in a single preparation.

2. Immunization of livestock animals

2.1 Active/passive immunization

In contrast to humans, newborn farm animals (foals, piglets, calves, lambs, kids) depend totally, and companion animals (kittens, puppies) almost completely upon uptake of colostral antibodies for their systemic maternal immunity against pathogens [5]. Intestinal uptake occurs via endocytosis, involving the neonatal Fc receptor (FcRn) and is highest immediately after birth and declines rapidly within 24 h as intestinal cells mature and intestinal flora are established. The time of cessation of this macromolecular transport (gut closure) varies by species and immunoglobulin type, ranging between 20 to 36 h of age [6]. For multiparous animal species, the degree of passive immunity can be heterogeneous between litters and among members of a same litter because of variability in colostral absorption. This is true for piglets, puppies and kittens, whose levels of passive antibodies are maximum 36-48 h after birth. From this time on, the immunoglobulin concentrations decline in the serum of the newborn animal. The half-life depends on immunoglobulin isotype, and on the species, varying between 1 to 4 days for IgA and IgM, to approximately 8 to 22 days for canine and equine IgG, respectively [7]. The affinity of IgG for endothelial FcRn most likely accounts for these differences observed in serum half-life among species and different IgG subclasses [7,8]. Also, the growth rate of the animal influences the rate of decline in the level of the maternally-derived antibodies. This is particularly clear in canine species, where dogs belonging to rapid growth breeds eliminate their maternally-derived antibodies more quickly than slow-growth breeds. In addition to differences in uptake of maternal antibodies, the degree of passive immunity is not equal for all tissues. For instance, colostral immunity protects young animals against systemic infection during the first months of life, whereas the respiratory tract mucus is protected only for a few weeks [9].

Shortly after parturition, drastic changes occur in the composition of colostrum with a drastic drop in IgG and IgA. In most domestic animals, the drop in IgA is less pronounced than IgG, so that IgA becomes the most important immunoglobulin in milk [10]. Milk antibodies are essential to protect young animals against intestinal infections. The IgA in the milk is dimeric secretory IgA (SIgA). The dimeric IgA is secreted in the mammary gland tissue by plasma cells, binds with its J chain to the polymeric immunoglobulin receptor (pIgR) expressed at the basolateral site of the alveolar epithelial cells and is endocytosed, transcytosed and exocytosed to the interstitial space after cleavage of the receptor. The extracellular 80 kDa part of pIgR is exceptionally carbohydrate-rich, and when incorporated into the Ig molecules as bound secretory component (SC), it endows SIgA with resistance against proteolytic degradation [11]. In ruminants, IgG concentrations remain higher than IgA, and IgG1 is specifically enriched in colostrum and milk, with levels approximately 10 times higher than IgA or IgG2. The role of FcRn in this transport has not been completely clarified [7,8].

2.2 Induction of protective immunity

At weaning, lactogenic protection disappears, making the young animals highly susceptible to infections with enteropathogens. Most pathogens either colonize the mucosa or invade the host at a mucosal surface. Optimal protection against these pathogens most often involves the induction of pathogen-specific SIgA at the infection site [12]. As such, an optimal vaccine should induce robust mucosal SIgA immune responses.

Parenteral vaccines typically induce IgG, a response that is not particularly effective against these types of infections. The best way to elicit pathogen-specific SIgA is to activate the local mucosa-associated lymphoid tissue (MALT) at the site of colonization or invasion through mucosal vaccination. This necessity to administer vaccines at the mucosal site relating to the pathogen's tropism is further highlighted by the compartmentalization of the mucosal immune system. For example, stimulation of gut-associated lymphoid tissue (GALT) does not induce a protective SIgA response in the respiratory tract, while induction of an immune response at the nasal mucosa fails to induce intestinal protection [11,13]. Taking this into account, the induction of mucosal immunity further requires the vaccine to pass several physiological barriers and defence mechanisms. To reach the inductive sites of the mucosal immune system, whether it is upon oral, intranasal, rectal or urogenital administration, the vaccine has to surmount mucus and antimicrobial peptides and traverse the epithelial barrier. In case of oral administration, the vaccine also needs to survive the low pH in the stomach, digestive enzymes and bile salts and be transported via peristalsis to the GALT. Furthermore, the vaccine has to trigger protective mucosal immunity instead of tolerance, which is the dominant response mode of the mucosal immune system, and this without causing severe inflammation [13]. Fusing vaccine antigens to antibody or antibody fragment to target the subunit vaccine to antigen-sampling routes at the mucosal surfaces, such as transcytotic epithelial receptors, could drastically improve oral vaccine efficacy [14].

Only a limited number of mucosal vaccines have been shown to meet these criteria and, consequently, only a few have been internationally licensed. Of those that have been licensed, most are based on live-attenuated pathogens and a few are inactivated pathogens [15]. No mucosal subunit vaccines have been licensed so far. Whereas many particle systems, such as virus-like particles (VLPs, see text) or other particles have been shown to be immunogenic in mice via the oral route, almost none of these were successful in larger animals or humans [3]. This could be explained by the longer intestinal transit time for these particles to reach the inductive sites in larger mammalian species in contrast with mice. As a result, in larger animals, only a small portion of the particles will reach the GALT, resulting in fewer particles being taken up by M cells and subsequently no or low induction of intestinal mucosal immune responses.

In contrast to particulate systems, soluble antigens are not immunogenic and in general induce tolerance upon mucosal administration even in mice. However, a few soluble antigens have been shown to be immunogenic via the mucosal route, such as cholera toxin (CT), thermolabile enterotoxin (LT) and their B subunits (CTB and LTB) [16], and the purified F4 fimbriae of enterotoxigenic *E. coli* in pigs [17]. These antigens are characterized by the ability to bind to receptors on enterocytes in the small intestine and to be taken up by these epithelial cells [18], followed by induction of an antigen-specific IgA response. Whereas microgram quantities of CTB and LTB are immunogenic, F4 has to be given in milligram amounts [17]. The oral route has the advantage over other routes in that the vaccine antigens can be administered in the feed, eliminating the need to restrain livestock during administration and allowing the use of less-purified antigens.

2.3 Modes of vaccination

2.3.1 Subcutaneous and intramuscular

The delivery of veterinary vaccines, in general, is by injection although there are variations depending upon the animal species being immunized, management practices and age of the animal. For example, virtually all vaccines for cattle are delivered parenterally, while those for use in poultry are delivered by injection, orally, or by aerosol. Ultimately, the route of delivery is dictated largely by the various management systems employed, as well as the ease of handling of individual animals.

There are a number of issues associated with invasive vaccine delivery in food-producing animals, one of which is the economic loss associated with trimming of area surrounding injection site lesions. Many veterinary vaccines are extremely pro-inflammatory in nature, an example being Clostridial vaccines used in cattle. When delivered subcutaneously, these vaccines tend to result in a large swelling which can persist for months. On the other hand, intramuscular injection does not result in overt swelling but causes significant tissue damage near the injection site. The cost associated with carcass trimming has been estimated to be between $1.46 and $40.00 per animal [19]. In addition, it is not uncommon for needles to break during intramuscular delivery, causing problems at processing, as well as the retail level. While injection of the antigens themselves can result in tissue damage, most killed vaccines also contain strong adjuvants which contribute to this damage. Adjuvants significantly increase the cost of the vaccines and also dictate both the quality and magnitude of the immune response, the former of which has been biased towards Th2 immune responses. Adjuvants currently in use are suitable for injection, but most are not compatible with mucosal delivery [20]. To maintain their efficacy, most injectable vaccines require proper refrigeration and storage, a need that can be challenging in extensive livestock operations especially in developing nations.

2.3.2 Intranasal

The delivery of modified live viral vaccines via the intranasal route or in drinking water has been effective. However, live bacterial vaccines are not commonly used, in part due to the use of antibiotics in the industry. Mucosal vaccines are available for swine, including those for *Bordetella bronchiseptica*, where they have been shown to result in enhanced SIgA production following a single administration by the intranasal route [21]. A novel adjuvant platform consisting of CpG ODNs, polyphosphazenes and cationic innate defense regulator peptide (IDR) 1002, has also been tested for efficacy in a swine model and shown to provide a long duration of immunity against *Bordetella pertussis* in mice following a single intranasal administration [22]. Interestingly, this formulation also works in the presence of maternal antibodies [23], making it ideal for mucosal immunization of neonates.

All presently available commercial vaccines targeting the respiratory tract via intranasal, aerosol or conjunctival application are live attenuated or vector vaccines [24]. Nevertheless, there is the potential for using protein vaccines consisting of dead microorganisms or subunits (virulence factors). Immunization of the respiratory tract has been experimentally demonstrated by i) using particulate delivery systems, which are either lipophilic, mucoadhesive and/or contain immunomodulating molecules, ii) using soluble conjugates of antigens (or epitopes) and a carrier, targeting the antigens to the mucosa of the respiratory tract or iii) using soluble antigens. Often, adjuvants are needed for strong mucosal immune responses [25]. Whereas experimental results have been promising in many studies, no dead vaccines for immunization of the respiratory tract have been commercialized, as adverse reactions have hampered their development. Indeed, anaphylaxis due to impurities, or Bell's palsy due to vaccine components have been described [26]. Results from animal studies suggest that the intranasal route may itself facilitate transport of proteins, inactivated vaccines, live viruses or other particles into the central nervous system [27]. Therefore, candidate vaccines targeting the respiratory tract mucosa have to be thoroughly evaluated for adverse effects.

2.3.3 Oral

Oral vaccination, or so called "edible vaccines", have been traditionally viewed as the panacea of plant-produced vaccines in terms of their use as an approach to disease control [28]. Edible vaccines offer several advantages over conventional methods of vaccine delivery. Edible vaccines come in contact with the lining of the digestive tract, thus giving them the potential to stimulate both mucosal and systemic immunity, the former of which is a response that is notoriously difficult to achieve through injections, which bypass mucosal barriers. In part, this accounts for the reason as to why the efficacy of injectable vaccines against intestinal pathogens has generally been quite poor.

Edible vaccines also have positive implications for livestock welfare, as they could be administered directly in the diet, eliminating the need to confine the animal, or the need to breach the skin through injection, a practice that can promote secondary infections. Oral administration of vaccines eliminates the risks that injection-based methods pose on meat quality as a result of intramuscular administration.

3. Plant-based bioreactors

Being eukaryotic organisms, plants can express, synthesize and process complex heterologous proteins similarly to "conventional", fermentation-based expression systems, such as mammalian, insect and yeast cell cultures. Yet, plants have some variances in the pattern of protein glycosylation [29]. Production of recombinant therapeutic proteins has been demonstrated in a variety of plant species. Plant cells contain genomes of three types: nuclear, chloroplast (plastome) and mitochondrial genomes. Generation of stable transgenic plants that produce recombinant proteins can be efficiently achieved through genetic engineering of the nuclear genome or the plastome. In addition, transient expression methods allow quick and robust production of recombinant proteins by way of infiltration of plant leaf tissue with transgene-harboring agrobacteria [30].

Recombinant proteins produced in nuclear-transformed plants are synthesized in the cytoplasm and can be secreted, or accumulated in different sub-cellular organelles with the use of appropriate transit or signal peptides. Using tissue-specific promoters enables spatially-defined expression of the transgene in applicable plant organs, such as leaves, seeds, fruits or tubers [31]. Nuclear-transformed plants offer tremendous simplicity for production of a vaccine product, as seed lines can be developed and propagation of plant biomass can utilize traditional agricultural technologies and infrastructure. Note, however, that nuclear-transformed plants typically express lower yields of recombinant proteins compared with transient expression, require prolonged timeframes for generation and selection of transgenic seed lines, and require measures to prevent environmental contamination due to transgene flow via open field cross-pollination [32].

Transgenic plants with transformed plastome (transplastomic plants) possess several beneficial traits, such as i) high-ploidy of plastome and lack of positional effects or transgene silencing, leading to synthesis of typically very high levels of recombinant proteins, ii) the ability to express artificial operons, thus allowing expression of several proteins in one transformational step, and iii) tight transgene containment due to maternal inheritance of plastid DNA in most cultivated plants [33]. The absence of a glycosylation machinery in chloroplasts thwarts the expression of proteins where glycans are essential for structure/conformation; however, this technology eliminates risks of addition of potentially allergenic non-mammalian glycans and offers advantages for expression of non-glycosylated proteins of prokaryotic origin [34].

High yields of recombinant proteins can be obtained quickly with transient expression systems through use of viral, virus-derived and non-viral expression vectors [30]. Infiltration of the leaf tissue with an *Agrobacterium* intermediate host containing any of these types of expression vectors (agroinfiltration) is the most common method used for delivery of foreign DNA into plant cells. The main advantage of the transient expression systems is the production speed that enables vaccines to be manufactured within periods as short as one month after obtaining the sequence of the antigen [35]. However, transient expression systems are labor- and material-intensive procedures involving growing *Agrobacterium* cultures, and diluting them in infiltration cocktails, immersion of plant aerial biomass into the Agrobacterium suspension, infiltrating the agrobacteria into leaves by pulling and releasing a vacuum to allow entry of *Agrobacterium* into the plant tissues [36]. These manipulations add cost to recombinant protein production, but have the advantage of using wild type plants, which is viewed by regulatory authorities favorably. The US Defense Advanced Research Program Agency (DARPA) has funded major infrastructure projects, such as Medicago's [37] commercial-scale production facility in the Research Triangle Park, NC, and Kentucky BioProcessing's [38] production facility in Owensboro, KY. Also, an improved viral vector-based inducible system that can be deployed for field production has recently been developed [39].

Other plant-based production systems include algae and moss cell-suspension cultures grown in bioreactors. High-level containment and sterile growth conditions are advantages of these systems, compared to whole plants in terms of good manufacturing practice (GMP) for recombinant protein production, though the cost of these systems is high, while scale-up ability is limited [40].

4. Post-translational protein modifications in plants

Although the genetic code is universal and a given nucleotide sequence results in the same order of amino acids in the polypeptide regardless of what organism is translating the RNA message, proteins differ in structure depending on the organism they are produced in. This is due to the fact that a multitude of modifications can take place after the ribosomal synthesis of the polypeptide, so called post-translational modifications (PTMs). In the case of therapeutic proteins these PTMs are of high importance, since they might alter the structure of the protein, its functionality and especially its immunogenicity [41]. PTMs include glycosylation, phosphorylation, lipidation, disulfide-bridging (to name only the most prominent), which basically occur in vivo, but some might also occur during downstream processing of a given therapeutic protein. Different organisms are capable of various PTMs, e.g. bacteria do not glycosylate proteins, while eukaryotic organisms perform extensive glycomodifications. Moreover, type and linkage of sugars vary considerably among cell types and organs, as well as at different developmental stages and environmental conditions, making this particular modification highly diverse. In the case of recombinant therapeutics for parenteral administration, it is of importance to retain the native glycosylation pattern to avoid shortened half-life and unintended immunogenicity. Plants do glycosylate recombinant proteins in a manner that differs from that in mammalian cell systems, and glycosylation may even vary among plant species, organs and cell types. In some cases this can even be an advantage, exemplified by a recombinant glucocerebrosidase (taliglucerase alfa) made in carrot cells. Here, the sugars added to the produced recombinant enzyme more closely resemble the native structure with terminal mannose, making this product superior or "biobetter", compared to the CHO cells-derived product [42]. As a further improvement, glycosylation machinery in plants can be engineered to produce mammalian-like glycan patterns with terminal sialic acid, making the recombinant proteins almost indistinguishable from those produced in mammalian cell lines (see "Glycoengineering" in text).

5. Opportunities and advantages of plant systems

5.1 Storage/Shelf life/Purification

Plant-based expression systems raise the possibility that antigens or antibodies can be produced in a form that is stable during storage and is amenable to extraction and purification procedures [43]. Dried or lyophilized leafy biomass, as well as plant storage tissues, such as seeds, retain unchanged levels of accumulated recombinant proteins for years at normal room temperatures, thus reducing stowing costs and facilitating distribution without need for a cold chain [44,45]. Such a production system would allow stockpiling of the transgenic plant material (lyophilized leaf biomass or seeds) for manufacturing of rapid-response veterinary biologics targeted against pathogens of epidemiological relevance. The time to product would then only be dependent on the speed of extraction and downstream processing, if purification is required, or immediate, if formulated lyophilized biomass or whole seeds can be administered in feed [46]. Some plant-based expression strategies, such as the expression of recombinant antigens in oil bodies or implementation of particular protein tags are specifically focused at overcoming the complexities of purification procedures (reviewed in [47]). Although purified plant-derived biologics are functional and effective, a key benefit of plants is the ability to deliver recombinant pharmaceuticals as minimally processed feed, such as flour paste from edible tissues [48]. Expression in seeds may also help protect antigens from digestion within the intestinal tract, especially if they target the formation of protein bodies, which can increase the delivery of antigens to the mucosal surface [49]. Remarkably, the formation of ectopic storage organelles as sink compartments for recombinant proteins can be induced in tissues that are not adapted for storage functions [50].

5.2 Glycoengineering

Glycosylation affects the quality of recombinant pharmaceuticals as different glycan structures can potentially influence stability, subcellular targeting, immunogenicity, pharmacokinetics and biological activity. The precise control and optimization of glycan modification to manufacture homogeneous protein therapeutics with specific designer glycoforms that confer superior efficacy has therefore become an important issue for all production platforms, including mammalian cells.

The mechanisms of N-glycosylation in plants and mammals differ in Golgi-specific modifications, such as the addition of β(1,2)-linked xylose and core α(1,3)-linked fucose residues in plants, and the addition of β(1,4)-linked galactose and sialic acid residues in mammals [51]. Therefore, strategies to control the glycosylation of recombinant proteins were established in plants early on, such as subcellular targeting to prevent the addition of certain sugar residues [52] and glycoengineering to replace sugars with more desirable counterparts [53]. A key example of glycan control by targeting is the first commercially available plant-derived human therapeutic protein, taliglucerase alfa, indicated for the lysosomal storage disorder called Gaucher's disease. In this case targeting to the plant vacuole resulted in the formation of glycan structures with terminal mannose residues promoting uptake of the recombinant protein via mannose-specific surface receptors on macrophages [54].

Engineering the plant N-glycosylation pathway has been achieved by various approaches including conventional mutagenesis or homologous recombination, RNA interference and transgene expression [53]. The versatility of plants for the production of specific N-glycoforms has turned a perceived disadvantage into one of the major strengths of plant production platforms. In addition to the abolition of β(1,2)-linked xylose and core α(1,3)-linked fucose residues, and the complete reconstruction of mammalian glycosylation pathways in plants [55], product-specific designer N-glycans have been engineered for improved efficacy. For example, glycoengineered plants can be used to produce glyco-optimized antibody versions with improved pharmacokinetic properties due to greater receptor affinity [56].

Another type of glycosylation whose impact is less widely known is the mucin-like O-glycosylation of serine, threonine and hydroxyproline residues, the latter being unique to plants. However, recent efforts have addressed the engineering of O-linked glycans [57]. It has been suggested that O-glycan structures may function as adjuvants, or may increase serum stability [51]. Tailored mammal-like O-glycan structures could also improve the stability and activity of proteins such as erythropoietin and secretory IgA, giving plants a competitive edge for the production of these compounds.

5.3 Vaccine bioencapsulation and delivery

Although plants have been shown to manufacture biologically-active therapeutics in amounts sufficient for oral administration to livestock, plant-derived antigens require a formulation to protect them from the hostile environment of the gastro-intestinal tract, without interfering with the immunogenicity of the antigen. Depending on the plant species and the plant tissue in which the subunit proteins are expressed, the plant matrix could provide some protection against these harsh conditions. Not only does this eliminate the need for costly purification, but the provision of a durable matrix offers a protective and stabilizing effect beyond harvest and upon mucosal administration [58]. Any plant cell matrix can be effective to enhance resistance against digestion, thereby increasing exposure of a vaccine to immune effector cells, but the protective effect can be further enhanced by incorporation of the vaccine proteins into storage organelles [59]. The use of seeds is particularly suitable to achieve bioencapsulation of recombinant proteins in specialized storage organelles that are derived from the endomembrane system and allow proteins to accumulate within a protective matrix [52]. Clear benefits have been demonstrated in seed-based production systems as recombinant proteins expressed in rice or pea seeds were better protected from degradation than their purified counterparts upon oral delivery [60,61]. Nevertheless, plant-based production could also negatively influence the immunogenicity of the antigen by influencing antigen folding, glycosylation and/or by interaction with the antigen, interfering with its capacity to target the mucosa [46]. The latter could be one of the reasons why F4 fimbriae to which alfalfa crushed leaf biomass was added, showed a decreased immune response in pigs in comparison with F4 without this plant material (Cox et al., unpublished results).

5.4 Scale-up and speed

Scaling up production of recombinant proteins in transgenic or transplastomic plants is much easier and less costly than similar scaling up in mammalian or microbial cells for the simple reason that each plant could be considered as a bioreactor and all that is required is sowing a seed and providing light, water and fertilizer, as opposed to an expensive upfront investment in infrastructure and bioreactor facilities for cell cultures and the formulation of complex cell culture media. Therefore, scaling up or down can be achieved quickly with no major investment. A single tobacco plant can produce over 150 000 seeds, allowing fast scale-up within a few months. Tobacco biomass yields can reach up to 100 tons/ha in a single field season [62]. If containment is necessary, a similar or higher yield is achievable in greenhouses; and high level accumulation of the desired protein at 1 g/kg fresh leaf weight means that 100 kg of a protein can be produced in a single hectare (Menassa et al., unpublished data). However, using stable transgenic/transplastomic lines implies a lag time in producing a high expressing line and obtaining seed. In the case of a catastrophic epidemic or pandemic, much faster timelines are required. For this, transient production in *Nicotiana benthamiana* is ideal with a timeline from cloning of the genes to vaccine production of only a few weeks [35]. As well, this system obviates the need for production of transgenic plants, thus easing the regulatory framework for scale up. In this system, wild type *Nicotiana benthamiana* plants are grown in greenhouses and infiltrated with *Agrobacterium* cultures containing the expression construct required for recombinant protein production. The infiltrated plants are harvested 4-10 days post-infiltration, and the protein is purified. Several companies (Medicago Inc., Fraunhofer USA, Kentucky BioProcessing LLC) have adopted this system for production of influenza vaccines and monoclonal antibodies [35,63,64]. The MagnICON® system developed by ICON Genetics GmbH [65] allows the production and purification of monoclonal antibodies at an expected yield of 250 mg/kg plant fresh weight [63], and Medicago Inc. was able to produce 10 million doses of influenza vaccine within one month in their 97 000 square foot facility in North Carolina.

6. Examples of therapeutic proteins produced in plants

6.1 Antibodies

It has been more than 25 years since the first IgG antibody was expressed in plants. Since then, there have been numerous publications in the scientific literature on the production of antibodies in plants, such as those targeting bacteria, cancer targets and highly pathogenic viruses such as HIV and Ebola [66]. The current epidemic caused by the Ebola virus in West Africa has brought attention to a plant-produced antibody cocktail. This cocktail, called ZMAPP, was recently shown to reverse advanced Ebola disease in 100% of tested Rhesus macaques [67]. Six publications describe the production of five of 38 approved therapeutic antibodies in plants (Table 1).

Therapeutic and prophylactic antibodies are required in massive amounts and on a constant basis, and might therefore be produced more economically by using transgenic plants rather than fermentation. In addition, neutralizing antibodies indicated as topical or oral microbicides can also be delivered in plant material such as seeds, as demonstrated by the administration of peas containing single-chain antibodies with high sporozoite-neutralizing activity against the coccidiosis parasite, *Eimeria tenella,* for the prevention of gastrointestinal infections in chickens [60]. In another, more recent study the protection of weaned piglets against enterotoxigenic *E. coli* infection was achieved by the oral administration of seeds producing IgA [72].

Whereas simple proteins such as single chain antibody fragments tend to be easily expressed in bacteria, complex glycoproteins such as monoclonal antibodies usually require eukaryotic production systems. Full size antibodies tend to be expressed well in plants because the secretory pathway in plant cells contains an extensive molecular chaperone system. Plants are particularly beneficial for the production of secretory IgA molecules because they can produce all four of the polypeptide components and assemble a fully functional molecule [73]. In contrast, three of the protein components are produced by plasma cells in mammals, but the fourth is produced by epithelial cells,

Table 1 PubMed listings for therapeutic antibodies produced in plants

Antibody (generic name)	Antibody (commercial name)	Plant species	Reference
Cetuximab	Erbitux	*Zea mays*	[68]
Nimotuzumab	BIOMAb EGFR, TheraCIM, Theraloc, CIMAher	*Nicotiana tabacum*	[69]
Palivizumab	Synagis	*Nicotiana benthamiana*	[70]
Rituximab	Rituxan, Mabthera	*Lemna minor*	[56]
Trastuzumab	Herceptin	*Nicotiana benthamiana*	[71]
ZMAPP	-	*Nicotiana benthamiana*	[67]

and assembly can only occur in the extracellular environment. Secretory IgA assembly can also be achieved in CHO cells carrying the four different transgenes, but the efficiency of assembly is low [74]. Therefore, plants offer a valuable and superior large-scale production system for this preferred format of mucosal antibodies.

6.2 Antigens: VLPs

Viral diseases are probably the most important culprit for the severe economic losses in livestock production worldwide. Although antibiotics are not used to treat or prevent viral infection outbreaks, pathogenic viruses often predispose infected animals for secondary bacterial infections, which do require antibiotic treatment. Thus, preventive vaccinations to control primary viral infections help to reduce the need for antibiotics application in livestock production.

Virus-like particles (VLPs) are defined as multisubunit protein structures with self-assembling competence that show an identical or highly similar overall structure to the corresponding native viruses [75]. Studies document a high immunogenic capacity of VLPs due to their display of multiple repeated antigenic motifs, which trigger B cell activation and elicit higher antibody titers compared to monomeric antigens. Strong humoral immune responses could be induced by VLPs without adjuvants, while avoiding stimulation of inflammatory T cell responses [76]. Many different VLPs (more than 100) originating from phages and plant, insect, and vertebrate viruses have been described and summarized in an excellent review [75], including examples of the preparative and large-scale manufacturing of VLPs in bacteria, yeast cells, insect cells and mammalian cells.

Mason et al. first demonstrated that the expression of human hepatitis B virus structural proteins in plants results in enveloped VLPs that "bud-out" as spherical particles of 22 nm in diameter off the intracellular membranes [77]. The further engineering of enveloped hepatitis B virus VLPs into nanoparticles allowed the display of large foreign antigens or the development of bivalent vaccines [78]. Simultaneous transient expression of four distinct structural proteins of Bluetongue virus (BTV) led to assembly of heteromultimeric VLPs able to elicit a strong antibody response in sheep, which provided protective immunity against BTV challenge [79]. Another example of VLPs produced in plants with improved transient expression is Norwalk virus-derived non-enveloped VLPs [80]. Lettuce containing low levels of secondary metabolites has been used to develop a robust plant virus-based production platform for VLPs derived from the Norwalk virus capsid and combined with a scalable processing method [81].

The concept of producing VLPs in plants is generally connected to the idea of edible vaccines [75]. However, there are several hurdles to resolve before this concept could be implemented, despite all of its obvious benefits. Quality control issues and precise formulation of vaccine products, as well as documented control by the relevant regulatory bodies would preclude easy on-site production in food/feed plant organs. The administration of such vaccines has to be regulated to avoid insufficient antigen application or, vice versa, to avoid the development of immune tolerance. Even orally administered VLP-type vaccines will have to be at least processed, enriched, formulated and applied under supervision, to ensure reproducible results [29].

Both the most recent and the most successful application of the plant-based VLP concept has been by Medicago Inc. (for review see [35]). A proprietary, plant-based transient expression system has been developed to produce vaccines made of budded influenza hemagglutinin particles [82]. The developed platform allowed the vaccine to be produced within one month of the disclosure of hemagglutinin sequences, from identified strains as H1N1 [82]. Because many influenza types (i.e. H5N1, H1N1) are zoonotic diseases, vaccination with plant-based VLPs has to be further developed especially in terms of lowering down-stream processing costs to fit into the economic constraints associated with a veterinary vaccine. An excellent comparative summary of different plant-based vaccines including expression levels, immunogenicity, VLP strategies and anticipated cost is given in a review by Scotti and Rybicki [83]. The authors conclude that proof of efficacy was demonstrated for several plant-based VLP vaccines and plant-based expression systems could do as well as conventional production systems based on fermentation. They claim a rather optimistic future of plant-based VLPs, if real costs are in the predicted range.

6.3 Subunit vaccines

The concept of using plants as expression hosts for veterinary subunit vaccines has been studied extensively within the past two decades. However, only a few studies have tested the efficacy of plant-made subunit vaccines in farm animals. This section summarizes examples showing immunization data with host species.

6.3.1 Poultry

In 2006 Dow Agro Sciences obtained USDA approval for a plant cell culture-based vaccine for poultry against Newcastle disease virus [84]. This vaccine was composed of recombinant hemagglutinin-neuraminidase protein expressed in transgenic tobacco suspension cells and formulated as an injectable vaccine. Other studies on Newcastle disease virus include expression of full-size glycoproteins in transgenic potato and tobacco leaves, maize and rice seeds (reviewed in [85]). The antigens were shown to be immunogenic and protective in chickens after oral delivery.

An edible potato-based vaccine has been developed against chicken infectious bronchitis virus (IBV) [86]. Sliced tubers expressing viral S1 glycoprotein were administered in three doses over two weeks; chickens were challenged with IBV one week after the last administration. Orally immunized chickens developed a virus-specific antibody response and were protected against IBV. Another research group succeeded in vaccinating chickens against infectious bursal disease virus (IBDV) with plant-made VP2 protein. Chickens orally immunized with *Arabidopsis* crude leaf extracts or transgenic rice seeds were protected to a similar level achieved with a commercial injectable vaccine [87]. Recently, the VP2 antigen was produced transiently in *Nicotiana benthamiana* and induced neutralizing antibodies in immunized chickens [88].

6.3.2 Swine

The use of maize seeds as an edible delivery vehicle against porcine Transmissible gastroenteritis coronavirus (TGEV) has been extensively studied. The envelope spike protein was used as an antigen to raise neutralizing antibodies and the efficacy of this plant-made vaccine has been presented in experiments with piglets [89]. In addition, it was found that the antigen was stable during storage in various conditions and authors were able to concentrate the antigen using milling techniques.

Enterotoxigenic *E. coli* (ETEC) causing post-weaning diarrhea in piglets has been a target for a plant-made vaccine. The major subunit protein of ETEC F4 fimbriae has been expressed in the leaves of tobacco [90], alfalfa [46] and in seeds of barley [91]. This subunit vaccine was shown to be immunogenic and partially protective after oral delivery to weaned piglets [46].

Capsid protein VP1 antigenic epitope of the of Foot-and-mouth disease virus (FMDV) was used to substitute a part of Bamboo mosaic virus coat protein, resulting in display of the epitope on virions that retained their infectivity and could be propagated in plants [92]. It was demonstrated that immunization with the extracted chimeric virions by intramuscular injection could fully protect pigs against FMDV challenge by effectively inducing humoral and cell-mediated immune responses.

6.3.3 Cattle

Transgenic peanut plants expressing bovine Rinderpest virus hemaglutinin raised immune responses in cattle [93]. This oral vaccine was able to raise virus-specific antibodies which also neutralized the virus in vitro. Immunogenicity of a Tobacco mosaic virus (TMV)-based vaccine against bovine herpes virus (BHV) was studied in cattle [94]. Immunogenic glycoprotein D was produced as a by-product in TMV-inoculated tobacco plants, and the crude plant extract emulsified in oil and subsequently injected into cattle was able to raise specific humoral and cellular immune responses. Most importantly, cattle were protected against BHV to similar levels as those vaccinated with the commercial vaccine.

A plant-made subunit vaccine against Bovine viral diarrhea virus (BVDV) has been developed in Argentina. The structural protein E2 of BVDV was expressed in transgenic alfalfa as a fusion to a peptide for targeting the product to antigen-presenting cells [95]. Partially purified antigen was administered intramuscularly to calves and protected them against BVDV challenge.

6.4 Toxic proteins

Although the efficacy of treatments with classical antibiotics is declining due to the widespread development of antibiotic resistance among major pathogenic bacteria, there are very little alternatives for fighting infections. One novel therapeutic option could be the use of phage lysins - enzymes that target and hydrolyze bacterial cell walls, efficiently killing a large array of bacteria [96]. However, due to the toxic nature of these proteins, their production in bacteria cannot be achieved, limiting the availability for testing or manufacture. The lack of the specific, bacterial-type cell wall structures targeted by lysins makes plants an alternative platform for production of therapeutic proteins which are highly toxic to bacteria. In a promising report [97], Oey et al. showed that by targeting the genes encoding the lysozyme Cpl-1 and the amidase Pal to the tobacco plastome, functional lysins could be synthesized and accumulated at high levels in chloroplasts. Several reports described successful transplastomic as well as transient expression-mediated production of short anti-microbial peptides, analogs of secreted defensins, which can be used for control of bacterial, viral and fungal infections [98-100]. Hence, plants represent a valuable production system for anti-microbial toxic proteins, offering cost-effective solution to obtain large quantities of proteinaceous antibiotics that could be administered through feed.

7. Conclusions

The use of vaccines and prophylactics for the control of infectious diseases in the livestock industry will grow as antibiotics applications diminish. Plants as bioreactors comprise a valuable option for production of recombinant protein therapeutics for animal health. In recent years numerous studies demonstrated the feasibility and advantages of plant-based production platforms for various proteins with therapeutic use, including complex antibodies, subunit vaccines and immunogenic virus-like particles. Plant-made therapeutic products are currently on the cusp of widely entering biotechnology markets. Interaction and concerted actions of the plant biotechnology sector with veterinarians and regulatory authorities will facilitate development of novel approaches to sustainable, antibiotic-free livestock agriculture.

8. List of abbreviations

BHV: Bovine herpes virus; BVDV: Bovine viral diarrhea virus; CT: Cholera toxin; CTB: B subunit of CT; DARPA: Defense advanced research program agency; ETEC: Enterotoxigenic *E. coli*; FcRn: Neonatal Fc receptor; FMDV: Foot-and-mouth disease virus; GALT: Gut-associated lymphoid tissue; GMP: Good Manufacturing Practice; IBV: Infectious bronchitis virus; Ig: Immunoglobulin; LT: Thermolabile enterotoxin; LTB: B subunit of LT; MALT: Mucosa-associated lymphoid tissue; PTMs: Post-translational modifications; scFv: Single-chain variable antibody fragments; TGEV: Transmissible gastroenteritis coronavirus; TMV: Tobacco mosaic virus; VLPs: Virus-like particles.

9. Competing interests

The authors declare that they have no competing interests.

10. Authors' contributions

IK, ET, EC, BD, UC, JJ, ES, HW, TM, AP, MDM, JCH, RM – all contributed equally in writing the manuscript. IK coordinated the drafting and IK and RM edited the manuscript. All authors read and approved the final manuscript.

11. Acknowledgements

We gratefully acknowledge the help form Tanja Patry and Dorothy Drew in manuscript preparation and formatting. This collaborative manuscript is an output from a workshop held in London, Ontario on September 23-25, 2013 and sponsored by the OECD Co-operative Research Programme on Biological Resource Management for Sustainable Agricultural Systems, whose financial support made it possible for some of the invited speakers to attend. We apologize to those authors whose work was not cited here, as many relevant references were omitted due to space restrictions.

Author details

[1]Department of Biology, University of Western Ontario, 1151 Richmond St, London, ON, Canada. [2]AAFC, Southern Crop Protection and Food Research Centre, 1391 Sandford St, London, ON, Canada. [3]Laboratory of Immunology, Faculty of Veterinary Medicine, Ghent University, Salisburylaan 133, 9820 Merelbeke, Belgium. [4]Leibniz Institute of Plant Genetics and Crop Plant Research, Gatersleben, Germany. [5]VTT Technical Research Centre of Finland, Espoo, Finland. [6]Department for Applied Genetics and Cell Biology, University of Natural Resources and Life Sciences, Vienna, Austria. [7]Technische Universität Darmstadt, FB Biologie, Schnittspahnstr. 5, D-64287 Darmstadt, Germany. [8]AAFC, Lethbridge Research Centre, 5403, 1 Avenue South, Lethbridge, Alberta, Canada. [9]Vaccine and Infectious Disease Organization (VIDO), University of Saskatchewan, 120 Veterinary Road, Saskatoon, Saskatchewan, Canada. [10]Department of Veterinary Microbiology, University of Saskatchewan, 120 Veterinary Road, Saskatoon, Saskatchewan, Canada. [11]PlantForm Corp., c/o Room 2218, E.C. Bovey Bldg, University of Guelph, Guelph, Ontario N1G 2 W1, Canada. [12]School of Environmental Sciences, University of Guelph, 50 Stone Road East, Guelph, Ontario N1G 2 W1, Canada.

12. References

1. Scallan E, Hoekstra RM, Angulo FJ, Tauxe RV, Widdowson MA, Roy SL, Jones JL, Griffin PM: **Foodborne illness acquired in the United States–major pathogens.** *Emerg Infect Dis* 2011, **17**:7–15.
2. One Health Initiative: **One Health Initiative will unite human and veterinary medicine.** 2014. [http://www.onehealthinitiative.com/index.php] (accessed 2014/08/29).
3. Potter A, Gerdts V, Litte-van den Hurk S: **Veterinary vaccines: alternatives to antibiotics?** *Anim Health Res Rev* 2008, **9**:187–199.
4. Research and Markets: **Animal/Veterinary Vaccines Market by Products, Diseases & Technology – Global Forecast to 2018.** 2013. [http://www.researchandmarkets.com/research/gcksr4/animalveterinary] (accessed 2014/08/29).
5. Chappuis G: **Neonatal immunity and immunisation in early age: lessons from veterinary medicine.** *Vaccine* 1998, **16**:1468–1472.
6. Sangild PT: **Uptake of colostral immunoglobulins by the compromised newborn farm animal.** *Acta Vet Scand Suppl* 2003, **98**:105–122.
7. Hurley WL, Theil PK: **Perspectives on immunoglobulins in colostrum and milk.** *Nutrients* 2011, **3**:442–474.
8. Cervenak J, Kacskovics I: **The neonatal Fc receptor plays a crucial role in the metabolism of IgG in livestock animals.** *Vet Immunol Immunopathol* 2009, **128**:171–177.
9. Mayer B, Kis Z, Kajan G, Frenyo LV, Hammarstrom L, Kacskovics I: **The neonatal Fc receptor (FcRn) is expressed in the bovine lung.** *Vet Immunol Immunopathol* 2004, **98**:85–89.
10. Porter P, Noakes DE, Allen WD: **Secretory IgA and antibodies to Escherichia coli in porcine colostrum and milk and their significance in the alimentary tract of the young pig.** *Immunology* 1970, **18**:245–257.
11. Brandtzaeg P: **Secretory immunity with special reference to the oral cavity.** *J Oral Microbiol* 2013, **5**:20401.
12. Snoeck V, Peters IR, Cox E: **The IgA system: a comparison of structure and function in different species.** *Vet Res* 2006, **37**:455–467.
13. Holmgren J, Czerkinsky C: **Mucosal immunity and vaccines.** *Nat Med* 2005, **11**:S45–S53.
14. Devriendt B, De Geest BG, Goddeeris BM, Cox E: **Crossing the barrier: Targeting epithelial receptors for enhanced oral vaccine delivery.** *J Control Release* 2012, **160**:431–439.
15. Holmgren J, Svennerholm AM: **Vaccines against mucosal infections.** *Curr Opin Immunol* 2012, **24**:343–353.
16. Cox E, Verdonck F, Vanrompay D, Goddeeris B: **Adjuvants modulating mucosal immune responses or directing systemic responses towards the mucosa.** *Vet Res* 2006, **37**:511–539.
17. Van den Broeck W, Cox E, Goddeeris BM: **Receptor-dependent immune responses in pigs after oral immunization with F4 fimbriae.** *Infect Immun* 1999, **67**:520–526.
18. Snoeck V, Van den Broeck W, De Colvenaer V, Verdonck F, Goddeeris B, Cox E: **Transcytosis of F4 fimbriae by villous and dome epithelia in F4-receptor positive pigs supports importance of receptor-dependent endocytosis in oral immunization strategies.** *Vet Immunol Immunopathol* 2008, **124**:29–40.
19. Boleman SL, Boleman SJ, Morgan WW, Hale DS, Griffin DB, Savell JW, Ames RP, Smith MT, Tatum JD, Field TG, Smith GC, Gardner BA, Morgan JB, Northcutt SL, Dolezal HG, Gill DR, Ray FK: **National Beef Quality Audit-1995: survey of producer-related defects and carcass quality and quantity attributes.** *J Anim Sci* 1998, **76**:96–103.
20. Wilson-Welder JH, Torres MP, Kipper MJ, Mallapragada SK, Wannemuehler MJ, Narasimhan B: **Vaccine adjuvants: current challenges and future approaches.** *J Pharm Sci* 2009, **98**:1278–1316.
21. Lawhorn DB: **Atrophic rhinitis.** In *Texas A&M AgriLife Extension Service.* 2002. [http://hdl.handle.net/1969.1/87644]. (accessed 2014/10/28).
22. Garlapati S, Eng NF, Kiros T, Kindrachuk J, Mutwiri G, Hancock RE, Potter A, Babiuk LA, Gerdts V: **Immunization with PCEP microparticles containing pertussis toxoid, CpG ODN and a synthetic innate defense regulator peptide induce protective immunity against pertussis.** *Vaccine* 2011, **29**:6540–6548.
23. Polewicz M, Gracia A, Garlapati S, van Kessel J, Strom S, Halperin S, Hancock RE, Potter A, Babiuk LA, Gerdts V: **Novel vaccine formulations against pertussis**

offer earlier onset of immunity and provide protection in the presence of maternal antibodies. *Vaccine* 2013, **31**:3148–3155.

24. Lycke N: **Recent progress in mucosal vaccine development: potential and limitations.** *Nat Rev Immunol* 2012, **12**:592–605.
25. Zaman M, Chandrudu S, Toth I: **Strategies for intranasal delivery of vaccines.** *Drug Deliv Transl Res* 2013, **3**:100–109.
26. Mutsch M, Zhou W, Rhodes P, Bopp M, Chen RT, Linder T, Spyr C, Steffen R: **Use of the inactivated intranasal influenza vaccine and the risk of Bell's palsy in Switzerland.** *N Engl J Med* 2004, **350**:896–903.
27. Johnston M, Zakharov A, Papaiconomou C, Salmasi G, Armstrong D: **Evidence of connections between cerebrospinal fluid and nasal lymphatic vessels in humans, non-human primates and other mammalian species.** *Cerebrospinal Fluid Res* 2004, **1**:2.
28. Langridge WH: **Edible vaccines.** *Sci Am* 2000, **283**:66–71.
29. Rybicki EP: **Plant-made vaccines for humans and animals.** *Plant Biotechnol J* 2010, **8**:620–637.
30. Komarova TV, Baschieri S, Donini M, Marusic C, Benvenuto E, Dorokhov YL: **Transient expression systems for plant-derived biopharmaceuticals.** *Expert Rev Vaccines* 2010, **9**:859–876.
31. Desai PN, Shrivastava N, Padh H: **Production of heterologous proteins in plants: strategies for optimal expression.** *Biotechnol Adv* 2010, **28**:427–435.
32. Sharma AK, Sharma MK: **Plants as bioreactors: Recent developments and emerging opportunities.** *Biotechnol Adv* 2009, **27**:811–832.
33. Bock R, Warzecha H: **Solar-powered factories for new vaccines and antibiotics.** *Trends Biotechnol* 2010, **28**:246–252.
34. Tregoning JS, Nixon P, Kuroda H, Svab Z, Clare S, Bowe F, Fairweather N, Ytterberg J, van Wijk KJ, Dougan G, Maliga P: **Expression of tetanus toxin Fragment C in tobacco chloroplasts.** *Nucleic Acids Res* 2003, **31**:1174–1179.
35. D'Aoust M, Couture MM, Charland N, Trépanier S, Landry N, Ors F, Vézina L: **The production of hemagglutinin-based virus-like particles in plants: a rapid, efficient and safe response to pandemic influenza.** *Plant Biotechnol J* 2010, **8**:607–619.
36. Gleba Y, Klimyuk V, Marillonnet S: **Viral vectors for the expression of proteins in plants.** *Curr Opin Biotechnol* 2007, **18**:134–141.
37. Medicago Inc: 2014. [http://www.medicago.com/English/Home/default.aspx] (accessed 2014/08/29).
38. Kentucky Bioprocessing LLC: 2014. [http://www.kbpllc.com/] (accessed 2014/08/29).
39. Werner S, Breus O, Symonenko Y, Marillonnet S, Gleba Y: **High-level recombinant protein expression in transgenic plants by using a double-inducible viral vector.** *Proc Natl Acad Sci U S A* 2011, **108**:14061–14066.
40. Xu J, Ge X, Dolan MC: **Towards high-yield production of pharmaceutical proteins with plant cell suspension cultures.** *Biotechnol Adv* 2011, **29**:278–299.
41. Walsh G: **Post-translational modifications of protein biopharmaceuticals.** *Drug Discov Today* 2010, **15**:773–780.
42. Aviezer D, Brill-Almon E, Shaaltiel Y, Hashmueli S, Bartfeld D, Mizrachi S, Liberman Y, Freeman A, Zimran A, Galun E: **A plant-derived recombinant human glucocerebrosidase enzyme - a preclinical and phase I investigation.** *PLoS One* 2009, **4**:e4792.
43. Peters J, Stoger E: **Transgenic crops for the production of recombinant vaccines and anti-microbial antibodies.** *Hum Vaccin* 2011, **7**:367–374.
44. Stoger E, Ma JK, Fischer R, Christou P: **Sowing the seeds of success: pharmaceutical proteins from plants.** *Curr Opin Biotechnol* 2005, **16**:167–173.
45. Lakshmi PS, Verma D, Yang X, Lloyd B, Daniell H: **Low cost tuberculosis vaccine antigens in capsules: expression in chloroplasts, bio-encapsulation, stability and functional evaluation in vitro.** *PLoS One* 2013, **8**:e54708.
46. Joensuu JJ, Verdonck F, Ehrstrom A, Peltola M, Siljander-Rasi H, Nuutila AM, Oksman-Caldentey KM, Teeri TH, Cox E, Goddeeris BM, Niklander-Teeri V: **F4 (K88) fimbrial adhesin FaeG expressed in alfalfa reduces F4+ enterotoxigenic *Escherichia coli* excretion in weaned piglets.** *Vaccine* 2006, **24**:2387–2394.
47. Wilken LR, Nikolov ZL: **Recovery and purification of plant-made recombinant proteins.** *Biotechnol Adv* 2012, **30**:419–433.
48. Jacob SS, Cherian S, Sumithra TG, Raina OK, Sankar M: **Edible vaccines against veterinary parasitic diseases–current status and future prospects.** *Vaccine* 2013, **31**:1879–1885.
49. Streatfield SJ: **Plant-based vaccines for animal health.** *Rev Sci Tech* 2005, **24**:189–199.
50. Phan HT, Hause B, Hause G, Arcalis E, Stoger E, Maresch D, Altmann F, Joensuu J, Conrad U: **Influence of elastin-like polypeptide and hydrophobin on recombinant hemagglutinin accumulations in transgenic tobacco plants.** *PLoS One* 2014, **9**:e99347.
51. Gomord V, Fitchette AC, Menu-Bouaouiche L, Saint-Jore-Dupas C, Plasson C, Michaud D, Faye L: **Plant-specific glycosylation patterns in the context of therapeutic protein production.** *Plant Biotechnol J* 2010, **8**:564–587.
52. Hofbauer A, Stoger E: **Subcellular accumulation and modification of pharmaceutical proteins in different plant tissues.** *Curr Pharm Des* 2013, **19**:5495–5502.
53. Bosch D, Castilho A, Loos A, Schots A, Steinkellner H: **N-glycosylation of plant-produced recombinant proteins.** *Curr Pharm Des* 2013, **19**:5503–5512.
54. Shaaltiel Y, Bartfeld D, Hashmueli S, Baum G, Brill-Almon E, Galili G, Dym O, Boldin-Adamsky SA, Silman I, Sussman JL, Futerman AH, Aviezer D: **Production of glucocerebrosidase with terminal mannose glycans for enzyme replacement therapy of Gaucher's disease using a plant cell system.** *Plant Biotechnol J* 2007, **5**:579–590.
55. Castilho A, Strasser R, Stadlmann J, Grass J, Jez J, Gattinger P, Kunert R, Quendler H, Pabst M, Leonard R, Altmann F, Steinkellner H: **In planta protein sialylation through overexpression of the respective mammalian pathway.** *J Biol Chem* 2010, **285**:15923–15930.
56. Gasdaska JR, Sherwood S, Regan JT, Dickey LF: **An afucosylated anti-CD20 monoclonal antibody with greater antibody-dependent cellular cytotoxicity and B-cell depletion and lower complement-dependent cytotoxicity than rituximab.** *Mol Immunol* 2012, **50**:134–141.
57. Yang Z, Drew DP, Jorgensen B, Mandel U, Bach SS, Ulvskov P, Levery SB, Bennett EP, Clausen H, Petersen BL: **Engineering mammalian mucin-type O-glycosylation in plants.** *J Biol Chem* 2012, **287**:11911–11923.
58. Takaiwa F: **Update on the use of transgenic rice seeds in oral immunotherapy.** *Immunotherapy* 2013, **5**:301–312.
59. Khan I, Twyman RM, Arcalis E, Stoger E: **Using storage organelles for the accumulation and encapsulation of recombinant proteins.** *Biotechol J* 2012, **7**:1099–1108.
60. Zimmermann J, Saalbach I, Jahn D, Giersberg M, Haehnel S, Wedel J, Macek J, Zoufal K, Glunder G, Falkenburg D, Kipriyanov S: **Antibody expressing pea seeds as fodder for prevention of gastrointestinal parasitic infections in chickens.** *BMC Biotechnol* 2009, **9**:79.
61. Nochi T, Takagi H, Yuki Y, Yang L, Masumura T, Mejima M, Nakanishi U, Matsumura A, Uozumi A, Hiroi T, Morita S, Tanaka K, Takaiwa F, Kiyono H: **Rice-based mucosal vaccine as a global strategy for cold-chain- and needle-free vaccination.** *Proc Natl Acad Sci U S A* 2007, **104**:10986–10991.
62. Woodleif WG, Chaplin JF, Cambell CR, Dejong DW: **Effect of variety and harvest treatments on protein yield of close grown tobacco.** *Tobacco Sci* 1981, **25**:83–86.
63. Pogue GP, Vojdani F, Palmer KE, Hiatt E, Hume S, Phelps J, Long L, Bohorova N, Kim D, Pauly M, Velasco J, Whaley K, Zeitlin L, Garger SJ, White E, Bai Y, Haydon H, Bratcher B: **Production of pharmaceutical-grade recombinant aprotinin and a monoclonal antibody product using plant-based transient expression systems.** *Plant Biotechnol J* 2010, **8**:638–654.
64. Cummings JF, Guerrero ML, Moon JE, Waterman P, Nielsen RK, Jefferson S, Gross FL, Hancock K, Katz JM, Yusibov V, Fraunhofer USACfMBSG: **Safety and immunogenicity of a plant-produced recombinant monomer hemagglutinin-based influenza vaccine derived from influenza A (H1N1) pdm09 virus: a Phase 1 dose-escalation study in healthy adults.** *Vaccine* 2014, **32**:2251–2259.
65. ICON Genetics GmbH: 2014. [http://www.icongenetics.com/html/home.htm] (accessed 2014/08/29).
66. Melnik S, Stoger E: **Green factories for biopharmaceuticals.** *Curr Med Chem* 2013, **20**:1038–1046.
67. Qiu X, Wong G, Audet J, Bello A, Fernando L, Alimonti JB, Fausther-Bovendo H, Wei H, Aviles J, Hiatt E, Johnson A, Morton J, Swope K, Bohorov O, Bohorova N, Goodman C, Kim D, Pauly MH, Velasco J, Pettitt J, Olinger GG, Whaley K, Xu B, Strong JE, Zeitlin L, Kobinger GP: **Reversion of advanced Ebola virus disease in nonhuman primates with ZMapp.** *Nature* 2014, **514**:47–53.
68. Lentz EM, Garaicoechea L, Alfano EF, Parreno V, Wigdorovitz A, Bravo-Almonacid FF: **Translational fusion and redirection to thylakoid lumen as strategies to improve the accumulation of a camelid antibody fragment in transplastomic tobacco.** *Planta* 2012, **236**:703–714.
69. Rodriguez M, Ramirez NI, Ayala M, Freyre F, Perez L, Triguero A, Mateo C, Selman-Housein G, Gavilondo JV, Pujol M: **Transient expression in tobacco leaves of an aglycosylated recombinant antibody against the epidermal growth factor receptor.** *Biotechnol Bioeng* 2005, **89**:188–194.

70. Zeitlin L, Bohorov O, Bohorova N, Hiatt A, do Kim H, Pauly MH, Velasco J, Whaley KJ, Barnard DL, Bates JT, Crowe JE Jr, Piedra PA, Gilbert BE: **Prophylactic and therapeutic testing of Nicotiana-derived RSV-neutralizing human monoclonal antibodies in the cotton rat model.** *MAbs* 2013, **5:**263–269.
71. Grohs BM, Niu Y, Veldhuis LJ, Trabelsi S, Garabagi F, Hassell JA, McLean MD, Hall JC: **Plant-produced trastuzumab inhibits the growth of HER2 positive cancer cells.** *J Agric Food Chem* 2010, **58:**10056–10063.
72. Virdi V, Coddens A, De Buck S, Millet S, Goddeeris BM, Cox E, De Greve H, Depicker A: **Orally fed seeds producing designer IgAs protect weaned piglets against enterotoxigenic *Escherichia coli* infection.** *Proc Natl Acad Sci U S A* 2013, **110:**11809–11814.
73. Ma JK, Hiatt A, Hein M, Vine ND, Wang F, Stabila P, van Dolleweerd C, Mostov K, Lehner T: **Generation and assembly of secretory antibodies in plants.** *Science* 1995, **268:**716–719.
74. Corthesy B: **Recombinant secretory IgA for immune intervention against mucosal pathogens.** *Biochem Soc Trans* 1997, **25:**471–475.
75. Zeltins A: **Construction and characterization of virus-like particles: a review.** *Mol Biotechnol* 2013, **53:**92–107.
76. Spohn G, Bachmann MF: **Exploiting viral properties for the rational design of modern vaccines.** *Expert Rev Vaccines* 2008, **7:**43–54.
77. Mason HS, Lam DM, Arntzen CJ: **Expression of hepatitis B surface antigen in transgenic plants.** *Proc Natl Acad Sci U S A* 1992, **89:**11745–11749.
78. Greco R, Michel M, Guetard D, Cervantes-Gonzalez M, Pelucchi N, Wain-Hobson S, Sala F, Sala M: **Production of recombinant HIV-1/HBV virus-like particles in Nicotiana tabacum and Arabidopsis thaliana plants for a bivalent plant-based vaccine.** *Vaccine* 2007, **25:**8228–8240.
79. Thuenemann EC, Meyers AE, Verwey J, Rybicki EP, Lomonossoff GP: **A method for rapid production of heteromultimeric protein complexes in plants: assembly of protective bluetongue virus-like particles.** *Plant Biotechnol J* 2013, **11:**839–846.
80. Santi L, Batchelor L, Huang Z, Hjelm B, Kilbourne J, Arntzen CJ, Chen Q, Mason HS: **An efficient plant viral expression system generating orally immunogenic Norwalk virus-like particles.** *Vaccine* 2008, **26:**1846–1854.
81. Lai H, He J, Engle M, Diamond MS, Chen Q: **Robust production of virus-like particles and monoclonal antibodies with geminiviral replicon vectors in lettuce.** *Plant Biotechnol J* 2012, **10:**95–104.
82. Vézina L-P, D'Aoust M-A, Landry N, Couture MMJ, Charland N, Ors F, Barbeau B, Sheldon AJ: **Plants as an innovative and accelerated vaccine-manufacturing solution.** *Bio Pharm Int* 2011, Santa Monica, CA: Advanstar Communications Inc. S27–S30.
83. Scotti N, Rybicki EP: **Plant-produced virus-like particle vaccines.** In *Virus-like Particles in Vaccine Development.* Edited by Buonaguro FM, Buonaguro L. London, UK: Future Medicine Ltd; 2014:102–118.
84. Vermij P: **USDA approves the first plant-based vaccine.** *Nat Biotechnol* 2006, **24:**233–234.
85. Joensuu JJ, Niklander-Teeri V, Brandle JE: **Transgenic plants for animal health: Plant-made vaccine antigens for animal infectious disease control.** *Phytochem Rev* 2008, **7:**553–577.
86. Zhou JY, Cheng LQ, Zheng XJ, Wu JX, Shang SB, Wang JY, Chen JG: **Generation of the transgenic potato expressing full-length spike protein of infectious bronchitis virus.** *J Biotechnol* 2004, **111:**121–130.
87. Wu J, Yu L, Li L, Hu J, Zhou J, Zhou X: **Oral immunization with transgenic rice seeds expressing VP2 protein of infectious bursal disease virus induces protective immune responses in chickens.** *Plant Biotechnol J* 2007, **5:**570–578.
88. Gomez E, Lucero MS, Chimeno Zoth S, Carballeda JM, Gravisaco MJ, Berinstein A: **Transient expression of VP2 in Nicotiana benthamiana and its use as a plant-based vaccine against infectious bursal disease virus.** *Vaccine* 2013, **31:**2623–2627.
89. Lamphear BJ, Jilka JM, Kesl L, Welter M, Howard JA, Streatfield SJ: **A corn-based delivery system for animal vaccines: an oral transmissible gastroenteritis virus vaccine boosts lactogenic immunity in swine.** *Vaccine* 2004, **22:**2420–2424.
90. Kolotilin I, Kaldis A, Devriendt B, Joensuu J, Cox E, Menassa R: **Production of a subunit vaccine candidate against porcine post-weaning diarrhea in high-biomass transplastomic tobacco.** *PLoS One* 2012, **7:**e42405.
91. Joensuu JJ, Kotiaho M, Teeri TH, Valmu L, Nuutila AM, Oksman-Caldentey KM, Niklander-Teeri V: **Glycosylated F4 (K88) fimbrial adhesin FaeG expressed in barley endosperm induces ETEC-neutralizing antibodies in mice.** *Transgenic Res* 2006, **15:**359–373.
92. Yang CD, Liao JT, Lai CY, Jong MH, Liang CM, Lin YL, Lin NS, Hsu YH, Liang SM: **Induction of protective immunity in swine by recombinant bamboo mosaic virus expressing foot-and-mouth disease virus epitopes.** *BMC Biotechnol* 2007, **7:**62.
93. Khandelwal A, Lakshmi Sita G, Shaila MS: **Oral immunization of cattle with hemagglutinin protein of rinderpest virus expressed in transgenic peanut induces specific immune responses.** *Vaccine* 2003, **21:**3282–3289.
94. Perez Filgueira DM, Zamorano PI, Dominguez MG, Taboga O, Del Medico Zajac MP, Puntel M, Romera SA, Morris TJ, Borca MV, Sadir AM: **Bovine herpes virus gD protein produced in plants using a recombinant tobacco mosaic virus (TMV) vector possesses authentic antigenicity.** *Vaccine* 2003, **21:**4201–4209.
95. Aguirreburualde MS, Gomez MC, Ostachuk A, Wolman F, Albanesi G, Pecora A, Odeon A, Ardila F, Escribano JM, Dus Santos MJ, Wigdorovitz A: **Efficacy of a BVDV subunit vaccine produced in alfalfa transgenic plants.** *Vet Immunol Immunopathol* 2013, **151:**315–324.
96. Pastagia M, Schuch R, Fischetti VA, Huang DB: **Lysins: the arrival of pathogen-directed anti-infectives.** *J Med Microbiol* 2013, **62:**1506–1516.
97. Oey M, Lohse M, Scharff LB, Kreikemeyer B, Bock R: **Plastid production of protein antibiotics against pneumonia via a new strategy for high-level expression of antimicrobial proteins.** *Proc Natl Acad Sci U S A* 2009, **106:**6579–6584.
98. Zeitler B, Bernhard A, Meyer H, Sattler M, Koop HU, Lindermayr C: **Production of a *de-novo* designed antimicrobial peptide in *Nicotiana benthamiana*.** *Plant Mol Biol* 2013, **81:**259–272.
99. Lee SB, Li B, Jin S, Daniell H: **Expression and characterization of antimicrobial peptides Retrocyclin-101 and Protegrin-1 in chloroplasts to control viral and bacterial infections.** *Plant Biotechnol J* 2011, **9:**100–115.
100. Company N, Nadal A, La Paz JL, Martinez S, Rasche S, Schillberg S, Montesinos E, Pla M: **The production of recombinant cationic alpha-helical antimicrobial peptides in plant cells induces the formation of protein bodies derived from the endoplasmic reticulum.** *Plant Biotechnol J* 2014, **12:**81–92.

2

Localization of annexins A1 and A2 in the respiratory tract of healthy calves and those experimentally infected with *Mannheimia haemolytica*

Chandrika Senthilkumaran[1], Joanne Hewson[3], Theresa L Ollivett[2], Dorothee Bienzle[1], Brandon N Lillie[1], Mary Ellen Clark[1] and Jeff L Caswell[1*]

Abstract

Annexins A1 and A2 are proteins known to function in the stress response, dampening inflammatory responses and mediating fibrinolysis. We found, in healthy cattle recently arrived to a feedlot, that lower levels of these proteins correlated with later development of pneumonia. Here we determine the localization of annexin A1 and A2 proteins in the respiratory tract and in leukocytes, in healthy calves and those with *Mannheimia haemolytica* pneumonia. In healthy calves, immunohistochemistry revealed cytoplasmic expression of annexin A1 in the surface epithelium of large airways, tracheobronchial glands and goblet cells, to a lesser degree in small airways, but not in alveolar epithelium. Immunocytochemistry labeled annexin A1 in the cytoplasm of neutrophils from blood and bronchoalveolar lavage fluid, while minimal surface expression was detected by flow cytometry in monocytes, macrophages and lymphocytes. Annexin A2 expression was detected in surface epithelium of small airways, some mucosal lymphocytes, and endothelium, with weak expression in large airways, tracheobronchial glands and alveolar septa. For both proteins, the level of expression was similar in tissues collected five days after intrabronchial challenge with *M. haemolytica* compared to that from sham-inoculated calves. Annexins A1 and A2 were both detected in leukocytes around foci of coagulative necrosis, and in necrotic cells in the center of these foci, as well as in areas outlined above. Thus, annexins A1 and A2 are proteins produced by airway epithelial cells that may prevent inflammation in the healthy lung and be relevant to development of pneumonia in stressed cattle.

Introduction

Annexins A1 and A2 are abundant proteins in bronchoalveolar lavage (BALF) of healthy calves, and lower levels in healthy at-risk calves were recently found to correlate with later development of bovine respiratory disease [1]. Annexin A1 and A2 are thought to quell inflammatory responses, and may thus promote resolution of inflammation and limit its injurious effects. Specifically, annexin A1 inhibits phospholipase A2 and eicosanoid synthesis, dampens neutrophil inflammatory responses, promotes neutrophil apoptosis, and stimulates interleukin-10 secretion from macrophages [2-7]. Annexin A2 activates plasminogen and thereby leads to fibrinolysis, enhances macrophage-mediated phagocytosis of apoptotic cells, and promotes airway epithelial cell repair [8-10]. Annexin A1 and A2 expression levels vary in different tissues [11]. An in vitro study of bovine tracheal epithelial cell cultures showed that annexin A1 was mostly expressed in differentiated cells and annexin A2 in undifferentiated cells, perhaps reflecting the anti-inflammatory and regenerative functions, respectively, of these proteins [12].

Annexin A1 levels increase with transportation stress [13], consistent with in vitro findings of increased annexin A1 and A2 expression after corticosteroid treatment of cultured bovine tracheal epithelial cells [12]. Recently, we found that as calves that were stressed by weaning and transportation arrived to a feedlot, those with higher levels of annexin A1 and A2 were less likely to later develop

* Correspondence: jcaswell@uoguelph.ca
[1]Department of Pathobiology, University of Guelph, Guelph, ON, N1G 2W1, Canada
Full list of author information is available at the end of the article

bacterial pneumonia [1]. Thus, the major objective of the present study was to determine the localization of annexins A1 and A2 in the respiratory tract of healthy calves, as well as to characterize differences that occur in inflamed lungs as a result of bacterial infection. This knowledge is necessary to understand how anti-inflammatory responses develop in the lung, and for development of methods to modulate these responses for prevention of bovine respiratory disease.

Materials and methods

Animals and sample collection

Samples of normal respiratory tissues were collected from two 2-month-old healthy male Holstein calves within 3 h of euthanasia. Samples of nasal tissue, trachea, bronchi, and lung containing alveoli and bronchioles were fixed in formalin overnight and processed routinely.

Further samples were collected from Holstein bull calves that were experimentally infected with *M. haemolytica* and from sham-inoculated control calves. Procedures were approved by the University of Guelph Animal Care Committee (AUP #12R055). Six Holstein bull calves, 102–139 days of age, were randomly assigned to two groups. *M. haemolytica*, isolated originally from a calf with pneumonia, was grown to log phase and diluted in PBS to optical density of 0.74 (shown to contain 2.8×10^8 CFU/mL as determined by follow-up colony counts). Three calves were sedated with xylazine, and inoculated with 25 mL of inoculum (total dose of 7×10^9 colony-forming units of *M. haemolytica* in phosphate-buffered saline) using a bronchoscope passed to the tracheal bifurcation. The 3 other calves, serving as uninfected controls, were similarly inoculated with 25 mL PBS. All infected calves developed moderately severe depression, reduced appetite and fever, as well as ultrasonographic evidence of consolidation within 2 hours of challenge that was maximal at 24 h, and elevated serum haptoglobin levels that peaked at 60 – 72 h after experimental challenge (data not shown). Calves were euthanized after 5 days. Tracheal, bronchial and lung tissues were fixed overnight in formalin and processed routinely.

Blood and BALF cells were collected from two healthy 2-3 month old Holstein male calves for immunocytochemistry. For flow cytometry, peripheral blood was collected from eight healthy adult Holstein cows after their first parturition.

Immunohistochemistry and immunocytochemistry

For immunohistochemistry (IHC), tissue sections were prepared routinely, deparaffinized and rehydrated. Heat-induced epitope retrieval was performed using a pressure cooker with sodium citrate buffer (pH 6.0) at a pressure of 18 pounds per square inch to achieve a temperature of approximately 120 °C at full pressure (Dako North America, California, USA). Cooled slides were washed and treated with endogenous enzyme blocker and serum-free protein blocker (S2003 and X0909, Dako). The slides were incubated overnight with the primary antibody in a humidified chamber at 4 °C, using either rabbit polyclonal anti-human annexin A1 primary antibody (2 μg/150 μL; H00000301-D01P, Novus Biologicals, Oakville, ON, Canada) or goat polyclonal anti-human annexin A2 primary antibody (1 μg/150 μL; NB 100-881, Novus Biologicals). Slides were then washed and incubated with secondary antibody for 30 min, using peroxidase-based EnVision™+ Dual Link Kit (#K406511-2, Dako Cytomation, Carpinteria, California, USA) for annexin A1, or HRP-conjugated rabbit anti-goat immunoglobulin (1:2000, Dako Cytomation) for annexin A2. NovaRED (Vector Laboratories, Burlingame, California, USA) was used as chromogen with Harris hematoxylin counterstain.

For immunocytochemistry (ICC), leukocytes were separated from whole blood by hypotonic lysis and cytocentrifuge preparations were made on charged slides. Preparations of BALF leukocytes were made in the same way. The cell preparations were fixed in acetone, and annexin A1 was detected as described above.

As negative controls for IHC and ICC, rabbit polyclonal anti-Toxoplasma antibody (2 μg/150 μL) was used in place of primary antibody for annexin A1, and goat polyclonal anti-influenza antibody (1 μg/150 μL) was similarly used as the negative control for annexin A2. As a further negative control, annexin A1 antibody was pre-incubated with bovine native annexin A1 protein (MBS318252, MybioSource, San Diego, CA, USA) for 1 h, using 1 μg antibody per 2.5 μg antigen for IHC, or 1 μg antibody per 1.5 μg antigen for 1 h for ICC. The IHC and ICC procedures were completed as above.

Immunolabeled slides were randomized and masked so that the assessment was done without knowledge of animal identity or treatment group. A semi-quantitative system was used to score each component of the respiratory system for intensity of immunolabeling (0, no staining; 1, equivocal; 2, minimal; 3, moderate; 4, abundant).

Flow cytometry

Leukocytes were separated from red blood cells as above then incubated with rabbit polyclonal anti-human annexin A1 antibody (H00000301-D01P, Novus Biologicals) at a concentration of 0.1 mg/mL, for 2 h at 4 °C. Cells were washed once then incubated for 15 min with sheep anti-rabbit immunoglobulin antibody conjugated to R-phycoerythrin (1:5 dilution, STAR35A, AbD Serotec, Raleigh, USA) at 4 °C for 15 min. After washing, the cells were evaluated using a BD FACScanTM (BD Biosciences, USA) with acquisition of 300 000 events and analyzed using FlowJo software (version 7.6, Treestar Inc, Standord, CA) [14].

Statistical analysis

The median fluorescence intensity (MFI) of leukocytes (neutrophils, lymphocytes and monocytes) was compared using Student's t test (GraphPad, Prism 6) and considered significant at $P < 0.05$.

Results

Annexin A1 and A2 expression in respiratory tissues of healthy calves

Immunohistochemistry findings were similar in sections of respiratory tissues from the two healthy calves (see Additional file 1). Annexin A1 immunolabeling was detected in the surface epithelium of the nasal cavity, trachea, bronchi and bronchioles, in both the apical and basal areas of the cytoplasm. The signal intensity was highest in the epithelium lining the nasal cavity, trachea (Figure 1A) and large bronchi (Figure 1B), lower in small bronchi and large bronchioles (Figure 1C), and infrequent in the terminal bronchioles. Labeling was also detected in cilia, goblet cells, and glandular and ductular epithelium of tracheobronchial glands (Figures 1A and B). Alveolar macrophages and some tracheobronchial mucosal lymphocytes were positively labeled, but cells in the alveolar septa were not labeled (Additional file 1F). Immunolabeling was noted in the airway smooth muscle and nerve terminals, but no labeling of connective tissue was observed in the bronchial adventitia or the lamina propria. Pre-incubation of annexin A1 antibody with annexin native protein abrogated the signal intensity (Additional file 1E). Labeling was not observed in sections treated with the control antibody in place of the primary antibody (Additional file 1B).

Annexin A2 immunolabeling was detected in epithelial cells lining the trachea, bronchi, bronchioles and alveoli, in both apical and basal areas of the cytoplasm (Additional file 2 and Additional file 3). The intensity of the signal was weak in the surface epithelium of the trachea and bronchi (Figure 2A). Bronchioles in most areas had intense labeling that was greater than that seen in the large airways, but this was not uniform throughout the sections (Figures 2B and D). The tracheobronchial glands were weakly labeled, and goblet cells or cilia were not labeled (Additional file 2A and Additional file 3A). Large lymphocytes in the tracheobronchial lamina propria were positively labeled (Figure 2A). Although the alveolar epithelium appeared negative, individual cells (suggestive of macrophages and endothelial cells) in alveolar septa were labeled (Figure 2C). Intense immunolabeling was observed in the endothelium of blood vessels (Figure 2D) and in plasma. Weak immunolabeling was noted in the airway smooth muscle and nerve terminals, and no labeling was observed in connective tissue of the bronchial adventitia or lamina propria. Labeling was not observed in sections treated with the negative control antibody in place of the primary antibody (Additional file 2C).

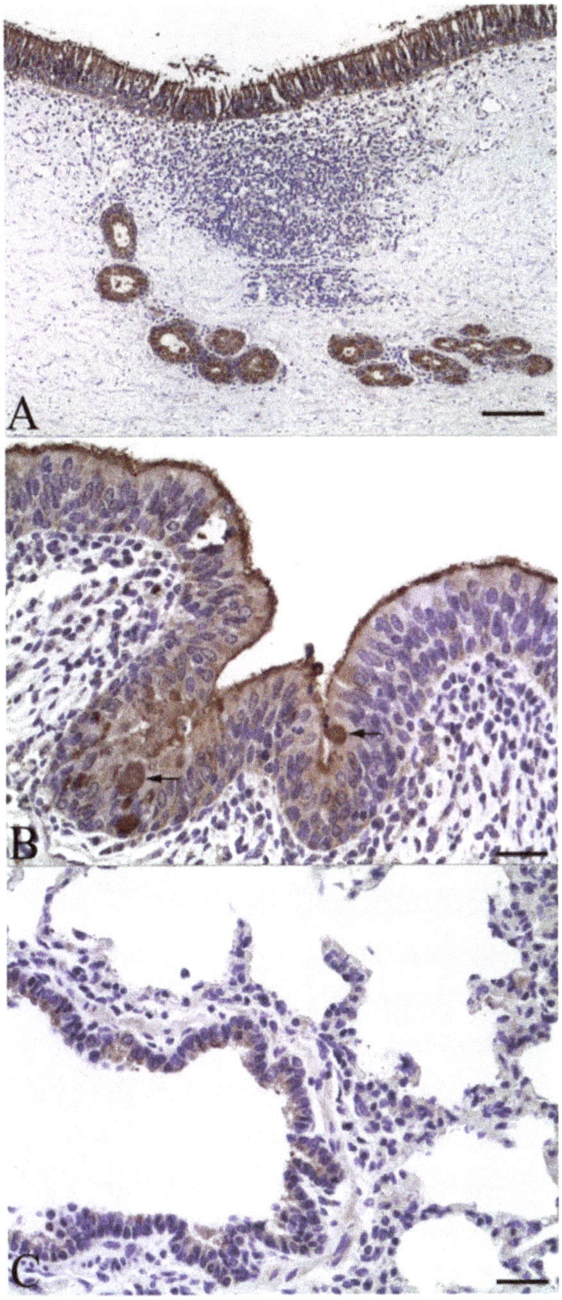

Figure 1 Immunohistochemistry for annexin A1 in normal tissues. (A) Trachea, with intense labeling of surface epithelium and mucosal glands. Bar = 100 µm. **(B)** Bronchus, with labeling of surface epithelium including cilia and goblet cells (arrows). Bar = 70 µm. **(C)** Weaker labeling of bronchiolar epithelium. Bar = 50 µm.

Annexin A1 and A2 expression in lung following *M. haemolytica* challenge

Immunohistochemical labeling of annexins A1 and A2 were compared in calves challenged with *M. haemolytica*

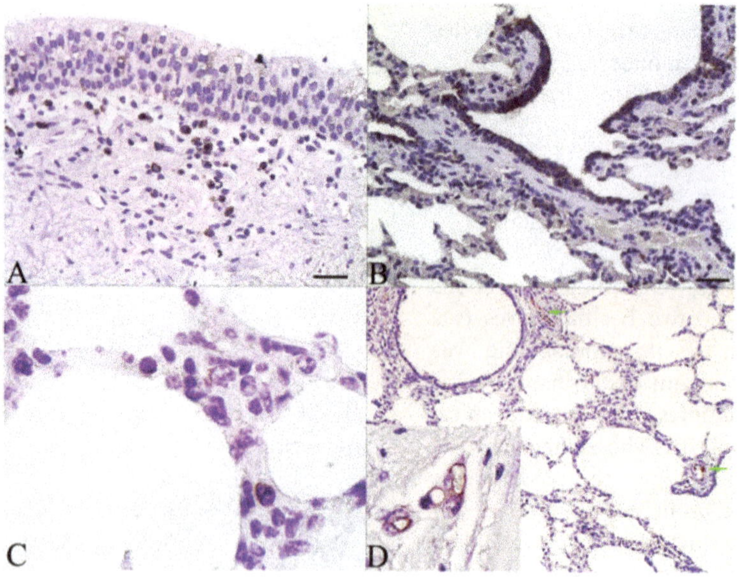

Figure 2 Immunohistochemistry for annexin A2 in normal tissues. (A) Trachea, with strong labeling of leukocytes but weak labeling of epithelium. Bar = 30 μm. **(B)** Bronchiole, with prominent labeling of epithelial cells. Bar = 30 μm **(C)** Labeling of individual cells in an alveolar septum consistent with macrophages or endothelial cells. **(D)** Absence of labeling of alveolar septa. Blood vessels (arrows) and bronchiolar epithelium are labeled. Bar = 50 μm. Inset: Intense labeling of endothelial cells in the lamina propria of a bronchus.

and sham-challenged animals (Additional file 4 and Additional file 5). The histopathologic findings included foci of coagulative necrosis surrounded by a rim of necrotic leukocytes, the presence of fibrin and neutrophils within alveoli, and sloughed epithelial cells and infiltration of leukocytes into the lumen of airways. The necrotic foci and the leukocytes around the necrotic foci had patchy areas of immunolabeling for annexin A1 and to a minor extent for annexin A2 (Figures 3A and B). Annexin A1 labeling was intense within neutrophils at the center of

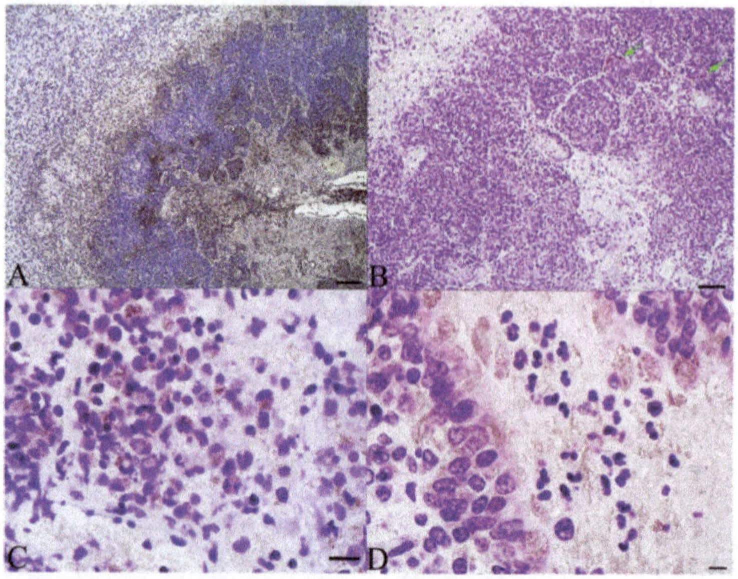

Figure 3 Immunohistochemistry for annexins A1 and A2 in calves challenged with *M. haemolytica*. (A) Annexin A1 expression in leukocytes within a focal area of coagulation necrosis (lower right) and in the band of leukocytes surrounding it. Bar = 100 μm. **(B)** Scant annexin A2 expression within necrotic cells, probably leukocytes (arrows), surrounding the focal area of necrosis. Bar = 50 μm. **(C)** Labeling of annexin A1 in necrotic leukocytes bordering an area of necrosis. Bar = 25 μm. **(D)** In an inflamed bronchiole, there is annexin A1 labeling of goblet cells including those that have been shed from the epithelium, but exudate neutrophils are unlabeled. Bar = 15 μm.

the necrotic foci (Figure 3C). In contrast, neutrophils within bronchioles and alveoli were weakly and inconsistently labeled (Figure 3D). There was shedding of goblet cells from the bronchial epithelium and these goblet cells were intensely labeled for annexin A1 (Figure 3D). Subjectively, annexin A1 labeling of the epithelium of terminal bronchioles was more frequently detected in *M. haemolytica-* vs. sham-challenged animals, but this was not confirmed by the blinded objective evaluation (Additional file 6). Labeling for annexins A1 and A2 in the large airways was not significantly different between the calves challenged with *M. haemolytica* compared to the sham-challenged calves. Use of the negative control antibody did not result in labeling (Additional file 4C and E).

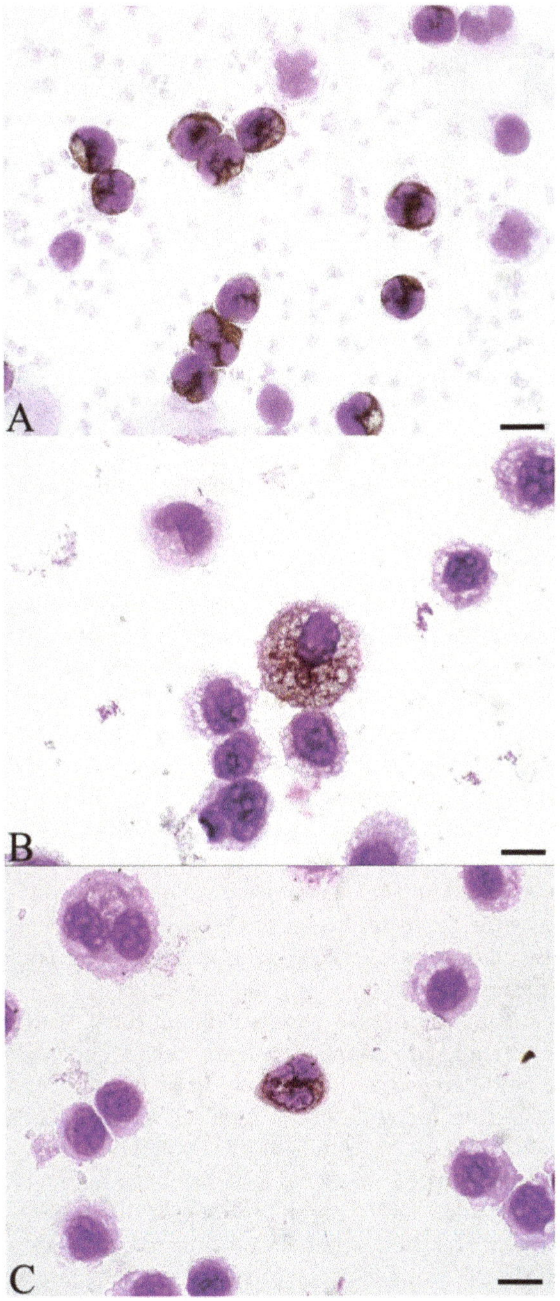

Figure 4 Immunocytochemistry for annexin A1. (A) Neutrophils in blood labeled for annexin A1; monocytes, lymphocytes and platelets are unlabeled. Bar = 10 μm. **(B)** Bronchoalveolar lavage fluid (BALF); Annexin A1 labeling in the cytoplasm of large foamy macrophages, but not in other macrophages. Bar = 10 μm. **(C)** BALF; neutrophils are rare in normal BALF but those present are labeled for annexin A1. Bar = 10 μm.

Annexin A1 expression in blood and BALF leukocytes

In normal blood leukocytes, immunocytochemistry showed positive labeling for annexin A1 in 100% of neutrophils (Figure 4A). The signal was detected in the cytoplasm, and cell membrane labeling was not observed. Lymphocytes, monocytes and platelets were not labeled. Adsorption of the primary antibody with annexin A1 protein abrogated the immunolabeling of the neutrophils (Additional file 7C).

In BALF, annexin A1 was not detected in most macrophages, nor in any lymphocytes (Additional file 7). However, annexin A1 signal was detected in low numbers of large BAL macrophages with abundant vacuolated cytoplasm (Figure 4B) and in large macrophages with features suggestive of apoptosis. Neutrophils were rare in cytocentrifuge preparations from the BALF of healthy calves, but those neutrophils present had intense labeling for annexin A1 (Figure 4C).

Blood leukocytes were analyzed by flow cytometry for cell-surface expression of annexin A1 (Figure 5, Additional file 8). Among the leukocytes, 26% of lymphocytes and 18% of monocytes had median fluorescence intensity (MFI) above that seen in the negative control. The difference in MFI was significant in lymphocytes and monocytes ($P < 0.0001$ and $P = 0.0003$, Student's t-test). In contrast, neutrophils had little or no shift in the MFI ($P = 0.366$) indicating lack of surface expression of annexin A1.

Discussion

We investigated the distribution of annexin A1 and A2 protein within the respiratory tract of healthy cattle, and compared this to the levels found after experimental infection with *M. haemolytica*. In healthy calves, immunolabeling for annexins A1 and A2 was detected throughout the respiratory tract, especially in the airway surface epithelium and submucosal glands. Subtle differences in distribution and intensity of expression were noted for these two proteins: annexin A1 labeling was greatest in the surface and glandular epithelium of large proximal airways, and was present in goblet cells but not alveoli or endothelium; whereas annexin A2 labeling was weak in both surface epithelium of proximal and distal small airways, and was more intense in leukocytes and in endothelial cells. We found similar levels of both annexins A1 and A2 in undifferentiated club cells compared

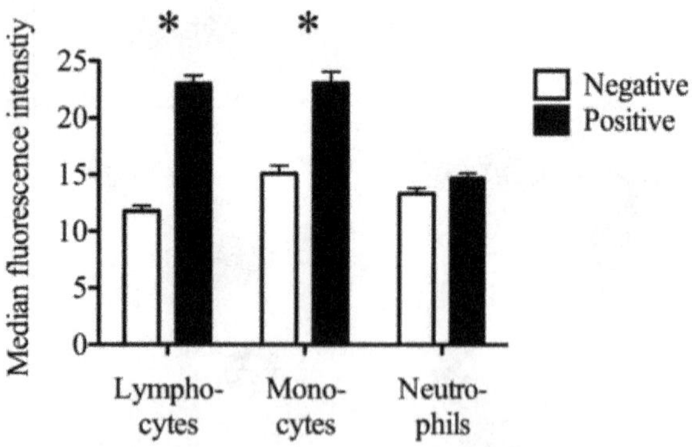

Figure 5 Flow cytometric detection of annexin A1 on the surface of blood leukocytes. Positive: antibody against annexin A1; negative: omission of the primary antibody. Median ± SEM from 8 animals. The MFI was significantly different from the negative control for lymphocytes ($P < 0.0001$) and monocytes ($P = 0.0003$) but not for neutrophils ($P = 0.366$).

to differentiated ciliated epithelial cells and goblet cells of the trachea and bronchi, in contrast to previous work that was based on undifferentiated and differentiated (secretory) cells cultured in vitro [12]. The findings imply that the annexin A1 and A2 protein detected in bronchoalveolar lavage fluid of healthy calves is secreted by airway epithelial cells, since neutrophils are rare in the lumen of normal airways. Thus, annexin A1 and A2 are among the products secreted by airway epithelial cells that maintain an anti-inflammatory state in the healthy respiratory tract, and regulation of these responses may influence clinical outcome in cattle experiencing risk factors for pneumonia.

Comparison of calves experimentally infected with *M. haemolytica* and sham-inoculated calves showed little or no difference in the localization or intensity of immunolabeling for annexin A1 and A2. This argues against but does not eliminate the possibility that annexin gene expression is induced by inflammation, since steady state levels could be achieved if protein synthesis and secretion were both upregulated. Measuring annexin A1 levels in BALF of calves with pneumonia would address this possibility. However, the calves infected with *M. haemolytica* showed intense labeling of annexin A1 in leukocytes (mainly degenerating neutrophils) and BALF cells undergoing apoptosis. Conversely, exudate neutrophils within the lumen of airways were not labeled, perhaps as a result of activation-induced secretion of this protein. These findings suggest that during inflammation, annexin A1 released from leukocytes may contribute to the amount of this protein present in the inflamed tissue. The findings show no change in annexin A1 immunolabeling in lung parenchymal cells during pneumonia, but suggest increased levels of annexin A1 protein in the lung as a result of leukocyte infiltration. These data are consistent with prior detection of annexin A1 in the BALF of normal calves and those with experimentally induced bacterial and viral pneumonia [15,16].

The immunocytochemistry and flow cytometry results showed annexin A1 immunolabeling in the cytoplasm of normal blood and BALF neutrophils, but not on the cell surface. These findings concur with findings in human blood leukocytes [17], where annexin A1 was abundant in the cytoplasm of neutrophils, monocytes and natural killer cells but surface expression was not detected, and both surface and cytoplasmic expression was low in lymphocytes.

The flow cytometric analysis showed that, in the resting state, only a small amount of annexin A1 was present on the surface of lymphocytes and monocytes, and neutrophils had no detectable cell-surface expression of annexin A1. In contrast, studies of human leukocytes have shown low but detectable surface expression of annexin A1 on neutrophils [18]. The detection of annexin A1 in the cytoplasm of a subset of BAL macrophages does not necessarily indicate synthesis by these cells. Instead, annexin A1 immunolabeling in large foamy macrophages may have resulted from pinocytosis of airway secretions or phagocytosis of epithelial cells or neutrophils that contained this protein.

Annexin A1 has several known anti-inflammatory functions: it inhibits transendothelial migration and activation of neutrophils, enhances neutrophil apoptosis, inhibits activation of MAP kinase-mediated signal transduction, downregulates synthesis of inflammatory eicosanoids, and enhances secretion of the anti-inflammatory cytokine interleukin-10 from macrophages [2-7]. Similarly, the functions of annexin A2 include activation of plasminogen to initiate fibrinolysis, enhancing macrophage-mediated phagocytosis of apoptotic leukocytes, and enhancing repair of airway epithelial cells [8-10]. The finding that annexins A1 and A2 are mainly derived from airway epithelial cells in healthy individuals furthers understanding of how these cells dampen inflammation in the healthy airway and lung. Thus, although airway epithelial cells are capable of producing pro-inflammatory mediators and initiating airway host defenses, the resting airway epithelium appears to maintain homeostasis and the non-inflamed state of the healthy lung. Despite constant inhalation of organic dusts and bacteria, inflammation in the lung appears to be limited by secretion of annexins A1 and A2, club cell secretory protein, odorant binding protein, chitinase-like proteins, surfactant proteins A and D, lipoxins and resolvins, as well as epithelial cell surface expression of integrins and CD200 [19-21]. This concept suggests that dysregulation of these effects in airway epithelial cells could lead to tissue damage from the ensuing inflammatory response.

This may explain the prior findings that calves with higher levels of annexins A1 and A2 in BALF had reduced prevalence of clinically apparent pneumonia.

In conclusion, annexin A1 immunolabeling was found to be most prominent in the surface epithelium, goblet cells and submucosal glands of the large proximal airways, and was also detected in the epithelium of distal airways, blood and BALF neutrophils, and large foamy macrophages in BALF. Annexin A2 immunolabeling was most abundant in the epithelial cells of the distal airways and in endothelial cells, with labeling also detected in alveoli and proximal airways, as well as in leukocytes and endothelial cells. The pattern and intensity of expression in the lung parenchyma was similar in calves with experimentally induced *M. haemolytica* pneumonia as in sham-inoculated calves, for both annexin A1 and A2. These findings imply that annexin A1 in the BALF of healthy calves mainly originates from the airway epithelium, whereas annexin A2 in BALF arises from airway epithelium and mucosal leukocytes. In BALF from inflamed lung, annexins A1 and A2 may also originate from leukocytes.

Additional files

Additional file 1: Immunohistochemistry for annexin A1 in normal tissues. (A) Trachea, with intense labeling of surface epithelium and tracheal glands. (B) Trachea; absence of labeling with the control antibody against *Toxoplasma*. (C) Bronchus, with labeling of surface epithelium including cilia and goblet cells (arrows). Inset: negative control (pre-incubation of antibody with antigen). (D) Weaker labeling of bronchiolar epithelium. (E) Bronchiole, negative control (prior adsorption of primary antibody with annexin protein) with partially abrogated labeling. (F) Absence of labeling of alveolar septa; minor labeling of bronchiolar epithelium.

Additional file 2: Immunohistochemistry for annexin A2 in normal tissues. (A) Trachea, with labeling of surface epithelium, mucosal glands, and lymphocytes in the lamina propria. Goblet cells or cilia of the respiratory epithelium were not labeled (arrow). (B) Bronchus, similar labeling as in the trachea. (C) Bronchus. Absence of labeling in the negative control using antibody against influenza virus. (D) Trachea, with strong labeling of leukocytes but weak labeling of epithelium. (E) Bronchus, similar labeling as in the trachea. (F) Bronchiole, with prominent labeling of the epithelium.

Additional file 3: Immunohistochemistry for annexin A2 in normal tissues. (A) Trachea, with labeling of tracheal glands. (B) Absence of labeling of alveolar septa. Blood vessels (arrows) and bronchiolar epithelium is labeled. (C, D) Labeling of individual cells in the alveolar septa consistent with macrophages or endothelium. (E) Intense labeling of endothelial cells in the lamina propria of a bronchus.

Additional file 4: Focal coagulation necrosis and inflammation in the lung of a calf challenged with *M. haemolytica*. (A) Focal necrosis (lower right) separated from more normal lung (upper left) by a dense band of necrotic leukocytes. Hematoxylin and eosin. (B) Annexin A1 expression in leukocytes in the necrotic lesion and in the band of leukocytes surrounding it. (C) Negative control for annexin A1 immunostain, using a primary antibody against Toxoplasma. (D) Scant annexin A2 expression in exudate surrounding the focal area of necrosis. (E) Negative control for annexin A2 immunostain, using a primary antibody against influenza virus.

Additional file 5: Immunohistochemistry for annexin A1 and A2 in the lung of a calf challenged with *M. haemolytica*. (A) Strong labelling of annexin A1 in necrotic leukocytes bordering an area of necrosis. (B) Weak labelling of annexin A2 in necrotic leukocytes bordering an area of necrosis. (C) Inflamed bronchiole, with moderate labeling for annexin A1. (D) Inflamed bronchiole, with weak labeling for annexin A2. (E) Inflamed bronchiole. There is annexin A1 labeling of goblet cells including those that have been shed from the epithelium, but exudate neutrophils are unlabeled. (F) Inflamed bronchiole. Annexin A2 labeling of bronchiolar exudate, but not of goblet cells or neutrophils.

Additional file 6: Semi-quantitative scoring of immunohistochemical labeling of annexins A1 and A2 in the respiratory tract of six calves. Three calves had been infected with *Mannheimia haemolytica* by intrabronchial challenge, and three were unchallenged controls.

Additional file 7: Immunocytochemistry for annexin A1 in normal blood leukocytes and normal bronchoalveolar lavage fluid (BALF). (A) Blood smear, Wright's stain. (B) Neutrophils in blood labeled for annexin A1; monocytes and lymphocytes are unlabeled. (C) Negative control, using an antibody against Toxoplasma. (D) Wright's stain of BALF leukocytes, showing macrophages and a single neutrophil. (E) BALF; Annexin A1 labeling in the cytoplasm of large foamy macrophages, but not in other macrophages. (F) BALF; neutrophils are rare in normal BALF but those present are labeled for annexin A1.

Additional file 8: Flow cytometry for surface expression of annexin A1 in normal bovine blood leukocytes. (A) Scatterplot, indicating forward- and side-scatter characteristics of neutrophils, lymphocytes and monocytes. (B, C, D) Histograms of fluorescence (annexin A1) vs. cell count for cells gated as neutrophils (B), lymphocytes (C) and monocytes (D). Blue: labeled with antibody against annexin A1; red: negative control (primary antibody omitted). (E) Flow cytometric detection of annexin A1 on the surface of blood leukocytes. Positive: antibody against annexin A1; negative: omission of the primary antibody. Median ± SEM from 8 animals. The MFI was significantly different from the negative control for lymphocytes ($P < 0.0001$) and monocytes ($P = 0.0003$) but not for neutrophils ($P = 0.366$).

Abbreviations
ICC: Immunocytochemistry; IHC: Immunohistochemistry; MFI: Median fluorescence intensity.

Competing interests
The authors declare that they have no competing interests.

Authors' contributions
CS carried out the studies and prepared the manuscript. JH participated in study design, acquisition and analysis of data. MEC and TLO contributed to study design, acquisition and analysis of the data. BNL participated in study design and analysis of data. JLC conceived of the study and participated in its design and coordination and helped to draft the manuscript. All authors read and approved the final manuscript.

Acknowledgements
This work was supported by the Natural Sciences and Engineering Research Council of Canada (NSERC), the Beef Cattle Research Council (Canadian Cattlemen's Association), the Ontario Ministry of Agriculture and Food, and the Ontario Veterinary College Fellowship program. This project was funded in part through Growing Forward, a federal-provincial-territorial initiative; the Agricultural Adaptation Council assists in the delivery of Growing Forward programs in Ontario. We thank Dr Cynthia Miltenburg, University of Guelph for providing samples for flow cytometry and Dr Josepha Delay, Animal Health Laboratory, University of Guelph for providing control antibodies.

Author details
[1]Department of Pathobiology, University of Guelph, Guelph, ON, N1G 2W1, Canada. [2]Department of Population Medicine, University of Guelph, Guelph, ON, N1G 2W1, Canada. [3]Department of Clinical Studies, University of Guelph, Guelph, ON, N1G 2W1, Canada.

References

1. Senthilkumaran C, Clark ME, Abdelaziz K, Bateman KG, Mackay A, Hewson J, Caswell JL (2013) Increased annexin A1 and A2 levels in bronchoalveolar lavage fluid are associated with resistance to respiratory disease in beef calves. Vet Res 44:24
2. Ferlazzo V, D'Agostino P, Milano S, Caruso R, Feo S, Cillari E, Parente L (2003) Anti-inflammatory effects of annexin-1: stimulation of IL-10 release and inhibition of nitric oxide synthesis. Int Immunopharmacol 3:1363–1369
3. da Cunha EE, Oliani SM, Damazo AS (2012) Effect of annexin-A1 peptide treatment during lung inflammation induced by lipopolysaccharide. Pulm Pharmacol Ther 25:303–311
4. Croxtall JD, Gilroy DW, Solito E, Choudhury Q, Ward BJ, Buckingham JC, Flower RJ (2003) Attenuation of glucocorticoid functions in an Anx-A1-/- cell line. Biochem J 371:927–935
5. Gavins FN, Hickey MJ (2012) Annexin A1 and the regulation of innate and adaptive immunity. Front Immunol 3:354
6. Vago JP, Nogueira CR, Tavares LP, Soriani FM, Lopes F, Russo RC, Pinho V, Teixeira MM, Sousa LP (2012) Annexin A1 modulates natural and glucocorticoid-induced resolution of inflammation by enhancing neutrophil apoptosis. J Leukoc Biol 92:249–258
7. Yang YH, Toh ML, Clyne CD, Leech M, Aeberli D, Xue J, Dacumos A, Sharma L, Morand EF (2006) Annexin 1 negatively regulates IL-6 expression via effects on p38 MAPK and MAPK phosphatase-1. J Immunol 177:8148–8153
8. Ling Q, Jacovina AT, Deora A, Febbraio M, Simantov R, Silverstein RL, Hempstead B, Mark WH, Hajjar KA (2004) Annexin II regulates fibrin homeostasis and neoangiogenesis in vivo. J Clin Invest 113:38–48
9. Patchell BJ, Wojcik KR, Yang TL, White SR, Dorscheid DR (2007) Glycosylation and annexin II cell surface translocation mediate airway epithelial wound repair. Am J Physiol Lung Cell Mol Physiol 293:L354–363
10. Swisher JF, Khatri U, Feldman GM (2007) Annexin A2 is a soluble mediator of macrophage activation. J Leukoc Biol 82:1174–1184
11. Dreier R, Schmid KW, Gerke V, Riehemann K (1998) Differential expression of annexins I, II and IV in human tissues: an immunohistochemical study. Histochem Cell Biol 110:137–148
12. Vishwanatha JK, Muns G, Beckmann JD, Davis RG, Rubinstein I (1995) Differential expression of annexins I and II in bovine bronchial epithelial cells. Am J Respir Cell Mol Biol 12:280–286
13. Mitchell GB, Clark ME, Siwicky M, Caswell JL (2008) Stress alters the cellular and proteomic compartments of bovine bronchoalveolar lavage fluid. Vet Immunol Immunopathol 125:111–125
14. Reggeti F, Bienzle D (2011) Flow cytometry in veterinary oncology. Vet Pathol 48:223–235
15. Katoh N, Miyamoto T, Nakagawa H, Watanabe A (1999) Detection of annexin I and IV and haptoglobin in bronchoalveolar lavage fluid from calves experimentally inoculated with Pasteurella haemolytica. Am J Vet Res 60:1390–1395
16. Katoh N (2000) Detection of annexins I and IV in bronchoalveolar lavage fluids from calves inoculated with bovine herpes virus-1. J Vet Med Sci 62:37–41
17. Spurr L, Nadkarni S, Pederzoli-Ribeil M, Goulding NJ, Perretti M, D'Acquisto F (2011) Comparative analysis of Annexin A1-formyl peptide receptor 2/ALX expression in human leukocyte subsets. Int Immunopharmacol 11:55–66
18. Perretti M, Flower RJ (2004) Annexin 1 and the biology of the neutrophil. J Leukoc Biol 76:25–29
19. Katavolos P, Ackerley CA, Viel L, Clark ME, Wen X, Bienzle D (2009) Clara cell secretory protein is reduced in equine recurrent airway obstruction. Vet Pathol 46:604–613
20. Mitchell GB, Clark ME, Caswell JL (2007) Alterations in the bovine bronchoalveolar lavage proteome induced by dexamethasone. Vet Immunol Immunopathol 118:283–293
21. Holt PG, Strickland DH (2008) The CD200-CD200R axis in local control of lung inflammation. Nat Immunol 9:1011–1013

3

The early intestinal immune response in experimental neonatal ovine cryptosporidiosis is characterized by an increased frequency of perforin expressing NCR1$^+$ NK cells and by NCR1$^-$ CD8$^+$ cell recruitment

Line Olsen[1*], Caroline Piercey Åkesson[1], Anne K Storset[2], Sonia Lacroix-Lamandé[3], Preben Boysen[2], Coralie Metton[3], Timothy Connelley[4], Arild Espenes[1], Fabrice Laurent[3] and Françoise Drouet[3*]

Abstract

Cryptosporidium parvum, a zoonotic protozoan parasite, causes important losses in neonatal ruminants. Innate immunity plays a key role in controlling the acute phase of this infection. The participation of NCR1+ Natural Killer (NK) cells in the early intestinal innate immune response to the parasite was investigated in neonatal lambs inoculated at birth. The observed increase in the lymphocyte infiltration was further studied by immunohistology and flow cytometry with focus on distribution, density, cellular phenotype related to cytotoxic function and activation status. The frequency of NCR1+ cells did not change with infection, while their absolute number slightly increased in the jejunum and the CD8+/NCR1- T cell density increased markedly. The frequency of perforin+ cells increased significantly with infection in the NCR1+ population (in both NCR1+/CD16+ and NCR1+/CD16- populations) but not in the NCR1-/CD8+ population. The proportion of NCR1+ cells co-expressing CD16+ also increased. The fraction of cells expressing IL2 receptor (CD25), higher in the NCR1+/CD8+ population than among the CD8+/NCR1- cells in jejunal Peyer's patches, remained unchanged during infection. However, contrary to CD8+/NCR1- lymphocytes, the intensity of CD25 expressed by NCR1+ lymphocytes increased in infected lambs. Altogether, the data demonstrating that NK cells are highly activated and possess a high cytotoxic potential very early during infection, concomitant with an up-regulation of the interferon gamma gene in the gut segments, support the hypothesis that they are involved in the innate immune response against *C. parvum*. The early significant recruitment of CD8+/NCR1- T cells in the small intestine suggests that they could rapidly drive the establishment of the acquired immune response.

Introduction

As with all neonatal mammals, the new-born ruminant is challenged by infections at vulnerable mucosal sites like the gut mucosa, frequently leading to enteritis. *Cryptosporidium parvum* (*C. parvum*), a protozoan parasite highly prevalent in cattle and small ruminant flocks throughout the world is a zoonotic agent. In sheep, *C. parvum* causes moderate to severe, but usually self-limiting enteric neonatal disease [1,2] with low mortality. However, in very young ruminants, this parasite may cause profuse diarrhoea and can lead to death by dehydration if combined with co-infections or deficiencies in nutrition and husbandry [3]. The parasite cycle ends with either thin-walled oocysts that auto-infect the host or thick-walled oocysts that are released in the environment [4]. Both animal health and welfare, economic impact and the zoonotic aspect make cryptosporidiosis one of the most important gastro-intestinal diseases in ruminant production. To date there is no vaccine available, and halofuginone lactate is the only drug with marketing

* Correspondence: l.olsen@nmbu.no; francoise.drouet@tours.inra.fr
[1]Department of Basic Sciences and Aquatic Medicine, Faculty of Veterinary Medicine and Biosciences, Norwegian University of Life Sciences, Oslo, Norway
[3]Institut National de la Recherche Agronomique, UMR1282, Infectiologie et Santé Publique, Laboratoire Apicomplexes et Immunité Muqueuse, Nouzilly, France
Full list of author information is available at the end of the article

authorization for preventive treatment of cryptosporidiosis [5,6]. To develop an adequate immunoprophylaxis strategy, it is therefore important to clarify the early immune events leading to a protective response against this parasite as neonates frequently become infected within the few hours following birth.

Only limited information is available on the neonatal ruminant intestinal immune response to *C. parvum* during the early stages of the infection. Pathogenicity and brief pathology of ovine cryptosporidiosis were described in lambs for the first time [1,2,7] more than three decades ago and more recent data were obtained in calves describing the intestinal response to the parasite with an increase of T cell subsets [8-12]. Nevertheless, our understanding of the immuno-pathological response to *C. parvum* remains poor in these species.

Recovery and protection from reinfection have been associated with a CD4+ T cell response starting from the second week post inoculation [13-15]. In cattle, this response has been associated with a production of gamma interferon (IFNγ) [11,12]. SCID mice lacking B and T cells develop chronic inflammation upon *C. parvum* infection, which progressively becomes fatal [13,15,16]. More recent experiments performed with mice tend to demonstrate that the innate immune system could be sufficient to resolve the infection [17] and we recently showed in neonatal mice that innate immunity can control the acute phase of the disease [18]. As Natural Killer (NK) cells are key players in innate immune responses they might play a role in the early host immune response against this parasite in young lambs. NK cells have been suggested to be important participants in the immune response against *C. parvum* infection; Barakat et al. [19] found that NK cells had an important role for the innate control of *C. parvum* infection in mice and Dann et al. [20] showed that NK cells lead to clearance of cryptosporidia from the intestine of humans.

Most of the studies on the role of NK cells in *C. parvum* infections have been performed with adult murine models which are not the most suitable species for studying *C. parvum* pathogenesis; indeed they are not naturally susceptible, rarely develop diarrhoea and do not develop the same mucosal pathology as observed in larger animals and humans [21,22].

The jejunum and ileum contain Peyer's patches (PPs) that are considered as immune sensors of the intestine and are important for immune protection at mucosal surfaces and the induction of mucosal immune responses in the intestine [23,24]. Whereas the PPs of the jejunum (JPPs) are recognized as secondary lymphoid organs of the intestinal wall, the continuous ileal PP (IPP) is also responsible for the generation of B cells and is thus considered as a primary lymphoid tissue [25-28]. The specialized follicle associated epithelium (FAE) that overlies PPs is capable of transporting luminal antigens [29] to the underlying immune cells to promote a tolerogenic or an inflammatory response, which will be set in action in the lamina propria. Our aim was to get an insight into the early local immune response in the different sections of the small intestine and associated lymphoid tissues of lambs during the neonatal period with a particular focus on NK cells, which we have shown to be active in neonatal calves [30], and CD8 T lymphocytes, that have been shown to be important in controlling *C. parvum* infection in humans [31].

In lambs inoculated soon after birth, we observed an activation of the NCR1+ NK population in the gut with increased expression of perforin, CD16 and CD25. In contrast, the expression of perforin and CD25 by CD8+/NCR1- T lymphocytes did not increase in infected lambs although the density and percentages of this population increased from day 3 post-inoculation (pi) in both the inductive and effector sites of the small intestine.

Materials and methods

Animals and experimental design

The lambs used for this study were born from Préalpes ewes maintained in protected facilities with a conventional status (PFIE-INRA-37380 Nouzilly). At birth the lambs were allowed to suckle the colostrum and then received artificial milk *ad libitum* until euthanasia. Within 24 h, age-matched "pairs of lambs" (occasionally triplets), i.e. lambs born within a 12 h interval, were relocated to two identical rooms, one for the inoculated lambs and one for the controls. The day following birth, the animals were inoculated *per os* with 2×10^6 oocysts of *C. parvum* (day 0 pi). During the experiment, symptoms were registered and pathological signs briefly recorded at the time of slaughter. Animals were slaughtered at various days pi (dpi), i.e. 0, 1, 2, 3, 6 and 11 dpi by electric stunning and bleeding according to the AMVA guideline on euthanasia; matched pairs of lambs were slaughtered the same day and their organs processed simultaneously. All experimental protocols were conducted in compliance with French legislation (Décret: 2001–464 29/05/01) and EEC regulations (86/609/CEE) governing the care and use of laboratory animals, after validation by the local ethics committee for animal experimentation (CEEA VdL: 2011-05-2).

Parasite and infection

Collection of oocysts

C. parvum oocysts were isolated from the faeces of neonatal calves infected with oocysts initially obtained from an infected child and maintained by repeated passage in calves. Oocysts were purified as previously described [32].

Parasitic load detection

In a set of animals, faeces were collected daily to assess the oocyst excretion pattern (Figure 1A). The first oocysts pass in the faeces at day 3 or 4 pi. Therefore, to assess the parasitized status of the inoculated lambs slaughtered early after inoculation (before parasite excretion) and the uninfected status of their controls, the presence of *C. parvum* in the mucosa was tested on fragments of intestine by assessing the expression of a cryptosporidium-specific gene by real time RT-PCR as previously described [32]. From day 4 pi the level of infection was also assessed by counting oocysts in the faeces as described by Naciri et al. [5].

Collection of tissue specimens

Samples of jejunum, JPPs, IPP, spleen and small intestinal mesenteric lymph nodes (MLN) were taken. Tissue sampling for cryostat sectioning was performed as previously described [33]. In short, tissues were chilled in isopentane before freezing in liquid nitrogen and storage at −70 °C. In addition, tissues were fixed in formalin and embedded in paraffin wax (FFPE). Some tissues were snap frozen in liquid nitrogen for RNA analyses. In pairs of age matched control and inoculated lambs, fresh tissues were collected in ice-cold RPMI medium supplemented with 5% foetal calf serum (FCS) and 1% penicillin streptomycin (P/S) for extraction of the cells.

Antibodies used for labelling

The antibodies (Abs) used in this study were against: ovine NCR1/NKp46 (EC1.1; IgG1 [34]), bovine NCR1/NKp46 (AKS6; IgG2b [35]), bovine TcR1-N7 (86D; IgG1) that labels γδ-T lymphocytes, bovine CD25 (CACT116A; IgG1), from VMRD/WSU (Pullman, USA), human CD16 (KD1; IgG2a, [36,37]), human CD3 (A0452; pAb) from Dako (Trappes, France), ovine CD8 (38.65; IgG2a) from Serotec (UK) and Ki67 (ab15580; pAb and NCL-L-Ki67-MM1; IgG1) from Abcam (Cambridge, UK) and Novocastra Laboratories-Leica (UK) respectively. The anti-human perforin-FITC kit (δG9; IgG2b) was from BD Pharmingen (France). IgG1, IgG2a, IgM mouse isotype controls for flow cytometry were from Dako and IgG2b from Caltag- Invitrogen (France). Isotype controls for IHC against IgG1, IgG2a and IgG2b were from BD Biosciences (USA). Subtype-specific secondary Abs conjugated with Tricolor (TC) or R-Phycoerythrin (PE) were from Caltag. Goat anti-mouse IgG Fab'2 secondary Abs conjugated with Fluo Probe (FP) 488 were from Fluo Probes- Interchim (France). Alexa Fluor-conjugated secondary Abs AF 350, 488, 546, 594 and 633 for indirect immunofluorescence were from Molecular Probes-Invitrogen.

Histology techniques

All FFPE tissues were stained and examined with haematoxylin and eosin (H&E) according to standard histological techniques [38] for routine histological examination. Samples of intestine for electron microscopy (EM) were fixed with 3% glutaraldehyde in 0.1 M cacodylate buffer, then processed as previously described for transmission EM [39] and scanning EM [40]. The samples were examined with a Jeol 1010 transmission electron microscope (Jeol, Croissy-sur-Seine, France) and a FEG Gemini 982 scanning electron microscope (Carl Zeiss, Jena, Germany). For in situ immunolabelling, standard indirect methods with avidin-biotin complex peroxidase (Vectastain® ABC Kit, Vector Laboratories, USA) were used against *C. parvum*. Prior to immunolabelling of the FFPE sections, 4 μm thick sections were placed on positively charged slides and dried at 59 °C. After a standard dewaxing procedure, sections were treated for antigen retrieval in citrate buffer (0.01 M citric acid monohydrate, pH 6.0) in a microwave. Endogenous peroxidase was inhibited by treatment with 3% H_2O_2 in methanol for 10 min. Further blocking of unspecific binding and incubation with antibodies were performed as described by the manufacturer. The specific binding of the antibodies was visualized by using ImmPACT™ AEC after counter staining with Mayer's haematoxylin. Indirect immunolabelling was performed on cryosections, according to a protocol described earlier [33,41]. Fluorescent sections were examined under a Leica DM RXA fluorescence microscope (Germany), and images were captured using a SPOT RT Slider™ camera (Diagnostic Instruments, USA) with SPOT 5.0 Advanced Software (Diagnostic Instruments). In addition, images were captured using a Zeiss Axiovert 100 inverted microscope, equipped with an LSM 510 laser confocal unit with the Zeiss ZEN 2009 Software (Carl Zeiss).

Microscopic evaluation of immuno-labelled slides

To ascertain whether morphological features observed on H&E sections were related to *C. parvum* infection in the gut, the sections were blind coded. Features present in each section were listed and each feature was subjectively recorded in a visual analogue scale (VAS) ranging from 0 to 100. For immunofluorescent qualitative analysis of NCR1+ cells, single-blinded analysis was done. For quantitative analysis of CD8+ cells in the IPP, images were taken and processed as previously described [33]. Briefly, images of 400× from at least 5 individual villi and domes from the ileal segment were taken. A pixel-to-millimetre calibration was performed and the areas were defined in mm^2.

Extraction and purification of mononuclear cells from the organs

Spleen and MLN tissues were processed as previously described [42]. The whole organs were treated to assess the absolute number of mononuclear cells (MNC). All mediums and chemicals were from Sigma-Aldrich (Lyon, France) unless otherwise stated. Briefly, the tissues were

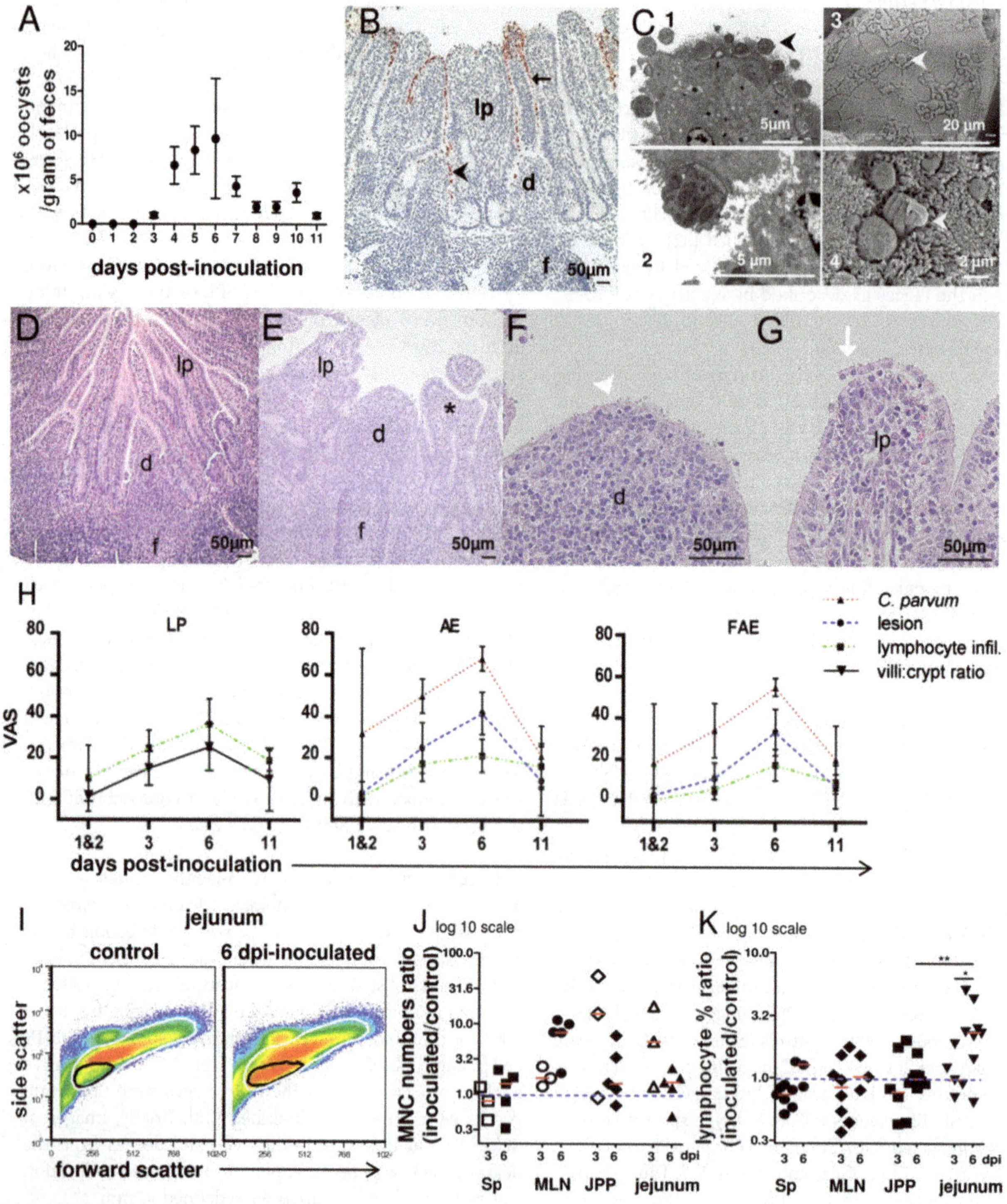

Figure 1 (See legend on next page.)

(See figure on previous page.)

Figure 1 *C. parvum* oocyst excretion, lesions and lymphocyte infiltration during infection. (A) *C. parvum* oocyst excretion: mean/gram of faeces ± standard error (10 to 15 animals). **(B)** *C. parvum* parasitic stages immunolabelled in brown in a 3 dpi ileal Peyer's patch (IPP): on the brush border of absorptive epithelium (AE) (arrow) and follicle-associated epithelium (fae/FAE) (arrowhead) covering the lamina propria (lp/LP) and dome (d). Lymphoid follicle (f). **(C)** Trophozoites and meronts at 6 dpi, in the JPP AE (arrowhead) observed by transmission EM (C1, C2) and scanning EM of meronts in infected FAE (C3; arrowhead) and merozoite leaving a meront (C4; arrowhead). **(D-G)** PPs representative changes during infection (HE staining). JPPs of control **(D)** and 6 dpi inoculated lambs **(E)** with villous atrophy and fusion (*) and lymphocyte infiltration in lp. **(F-G)** Attenuation, lymphocyte infiltration, detachment of fae (arrowhead) and absorptive epithelium (AE) (arrow) in an infected IPP. **(H)** Semi quantitative scoring of histopathological changes in IPP during infection. Sections from control lambs were used as a baseline and each change was rated according to severity on a 0 to 100 visual analogue scale (VAS). Values represent mean with 95% confidence intervals for 4 to 8 animals. **(I-K)** Cells extracted of spleen (Sp), mesenteric lymph nodes (MLN), JPPs and jejunum from matched pairs of lambs were purified on density gradients and mononuclear cell (MNC) and lymphocyte percentages were determined by flow cytometry on morphology parameters. **(I)** Plots show the gating of lymphocytes (black gate) and MNC (white gate) in the jejunum. In this example, lymphocytes represented 11 and 38% of MNC (88 and 84% of the cells analyzed) in control versus matched inoculated lamb, respectively. **(J)** The MNC absolute number ratio and **(K)** the lymphocyte percentage ratio were determined for each pair of lambs at 3 or 6 dpi. The red bars indicate the median values. Mann–Whitney statistic test: significance * $p < 0.05$, ** for $p < 0.01$.

disrupted in Hanks medium (HBSS) containing 2% FCS and 1% P/S by crushing on a 200 μm nylon gauze with a syringe piston. Splenic red blood cells were lysed with ammonium chloride solution (0.155 M NH_4Cl, pH 7.4) then resuspended in HBSS medium. MNC were then purified on Histopaque^{TM} d = 1.077, washed and stored in ice cold RPMI medium supplemented with 10% FCS and 1% P/S until labelling.

Gut tissues were processed with a technique adapted from Renaux et al. [43] and Pérez-Cano et al. [44] to recover lamina propria MNC. Briefly, the gut tract was emptied of faecal content and rinsed with Phosphate Buffer Saline (PBS) buffer. The JPPs were dissected carefully, pooled then processed as the jejunal tissue. The whole jejunum and the JPPs were weighed separately before 30-gram samples of jejunum were taken for extraction of cells. The gut was opened and cut into 1 cm^2 fragments. The epithelial cells and intra-epithelial lymphocytes were extracted by incubation for 20 min at 37 °C in HBSS without Ca and Mg containing 3 mM ethylene diamine tetraacetic acid disodium salt (EDTA), 2 mM dithioerythritol, 10% FCS and 1% P/S under magnetic stirring and discarded. Then the lamina propria lymphocytes were extracted. The EDTA treated intestinal pieces were washed with HBSS, then incubated at 37 °C for 45 mn under magnetic stirring in RPMI medium containing 9.25U/mL type I collagenase, 30U/mL dispase II (Roche, Rosny sous Bois, France) and 2500U/mL bovine pancreas DNase I (Calbiochem, USA). The cell suspension was filtered on a 500 μM nylon mesh and the cells were washed with RPMI-10% SVF. The MNC were purified on a 75%/40% Percoll (GE Healthcare - Bio-Sciences, Sweden) gradient, washed and stored in ice cold RPMI-10% FCS until labelling. The living cells were counted with Thoma chambers and the absolute number in the organ (spleen, MLNs or JPPs) was calculated as follows: number of cells per mL multiplied by number of mL of cell suspension for the whole organ. For the jejunum, as the cells were extracted from 30 grams of tissue, the latter result was multiplied by the ratio: jejunum total weight (in grams)/30. For all the analyses and comparisons reported, the organs from age-matched control and inoculated pairs of lambs were processed simultaneously to minimize technical induced variations.

Cell labelling and flow cytometry

Single or multiple indirect labelling of surface receptors was performed on purified ovine cells using Abs against the molecules NCR1, CD8, TCR1, CD16 and CD25 revealed by subtype-specific secondary Abs. Direct intracellular perforin labelling was performed with the perforin-FITC kit and the Cytofix/Cytoperm and Permwash solutions (BD Pharmingen). The samples were analysed on a FACS CALIBUR flow cytometer (Becton Dickinson), equipped with Cell-Quest Pro software. At least 2×10^5 viable cells were analysed for spleen, MLN and PPs and at least 10^6 cells for the jejunum. The analyses of labelling were performed with the FCS express software; percentages of perforin+ and CD25+ cells and median fluorescence intensity (MFI) were determined using the histogram subtraction and statistics functions of the software. Relative numbers of cell subsets determined by flow cytometry (subset %) were converted into absolute numbers per organ according to the formula: (subset% × MNC%)/100 × total number of cells in organ (as calculated above).

RNA isolation and real-time RT-PCR

RNA was extracted from tissues with TRIZOL solution (Invitrogen), according to the manufacturer's instructions. Purified RNA was reverse-transcribed using oligo (dT) primers and M-MLV reverse transcriptase (Promega, France). For PCR experiments, primer pairs were designed using Primer 3 software (Additional file 1). Each primer was designed on different exons to span the intervening intron and thus avoid amplification from contaminating genomic DNA. Q-RT-PCR assays were carried out by combining cDNA with primers and IQ SYBRGreen Supermix (Bio-Rad, USA) and were run on a Chromo4 (Bio-Rad). Samples were normalized internally using the average cycle quantification (Cq) of three reference genes Hypoxanthine phosphoribosyltransferase (HPRT), b-Actin and Glyceraldehyde-3-phosphate dehydrogenase (GAPDH). Gene expression values are expressed as relative values after Genex macro analysis (Bio-Rad).

Statistical analyses

For the morphometric analysis of the density of CD8+ cells, it was necessary to compensate for natural variability between individuals; therefore the non-parametric Wilcoxon-van Elteren [45] test was used to calculate the significance of differences between the two groups. Two-tailed tests were performed and differences considered significant for p-values < 0.05. Flow cytometry data were analysed with GraphPad software: the nonparametric Mann–Whitney test was used to test the significance of differences between means from inoculated lambs and matched controls, the Wilcoxon test to compare different subsets of cells from the same animals and the paired t test to compare groups of paired lambs.

Results

C. parvum induces typical enteritis lesions with immune cell recruitment in the segments of the neonatal ovine small intestine

In neonatal lambs infected on the day of birth, the kinetics of *C. parvum* oocyst excretion was evaluated daily (Figure 1A). The *C. parvum* infected or uninfected status was verified by measuring the expression of a cryptosporidium specific gene in gut tissues by RT-PCR (data not shown). The excretion of oocysts started from day 3 pi coinciding with the onset of watery diarrhoea and mild dehydration and reached a peak at 6 dpi (Figure 1A). At necropsy, there was a mild to moderate enlargement of mesenteric lymph nodes (MLN) in the inoculated lambs from day 2 pi (1.5-3 fold weight increase on average compared to controls) while no visible change of the spleen was observed. Histopathological observations confirmed the macroscopical findings demonstrating a mild to moderate, diffuse and catarrhal enteritis. Parasites were observed in the brush border throughout the whole gut, with increased density in distal jejunum and ileum. In all PPs, the FAE was also infected (Figures 1B, 1C-F) but, as previously observed in the mouse model (unpublished data), we could not observe developing parasites in M cells. The lesions of superficial, lymphocytic and granulocytic diffuse enteritis, with shortening and bridging of the villi (Figures 1D-G) affected not only the absorptive epithelium, but also the FAE of the dome in which attenuation and sloughing and, to a lesser degree necrosis, could be observed. The pathological changes and the amount of *C. parvum* found on the epithelium increased gradually, reaching a peak at 6 dpi, and were partly resolved by day 11 pi (Figure 1H). In gut sections from JPPs and IPP, the mononuclear cell (MNC) infiltration (identified mainly as lymphocytes with small round and dense nuclei surrounded by narrow eosinophilic cytoplasm) was observed from day 3 pi in both villi and dome and their respective epitheliums (Figures 1E-H). Using flow cytometry, we analysed the recruitment of lymphoid cells in MLNs, the jejunum and JPPs, and spleen as a reference of a systemic organ (Figures 1I-J). There was a tendency towards an increase in the absolute number of MNCs in the gut and MLNs at 3–6 dpi: the ratio between the absolute numbers of MNCs in inoculated lambs and their matched controls was superior to one in most pairs i.e. 6 of 8 in JPPs, 7 of 8 in the jejunum and 8 of 8 in the MLNs (Figure 1J). This was consistent with the necropsy and histology findings, and suggested that the immune response to this infection occurs locally and within the draining lymph nodes. Considering the percentage of total lymphocytes in the different tissues, we found that in most (10 of 13) pairs of lambs at 3 and 6 dpi, there was an increase in the lymphocyte proportion in the jejunum of the inoculated lamb (ratio significantly superior to 1, $p < 0.01$) (Figure 1K) and this local increase could already be observed as early as 1 and 2 dpi (data not included in Figures 1J and K).

We and others have shown that interferon gamma (IFNγ) is a key cytokine for controlling infected enterocytes in the mouse model [32,46]. In contrast, interleukin 22 (IL22), that is now considered to play an important role in intestinal tissue repair [47,48], has not been investigated in response to *C. parvum* infection. Infection of lambs was associated with an increase in the expression of the IFNγ and IL22 genes which was evident from as early as 1 dpi with a further increase observed at 3 and 6 dpi (Figure 2). The up-regulation of IFNγ and IL22 during the infection may participate in the clearance of the infection and the recovery of the epithelial integrity, respectively.

The proportion of NCR1+ lymphocytes did not change with infection although a slight increase in their absolute numbers was observed in the small intestine of infected lambs

NCR1+ lymphocytes are known to be IFNγ producing cells and important players of the innate response. As an increase of lymphocytes in the gut segments was observed early in the infection at 3 and 6 dpi (Figures 1E-H, K) and even earlier at 1–2 dpi (data not included in Figure 1K), we analysed the local changes of NCR1+ lymphocytes in the GALTs at different time-points of infection. Preliminary studies revealed that the proportion of NCR1+ cells was rather low in the ileum compared to jejunum and JPPs; consequently immunohistology was

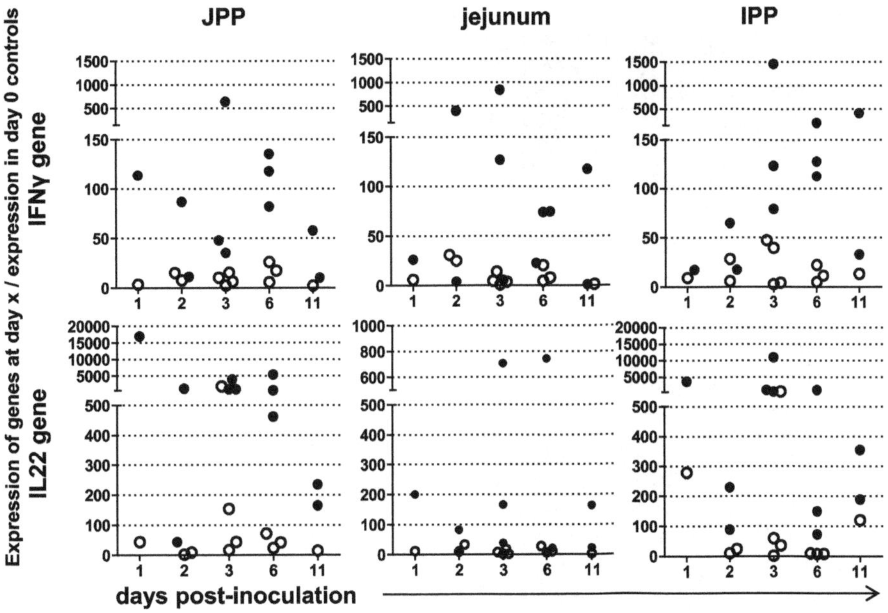

Figure 2 IFNγ and IL22 gene expression in samples from intestinal tissues. At slaughter, fragments of the small intestine were frozen in nitrogen and processed for quantification of IFNγ and IL22 gene expression by qRT-PCR. Each point represents the ratio of the number of gene copies in one individual (Ct) to the reference corresponding to the mean of the number of copies in two control animals slaughtered at birth (Ct0). The open and filled circles correspond to control and inoculated lambs respectively. JPP; jejunal Peyer's patch, IPP; ileal Peyer's patch.

preferred to flow cytometry to assess the cell recruitment in the IPP.

As previously found in the GALTs of other healthy 1–2 month-old lambs [33,34,49], NCR1 labelling of IPP sections (Figure 3A) revealed the presence of NCR1+ cells in the interfollicular T cell areas and domes, and to a lesser degree in the lamina propria and intraepithelial compartment, while few or none were observed in the follicles. There was neither a difference in the density (number of labelled cells per area) nor a change in localization of NCR1+ cells in the infected lambs compared to the controls at any time during the infection (Figure 3A). The NCR1+ lymphocyte proportions were also examined by flow cytometry in gut segments, MLN and spleen (Figures 3B-D). No difference in the proportion of NCR1+ lymphocytes (Figure 3C) or in the percentages ratio (inoculated/matched control) (Figure 3D) could be detected in any organ at any time-point. Also, no difference was detected in the level of expression of the NCR1 gene in the different gut segments (Additional file 2). However, both the absolute number of mononuclear cells and the lymphocyte percentage were higher in the jejunum of inoculated lambs (Figures 1H, J, K). In addition, when specifically examining the absolute numbers of NCR1+ lymphocytes in gut segments of paired lambs, a statistics test could only be applied to data from JPPs at day 6 pi ($p < 0.05$), but a similar tendency to an increase in infected lambs was seen at other time points and in the jejunum (Additional file 3). We conclude that in small intestinal segments, NCR1+ lymphocytes do not increase in relative numbers, although they most likely increase in absolute numbers during the early stages of infection.

The frequency of NCR1+ lymphocytes expressing perforin increases with infection and is concurrent with a preferential increase of the NCR1+/CD16+ subpopulation in JPPs and jejunum

Of the two subsets of NK cells described in humans, the CD56^{dim}CD16+ population is considered to have strong cytotoxic properties. Recently, the presence of two populations of NK cells with different CD16 expression were described in the sheep intestine [33,50]. Since the expression of CD16 might reflect the cytotoxic potential of NK cells, we analysed the balance between the NCR1+/CD16+ and NCR1+/CD16- subpopulations during the course of infection (Figures 4A-C). In control animals more than 55-60% NCR1+ lymphocytes expressed the CD16 receptor in spleen and MLN (Figure 4B) while, in JPPs and jejunum, they represented only 20-40% of NCR1+ lymphocytes (Figure 4B). In inoculated animals an increase in the NCR1+/CD16+ subpopulation (2 fold on average) was observed at 3–6 dpi in the cells extracted from JPPs and jejunum ($p < 0.01$) (Figure 4C). In addition, in around half of the inoculated lambs an increase in the level of expression of the CD16 receptor was observed (MFI), (data not shown).

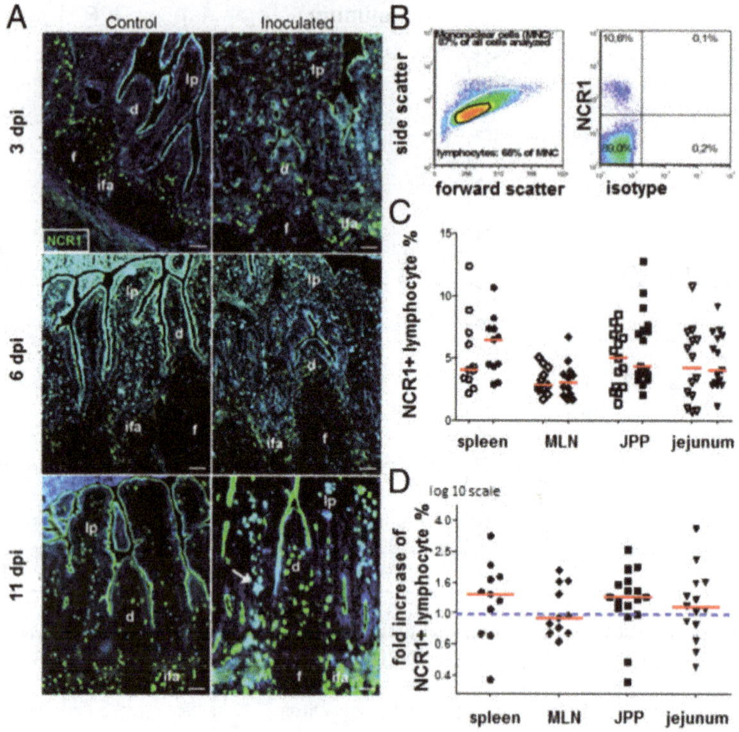

Figure 3 Proportions of NCR1+ lymphocytes in different tissues during *C. parvum* infection. (A) Sections from ileal Peyer's patches of lambs 3, 6 and 11 dpi and their age-matched controls were labelled with NCR1 (green) mAb. NCR1+ cells changed neither in density nor location during infection. Diffuse light blue spots were identified as autofluorescence using the blue filter, especially in the lamina propria (lp). Dome (d), interfollicular area (ifa), follicle (f). Bar 50 μm. **(B-D)** The NCR1+ lymphocyte percentage within the mononuclear cell population (MNC) was determined by flow cytometry. **(B)** The plots show the example of the NCR1 labelling in cells purified from jejunal Peyers'patches (JPP) at 6 dpi and gated as indicated (black gate); the right plot shows the labelling with both the anti-ovine NCR1 mAb and the isotype control of the CD8 mAb. **(C)** The NCR1+ lymphocyte percentage is shown in the different organs of lambs from 1 to 6 or 7 days of age: each dot represents one animal and the bars indicate the mean values. Control lambs (open symbols) inoculated lambs (filled symbols). Mesenteric lymph nodes (MLN). **(D)** The points represent the fold increase of NCR1+ lymphocytes (i.e. ratio inoculated/control NCR1+ lymphocyte percentage) for each pair of age-matched lambs shown in graph C, and the red bars show the medians. The mean ratio was significantly superior to one with a confidence interval of 1.21-1.57 for spleen, 1.05-1.15 for MLN, 1.17-1.55 for JPP and 1.28-1.34 for jejunum ($p < 0.01$).

The perforin content, which directly reflects the cytotoxic potential of the NCR1+ lymphocytes, was examined in the same two subpopulations at 6 dpi (Figure 4D). In both subpopulations, the percentage of perforin+ cells (Figure 4D) and their mean perforin content (MFI shown in the representative example (Figure 4E)) were increased in infected lambs.

C. parvum infection induces a strong increase of the CD8 + NCR1- cell population in the intestine

Circulating NCR1 lymphocytes from ruminants are known to express the CD8 marker, also expressed by subsets of both αβ and γδ T lymphocytes [30,34,51]. We therefore examined the expression of this marker in JPPs and jejunum and found that the vast majority of NCR1 lymphocytes expressed CD8 (Figure 5A). In addition, a large population of CD8+ NCR1- lymphocytes was also observed (Figure 5A). Three populations of CD8+ lymphocytes could be distinguished: NCR1+/CD8+ NK cells, $CD8^{tot}$/NCR1-, with a $CD8^{hi}$/NCR1- cell population included in the latter. The proportion of NCR1+/CD8+ NK cells was similar in JPPs and jejunum and did not change during the infection (Figure 5B), which was in agreement with the results shown in Figures 3C and D. However, the $CD8^{tot}$/NCR1- cells that already predominated in JPPs and particularly in the jejunum at homeostasis increased significantly during infection (3–6 dpi); this increase was not due to a specific increase of the included $CD8^{hi}$/NCR1- sub population (shown in Figure 5A). We sought to elucidate if this global increase of the $CD8^{tot}$/NCR1- population was caused by a recruitment or local proliferation of CD8+ lymphocytes. Double immunofluorescent labelling against CD8 and Ki-67 on gut sections (Figures 5C and D) showed that although the density of CD8+ cells increased in the inoculated lambs, the proportion of CD8+/Ki-67+ proliferating cells remained the same as in the controls, indicating that only a minor fraction of the local CD8+ cell population was proliferating in situ and that the increase in the CD8+ cells most probably was caused by cells recruited from blood. As several cell types

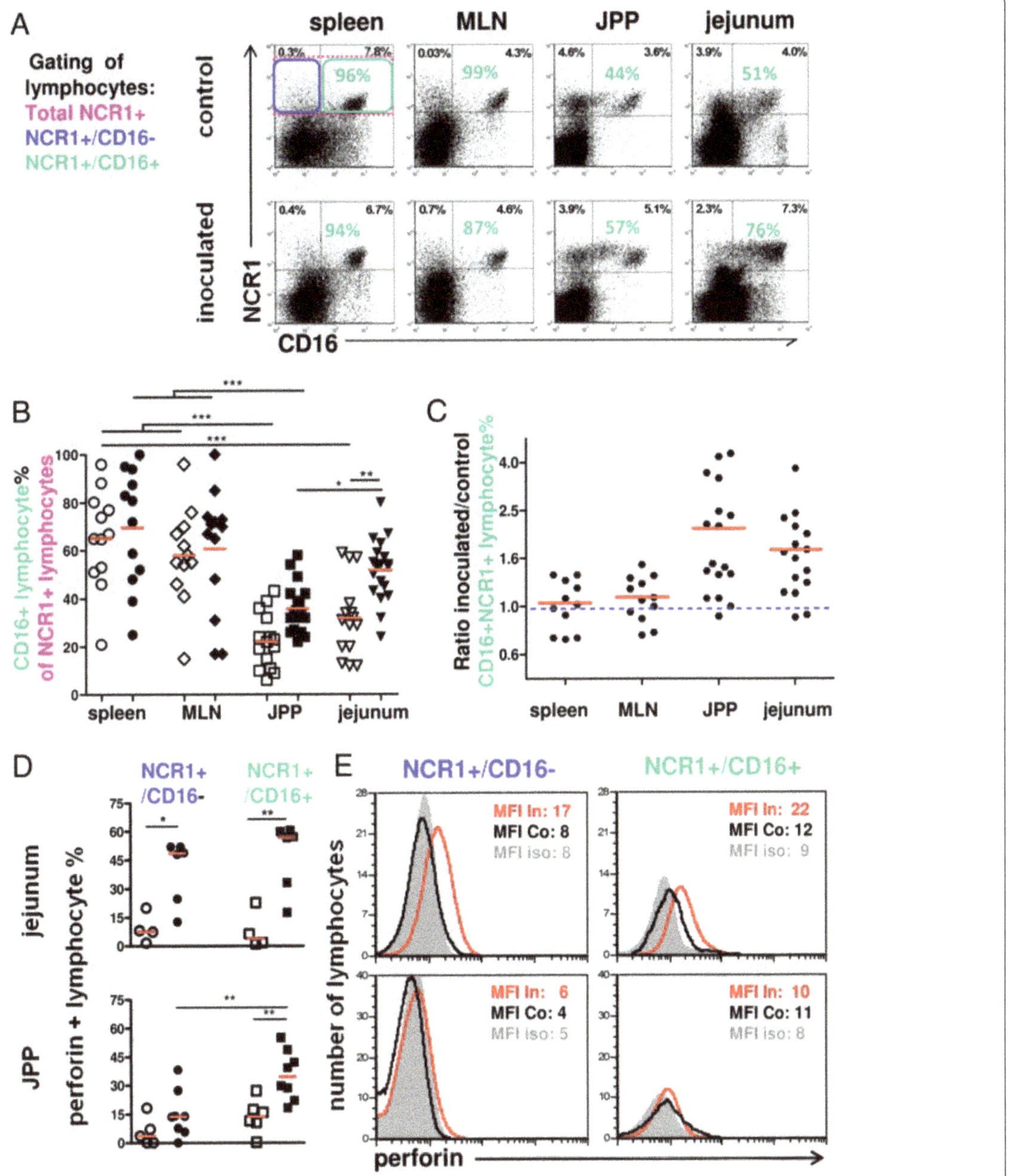

Figure 4 Increase in NCR1+/CD16+ lymphocyte percentage and perforin+ cell percentage in the jejunum during infection. (A) Cells labelled with anti NCR1 and CD16 mAbs and gated on the lymphocyte gate (shown in Figure 1I) were analyzed by flow cytometry in spleen, mesenteric lymph nodes (MLN), jejunal Peyer's patches (JPP) and jejunum. The quadrants were set according to the labelling obtained with the isotype controls for the same number of cells analyzed. Percentages indicated in black represent the CD16-/NCR1+ and CD16+/NCR1+ lymphocyte percentages of which the non-specific labelling was subtracted. Percentages of CD16+ cells among NCR1+ lymphocytes are indicated in green. Data are from an inoculated lamb at 6 dpi and its control. **(B)** Individual CD16+ percentages of NCR1+ lymphocytes are indicated for animals 2–6 dpi, control lambs (open symbols), inoculated lambs (filled symbols). The red bars indicate the mean values. **(C)** The points represent the inoculated/control ratio of NCR1+/CD16+ lymphocytes for each pair of age-matched lambs. **(D-E)** NCR1 and CD16 double labelled cells were permeabilized for intracellular labelling with an anti-human perforin mAb or isotype control to determine the perforin+ cell percentage in both NCR1+ subpopulations by histogram subtraction at 6 dpi. Control lambs (open symbols), inoculated lambs (filled symbols). **(E)** The data shown are representative of the lambs whose individual percentages of perforin+ cells are shown in Figure 4D. The red and black line limited histograms correspond to the inoculated lamb (In) and its matched control (Co) respectively, the gray filled histogram to the isotype control of the perforin mAb (iso); the mean fluorescence intensity (MFI) is indicated for each histogram. The comparisons were made with the Mann-Whitney (control/inoculated) and Wilcoxon tests (paired data). Significant difference probability: * $p < 0.05$, ** $p < 0.01$, *** $p < 0.001$. The inoculated/control CD16+/NCR1+ lymphocyte ratio was calculated for each pair of lambs **(C)**; the mean was significantly superior to 1 with confidence interval of 1.4-2.82 for JPPs and 1.48-2.32 for jejunum ($p < 0.01$).

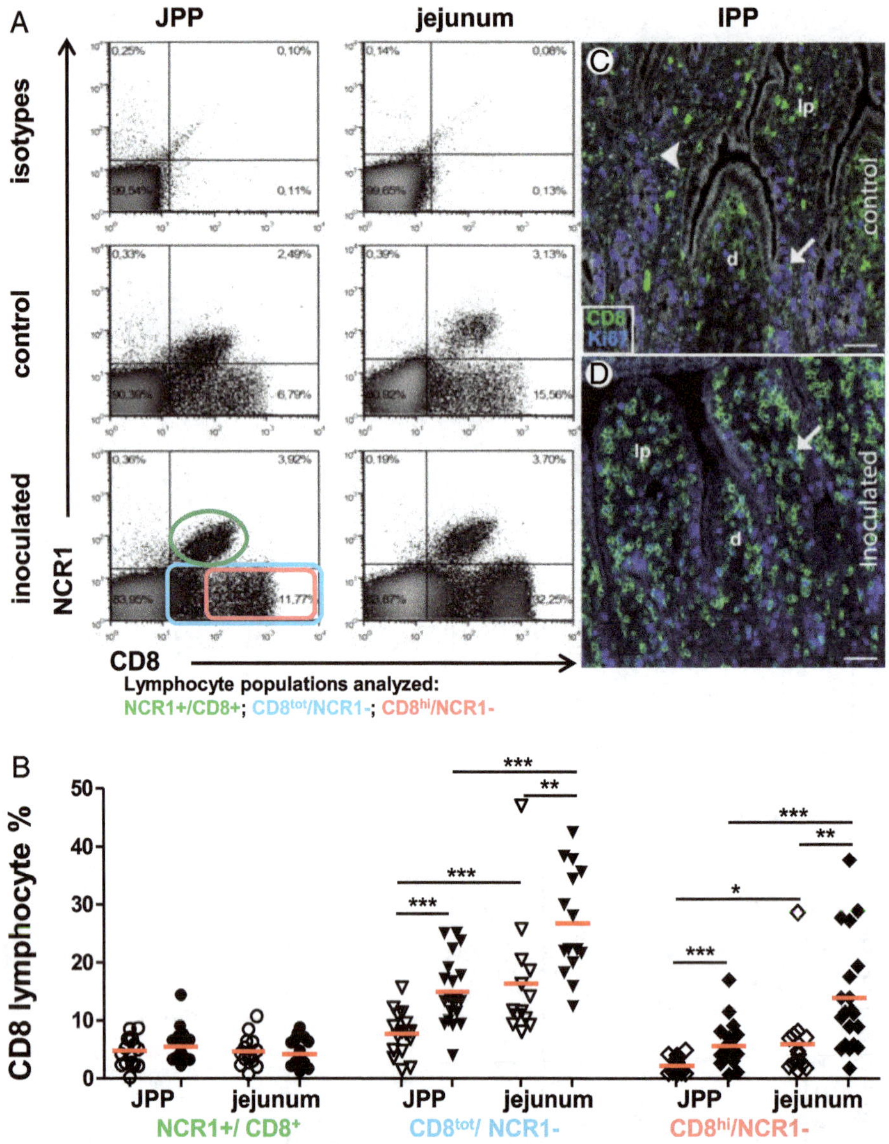

Figure 5 CD8+ lymphocyte increase in the jejunum and jejunal Peyer's patches. (A) Cells isolated from jejunal Peyer's patches (JPP) and jejunum were double labelled with anti CD8 and NCR1 mAbs and analyzed by flow cytometry. The plots show data from a 6 dpi inoculated lamb and its 7 day-old matched control and are representative of 8 matched pairs of 7 day-old lambs. The gating used for the analyses shown in B is indicated with the corresponding colours. **(B)** The percentages of the 3 different populations of CD8+ lymphocytes corresponding to the 3 gates shown in **(A)** were analyzed in jejunum and JPP from lambs 2–6 dpi. Control lambs (open symbols), inoculated lambs (filled symbols). The means are indicated in red. The comparisons were made with the Mann–Whitney (control/inoculated) and Wilcoxon tests (paired data). Statistically significant differences are indicated with * $p < 0.05$, ** $p < 0.01$, *** $p < 0.001$. **(C-D)** Section of an ileal Peyer's patch (IPP) from a 7 day old control **(C)** and a 6 dpi lamb **(D)** were double labelled with anti CD8 (green) and Ki-67 (blue) antibodies. The images shown are obtained by merging these images with the white light image. The double positive cells (arrow) display CD8 cytoplasmic staining and Ki67 nuclear staining. Pinpoint sized spots (arrowhead) are identified as autofluorescence. Dome (d), lamina propria (lp). Bar 50 μm.

may express CD8, we sought to clarify the identity of the CD8+ cells in sections. In gut sections, the vast majority of CD8+ cells were also CD3+ (Figures 6A and B) and thus represent CD8 T lymphocytes. As the CD8^{low} labelling of NCR1+ cells was not perceptible in immunohistology (not shown), we conclude that we only could visualize the CD8^{high} population of the NCR1- cells with this technique. Their density increased in villi, dome and their respective epitheliums in both JPPs and IPP. As the changes were observed to be similar in the jejunal and ileal segments, IPP was chosen for quantification to verify the observations in the sections (Figure 6C). CD8+ cell density increased significantly at days 3 and 6 pi, in the lamina propria and absorptive epithelium of the villi and at 6 dpi in the dome including FAE which supported the flow cytometry data (Figure 5B). To discriminate between αβ and γδ T cells

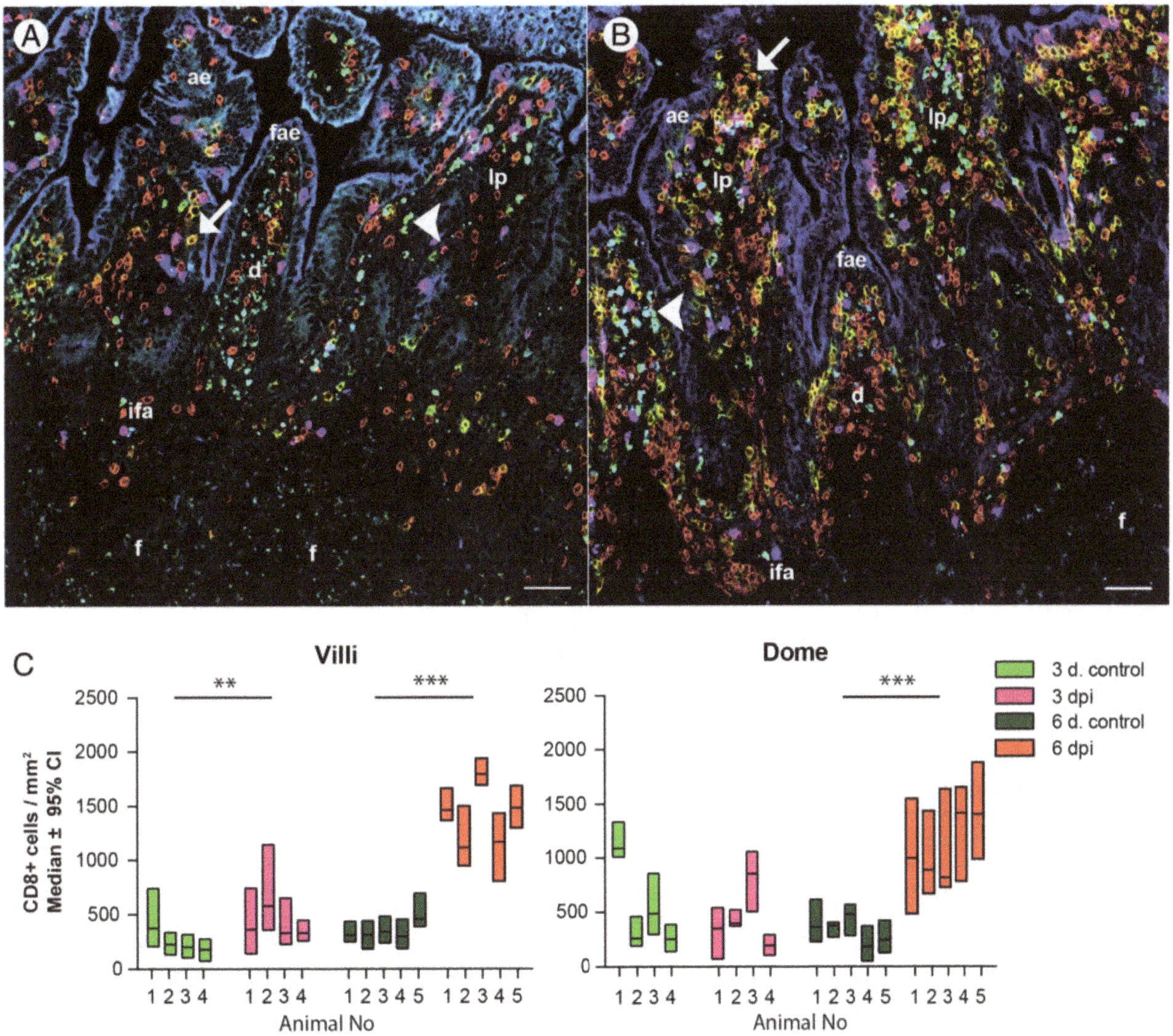

Figure 6 Significant increase of CD8+ cells in the ileum of infected lambs. Ileal Peyer's patches sections from a pair of 6 day-old matched lambs, control **(A)** and inoculated **(B)**, were labelled with Ab against CD3 (red), CD8 (green) and γδTCR (blue). Increased numbers of yellow CD3+/CD8+ cells (arrow) in the lamina propria (lp) and dome (d) were seen in the inoculated animals compared with the controls. Few or no CD3+/CD8+/γδTCR+ cells were observed. Light blue dots (arrowhead) were identified as autofluorescence and thus differentiated from the specific labelling which was localised in the cell membrane. Absorptive epithelium (ae), follicle-associated epithelium (fae), follicle (f), interfollicular area (ifa). Bar 50 μm. **(C)** The increase of CD3+/CD8+ cells in the ileal Peyer's patch was demonstrated by quantitative analysis of positive cells per mm^2 in villi and dome, including the covering epithelium. The graphs show the median with 95% confidence interval constructed using the Bernoulli-Wilcoxon procedure. Statistically significant differences are indicated as ** $p < 0.01$ and *** $p < 0.001$.

and to better characterize the CD8+/NCR1- population, we analyzed the expression of TCR1, the γδ T cell receptor, on CD8+ cells. TCR1+ T cells were scarce in gut sections of JPPs and IPP (Figures 6A and B), and no obvious increase of density was observed in infected animals compared to controls. Similar results were found with flow cytometry (Additional file 4) although this method indicated a 2–3 fold increase of γδ T cell percentage in jejunum. Only 3 to 12% of CD8+ cells co-expressed TCR1. Thus the vast majority of CD8+/NCR1- lymphocytes recruited during the infection are most probably conventional αβ CD8+ T cells.

The proportion of perforin+ cells within the intestinal NCR1+ population and their activation (CD25 MFI) increase with infection while they remain stable in the CD8+/NCR1- population

To determine the functional potential of the CD8+ subpopulations, the perforin content (Figure 7) and the activation status (Figure 8) were analyzed by flow cytometry. The

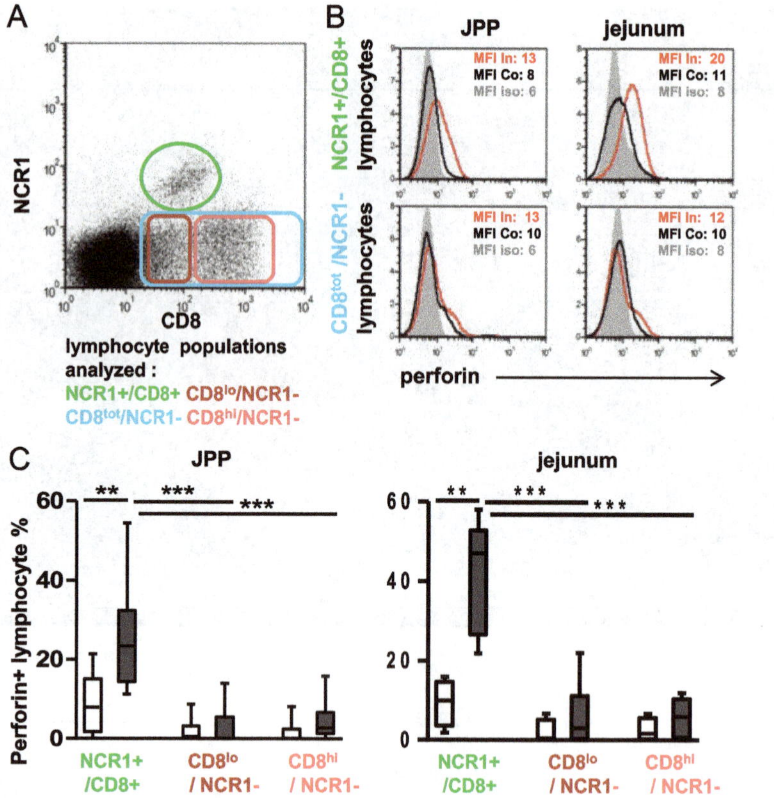

Figure 7 Perforin+ lymphocytes among CD8+ lymphocytes in the gut. (A) Cells extracted from gut tissues were double labelled with anti NCR1 and CD8 mAbs then fixed and permeabilized and labelled with an anti perforin mAb. The plot shows (example of jejunum at 6 dpi) the gating of the lymphocyte populations analyzed. **(B)** Lymphocytes from an inoculated lamb (3 dpi) and its control were gated either on the CD8+/NCR1+ or the $CD8^{tot}$/NCR1- populations then analyzed for the perforin content. The red line limited histogram corresponds to the inoculated lamb (In), the black line limited histogram to its matched control (Co) and the gray filled histogram to the isotype control of the perforin mAb (iso) and the mean fluorescence intensity (MFI) is indicated for each histogram. **(C)** The analysis of the perforin expression by CD8+ lymphocyte sub-populations (gates shown on Figure 7A) was performed in 3 control and 4 age-matched 6 dpi inoculated lambs. The comparisons were made with the Mann–Whitney (control/inoculated) and Wilcoxon tests (paired data). Statistically significant differences are indicated with ** $p < 0.01$ and *** $p < 0.001$.

percentage of perforin+ cells among the NCR1+/CD8+ population was already noticeably increased in both JPPs and jejunum while it was low in the CD8+/NCR1- population in the age-matched pair tested at 3 dpi (Figures 7A and B). At 6 dpi, this feature was confirmed (Figure 7C). The activation status of the same populations was also assessed through the expression of the IL2 receptor (CD25) (Figure 8). In JPPs of control animals, around 70% the NCR1+ lymphocytes expressed CD25 compared with 40% of the $CD8^{lo}$ and less than 30% of the $CD8^{hi}$ population. This latter population was also the less activated in the jejunum. Surprisingly, the proportion of CD25+ cells did not increase during the infection in any of the populations analysed. However, considering the higher level of expression of the CD25 marker (MFI) on the NCR1+ lymphocytes of JPPs from the inoculated lambs at day 6 pi, these cells were significantly more activated than in the controls (Additional file 5).

Discussion

The early immune response of neonatal ruminants to *C. parvum* infection is still largely unknown although some insight has been gained on the recruitment of CD8 lymphocytes by Wyatt et al. [10,52] and of mast cells by Li et al. [53] in the gut of infected calves. Natural Killer (NK) cells have been known for a long time to be important actors of the primary innate immune response through cytotoxicity and IFNγ production and also through a regulatory role in the immune response via their interaction with other cells and their ability to produce various cytokines once activated. The objective of this work was to investigate the participation of NK cells in the first steps of the innate immune response to *C. parvum* in a natural host, the neonatal lamb, in response to a controlled experimental infection. NK cells express several receptors, including CD8, that are common to several lymphocyte types. Over the last decade, the activating receptor NKp46, renamed Natural Cytotoxicity Receptor

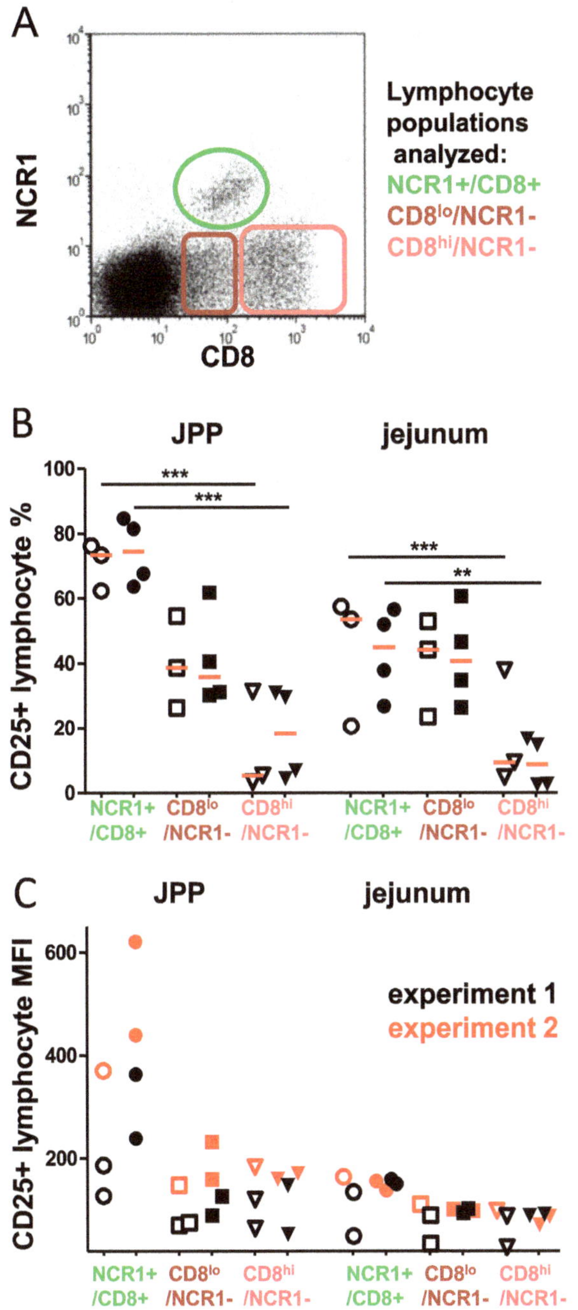

Figure 8 Expression of CD25 on small intestinal NCR1+ and CD8+ lymphocytes. (A) The expression of the activation marker CD25 was analyzed at 6 dpi in the populations gated as indicated. The individual percentages **(B)** and the mean fluorescence intensity (MFI) of CD25+ cells **(C)** are shown for the 3 populations. Medians are shown with red bars. Control lambs (open symbols), inoculated lambs (filled symbols). In C, the results of the two experiments are shown with red or black symbols. The comparisons were made with the Mann-Whitney (control/inoculated) and Wilcoxon tests (paired data). Statistically significant differences are indicated with ** $p < 0.01$ and *** $p < 0.001$.

1 (NCR1) in the new nomenclature, had come to be considered as the prototypal marker to define NK cells in most species [35,54,55]. However, various recent studies on innate immune cells in mice and humans led to the discovery that NCR1+ cells not only include conventional NK cells (cNK) but also innate lymphoid cells (ILC) of groups 1 and 3 (including NK22/ILC22) [56]. In mouse and human, ILCs participate in the intestinal defence and homeostasis but, to date, these cells have not been characterized in ruminants and their presence in this species is therefore still speculative. We examined the changes in the NCR1+ lymphocytes, in two inductive sites of the small intestine, the ileal (IPP) and jejunal Peyer's patches (JPPs), both known for playing distinct roles in the mucosal immunity of sheep, and the jejunum which is considered a major effector site with a special focus on days 3 and 6 pi [28,57,58]. The two techniques used for this study (immunohistology and flow cytometry) brought concordant and complementary results. The histopathological findings revealed a marked lymphocyte infiltration and proliferation in the intestinal mucosa already by day 3 pi (end of the parasite prepatent period) and at day 6 pi (around the peak of infection). Some Ki-67+ proliferating cells were CD8+ cells suggesting a proliferation in situ beside recruitment from blood and secondary lymphoid organs. CD8 is expressed both by T cells and most mucosal NK cells in ruminants, and both of these lymphocytes are known to be recruited in inflammatory conditions and several infections in human and mice [59,60]. NCR1+/CD8+ lymphocytes representing NK cells were part of the early lymphocyte infiltration observed in MLN and all the small intestine and the CD3+/CD8+/NCR1- population (corresponding to CD8+ T lymphocytes) also presented a marked increase in the lamina propria and absorptive epithelium of the villi and, with a short delay, within the dome and FAE of inoculated lambs during this period as previously observed by Wyatt et al. in calves [52]. Flow cytometry revealed that only a scarce proportion of the CD8+/NCR1- lymphocytes expressed the γδ TCR1 suggesting that the vast majority of these cells were conventional CD8 T lymphocytes. The increase of CD8+ T cells at the onset of oocyst shedding may indicate that the adaptive immune response was initiated in the gut tissue at that time.

As the NCR1+ cell proportion within the lymphocyte population is rather low (5% on average) and the individual variability is high in very young animals, the variations due to infection were less conspicuous for NK cells than for CD8 T lymphocytes.

However, exploring the functional potential of NK cells we found that they are likely participating in the early response to this infection. The cytotoxic potential of NCR1+ lymphocytes was explored through their perforin content. Importantly, the proportion of perforin+ cells within the total NCR1+/CD8+ NK cell population, already higher than in the CD8+/NCR1- T cell population at homeostasis, increased from day 3 of infection. The higher cytotoxicity of purified jejunal and JPP NCR1+ cells from a 6 dpi-infected lamb compared to its control (Drouet unpublished data, Additional file 6) is in agreement with these data. Moreover, NCR1+ cells expressed high levels of the IL2 receptor (CD25 MFI) especially in infected lambs and their percentage was particularly high in JPPs, indicating that NCR1+ NK cells are activated in all the gut and especially in this inductive lymphoid tissue. In contrast, the proportion of perforin+ cells remained stable within the CD8+/NCR1- T cell population at 6 dpi. Analysing the cytotoxicity of CD8 T lymphocytes derived from healthy cryptosporidium seropositive and negative donors sensitized in vitro with a cryptosporidium antigen, on an intestinal cell line (CaCo2) infected with the parasite, Pantenbourg et al. [31] found that those from the seropositive donor were more cytotoxic. Comparing our in vivo results with those of Pantenbourg et al. we may hypothesize that in the present study, at 6 dpi, the CD8 T lymphocytes are likely still in the situation of a primary response in which they have a poor cytolytic potential because they are not yet fully sensitized to the parasitic antigens. Supporting this hypothesis, the CD8+ T cells were also globally less activated (low CD25 MFI) than the NCR1+ cells and surprisingly the level of expression of CD8 is not correlated with a higher activation status since $CD8^{hi}$ T cells expressed less CD25 than the whole CD8+ population. $CD8^{hi}$/NCR1- cells may represent cells at a different stage of differentiation.

The expression of the CD16 marker has long been associated with enhanced cytotoxic properties in human NK cells. Concerning the expression of the CD16 marker on lamb NCR1+ NK cells, we confirmed in week-old lambs the presence of CD16- and CD16+ subpopulations similar to those we have previously described in the gut of older lambs [33,49] and adults [34] and in which there was a tendency to a higher representation of the CD16+/NCR1+ NK subpopulation in older lambs [49]. The *C. parvum* infection in this study was associated with an increase in the frequency of the NCR1+/CD16+ subpopulation among total NK cells, which could indicate a higher cytotoxicity of intestinal NK cells in the infected lambs. Therefore we sought to find out if the CD16+ subpopulation displayed a higher perforin content, reflecting a higher cytotoxic potential, but the proportion of perforin+/NCR1+ lymphocytes increased in both CD16- and CD16+ subpopulations (up to 60%) with infection, especially in the jejunum. Interestingly, a cytotoxicity assay probe trial performed with CD16-/NCR1+ and CD16+/NCR1+ FACS-sorted subpopulations, failed to show any difference between the two subpopulations (Drouet unpublished data). These data suggest that the expression of CD16 on sheep NK cells might be associated with a function different from that of their human homologs, perhaps more linked with antibody dependent cell cytotoxicity than direct cytotoxicity.

Finally, considering the cytokine profile during the first days of infection, the up-regulation of IFNγ gene expression observed in inoculated lambs, is in agreement with our data obtained from rodent neonates where an early production of IFNγ is known to be a determinant for the resolution of the infection in neonatal mice [32]. Both cNK cells and T lymphocytes are known to be significant producers of IFNγ and it will be of interest to ascertain in future studies their relative contributions to its production during the course of *C. parvum* infection and resolution in sheep. The increased expression of the IL22 gene observed in all segments of the small intestine of the inoculated lambs from the very first days of infection, could come from NK22/ILC22 cells (ILC3) and/or lymphoid tissue inducers (LTi) known to produce this cytokine in mice and humans [48]. However, a recent publication [61] shows that cNK cell depletion in mouse leads to a decreased production of IL22 in the lung during *Klebsiella pneumoniae* infection, suggesting that mucosal cNK may also produce IL22. As in mouse, ovine NCR1+ cells isolated from jejunum (magnetic sorting) were able to up-regulate the expression of the IL22 gene upon in vitro stimulation by rh IL23 [50]. When more antibodies cross reactive with sheep become available, it will be of great interest to further analyse the NCR1+ together with CD8+ NCR1- lymphocytes, to study their crosstalk and characterize their subsets and respective participation in the cytokine production and resolution of cryptosporidiosis.

In the mouse model the involvement of NK cells is debated; whereas works from the team of MacDonald [19,62] support an involvement of NK1.1+ NK cells in the protective response, we recently failed [18] to demonstrate a potent role for NCR1+ NK cells in the immune response of neonatal mice to the infection with *C. parvum*. The use of different markers to analyse NK cells makes it difficult to compare results from different studies but, more importantly, the distribution of the different lymphoid cell types within the gut mucosa of neonates differs notably between ruminants and mice. The dramatic difference in their developmental status at birth is illustrated by the presence of very scarce NK cells in the gut of mice [18] and rat [44,63], while we have shown here that they are already well represented in the gut of neonatal lambs.

Altogether, the experimental data presented here demonstrate that activated NK cells that possess a high cytotoxic potential are present very early in the small intestine and likely involved in the innate response to this infection. We recently demonstrated in neonatal mice [18] that dendritic cells play a key role in the resolution of *C. parvum* infection. Dendritic cells are known to produce both IL23 and IL12 that contribute to the production of IL22 by ILC22, and IFNγ by activated cNK cells, respectively. The crosstalk between NK cells and dendritic cells warrants further study since cooperation between these two cell types, as described for other infections in human and murine species, is a key mechanism governing innate immunity against intracellular parasites. The adaptive immune response is often required for complete control of infection [18,64]. The early increase in the CD8 + T cell population that we observed in infected lambs probably coincides with the onset of the adaptive immune response and further studies are needed for better comprehension of cell interactions during this important stage of the immune response. As a specific acquired immune response requires processing and presentation of antigens to effector cells, it would be interesting to investigate the sampling of cryptosporidium antigens from the gut lumen by FAE and dendritic cells; indeed, in this study, we did not observe any cryptosporidium labelling below the epithelium, contrary to what Landsverk [29] and Åkesson et al. [65] observed with other pathogens. More specific studies on presentation of the parasite antigens to lymphocytes in the GALT would therefore be useful.

Additional files

Additional file 1: Primer sequences. For PCR experiments, primer pairs were designed using Primer 3 software. Crypto = *Cryptosporidium parvum*.

Additional file 2: Expression of the NCR1 gene in the gut during infection. At slaughter, fragments of the small intestine were frozen in nitrogen and processed for quantification of the expression of the NCR1 gene by qRT-PCR. The individual data represent the ratio of the number of gene copies to the mean number of copies of two control animals slaughtered at birth. Control lambs (open symbols), inoculated lambs (filled symbols).

Additional file 3: Absolute numbers of NCR1+ lymphocytes in the small intestine. Cells extracted from jejunal Peyer's patches (JPP) and jejunum from matched pairs of lambs were purified on density gradients and the numbers of MNC and lymphocyte percentages were determined by flow cytometry on morphology parameters as shown in Figure 1I. The MNC absolute number, the lymphocyte percentage and the NCR1+ cell percentage of lymphocytes were determined for each pair of lambs at 3 or 6 dpi to calculate the absolute number of NCR1+ lymphocytes (log 10 transformed) in the tissues of each animal. The matched colour symbols correspond to paired lambs; control lambs (open symbols), inoculated lambs (filled symbols). The paired *t* test performed on log 10 transformed data from JPP at day 6 pi was significant (** $p < 0.01$).

Additional file 4: Gamma delta lymphocytes in the gut lamina propria. Cells isolated from jejunal Peyer's patches (JPP) and jejunum, were double labelled with anti TCR1 and CD8 mAbs. Cells with lymphocyte morphology were gated. The plots show data from a 7 day-old lamb at 6 dpi and its age-matched control. Representative plot of 3 matched pairs of 7 day-old lambs. The percentages indicated in red represent the percentage of positive cells in the dotted rectangle minus the percentage of non-specific labelling obtained with the isotype control antibody.

Additional file 5: Expression of CD25 on small intestinal NCR1+ lymphocytes. The expression of the activation marker CD25 was analyzed in the NCR1+ population and gated as indicated in Figure 8. The individual percentages and the mean fluorescence intensity (MFI) of CD25+ cells are shown in jejunal Peyer's patches (JPP) and jejunum. Medians are shown with black bars. The matched color symbols correspond to paired lambs; control lambs (open symbols), inoculated lambs (filled symbols). A paired *t* test was performed on CD25-MFI data. Statistically significant differences are indicated with ** $p < 0.01$.

Additional file 6: Cytotoxicity of small intestinal NCR1+ cells from a *C. parvum* infected lamb and its control. At six days post-inoculation, the NCR1+ cells were isolated from Jejunal Peyer's patches (JPP) and jejunum from an inoculated lamb and its age-matched control by magnetic sorting. The isolated cells were cultured for 4 days in the presence of recombinant ovine IL2 and recombinant human IL15. Their cytotoxicity was assessed against the ovine fibroblast line IDO5 as described by Elhmouzi et al. [51].

Abbreviations
MLN: Mesenteric lymph node; GALT: Gut associated lymphoid tissues; IPP: Ileal Peyer's patch; JPPs: Jejunal Peyer's patches; FAE: Follicle associated epithelium; MNC: Mononuclear cell; NK cells: Natural killer cells; IL: Interleukin; IFNγ: Gamma interferon; CD: Cluster of differentiation; dpi: Days post-inoculation.

Competing interests
The authors declare that they have no competing interests.

Authors' contributions
Conceived and designed the experiments: FD, AE, LO. Performed the experiments: LO, CPA (necropsies, histology), FD (necropsies, flow cytometry), SL and CM (real time PCR). Analysed the data: FD and LO, AE, SL, CM, CPÅ. Contributed to animals/reagents/materials/analysis tools: FD, FL, TC, AS. Wrote the paper: FD and LO, FL, SL, AS, PB, AE, CPÅ, TC. All authors read and approved the final manuscript.

Authors' information
Fabrice Laurent and Françoise Drouet share co-seniorship.

Acknowledgements
The authors thank Thierry Chaumeil (INRA-PFIE) for the practical organization of the animal experimentations, Tore Engen, Kristian Franer, Vanessa Rong, Gaëtan Brunet, Laila Aune and Lene Hermansen for excellent technical support, Yves Le Vern (INRA cytometry platform) for his advice, Muriel Naciri and Geneviève Fort for their parasitology expertise and support, Jacques Cabaret for his expertise of statistical analyses and Daniela Pende for her kind supply of the KD1 monoclonal antibody. This work was supported by the bilateral mobility Aurora program (N°27417ND), financed by the Norwegian Research Council and the French Ministry of Foreign Affairs.

Author details
[1]Department of Basic Sciences and Aquatic Medicine, Faculty of Veterinary Medicine and Biosciences, Norwegian University of Life Sciences, Oslo, Norway. [2]Department of Food Safety & Infection Biology, Faculty of Veterinary Medicine and Biosciences, Norwegian University of Life Sciences, Oslo, Norway. [3]Institut National de la Recherche Agronomique, UMR1282, Infectiologie et Santé Publique, Laboratoire Apicomplexes et Immunité Muqueuse, Nouzilly, France. [4]The Roslin Institute, Royal (Dick) School of Veterinary Studies, University of Edinburgh, Edinburgh, UK.

References
1. Angus KW, Tzipori S, Gray EW (1982) Intestinal lesions in specific-pathogen-free lambs associated with a cryptosporidium from calves with diarrhea. Vet Pathol 19:67–78
2. Snodgrass DR, Angus KW, Gray EW (1984) Experimental cryptosporidiosis in germfree lambs. J Comp Pathol 94:141–152
3. de Graaf DC, Vanopdenbosch E, Ortega-Mora LM, Abbassi H, Peeters JE (1999) A review of the importance of cryptosporidiosis in farm animals. Int J Parasitol 29:1269–1287
4. Chen XM, Keithly JS, Paya CV, LaRusso NF (2002) Cryptosporidiosis. N Engl J Med 346:1723–1731

5. Naciri M, Mancassola R, Fort G, Danneels B, Verhaeghe J (2011) Efficacy of amine-based disinfectant KENOCOX on the infectivity of Cryptosporidium parvum oocysts. Vet Parasitol 179:43–49
6. Lefay D, Naciri M, Poirier P, Chermette R (2001) Efficacy of halofuginone lactate in the prevention of cryptosporidiosis in suckling calves. Vet Rec 148:108–112
7. Tzipori S, Angus KW, Campbell I, Clerihew LW (1981) Diarrhea due to Cryptosporidium infection in artificially reared lambs. J Clin Microbiol 14:100–105
8. Abrahamsen MS, Lancto CA, Walcheck B, Layton W, Jutila MA (1997) Localization of alpha/beta and gamma/delta T lymphocytes in Cryptosporidium parvum-infected tissues in naive and immune calves. Infect Immun 65:2428–2433
9. Fayer R, Gasbarre L, Pasquali P, Canals A, Almeria S, Zarlenga D (1998) Cryptosporidium parvum infection in bovine neonates: dynamic clinical, parasitic and immunologic patterns. Int J Parasitol 28:49–56
10. Wyatt CR, Brackett EJ, Barrett WJ (1999) Accumulation of mucosal T lymphocytes around epithelial cells after in vitro infection with Cryptosporidium parvum. J Parasitol 85:765–768
11. Wyatt CR, Brackett EJ, Perryman LE, Rice-Ficht AC, Brown WC, O'Rourke KI (1997) Activation of intestinal intraepithelial T lymphocytes in calves infected with Cryptosporidium parvum. Infect Immun 65:185–190
12. Wyatt CR, Brackett EJ, Savidge J (2001) Evidence for the emergence of a type-1-like immune response in intestinal mucosa of calves recovering from cryptosporidiosis. J Parasitol 87:90–95
13. McDonald V, Bancroft GJ (1994) Mechanisms of innate and acquired resistance to Cryptosporidium parvum infection in SCID mice. Parasite Immunol 16:315–320
14. McDonald V, Deer R, Uni S, Iseki M, Bancroft GJ (1992) Immune responses to Cryptosporidium muris and Cryptosporidium parvum in adult immunocompetent or immunocompromised (nude and SCID) mice. Infect Immun 60:3325–3331
15. McDonald V, Robinson HA, Kelly JP, Bancroft GJ (1994) Cryptosporidium muris in adult mice: adoptive transfer of immunity and protective roles of CD4 versus CD8 cells. Infect Immun 62:2289–2294
16. Ungar BL, Kao TC, Burris JA, Finkelman FD (1991) Cryptosporidium infection in an adult mouse model. Independent roles for IFN-gamma and CD4+ T lymphocytes in protective immunity. J Immunol 147:1014–1022
17. Korbel DS, Barakat FM, Di Santo JP, McDonald V (2011) CD4+ T cells are not essential for control of early acute Cryptosporidium parvum infection in neonatal mice. Infect Immun 79:1647–1653
18. Lantier L, Lacroix-Lamande S, Potiron L, Metton C, Drouet F, Guesdon W, Gnahoui-David A, Le Vern Y, Deriaud F, Fenis A, Rabot S, Descamps A, Werts C, Laurent F (2013) Intestinal CD103+ dendritic cells are key players in the innate immune control of Cryptosporidium parvum infection in neonatal mice. PLoS Pathog 9:e1003801
19. Barakat FM, McDonald V, Di Santo JP, Korbel DS (2009) Roles for NK cells and an NK cell-independent source of intestinal gamma interferon for innate immunity to Cryptosporidium parvum infection. Infect Immun 77:5044–5049
20. Dann SM, Wang HC, Gambarin KJ, Actor JK, Robinson P, Lewis DE, Caillat-Zucman S, White AC, Jr (2005) Interleukin-15 activates human natural killer cells to clear the intestinal protozoan cryptosporidium. J Infect Dis 192:1294–1302
21. Laurent F, McCole D, Eckmann L, Kagnoff MF (1999) Pathogenesis of Cryptosporidium parvum infection. Microbes Infect 1:141–148
22. McDonald V (2000) Host cell-mediated responses to infection with Cryptosporidium. Parasite Immunol 22:597–604
23. Jung C, Hugot JP, Barreau F (2010) Peyer's patches: the immune sensors of the intestine. Int J Inflam 2010:823710
24. Makala LH, Suzuki N, Nagasawa H (2002) Peyer's patches: organized lymphoid structures for the induction of mucosal immune responses in the intestine. Pathobiology 70:55–68
25. Aleksandersen M, Hein WR, Landsverk T, McClure S (1990) Distribution of lymphocyte subsets in the large intestinal lymphoid follicles of lambs. Immunology 70:391–397
26. Reynolds JD, Morris B (1983) The evolution and involution of Peyer's patches in fetal and postnatal sheep. Eur J Immunol 13:627–635
27. Landsverk T (1984) Is the ileo-caecal Peyer's patch in ruminants a mammalian "bursa-equivalent"? Acta Pathol Microbiol Immunol Scand A 92:77–79
28. Yasuda M, Jenne CN, Kennedy LJ, Reynolds JD (2006) The sheep and cattle Peyer's patch as a site of B-cell development. Vet Res 37:401–415
29. Landsverk T (1987) Cryptosporidiosis and the follicle-associated epithelium over the ileal Peyer's patch in calves. Res Vet Sci 42:299–306
30. Elhmouzi-Younes J, Storset AK, Boysen P, Laurent F, Drouet F (2009) Bovine neonate natural killer cells are fully functional and highly responsive to interleukin-15 and to NKp46 receptor stimulation. Vet Res 40:54
31. Pantenburg B, Castellanos-Gonzalez A, Dann SM, Connelly RL, Lewis DE, Ward HD, White AC, Jr (2010) Human CD8(+) T cells clear Cryptosporidium parvum from infected intestinal epithelial cells. Am J Trop Med Hyg 82:600–607
32. Lacroix-Lamande S, Mancassola R, Naciri M, Laurent F (2002) Role of gamma interferon in chemokine expression in the ileum of mice and in a murine intestinal epithelial cell line after Cryptosporidium parvum infection. Infect Immun 70:2090–2099
33. Olsen L, Boysen P, Akesson CP, Gunnes G, Connelley T, Storset AK, Espenes A (2013) Characterization of NCR1+ cells residing in lymphoid tissues in the gut of lambs indicates that the majority are NK cells. Vet Res 44:109
34. Connelley T, Storset AK, Pemberton A, MacHugh N, Brown J, Lund H, Morrison IW (2011) NKp46 defines ovine cells that have characteristics corresponding to NK cells. Vet Res 42:37
35. Storset AK, Kulberg S, Berg I, Boysen P, Hope JC, Dissen E (2004) NKp46 defines a subset of bovine leukocytes with natural killer cell characteristics. Eur J Immunol 34:669–676
36. Moretta A, Ciccone E, Pantaleo G, Tambussi G, Bottino C, Melioli G, Mingari MC, Moretta L (1989) Surface molecules involved in the activation and regulation of T or natural killer lymphocytes in humans. Immunol Rev 111:145–175
37. Moretta A, Ciccone E, Tambussi G, Bottino C, Viale O, Pende D, Santoni A, Mingari MC (1989) Surface molecules involved in CD3-negative NK cell function. A novel molecule which regulates the activation of a subset of human NK cells. Int J Cancer Suppl 4:48–52
38. Suvarna K, Layton C, Bancroft JD (2012) Bancroft's theory and practice of histological techniques. Elsevier. ISBN: 978-0-7020-4226-3
39. Pakandl M, Sewald B, Drouet-Viard F (2006) Invasion of the intestinal tract by sporozoites of Eimeria coecicola and Eimeria intestinalis in naive and immune rabbits. Parasitol Res 98:310–316
40. Ferret-Bernard S, Remot A, Lacroix-Lamande S, Metton C, Bernardet N, Drouet F, Laurent F (2010) Cellular and molecular mechanisms underlying the strong neonatal IL-12 response of lamb mesenteric lymph node cells to R-848. PLoS One 5:e13705
41. Akesson CP, McL Press C, Espenes A, Aleksandersen M (2008) Phenotypic characterisation of intestinal dendritic cells in sheep. Dev Comp Immunol 32:837–849
42. Tourais-Esteves I, Bernardet N, Lacroix-Lamande S, Ferret-Bernard S, Laurent F (2008) Neonatal goats display a stronger TH1-type cytokine response to TLR ligands than adults. Dev Comp Immunol 32:1231–1241
43. Renaux S, Quere P, Buzoni-Gatel D, Sewald B, Le Vern Y, Coudert P, Drouet-Viard F (2003) Dynamics and responsiveness of T-lymphocytes in secondary lymphoid organs of rabbits developing immunity to Eimeria intestinalis. Vet Parasitol 110:181–195
44. Perez-Cano FJ, Castellote C, Gonzalez-Castro AM, Pelegri C, Castell M, Franch A (2005) Developmental changes in intraepithelial T lymphocytes and NK cells in the small intestine of neonatal rats. Pediatr Res 58:885–891
45. van Elteren PH (1960) On the combination of independent two-sample tests of Wicoxon. Bull Int Statist Inst 37:351–361
46. Theodos CM, Sullivan KL, Griffiths JK, Tzipori S (1997) Profiles of healing and nonhealing Cryptosporidium parvum infection in C57BL/6 mice with functional B and T lymphocytes: the extent of gamma interferon modulation determines the outcome of infection. Infect Immun 65:4761–4769
47. Fuchs A, Colonna M (2011) Natural killer (NK) and NK-like cells at mucosal epithelia: Mediators of anti-microbial defense and maintenance of tissue integrity. Eur J Microbiol Immunol (Bp) 1:257–266
48. Vivier E, Spits H, Cupedo T (2009) Interleukin-22-producing innate immune cells: new players in mucosal immunity and tissue repair? Nat Rev Immunol 9:229–234
49. Drouet F, Connelley T, Brunet G, Boysen P, Pende D, Storset AK, Laurent F (2010) Ovine Natural Killer cells from the intestinal mucosal system. In: Boysen ASP (ed) Proceedings of NK cells in veterinary species; satellite

symposium to the 12th meeting of the Society for Natural Immunity & NK 2010: 11th September 2010; Cavtat, Croatia

50. Drouet F, Connelley T, Boysen P, Pende D, Storset AK, Laurent F (2011) Sheep, a model to study intestinal NKp46+ cell subset functions in neonatal infections. In: Immunology S.f.M (ed) Proceedings of 15th International Congress of Mucosal Immunology: 5–9 July 2011; Paris
51. Elhmouzi-Younes J, Boysen P, Pende D, Storset AK, Le Vern Y, Laurent F, Drouet F (2010) Ovine CD16+/CD14- blood lymphocytes present all the major characteristics of natural killer cells. Vet Res 41:4
52. Wyatt CR, Brackett EJ, Perryman LE (1996) Characterization of small intestine mucosal lymphocytes during cryptosporidiosis. J Eukaryot Microbiol 43:66S
53. Li S, Li W, Yang Z, Song S, Yang J, Gong P, Zhang W, Liu K, Li J, Zhang G, Zhang X (2013) Infection of cattle with Cryptosporidium parvum: mast cell accumulation in small intestine mucosa. Vet Pathol 50:842–848
54. Boysen P, Storset AK (2009) Bovine natural killer cells. Vet Immunol Immunopathol 130:163–177
55. Walzer T, Jaeger S, Chaix J, Vivier E (2007) Natural killer cells: from CD3 – NKp46+ to post-genomics meta-analyses. Curr Opin Immunol 19:365–372
56. Cherrier M (2014) [Innate lymphoid cells: new players of the mucosal immune response]. Med Sci (Paris) 30:280–288. (in French)
57. Landsverk T, Halleraker M, Aleksandersen M, McClure S, Hein W, Nicander L (1991) The intestinal habitat for organized lymphoid tissues in ruminants; comparative aspects of structure, function and development. Vet Immunol Immunopathol 28:1–16
58. Mutwiri G, Watts T, Lew L, Beskorwayne T, Papp Z, Baca-Estrada ME, Griebel P (1999) Ileal and jejunal Peyer's patches play distinct roles in mucosal immunity of sheep. Immunology 97:455–461
59. Gregoire C, Chasson L, Luci C, Tomasello E, Geissmann F, Vivier E, Walzer T (2007) The trafficking of natural killer cells. Immunol Rev 220:169–182
60. Shi FD, Ljunggren HG, La Cava A, Van Kaer L (2011) Organ-specific features of natural killer cells. Nat Rev Immunol 11:658–671
61. Xu X, Weiss ID, Zhang HH, Singh SP, Wynn TA, Wilson MS, Farber JM (2014) Conventional NK cells can produce IL-22 and promote host defense in Klebsiella pneumoniae pneumonia. J Immunol 192:1778–1786
62. McDonald V, Korbel DS, Barakat FM, Choudhry N, Petry F (2013) Innate immune responses against Cryptosporidium parvum infection. Parasite Immunol 35:55–64
63. Drouet F, Lemoine R, El Hmouzi J, Le Vern Y, Lacroix-Lamandé S, Laurent F (2007) Cellules impliquées dans la production précoce d'interféron gamma au cours de l'infection de l'animal nouveau-né par *Cryptosporidium parvum*: participation des cellules NK? In: INRA (ed) Proceedings of Animal Health department conference; Tours, France
64. McDonald V (2011) Cryptosporidiosis: host immune responses and the prospects for effective immunotherapies. Expert Rev Anti Infect Ther 9:1077–1086
65. Akesson CP, McGovern G, Dagleish MP, Espenes A, Mc LPC, Landsverk T, Jeffrey M (2011) Exosome-producing follicle associated epithelium is not involved in uptake of PrPd from the gut of sheep (Ovis aries): an ultrastructural study. PLoS One 6:e22180

4

Immune responses associated with homologous protection conferred by commercial vaccines for control of avian pathogenic *Escherichia coli* in turkeys

Jean-Rémy Sadeyen[1], Zhiguang Wu[2], Holly Davies[1], Pauline M van Diemen[3], Anita Milicic[3], Roberto M La Ragione[4,5], Pete Kaiser[2], Mark P Stevens[2] and Francis Dziva[1,6*]

Abstract

Avian pathogenic *Escherichia coli* (APEC) infections are a serious impediment to sustainable poultry production worldwide. Licensed vaccines are available, but the immunological basis of protection is ill-defined and a need exists to extend cross-serotype efficacy. Here, we analysed innate and adaptive responses induced by commercial vaccines in turkeys. Both a live-attenuated APEC O78 Δ*aroA* vaccine (Poulvac® *E. coli*) and a formalin-inactivated APEC O78 bacterin conferred significant protection against homologous intra-airsac challenge in a model of acute colibacillosis. Analysis of expression levels of signature cytokine mRNAs indicated that both vaccines induced a predominantly Th2 response in the spleen. Both vaccines resulted in increased levels of serum O78-specific IgY detected by ELISA and significant splenocyte recall responses to soluble APEC antigens at post-vaccination and post-challenge periods. Supplementing a non-adjuvanted inactivated vaccine with Th2-biasing (Titermax® Gold or aluminium hydroxide) or Th1-biasing (CASAC or CpG motifs) adjuvants, suggested that Th2-biasing adjuvants may give more protection. However, all adjuvants tested augmented humoral responses and protection relative to controls. Our data highlight the importance of both cell-mediated and antibody responses in APEC vaccine-mediated protection toward the control of a key avian endemic disease.

Introduction

Avian pathogenic *Escherichia coli* (APEC) cause colibacillosis, a complex of respiratory and systemic diseases that exert substantial welfare and economic costs on poultry producers worldwide. Losses are incurred through premature deaths, condemnation of carcasses at slaughter, reduced productivity and recurring costs associated with antibiotic prophylaxis and therapy. A recent longitudinal survey of broiler flocks in the United Kingdom found evidence of colibacillosis in 39% of dead birds [1], and the same authors implicated colibacillosis in 70% of deaths of broiler chicks 2–3 days after placement [2]. A number of risk factors are known, including prior or concurrent infection with respiratory viruses or *Mycoplasma*, stress and injury associated with formation of a social hierarchy, onset of sexual maturity and intense laying, and poor biosecurity, hygiene and ventilation. The control of colibacillosis requires the mitigation of such risk factors, but can also be partly achieved through vaccination.

A major impediment to the design of effective vaccines is the remarkable diversity of *E. coli* associated with avian disease. Though serogroups O1, O2 and O78 and sequence types ST23 and ST95 are commonly observed, it is clear that *E. coli* has evolved to cause avian disease from diverse lineages via the acquisition of distinct virulence genes [3,4]. Indeed, we recently reported that a ST23 serogroup O78 strain differed from the prototype ST95 serogroup O1 strain by over 1100 chromosomal genes and marked variation exists in their plasmid repertoire and content [4-6]. Recent analysis of APEC genome sequences

* Correspondence: francis.dziva@sta.uwi.edu
[1]Avian Infectious Diseases Programme, The Pirbright Institute, Compton, Berkshire, RG20 7NN, UK
[6]Present address: School of Veterinary Medicine, The University of the West Indies, St Augustine, Trinidad and Tobago
Full list of author information is available at the end of the article

indicates that they may also possess zoonotic potential owing to their similarity to *E. coli* that cause human extra-intestinal infections, such as ascending urinary tract infections, sepsis and neonatal meningitis [7-10]. Of further concern is the emergence of multi-drug resistant *E. coli* strains in poultry, including those encoding extended spectrum beta-lactamases (ESBLs), cephalosporin-resistance and plasmid-mediated quinolone resistance (PMQR) [11-15]. This is compounded by evidence of direct transmission of poultry *E. coli* strains to humans [16,17]. Taken together with the burden of avian disease, a need exists to improve control of APEC in reservoir hosts.

The control of APEC has been largely reliant upon vaccination with autologous bacterins [18-20], but these confer short-lived serotype-specific protection and their effectiveness is blunted by the diversity of *E. coli* capable of infecting poultry. Live-attenuated vaccines are preferable owing to ease of administration and improved cross-serotype protection and hence are entering the market [21,22]. Numerous attenuated mutants have been described and evaluated as candidate live vaccines in experimental models, though direct comparisons of these are lacking and their mode of action is not understood [21,23-25].

In a subacute model of APEC O78 infection in turkeys, we have shown that clearance of primary infection is associated with the induction of both humoral and cell-mediated responses [26]. It is unclear whether such events are also induced by existing commercial vaccines. Passively administered antibody either acquired vertically via egg-yolk [27-29] or administered intravenously [30-32] can be protective against APEC infection. Vaccination of turkeys with a low dose of a live virulent strain appeared to give better protection compared to a heat- or formalin-inactivated non-adjuvanted vaccine [30]. Whilst such protection was associated with humoral responses, innate responses leading to adaptive immunity were not analysed, and the contribution of cell-mediated immunity in protection was not measured. Moreover, the use of a virulent strain or inactivated vaccine without adjuvant does not reflect commercial practice in poultry production. We therefore sought to define the innate and adaptive responses associated with protection conferred by licensed inactivated and live-attenuated vaccines.

Materials and methods

Bacterial strains, growth media and preparation of vaccines

E. coli serogroup O78:K80 strain EC34195 was isolated from a chicken that died of colibacillosis and has been extensively studied [33]. Deletion of 100 bp of the *aroA* gene of this strain gave rise to the live-attenuated vaccine Poulvac® *E. coli* presently commercialized by Zoetis for the control of avian colibacillosis [22]. The lyophilized Poulvac® *E. coli* vaccine strain was re-constituted in sterile water to ca. 10^9 colony-forming units (CFU) per mL prior to use. A whole cell formalin-inactivated vaccine based on strain EC34195 was prepared without adjuvant (hereafter designated bacterin), or with a licensed aluminium hydroxide adjuvant, by a supplier of emergency poultry vaccines according to standard procedures (Ridgeway Biologicals Ltd., Compton, UK). A spontaneous nalidixic acid resistant derivative of EC34195 was produced by plating approximately 10 $\log_{10}$ colony-forming units (CFU) of EC34195 on MacConkey agar (Oxoid, Basingstoke, UK) supplemented with 25 μg/mL nalidixic acid (Mac + Nal). The subsequent derivative (EC34195nal^R) was passaged in pure culture and confirmed to possess an identical growth rate, phenotypic characteristics and panel of virulence-associated genes (*cvi/cvaC iss*, *iucD* and *tsh*) to the parent strain. Strain EC34195nal^R was stored at −70 °C in 15% (v/v) glycerol in Luria Bertani (LB) broth until required. The inoculum of this strain was prepared as described [26].

Experimental animals

Animal experiments were conducted according to the requirements of the Animal (Scientific Procedures) Act 1986 (licence no. 30/2463) with the approval of the Local Ethical Review Committee. Male Big5FLX turkeys were obtained from Aviagen Ltd. (Tattenhall, Cheshire, UK) as day-old poults, housed and reared as previously described [26].

Analysis of protection conferred by licensed live-attenuated and whole cell formalin-inactivated APEC O78 vaccines in turkeys

Thirty 1-day old turkey poults were randomly housed in groups of 10 birds per room on floor pens to simulate commercial practice. For the delivery of a coarse aerosol spray of live vaccine, birds were restrained in one corner of the room at a density of 10 birds per 0.25 m^2, and the vaccine was administered with a syringe fitted with a device that creates a coarse aerosol directed at the faces of individual birds. Group A (control) received 10 mL sterile saline as coarse spray (per group, not individually) while group B received 10 mL of saline containing 10^7 CFU per mL of the Poulvac® *E. coli* live-attenuated vaccine. Each bird in group C received 0.2 mL (containing the equivalent of approximately 2×10^9 CFU) of the EC34195 inactivated vaccine via the subcutaneous route as per commercial practice and recommended by the manufacturer. Birds were monitored for adverse reactions every 3 h for the first 24 h and thereafter twice daily until the booster vaccinations. Birds in group B were given a booster of ca. 10^7 CFU per mL in drinking water at 7 days of age. Excess vaccine-treated water was discarded after 18 h. Birds in group C were given a booster (0.4 mL) of the same inactivated vaccine at 14 days of age via the subcutaneous route in the neck region. The control group was given sterile saline in drinking water mixed at the same proportions as for the live vaccine. Birds were monitored twice daily for the remainder of the experiment. On day 41 post-primary vaccination, all the birds were inoculated into the left caudal thoracic airsac with 10^7 CFU of the EC34195nal^R strain, on which both vaccines are based, in 100 μL of saline and monitored overnight for clinical signs. After 24 h, all the birds were killed humanely and subjected to *post-mortem* examination essentially as described [26]. Part of the spleen was collected for T cell re-stimulation assays. Lung, liver, kidney and the remaining spleen tissue were sampled to enumerate tissue-associated bacteria whilst blood and bile were collected for serology.

Analysis of innate and adaptive responses upon vaccination with licensed live-attenuated and inactivated APEC O78 vaccines in turkeys

Having established vaccine efficacy in pilot studies (above), one hundred and thirty-five 1-day old turkey poults were randomly divided into 3 groups of 45 birds and housed separately. Birds were vaccinated as described above with sterile saline (control group), Poulvac® *E. coli* or inactivated vaccine with aluminium hydroxide adjuvant. Boosters were given at the respective time-points as above. On days 1, 3, 5, 7, 14, 21 and 28 post-primary vaccination, five birds were randomly removed from each group, killed humanely and subjected to *post-mortem* examination. From each bird, sections of liver, lung and spleen were collected in RNAlater (Ambion, Warrington, UK) for cytokine analysis. In the live vaccine group, the remainder of the lung was used to enumerate the vaccine strain as described below. Selected colonies were subjected to PCR analysis spanning the *aroA* gene using the primers (*aroA*-F-TTGAGTTCGAACGTCGTCAC and *aroA*-R-GCAA TGTGCCGACGTCTTTG) and agglutination with specific anti-O78 serum (AHVLA, Weybridge, UK) to confirm recovery of the vaccine strain. At day 28 post-primary vaccination, the spleen was collected into ice-cold RPMI1640 medium for use in T cell re-stimulation assays and blood and bile were collected for serology. On day 41 post-primary vaccination, all the remaining birds were challenged, subjected to *post-mortem* examination 24 h later and tissues sampled as described above.

Total RNA extraction and real-time quantitative RT-PCR for cytokine mRNA

Total RNA extraction and cytokine mRNA analyses were performed essentially as described [26]. Data are expressed in terms of the cycle threshold value (Ct), normalised for each sample using the Ct value of 28S rRNA product for the same sample, as described previously [34,35]. Final results are shown as corrected ΔCt, using the normalised value.

Enumeration of tissue-associated bacteria

Viable tissue-associated bacteria were enumerated essentially as described [4]. The lower limit of detection by this method was 1.79 $\log_{10}$ CFU/g of tissue. Enrichment cultures were also performed in which 1 mL of tissue homogenate was cultured in 9 mL brain heart infusion (BHI) broth for 18 h at 37 °C aerobically, prior to plating on Mac + Nal, giving a theoretical lower limit of detection by enrichment of 1 $\log_{10}$ CFU/g of tissue.

Measurement of antibody and cell-mediated responses

Preparation of APEC soluble antigens for ELISA, quantification of total protein content, storage and subsequent antibody assays were performed essentially as described [26]. Cell-mediated responses were determined by splenocyte proliferation assays again as previously described [26] and data is expressed as mean counts per minute (cpm).

Analysis of a bacterin mixed with Th1- or Th2-biasing adjuvants

The Th1-stimulating adjuvant CASAC: (combined **a**djuvant **s**ynergistic **a**ctivation of **c**ellular immunity) was formulated by an adaptation of the method described [36]. Briefly, the first dose comprised 50 μg of monophosphoryl lipid A (MPL; Invivogen, Toulouse, France), 50 μg of Pam3CysSerLys4 (Pam3CSK4; EMC Microcollections, Tuebingen, Germany) and 50 μg of chicken interferon-γ (2B Scientific, Upper Heyford, UK) homogenized with 100 μL (same dose as previously used) of formalin-inactivated EC34195 supplied to commercial specification by Ridgeway Biologicals Ltd. but without adjuvant (bacterin). The booster comprised the same ingredients of CASAC mixed with 200 μL of bacterin. Bacterin formulated with a second Th1-biasing adjuvant was separately prepared using synthetic cytosine phosphodiester-guanine (CpG)-containing oligodeoxynucleotides (ODN) as described [37]. The sequence for CpG-ODN, TC**GTCGTT**T**GTCGTT**T**TGTCGTT** (bold motifs enhance CpG-ODN activity), was synthesized with a phosphothionate backbone (Sigma). The first dose was prepared by mixing 20 μg of synthetic CpG-ODN (in sterile pyrogen-free water) with 100 μL of the non-adjuvanted EC34195 bacterin. The booster dose comprised the same amount of CpG-ODN in 200 μL of non-adjuvanted EC34195 bacterin.

For comparison, the formalin-inactivated bacterin without adjuvant was also formulated with Th2-stimulating adjuvants. The first of these comprised a dose of 100 μL of EC34195 bacterin thoroughly mixed with an equal volume (ratio of 1:1) of Titermax® Gold (Sigma) as per manufacturer's instructions. The booster dose was 200 μL of the homogenous mixture. EC34195 bacterin formulated with aluminium hydroxide adjuvant was also tested as another Th2-stimulating adjuvant; 100 μL for primary vaccination and 200 μL for the booster (same dose as in the pilot studies).

For vaccination, thirty 1-day old turkey poults were randomly divided into 6 groups of 5 birds and housed separately as before. Group 1 received sterile saline (negative control group), group 2 received formalin-inactivated EC34195 bacterin without adjuvant (control group), group 3 received the same bacterin formulated with CpG-ODN, group 4 received the same bacterin with CASAC, group 5 received the same bacterin mixed with aluminium hydroxide, group 6 received the same bacterin mixed with Titermax® gold. All vaccines were administered by the subcutaneous route with booster doses for the respective vaccine formulations given at 14 days of age via the same route. Birds were monitored twice daily for the duration of the experiment. On day 41 post-primary vaccination, all the birds were inoculated with 10^7 CFU of strain EC34195nal^R in 100 μL of saline into the left caudal thoracic airsac as above and monitored overnight for clinical signs. All the birds were killed humanely and subjected to *post-mortem* examination and collection of organs and blood as above.

Statistical analyses

Cytokine data was analysed for statistical significance using a one-way ANOVA test with an *ad hoc* Tukey's test. Bacterial counts recovered from tissues, antibody levels and splenocyte recall responses were analysed by Student's *t*-test. P values ≤ 0.05 were considered significant.

Results

Licensed live-attenuated and formalin-inactivated vaccines based on APEC O78 are protective against homologous challenge in turkeys

To evaluate the protective efficacy of existing vaccines and establish models in which the basis of protection can be dissected, turkeys were vaccinated using Poulvac® *E. coli* or an inactivated vaccine based on the parent strain of Poulvac® *E. coli* and compared to mock-vaccinated turkeys. In birds given the live vaccine, up to ca. 4 $\log_{10}$ CFU per gram lung tissue of the vaccine strain was detected 1, 3, 5 and 7 days post-primary vaccination (data not shown). Recovery of the vaccine strain was confirmed by a specific PCR for the *aroA* gene in *E. coli* isolated from the lung homogenates at these times (data not shown). The live-attenuated vaccine strain was not detectable at any other time-points in any group.

Upon intra-airsac challenge of vaccinated birds with a nalidixic acid resistant derivative of the strain used to prepare the vaccines, significant protection was observed in the groups that received either Poulvac® *E. coli* or the inactivated vaccine (Figure 1). Approximately 4 $\log_{10}$ CFU/g EC34195nal^R were recovered from the lung, liver, spleen and kidney of mock-vaccinated turkeys. In contrast, nalidixic acid resistant *E. coli* were only detectable in the spleens, livers and kidneys of turkeys that received the inactivated vaccine by enrichment, where the theoretical lower limit of detection was 1 $\log_{10}$ CFU/g (Figure 1; $P < 0.05$). The number of nalidixic acid resistant *E. coli* recovered from the lung, liver, spleen and kidney of turkeys that received the live vaccine was significantly reduced by around 2 $\log_{10}$ CFU/g (Figure 1; $P < 0.05$). Consistent with the lower numbers of bacteria recovered from the organs of vaccinated birds after challenge with EC34195nal^R, none of the vaccinated birds exhibited clinical signs or pathological lesions indicative of colibacillosis as previously defined [26]. By contrast, all mock-vaccinated birds challenged with EC34195nal^R exhibited clinical signs typical of colibacillosis (respiratory distress, hunched posture, ruffled feathers, reduced response to stimulus) and gross *post-mortem* lesions including airsacculitis, pericarditis, perihepatitis and fibrin deposits on serosal surfaces at 24 h post-challenge. It can therefore be inferred that the strain is virulent and that live-attenuated or inactivated vaccines derived from it confer protection against homologous re-challenge.

Quantification of cytokine transcripts indicates that licensed live-attenuated and inactivated APEC O78 vaccines predominantly induce a Th2 response in the spleen of turkeys

To assess cytokine responses as signatures of innate and adaptive immune responses induced by the live-attenuated and inactivated vaccines, turkey poults were vaccinated as above and killed at intervals. We analysed the levels of transcripts encoding a pro-inflammatory cytokine (IL-1β), a pro-inflammatory chemokine (CXCLi2), a signature Th1 cytokine (IFN-γ), a signature Th2 cytokine (IL-13) and two signature T regulatory cytokines (IL-10 and TGF-β4), at intervals post-primary and -secondary vaccination.

The normalised levels of transcripts encoding these cytokines are shown over time in the spleen (Figure 2), liver (Figure 3) and lung (Figure 4). In the spleen, the live-attenuated and inactivated vaccines significantly induced transcription of IL-13 in the first week post-primary vaccination (Figure 2; $P < 0.05$). In the same period, transcription of the signature Th1 cytokine IFN-γ was significantly repressed following vaccination relative to levels in the mock-vaccinated controls (Figure 2; $P < 0.05$), and transcription levels of the anti-inflammatory cytokine TGF-β4 (the chicken equivalent of mammalian TGF-β1) were significantly induced following vaccination (Figure 2; $p < 0.05$). Together, these data indicate a bias towards a Th2 response at a key site of immune priming

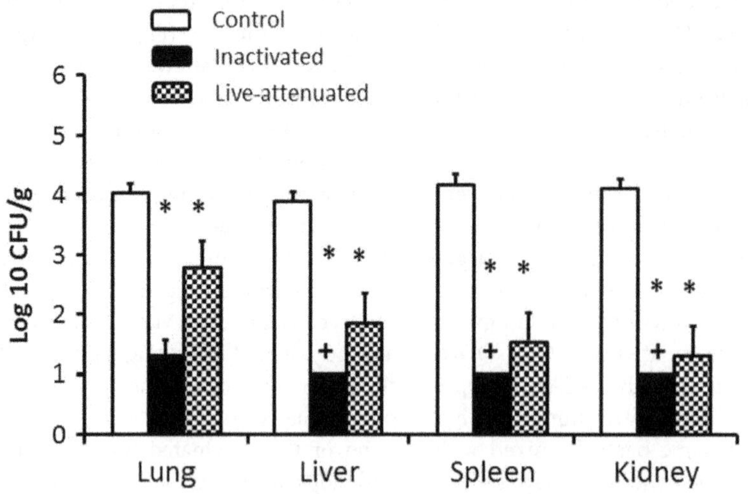

Figure 1 Recoveries of strain EC34195nal^R from organs of vaccinated turkeys at 24 h post-challenge. Turkey poults were given sterile saline (mock) as a coarse spray (open bars), a formalin-inactivated vaccine of the parent strain EC34195 formulated in aluminium hydroxide adjuvant via the subcutaneous route (black bars) or Poulvac® *E. coli* as a coarse spray (checked black and white bars) starting at one day-old as indicated in the Materials and methods. All turkeys were challenged via the intra-airsac route at day 41 post-primary vaccination with EC34195nal^R and the indicated tissues recovered 24 h later. The data are expressed as mean $\log_{10}$ CFU/g tissue ± standard error of the mean. The limit of detection by direct plating was 1.79 and limit of detection by enrichment was 1 $\log_{10}$ CFU/g tissue; + denotes values after enrichment of tissue homogenates. *denotes $P \leq 0.05$ relative to mock-vaccinated controls.

during the typical period of induction of an adaptive immune response to primary vaccination.

In the other two organs, the pattern is less clear. Elevated IL-13 mRNA expression levels were also detected in the liver (Figure 3) and lung (Figure 4), but only at a couple of time-points and with no discernible pattern in the first week post-primary vaccination with live-attenuated or inactivated vaccines. In the lung, IFN-γ transcription was generally lower in turkeys given the live-attenuated vaccine compared to mock-vaccinated birds, significantly so at multiple time-points (Figure 4). However, the inactivated vaccine only significantly repressed IFN-γ transcription in the lung at 21 and 28 days post-primary vaccination, time-points which would represent the resolution of a normal adaptive immune response to primary vaccination (Figure 4). No repression of IFN-γ transcription was detected in the liver at any time-point (Figure 3). In both organs, we detected significant induction of TGF-β4 mRNA expression in turkeys vaccinated with the live-attenuated or inactivated vaccines, particularly in the first two weeks post-primary vaccination (Figures 3 and 4; $P < 0.05$).

Differences between groups in transcription of the other cytokines analysed did not show consistent trends across organs or time in vaccinated turkeys relative to controls, with the exception of CXCLi2 expression, which was unaltered following vaccination in the spleen (Figure 2), consistently down-regulated in the lung (Figure 4; $P < 0.05$) and generally up-regulated in the liver (Figure 3; $P < 0.05$). CXCLi2 mainly chemo-attracts monocytes [35], and this differential expression may reflect traffic of these cells in response to vaccination.

Vaccine-induced protection against homologous challenge is associated with elevated adaptive responses

To identify adaptive immune responses associated with protection against homologous challenge induced by each vaccine, we measured humoral and cellular responses at intervals after primary and secondary vaccination of turkeys using samples from the same birds as used for cytokine analysis. Immunoglobin Y (IgY) levels and splenocyte proliferation responses were measured in birds killed at day 28 and after challenge (day 42) whereas IgA in bile was measured 24 h after challenge. Both vaccines induced elevated IgY levels post-primary vaccination relative to the mock-vaccinated group, for the inactivated vaccine at both intervals and for the live-attenuated vaccine at day 42 (Figure 5A; $P \leq 0.05$). APEC-specific IgA was elevated in bile from poults given the inactivated vaccine relative to the mock-vaccinated group (Figure 5B; $P \leq 0.05$).

The ability of splenocytes recovered from each group to proliferate in response to mitogen or soluble EC34195 antigen was also evaluated at day 28 post-primary vaccination and at *post-mortem* examination on day 42 (24 h after challenge). The response to ConA was comparable between the birds given mock- or inactivated vaccine at day 28, and was not significantly different from control birds in the group given Poulvac® *E. coli* (Figure 6A). After challenge, almost no proliferation of splenocytes from the control group was seen in response to ConA (Figure 6A),

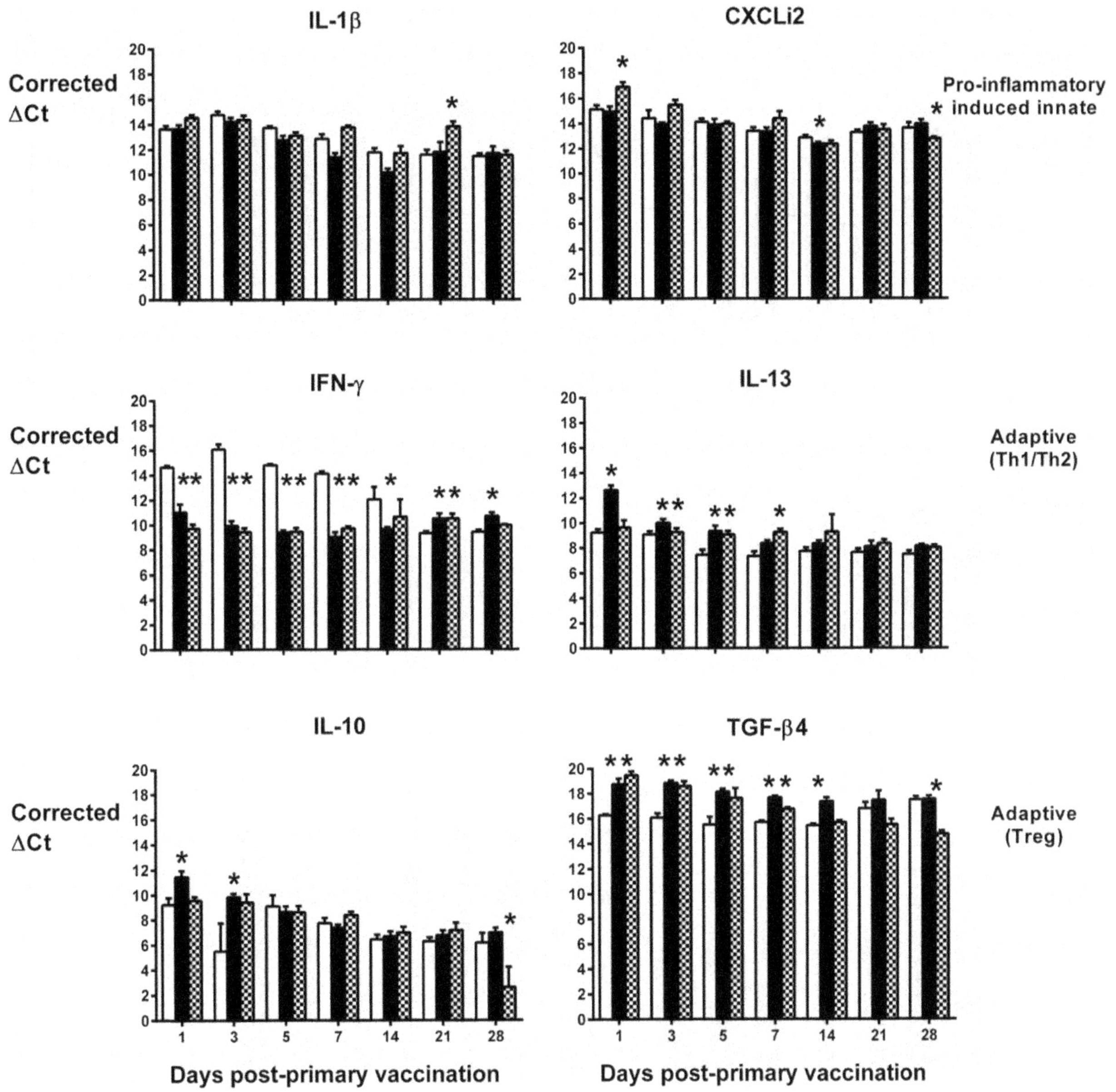

Figure 2 Levels of cytokine transcripts in the spleens of vaccinated turkeys as measured by real-time qRT-PCR. Results are expressed as corrected ΔCt values ± standard error of the mean after normalization with the Ct value of 28S rRNA product of each sample. Turkey poults were given sterile saline (mock) as a coarse spray (open bars), a formalin-inactivated vaccine based on the parent strain EC34195 formulated in aluminium hydroxide adjuvant via the subcutaneous route (black bars) or Poulvac® *E. coli* as a coarse spray (checked black and white bars) starting at one day-old. Five birds from each group were sampled per time-point. *denotes $P \leq 0.05$ relative to mock-vaccinated controls.

consistent with a suppressive effect of APEC O78 infection detected following primary and secondary infection [26]. Splenocytes recovered from birds given live-attenuated or inactivated vaccines at day 42 proliferated in response to ConA (Figure 6A).

Splenocyte proliferation in response to APEC soluble antigen was significantly elevated both vaccinated groups at day 42 relative to levels in the mock-vaccinated group (Figure 6B, $P < 0.05$). Responses were lower in the group given the live-attenuated vaccine relative to the control group at day 28 and relative to the inactivated vaccine group at both time-points. At day 42, no response to EC34195 soluble antigen was seen in the control group.

Impact of Th1- and Th2-stimulating adjuvants on protection conferred by the APEC O78 inactivated bacterin

To examine the effects of Th1- and Th2-stimulating adjuvants, we formulated the EC34195 inactivated bacterin with two compounds with a reported bias toward Th1 responses (CASAC or CpG) and two with a reported

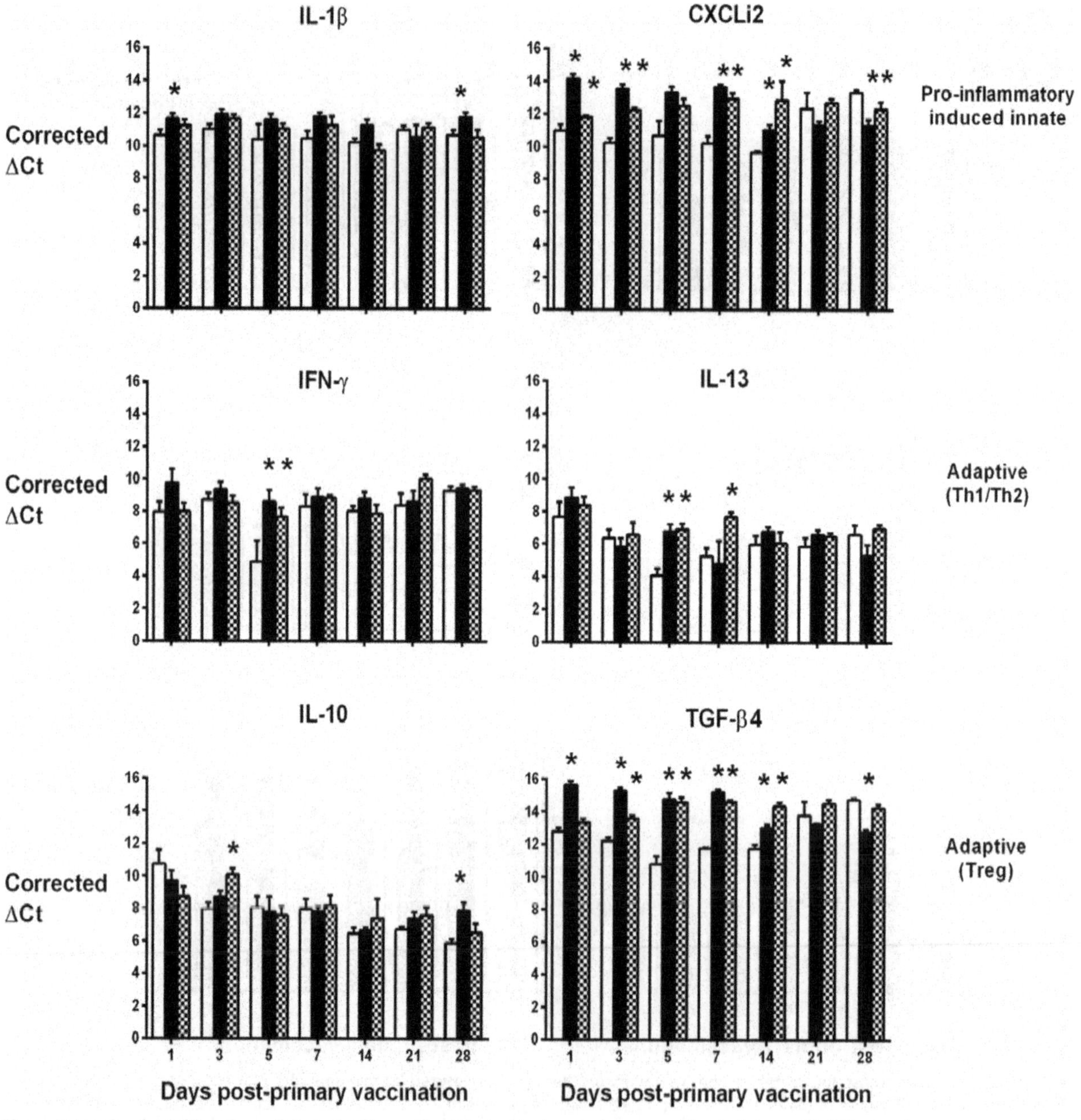

Figure 3 Levels of cytokine transcripts in the livers of vaccinated turkeys as measured by real-time qRT-PCR. Details are as in the legend to Figure 2.

bias to Th2 responses (aluminium hydroxide or TiterMax® Gold) [36,38,39]. The vaccines were given to day-old turkey poults and again 14 days later by the subcutaneous route, with intra-airsac challenge with EC34195nal^R at day 41, as described in pilot studies where protection conferred by the inactivated vaccine was shown (Figure 1). A bacterin without adjuvant and mock-vaccination with saline were used as controls.

At 24 h post-challenge, statistically significant reductions in the numbers of EC34195nal^R recovered from the liver and kidney were observed in birds vaccinated with bacterin formulated with either CASAC or CpG oligonucleotides as adjuvants, and in the spleen of birds vaccinated with CpG oligonucleotides, relative to levels in the mock-vaccinated group (Figure 7A; $P < 0.05$). In the groups that received the bacterin formulated with CASAC or CpG, there was also a significant reduction in bacterial numbers in the liver relative to the group that received the bacterin alone, but this difference was not seen in the spleen, kidney or lung (Figure 7A).

In the turkeys vaccinated with the bacterin formulated with the Th2-stimulating adjuvants aluminium hydroxide

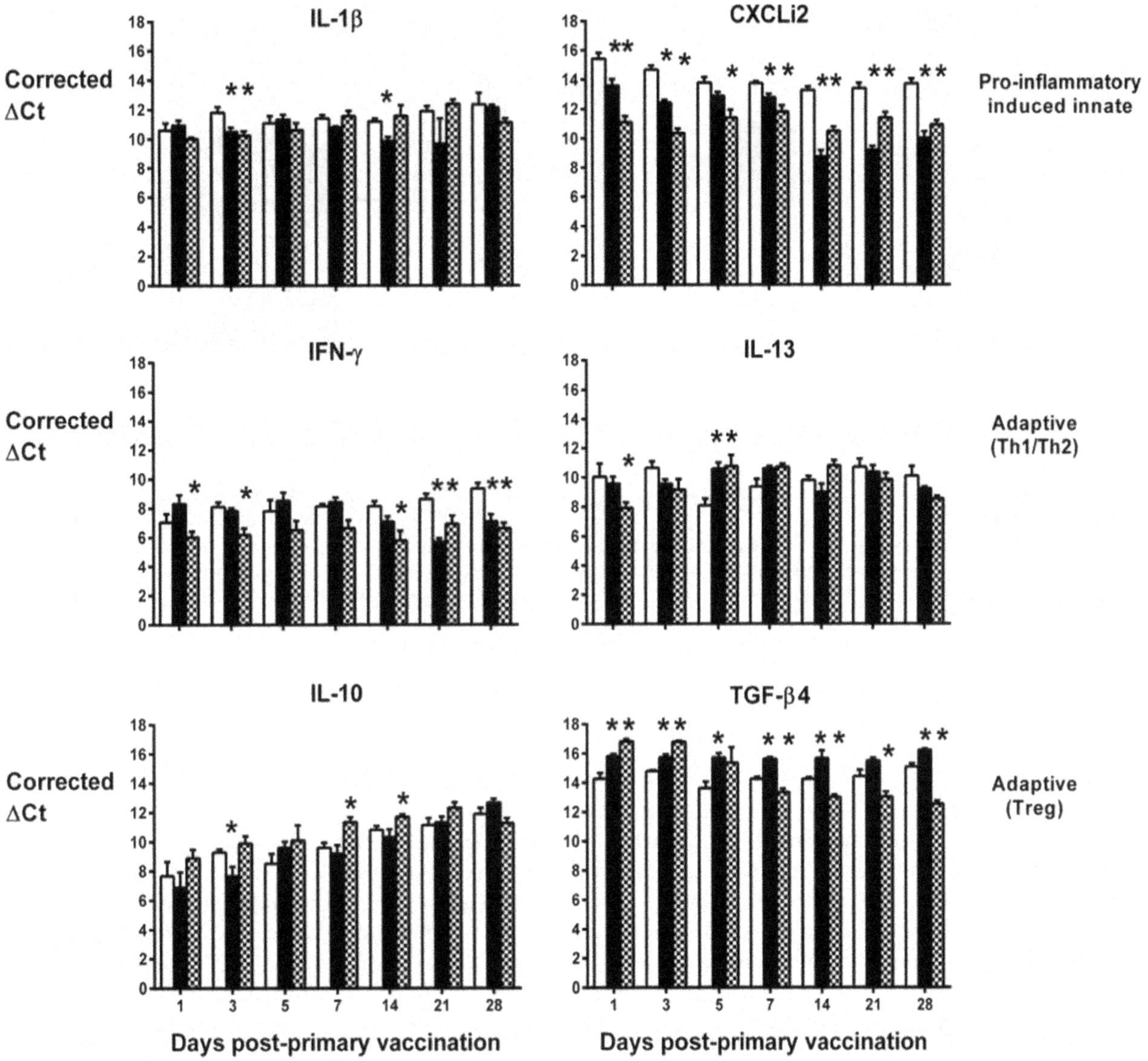

Figure 4 Levels of cytokine transcripts in the lungs of vaccinated turkeys as measured by real-time qRT-PCR. Details are as in the legend to Figure 2.

or TiterMax®, no nalidixic acid resistant *E. coli* were isolated from the liver, kidney and spleen on direct plating (Figure 7B), but they were detected by enrichment of homogenates of these organs (a theoretical limit of detection of 1 $\log_{10}$ CFU/g). Differences in bacterial numbers were statistically significant in all organs from the group that received bacterin formulated with TiterMax® relative to either the bacterin alone or mock-vaccinated control groups ($P < 0.05$). Significant reductions in bacterial numbers were also seen in the liver, spleen and kidney of birds that received the bacterin with aluminium hydroxide relative to the groups that received mock, bacterin alone, or bacterin formulated with CASAC or CpG (Figure 7A and B).

On analysis of APEC-specific IgY at 42 days post-primary vaccination, the bacterin alone induced significantly elevated APEC-specific IgY levels relative to mock vaccinated birds (Figure 7C; $P < 0.05$). The magnitude of the APEC-specific IgY response was no greater when the bacterin was formulated with CpG and marginally lower when formulated with CASAC relative to bacterin alone (Figure 7C). Levels of APEC-specific IgY were no greater in the groups that received the bacterin formulated with aluminium hydroxide and marginally greater when formulated with TiterMax® compared to the bacterin alone (Figure 7D). There is therefore a suggestion that these Th2-biasing adjuvants might generate greater levels of APEC-specific IgY response than Th1-biasing adjuvants.

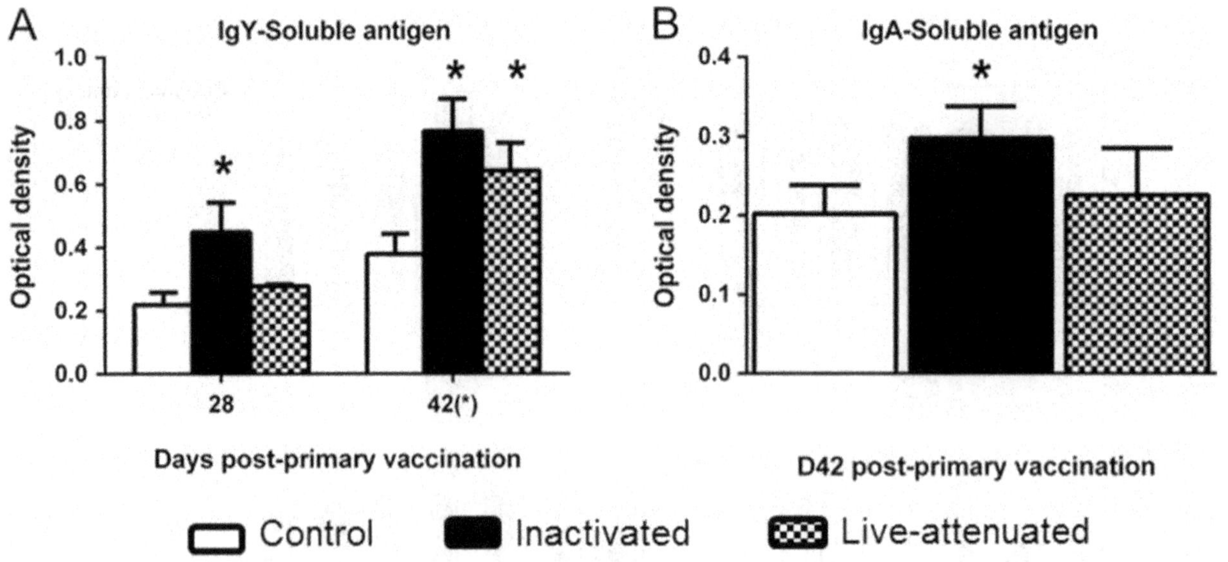

Figure 5 APEC-specific antibody responses in vaccinated turkeys before and after challenge. Turkey poults were given sterile saline (mock) as a coarse spray (open bars), a formalin-inactivated vaccine based on the parent strain EC34195 formulated in aluminium hydroxide adjuvant via the subcutaneous route (black bars) or Poulvac® *E. coli* as a coarse spray (checked black and white bars) starting at one day-old. Five birds from each group were sampled at day 28 post-primary vaccination and 10 birds per group at day 42 post-primary vaccination (24 h after intra-airsac challenge with EC34195nal^R) and serum IgY **(A)** and bile IgA **(B)** levels determined by an APEC-specific ELISA. *denotes $P \leq 0.05$ relative to mock-vaccinated controls.

Discussion

We recently analysed innate and adaptive responses induced by primary APEC O78 infection and demonstrated an association of these with protection against homologous re-challenge [26]. Here, we extended our studies to dissect the immune responses induced by licensed APEC O78-based live-attenuated and inactivated vaccines and their association with protection. We verified that the two vaccines (Poulvac® *E. coli* and a formalin-inactivated vaccine based on its parent strain prepared to commercial specifications) were protective against homologous intra-airsac challenge with EC34195nal^R of turkeys (Figure 1) before examining vaccine-induced innate and adaptive responses. Protection was observed both at the level of clinical signs and the appearance of gross *post-mortem* lesions typical of colibacillosis, as well as the burden of the challenge strain in the lungs and visceral organs. Whilst we were reliably able to detect vaccine-mediated protection against systemic disease and lung colonisation in the turkey model, we acknowledge that it relies on homologous challenge with high doses instilled directly into the left caudal airsac. The basis of protection may therefore differ when turkeys are challenged by heterologous APEC via other routes or natural exposure, and indeed may differ in other avian species. We also acknowledge that the protection observed is largely against bacterial replication in internal organs after systemic translocation of APEC rather than at mucosal surfaces, as the model mimics the often fatal form of avian colibacillosis but not superficial or subacute infections where limited invasion occurs.

Variance between the birds receiving the live-attenuated vaccine by coarse spray and in the drinking water was limited, implying that reasonably uniform doses were given despite the inherent limitations of the mode of delivery. We recovered consistent numbers of the Poulvac® *E. coli* strain from the lung and internal organs of vaccinated birds, and confirmed isolates had the expected genotype. The protection observed is consistent with a recent study by the producers of the vaccine strain [22]. Although vaccination of birds less than 2 weeks of age against *E. coli* can lead to poor protection, which is thought to be due to the relative immaturity of their immune system at that point [27], our protocol adhered to the recommended practice described for Poulvac® *E. coli* [22], and we believe that the protective responses observed in our models are such that an evaluation of the role of innate and adaptive responses in the protection observed is justified.

Inactivated vaccines based on formalin- or heat-inactivated *E. coli* are generally believed to confer protection against avian colibacillosis in an antibody-dependent manner [30,40]. This has been partly established through passive transfer of hyper-immune serum [29-32] or egg-yolk antibody [27,28,41]. However, cytokine responses to APEC vaccination have not previously been analysed. Similarly, whilst live-attenuated mutants of various kinds can confer resistance against APEC in target host species

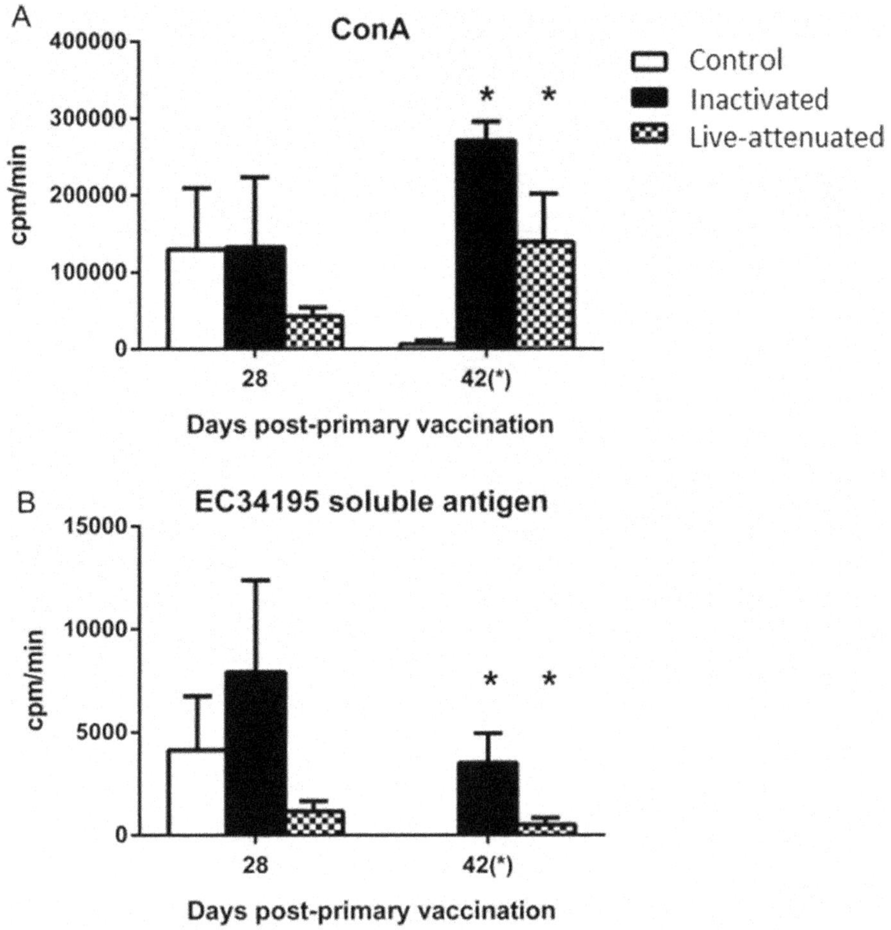

Figure 6 Turkey splenocyte proliferation responses to Concanavalin A and EC34195 soluble lysate in vaccinated turkeys before and after challenge. Turkey poults were given sterile saline (mock) as a coarse spray (open bars), a formalin-inactivated vaccine based on the parent strain EC34195 formulated in aluminium hydroxide adjuvant via the subcutaneous route (black bars) or Poulvac® *E. coli* as a coarse spray (checked black and white bars) starting at one day-old. Five birds were sampled from each group at each time and splenocytes re-stimulated with ConA **(A)** or EC43195 soluble lysate **(B)**. The data are presented as mean counts per minute ± standard error of the mean. *denotes $P \leq 0.05$ relative to mock-vaccinated controls.

[21,22,30,42-44], the innate and cell-mediated responses they elicit are ill-defined. Studies by Fernandez Filho et al. [43] with Poulvac® *E. coli* only examined peripheral cellular responses to vaccination, with a fine spray, of day-old chicks. No booster was given to those birds at 7 days of age via drinking water as is recommended [22]. A recent field trial of Poulvac® *E. coli* [42] also supports that giving a booster in drinking water is not necessary. Interestingly, a higher level of peripheral B lymphocytes was detected in the control than the vaccinated group and the authors speculated that Poulvac® *E. coli* may suppress humoral responses and that they may therefore be dispensable in protection [43]. In support of this, Salehi et al. [44] also reported a lack of significant induction of antibody response in chickens after aerosol administration of an independent *aroA* mutant of *E. coli*. In contrast, we observed that Poulvac® *E. coli* elicited significantly elevated APEC-specific serum IgY in turkeys relative to mock-vaccinated poults. Differences between this study and earlier reports could of course be due to variations in the vaccination protocols, in particular the administration of single dose of the vaccine when birds are still immunologically immature.

The induction of APEC-specific humoral responses by both vaccines in this study is supported by analysis of transcription of cytokines and chemokines at a key site of immune priming, the spleen. In the spleen, during the first week post-vaccination, transcription of the signature Th1 cytokine IFN-γ was repressed, whereas that of the signature Th2 cytokine IL-13 was significantly induced by both vaccines. Reduced transcription of IFN-γ was also seen in the lung at multiple time-points after vaccination with the live-attenuated vaccine but was not evident in the liver. IL-13 mRNA expression levels in the lung and liver in the first week post-primary vaccination showed no

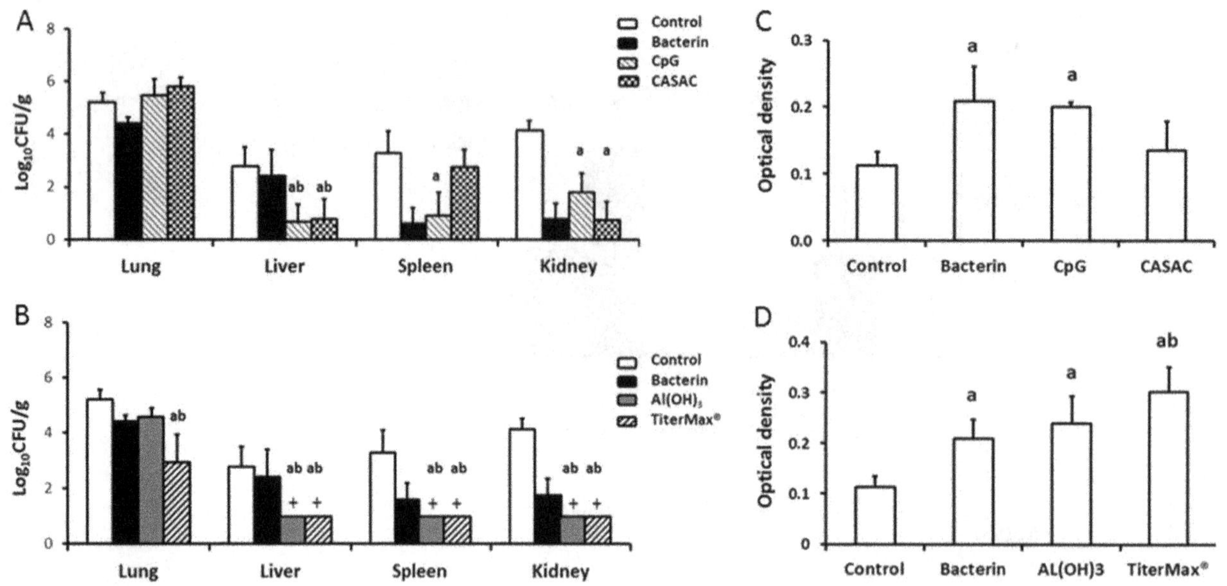

Figure 7 Recoveries of strain EC34195nal[R] from organs of turkeys vaccinated with a formalin-inactivated bacterin formulated with different adjuvants at 24 h post-challenge. Turkey poults were given sterile saline (negative control), an EC34915-based inactivated bacterin without adjuvant, or formulated with adjuvants that promote a Th1 response (CASAC or CpG-oligonucleotides **(A)**), or Th2 response (Titermax® Gold or aluminium hydroxide **(B)**). All vaccines were given by the subcutaneous route at 1 day-old and boosted at day 14. All the birds were challenged at day 41 post-primary vaccination via the intra-airsac route with EC34195nal[R] and sampled after 24 h. The data are presented as mean log_{10} CFU/g tissue ± standard error of the mean. APEC-specific serum IgY levels for corresponding birds at post-mortem examination were measured by ELISA compared to mock- and bacterin-vaccinated groups, Th1- **(C)** and Th2-stimulating adjuvants **(D)**. + denotes value of EC34195nal[R] after enrichment. "a" denotes $P \leq 0.05$ relative to turkey poults that received sterile saline (mock-vaccinated group), "b" denotes $P \leq 0.05$ relative to bacterin alone, and "ab" is significance relative to both mock- and bacterin-vaccinated groups.

discernible pattern. The expression of TGF-β4 in all organs could be suggestive of a proliferative cellular response that requires some kind of regulation. Transient expression of IL-6 was observed in the first 5 days in the spleen, but not liver or lung (data not shown). Since the nature of such proliferative cellular responses could not be discerned, we reasoned that TGF-β4 acted primarily as an anti-inflammatory suppressing the expression of IL-6 in all organs. Overall, the data are indicative of a Th2-biased response to vaccination in the spleen, albeit this is less evident in the liver and lung. The magnitude of cytokine responses was not markedly different between the live-attenuated and inactivated vaccine groups and therefore cannot readily be associated with the magnitude of the adaptive responses measured.

After challenge, splenocyte recall responses to ConA or APEC-specific antigens in the control group (with a high bacterial recovery in the spleen) were poor and absent respectively. These data are consistent with the suppressive effect of APEC O78 on proliferative responses detected in our earlier studies [26], and may imply that the live-attenuated vaccine also has a negative effect on the capacity of splenocytes to proliferate in response to mitogen. As the live-attenuated vaccine could not be recovered from vaccinated turkey poults at day 28, it is difficult to separate the extent to which proliferative responses are an accurate reflection of recall responses, or were compromised owing to presence of low numbers of bacteria or their products. The possibility of suppressive effects makes it difficult to interpret the response in the group given the inactivated vaccine at day 42, as the spleen was recovered after challenge of such birds. Earlier evidence suggests that inactivated vaccines are poor inducers of T cell-mediated immunity [45]. However, we detected significantly elevated splenocyte proliferative responses to APEC-specific antigens induced by the inactivated vaccine after challenge. Studies with a killed *Salmonella* vaccine have also shown a significant induction of lympho-proliferative responses, though these were age- and antigen-dependent [46]. APEC membrane vesicles can evoke both antibody production and T cell proliferation and specifically stimulate T cytotoxic cells to confer resistance against APEC [47], further indicating that inert APEC vaccines can stimulate both adaptive pathways.

Given the potential importance of the Th2 pathway in protection conferred by the vaccines tested, we evaluated the effects of Th1- and Th2-stimulating adjuvants using an EC34195-based bacterin. This enabled us to standardize the dose and timing and compare protection observed without adjuvant with that given by bacterin formulated with aluminium hydroxide that had already proven to be protective throughout. Although the use of Th1 adjuvants resulted in significant reduction in bacterial numbers recovered from internal organs relative to the control (mock-vaccinated) group, the Th2 adjuvants elicited better protective responses in the lungs (especially TiterMax®) and internal organs. CpG-ODN induce predominantly a Th1 response [38,39,48], and administration of these on their own 3 days prior to challenge confers protection against *E. coli* infections in neonatal and adult chickens [49,50]. Furthermore, formulating an inactivated vaccine with these motifs imparted a more potent effect in halting the spread of a lethal APEC strain [51], implying the importance of Th1 responses in resistance against APEC. In this study CpG-ODN did not significantly augment humoral responses or protection relative to the bacterin alone, except in the liver. CASAC is a recently described potent Th1-stimulating adjuvant consisting of three components [36], including interferon-gamma (IFN-γ). We used chicken IFN-γ owing to its commercial availability, and is biologically cross-reactive in the turkey [52]. As with CpG, CASAC did not potentiate humoral responses or protection relative to those seen with the bacterin alone, except in the liver. One of the Th2-biasing adjuvants (TiterMax®) gave significantly improved protection relative to the bacterin alone as well as significantly elevated APEC-specific IgY levels, whereas the other (aluminium hydroxide) was not different to responses to the bacterin alone, in accordance with earlier reports [18,20]. While it is not conclusively clear if Th2 adjuvants stimulate more potent antibody responses and protection than Th1 adjuvants in the context of inactivated APEC vaccines, the data suggest that further research to augment Th2 responses has merit.

In conclusion, we show that live and inactivated APEC vaccines are protective against experimental intra-airsac challenge in a turkey model of acute colibacillosis and that they both induce predominantly a Th2 response in the spleen that correlates with elevated APEC-specific antibody levels. Whilst we have defined the responses associated with vaccine-mediated protection against homologous challenge, the relative contribution of humoral and cell-mediated immunity in protection against heterologous APEC infection requires further study. Demonstration of a key role for antibody will help to prime reverse vaccinology to identify conserved surface-exposed constituents of APEC that can elicit antibody to fix complement and prime phagocytosis. Although our recent sequencing of APEC indicates that *E. coli* evolve to cause avian disease from varied lineages via acquisition of distinct sets of virulence genes, we also revealed a core genome encoding of over 3000 conserved factors [4]. Mining of the core genome of human extraintestinal pathogenic *E. coli* strains has yielded a subset of factors that show promise as cross-protective vaccines for control of sepsis and urinary tract infections [53,54], and a similar approach for avian colibacillosis has merit. The models and data presented here will help to inform and evaluate improved vaccines in target hosts.

Competing interests
The authors declare that they have no competing interests.

Authors' contributions
JRS and FD designed, conducted and supervised the experiments. ZW and PvD assisted in animal experiments and assays. AM and FD supervised adjuvant studies. RML and FD supervised the vaccine studies. FD, PK and MPS secured funding, analysed and interpreted the data and wrote the manuscript. All authors read and approved the manuscript.

Acknowledgements
We gratefully acknowledge the support of the Biotechnology and Biological Sciences Research Council (BB/E001859/1 and Institute Strategic Programme grants to The Pirbright Institute and The Roslin Institute), the British Poultry Council (Turkey R&D Sector) and Aviagen Ltd.

Author details
[1]Avian Infectious Diseases Programme, The Pirbright Institute, Compton, Berkshire, RG20 7NN, UK. [2]The Roslin Institute and Royal (Dick) School of Veterinary Studies, University of Edinburgh, Easter Bush, Midlothian EH25 9RG, UK. [3]The Jenner Institute, University of Oxford, Oxford OX3 7DQ, UK. [4]School of Veterinary Medicine, University of Surrey, Guildford, GU2 7TE, UK. [5]Department of Bacteriology, AHVLA, Weybridge, Surrey, KT15 3NB, UK. [6]Present address: School of Veterinary Medicine, The University of the West Indies, St Augustine, Trinidad and Tobago.

References
1. Kemmett K, Williams NJ, Chaloner G, Humphrey S, Wigley P, Humphrey T: **The contribution of systemic *Escherichia coli* infection to the early mortalities of commercial broiler chickens.** *Avian Pathol* 2014, **43**:37–42.
2. Kemmett K, Humphrey T, Rushton S, Close A, Wigley P, Williams NJ: **A longitudinal study simultaneously exploring the carriage of APEC virulence associated genes and the molecular epidemiology of faecal and systemic E. coli in commercial broiler chickens.** *PLoS One* 2013, **8**:e67749.
3. Dziva F, Stevens MP: **Colibacillosis in poultry: unravelling the molecular basis of virulence of avian pathogenic *Escherichia coli* in their natural hosts.** *Avian Pathol* 2008, **37**:355–366.
4. Dziva F, Hauser H, Connor TR, van Diemen PM, Prescott G, Langridge GC, Eckert S, Chaudhuri RR, Ewers E, Mellata M, Mukhopadhyay S, Curtiss R 3rd, Dougan G, Wieler LH, Thomson NR, Pickard DJ, Stevens MP: **Sequencing and functional annotation of avian pathogenic *Escherichia coli* serogroup O78 strains reveal the evolution of *E. coli* lineages pathogenic for poultry via distinct mechanisms.** *Infect Immun* 2013, **81**:838–849.
5. Mellata M, Maddux JT, Nam T, Thomson N, Hauser H, Stevens MP, Mukhopadhyay S, Sarker S, Crabbé A, Nickerson CA, Santander J, Curtiss R III: **New insights into the bacterial fitness-associated mechanisms revealed by the characterization of large plasmids of an avian pathogenic E. coli.** *PLoS One* 2012, **7**:e29481.
6. Mellata M, Touchman JW, Curtiss R: **Full sequence and comparative plasmid pAPEC-1 of avian pathogenic *Escherichia coli* chi7122 (O78:K80:H9).** *PLoS One* 2009, **7**:e4232.
7. Mellata M: **Human and avian extraintestinal pathogenic *Escherichia coli*: infections, zoonotic risks, and antibiotic resistance trends.** *Foodborne Pathog Dis* 2013, **10**:916–932.
8. Ewers C, Li G, Wilking H, Kiessling S, Alt K, Antáo EM, Laturnus C, Diehl I, Glodde S, Homeier T, Böhnke U, Steinrück H, Philipp HC, Wieler LH: **Avian pathogenic, uropathogenic, and newborn meningitis-causing *Escherichia coli*: how closely related are they?** *Int J Med Microbiol* 2007, **297**:163–176.
9. Johnson TJ, Kariyawasam S, Wannemuehler Y, Mangiamele P, Johnson SJ, Doetkott C, Skyberg JA, Lynne AM, Johnson JR, Nolan LK: **The genome sequence of avian pathogenic *Escherichia coli* strain O1:K1:H7 shares**

strong similarities with human extra-intestinal pathogenic *E. coli* genomes. *J Bacteriol* 2007, **189**:3228–3236.

10. Johnson TJ, Wannemuehler Y, Johnson SJ, Stell AL, Doetkott C, Johnson JR, Kim KS, Spanjaard L, Nolan LK: **Comparison of extraintestinal pathogenic *Escherichia coli* strains from human and avian sources reveals a mixed subset representing potential zoonotic pathogens.** *Appl Environ Microbiol* 2008, **74**:7043–7050.
11. Cortés P, Blanc VMora A, Dahbi G, Blanco JE, Blanco M, López C, Andreu A, Navarro F, Alonso MP, Bou G, Blanco J, Llagostera M: **Isolation and characterization of potentially pathogenic antimicrobial-resistant *Escherichia coli* strains from chicken and pig farms in Spain.** *Appl Environ Microbiol* 2010, **76**:2799–2805.
12. Costa D, Vinué L, Poeta P, Coelho AC, Matos M, Sáenz Y, Somalo S, Zarazaga M, Rodrigues J, Torres C: **Prevalence of extended-spectrum beta-lactamase-producing *Escherichia coli* isolates in faecal samples of broilers.** *Vet Microbiol* 2009, **138**:339–344.
13. Jakobsen L, Spangholm DJ, Pedersen K, Jensen LB, Emborg HD, Agerso Y, Aarestrup FM, Hammerum AM, Frimodt-Møller N: **Broiler chickens, broiler chicken meat, pigs and pork as sources of ExPEC related virulence genes and resistance in *Escherichia coli* isolates from community-dwelling humans and UTI patients.** *Int J Food Microbiol* 2010, **142**:264–272.
14. Overdevest I, Willemsen I, Rijnsburger M, Eustace A, Xu L, Hawkey P, Heck M, Savelkoul P, Vandenbroucke-Grauls C, van der Zwaluw K, Huijsdens X, Kluytmans J: **Extended-spectrum β-Lactamase genes of *Escherichia coli* in chicken, meat and humans, the Netherlands.** *Emerg Infect Dis* 2011, **17**:1216–1222.
15. Wang XM, Liao XP, Zhang WJ, Jiang HX, Sun J, Zhang MJ, He XF, Lao DX, Liu YH: **Prevalence of serogroups, virulence genotypes, antimicrobial resistance, and phylogenetic background of avian pathogenic *Escherichia coli* in south of China.** *Foodborne Pathog Dis* 2010, **7**:1099–1106.
16. Linton AH, Howe K, Bennett PM, Richmond MH, Whiteside EJ: **The colonization of the human gut by antibiotic resistant *Escherichia coli* from chickens.** *J Appl Bacteriol* 1977, **43**:465–469.
17. Ojeniyi AA: **Direct transmission of *Escherichia coli* from poultry to humans.** *Epidemiol Infect* 1989, **103**:513–522.
18. Deb JR, Harry EG: **Laboratory trials with inactivated vaccines against *Escherichia coli* (O78:K80) infection in fowls.** *Res Vet Sci* 1976, **20**:131–138.
19. Deb JR, Harry EG: **Laboratory trials with inactivated vaccines against *Escherichia coli* (O2:K1) infection in fowls.** *Res Vet Sci* 1978, **24**:308–313.
20. Trampel DW, Griffith RW: **Efficacy of aluminium hydroxide-adjuvanted *Escherichia coli* bacterin in turkey poults.** *Avian Dis* 1997, **41**:263–268.
21. Frommer A, Freidlin PJ, Bock RR, Leitner G, Chaffer M, Heller ED: **Experimental vaccination of young chickens with a live, non-pathogenic strain of *Escherichia coli*.** *Avian Pathol* 1994, **23**:425–433.
22. La Ragione RM, Woodward MJ, Kumar M, Rodenberg J, Fan H, Wales AD, Karaca K: **Efficacy of a live attenuated *Escherichia coli* O78 : K80 vaccine in chickens and turkeys.** *Avian Dis* 2013, **57**:273–279.
23. Kariyawasam S, Wilkie BN, Gyles CL: **Construction, characterization and evaluation of the vaccine potential of three genetically defined mutants of avian pathogenic *Escherichia coli*.** *Avian Dis* 2004, **48**:287–299.
24. Kwaga JP, Allan BJ, van den Hurk JV, Seida H, Potter AA: **A *carAB* mutant of avian pathogenic *Escherichia coli* sergroup O2 is attenuated and effective as a live oral vaccine against colibacillosis in turkeys.** *Infect Immun* 1994, **62**:3766–3772.
25. Peighambari SM, Hunter DB, Shewen PE, Gyles CL: **Safety, immunogenicity and efficacy of two *Escherichia coli cya crp* mutants as vaccines for broilers.** *Avian Dis* 2002, **46**:287–297.
26. Sadeyen JR, Kaiser P, Stevens MP, Dziva F: **Analysis of immune responses induced by avian pathogenic *Escherichia coli* infection in turkeys and their association with resistance to homologous re-challenge.** *Vet Res* 2014, **45**:19.
27. Heller ED, Leitner G, Drabkin N, Melamed D: **Passive immunization of chicks against *Escherichia coli*.** *Avian Pathol* 1990, **19**:345–354.
28. Kariyawasam S, Wilkie BN, Gyles CL: **Resistance of broiler chickens to *Escherichia coli* respiratory tract infection induced by passively transferred egg-yolk antibodies.** *Vet Microbiol* 2004, **98**:273–284.
29. Rosenberger JK, Fries PA, Cloud SS: **In vitro and in vivo characterization of avian *Escherichia coli*. III. Immunization.** *Avian Dis* 1985, **29**:1108–1117.
30. Arp LH: **Consequences of active and passive immunization of turkeys against *Escherichia coli* O78.** *Avian Dis* 1980, **24**:808–815.
31. Arp LH: **Effect of passive immunization on phagocytosis of blood-borne *Escherichia coli* in spleen and liver of turkeys.** *Am J Vet Res* 1982, **43**:1034–1040.
32. Bolin CA, Jensen AE: **Passive immunization with antibodies against iron-regulated outer membrane proteins protects turkeys from *Escherichia coli* septicaemia.** *Infect Immun* 1987, **55**:1239–1242.
33. La Ragione RM, Collighan RJ, Woodward MJ: **Non-curliation of *Escherichia coli* O78:K80 isolates associated with IS1 in *csgB* and reduced persistence in poultry infection.** *FEMS Microbiol Lett* 1999, **175**:247–254.
34. Gibson MS, Fife M, Bird S, Salmon N, Kaiser P: **Identification, cloning, and functional characterization of the IL-1 receptor antagonist in the chicken reveal important differences between the chicken and mammals.** *J Immunol* 2012, **189**:539–550.
35. Poh TY, Pease J, Young JR, Bumstead N, Kaiser P: **Re-evaluation of chicken CXCR1 determines the true gene structure: CXCLi1 (K60) and CXCLi2 (CAF/interleukin-8) are ligands for this receptor.** *J Biol Chem* 2008, **283**:16408–16415.
36. Wells JW, Cowled CJ, Farzaneh F, Noble A: **Combined triggering of dendritic cell receptors results in synergistic activation and potent cytotoxic immunity.** *J Immunol* 2008, **181**:3422–3431.
37. Loots K, van Loock M, Vanrompay D, Goddeeris BM: **CpG motifs as adjuvant in DNA vaccination against *Chlamydophila psittaci* in turkeys.** *Vaccine* 2006, **24**:4598–4601.
38. Chu RS, Targoni OS, Krieg AM, Lehmann PV, Harding CV: **CpG oligonucleotides act as adjuvants that switch on T helper 1 (Th1) immunity.** *J Exp Med* 1997, **186**:1623–1631.
39. Weeratna RD, McCluskie MJ, Xu Y, Davies HL: **CpG DNA induces stronger immune responses with less toxicity than other adjuvants.** *Vaccine* 2000, **18**:1755–1762.
40. Leitner G, Melamed D, Drabkin N, Heller ED: **An enzyme-linked immunosorbent assay for detection of antibodies against *Escherichia coli*: association between indirect hemagglutination test and survival.** *Avian Dis* 1990, **34**:58–62.
41. Heller ED: **The immune response of hens to multiple *Escherichia coli* injections and transfer of immunoglobulins to the egg and hatched chick.** *Res Vet Sci* 1975, **18**:117–120.
42. Mombarg M, Bouzoubaa K, Andrews S, Vanimisetti HB, Rodenberg J, Karaca K: **Safety and efficacy of an *aroA*-deleted live vaccine against avian colibacillosis in a multicentre field trial in broilers in Morocco.** *Avian Pathol* 2014, **43**:276–281.
43. Fernandez Filho T, Favaro C Jr, Ingberman M, Beirao BCB, Inoue A, Gomes L, Caron LF: **Effect of spray *Escherichia coli* vaccine on the immunity of poultry.** *Avian Dis* 2013, **57**:671–676.
44. Salehi TZ, Tabatabaei S, Karimi V, Fasaei BN, Derakhshandeh A, Jahromi OAN: **Assessment of immunity against avian colibacillosis induced by an *aroA* mutant containing increased serum survival gene in broilers.** *Braz J Microbiol* 2012, **43**:363–370.
45. Collins FM: **Vaccines and cell-mediated immunity.** *Bacteriol Rev* 1974, **38**:371–402.
46. Okamura M, Lillehoj HS, Raybourne RB, Babu US, Heckert RA: **Cell-mediated immune responses to a killed *Salmonella enteritidis* vaccine: lymphocyte proliferation, T-cell changes and interfleukin-6 (IL-6), IL-1, IL-2 and IFN-γ production.** *Comp Immunol Microbiol Infect Dis* 2004, **27**:255–272.
47. Chaffer M, Schwartsburd B, Heller ED: **Vaccination of turkey poults against pathogenic *Escherichia coli*.** *Avian Pathol* 1997, **26**:377–390.
48. Patel BA, Gomis S, Dar A, Willson PJ, Babiuk LA, Potter A, Mutwiri G, Tikoo SK: **Oligodeoxynucleotides containing CpG motifs (CpG-ODN) predominantly induce Th1-type immune response in neonatal chicks.** *Dev Comp Immunol* 2008, **32**:1041–1049.
49. Gomis S, Babiuk L, Allan B, Willson P, Waters E, Ambrose N, Hecker R, Potter A: **Protection of neonatal chicks against a lethal challenge of *Escherichia coli* using DNA containing cytosine-phosphodiester-guanine motifs.** *Avian Dis* 2004, **48**:813–822.
50. Gomis S, Babiuk L, Allan B, Wilson P, Waters E, Hecker R, Potter A: **Protection of chickens against a lethal challenge of *Escherichia coli* by a vaccine containing CpG oligonucleotides as an adjuvant.** *Avian Dis* 2007, **51**:78–83.
51. Gomis S, Babiuk L, Godson DL, Allen B, Thrush T, Townsend H, Willson P, Waters E, Hecker R, Potter A: **Protection of chickens against *Escherichia coli* infections by DNA containing CpG motifs.** *Infect Immun* 2003, **71**:857–863.

52. Lawson S, Rothwell L, Lambrecht B, Howes K, Venugopal K, Kaiser P: **Turkey and chicken interferon-γ, which share high sequence identity, are biologically cross-reactive.** *Dev Comp Immunol* 2001, **25**:69–82.
53. Moriel DG, Bertoldi I, Spagnuolo A, Marchi S, Rosini R, Nesta B, Pastorello I, Corea VA, Torricelli G, Cartocci E, Savino S, Scarselli M, Dobrindt U, Hacker J, Tettelin H, Tallon LJ, Sullivan S, Wieler LH, Ewers C, Pickard D, Dougan G, Fontana MR, Rappuoli R, Pizza M, Serino L: **Identification of protective and broadly conserved vaccine antigens from the genome of extraintestinal pathogenic *Escherichia coli*.** *Proc Natl Acad Sci U S A* 2010, **107**:9072–9077.
54. Nesta B, Spraggon G, Alteri C, Moriel DG, Rosini R, Veggi D, Smith S, Bertoldi I, Pastorello I, Ferlenghi I, Fontana MR, Frankel G, Mobley HL, Rappuoli R, Pizza M, Serino L, Soriani M: **FdeC, a novel broadly conserved *Escherichia coli* adhesin eliciting protection against urinary tract infections.** *MBio* 2012, **3**:e00010–e00012.

TGF-β superfamily members from the helminth *Fasciola hepatica* show intrinsic effects on viability and development

Ornampai Japa[1], Jane E Hodgkinson[3], Richard D Emes[1,2] and Robin J Flynn[1*]

Abstract

The helminth *Fasciola hepatica* causes fasciolosis throughout the world, a major disease of livestock and an emerging zoonotic disease in humans. Sustainable control mechanisms such as vaccination are urgently required. To discover potential vaccine targets we undertook a genome screen to identify members of the transforming growth factor (TGF) family of proteins. Herein we describe the discovery of three ligands belonging to this superfamily and the cloning and characterisation of an activin/TGF like molecule we term FhTLM. FhTLM has a limited expression pattern both temporally across the parasite stages but also spatially within the worm. Furthermore, a recombinant form of this protein is able to enhance the rate (or magnitude) of multiple developmental processes of the parasite indicating a conserved role for this protein superfamily in the developmental biology of a major trematode parasite. Our study demonstrates for the first time the existence of this protein superfamily within *F. hepatica* and assigns a function to one of the three identified ligands. Moreover further exploration of this superfamily may yield future targets for diagnostic or vaccination purposes due to its stage restricted expression and functional role.

Introduction

Transforming growth factor (TGF)–β1 is a multifaceted cytokine belonging to the TGF-β superfamily of proteins composed of the TGF and bone morphogenic proteins (BMP) subfamilies. Structurally TGF subfamily members are characterised by the presence of 9 cysteine residues while 7 residues are found in BMP proteins. TGF-β1 signalling is involved in the development and differentiation of animal tissues and organs [1,2] and its pathway components are very well conserved and seemingly evolved early in the history of animals [3]. Members of the TGF superfamily have been described in both higher and lower animals. Despite their pivotal role in animal development there is no apparent correlation regarding the complexity of morphology and the number of the signalling pathway members present [4]. Regardless, this protein superfamily has enormous diversity and specificity of signalling is defined through a combination of receptors and cognate intracellular signalling components. Upon ligation, TGF-β serine threonine kinase (STK) receptors directly activate the relevant receptor-activated Smad (R-Smad) signalling component. Smad2 and 3 transduce the TGF-β/activin signal and while Smad1, 5 and 8 mediate the BMP signal. Smad4 is subsequently joined to the activated R-Smad complex and this migrates into the nucleus to regulate expression of target genes [5].

In the model organism *Caenorhabditis elegans*, TGF-β-like ligands, Decapentaplegic BMP-like (DBL)-1 and Dauer formation abnormal (DAF)-7 have been well characterized [6]. Ce-DBL-1, a homolog of BMPs, was found to influence body size and tail formation of male worms. Mutant worms lacking DBL-1 have been shown to be smaller than wild type worms while reintroduction and overexpression of a DBL-1 expressing plasmid was found to result in longer worms [7]. Signalling by the TGF-β subfamily member DAF-7, was shown to be involved in the control of the dauer stage and mutant DAF-7 worms were found to be more susceptible to temperature change. Mutant DAF-7 worms have also been shown to enter into the arrest stage under inappropriate conditions or fail to enter the dauer stage entirely [8].

* Correspondence: robin.flynn@nottingham.ac.uk
[1]School of Veterinary Medicine and Science, University of Nottingham, Sutton Bonington, Nottingham LE12 5RD, UK
Full list of author information is available at the end of the article

Several studies have examined the expression and localization of TGF-β homologues during the life cycle of parasitic helminths and homologues of DAF-7 have been extensively investigated amongst parasitic nematodes. It has been suggested that this ligand controls arrested development of parasitic nematodes particularly during the infective L3 stage [9]. A wide array of intestinal nematodes exhibit a high level of expression of DAF-7 homologue in their L3 stages including *Ancylostoma caninum*, [10,11], *Strongyloides ratti*, *Parastrongyloides trichosuri* [12,13], *Heligmosomoides polygyrus* and *Teladorsagia circumcincta* [14].

Within trematodes, TGF-β proteins have only been extensively studied in *Schistosoma* spp., where expression of TGF-β or BMP family members has been detected throughout the life cycle [15-17]. SmInAct is a TGF-β/Activin-like ligand, expressed in female *S. mansoni* worms and their eggs. Reduction in levels of SmInAct by RNAi resulted in stunting of the female worms and incomplete development of eggs. SmInAct was localised to embryonated eggs and female reproductive organs supporting its role in worm development [15]. Homologues of BMP proteins have also been demonstrated in *S. mansoni* (SmBMP) and *S. japonicum* (SjBMP), with levels of SjBMP expression were greatest in early larval stages and eggs of *S. japonicum* [17]. The transcript was localized to the tegument and epithelium of adults; furthermore it was also present in the ovary of the female worm. RNAi knockdown resulted in a phenotype with low egg output and stunted egg development.

Fasciola hepatica is a major trematode parasite of livestock and an emerging human zoonotic disease found throughout the world. *F. hepatica* completes its lifecycle through the utilisation of a mud-snail intermediate host before reaching maturity, as a hermaphrodite, within the liver and bile ducts of ruminants. Control is centred on chemotherapy but mounting drug resistance and shifting patterns of disease underline the need for novel and sustainable strategies for control. In order to develop effective novel therapeutic targets, it is important to understand parasite biology and immune evasion mechanisms. Genes previously identified as encoding for homologues of the TGF-β family are present in a number of parasitic worms and these molecules may offer novel therapeutic approaches for the control of multiple species of veterinary and medical importance, e.g. *A. caninum*, *S. stercoralis* and *H. contortus* [18]. Herein, we sought to identify any gene(s) encoding TGF-β homologues present in the *F. hepatica* genome given that any TGF-β molecules present may control parasite development, thus presenting an attractive target for parasite control or diagnosis.

Materials and methods

Genome analysis

Genome analysis was conducted using the putative *F. hepatica* genome produced in the laboratory of Dr Jane Hodgkinson University of Liverpool [19]. TGF-β like sequences were identified in the *F. hepatica* genome through a tBlastn search of the draft genome contigs using protein sequences of TGF-β1-3 from mammalian hosts and SmInAct, a TGF-β like protein from *S. mansoni* as queries. All translated potential matching regions were compared to both the non-redundant (nr) database and a database of translated bovine genes using the Blastp algorithm. An E-value cut off of 1×10^{-4} was used to define a significant hit. Candidate genes were identified from genomic DNA using the exonerate software (scripts available at [20]. The deduced amino acid sequences of TGF-β like proteins of *F. hepatica* and other helminths identified from PSI Blast (Position Specific Iterated Blast) and with mammalian TGF-β and BMP subfamily were aligned using MUSCLE [21] implemented in the Seaview program [22,23].

RACE cloning, recombinant expression vector construction and protein production

First strand cDNA from adult *F. hepatica* was prepared as template for RACE using GeneRacer™ Kit (Invitrogen, UK) following the manufacturers' protocol. 5' and 3' RACE was completed to as outlined by manufacturers' protocols. To construct the recombinant plasmid, primers incorporating restriction sites were used to amplify the entire FhTLM ORF before cloning into a pET28a (Novagen) plasmid containing a 6X-His Tag as follows: Forward 5- GCGGCTAGC ATGTGCAATTATGTGCCCGTTTTG-3 where the underlined sequence represents the NheI restriction site and Reverse 5- GCGCTCGAGTCAGATGACATTTGTTCCGGC AAG-3 where the underlined sequence represents the XhoI restriction site. The pET28aFhTLM plasmid was chemically transformed into *E. coli* Rosetta BL21 DE3/pLysS (Novagen, USA) and seeded onto LB agar supplemented with 30 μg/mL of kanamycin and 34 μg/mL of chloramphenicol. Positive clones were confirmed by colony PCR and individual sequencing. Thereafter bulk cultures were produced by inoculating 10 mL of LB with a single colony overnight and subsequently sub-culturing this into 500 mL of LB broth. Protein expression was induced by addition of IPTG at a final concentration of 1 mM, thereafter His-tagged FhTLM supernatant was purified over a Nickel resin column (Sigma-Aldrich). Before use recombinant protein was subject to phase separation to remove endotoxin residues [24]. Briefly, proteins were adjusted to 0.5 μg/mL concentration in a final volume of 5% Trition X-114. Samples were vortexed, incubated on ice for 5 min, incubated at 37 °C for 5 min and centrifuged at 5000 × *g* for 7 min. The lipid free fraction in the upper aqueous phase was retained and dialysed into PBS before further use.

Functional assays

Unembryonated eggs released from fresh adult worms were collected and washed several times with dH_2O. The egg suspension was adjusted to 1000 eggs/mL and 100 µL was distributed in 96-well plates. The eggs were then incubated with rFhTLM and human TGF-β (Peprotech) at 2.5 and 250 pg/mL containing penicillin (50 U/mL) and streptomycin (50 µg/mL) and gentamycin (10 µg/mL). The plate was covered with foil to prevent light activation and kept in a 30 °C dark incubator. At day 2, and 7 of incubation, the egg culture plate was removed and egg development was examined under an inverted microscope (Medline Scientific, UK). To assess egg production in adult worms, they were stimulated as above and eggs were counted in aliquots of culture supernatant under a stereomicroscope. Egg number was presented as eggs/gram of tissue wet weight for each fluke.

For an in vitro assessment of the rFhTLM effect on the newly excysted juveniles (NEJs) they were prepared as described elsewhere [25]. NEJs were cultured in RPMI-1640 containing 250 ng/mL of rFhTLM, or TGF-β at 37 °C with 5% CO_2. Control worms were treated with PBS. After 24 h of cultivation, parasites were subsequently evaluated for viability and motility. Motility was observed under a stereo microscope and scored as +, ++, and +++. NEJs viability was determined by the MTT (3-[4, 5-dimethylthiazol-2-yl]-2, 5- diphenyltetrazolium bromide) assay according to manufacturers' instructions (Sigma-Aldrich). Briefly, 100 µL of MTT (5 mg/mL) was added to cultures containing parasites and incubated for 30 min at 37 °C. The solution was then replaced with DMSO and incubated at RT for 1 h. Optical density (OD) was read at 540 nm of solutions in an ELISA plate after this.

Lifestage PCR and in situ hybridisation

FhTLM gene expression was determined using cDNA prepared from various parasite life stages by conventional RT-PCR using *Taq* DNA Polymerase (Qiagen, UK) according to manufacturer's instruction briefly, 5 µL of cDNA was used as template in a 50 µL PCR. FhTLM primers (5'-3') were Forward GCTTGCCAATCGGGTGGACAGCAATTCA and Reverse CTGCATCCACATCCGAGAACAATGAG giving a band size of 342 bp. β-tubulin used as a housekeeping Forward GTATTGCATCGACAACGAAGCT and Reverse GTGCAAACGGGGGAACGG giving a band size of 192 bp.

To perform in situ hybridization the method of Pearson [26] was used in combination with a specific FhTLM DIG-labelled riboprobe (Roche UK). After fixing in 4% PFA specimens were moved to PBS with 0.5% Triton X-100 (PBSTx). Specimens were placed in 6% h2o2 followed by washing in 100% methanol; thereafter samples were rehydrated in a gradient of decreasing methanol. Specimens were incubated in PCR-grade proteinase K 10 µg/mL (Roche), re-fixed in 4% PFA and rinsed twice with PBSTx. Specimens were incubated in hybridization buffer (Sigma-Aldrich) for 2 h at 56 °C. This solution was refreshed and 1 µg/mL of hydrolysed DIG labelled probe was added and specimens incubated at 56 °C overnight. Thereafter specimens were washed with fresh hybridisation solution, saline sodium citrate buffer and maleic acid buffer with 0.1% Tween-20 (MABT). Specimens were then blocked in 1% Roche blocking solution and 20% horse serum for 2 h at RT and then incubated overnight with anti-DIG AP conjugated antibody at 4 °C overnight. Specimens were then washed in MABT 6 times for 20 min, colour was developed by the addition of NBT/BCIP substrate (Sigma-Aldrich), and PBSTx was used to stop signal development. Specimens were then cleared and mounted prior to examination. The sequences of the probes are as follows; sense - GCTTGCCAATCGGGTGGACAGCAATTCACATGTTGCACGCAATCGTTGAAAATTTACTTCTCCGAGATTGGGTGGGATCGTTGGATTATTCATCCGAAAAAATTCGAACCAAACTACTGCCGAGGATCCTGTCAAGTGAACGGTTTCCAGAGTACACACTACGAAGTGCTCAATCTTTTGTCACACAAAAATCTGACACAGCTGAAAGATGTGCCGCGTGGAACAATACAGTCTTGTTGTTATCCGACACGACGAA; anti-sense - CTGCATCCACATCCGAGAACAATGAGATTATGCAATGTGTGCATTCGCACGTCTTTATTTCGATCCAAATAGAGTAACGTGAACGTGGTTCGTCGTGTCGGATAACAACAAGACTGTATTGTTCCACGCGGCACATCTTTCAGCTGTGTCAGATTTTTGTGTGACAAAAGATTGAGCACTTCGTAGTGTGTACTCTGGAAACCGTTCACTTGACAGGATCCTCGGCAGTAGTTTGGTTCGAATTTTTTCGGATGAATAATCCAACGATCCCACCCAATCTCGGAGAAGTAAATTTTCAACGATTGCGTGCAACATGTGAATTGCTGTCCACCCGATTGGCAAGC.

Statistical analysis

Statistical analysis was conducted using Prism 6.04 (Graphpad Software Inc.) details of the test used is indicated in figure legends along with *p*-values. A *p*-value of < 0.05 was taken to indicate significance.

Results

Identification of TGF-β superfamily members

To identify potential *F. hepatica* TGF-like sequences we screened for mammalian TGF-β-like sequences in the available *F. hepatica* Sanger EST database, however none were detectable. Conversely, TGF-β homologues were widespread in Platyhelminthes and nematode species. A PSI-Blast search using *Bos taurus* TGF-β1-3 identified 61 potential TGF-β homologues in nematodes and 11 in platyhelminths.

Identification of putative TGF-β superfamily members of *F. hepatica* was carried out by tBlastn searching of an unpublished genome database [19] using TGF-β protein sequences from closely related mammalian hosts of *F. hepatica* and the closely related helminth parasite, *S. mansoni*. The tBlastn search returned 4 hits for each of the *B. taurus* and *S. mansoni* queries; the top 3 hits originated from the same scaffolds numbered 40128, 30949 and 35064 (Additional file 1).

Sequence similarity was low between *F. hepatica* TGF-β-like candidates and mammalian TGF-β superfamily members. In contrast, the tBlastn query using SmInAct of *S. mansoni* identified mammalian homologs with high similarity particularly over approximately 100 amino acids of the C-terminal region.

This analysis showed at least 3 potential members of the TGF-β superfamily existed in the *F. hepatica* genome. To further confirm the presence of the hypothetical TGF-β superfamily, the translated peptide sequences retrieved from tBlastn were individually searched for the conserved TGF-β domain. The results showed that the three translated peptides were identified as possibly encoding proteins containing the TGF-β conserved domain. Subsequent Blastp searching against the bovine genome showed that scaffold 35064 (hereafter referred to as *Fasciola hepatica* TGF Like Molecule FhTLM) displayed 32% similarity to bovine inhibinβ chain (NP_001192912), a member of TGF-β subfamily. Furthermore, the deduced protein from scaffold 35064 was 59% similar to SmInAct of *S. mansoni* and inhibin-β B chain of *C. sinensis*. The remaining 2 scaffolds displayed most similarity to the members of BMP subfamily and were subsequently referred to as FhBMP1 FhBMP2.

Phylogenetic analysis

To examine sequence features of the candidate TGF-β superfamily members, we performed a multiple sequence alignment of known TGF-β proteins from both mammalian hosts and helminths. Bovine TGF-β1-3 and BMP4-7 were included as reference sequences for both protein subfamiles. The alignment indicated that all TGF-β superfamily members contain 7 conserved cysteine residues in their C-terminal region. Furthermore, mammalian and helminths TGF-β subfamily members contained an additional 2 cysteine residues. As expected, the putative FhTLM sequence contained 9 cysteine residues while FhBMP1 and FhBMP2 contained 7 cysteine residues. An alignment of protein sequences of the candidate *F. hepatica* TGF-β subfamily member and known TGF-β of other organisms is shown in Figure 1.

The evolutionary relationship between the putative TGF-β *F. hepatica* ligands and other members of TGF-β superfamily from helminths and mammalian hosts was

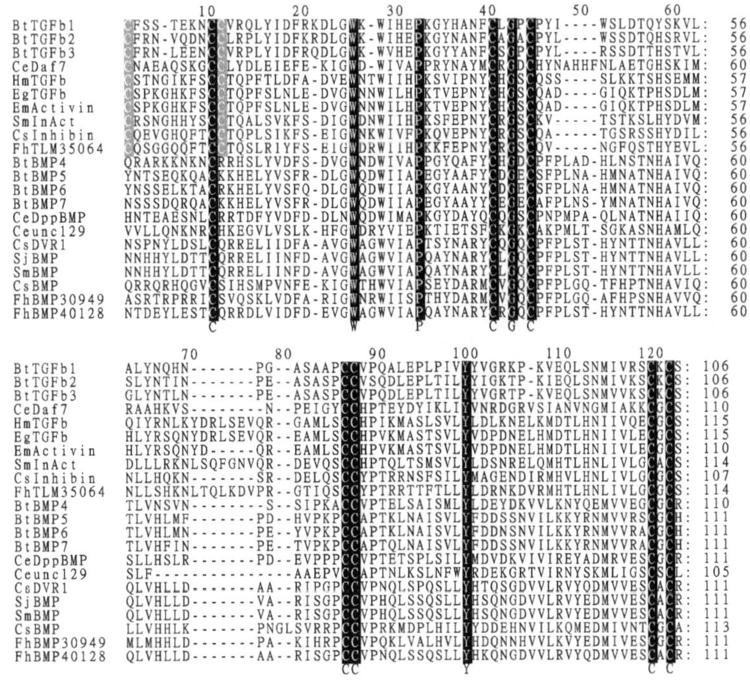

Figure 1 Multiple sequence alignment of the deduced amino acid sequence at C-terminal region of the TGF-β superfamily members from *F. hepatica* and known TGF-β proteins. Conserved residues among TGF-β superfamily are shaded in black background, additional cysteine residues conserved among TGF-β subfamily member are shaded in grey. Accession numbers for sequences used in this analysis are: *Bos taurus* TGF-β1 (BtTGFb1), NP_001159540; *B. taurus* TGF-β2 (BtTGFb2), DAA21445.1; *B. taurus* TGF-β3 (BtTGFb3), DAA25016; *B. taurus* BMP4 (BtBMP4), NP_001039342; *B. taurus* BMP5 (BtBMP5), DAA16713.1; *B. taurus* BMP6 (BtBMP6), DAA16077.1; *B. taurus* BMP7 (BtBMP7), DAA23024.1; *C. elegans* DAF-7 (CeDaf7), NP497265.1; *C. elegans* Dpp BMP (CeDppBMP), AAB04986.2; *C. elegans* unc129 (Ceunc129), NP501566.1; *C. sinensis* inhibin β B chain (CsInhibin), GAA54687.1; *C. sinensis* BMP (CsBMP), GAA53092.1; *C. sinensis* DVR1 (CsDVR1), GAA43145.2; *S. mansoni* InAct (SmInAct), XP_002577586.1; *S. mansoni* BMP (SmBMP), ABL74278.1; *S. japonicum* BMP (SjBMP), ADM48811.1; *H. microstoma* TGF-β family (HmTGFb), CDJ10022.1; *E. multilocularis* activin (EmActivin), CCV01195.1; *E. granulosus* TGF-β (EgTGFb), CDJ22078.1.

investigated by multiple alignment and subsequent phylogenetic tree construction by PhyML software [27] using the WAG model [28]. Phylogenetic analysis of the conserved TGF-β domain was carried out on a total of 87 sequences of helminth and mammal TGF-β proteins. The phylogenetic tree displayed two major subfamilies of TGF-β members; one subfamily included 38 sequences of identified host and helminth TGF-β subfamily members. The second subfamily included 49 sequences from the BMP protein subfamily (Additional file 2).

Platyhelminth TGF-β homologues represented an individual phylogenetic clade. Inside this clade, three subclades of TGF-β homologues were clearly distinguished as belonging to free living flatworms, cestodes and trematodes. The trematode TGF-β subclade contained 2 branches; blood flukes and liver flukes. The FhTLM sequence was located in the liver fluke branch which showed greatest similarity to *C. sinensis* inhibin-β B chain.

Cloning, gene structure, protein structure

The complete sequence of FhTLM was identified by means of rapid amplification of cDNA ends (RACE). Based on the partial sequence obtained from gene exonerate, primers were designed for amplifying the 5' and 3' ends of the FhTLM cDNA. 5' RACE amplification of the *F. hepatica* RACE cDNA produced 3 products ranging from 800 bp-1.9 kb (Figure 2A). A Blastn search of the sequenced 1860 bp PCR product against the *F. hepatica* genome database showed that the sequence of a 1860 bp fragment aligned with the sequence of *F. hepatica* genome scaffold 35064 representing the 5' end of FhTLM containing a 5'UTR and N-terminal region. The 3' portion of FhTLM was amplified using primers specific to the conserved C-terminal domain of TGF-β. An amplicon of approximately 1994 bp (Figure 3A) was found to compromise the 3' end of FhTLM, a 3'UTR and polyA tail. When sequenced this fragment mapped to scaffold 35064 of the *F. hepatica* genome. An overlapping sequence of approximately 420 bp between the 5' and 3' fragments displayed identical sequence. Manual compiling of these two cDNA ends resulted in a 3403 bp full-length sequence. The full length of FhTLM transcript was 3403 bp including a 192 bp 5'UTR, 1665 nt of coding region, and a 1547 nt of 3' UTR including a poly A tail. The putative ORF of FhTLM ranges from the 193 nt to the 1857 nt bases. Recombinant FhTLM (rFhTLM) was generated by cloning the

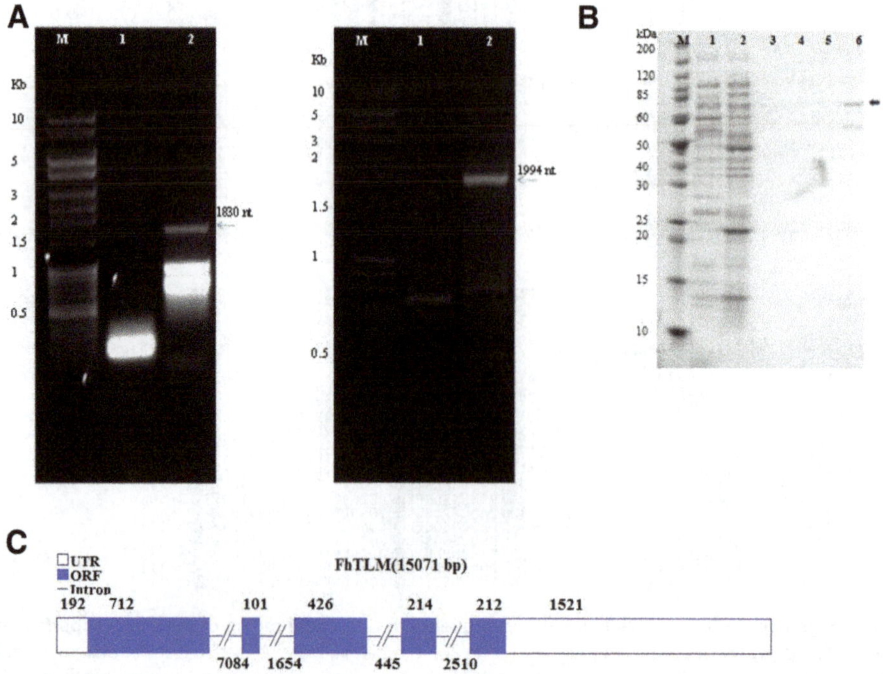

Figure 2 Amplication, cloning and expression of FhTLM. (A) 1.5% Agarose gel electrophoresis of amplified PCR fragments from 5' RACE (left panel) and 3' RACE (right panel). 5'-RACE product of 1830 bp and 3'-RACE product of 1994 bp were obtained from nested PCR, M, 1 Kb DNA ladder. **(B)** Coomassie stained SDS PAGE of protein expression from transformed Rosetta BL21 induced by 1 mM IPTG. Image represents native conditions. M; Protein marker, Lane 1; Supernatant uninduced Rosetta BL21, Lane2; Supernatant induced Rosetta BL21, Lane 3; Elution buffer 20 mM imidazole, Lane 4; Elution buffer 40 mM imidazole, Lane 5; Elution buffer 60 mM imidazole, Lane 6; Elution buffer 80 mM imidazole. **(C)** Organisation of the FhTLM gene depicting regions of the ORF (blue), exons (dashed lines), and UTRs (white) and their size in bases.

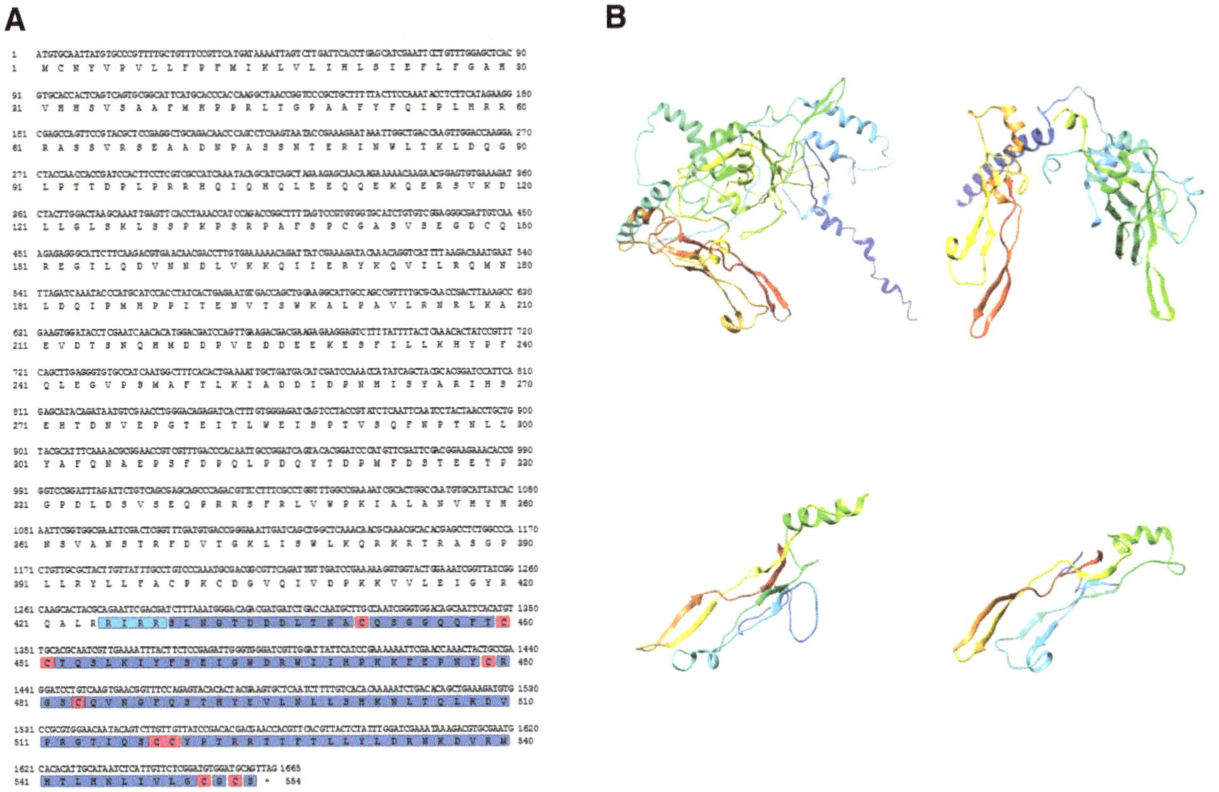

Figure 3 Amino acid sequence and predicted 3D structure of FhTLM. (A) Amino acid sequence showing corresponding nucleotide sequence along the putative cleavage site is shaded in light blue. The active TGF-β domain is shown blue shaded and sequences in pink background indicate the conserved cysteine residues in the active domain. **(B)** 3D structure of predicted FhTLM from Phyre2 by homology search modelling based on template 3rjrD (*Sus scrofa* TGF-β1). Full FhTLM protein; Full 3rjrD protein; FhTLM active domain; active domain of 3rjrD. On the models blue indicates the N-terminus and red indicates the C-terminus. The secondary structure components of FhTLM are composed of 13 α-helices and 16 β-sheets and 3rjrD are composed of 7 α-helices and 19 β-sheets.

ORF sequence in pET28a at a NheI/XhoI site and transforming the vector into Rosetta blue cells. Purified rFhTLM appeared as a 65-70 kDa band on native SDS-PAGE gels (Figure 2B). A local Blastn search of FhTLM sequence against the *F. hepatica* genome allowed us to determine the structure of the gene encoding for FhTLM (Figure 2C).

The ORF encodes a deduced protein of 554 amino acid residues (Figure 3A), containing a conserved 126 amino acid long C-terminal domain. A furin proteolytic cleavage site, RIRR, was present at position 425–428 of the FhTLM molecule. Downstream of the cleavage site the C-terminal region contained 9 conserved cysteine residues characteristic of the TGF subfamily. No signal peptide sequences were detected. Within the active domain FhTLM is 60% identical (at the amino acid level) to *C. sinensis* inhibin-β B chain and 58% identical to SmInAct of *S. mansoni*. While, FhTLM is 35% similar to inhibin-β of human and cow and 32% similar to human and bovine TGF-β1 (Table 1).

Protein models of FhTLM were constructed by searching against the Protein Data Bank (PDB) on Phyre2 [29]. The results showed that predicted FhTLM models of the propeptide and conserved active domain share fold structure with *Sus scrofa* TGF-β1 PDB crystal structure (c3rjrD). The predicted structure consists of 13 α-helices and 16 β-sheets present in the secondary structure of FhTLM (Figure 3B). The final model for FhTLM precursor was built from 65% coverage sequence based on the c3rjrD template corresponding to the sequence at the C-terminal with >90% confidence. The predicted model of active domain sequence was constructed from 87% of the FhTLM sequence (109 amino acids) and demonstrated 2 α-helices and 7 β-sheets. The confidence score of this model was 100% indicating that the model was correct and the FhTLM and TGF-β1 are truly homologous.

Lifestage expression and localisation

Semi-quantitative PCR analysis was used to assess the expression of FhTLM mRNA throughout liver fluke development. Gene specific primers were designed against regions flanking introns in FhTLM mRNA using β-tubulin as a house-keeping gene. The predicted size of PCR products

Table 1 Amino acid Sequence similarities between FhTLM and selected TGF-β homologues

Gene ID	Subject length	Max score	Query cover	E-value	Identity (%)
TGF-β1 [*H. sapiens*]	116	52.8	99	$9e^{-15}$	32
TGF-β1 [*B. taurus*]	116	52.8	99	$9e^{-15}$	32
Inhibin beta B chain [*B. taurus*]	122	75.5	83	$7e^{-23}$	35
Inhibin beta B chain [*H. sapiens*]	122	75.5	83	$7e^{-23}$	35
DAF-7 [*C. elegans*]	120	72.0	87	$2e^{-21}$	32
TGF-β1 family [*H. microstoma*]	132	120	99	$4e^{-40}$	40
TGF-β1 family [*E. granulosus*]	135	130	100	$9e^{-44}$	43
Activin [*E. multilocularis*]	135	130	100	$9e^{-44}$	43
Inhibin beta B chain [*C. sinensis*]	130	179	99	$63e^{-63}$	60
SmInAct [*S. mansoni*]	130	174	99	$42e^{-61}$	58

for FhTLM and β-tubulin are 342 and 192 bp, respectively. FhTLM and β-tubulin transcripts were detected at all parasite stages examined. However, FhTLM and β-tubulin mRNA were expressed at varying levels within different lifestages. Using ImageJ software, values for FhTLM expression were normalized to β-tubulin expression levels. Relative quantification revealed that highest levels of FhTLM were detected in NEJ and unembryonated eggs whereas adult and miracidial stages displayed the lowest levels of expression (Figure 4).

We next conducted in situ hybridization to confirm our PCR results above and establish the location of the mRNA within parasite tissues. In adult specimens we detected the transcript widely spread on the tegument and sub-tegumental region of the adult fluke (Figure 5A). A strong signal was present in the anterior and posterior end (Figure 5A). A faint staining pattern along the lateral part of worm starting from shoulder to tail was also seen. A positive reaction could also be observed as a fine dot pattern spread over the ventral surface of the treated flukes (Figure 5C). In situ hybridization of adult liver fluke showed no signal within the reproductive organs. In NEJs (Figure 5E), the FhTLM transcript was widely dispersed throughout the internal structures with an intense signal around the centre of the body. No signal was present within the pharynx, or the anterior and posterior ends of NEJs. The overall intensity of in situ hybridisation staining within NEJs confirmed the expression analysis above. Sparse staining was seen in metacercariae, eggs, and miracidium.

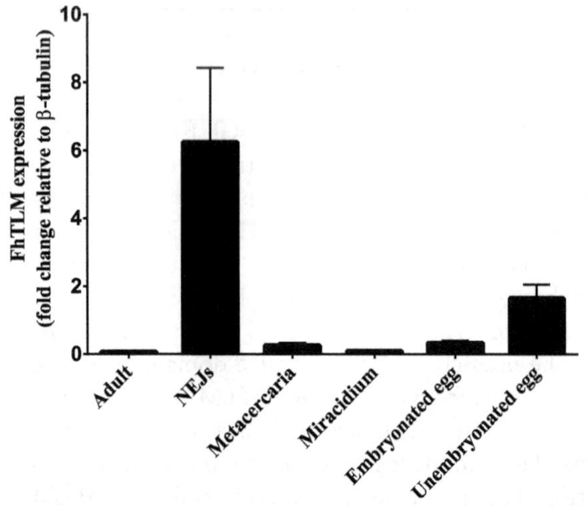

Figure 4 Life stage PCR detection of FhTLM transcript by PCR using cDNA template form the indicated stages of *F. hepatica*. The FhTLM product is 342 bp while β-tubulin is 196 bp. Relative quantification (fold change) of FhTLM mRNA expression compared to the corresponding of the β-tubulin control from the identical developmental stage of *F. hepatica* including adult, NEJ, metaceracaria, miracidium, embryonated egg and unembryonated egg. Values were analyzed from three independent PCRs, with similar results and values shown are representative means ± SD from a single experiment.

Intrinsic effects of FhTLM in *F. hepatica*

The effect of rFhTLM on adult liver flukes was tested by incubating specimens with recombinant protein and conducting observations after 24 h. Measurements of viability (Figure 6A), via MTT assay, and egg production (Table 2) showed no significant differences in the viability of flukes and number of eggs detected between specimens from all treatments. As controls, adult worms were also exposed to mammalian TGF-β with similarly negative results.

Similar experiments with NEJs producing strikingly contrasting results, all NEJs remained viable after 24 h. Their motility was examined by observation and assigned semi-quantitative scores. NEJs treated with rFhTLM were the most active (i.e. exhibited most movement) compared to those observed that were treated with TGF-β, however both of these groups contained parasites with greater motility when compared to PBS treated NEJs (Figure 6B). This data would appear to correlate with our MTT results, as TGF-β treated NEJs displayed enhanced viability compared to PBS treated NEJs but this was still lower than the

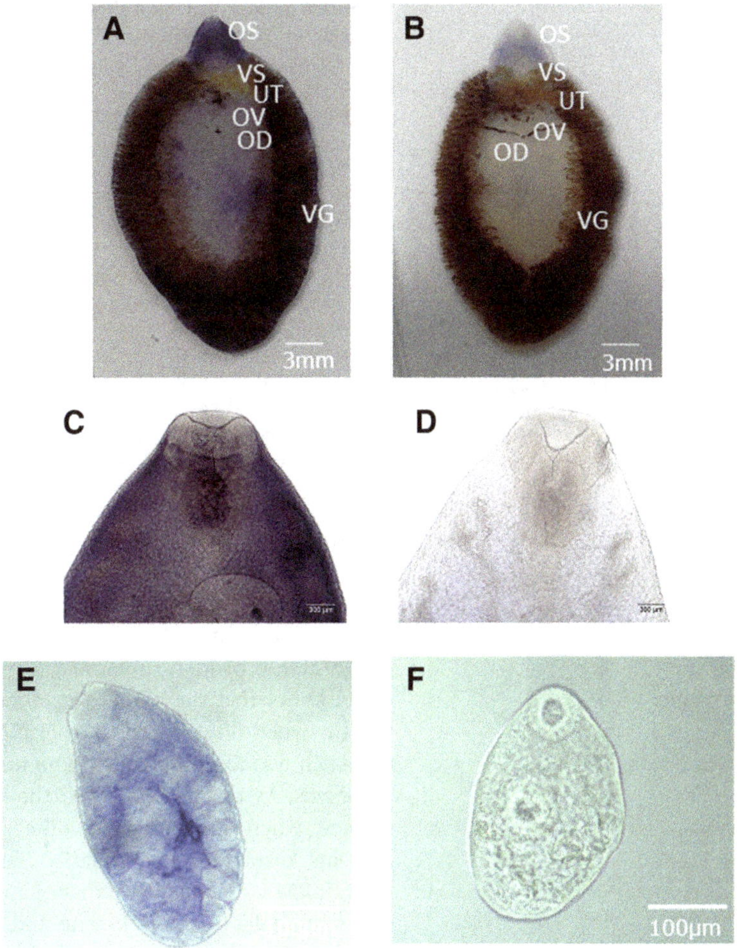

Figure 5 Whole mount in situ hybridization of FhTLM in adult liver fluke. (A) Adult stage treated with antisense FhTLM probe showing a blue precipitate at several parts of the worm cephalic cone including oral sucker (OR), ventral sucker (VS), no staining detected in uterus (UT), oviduct (OV) and vitelline gland (VG). **(B)** Sense control showing unstained worm. Scale bar, **A** & **B**, indicates 3 mm. Localization of FhTLM transcript on the cephalic cone of the adult worms **(C)**. Control worm with no visible signal **(D)**. Scale bar, **C** & **D**, indicates 300 μm. NEJ stained showing extensive straining except in the pharynx, oral and ventral suckers **(E)**. **(F)** control NEJs. Scale bar indicates 100 μm.

group treated with rFhTLM who displayed the greatest levels of viability (Figure 6C).

We next sought to test the effects of rFhTLM on egg development as we had noticed a peak in expression in unembryonated eggs. Unembryonated eggs can be cultured in vitro to develop the egg mass to an embryonated state and hatch after 7–9 days. Batches of eggs were incubated with rFhTLM, TGF-β, or control for 7 days before examination. A significant difference in egg development was observed between treated and non-treated groups. rFhTLM and TGF-β1 showed similar effects in that they increased embryonation of eggs and development of the egg mass (Figure 6C). There was slightly higher percentage of embryonation induced by rFhTLM when compared to TGF-β. In control groups only 25% of egg showed signs of development while eggs treated with 250 ng/mL of TGF-β or rFhTLM had 78.21% and 84.30% of eggs developed, respectively. At a low concentration of both TGF-β and rFhTLM development levels were similar to control group with no statistical differences detected.

Discussion

In this study, we have identified mammalian TGF-β homologues from the *F. hepatica* genome database using a bioinformatics approach. Our analysis suggests that there are three TGF-β superfamily members present in the *F. hepatica* genome. Upon further characterisation we found that two of these correspond to BMP homologues and one is a TGF-β homologue which we termed FhTLM. A full sequence of the cDNA encoding this protein was isolated using RACE. The putative FhTLM contains a prodomain and conserved TGF-β protein domain without a signal peptide. Similar to other TGF-β

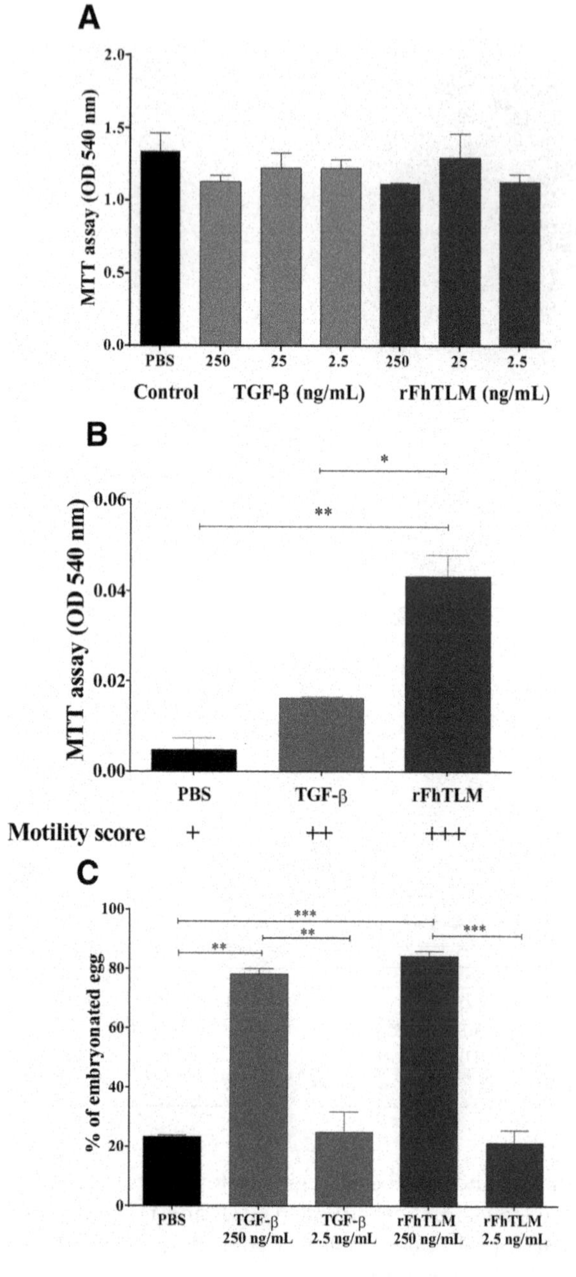

Figure 6 Intrinsic biological effects of FhTLM are lifestage specific. (A) Effect of rFhTLM on the viability of adult liver flukes. Viability was determined by MTT reduction after of 24 hours of incubation. Results are plotted as mean ± SEM of triplicate readings. from one of two independent experiments. **(B)** Effects of rFhTLM on the motility and viability of NEJs. Viability of the NEJs was determined by MTT reduction at 24 h of incubation 250 ng/mL of rFhTLM and TGF-β, or PBS. Results are plotted as the mean OD reading values ± SEM from three replicates from one of two independent experiments. Motility was recorded in the same experiments is indicated underneath using a semi-quantitative scale. **(C)** Biological effect of rFhTLM on egg embryonation. Unembryonated eggs were incubated with rFhTLM and TGF-β at the indicated dose, or dH2O for 7 days and the egg development was examined microscopically. Results are represented as mean ± SEM of % embryonated egg. Data in panel **B** is analysed by 1-way anova and data in panel **C** is analysed using 2-way anova. Significant differences are $*P < 0.05$, $**P < 0.01$ and $***P < 0.001$. All results are representative of one of two independent experiments.

subfamily members, FhTLM contains a highly conserved region in the C-terminal with 9 cysteine residues which are involved in the formation of the disulfide bridges in the cysteine knot within and between chains, a hallmark of the TGF-β protein subfamily.

We found that the cDNA sequence displays a very low identity when Blasted against available datasets, the top hit by Blastn was found to be the *S. mansoni* SmInAct mRNA sequence. At the protein level, the deduced FhTLM sequence when compared to other mammalian TGF-β proteins, displayed low similarity. The similarity between the FhTLM C-terminal and that of a nematode, *C. elegans*, and mammalian TGF-β, bovine and human, are between 32-35%. However, FhTLM exhibits a high degree of conservation to TGF-β homologues from trematodes and cestodes. Sequence analysis revealed over 50% similarity between the conserved domains of TGF-β members of the plathyhelminths. The amino acid sequence of FhTLM shares 60% identity with *C. sinensis* inhibin-β B chain and 58% identity to *S. mansoni* SmInAct.

Phylogenetic analysis of the TGF-β members demonstrated that FhTLM clustered within the platyhelminth group consisting of TGF-β homologues from the subclasses Turbellaria, Cestoda and Trematoda. Our phylogenetic tree was reproducible confirming the described relationship between free living worms and parasitic worms. The parasitic flatworm TGF-βs are clustered in the same group, separate from free living planaria inferring that the TGF-β of the parasitic worms share common function (s) which might be specific and vital to establishing a parasitic life cycle. To date only 5 TGF-β homologous ligands have been reported in parasitic flatworms including *S. mansoni* [15], *C. sinensis* [30], *E. multilocularis* [31], *E. granulosus* and *H. microstoma* [32]. We observed that all parasitic flatworms including *F. hepatica* contain only one TGF-β homologue but vary in the number of BMP homologues whereas free living planaria have 2 TGF-β like proteins [33].

Table 2 Biological effects of rFhTLM on egg production of the adult liver fluke – displayed as average egg no./gram of fluke weight

Treatment (ng/mL)		Average egg no./g
PBS		40332.92
TGF-β	*250*	15626.23
	25	14851.90
	2.5	27917.94
rFhTLM	*250*	14790.10
	25	16414.05
	2.5	10833.33

The major conserved developmental signalling pathways including Wingless related (Wnt), Delta/Notch, Hedgehog (Hh) and TGF-β have been identified in all bilateral animals studied. It is very clear that the components of these signalling pathways are evolutionary conserved amongst animal species in terms of structure and function [2]. TGF-β super family proteins (particularly Nodal/Activin and BMPs) are essential during early embryogenesis and developmental processes. These pathways operate continuously in fully developed animals playing important roles in tissue morphogenesis and homeostasis [3]. Defects in TGF-β signalling pathways can result in remarkable changes in the phenotype of multiple model animals [7,34] and lead to serious clinical diseases in humans [3,5]. Herein we show a conservation of these processes within the *F. hepatica* TGF family member, FhTLM. Our results indicate that rFhTLM can increase the process of embryonation within eggs and increase the viability and motility of NEJs. Interestingly our results demonstrated that there was no effect of rFhTLM on adult worms. This stage restricted mode of action also aligns with the results we obtained when investigating the pattern of FhTLM expression within different lifestages, where NEJs demonstrated the greatest levels of expression and levels within adults were relatively low. The next highest levels of expression after those seen in NEJs were seen in unembryonated eggs which would confirm that the actions of FhTLM seen here in our experiments could arise from endogenous protein. Most likely, in our in vitro experiments using recombinant FhTLM and human TGF-β these proteins were actively scavenged from the environment. Our previous work has shown that eggs interact with their surroundings [35]. Our results are in line with the reported function of SmInAct which is also involved in embryonation of eggs in *S. mansoni* [15]. However contrary to findings in *S. mansoni* we did not find FhTLM to be highly expressed within the reproductive organs of adult worms, this may be due to *F. hepatica* being hermaphrodite in nature or a more species-intrinsic function of SmInAct.

During our initial screening for a TGF-like molecule within *F. hepatica* antigens we demonstrated the ability of native and recombinant FhTLM to bind the mammalian receptor complex and initiate signalling. This is interesting given the reported cross-talk between parasite and host ligands for TGF-like molecules in other parasite species *H. polygyrus* [36] and *B. malayi* [37]. Whether this cross-talk occurs in the case of *F. hepatica* infection remains to be investigated, but could yet yield further control targets.

In conclusion we have identified for the first time members of the *F. hepatica* TGF protein superfamily. Cloning and further characterisation of a TGF-β/activin like member of this family, FhTLM, revealed a distinct expression pattern. The biological effects of a recombinant form of this protein demonstrated activities that were limited to enhanced embryonation and survival of juvenile parasites. Further analysis using RNAi will determine the full phenotype of FhTLM and the function of other TGF superfamily members from *F. hepatica*. FhTLM may yet be a promising diagnostic target for the identification of animals harbouring pre-patent infections due to the high, and specific, levels of expression of FhTLM seen in NEJs. Likewise characterisation of the function of FhTLM would indicate that it is essential to NEJ survival and motility, and thus possibly peritoneal migration making it a target in terms of a vaccine designed to halt NEJ migration and establishment.

Additional files

Additional file 1: BLASTn output from genome wide analysis of *F. hepatica*. tBlastn output window from genome wide analysis using SmInAct as a query sequence, displaying matching to scaffolds 35064, 40128, 30949. These scaffolds contained the putative FhTLM sequence.

Additional file 2: Phylogenetic relationships of mammalian TGF-β and helminth TGF-β homologues. The phylogenetic tree represents the relationship of the representative sequences of mammalian TGF-β family members and TGF-β homologues of helminths. Numbers at nodes are boostrap value based on 1000 bootstrap replicates.

Competing interests
The authors declare that they have no competing interests.

Authors' contributions
RJF, RDE and OJ conceived and designed the experiments and analysed the data; JEH contributed novel reagents and resources; OJ and RJF performed experiments; RJF and OJ wrote the paper. All authors contributed to the final draft of the manuscript. All authors read and approved the final manuscript.

Acknowledgements
We would like to thank Prof Mike Doenhoff and members of the Flynn group for helpful discussions. OJ was funded through a University of Nottingham International Office Scholarship and The University of Phayao Thailand. RDE is supported by the Advanced Data Analysis Centre through the University of Nottingham. Work in the Flynn group is funded through the Technology Strategy Board (BB/L011530/1).

Author details
[1]School of Veterinary Medicine and Science, University of Nottingham, Sutton Bonington, Nottingham LE12 5RD, UK. [2]Advanced Data Analysis

Centre, University of Nottingham, Sutton Bonington, Nottingham LE12 5RD, UK. [3]Department of Infection Biology, Institute of Infection and Global Health, University of Liverpool, Liverpool L3 5RF, UK.

References

1. Huminiecki L, Goldovsky L, Freilich S, Moustakas A, Ouzounis C, Heldin CH (2009) Emergence, development and diversification of the TGF-βsignalling pathway within the animal kingdom. BMC Evol Biol 9:28
2. Richards GS, Degnan BM (2009) The dawn of developmental signaling in the metazoa. Cold Spring Harb Symp Quant Biol 74:81–90
3. Wu MY, Hill CS (2009) TGF-β superfamily signaling in embryonic development and homeostasis. Dev Cell 16:329–343
4. Kusserow A, Pang K, Sturm C, Hrouda M, Lentfer J, Schmidt HA, Technau U, von Haeseler A, Hobmayer B, Martindale MQ, Holstein TW (2005) Unexpected complexity of the Wnt gene family in a sea anemone. Nature 433:156–160
5. ten Dijke P, Arthur HM (2007) Extracellular control of TGF-β signalling in vascular development and disease. Nat Rev Mol Cell Biol 8:857–869
6. Zhang X, Zhang Y (2012) DBL-1, a TGF-β, is essential for *Caenorhabditis elegans* aversive olfactory learning. Proc Natl Acad Sci U S A 109:17081–17086
7. Morita K, Chow KL, Ueno N (1999) Regulation of body length and male tail ray pattern formation of *Caenorhabditis elegans* by a member of TGF-β family. Development 126:1337–1347
8. Gumienny TL, Savage-Dunn C (2013) TGF-β signaling in *C. elegans*. In: The *C. elegans* Research Community (eds) WormBook doi/10.1895/wormbook.1.22.2.
9. Viney ME, Thompson FJ, Crook M (2005) TGF-β and the evolution of nematode parasitism. Int J Parasitol 35:1473–1475
10. Brand AM, Varghese G, Majewski W, Hawdon JM (2005) Identification of a DAF-7 ortholog from the hookworm *Ancylostoma caninum*. Int J Parasitol 35:1489–1498
11. Freitas TC, Arasu P (2005) Cloning and characterisation of genes encoding two transforming growth factor-beta-like ligands from the hookworm, Ancylostoma caninum. Int J Parasitol 35:1477–1487
12. Crook M, Thompson FJ, Grant WN, Viney ME (2005) daf-7 and the development of *Strongyloides ratti* and *Parastrongyloides trichosuri*. Mol Biochem Parasitol 139:213–223
13. Massey HC, Castelletto ML, Bhopale VM, Schad GA, Lok JB (2005) Sst-tgh-1 from Strongyloides stercoralis encodes a proposed ortholog of daf-7 in *Caenorhabditis elegans*. Mol Biochem Parasitol 142:116–120
14. McSorley HJ, Grainger JR, Harcus Y, Murray J, Nisbet AJ, Knox DP, Maizels RM (2010) daf-7-related TGF-β homologues from Trichostrongyloid nematodes show contrasting life-cycle expression patterns. Parasitology 137:159–171
15. Freitas TC, Jung E, Pearce EJ (2007) TGF-β signaling controls embryo development in the parasitic flatworm *Schistosoma mansoni*. PLoS Pathog 3:e52
16. Freitas TC, Pearce EJ (2010) Growth factors and chemotactic factors from parasitic helminths: molecular evidence for roles in host-parasite interactions versus parasite development. Int J Parasitol 40:761–773
17. Liu R, Zhao QP, Ye Q, Xiong T, Tang CL, Dong HF, Jiang MS (2013) Cloning and characterization of a bone morphogenetic protein homologue of *Schistosoma japonicum*. Exp Parasitol 135:64–71
18. Hewitson JP, Grainger JR, Maizels RM (2009) Helminth immunoregulation: the role of parasite secreted proteins in modulating host immunity. Mol Biochem Parasitol 167:1–11
19. Hodgkinson J, Cwiklinski K, Beesley NJ, Paterson S, Williams DJ (2013) Identification of putative markers of triclabendazole resistance by a genome-wide analysis of genetically recombinant *Fasciola hepatica*. Parasitology 140:1523–1533
20. Predication of Genes based on Exonerate. https://github.com/ADAC-UoN/predict.genes.by.exonerate.pipeline. Accessed on 14 March 2013
21. Edgar RC (2004) MUSCLE: multiple sequence alignment with high accuracy and high throughput. Nucleic Acids Res 32:1792–1797
22. Galtier N, Gouy M, Gautier C (1996) SEAVIEW and PHYLO_WIN: two graphic tools for sequence alignment and molecular phylogeny. Comput Appl Biosci 12:543–548
23. Gouy M, Guindon S, Gascuel O (2010) SeaView version 4: A multiplatform graphical user interface for sequence alignment and phylogenetic tree building. Mol Biol Evol 27:221–224
24. Aida Y, Pabst MJ (1990) Removal of endotoxin from protein solutions by phase separation using Triton X-114. J Immunol Methods 132:191–195
25. Wilson LR, Good RT, Panaccio M, Wijffels GL, Sandeman RM, Spithill TW (1998) *Fasciola hepatica*: characterization and cloning of the major cathepsin B protease secreted by newly excysted juvenile liver fluke. Exp Parasitol 88:85–94
26. Pearson BJ, Eisenhoffer GT, Gurley KA, Rink JC, Miller DE, Sanchez Alvarado A (2009) Formaldehyde-based whole-mount *in situ* hybridization method for planarians. Dev Dyn 238:443–450
27. Guindon S, Dufayard JF, Lefort V, Anisimova M, Hordijk W, Gascuel O (2010) New algorithms and methods to estimate maximum-likelihood phylogenies: assessing the performance of PhyML 3.0. Syst Biol 59:307–321
28. Whelan S, Goldman N (2001) A general empirical model of protein evolution derived from multiple protein families using a maximum-likelihood approach. Mol Biol Evol 18:691–699
29. Kelley LA, Sternberg MJ (2009) Protein structure prediction on the Web: a case study using the Phyre server. Nat Protoc 4:363–371
30. Wang X, Chen W, Huang Y, Sun J, Men J, Liu H, Luo F, Guo L, Lv X, Deng C, Zhou C, Fan Y, Li X, Huang L, Hu Y, Liang C, Hu X, Xu J, Yu X (2011) The draft genome of the carcinogenic human liver fluke *Clonorchis sinensis*. Genome Biol 12:R107
31. Brehm K (2010) *Echinococcus multilocularis* as an experimental model in stem cell research and molecular host-parasite interaction. Parasitology 137:537–555
32. Tsai IJ, Zarowiecki M, Holroyd N, Garciarrubio A, Sanchez-Flores A, Brooks KL, Tracey A, Bobes RJ, Fragoso G, Sciutto E, Aslett M, Beasley H, Bennett HM, Cai J, Camicia F, Clark R, Cucher M, De Silva N, Day TA, Deplazes P, Estrada K, Fernandez C, Holland PW, Hou J, Hu S, Huckvale T, Hung SS, Kamenetzky L, Keane JA, Kiss F, et al. (2013) The genomes of four tapeworm species reveal adaptations to parasitism. Nature 496:57–63
33. Gavino MA, Wenemoser D, Wang IE, Reddien PW (2013) Tissue absence initiates regeneration through Follistatin-mediated inhibition of Activin signaling. Elife 2:e00247
34. Lehmann P, Rank P, Hallfeldt KL, Krebs B, Gartner R (2006) Dose-related influence of sodium selenite on apoptosis in human thyroid follicles in vitro induced by iodine, EGF, TGF-β, and H_2O_2. Biol Trace Elem Res 112:119–130
35. Moxon JV, Flynn RJ, Golden O, Hamilton JV, Mulcahy G, Brophy PM (2010) Immune responses directed at egg proteins during experimental infection with the liver fluke *Fasciola hepatica*. Parasite Immunol 32:111–124
36. Grainger JR, Smith KA, Hewitson JP, McSorley HJ, Harcus Y, Filbey KJ, Finney CA, Greenwood EJ, Knox DP, Wilson MS, Belkaid Y, Rudensky AY, Maizels RM (2010) Helminth secretions induce *de novo* T cell Foxp3 expression and regulatory function through the TGF-β pathway. J Exp Med 207:2331–2341
37. Gomez-Escobar N, Gregory WF, Maizels RM (2000) Identification of tgh-2, a filarial nematode homolog of *Caenorhabditis elegans* daf-7 and human transforming growth factor beta, expressed in microfilarial and adult stages of *Brugia malayi*. Infect Immun 68:6402–6410

6

Immunoproteomic identification of immunodominant antigens independent of the time of infection in *Brucella abortus* 2308-challenged cattle

Jin Ju Lee[1], Hannah Leah Simborio[2], Alisha Wehdnesday Bernardo Reyes[2], Dae Geun Kim[2], Huynh Tan Hop[2], Wongi Min[2], Moon Her[1], Suk Chan Jung[1], Han Sang Yoo[3] and Suk Kim[2,4*]

Abstract

Brucellosis is a vital zoonotic disease caused by *Brucella*, which infects a wide range of animals and humans. Accurate diagnosis and reliable vaccination can control brucellosis in domestic animals. This study examined novel immunogenic proteins that can be used to detect *Brucella abortus* infection or as an effective subcellular vaccine. In an immunoproteomic assay, 55 immunodominant proteins from *B. abortus* 544 were observed using two dimensional electrophoresis (2DE) and immunoblot profiles with antisera from *B. abortus*-infected cattle at the early (week 3), middle (week 7), and late (week 10) periods, after excluding protein spots reacting with antisera from *Yersinia enterocolitica* O:9-infected and non-infected cattle. Twenty-three selected immunodominant proteins whose spots were observed at all three infection periods were identified using MALDI-MS/MS. Most of these proteins identified by immunoblot and mass spectrometry were determined by their subcellular localization and predicted function. We suggest that the detection of prominent immunogenic proteins during the infection period can support the development of advanced diagnostic methods with high specificity and accuracy; subsidiarily, these proteins can provide supporting data to aid in developing novel vaccine candidates.

Introduction

Brucella spp. are the etiological agents for brucellosis, a debilitating and chronic disease infecting a variety of domestic animals and humans. Brucellosis is characterized by abortion and sterility in livestock as well as undulant fever, arthritis and neurological disorders in humans [1]. Definitive diagnosis is commonly performed by isolation and identification of the causative organism(s), but because the isolation is time-consuming and dangerous, serological analysis is widely preferred [2]. Several specific serological tests have been developed for the definitive diagnosis of brucellosis, and these tests have been upgraded repeatedly to obtain reliable data [3]. However, a large number of tests still rely on presumptive evidence of infection. Most serological tests for *Brucella* infection use antibodies against common antigens of *Brucella* [4]. O-polysaccharide (OPS), a well-known immunodominant epitope in smooth lipopolysaccharide (SLPS) is a commonly used antigen in serological tests for the diagnosis of brucellosis [5,6]. Consequently, the serological diagnosis of brucellosis is complicated by cross-reactions of the antibodies against other Gram-negative bacteria, such as *Y. enterocolitica* O:9, which have conserved and highly analogous OPS structures [7,8]. Therefore, it is crucial to discover highly specific *Brucella* antigens that are immunogenic in the host. Several studies have focused on the use of antigenic proteins for alternative diagnostic methods and to improve vaccine efficacy. Recent studies have focused on the use of immunogenic proteins for serodiagnosis of brucellosis [9].

Several immunogenic proteins of *B. abortus* have been identified [10], but the antigens that are immunogenic at different stages of the infection have not been defined.

* Correspondence: kimsuk@gnu.ac.kr
[2]Institute of Animal Medicine, College of Veterinary Medicine, Gyeongsang National University, Jinju, 660-701, Republic of Korea
[4]Institute of Agriculture and Life Science, Gyeongsang National University, Jinju, 660-701, Republic of Korea
Full list of author information is available at the end of the article

Because *Brucella* causes latent infection, knowledge concerning the different stages of infection is important for the diagnosis and control of the disease. In this study, we obtained antisera against *B. abortus* from experimentally infected cattle at different stages of infection and studied unique immunogenic proteins to validate the immunogenic relationships and potential immunodominant markers at different stages of infection.

Materials and methods

Bacterial strains and culture conditions

The standard reference strains *B. abortus* 2308 and *B. abortus* 544, which are known as virulent biovar 1 strain, and *Y. enterocoitica* O:9 used in the present study were obtained from the Laboratory of Bacteriology Division in the Animal and Plant Quarantine Agency, Korea. The bacteria were cultured at 37 °C with aeration until the cells entered stationary phase. Subsequently, the number of viable bacteria was evaluated by plating 10-fold serial dilutions (made using PBS) on Brucella agar plates.

Preparation of antisera

Twenty-five apparently healthy Korean native heifers (Hanwoo) aged 18–20 months were used in this study. All animals were seronegative for brucellosis before immune challenge, as assessed by the standard tube agglutination test (STAT) and Rose Bengal test (RBT), which are internationally accepted serological tests for bovine brucellosis described by the OIE [5]. The cattle were divided into 3 groups: *B. abortus*-infected ($n = 10$), *Y. enterocoitica* O:9-infected ($n = 10$) and uninfected controls ($n = 5$). Bacterial inoculation was performed as described in previous methods [11]. Briefly, the first group was inoculated with 4×10^7 CFU of *B. abortus* 2308/head injecting a total of 100 μL (50 μL of inoculum per eye) via the intraconjunctival route. The second group was inoculated with 5×10^6 CFU of *Y. enterocoitica* O:9/head 3 times by 1 day interval via subcutaneous injection. The 5 cattle in the uninfected control group were inoculated with sterile PBS. After immune challenge, antisera against *B. abortus* were collected at three stages of infection; early (week 3), middle (week 7), and late (week 10). These time points in three stages of infection were determined based on low serological variations among individuals and high titer values. Samples were collected from all cattle in all groups. Using serological tests, 3 samples of each *B. abortus*-infected antisera (RBT-positive and STAT titers of > 1:400 at 3, 7, and 10 weeks post-challenge), *Y. enterocoitica*-infected antisera (RBT-negative and STAT titers of 1:200 against *Brucella* antigen at 3, 7 and 10 weeks post challenge), and non-infected sera were selected and used for immune analysis. The experimental procedures were approved by the ethical committee as NVRQS-AEC-2008-12, and the infected animals were euthanized according to the protocol of the Institution for Animal Care & Use Committee in Korea.

Preparations of antigens

Antigens were prepared as a protein mixture of whole cells including cell envelopes for proteomic analysis using a modification of a previously described procedure [10]. Briefly, *B. abortus* 544 cultures were centrifuged at $8000 \times g$ for 20 min at 4 °C and washed 3 times with ice-cold PBS (pH 7.6) by centrifugation. The bacterial pellet was resuspended in 50 mM Tris–HCl (pH 7.6) containing a complete protease inhibitor cocktail (PIC) and then sonicated on ice using a Sonifier 750 (Branson Ultrasonics, USA). The sonicated solution was centrifuged at $12\,000 \times g$ for 1 h at 4 °C, and the pellet was resuspended in lysis buffer (5 M urea, 2 M thiourea, 2% CHAPS, 1% SB 3–10, 1% DTT, and containing PIC) followed by incubation at 22 °C for 1 h with vigorous agitation. After centrifugation at $100\,000 \times g$ for 30 min, the supernatant was collected. The protein concentration was quantified using the Bradford assay [12].

Isoelectric focusing (IEF) and 2D SDS-PAGE

IEF and 2DE were conducted using a previously described method [13] with modifications. Eighteen-centimeter IPG strips (pH 3–10 and 4–7, GE Healthcare, USA) were rehydrated for 14 h at 22 °C with the lysed proteins and rehydration buffer (7 M urea, 2 M thiourea, 2% CHAPS, 0.2% DTT, 0.5% IPG buffer (pH 4–7), and 0.002% bromophenol blue). IEF was performed on a Protean IEF gel (GE Healthcare) at 20 °C for 14 h using the following conditions: 500 V for 1 h, gradient phase of 1000 V for 1 h, 1000 V for 3 h, gradient phase of 10 000 V for 3 h, 10 000 V for 5 h, 50 V for 30 min and a final phase of 50 V for 30 min. After IEF, each strip was equilibrated in 5 mL of equilibration buffer I (6 M urea, 50 mM Tris–HCl pH 8.8, 1% DTT, 30% glycerol, 2% SDS, and 0.002% bromophenol blue) for 15 min at 22 °C and then in equilibration buffer II (6 M urea, 50 mM Tris–HCl pH 8.8, 2.5% iodoacetamide, 30% glycerol, 2% SDS, and 0.002% bromophenol blue) under the same conditions. The equilibrated strips were loaded on the top of 12% SDS-polyacrylamide gels and sealed with melted 1% agarose solution. The proteins were two-dimensionally separated in resolving buffer (25 mM Tris pH 8.8, 192 mM glycine, 0.1% SDS) using Criterion electrophoresis equipment (Bio-Rad) equipped with a cooling device (Lauda E100, Germany), kept at 25 °C and supplied with regular power in two steps: 5 W/gel for 30 min and 20 W/gel until the protein dye reached the bottom of the gel (approximately 5 h). The separated proteins were transferred to PVDF membranes (Millipore, USA) for immunoblotting analysis; simultaneously, replicate gels containing the same protein samples were silver-stained to visualize the proteins. Three replicates of 2DE were performed in independent experiments.

Immunoblotting with antisera

The proteins were completely transferred to membranes using the TE70/77 PWR Semi-Dry Transfer Unit (GE Healthcare) according to the manufacturer's instructions. The membranes were blocked for 1 h at room temperature using 5% rabbit serum in Tris-buffered saline containing 0.1% Tween-20 (TBS-T) and then washed three times for 20 min in TBS-T. The blots were incubated overnight at 4 °C with a 1:500 dilution of the antisera derived from the immune-challenged and control cattle. The blots were then incubated for 1 h at room temperature with a 1:5000 dilution of goat anti-bovine IgG HRP-conjugated antibody (Sigma, USA). After washing, the immunolabeling was detected using ECL Western blotting reagents (GE Healthcare). Finally, specific immunogenic proteins were visualized using a ChemiDoc XRS Camera and the Quantity One 1D analysis software (Bio-Rad).

Gel image analysis and in-gel trypsin digestion

The silver-stained 2D gels were scanned using an ImageScanner™ (GE Healthcare) and cropped using ImageQuant TL (GE Healthcare). Automatic gel-image alignment and spot detection along with spot matching were performed using Progenesis SameSpots v 2.0 (Nonlinear Dynamics) to allow for more accurate spot identification [14]. Each gel was run in triplicate in parallel with three independent sample preparations. The spot matching across all gels without omitting values was set as a requirement for spot merging for data analysis. An average gel with best resolution was generated using the three independent replicates by including only those protein spots that were present in at least two of the replicates. The common spots, in keeping with shape and intensity over all replicates, were selected for normalization of spot volumes to equalize the probable variation in staining trait. The gel containing all spots on final average gel was used and transferred to the PVDF membrane which subsequently was subjected to react with antisera from cattle. In addition, image alignment and spot matching analyses were performed on the gel spots and the immunogenic protein spots detected by immunoblotting. The selected spots were manually excised from the gels, and the gel plugs containing the proteins were enzymatically digested with porcine trypsin (modified sequencing grade; Promega, USA) as described previously [13]. The spots were incubated with 50 mM ammonium bicarbonate (NH_4CO_3, pH 7.8)/50% acetonitrile (ACN) for 1 h at 22 °C to destain them and were washed and then dehydrated in ACN. The dehydrated spots were vacuum-dried to remove the solvent and then rehydrated overnight at 37 °C by digestion with trypsin (10 ng/μL) in 50 mM NH_4CO_3 (pH 7.8). The tryptic peptides were extracted with 0.1% trifluoroacetic acid (TFA)/50% can, and the combined extracts were vacuum-dried by centrifugation and resuspended in 0.5% TFA. The peptide mixture was desalted using ZipTip plates (Millipore) and then eluted with 0.2% TFA/50% ACN. Finally, the resulting solution was mixed with the matrix (10 mg/mL α-cyano-4-hydroxycinnamic acid in 50% ACN/1% TFA).

Protein identification by MALDI-TOF MS /MS analysis

All spectra were collected using an ABI 4700 proteomics analyzer Plus TOF-TOF Mass Spectrometer (Applied Biosystems, USA). MS/MS data were obtained using this instrument with a Nd:YAG laser with a 200 Hz repetition rate, and accumulation of up to 4000 shots were performed for each spectrum from which the three highest intense peaks were processed to an enhanced resolution. When the three intense peaks were subjected to downstream analysis, these were ignored for a period of 60 s. MS/MS mode was operated with 2 keV collision energy supplying air as the collision gas, which resulted in completion of nominally single collision conditions. MS/MS data were obtained using the default instrument calibration without internal or external calibration. The quality control parameters included based on the Mascot algorithm were the following: maximum of one missed cleavage permitted by trypsin, fixed modification (including residue specificity) of carbamidomethyl, variable modifications (including residue specificity) of oxidation, charge state of 12 to 14, mass tolerance for peptide ion (m/z) of 0.1 to 0.2 Da, cut-off score/expectation value for accepting individual MS spectra of highest expectation (probability on profound search, PPS). All protein identifications were made by only single protein spot and were collected using a score with the minimal number of high quality peptides per protein is 22. Peptide mass data were used to query the NCBI protein sequence and annotated genome databases of *Brucella* using the Mascot search engine (Matrix Science, London, UK) [15]. Based on the sequences identified using mass spectrometry, biological information on the chosen proteins was retrieved using the EXPASY database [16]. The sub-cellular localizations of bacterial proteins were predicted using PSORTb v. 2.0.4 [17]. Functional annotations were made based on the cluster of orthologous groups (COG) protein database generated by comparing all of the complete sequences of microbial genomes from the NCBI COG [18].

Results

2DE profiles of whole-cell antigens from *B. abortus* 544

The annotated 2DE proteome map of whole-cell proteins from *B. abortus* 544 is shown in Figure 1A. A total of 1181 protein spots were detected on the silver-stained

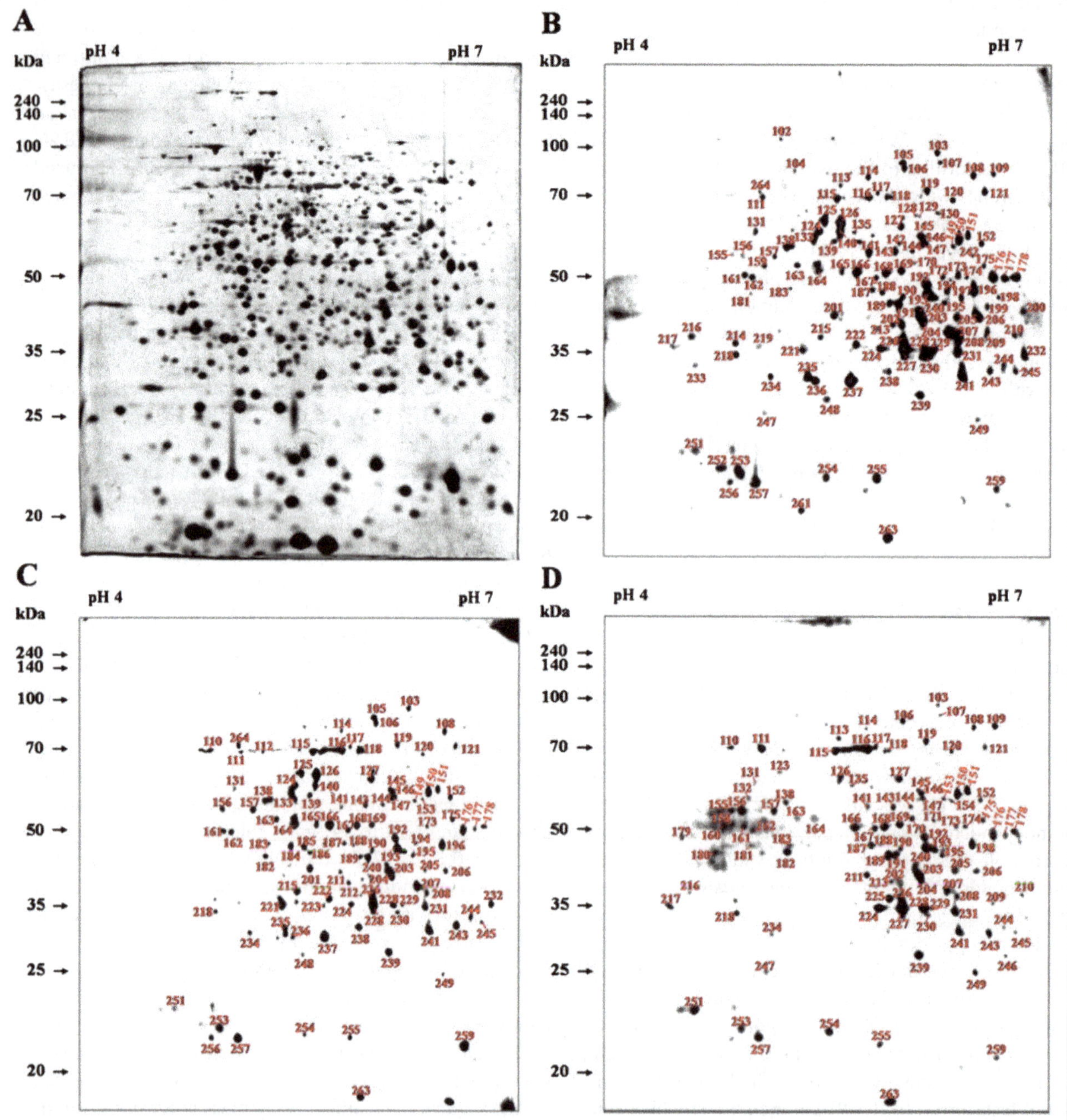

Figure 1 2DE profile of *B. abortus* proteins and immunoblotting with antisera from *B. abortus*-infected cattle. (A) 2DE profile of proteins from *B. abortus* detected on silver-stained 2DE gels within the p*I* range 4–7. Immunoblotting analyses were performed with antisera from cattle after 3 **(B)**, 7 **(C)**, and 10 weeks **(D)** of challenge with *B. abortus*. Three replicates of 2DE analysis were performed in the independent experiments.

2DE gels within the p*I* and molecular weight (M_r) ranges of 4–7 and 20–240 kDa, respectively. The 2DE map profiles of the best resolution were obtained from most of the detected spots in the 2DE gels of the three replicates from separate experiments. These replicates were selected based on equal 2D patterns and spot numbers reactive to individual serum from three different infection periods. The mean p*I* and M_r of all protein spots detected were 5.62 and 40.52 kDa, respectively. Using the broad pH range from 3–10, the protein spots with p$I < 4$ or p$I > 8$ were detected at relatively low resolution with few protein spots.

Immunogenic proteins in *B. abortus* at different infection periods and comparison with cross-reacting bacteria

By immunoblotting the diverse *B. abortus* proteins detected on 2DE gels, 134, 110, and 106 proteins were recognized using positive antisera from *B. abortus*-infected cattle at 3, 7, and 10 weeks of infection, respectively (Figures 1B-D). The negative sera from the non-infected cattle and the positive antisera from the cattle infected with *Y. enterocolitica* O:9 were also used for immunoblotting to exclude non-specific or cross reactions. Few reactions (25 protein spots) were observed using the negative control (NC) and *Y. enterocolitica* O:9-positive (YP) antisera (Table 1 and Figure 2). The spots reacting to the *B. abortus*-positive (BP) antisera that overlapped with those reacting to the NC (13 spots) and YP (13 spots) antisera were excluded (Figure 3). Among the immunogenic proteins that were not from non-specific and cross-reacting spots, 120 immunodominant proteins (Table 1) were observed using the antisera collected during at least one of the three infection periods, whereas 101, 84, and 78 proteins were specifically observed using BP antisera collected at weeks 3, 7, and 10, respectively (Table 2 and Figure 4). Fifty-five common antigens were predominantly specific to the BP antisera at all three stages of infection (Figure 5A). The percent similarity, calculated as the number of proteins that reacted to the antisera, was 45.83%, suggesting that highly immunogenic proteins were present in the bovine serum within 10 weeks of infection (Table 1). In addition, 19, 10, and 4 common immunoreactive spots were observed at 3 and 7 (Figure 5B), 3 and 10 (Figure 5C), and 7 and 10 weeks (Figure 5D), respectively. Furthermore, 17, 6, and 9 non-matched immunoreactive protein spots were observed, and the percent independence of these immunoreactions were 16.84%, 7.14%, and 11.54% at 3, 7, and 10 weeks, respectively (Table 2).

Identification of immunogenic proteins at different infection stages

Amongst the 55 immunogenic proteins detected at all three stages of infection, the signal intensities of 23 immunogens were higher than the average when normalized to the total valid spot intensity; these 23 proteins were analyzed using MALDI- MS/MS. The data revealed that several novel immunogenic proteins with diverse ORF had varying values for M_r and p*I* in MALDI-MS/MS (Table 3). NCBI BLAST searches of the proteins identified using MALDI-MS/MS show that 10 (43.5%), 2 (8.7%) and 2 (8.7%) proteins were predicted to have cytoplasmic, outer membrane-bound periplasmic and ribosomal localization, respectively. However, 9 spots (39.1%) were unknown proteins. Analysis of each identified protein indicates that 13 of the 23 proteins participate in multiple enzymatic activities. Notably, three hypothetical proteins (spots 187, 218 and 257) encoded by different ORF had putative molecular functions such as catalytic and protein disulfide oxidoreductase activities. The experimental p*I* and M_r values from MALDI-MS/MS identification were consistent with the theoretical values for most identified proteins, with the exception of spot 146, which was identified as an ABC transporter substrate-binding protein; the experimental and theoretical M_r values for this spot had the highest deviations (6.4).

Multiple proteins that were immunoreactive at all stages of infection had varying p*I*, M_r and functions. The identified proteins were sorted into functional groups based on the classification of proteins encoded in complete genomes established by COG: 14 were related to transport and metabolism [4 for amino acids (spots 146, 178, 204, and 207), 3 to carbohydrates (spots 118, 164, and 231), 2 to inorganic ions (spots 239 and 240), 2 to nucleotides (spots 151 and 254), 2 to coenzymes (spots 161 and 169), and 1 to secondary metabolites (spot 218)]; 3 were involved in ribosomal structure and biogenesis related to protein translation (spots 162, 203, and 231), and 2 were associated with cellular processes and signaling, including post-translational modification, protein turnover, and chaperones (spots 228 and 253).

Table 1 Comparison of immunoreactive proteins of *B. abortus* after immune challenge in cattle

Antisera immunoreactions compared					No. of matched protein spots	Total no. of protein spots	Similarity (%)[a]
BP			NC	YP			
Week 3	Week 7	Week 10					
+[b]	+	+	+	+	8	162	4.94
+	+	+	+	-	5	137	3.65
+	+	+	-	+	5	137	3.65
+	+	+	-	-	55	120	45.83
+	+	-	-	-	19	42	45.24
+	-	+	-	-	10	36	27.78
-[c]	+	+	-	-	4	19	21.05

NC - negative control, YP - *Y. enterocolitica*-positive sera, BP - *B. abortus*-positive sera.
[a]The percent similarity was calculated as the number of proteins common to the compared antisera immunoreactions divided by the total number of proteins in these antisera immunoreactions × 100.
[b]Positive reaction detected in immunoblotting.
[c]Negative reaction detected in immunoblotting.

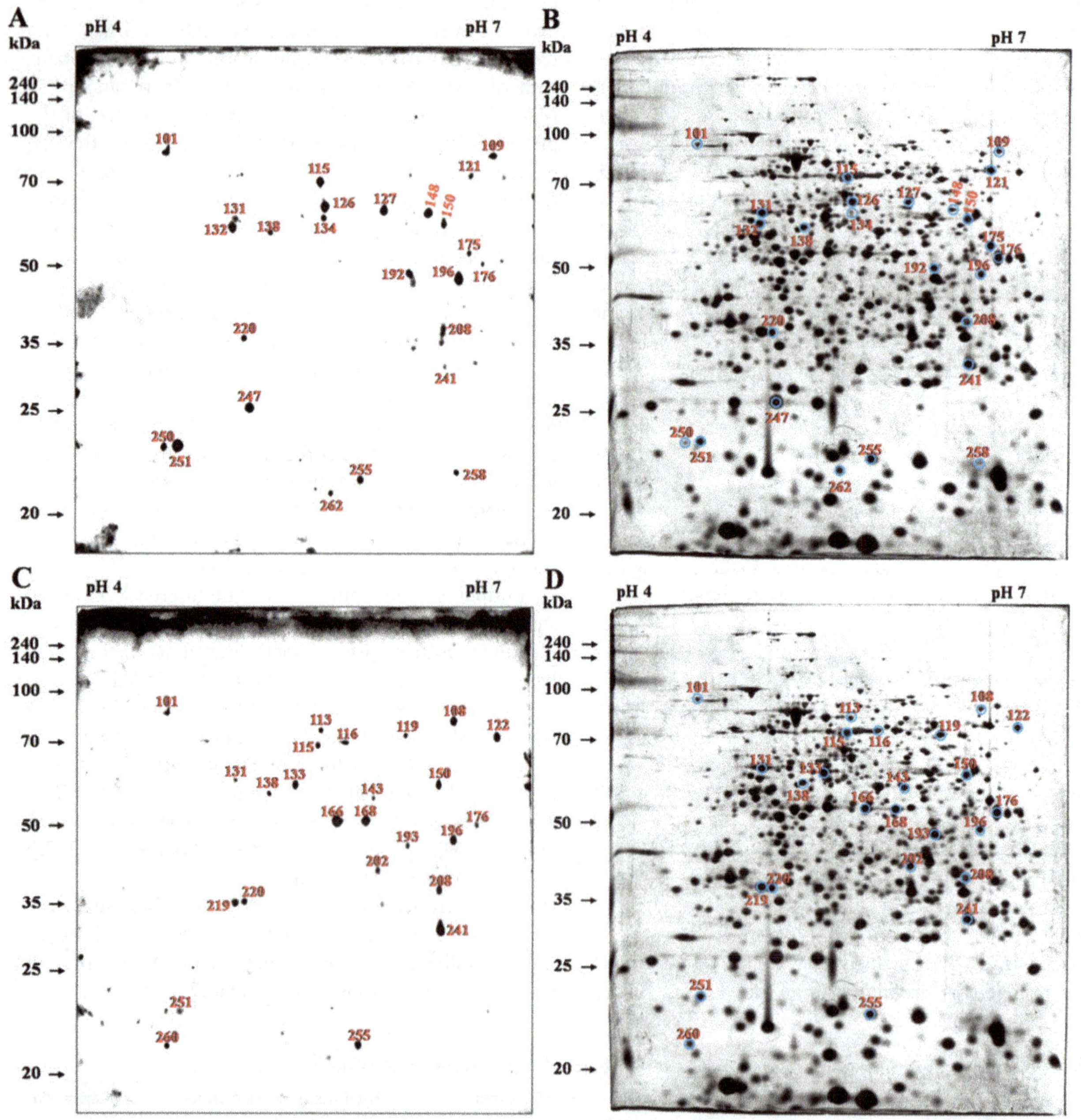

Figure 2 2DE analysis and the immunoblotting profile detected using sera from non-infected and *Y. enterocolitica*-infected cattle. A total of 25 immunoreactive dots were observed using the non-infected **(A)** and *Y. enterocolitica*-challenged **(C)** bovine sera, and the corresponding proteins are labeled on the 2DE gel [NC **(B)** and YP **(D)**]. The numbers represent the serial numbers of the immunoreactive proteins in immunoblotting analyses.

Discussion

Brucellosis is a re-emerging zoonosis that has regained scientific attention because its pathogenesis in human and animal disease has significantly evolved [1,19]. However, the overall burden of this disease remains underestimated and is not well studied. The disease ecology has evolved rapidly in recent years, and there are novel populations with high risk of exposure and the potential to develop chronic or latent infection [20]. Eradication of brucellosis in animals is important for prevention of this disease in human beings and requires optimal diagnosis and vaccination [3]. There are relatively efficient diagnostic tests for brucellosis, and vaccines have been consistently developed; however, there are still several limitations [21,22]. Furthermore, cross-reacting bacteria decrease the specificity of the tests, and this has impeded the control of brucellosis [7]. To address these problems, it is important to develop new strategies for

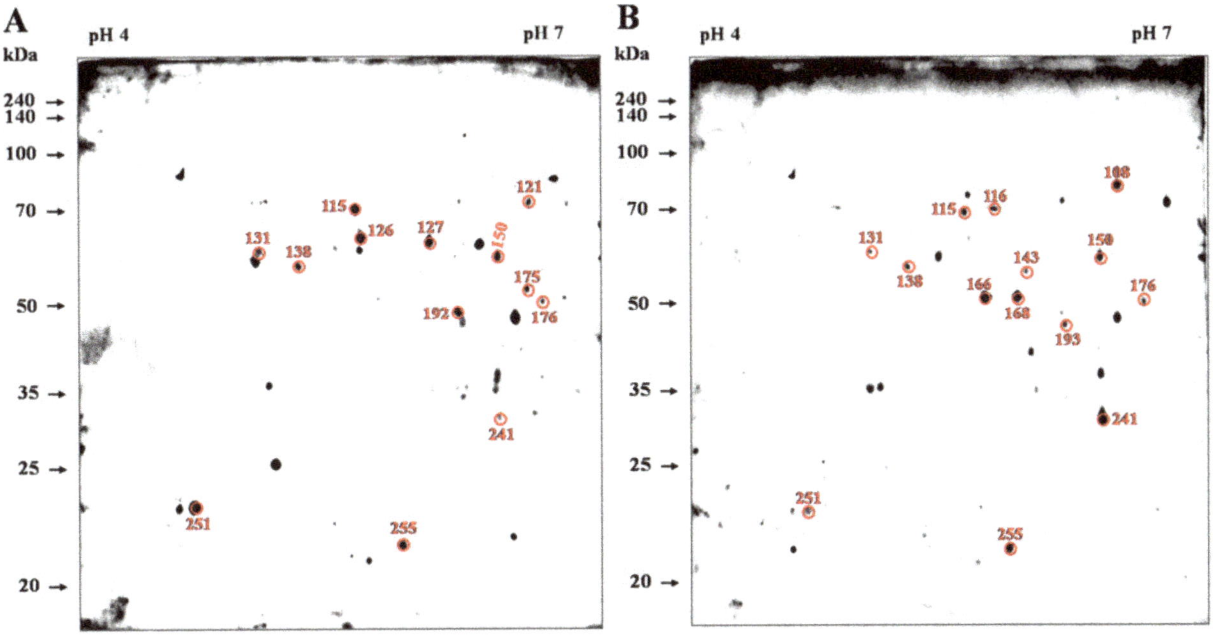

Figure 3 Comparative 2DE analysis of *B. abortus* proteins and immunoblotting profile of non-specific reactions. A total of 13 immunoreactive spots of common antigens that responded to the negative sera from non-infected cattle **(A)** and positive sera of *Y. enterocolitica* **(B)**, and three types of sera from cattle after 3, 7 and 10 weeks of challenge with *B. abortus* were selected. The numbers represent the serial numbers of the immunoreactive proteins in immunoblot analyses.

effective diagnosis with improved specificity. This study focused on identifying immunogenic proteins of *Brucella* from three different stages of infection (short-, middle-, and long-term) for the improvement of immunodiagnostics. Although distinct sets of *Brucella* antigens were only a limited set of proteins present at all three time points, these novel immunodominant proteins identified in our study might be suitable for the detection of *B. abortus* infection.

The 2DE gels containing *B. abortus* whole cell proteins were subjected to immunoblotting analysis using bovine antisera; the antisera were collected at three different phases of infection: the early (week 3), middle (week 7), and late (week 10) periods after challenge with *B. abortus*. An important diagnostic problem is the similarity of the O-antigenic side chains of *Brucella* and other Gram-negative bacteria such as *Y. enterocolitica* O:9 [7]. In this study, 25 protein spots reactive to *Y. enterocolitica* O:9-positive (YP) antisera and negative control (NC) sera in cattle were detected. By immunoblotting-linked gel image analysis of *B. abortus* proteins, the overlapping spots that were reactive to the YP and NC sera were excluded, and the spots that were reactive to the *B. abortus*-positive (BP) antisera at all stages of infection were selected; this analysis identified 120 distinct spots. The total number of spots reactive to the BP antisera at 3, 7, and 10 weeks post-challenge was comparable to the number of common spots (55) observed at all stages of infection. Furthermore, the common spots were 45.83% similar to those observed by immunoblotting using antisera from all three stages of infection; this suggests that the common immunoreactive spots might represent the proteins that are immunodominant at all stages of infection. The infection time-independent immunodominant proteins of *B. abortus* comprise proteins expressed from diverse genes encoding transport, metabolic functions and other

Table 2 Comparison of immunoreactive proteins of *B. abortus* that reacted independently with BP

	Antisera (BP) immunoreactions compared	No. of non-matched protein spots	Total no. of protein spots	Independence (%)[a]
Periods of challenge	week 3	17	101	16.84
	week 7	6	84	7.14
	week 10	9	78	11.54

BP - *B. abortus*-positive sera.
[a]The percent independence was calculated as the number of non-matched proteins to the antisera immunoreactions compared with others divided by the total number of proteins in these antisera immunoreactions × 100.

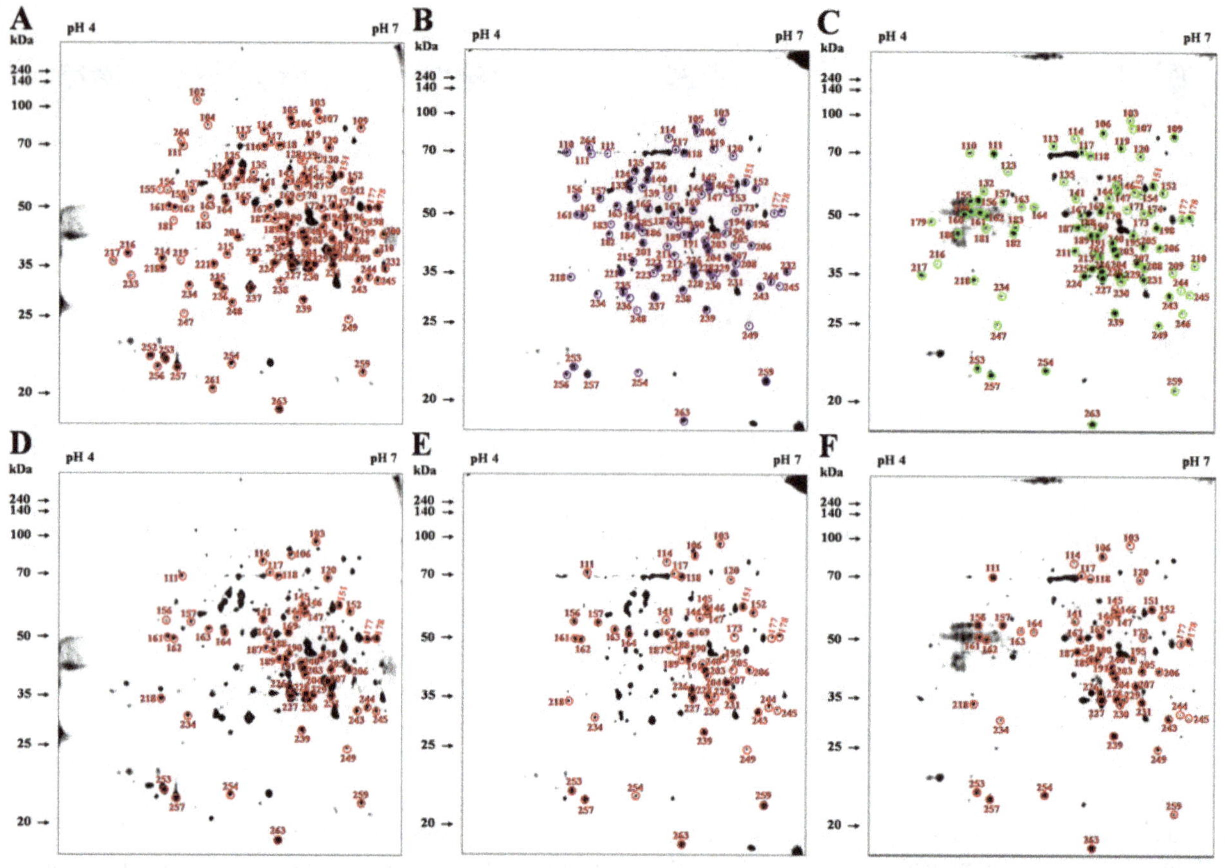

Figure 4 Immunoblotting profile of *B. abortus* proteins responded with *B. abortus*-infected bovine antisera excluding non-specific proteins. Immunoblotting analyses were performed with antisera from cattle after 3, 7, and 10 weeks of challenge with *B. abortus*. After excluding non-specific reactions, a total of 101 **(A)**, 84 **(B)**, and 78 **(C)** immunoreactive dots, as well as 55 protein spots that reacted with antisera at all 3 stages **(D, E, and F)**, were selected and labeled. The numbers represent the serial numbers of the immunoreactive proteins in immunoblot analyses.

immunogenic proteins. Previous studies have examined the immunogenicity of *Brucella* antigens but did not correlate this immunogenicity with the stage of infection. Therefore, this study identified several novel immunoreactive proteins in the bovine host based on the stage of infection.

Using the COG approach, most of the identified proteins were assigned functions related to the transport and metabolism of amino acids (60.9%). The 27.6 kDa DHDPR protein encoded by the *dapB* gene had the highest score value; DHDPR was proposed to function in the biosynthesis of lysine and diaminopimelate, but few proteomic studies have examined the role of this protein in *Brucella* infection [23]. The *dapB* in *Burkholderia pseudomallei* is an essential gene that was successfully mutagenized and identified as a beneficial marker [24]. Therefore, because the *B. abortus dapB*-encoded protein elicits an immunodominant response, this protein is a relevant candidate marker for infection. The predicted proteins involved in carbohydrate transport and metabolism included malate dehydrogenase (mdh), which functions in malate metabolism and the tricarboxylic acid cycle. mdh is expressed in response to acidic stress [25] and was broadly identified in *B. abortus* [10] and *B. melitensis* [26] using proteomic analyses. The second most frequent group included proteins related to ribosomal structure and protein translation. This group includes two ribosomal proteins, the 30S ribosomal protein S2 (RPS2) and the 50S ribosomal protein L25 (RPL25), and one translation elongation factor, EF-Ts (tsf). The RPS2 protein is highly conserved in prokaryotic-type ribosomes and is essential for binding of the ribosomal protein S1 to the 30S ribosomal subunit in *E. coli* [27]. In *Brucella*, RPS2 is repressed in response to oxidative stress [25] and is generally identified as the SSU ribosomal protein S1P of *B. melitensis* and *B. abortus* [10,26]. Additionally, elongation factor Ts (tsf), which is associated with protein translation, might be critical for the immunogenicity of *B. abortus*; this observation is consistent with previous data obtained by global protein analysis in *B. melitensis* [26]. Our study is the first to report that this protein is immunogenic at all stages of infection.

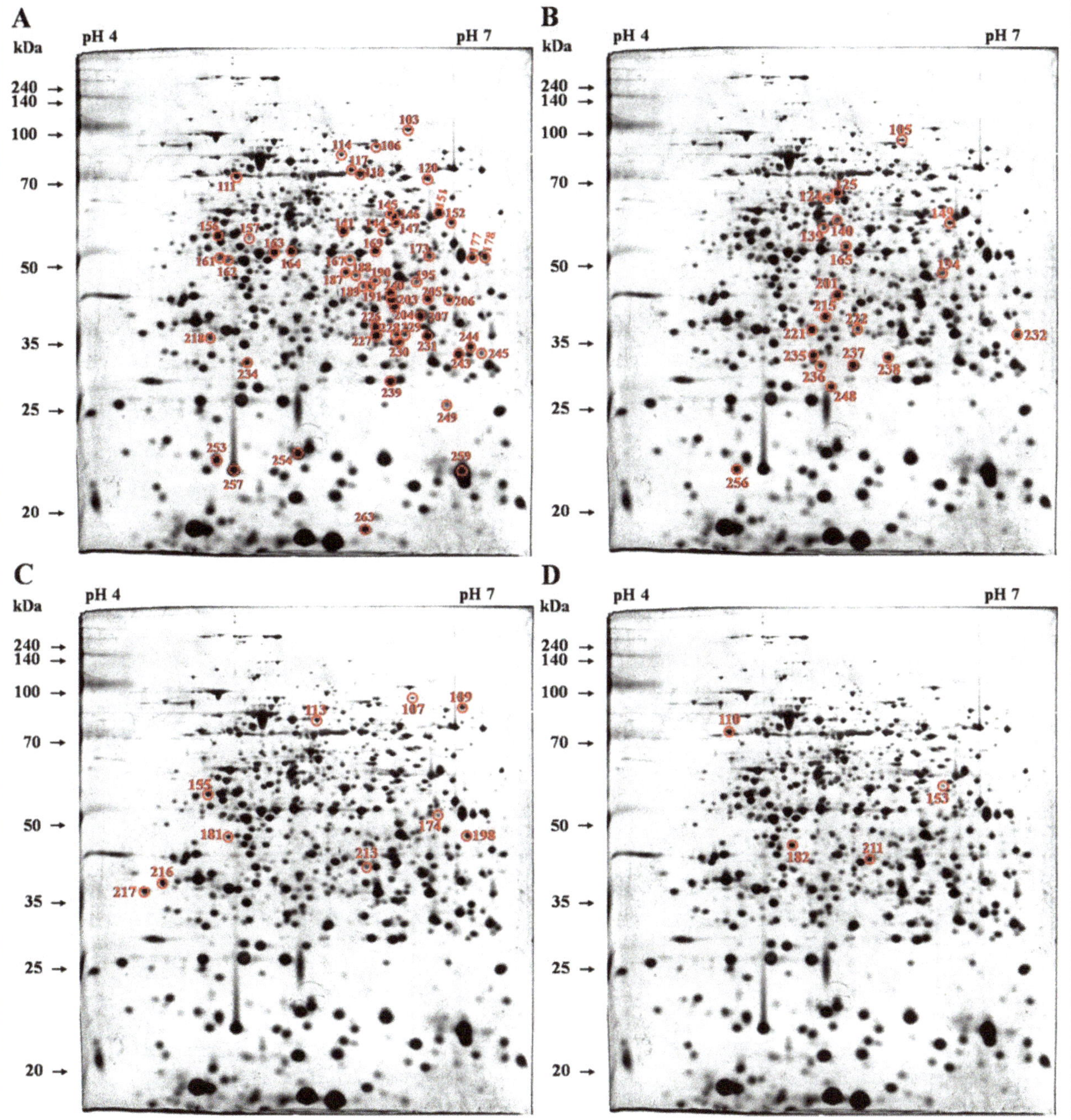

Figure 5 Comparative 2DE analysis of *B. abortus* proteins and immunoblotting profiles of specific reactions. (A) A total of 55 immunoreactive spots of antigen that responded to antisera from cattle after 3, 7 and 10 weeks of challenge with *B. abortus* were selected. A total of 19, 10, and 4 immunoreactive spots of antigen responded to antisera at 2 time-points: **(B)** after 3 and 7 weeks of challenge, **(C)** after 3 and 10 weeks, and **(D)** after 7 and 10 weeks; these spots were selected and labeled on the 2DE gel. The numbers represent the serial numbers of the immunoreactive proteins in immunoblot analyses.

In the group of proteins involved in inorganic ion transport and metabolism, the 22.5 kDa Fe-Mn super oxide dismutase (Fe-Mn-SOD) detected at the p*I* of 5.58 is an oxidoreductase with superoxide dismutase activity. The Fe-Mn-SOD protein of *B. melitensis* is correlated with regulation of the stress response and was identified as a heat-shock protein (Hsp) [25]. Furthermore, the role of metal ions such as Fe and Mn in the response to relatively stringent environments has been elucidated with respect to *Brucella* pathogenesis [28]. Similar to the regulation of Fe- and/or Mn-SOD in response to heat shock and oxidative stress in some bacteria [29], *B. abortus* Fe-Mn-SOD is an essential factor that regulates specific stress responses inside hosts. Several molecular

Table 3 Identification of matched immunoreactive proteins of *B. abortus* that reacted with *B. abortus*-positive bovine antisera

Spot no.	Gene name	Gene ID[a]	Protein identification	Protein ID[a]	Accession no[a]	Sequence length	Locus tag[a]	Score	M_r		p*I*	Sequence coverage (%)	Subcellular location[c]	COG functional category[d]
									Experimental	Theorectical[b]				
118	BruAb2_0325	3341905	aldehyde dehydrogenase	YP_223118.1	Q579C7	500	BruAb2_0325	249	53744	53435	5.64	29	unknown	G: Carbohydrate transport and metabolism
146	BruAb2_0024	3341776	branched chain amino-acid ABC transporter substrate-binding protein	YP_222837.1	Q57A58	471	BruAb2_0024	438	50740	44322	6.43	25	periplasmic space	E: Amino acid transport and metabolism
151	aspC	3339882	aspartate aminotransferase	YP_222177.1	Q57C18	400	BruAb1_1488	193	43812	43554	5.94	18	unknown	F: Nucleotide transport and metabolism
161	BruAb1_0775	3339474	3-hydroxyisobutyryl-CoA hydrolase	YP_221504.1	Q57DZ1	349	BruAb1_0775	258	38120	37802	4.84	27	unknown	H: Coenzyme transport and metabolism
162	tsf	3340671	elongation factor Ts	YP_221867.1	Q57CX8	305	BruAb1_1167	367	32061	31491	5.03	35	cytoplasm	J: Translation, ribosomal structure and biogenesis
164	mdh	3340925	malate dehydrogenase	YP_222574.1	Q57AX1	320	BruAb1_1903	76	33854	33704	5.24	7	cytoplasm	G: Carbohydrate transport and metabolism
169	tbpA	3340057	thiamine transporter substrate binding subunit	YP_222421.1	Q57BC4	334	BruAb1_1742	310	36843	36752	6.06	19	periplasmic space	H: Coenzyme transport and metabolism
178	BruAb1_1058	3341091	cysteine synthase A	YP_221767.1	Q57D78	342	BruAb1_1058	417	34445	36701	5.94	30	cytoplasm	E: Amino acid transport and metabolism
187	BruAb2_0291	3341871	hypothetical protein BruAb2_0291	YP_223086.1	Q579F9	330	BruAb2_0291	267	35457	35251	5.50	26	unknown	R: General function prediction only
203	rpsB	3340672	30S ribosomal protein S2	YP_221868.1	Q57CX7	256	BruAb1_1168	259	29308	27999	5.88	29	ribosome	J: Translation, ribosomal structure and biogenesis
204	ubiG	3340925	3-demethylubiquinone-9 3-methyltransferase	YP_415219.1	Q2YLN5	248	BAB1_1875	410	27653	27486	5.79	31	cytoplasm	E: Amino acid transport and metabolism
207	dapB	3341712	dihydrodipicolinate reductase	YP_223731.1	Q576R4	268	BruAb2_0991	536	28792	27605	5.92	45	cytoplasm	E: Amino acid transport and metabolism

Table 3 Identification of matched immunoreactive proteins of *B. abortus* that reacted with *B. abortus*-positive bovine antisera *(Continued)*

218	BruAb2_0647	3342272	hypothetical protein BruAb2_0647	YP_223419.1	Q577X6	224	BruAb2_0647	302	24961	24805	4.83	34	unknown	Q: Secondary metabolites biosynthesis, transport, and catabolism
227	BruAb2_0628	3342294	metal-dependent hydrolase	YP_223400.1	Q577Z5	237	BruAb2_0628	511	25223	25124	5.58	51	cytoplasm	R: General function prediction only
228	msrA	3341844	methionine sulfoxide reductase A	YP_223747.1	Q576P8	218	BruAb2_1009	167	24230	24017	5.65	20	cytoplasm	O: Posttranslational modification, protein turnover, chaperones
231	BruAb1_1470	3340810	50S ribosomal protein L25	YP_222213.1	Q57BY2	207	BruAb1_1470	171	22369	22383	5.91	47	ribosome	J: Translation, ribosomal structure and biogenesis
239	BruAb1_0588	3339410	Fe-Mn superoxide dismutase	YP_221327.1	Q57EG8	199	BruAb1_0588	359	22526	22540	5.83	37	unknown	P: Inorganic ion transport and metabolism
240	rocF	3341875	arginase	YP_223125.1	P0A2Y1	306	BruAb2_0333	188	33415	33182	5.63	24	unknown	P: Inorganic ion transport and metabolism
243	gpm	3341713	phosphoglyceromutase	YP_223732.1	Q576R3	206	BruAb2_0992	446	22929	22886	6.16	43	cytoplasm	G: Carbohydrate transport and metabolism
253	secB	3339678	preprotein translocase subunit SecB	YP_222709.1	P0C125	163	BruAb1_2047	343	17924	17878	4.89	46	cytoplasm	O: Posttranslational modification, protein turnover, chaperones
254	ndk	3339959	nucleoside diphosphate kinase	YP_221449.1	Q57E46	140	BruAb1_0713	58	15269	15278	5.27	20	cytoplasm	F: Nucleotide transport and metabolism
257	BruAb2_0845	3341366	hypothetical protein BruAb2_0845	YP_223598.1	Q577E7	177	BruAb2_0845	500	18506	18517	5.02	43	unknown	S: Function unknown
263	ohr	3341640	organic hydroperoxide resistance protein	YP_223139.1	Q579A6	140	BruAb2_0347	8	14337	14232	5.63	13	unknown	R: General function prediction only

[a]Gene ID, protein ID, accession no. and locus tag were retrieved from the NCBInr database.
[b]Theoretical molecular weight from the UniProtKB database entry.
[c]Subcellular locations were predicted using PSORTb v. 2.0.4.
[d]Cluster of orthologous groups (COG) protein database generated by comparing microbial genomes from the NCBI COG.

chaperones, including DnaK, GroEL and the HtrA protease, are known as stress proteins and virulence factors [25,30,31]; in our study, at least one chaperone protein, the pre-protein translocase subunit (SecB) was specific to a certain *B. abortus*-infection stage. SecB is a molecular chaperone specific to the proteobacteria, which comprises most gram-negative bacteria that are medically and industrially relevant [32]. SecB is required for the normal export of pre-proteins out of the cytoplasm, keeping them in a translocation-competent state.

Prevention of *Brucella* infections in livestock generally involves the use of live attenuated vaccines such as *B. abortus* (RB51 or S19) [33,34] and *B. melitensis* Rev1 [35]. S19 and Rev1 had the major disadvantage of inducing O-side chain-specific antibodies, which causes cross-reactivity during diagnosis; with RB51, the recovery of virulence was a major problem [36]. Consistently, several studies have focused on developing next-generation vaccines that are more safe and effective. Therefore, the immunogenic *Brucella* proteins identified in this study might provide supporting information for developing valid vaccine candidates that can elicit an efficient and specific immune response. Furthermore, it is important to consider the diagnostic method used depending on the animal and the stage of infection. Modern diagnostic methods are based on molecular approaches developed by proteomic analyses, and these advanced tools might soon replace the older, limited diagnostic methods. We suggest that the candidate proteins elucidated in this study might contribute a valuable solution to the present problems in the diagnosis of brucellosis, independent of the stage of infection. Ultimately, our investigation could provide helpful insight to advance the potential of immunogenic proteins as determinants for serological diagnosis and as novel tools for prevention of *Brucella* infection.

Competing interests

The authors declared that they have no competing interests.

Authors' contributions

LJJ carried out all experiments, contributed to data collection and analysis, and participated in drafting the manuscript; HLS and AWBR participated in the design of the study and contributed to the antigen preparation; DGK and HTH contributed to immunoblotting and participated in the design of the study; WM participated in the design of the study; MH, SCJ and HSY participated in the preparation of cattle infection; KS participated in the design of the study, carried out the data analysis, conceived the experiment and prepared the manuscript. All authors read and approved the final manuscript.

Acknowledgements

The work was supported by iPET (112012-3); Ministry of Agriculture, Food and Rural Affairs, and Animal and Plant Quarantine Agency, Korea.

Author details

[1]Animal and Plant Quarantine Agency, Anyang, Gyeonggi-do 430-757, Republic of Korea. [2]Institute of Animal Medicine, College of Veterinary Medicine, Gyeongsang National University, Jinju, 660-701, Republic of Korea. [3]Department of Infectious Diseases, College of Veterinary Medicine, Seoul National University, Seoul 151-742, Republic of Korea. [4]Institute of Agriculture and Life Science, Gyeongsang National University, Jinju, 660-701, Republic of Korea.

References

1. Seleem MN, Boyle SM, Sriranganathan N (2010) Brucellosis: a re-emerging zoonosis. Vet Microbiol 140:392–398
2. Al Dahouk S, Nockler K (2011) Implications of laboratory diagnosis on brucellosis therapy. Expert Rev Anti Infect Ther 9:833–845
3. McGiven JA (2013) New developments in the immunodiagnosis of brucellosis in livestock and wildlife. Rev Sci Tech 32:163–176
4. Nielsen K, Yu WL (2010) Serological diagnosis of brucellosis. Prilozi 31:65–89
5. McGiven JA, Stack JA, Perrett LL, Tucker JD, Brew SD, Stubberfield E, MacMillan AP (2006) Harmonisation of European tests for serological diagnosis of *Brucella* infection in bovines. Rev Sci Tech 25:1039–1053
6. Gall D, Nielsen K, Nicola A, Renteria T (2008) A proficiency testing method for detecting antibodies against *Brucella abortus* in quantitative and qualitative serological tests. Rev Sci Tech 27:819–828
7. Nielsen K, Smith P, Widdison J, Gall D, Kelly L, Kelly W, Nicoletti P (2004) Serological relationship between cattle exposed to *Brucella abortus*, *Yersinia enterocolitica* O:9 and *Escherichia coli* O157:H7. Vet Microbiol 100:25–30
8. Laurent TC, Mertens P, Dierick JF, Letesson JJ, Lambert C, De Bolle X (2004) Functional, molecular and structural characterisation of five anti-*Brucella* LPS mAb. Mol Immunol 40:1237–1247
9. Yang Y, Wang L, Yin J, Wang X, Cheng S, Lang X, Wang X, Qu H, Sun C, Wang J, Zhang R (2011) Immunoproteomic analysis of *Brucella melitensis* and identification of a new immunogenic candidate protein for the development of brucellosis subunit vaccine. Mol Immunol 49:175–184
10. Connolly JP, Comerci D, Alefantis TG, Walz A, Quan M, Chafin R, Grewal P, Mujer CV, Ugalde RA, DelVecchio VG (2006) Proteomic analysis of *Brucella abortus* cell envelope and identification of immunogenic candidate proteins for vaccine development. Proteomics 6:3767–3780
11. Ko KY, Kim JW, Her M, Kang SI, Jung SC, Cho DH, Kim JY (2012) Immunogenic proteins of *Brucella abortus* to minimize cross reactions in brucellosis diagnosis. Vet Microbiol 156:374–380
12. Bradford MM (1976) A rapid and sensitive method for the quantitation of microgram quantities of protein utilizing the principle of protein-dye binding. Anal Biochem 72:248–254
13. Gorg A, Weiss W, Dunn MJ (2004) Current two-dimensional electrophoresis technology for proteomics. Proteomics 4:3665–3685
14. Silva E, O'Gorman M, Becker S, Auer G, Eklund A, Grunewald J, Wheelock AM (2010) In the eye of the beholder: does the master see the SameSpots as the novice? J Proteome Res 9:1522–1532
15. Perkins DN, Pappin DJ, Creasy DM, Cottrell JS (1999) Probability-based protein identification by searching sequence databases using mass spectrometry data. Electrophoresis 20:3551–3567
16. The EXPASY Database [http://www.expasy.org/proteomics].
17. Gardy JL, Laird MR, Chen F, Rey S, Walsh CJ, Ester M, Brinkman FS (2005) PSORTb v. 2.0: expanded prediction of bacterial protein subcellular localization and insights gained from comparative proteome analysis. Bioinformatics 21:617–623
18. Makarova KS, Sorokin AV, Novichkov PS, Wolf YI, Koonin EV (2007) Clusters of orthologous genes for 41 archaeal genomes and implications for evolutionary genomics of archaea. Biol Direct 2:33
19. Pappas G (2010) The changing *Brucella* ecology: novel reservoirs, new threats. Int J Antimicrob Agents 36(Suppl 1):S8–11
20. Vrioni G, Pappas G, Priavali E, Gartzonika C, Levidiotou S (2008) An eternal microbe: *Brucella* DNA load persists for years after clinical cure. Clin Infect Dis 46:e131–136
21. Christopher S, Umapathy BL, Ravikumar KL (2010) Brucellosis: review on the recent trends in pathogenicity and laboratory diagnosis. J Lab Physicians 2:55–60
22. McGiven JA, Sawyer J, Perrett LL, Brew SD, Commander NJ, Fisher A, McLarnon S, Harper K, Stack JA (2008) A new homogeneous assay for high throughput serological diagnosis of brucellosis in ruminants. J Immunol Methods 337:7–15
23. Doytchinova IA, Flower DR (2007) Identifying candidate subunit vaccines using an alignment-independent method based on principal amino acid properties. Vaccine 25:856–866

24. Norris MH, Kang Y, Lu D, Wilcox BA, Hoang TT (2009) Glyphosate resistance as a novel select-agent-compliant, non-antibiotic-selectable marker in chromosomal mutagenesis of the essential genes asd and dapB of *Burkholderia pseudomallei*. Appl Environ Microbiol 75:6062–6075
25. Teixeira-Gomes AP, Cloeckaert A, Zygmunt MS (2000) Characterization of heat, oxidative, and acid stress responses in *Brucella melitensis*. Infect Immun 68:2954–2961
26. Wagner MA, Eschenbrenner M, Horn TA, Kraycer JA, Mujer CV, Hagius S, Elzer P, DelVecchio VG (2002) Global analysis of the *Brucella melitensis* proteome: Identification of proteins expressed in laboratory-grown culture. Proteomics 2:1047–1060
27. Byrgazov K, Manoharadas S, Kaberdina AC, Vesper O, Moll I (2012) Direct interaction of the N-terminal domain of ribosomal protein S1 with protein S2 in *Escherichia coli*. PLoS One 7:e32702
28. Barbier T, Nicolas C, Letesson JJ (2011) *Brucella* adaptation and survival at the crossroad of metabolism and virulence. FEBS Lett 585:2929–2934
29. Hantke K (2001) Iron and metal regulation in bacteria. Curr Opin Microbiol 4:172–177
30. Ghasemi A, Salari MH, Zarnani AH, Pourmand MR, Ahmadi H, Mirshafiey A, Jeddi-Tehrani M (2013) Immune reactivity of *Brucella melitensis*-vaccinated rabbit serum with recombinant Omp31 and DnaK proteins. Iran J Microbiol 5:19–23
31. Abbady AQ, Al-Daoude A, Al-Mariri A, Zarkawi M, Muyldermans S (2012) Chaperonin GroEL a *Brucella* immunodominant antigen identified using Nanobody and MALDI-TOF-MS technologies. Vet Immunol Immunopathol 146:254–263
32. Driessen AJ (2001) SecB, a molecular chaperone with two faces. Trends Microbiol 9:193–196
33. Moriyon I, Grillo MJ, Monreal D, Gonzalez D, Marin C, Lopez-Goni I, Mainar-Jaime RC, Moreno E, Blasco JM (2004) Rough vaccines in animal brucellosis: structural and genetic basis and present status. Vet Res 35:1–38
34. Thomas EL, Bracewell CD, Corbel MJ (1981) Characterisation of *Brucella abortus* strain 19 cultures isolated from vaccinated cattle. Vet Rec 108:90–93
35. Banai M (2002) Control of small ruminant brucellosis by use of *Brucella melitensis* Rev.1 vaccine: laboratory aspects and field observations. Vet Microbiol 90:497–519
36. Durward MA, Harms J, Magnani DM, Eskra L, Splitter GA (2010) Discordant *Brucella melitensis* antigens yield cognate CD8+ T cells in vivo. Infect Immun 78:168–176

Identification of microRNAs in PCV2 subclinically infected pigs by high throughput sequencing

Fernando Núñez-Hernández[1], Lester J Pérez[2], Marta Muñoz[1], Gonzalo Vera[3], Anna Tomás[4], Raquel Egea[3], Sarai Córdoba[3], Joaquim Segalés[1,5], Armand Sánchez[3,6] and José I Núñez[1*]

Abstract

Porcine circovirus type 2 (PCV2) is the essential etiological infectious agent of PCV2-systemic disease and has been associated with other swine diseases, all of them collectively known as porcine circovirus diseases. MicroRNAs (miRNAs) are a new class of small non-coding RNAs that regulate gene expression post-transcriptionally. miRNAs play an increasing role in many biological processes. The study of miRNA-mediated host-pathogen interactions has emerged in the last decade due to the important role that miRNAs play in antiviral defense. The objective of this study was to identify the miRNA expression pattern in PCV2 subclinically infected and non-infected pigs. For this purpose an experimental PCV2 infection was carried out and small-RNA libraries were constructed from tonsil and mediastinal lymph node (MLN) of infected and non-infected pigs. High throughput sequencing determined differences in miRNA expression in MLN between infected and non-infected while, in tonsil, a very conserved pattern was observed. In MLN, miRNA 126-3p, miRNA 126-5p, let-7d-3p, mir-129a and mir-let-7b-3p were up-regulated whereas mir-193a-5p, mir-574-5p and mir-34a down-regulated. Prediction of functional analysis showed that these miRNAs can be involved in pathways related to immune system and in processes related to the pathogenesis of PCV2, although functional assays are needed to support these predictions. This is the first study on miRNA gene expression in pigs infected with PCV2 using a high throughput sequencing approach in which several host miRNAs were differentially expressed in response to PCV2 infection.

Introduction

Porcine circovirus type 2 (PCV2) belongs to the *Circoviridae* family. The viral particle contains a single-strand circular DNA genome of 1768-9 nucleotides (nt), enclosed within a non-enveloped protein capsid with a diameter of 16- 18 nm. PCV2 is one of the smallest mammalian viruses encoding 11 potential reading frames, although expression has only been determined from 3 of them. ORF1 encodes the non-structural replication-associated protein Rep and its truncated variant Rep' [1], ORF2 encodes the structural capsid protein Cap [2] and a non-structural protein with an uncertain function is encoded by ORF3 [3]. Cap and Rep/Rep' carry out the two most elementary functions of a virus, copying and the successive packaging of the viral genome [4].

PCV2 is the etiological agent of PCV2-systemic disease (PCV2-SD), formerly known as postweaning multisystemic wasting syndrome, (PMWS) [5], an emerging disease in swine first described in 1991 [6]. PCV2 infection is widespread and its most frequent manifestation is by means of a subclinical infection. PCV2 is ubiquitous in swine livestock worldwide, but it has been demonstrated that PCV2 DNA load in serum is significantly higher in PCV2-SD affected pigs than in healthy pigs, which is considered an indicator of the disease [7]. PCV2-SD has a relatively high fatality rate among 5 to 12-week-old pigs. The disease from a clinical point of view causes dyspnea, a progressive loss of weight, anemia, tachypnea, diarrhea and jaundice. Microscopic lesions include lymphadenopathy, nephritis, pancreatitis, hepatitis and granulomatous interstitial pneumonia [6]. PCV2 is thought to be involved in the pathogenesis of porcine dermatitis and nephropathy syndrome (PDNS), and is linked with the occurrence of reproductive disease [5].

It has been suggested that PCV2 replicates firstly in the tonsil and in the regional lymph nodes [6]. PCV2 pathogenesis is related to the immunosuppression caused by the virus in pigs [8] and changes in cytokine production can

* Correspondence: ignacio.nunez@cresa.uab.cat
[1]Centre de Recerca en Sanitat Animal (CReSA), UAB-IRTA, Campus de la Universitat Autònoma de Barcelona, Bellaterra, Cerdanyola del Vallès, Spain
Full list of author information is available at the end of the article

play a role in this immunosuppression. Pigs with naturally acquired PCV2-SD had an altered cytokine mRNA expression pattern with overexpression of IL-10 mRNA in thymus and IFN-γ mRNA in tonsil, whereas a reduction in the expression of IFN-γ, IL-10, IL-12p40, IL-4 and IL-2 mRNA was observed in other lymphoid tissues [9]. Nevertheless, the mechanisms involved in these processes are poorly understood. This complexity is reflected, for example, in IL-10 expression where a feedback regulation between IL-10 and several microRNAs (miRNAs) has been described [10].

miRNAs are 19-24 nt long non-coding ssRNAs that regulate gene expression post-transcriptionally. Derived from hairpin precursors, they mediate the post-transcriptional silencing of an estimated 30% of protein coding genes in mammals by binding to complementary sites typically located in the 3′ untranslated regions (UTRs) of their target mRNAs [11,12]. This regulation of gene expression via microRNA-mediated RNA interference (RNAi) was first identified in *Caenorhabditis elegans* in 1998. Since this time, more than 21 000 miRNAs have been identified in all kind of species (miRNA registry at miRBase [13]) from mammals, to plants [14], and more recently in several viruses [15,16]. miRNAs have been shown to be implicated in several biological processes such as development, differentiation, homeostasis, carcinogenesis and a wide variety of diseases [17].

The biogenesis of miRNAs has been extensively described in the literature [12,18], but it is considered that there is a canonical pathway by which miRNAs are generated through consecutive cleavages of hairpin precursors by two RNase III enzymes, Drosha and Dicer. In the cell nucleus, the single strand-double strand junction of the pri-miRNA hairpin is recognized by Pasha (or DGCR8 in vertebrates), which is essential for the RNase III enzyme Drosha processing of the hairpin structure. This cleavage generates a 55–70 pre-miRNA hairpin that is exported to the cytoplasm assisted by exportin-5. Once in the cytoplasm, the terminal loop is split from the structure by the RNase III enzyme Dicer. Then, the duplexes are unwound to load the mature strand into an Argonaute containing RNA-induced silencing complex (RISC) [19,20]. The first 2-8 nucleotides (seed) of the miRNAs are essential in the recognition of the target, the complementarity can be complete or partial, and leads to mRNA translational repression or destabilization.

In this paper, the expression of microRNAs in subclinically PCV2 infected pigs was analysed using high throughput sequencing.

Material and methods

Animal infection

Six 6-week-old Landrace x Large White pigs were used. Four of them were intranasally inoculated with a total dose of 7 × $10^{4.8}$TCID$_{50}$ of PCV2 genotype b isolate Sp-10-7-54-13 [21], while 2 control pigs received PBS by the same route. At 21 days post-inoculation (dpi), animals were euthanized. Samples from eight tissues: spleen, inguinal lymph node, kidney, tonsil, thymus, mediastinal lymph node (MLN), lung and mesenterical lymph node, were collected in duplicate and immediately frozen in liquid nitrogen and stored at −80 °C. A third sample was collected in formalin for histopathological studies. Tissue sections were stained with haematoxylin and eosin, and in situ hybridization (ISH) was carried out in order to detect viral genome.

All animal experiments were performed in the CReSA facilities, and all procedures were carried out according to the guidelines of the institutional animal ethics committee of UAB, preserving the Spanish and European animal experimentation ethics law.

Homogenate and DNA- RNA extraction

Tissue samples of approximately 100 mg were homogenated with a pestle in 1 mL of Trizol (Invitrogen, Carlsbad, USA) to lyse the tissues and deactivate virus. Total RNA and DNA were isolated following the manufacturer's protocol and resuspended in 25 and 200 μL of RNAse-, DNAse- and proteinase free water (Sigma) for RNA and DNA, respectively.

Quantitative real time PCR to detect PCV2

A quantitative real-time PCR (qPCR) was performed in the 8 tissues from all animals to quantify PCV2 load. Probe and primers used for the procedure were those designed and used in [22]. The mix for the qPCR contained 900 nM primers PCV2F and PCV2R, 150 μM probe, 0.4 μL IC kit, 12.5 μL Taqman Universal Master Mix and 2.5 μL template. Nanopure autoclaved water was added to final volume of 25 μL. The conditions for the amplification were 10 min at 95 °C, 2 min at 50 °C and 40 cycles of 15 s at 95 °C and 1 min at 60 °C. Triplicates of each sample were used for the qPCR.

RNA integrity and quantification

Total RNA was quantified using ND 1000 Nanodrop® Spectrophotometer (Thermo Scientific, Wilmington, USA). RNA integrity and quality was analysed using the 2100 Expert Bioanalizer (Agilent Technologies, Santa Clara, USA). Total and low size RNA measurements were carried out. Total RNA was calculated using the Eukaryote total RNA Nano Series II software and specific chips (Agilent Technologies, Santa Clara, USA), while low size RNA was measured using the Small RNA Nano software and specific chips (Agilent Technologies, Santa Clara, USA).

Small RNA library construction

All procedures were carried out using the miRCat™ microRNA Cloning Kit (IDT, Iowa, USA) protocol as basis, with the modifications described in [23]. For the enrichment of the small RNA fraction, slices were cut from a 12% denaturing (7 M Urea) polyacrylamide gel, using a miSPIKE™ (IDT, Iowa, USA), as internal size marker. Small RNA fractions were purified using Performa DTR gel filtration cartridges (EdgeBio, Gaithersburg, USA). A double ligation was carried out using 3′ and 5′ linkers from miRCatTM kit (IDT, Coralville, USA) in two steps. The 3′ preadenylated linker was coupled to the small RNA fraction in a reaction in which the mix contained 1X Reaction Buffer for T4 Ligase (Thermo Fisher Scientific, Walthman, MA) without ATP, 0.1 mg BSA (Fermentas), 1U T4 RNA ligase (Fermentas) and 2.5 μM 3′ linker. 6.5 μL small RNA fraction was added and incubated at 37 °C for 2 h. The 5′ linker was coupled in a mix with 1X ligation buffer (Ambion), 1U T4 RNA ligase (Ambion) and 50 μM 5′ linker in presence of ATP. 7.5 μL 3′linked RNA was added to a final volume of 10 μL. The mixture was incubated for 2 h at 37 °C.

RT- PCR

RT was carried out with Super Script III Reverse Transcriptase (Life Technologies). Initial pre incubation at 65 °C for 5 min with 0.5 mM of each dNTP, 0.5 μM Primer mir5 and 11 μL RNA were carried out. In a second step a mix was prepared with 1X First-Strand Buffer, 5 mM DTT, 0.2 U RNaseOUT and 10 U SuperScript III RT in a final volume of 20 μL, the mix was incubated at 55 °C for 90 min, and 70 °C for 15 min.

PCR amplifications were performed using Expand High Fidelity Plus PCR System (Roche). Briefly, 0.05 U Expand High Fidelity Plus Enzyme Blend, 1X Expand High Fidelity Plus Reaction Buffer with 1.5 mM $MgCl_2$, 0.2 μM Primers A5 and B3, 0.2 μM of each dNTP, 4 μL cDNA and RNAse Free Water to a final volume of 50 μL. Primers A3 and B5 were designed as fused primers with sequence primers mir5 or mir3 (IDT, Iowa, USA) plus sequence primers A or B (454 GS-FLX Roche), respectively, labelled with a five nucleotide sequence tag for differentiating libraries. PCR conditions were 94 °C for 3 min, 20-25 cycles at 94 °C for 30 s, 57 °C for 45 s and 72 °C for 1 min followed by 71 °C for 7 min. The number of cycles was optimized for each library to avoid saturation. The resulting PCR was purified with the QIAquick PCR purification kit (Qiagen).

Cloning in pGEM-T Easy Vector System II Kit (Promega) and posterior Sanger sequencing with the ABI-PRISM 3700 (Applied Biosystems) were carried out to check the libraries construction prior to the high throughput sequencing.

High throughput sequencing

Amplicons were quantified using Qubit™ fluorometer, Quant-IT™ (Invitrogen™, Carlsbad, USA), prepared to a 10^{11} DNA molecules/μL and equimolecular pooled. Libraries were sequenced following the manufacturer's protocol with the 454 GS-FLX System (Roche) at the DNA sequencing facilities at CRAG (Centre de Recerca Agrogenòmica, Universitat Autònoma de Barcelona, Spain). Sequencing data have been submitted to the European Nucleotide Archive (ENA) [24] with the accession number PRJEB7603.

Sequence processing scheme

Primer sequences were trimmed and only those insert sequences between 15 and 29 nucleotides and with total number of sequences ≥3 were kept for further analysis.

For porcine miRNA profiling, sequences were compared to all available miRNA sequences (miRBase v20) using local Blast. Parameters were set to 100% identity and up to 4 mismatches allowed at the end of the sequences to solve the miRNA variability on 3′ and 5′ ends [25].

Differences in host miRNA expression were assessed. The total number of sequences obtained for each porcine miRNA was normalised by library size (in counts per thousand) and, then, averaged by group. Fold changes (FC) between groups were calculated using normalised data. Only miRNAs up or down-regulated for all individuals per group were taking into account.

miRNAs target prediction and biological functions

For the in silico study of the potential targets, the DIANA-microT v5.0 web server with an adjusted threshold of 0.7 was used [26,27]. There were no porcine genes in the databases, so the study was done using the human genome assuming sequence conservation [28]. In order to identify potential targets in the viral genome, miRanda program was used with the following parameters: -sc 140 –en 20. Potential targets were then studied employing Web-based Gene Set Analysis Toolkit (WebGestal) [29,30]. The analysis was done using the Kyoto Encyclopedia of Genes and Genomes Database (KEGG) to check the biological pathways in which miRNAs are involved. The selected parameters for the study were the multiple test adjustment by Benjamini and Hochberg [31] and the significance level set at 0.05.

Results

Experimental infection

Until 21 dpi no animals developed clinical signs. PCV2 infection was confirmed in inoculated animals by qPCR in 6 out of 8 tissues: Spleen, inguinal lymph node, tonsil, MLN, lung and mesenteric lymph node, confirming the subclinical nature of the infection (Table 1). No

Table 1 Genome copies/mg detected by qPCR in tissues of infected (number 3 to 6) and non-infected (number 1 and 2) pigs with PCV2

	Animal number					
Tissue	**1**	**2**	**3**	**4**	**5**	**6**
Spleen	-	-	3.2×10^2	2.9×10^2	7.2×10^1	4×10^2
Inguinal ln	-	-	1.2×10^4	3.3×10^2	1.7×10^3	8.9×10^2
Kidney	-	-	-	-	-	-
Tonsil	-	-	5.2×10^1	1.8×10^3	2.1×10^3	8×10^2
Thymus	-	-	-	-	-	-
Mediastinal ln	-	-	8.2×10^3	1.9×10^4	3.8×10^4	4.6×10^4
Lung	-	-	6×10^1	2.1×10^2	1.1×10^2	9.2×10^1
Mesenteric ln	-	-	2.5×10^2	7.6×10^2	7.2×10^1	1.1×10^3

amplification was observed in non-infected animals or in kidney and thymus of tested animals. PCV2 detection by in situ hybridization was negative for all samples tested. No histological lesions were observed at necropsy. MLN and tonsil were selected for small RNA library construction because of their viral load and because tonsil is the primary replication site.

miRNA sequence annotation

A total of 12 small RNA libraries were constructed and sequenced. From the total reads obtained (1 106 437), after trimming the adaptors sequences, and selecting inserts ranging from 15 to 29 nt, a total of 796 710 reads were obtained (Table 2). Reads were aligned to the miRBase database (v20), not allowing any changes inside but allowing a maximum of four changes in the sequence extremes. Finally, 562 483 reads (4700 unique sequences) were aligned to miRBase. A total of 508 miRNAs were described.

Differential expression analysis

miRNAs were considered differentially expressed (DE) when fold change (FC) difference between infected and non-infected animals was higher than 5 and when the up- or down-regulation was conserved for all animals per group. From the 119 miRNAs highly expressed (>80 reads) in MLN, 8 miRNAs were DE, five up-regulated (mir-126-3p, mir-126-5p, let-7d-3p, mir-129a, mir-let-7b-3p) and three down-regulated (mir-193a-5p, mir-574-5p and mir-34a) (Table 3). In tonsil, no miRNA was DE from the 115 miRNAs with more than 80 reads.

Table 2 High throughput sequencing reads

Total reads	1 106 437
Trimed, not empty reads, ranging from 15 to 29 nt	796 710
Aligned to miRBase	562 483
Unique sequences	4700
Number of miRNAs	508

Table 3 Differentially expressed miRNAs in the MLN

miRNA	Inf/non inf	Reads
ssc-miR-126-5p	6.28	18 794
ssc-miR-126-3p	7.51	17 050
ssc-miR-193a-5p	−54.29	3139
ssc-let-7d-3p	9.3	770
hsa-miR-574-5p	−19.9	310
ssc-miR-34a	−5.34	165
ssc-miR-129a	8.28	115
hsa-let-7b-3p	6.5	83

Target prediction and functional analysis

Diana micro-T was employed to identify putative targets for eight selected DE miRNAs. A list of 5502 target genes was identified (see Additional file 1). A gene ontology (GO) enrichment analysis was used to identify the functions of the target genes (Table 4). No significant related pathways were found for mir-let-7d-3p and ssc-miR-126-3p. Some pathways related to viral infection process and immune response were found to be significant, such as the T cell receptor signalling pathway, Fc gamma R-mediated phagocytosis and the Fc epsilon RI signalling pathway. The prediction of putative targets in viral genome indicated that two of the DE miRNAs targeted the PCV2 genome: mir-let-7d-3p and mir-129a, both targeting the Cap gene.

Discussion

miRNAs can be an important factor playing a role in virus/host interaction and in the immune response involved in the pathogenesis of PCV2 infection, in both subclinical and clinical scenarios. This work is the first study on miRNAs gene expression in pigs infected with PCV2 using a deep sequencing approach. In the experimental infection carried out, the lack of clinical signs, histological lesions and viral detection by ISH and the low viral load detected by qPCR is in agreement with previous studies where a subclinical infection has been developed [32].

Taking into account the comparison of the most expressed miRNAs in both tissues (CN > 80), 74.8% of the miRNAs were common. This is in concordance with the lymphoid origin of both tissues. When comparing the tissues analysed, the expression profile was affected differentially by the PCV2 infection. The miRNA expression was affected notably in MLN, whereas in tonsil, the miRNA expression pattern was less affected. A possible factor affecting this expression is the difference in viral load. However, differences in cytokine expression have

Table 4 Genome pathways predicted for selected miRNAs from Kyoto Encyclopedia of Genes and Genomes, related to the immune system and PCV2 pathogenesis

miRNA	Genome pathway
ssc-miR-126-3p	-
ssc-miR-126-5p	T cell receptor signalling pathway
	Natural killer cell mediated cytotoxicity
	B cell receptor signalling pathway
	Fc epsilon RI signalling pathway
	Chemokine signalling pathway
	mTor signalling pathway*
	MAPK signalling pathway*
ssc-miR-193a-5p	Cytosolic DNA-sensing pathway
ssc-let-7d-3p	-
ssc-miR-34a	Fc gamma R-mediated phagocytosis
	Hematopoietic cell lineage
	B cell receptor signalling pathway
	Fc epsilon RI signalling pathway
	T cell receptor signalling pathway
	Natural killer cell mediated cytotoxicity
	Leukocyte transendothelial migration
	MAPK signalling pathway*
hsa-miR-574-5p	T cell receptor signalling pathway
	MAPK signalling pathway*
hsa-let-7b-3p	T cell receptor signalling pathway
	Chemokine signalling pathway
	Fc gamma R-mediated phagocytosis
	Leukocyte transendothelial migration
	NOD-like receptor signalling pathway
	Hematopoietic cell lineage
	B cell receptor signalling pathway
	Toll-like receptor signalling pathway
	MAPK signalling pathway*
ssc-miR-129a	Fc epsilon RI signalling pathway
	B cell receptor signalling pathway
	Chemokine signalling pathway
	MAPK signalling pathway*

*Signal transduction.

been described between tonsil and others lymph nodes [9] although the basis of this differential expression is not clear. Thus, the conserved miRNA expression in tonsil could be associated to this different cytokine expression. On the other hand, tonsil has been suggested as a primary replication site for PCV2 [2]. Because all animals were euthanized at day 21, the expression of miRNA could be altered by the differences in the period of time when the tonsil and MLN were infected [33].

Differential expression of miRNAs in MLN is high due to the PCV2 infection; from the most represented miRNAs in both tissues (CN > 80): mir-126-3p, mir-126-5p, mir-let-7d-3p, miR-129-2-3p and mir-let-7b-3p were up-regulated in MLN of PCV2 infected animals, while miR-193a-5p, miR-574-5p and miR-34a-5p were down-regulated.

miRNAs DE could regulate genes that would be involved in the immune response, such as T cell receptor signalling pathways, natural killer cell mediated cytotoxicity, the B cell receptor signalling pathway, the chemokine signalling pathway, Fc gamma R- mediated phagocytosis, leukocyte transendothelial migration, the cytosolic DNA sensing pathway, the NOD-like receptor signalling pathway, hematopoietic cell lineage and also related to Fc epsilon R-I signalling pathways.

miR-126-5p is the most represented miRNA DE in MLN and has been involved in the intracellular expression of Toll-like receptors (TLRs) 7 and 9 by plasmacytoid dendritic cells, producing (anti-viral) type I interferons [34], thus, mir-126-5p can modulate the physiopathology of the immune response against PCV2. The extracellular signal-regulated kinase (ERK) signalling pathway, one of the three mitogen-activated protein kinase (MAPK), has been shown to be involved in the induction of autophagy by PCV2 [35] and the inhibition of ERK signalling pathways increases PCV2 replication [36]. In our functional analysis, miR-126-5p was associated with the MAPK signalling pathway, therefore, this miRNA could be involved in both processes.

TFPI (tissue factor pathway inhibitor) is one of the genes targeted by miR-126-5p. Comparison with a previous study [32] in which gene expression in response to PCV2 infection was analyzed by microarray hybridization, showed a TFPI gene down-regulation in MLN. This decreased expression could inhibit migration and cell proliferation and thus, could be involved in the inflammatory process developed in pigs with PCV2-SD [32]. On the other hand, in a coxsackievirus infection, miR-126 targets SPRED1, LRP6, and WRCH1 genes, mediating cross-talk between the ERK1/2 and Wnt/β-catenin pathways, enhancing viral replication and contributing to the viral cytopathogenicity [37].

Target prediction analysis indicated that miR-126-3p was potentially able to regulate only 20 genes but no related pathways were found. Interestingly, one of the targeted genes is the previously mentioned SPRED1, shared with miR-126-5p.

miR-let-7b-3p was up-regulated in MLN and has been shown to be able to potentially regulate a great number of genes, thereby several immunological pathways have been found for this miRNA. Besides this, this miRNA has also been associated with the MAPK signaling pathway. Target prediction analysis showed that miR-let-7b-3p can regulate the expression of the AP1S3 gene, which is involved in the modulation of Toll-like receptor 3 (TLR 3) signaling [38].

mir-let-7d-3p was up-regulated in MLN, although 13 genes were found as potentially regulated by this miRNA, no related immunological pathways were found. miR-193a-5p was down-regulated in medistinal lymph node, and could potentially regulate genes related to the cytosolic DNA- sensing pathway.

miR-34a-5p is down-regulated in MLN and this regulatory role was predicted to be involved in several immunological pathways and the MAPK signalling pathway. In this case, target prediction analysis revealed that miR-34a-5p targets KLRK1, killer cell lectin-like receptor subfamily K, member 1, which binds to a diverse family of ligands that include MHC class I chain-related A and B proteins and UL-16 binding proteins, where ligand-receptor interactions can result in the activation of NK and T cells [39]. It also regulates ARHGP6, a member of the Rho family that participates in endocytosis processes. PCV2 internalization is produced mainly by endocytosis, mainly through Rho- GTPase mediated dynamin- independent pathway [32].

miR-574-5p was down-regulated in MLN and was predicted to be involved in the regulation of the T cell receptor signalling and MAPK signalling pathways. miR-129-2-3p was down-regulated in MLN, predicted pathways in which this miRNA was involved were the Fc epsilon RI signalling, the MAPK signalling, the B cell receptor signalling, and chemokine signalling pathways. This miRNA has previously been described as targeting transcription factor SOX4 which has a critical function in normal B-cell ontogenesis [40].

Some of the predictions described in this work could be involved in the manifestation of the pathogenesis of the subclinically infected animals, but at this point, we want to indicate that further functional assays are needed to confirm the computational predictions of miRNAs target genes and the regulation of the pathways described.

The effect of host miRNAs on viral gene expression was analyzed using miRanda. Thus, mir-126-3p and mir-126-5p, the most represented DE miRNAs, showed no targets in the viral genome, while mir-let-7d-3p and mir-129a presented targets in the Cap gene of PCV2. Both miRNAs are up-regulated in MLN and can affect viral replication as has been seen for others viruses where several miRNAs can down-regulate the expression of viral proteins [41,42]. Nevertheless, the role of host miRNAs in the regulation of the viral replication is controversial as has been revealed in an extensive study [43]. The authors showed that many human viruses are refractory to inhibition by host miRNAs due to miRNA driven viral evolution. Thus, experimental assays are needed to clarify if PCV2 is regulated or not by porcine miRNAs.

The identification of the DE miRNAs and the prediction analysis regarding the functions of these miRNAs in an in vivo PCV2 infection in its natural host has been described in this study. The two tissues analysed presented a different behaviour in their miRNA expression pattern in response to the infection.

Additional file

Additional file 1: In silico target genes predicted for the eight selected DE porcine miRNAs in the infected and non-infected pigs. List of target genes predicted for the eight selected DE porcine miRNAs in animals infected and non-infected with PCV2, isolate Sp-10-7-54-13. Only ssc-miR-126-3p and ssc-let-7d-3p presented a low number of target genes (≤20).

Competing interests
The authors declare that they have no competing interests.

Authors' contributions
JIN and AS conceived and designed this study. FNH, LJP and MM performed the experiments. JIN and FNH analyzed data. JS, SC, and AT contributed reagents/material/analysis tools. JIN and FNH wrote the paper. GV and RE performed the bioinformatics analysis. AT and JS critically read the manuscript. All authors read and approved the final manuscript.

Acknowledgements
We thank all the personal from animal facilities of CReSA for their help with the animals. This research was supported by the projects AGL2007-66371-C02 and AGL2010-22358-C02 from Ministerio de Ciencia e Innovación. FN-H is the recipient of a PhD fellowship FI-DGR (AGAUR) from Generalitat de Catalunya. The manuscript has been edited by Dr Kevin Dalton.

Author details
[1]Centre de Recerca en Sanitat Animal (CReSA), UAB-IRTA, Campus de la Universitat Autònoma de Barcelona, Bellaterra, Cerdanyola del Vallès, Spain. [2]Centro Nacional de Sanidad Agropecuaria (CENSA), La Habana, Cuba. [3]Departament de Genètica Animal, Centre de Recerca en AgriGenòmica (CRAG), CSIC- IRTA-UAB-UB, Universitat Autònoma de Barcelona, Bellaterra, Barcelona, Spain. [4]Programa Infección e Inmunidad, Fundació d'Investigació Sanitària de les illes Balears, 07110 Buynola, Spain. [5]Departament de Sanitat i Anatomia Animals, Universitat Autònoma de Barcelona, Bellaterra, Barcelona, Spain. [6]Departament de Ciència Animal i dels Aliments, Universitat Autònoma de Barcelona (UAB), Bellaterra, Barcelona, Spain.

References
1. Cheung AK (2003) Transcriptional analysis of porcine circovirus type 2. Virology 305:168–180
2. Nawagitgul P, Morozov I, Bolin SR, Harms PA, Sorden SD, Paul PS (2000) Open reading frame 2 of porcine circovirus type 2 encodes a major capsid protein. J Gen Virol 81:2281–2287
3. Juhan NM, LeRoith T, Opriessnig T, Meng XJ (2010) The open reading frame 3 (ORF3) of porcine circovirus type 2 (PCV2) is dispensable for virus infection but evidence of reduced pathogenicity is limited in pigs infected by an ORF3-null PCV2 mutant. Virus Res 147:60–66
4. Finsterbusch T, Mankertz A (2009) Porcine circoviruses–small but powerful. Virus Res 143:177–183
5. Segales J (2012) Porcine circovirus type 2 (PCV2) infections: clinical signs, pathology and laboratory diagnosis. Virus Res 164:10–19
6. Rosell C, Segales J, Plana-Duran J, Balasch M, Rodriguez-Arrioja GM, Kennedy S, Allan GM, McNeilly F, Latimer KS, Domingo M (1999) Pathological, immunohistochemical, and in-situ hybridization studies of natural cases of

postweaning multisystemic wasting syndrome (PMWS) in pigs. J Comp Pathol 120:59–78
7. Fenaux M, Halbur PG, Gill M, Toth TE, Meng XJ (2000) Genetic characterization of type 2 porcine circovirus (PCV-2) from pigs with postweaning multisystemic wasting syndrome in different geographic regions of North America and development of a differential PCR-restriction fragment length polymorphism assay to detect and differentiate between infections with PCV-1 and PCV-2. J Clin Microbiol 38:2494–2503
8. Segales J, Domingo M, Chianini F, Majo N, Dominguez J, Darwich L, Mateu E (2004) Immunosuppression in postweaning multisystemic wasting syndrome affected pigs. Vet Microbiol 98:151–158
9. Darwich L, Pie S, Rovira A, Segales J, Domingo M, Oswald IP, Mateu E (2003) Cytokine mRNA expression profiles in lymphoid tissues of pigs naturally affected by postweaning multisystemic wasting syndrome. J Gen Virol 84:2117–2125
10. Quinn SR, O'Neill LA (2014) The role of microRNAs in the Control and mechanism of action of IL-10. Curr Top Microbiol Immunol 380:145–155
11. Zhang L, Hou D, Chen X, Li D, Zhu L, Zhang Y, Li J, Bian Z, Liang X, Cai X, Yin Y, Wang C, Zhang T, Zhu D, Zhang D, Xu J, Chen Q, Ba Y, Liu J, Wang Q, Chen J, Wang J, Wang M, Zhang Q, Zhang J, Zen K, Zhang CY (2012) Exogenous plant MIR168a specifically targets mammalian LDLRAP1: evidence of cross-kingdom regulation by microRNA. Cell Res 22:107–126
12. Bartel DP (2004) MicroRNAs: genomics, biogenesis, mechanism, and function. Cell 116:281–297
13. miRBase: the microRNA database [http://www.mirbase.org]
14. Reinhart BJ, Weinstein EG, Rhoades MW, Bartel B, Bartel DP (2002) MicroRNAs in plants. Genes Dev 16:1616–1626
15. Pfeffer S, Zavolan M, Grasser FA, Chien M, Russo JJ, Ju J, John B, Enright AJ, Marks D, Sander C, Tuschl T (2004) Identification of virus-encoded microRNAs. Science 304:734–736
16. Boss IW, Renne R (1809) Viral miRNAs and immune evasion. Biochim Biophys Acta 2011:708–714
17. Lindsay MA (2008) microRNAs and the immune response. Trends Immunol 29:343–351
18. Kim VN (2005) MicroRNA biogenesis: coordinated cropping and dicing. Nat Rev Mol Cell Biol 6:376–385
19. Tuddenham L, Pfeffer S (1809) Roles and regulation of microRNAs in cytomegalovirus infection. Biochim Biophys Acta 2011:613–622
20. Hammond SM, Boettcher S, Caudy AA, Kobayashi R, Hannon GJ (2001) Argonaute2, a link between genetic and biochemical analyses of RNAi. Science 293:1146–1150
21. Fort M, Sibila M, Nofrarias M, Perez-Martin E, Olvera A, Mateu E, Segales J (2010) Porcine circovirus type 2 (PCV2) Cap and Rep proteins are involved in the development of cell-mediated immunity upon PCV2 infection. Vet Immunol Immunopathol 137:226–234
22. Olvera A, Sibila M, Calsamiglia M, Segales J, Domingo M (2004) Comparison of porcine circovirus type 2 load in serum quantified by a real time PCR in postweaning multisystemic wasting syndrome and porcine dermatitis and nephropathy syndrome naturally affected pigs. J Virol Methods 117:75–80
23. Timoneda O, Nunez-Hernandez F, Balcells I, Munoz M, Castello A, Vera G, Perez LJ, Egea R, Mir G, Cordoba S, Rosell R, Segalés J, Tomàs A, Sánchez A, Núñez JI (2014) The role of viral and host microRNAs in the Aujeszky's disease virus during the infection process. PLoS One 9:e86965
24. European Nucleotide Archive [http://www.ebi.ac.uk/ena]
25. Lee LW, Zhang S, Etheridge A, Ma L, Martin D, Galas D, Wang K (2010) Complexity of the microRNA repertoire revealed by next-generation sequencing. RNA 16:2170–2180
26. Paraskevopoulou MD, Georgakilas G, Kostoulas N, Vlachos IS, Vergoulis T, Reczko M, Filippidis C, Dalamagas T, Hatzigeorgiou AG (2013) DIANA-microT web server v5.0: service integration into miRNA functional analysis workflows. Nucleic Acids Res 41:W169–173
27. Reczko M, Maragkakis M, Alexiou P, Grosse I, Hatzigeorgiou AG (2012) Functional microRNA targets in protein coding sequences. Bioinformatics 28:771–776
28. Shi B, Gao W, Wang J (2012) Sequence fingerprints of microRNA conservation. PLoS One 7:e48256
29. Zhang B, Kirov S, Snoddy J (2005) WebGestalt: an integrated system for exploring gene sets in various biological contexts. Nucleic Acids Res 33:W741–748
30. Wang J, Duncan D, Shi Z, Zhang B (2013) WEB-based GEne SeT AnaLysis Toolkit (WebGestalt): update 2013. Nucleic Acids Res 41:W77–83
31. Benjamini Y, Hochberg Y (1995) Controlling the false discovery rate: a practical and powerful approach to multiple testing. J Roy Stat Soc B Met 57:289–300
32. Tomas A, Fernandes LT, Sanchez A, Segales J (2010) Time course differential gene expression in response to porcine circovirus type 2 subclinical infection. Vet Res 41:12
33. Goher M, Hicks JA, Liu HC (2013) The interplay between MDV and HVT affects viral miRNa expression. Avian Dis 57:372–379
34. Ferretti C, La Cava A (2014) miR-126, a new modulator of innate immunity. Cell Mol Immunol 11:215–217
35. Zhu B, Zhou Y, Xu F, Shuai J, Li X, Fang W (2012) Porcine circovirus type 2 induces autophagy via the AMPK/ERK/TSC2/mTOR signaling pathway in PK-15 cells. J Virol 86:12003–12012
36. Wei L, Liu J (2009) Porcine circovirus type 2 replication is impaired by inhibition of the extracellular signal-regulated kinase (ERK) signaling pathway. Virology 386:203–209
37. Ye X, Hemida MG, Qiu Y, Hanson PJ, Zhang HM, Yang D (2013) MiR-126 promotes coxsackievirus replication by mediating cross-talk of ERK1/2 and Wnt/beta-catenin signal pathways. Cell Mol Life Sci 70:4631–4644
38. Setta-Kaffetzi N, Simpson MA, Navarini AA, Patel VM, Lu HC, Allen MH, Duckworth M, Bachelez H, Burden AD, Choon SE, Griffiths CE, Kirby B, Kolios A, Seyger MM, Prins C, Smahi A, Trembath RC, Fraternali F, Smith CH, Barker JN, Capon F (2014) AP1S3 mutations are associated with pustular psoriasis and impaired Toll-like receptor 3 trafficking. Am J Hum Genet 94:790–797
39. Fernandes LT, Tomas A, Bensaid A, Perez-Enciso M, Sibila M, Sanchez A, Segales J (2009) Exploratory study on the transcriptional profile of pigs subclinically infected with porcine circovirus type 2. Anim Biotechnol 20:96–109
40. Koens L, Qin YJ, Leung WY, Corver WE, Jansen PM, Willemze R, Vermeer MH, Tensen CP (2013) MicroRNA profiling of primary cutaneous large B-cell lymphomas. PLoS One 8:e82471
41. Cullen BR (2010) Five questions about viruses and microRNAs. PLoS Pathog 6:e1000787
42. Yan H, Zhou Y, Liu Y, Deng Y, Chen X (2014) miR-252 of the Asian tiger mosquito Aedes albopictus regulates dengue virus replication by suppressing the expression of the dengue virus envelope protein. J Med Virol 86:1428–1436
43. Bogerd HP, Skalsky RL, Kennedy EM, Furuse Y, Whisnant AW, Flores O, Schultz KL, Putnam N, Barrows NJ, Sherry B, Scholle F, Garcia-Blanco MA, Griffin DE, Cullen BR (2014) Replication of many human viruses is refractory to inhibition by endogenous cellular microRNAs. J Virol 88:8065–8076

Identification of systemic immune response markers through metabolomic profiling of plasma from calves given an intra-nasally delivered respiratory vaccine

Darren W Gray[1*], Michael D Welsh[2], Simon Doherty[2], Fawad Mansoor[2], Olivier P Chevallier[1], Christopher T Elliott[1] and Mark H Mooney[1]

Abstract

Vaccination procedures within the cattle industry are important disease control tools to minimize economic and welfare burdens associated with respiratory pathogens. However, new vaccine, antigen and carrier technologies are required to combat emerging viral strains and enhance the efficacy of respiratory vaccines, particularly at the point of pathogen entry. New technologies, specifically metabolomic profiling, could be applied to identify metabolite immune-correlates representative of immune protection following vaccination aiding in the design and screening of vaccine candidates. This study for the first time demonstrates the ability of untargeted UPLC-MS metabolomic profiling to identify metabolite immune correlates characteristic of immune responses following mucosal vaccination in calves. Male Holstein Friesian calves were vaccinated with Pfizer Rispoval® PI3 + RSV intranasal vaccine and metabolomic profiling of post-vaccination plasma revealed 12 metabolites whose peak intensities differed significantly from controls. Plasma levels of glycocholic acid, N-[(3α,5β,12α)-3,12-Dihydroxy-7,24-dioxocholan-24-yl]glycine, uric acid and biliverdin were found to be significantly elevated in vaccinated animals following secondary vaccine administration, whereas hippuric acid significantly decreased. In contrast, significant upregulation of taurodeoxycholic acid and propionylcarnitine levels were confined to primary vaccine administration. Assessment of such metabolite markers may provide greater information on the immune pathways stimulated from vaccine formulations and benchmarking early metabolomic responses to highly immunogenic vaccine formulations could provide a means for rapidly assessing new vaccine formulations. Furthermore, the identification of metabolic systemic immune response markers which relate to specific cell signaling pathways of the immune system could allow for targeted vaccine design to stimulate key pathways which can be assessed at the metabolic level.

Introduction

The vaccination of farm animals against endemic, genetically evolving and emerging pathogens is important not only to ensure animal health, but also to reduce the costs associated with disease losses, either clinical or subclinical. Successful vaccination leads to the production of specific T and B cell effector immune responses that assist in the control of infection within the animal. This results in the generation of virus neutralizing antibodies that recognize the pathogen, specific effector T-cell responses and the development of an immune memory response helping to protect against future exposure to the infection. Continuous vaccine development is required to address virus evolution, new and emerging viral threats and to improve vaccine efficacy against currently managed pathogens. However, assessment of new vaccine candidates, adjuvant and novel vaccine carrier systems (such as nanoparticles) using animal trials is extremely expensive and can take several months to years (investigation of short term immune responses, vaccine-challenge studies and field trials and long term immune protection against natural wildtype virus challenge) [1]. Although

* Correspondence: d.gray@qub.ac.uk
[1]Institute for Global Food Security (IGFS), School of Biological Sciences, Queen's University Belfast (QUB), Belfast, Northern Ireland, BT9 5AG, UK
Full list of author information is available at the end of the article

the expenditure associated with animal vaccine development is not fully disclosed, the estimated budget required to develop a single FDA approved vaccine for human studies is estimated in the region of $1-2 billion [2]. The majority of these costs are attributed to the high failure rate of vaccine candidates/formulations, with only 1 in every 10 000 vaccine formulations gaining approval by the FDA [3]. New vaccine candidates may initially be assessed in mice models, however this does not necessarily translate to performance in the target species and animal trials can have poor efficacy [4] or fail to induce immune protection at all [5] as a result of species differences in immune systems [3]. Furthermore, many factors such: as immune system maturity, vaccine delivery route, concurrent infections, poor nutrition and the presence of maternally derived antibodies can affect vaccine efficacy [6]. As the expenditure associated with candidate vaccine development escalates with clinical trial progression, rapid vaccine screening methods which can assess candidate vaccine effectiveness at early trial stages in vivo are required to minimize financial outlay and improve the speed of vaccine development pipelines.

In the agricultural industry the Bovine Respiratory Disease (BRD) complex is considered to be one of the most significant causes of economic loss in intensively reared cattle worldwide. The associated losses accruing from the elevated mortality and poor growth performance of infected animals [7] coupled with the need for costly therapeutic interventions have a significant negative impact on farm incomes. This disease complex is estimated to result in an annual total economic loss to the US agri-food industry of over $2 billion, with treatment and preventative costs approaching $3 billion [8]. Whilst vaccination against the infectious agents involved in BRD pathogenesis is currently employed to manage the disease [9,10], it has not significantly reduced BRD prevalence or severity. Furthermore, it has been observed that some animals fail to develop immune protection despite vaccine treatment, becoming infected with each new seasonal BRD outbreak [11]. Therefore, the development of new methods for screening BRD pathogen vaccine candidates, along with the clear understanding of the host immune response, would provide significant economic and animal welfare benefits to the agricultural industry by speeding up the vaccine development.

Current methods for determining viral vaccine effectiveness in mammalian species include assessment of neutralizing antibody titre [12,13], PCR-based detection of viral load in infected tissues at post-immunization challenge [12], expression of pro- and anti-inflammatory cytokines [13], duration of viral shedding after post-immunization challenge [14], and mortality/morbidity findings at post-mortem [15]. However, the quantitative analysis of pro- and anti-inflammatory cytokines is generally considered to be one of the important indicators of vaccine efficacy, but typically only occurs after preliminary candidate antigen or formulation screening [6], and may require a number of vaccines and challenge studies to fully elucidate the important factors associated with a protective immune response. A greater understanding of not only the proteomic responses to vaccination [16,17], but also the changes at the metabolic level in bio-fluids, such as plasma or serum, may help develop early marker-based screening tests. These can be used to assess the potential of new vaccine candidates and also may provide additional information to improve the rationale behind future vaccine approaches taking into account vaccine delivery routes, vaccine carrier technologies and animal genetics.

Untargeted metabolomic profiling refers to the top down global analysis of small molecules or "metabolites" with molecular weights less than 1 kDa and is typically performed by Nuclear Magnetic Resonance (NMR) or mass spectrometry (MS) techniques, with the later offering greater sensitivity. Ultra Performance Liquid Chromatography (UPLC) coupled to a highly accurate mass spectrometer allows for the separation and determination of elemental composition (and hence the identification) of 1000s of metabolites in a single sample. As metabolites are often end-stage products of biological processes, their analysis can provide a greater understanding of the physiological state of an organism at the time of sampling compared to genomic or proteomic analysis. The application of metabolomic techniques to the analysis of bio-fluids has been found to offer interesting new insights to the understanding of the physiological processes involved in disease development and diagnosis [18-21]. However, to date little emphasis has been placed on assessing the in vivo metabolomic changes induced by immunization procedures and foreign antigen exposure.

This study for the first time reports the metabolomic responses in plasma of calves vaccinated with an intranasal vaccine (Pfizer Rispoval® PI3 + RSV) composed of the modified live viruses Bovine Respiratory Syncytial Virus (BRSV) and Bovine Parainfluenza Virus-3 (BPI3V). BRSV and BPI3V are two of the major viral pathogens involved in the Bovine Respiratory Disease (BRD) complex [7]. The aims of the current study were to identify plasma metabolomic markers of the primary and secondary immune response in calves to administration of a commercial intranasal vaccine containing live modified virus. Importantly, it is well known that vaccination via the parenteral route leads to poor protection at mucosal surfaces. Therefore the studies undertaken here allow vaccine immunology and biomarkers to be identified through the natural route of infection for these respiratory viruses in order to identify the most suitable host defense mechanisms. This is the first untargeted UPLC-MS based metabolomics study to reveal metabolite markers of the immune response occurring during vaccination which may have potential use in the early screening of candidate vaccine effectiveness and aid new vaccine design by increasing the understanding of the processes involved in immune response development post vaccination.

Materials and methods

Chemicals and reagents

HPLC grade acetone was purchased from Sigma Aldrich (Dorset, UK). LC-MS grade acetonitrile, water, methanol and chloroform were purchased from Fisher Scientific (Loughborough, UK). All analytical standards for metabolite confirmation were purchased from Sigma Aldrich.

Experimental design and sample collection

All animal studies were carried out in accordance with the UK Animals (Scientific Procedures) Act 1986 and with the approval of the AFBI Ethical Review Committee. Figure 1 illustrates the experimental design and sample collection days throughout the study. Twelve male Holstein Friesian calves aged between 20 and 25 weeks were divided into two study groups ($n = 6$) and assigned as non-vaccinated or vaccinated calves. Vaccinated calves were treated with Pfizer Rispoval® PI3 + RSV intranasal vaccine (designated vaccinated animals) as per manufacturers instructions, and non-vaccinated calves were treated with empty poly(lactic-co-glycolic) acid PLGA nanoparticles (designated non-vaccinated) prepared using standard double emulsification solvent evaporation technique (w/o/w) [22]. Calves were dosed at day 0 and day 35, and screened weekly for the presence of BPI3V IgG in blood serum using Svanovir-PI3V-Ab kit (Boehringer Ingelheim Svanovir, Uppsala, Sweden) as per manufacturer's instructions. Calves were sampled at days 0 (pre-dosage), 7, 14, 28 (initial vaccine dosage), 42, 49 and 63 (booster dosage). One week after completion of the vaccination study (day 70) all calves were experimentally challenged with BPI3V through nasal inoculation with 2 mL of virus suspension ($TCID_{50}$ of $10^{6.78}$/mL) per nostril. Calves were sampled at days 70, 75, 82, 84 and 90 (days 0, 5, 12, 14 and 20 post-BPI3V challenge respectively). Serum was prepared from blood drawn by jugular venepuncture into 10 mL BD Vacutainer® glass serum tubes. The blood was allowed to clot at room temperature for 30 min prior to centrifugation at 2000 *g* to remove the clot. Samples were stored at 4 °C prior to analysis. Blood haematology was monitored weekly during vaccination stages and at days 70, 75, 82, 84 and 90 (post-BPI3V challenge stages). Rectal temperatures were taken at days 14, 28, 42 and 63. Blood was sampled from the calves by jugular venepuncture into 6 ml plastic K3 EDTA Vacuette tubes (Greiner bio-one, Stroudwater, UK) and processed to platelet poor plasma by the double centrifugation method previously described [23]. All samples were processed at random within 2 h of initial blood sampling and stored at −80 °C prior to use.

Sample preparation

600 μL of plasma was added to 2.4 mL of ice cold acetone, vortexed for 30 s and placed on ice for 15 min. The sample was then deproteinated by centrifugation at

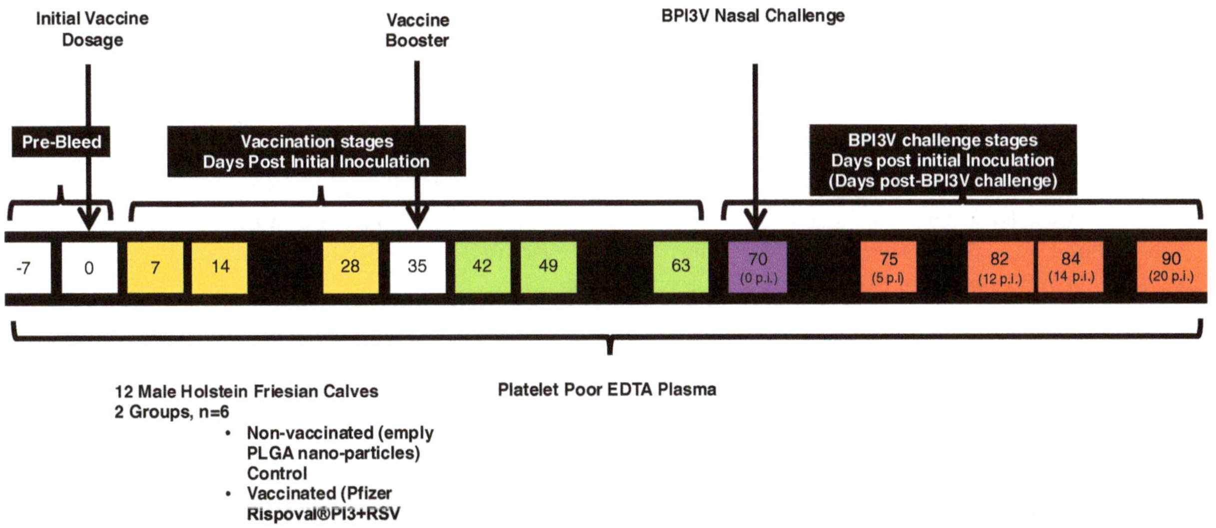

Figure 1 Sampling points for metabolomic profiling of plasma in calves following vaccination and subsequent BPI3V challenge. Male Holstein Friesian calves were dosed with Pfizer Rispoval®PI3 + RSV intranasal vaccine (vaccinated) or empty PLGA nanoparticles (non-vaccinated) at day 0. A secondary booster dosage was administered at day 35. At day 70 all animals were experimentally challenged with BPI3V via nasal inoculation. At day 6 during the BPI3V challenge study 3 calves per group were sacrificed for viral isolation and histology. Sampling points for metabolomic profiling of plasma are indicated throughout.

4000 *g* at 4 °C for 20 min. 2.4 mL of supernatant was removed and dried under nitrogen for 45 min at 40 °C using TurboVap LV (Caliper Life Sciences, Hopkinton, USA). Resulting residue was reconstituted in 500 µL of Ultra Pure H_2O and liquid/liquid extraction of lipids performed by addition of 500 µL of ice-cold Methanol: Chloroform (1:1 v/v) and vortexing for 30 s followed by centrifugation at 16 000 *g* at 4 °C for 15 min. liquid/ liquid extraction was repeated and after centrifugation 900 µL of the aqueous layer was removed and dried under nitrogen using TurboVap at 40 °C for 45 min. The residue was reconstituted in 300 µL Ultra Pure H_2O and filtered by centrifugation at 10 000 *g* at 4 °C using 0.22 µm Constar Spin-X® Centrifuge Tube Filter for 5 min.

UPLC-MS analysis of Bovine Plasma

UPLC-MS analysis was performed using an Acquity UPLC system coupled to a XEVO G2 Q-TOF (Waters Corporation, Milford, MA, USA. 8 µL of prepared sample extracts were injected onto an Acquity UPLC HSS-T3 C18 column (100 mm × 2.1 mm i.d., 1.8 µm; Waters Corporation, Milford, MA, USA). Column and autosampler temperature were maintained at 50 °C and 10 °C respectively. Chromatographic separation was carried out at a flow rate of 600 µL/min with mobile phase consisting of 99.9% H_2O/0.1% Formic Acid (A) and 99.9% Acetonitrile/0.1% Formic Acid (B). The elution gradient was as follows: 0–2 min isocratic at 1% of B, 2–14.5 min linear gradient from 1-100% of B, 14.5-17 min isocratic at 100% of B, 17–17.5 min linear gradient from 100-1% of B and finally 17.5-20 min isocratic at 1% of B. Mass spectrometry was performed using a Waters XEVO G2 QTOF operating in positive-ion mode (ESI+) with the capillary voltage set to 1500 V and the sampling cone voltage 30 V. The desolvation and cone gas flows were set at 750 L/h and 100 L/h respectively. Source and desolvation temperatures were 120 °C and 400 °C respectively. Leucine Enkephalin ($[M+H]^+$= 278.1141 Da, and [M+ H] = 556.2771 Da) was used for accurate lockmass calibration during data acquisition. Lockmass acquisition settings were: 0.5 s scan time, 30 s interval, 3 scan average, mass window +/− 0.5 Da. Collision energy was only applied on function 2, with ramping between 15 V and 30 V and centroid data was acquired using positive-ion, resolution mode.

Mass spectrometry data processing

Total Ion Count (TIC) chromatograms and spectra were acquired with MassLynx version 4.1 (Waters) in centroid format and metabolite data was processed using MarkerLynx software (Waters Corporation, Milford, MA, USA). The MarkerLynx method for data extraction and de-convolution was as follows: Ions were extracted from function 1 data using peak detection analysis of retention time window 0.30-14.50 min, with a mass range of 100 Da to 1200 Da. The extracted-ion chromatogram (XIC) window for data collection was 0.2 Da and apex peak tracking parameters were set to automatic with no smoothing. Data collection parameters consisted of an intensity threshold (counts) of 500 and a mass window of 0.02 Da with a retention time window of 0.20 min. A noise elimination level of 6 was applied and isotopes were removed. Peak heights for extracted ions were normalized against the total peak height of all extracted ions and standardized to a total ion count of 10 000. The results were exported in .csv format as a two dimensional data table in which rows and columns respectively represented analysed samples and the relative normalized peak heights of each detected mass spectrometric signal, i.e. as an Accurate Mass (m/z) and Retention Time (min) Pair (AMRTP).

Data analysis

Temporal changes in BPI3V antibody titre were analysed using two-tailed paired *T*-test, and significant differences between treatment groups at sampling stages was assessed using two-tailed heteroscedastic *T*-test. SIMCA-P+ version 13.0 (Umetrics, Sweden) was used for multivariate metabolite marker selection. For SIMCA-P+ analysis, data was prefiltered to exclude AMRTPs with coefficient of variation greater than 50% in replicate quality control pools. All centroid data were Pareto scaled and analysed by unsupervised Principle Component Analysis (PCA) and supervised discriminatory analysis by Orthogonal Projections of Latent Structures-Discriminant Analysis (OPLS-DA). Unsupervised PCA models were generated at each sampling day to reveal potential relationships between treatment groups. Supervised analysis by OPLS-DA was performed to reveal potential markers of response to treatment in vaccinated calves compared to non-vaccinated calves at each sampling day. Robustness of final OPLS-DA discriminative models was assessed by setting a predictive model of each case in which 2/3 of the data (known treatment) was used to predict the remaining 1/3 (unknown treatment).

Identification of potential metabolite markers

The elemental composition of selected parent compounds was determined in MassLynx using both positive and negative mode data. Mass uncertainty was set to 3mDa, odd and even electron state, carbon isotope filter of +/− 5% and elements included were C, H, O, N, P and S. Where applicable Na and K adduct elemental composition were determined with the respective element included in the analysis parameters. Elemental compositions were searched against PubChem and Chemspider online databases, and where possible Function 2 fragments were matched against Metlin, HMDB or Massbank databases. Where fragmentation spectra for the analyte in question was not available, in silico fragmentation was performed using Metfrag and Function 2 fragmentation data was validated against potential in silico fragments. Compounds revealed by database matching or in silico fragmentation had their identities confirmed against commercial analytical standards by UPLC-MS. Pooled plasma samples and individual standards (1 μM) were analysed under identical UPLC and mass spectrometric run conditions as utilized previously, and metabolite identities confirmed by matching retention time and Function 1 and Function 2 spectra (including low and high energy fragments and adducts).

Results

Haematological and immunological responses to vaccination

Calves were monitored throughout the study to ensure normal health status and assess immunological responses to vaccination. Rectal temperatures taken at days 14, 28, 42 and 63 were within the reference parameters 38.3 to 39.4 °C with no significant differences observed between study groups (as illustrated in Additional file 1). Serum was obtained from all calves to determine weekly IgG anti BPI3V sera titres during vaccination procedures and to perform routine blood hematology analysis to validate calve health. The results of BPI3V IgG antibody titre screening are shown in Figure 2 in addition to lymphocyte and neutrophil counts obtained from hematology results. Prior to vaccination no significant differences in the BPI3V IgG antibody titre between study groups were observed (Figure 2A). IgG BPI3V antibody titres were significantly elevated ($p < 0.05$) in vaccinated calves compared to non-vaccinated calves at days 14, 49, 56 and 63. The BPI3V IgG antibody titre in vaccinated calves was shown to increase significantly ($p < 0.05$) from days 7 to 14 and significantly ($p < 0.05$) declined from day 14 to 28 whilst remaining significantly ($p < 0.05$) elevated compared to day 0. On administration of the second vaccine dosage (day 35) BPI3V IgG antibody titre increased ($p < 0.05$) from days 42 to 56, and remained significantly elevated in the vaccinated study group relative to non-vaccinated calves until day 63. These IgG responses indicate that the booster immunization was necessary to further increase the titres of BPI3V specific antibodies. Upon BPI3V challenge at day 70, BPI3V IgG antibody titre was maintained at significantly higher ($p < 0.05$) levels at days 70 and 75 in vaccinated calves compared to non-vaccinated calves indicating an adaptive primed immune response to infection. There was an observed drop in BPI3V IgG titre in vaccinated calves from day 70 to day 75 but this level was still significantly higher than that found in non-vaccinated calves ($p < 0.05$). There were no significant changes in the levels of BPI3V IgG titre in vaccinated or non-vaccinated calves throughout the remaining infection stages, with mean BPI3V IgG titres remaining higher in vaccinated calves compared to non-vaccinated.

The haematology results are illustrated in Additional file 1. Red Blood Cell count (RCC), White Blood Cell count (WCC), Hemoglobin content (HG), Mean Corpuscular Volume (MCV), Mean Corpuscular Haemoglobin (MCH), Packed Cell Volume (PCV) and Platelet count (PLT) measurements for all calves were within the specified reference parameters based on data from Brun-Hansen et al. [24] for calves at corresponding ages which are known to differ from adults. However, significant differences in lymphocyte and neutrophil count were observed between study groups at a number of points throughout the vaccination stages of the study whilst remaining within reference parameters for healthy animals. Figure 2B reveals significantly ($p < 0.05$) higher lymphocyte counts at day 42 (2 weeks post-booster immunization) in vaccinated animals compared to non-vaccinated. Furthermore, lymphocyte counts in vaccinated animals were found to rise significantly ($p < 0.05$) from day 14 to 42 and decreased from day 49 to 63, with no significant temporal changes observed in non-vaccinated animals. Figure 2C illustrates that neutrophil counts were significantly higher at day 0 ($p < 0.01$) and day 14 ($p < 0.05$) and significantly lower ($p < 0.05$) at day 42 in vaccinated compared to non-vaccinated animals. Neutrophil counts decreased significantly ($p < 0.05$) in vaccinated animals from day 14 to 42 and increased significantly ($p < 0.05$) in non-vaccinated animals from day 14 to 42. At post-BPI3V challenge stages, WCC, RCC and lymphocyte counts were outside reference parameters. There was a significant ($p < 0.05$) rise in WCC in non-vaccinated animals after BPI3V infection from days 70 to day 75 and WCC was higher than reference parameters from days 75 to 90 in vaccinated calves, and significantly ($p < 0.05$) higher at day 90 in vaccinated calves compared to non-vaccinated. RCC was elevated outside reference parameters throughout the study and was significantly ($p < 0.05$) higher in vaccinated calves at day 75 compared to non-vaccinated. Whilst No significant differences were observed in lymphocyte counts between study groups, lymphocyte counts were above the reference parameters in both study groups at day 75. There was a significant increase in lymphocyte counts in non-vaccinated animals from day 70 to 75 and a significant decrease from days 75 between days 82, with no significant variations observed in lymphocyte counts of vaccinated animals. There were no observed significant differences in neutrophil counts between study groups at corresponding sampling points post-infection, however, significant ($p < 0.05$) temporal variations were observed with a decrease from day 70 to 75 in non-vaccinated animals, and an increase from day

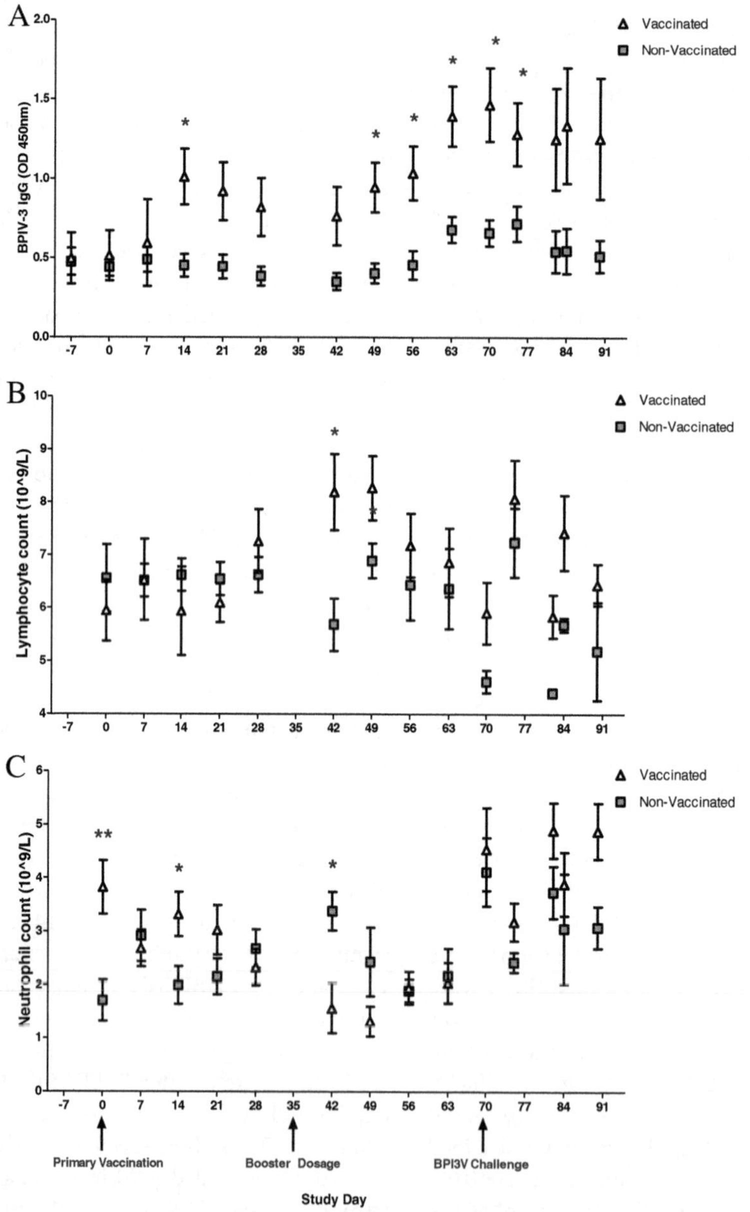

Figure 2 BPI3V-IgG, Lymphocyte and Neutrophil variations in response to vaccination and subsequent BPI3V challenge. (A) BPI3V antibody titre was determined in serum samples using Svanovir-PIV3 Ab Kit. **(B)** Lymphocyte and **(C)** neutrophil counts in blood. Significant differences in vaccinated animals compared to non-vaccinated animals at the same study day are indicated * $p < 0.05$, ** $p < 0.01$ and *** $p < 0.001$. Values represent mean ± S.E.M, $n = 6$.

75 to 82 in both study groups. Despite being within the reference parameters, significant differences were observed in PCV at day 75, MCV at day 82 and MCH at day 75 between study groups.

Selection of metabolomic markers of vaccine response via multivariate data analysis

Representative Base Peak Intensity (BPI) chromatograms of plasma from both a vaccinated and non-vaccinated calf at day 49 are presented in Figure 3. When observing the acquired chromatograms there is obvious poor column retention of polar compounds between 1 min and 2 min. Between 2 min and 14.5 min chromatographic separation was excellent, with no observable overlapping peaks and minor differences between the acquired profiles of respective study groups (e.g. peaks at 5.00 min and 7.73 min) can be determined by visual examination. 3224 features were extracted from raw data using MarkerLynx and normalized to reduce the effects of batch to batch variation in subsequent analysis steps. In order to validate

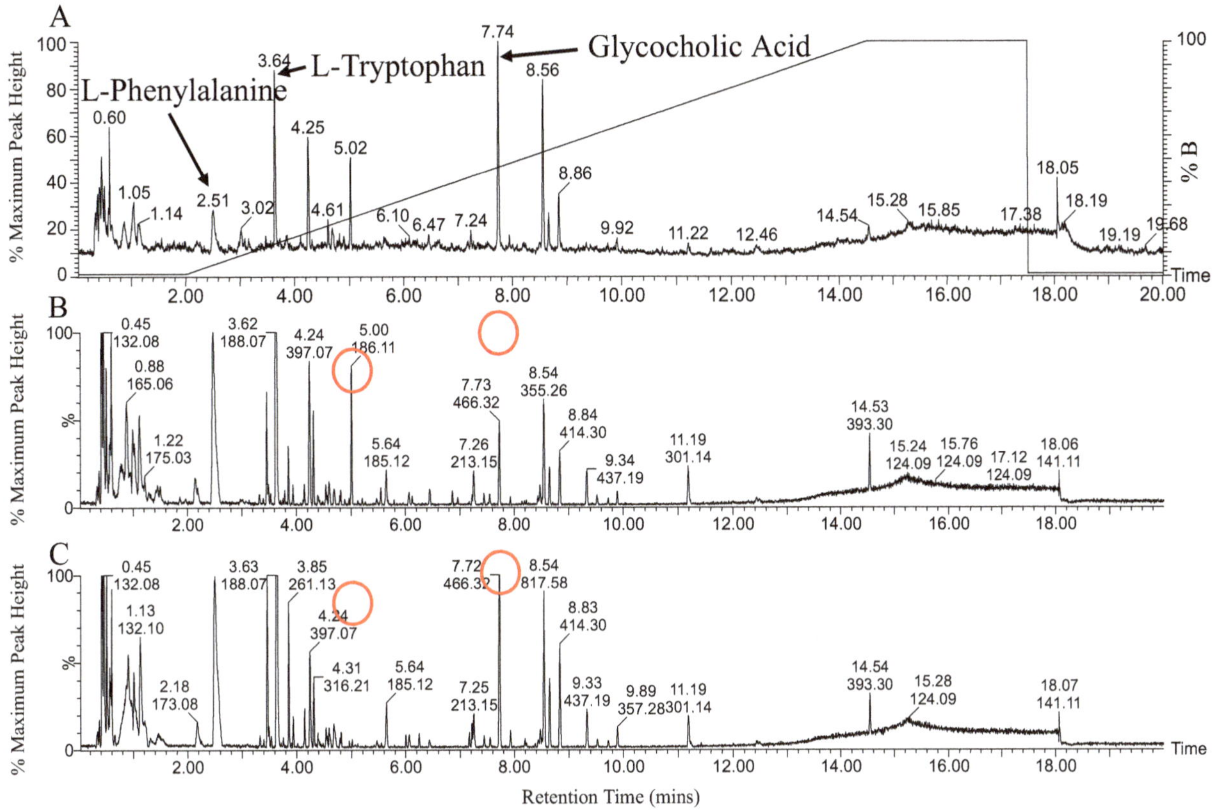

Figure 3 Metabolomic profiling of bovine plasma by positive ionization UPLC-MS. (A) Total Ion Chromatogram (TIC) of bovine plasma. Peaks relating to L-phenylalanine, L-tryptophan and glycocholic acid are indicated. The percentage of solvent B (99.9% acetonitrile, 0.1% formic acid) is indicated on right Y axis. **(B)** BPI chromatograms of plasma from a vaccinated calf at day 49 (two weeks after booster dosage), and **(C)** BPI chromatogram of plasma from a non-vaccinated calf at day 49. Representative differences between treatment groups are at the peaks indicated with retention times 5.00 and 7.73 min.

instrument performance landmark compounds in plasma (validated using pure standards) were used to analyse retention time deviation and mass accuracy between and within batch runs. The retention time deviation and mass accuracy of L-Phenylalanine, L-Tryptophan and Glycocholic Acid were determined in inter-run quality control pools and are presented in Additional file 2. Mass accuracy was consistent for all markers, with a maximum deviation of 2.26mDa. The maximum retention time deviation of peak top time was approximately 6 s. Maximum retention time deviation was observed with phenylalanine which can be accounted for by its wider elution time as illustrated in Figure 3. The excellent retention time stability and mass accuracy during and between separate analysis runs provides assurance in accuracy of the data collected.

Untargeted Principle Component Analysis (PCA) was performed in SIMCA-P+ v 13. The dataset was filtered to exclude variables with a coefficient of variation greater than 50% in replicate quality control pools. PCA models were constructed from 764 AMRTPs, and further divided into sub-models by sampling day. Replicate injections were tightly clustered on the PCA scores plot, indicating low inter-run variation in peak intensity. No injections were observed as having d-mox twice d-crit (possible outliers). The majority of variation explained by principle components (PC) 1 and 2 was due to variation between the three analysis runs (48.3 to 57.1%), and therefore for all stage PCA sub-models only PCs 3 and 4 were investigated. At days 7, 14, 42 and 49 there was separation on the PCA-scores plot between study groups when observing the variation in the data explained by principle components 3 and 4 shown in Figures 4B,C,E and F. Roughly 14 to 20% of the variation in the dataset was responsible for group separation in PCs 3 and 4 in substage PCA models. However, at days 28 and 63 there was a significant overlap between treatment groups (Figures 4D and G respectively). When the data from each analysis run was treated separately to remove run-to-run noise, group separation was achieved using principle components 1 and 2 only. Therefore, the only negative impact of combining data from separate analyses was

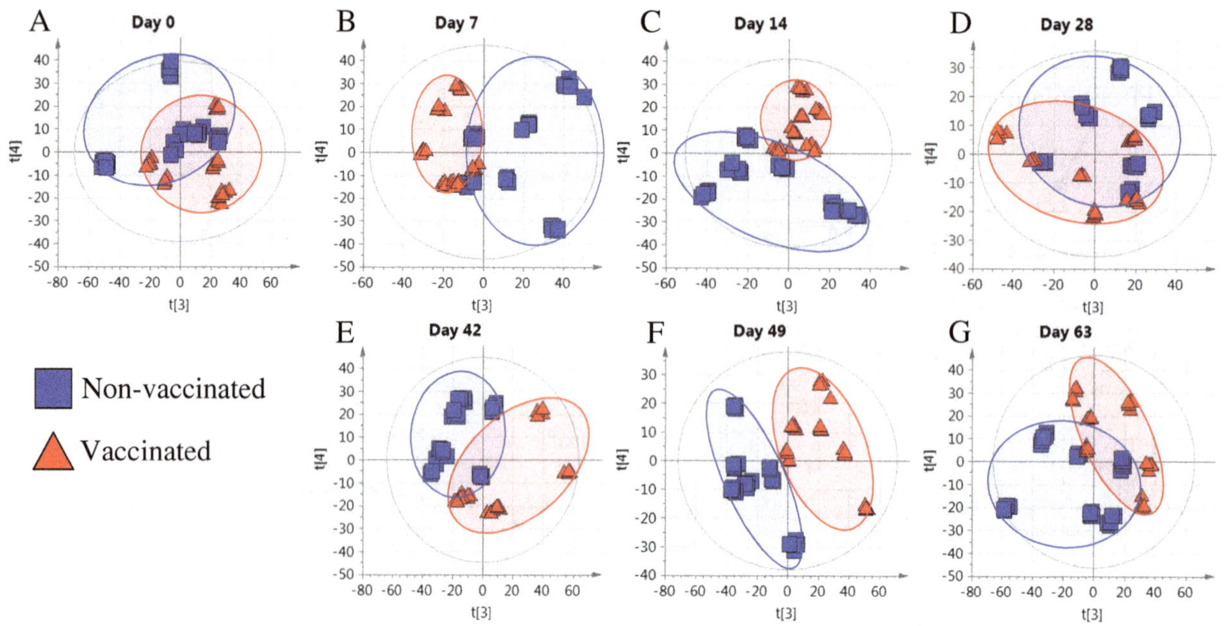

Figure 4 Unsupervised PCA scores plot of UPLC-MS profiled plasma from vaccinated and non-vaccinated calves. Unsupervised PCA scores plot of plasma from vaccinated and non-vaccinated calves at days 0, 7, 14, 28, 42, 49 and 63 are illustrated in Figures 4 **A-G** respectively.

that components representing analysis run separation could be ignored.

OPLS-DA was used for the selection of markers of immune response to vaccination. In order to validate OPLS-DA models, 2/3 of the randomly selected data (4 calves per group) was used to generate OPLS-DA models, with the remaining 1/3 used as a test set. The results from cross validation are illustrated in Additional file 3. At days 7, 14, 42 and 49 constructed models could accurately predict class allocation for the test set. At days 28 and 63 there was no correct classification for test samples, concurrent with the PCA scores plot in which there was no separation between study groups. Therefore, OPLS-DA models were constructed at days 7, 14, 42 and 49 for the selection of potential markers with all experimental calves used in the generation of these models. For all models the variables which contributed to study group discrimination in OPLS-DA models were selected on the criteria of a variable importance (V.I.P.) score > 1. The OPLS-DA S-plots of the metabolomic profiling of plasma from vaccinated and non-vaccinated calves at days 7, 14, 42 and 49 are illustrated in Figures 5A-D respectively. Many of the variables which contributed to the discrimination between study groups were related low energy fragments or adducts of parent compounds. 96 AMRTPs which demonstrated significant variation ($p < 0.05$, two-tailed heteroscedastic *T*-test) and a fold-change (FC) greater than 1.5 between treatment groups were selected (see Additional file 4). Significant AMRTPs were filtered to remove those with poorly consistent peak heights in replicate injections and high intergroup variability. Fragment ions and adducts were then identified by observing mass differences in co-eluting AMRTPS. Na and K adducts were observed as having mass differences of +22 and +38 respectively relative to the parent compound mass (M + H). Furthermore, by investigating function 2 fragmentation data, parent ions were selected as often having reduced peak intensity compared to Function 1.

Identification of parent ions and AMRTPs

Final selection for parent ions was based on raw data, not normalized intensity, reducing the chance of including normalization induced false positives. AMRTPs with poorly consistent peak intensity in replicate infections were also removed. Out of the 16 final parent ions selected, 4 were removed as being artifacts of the normalization process. The 12 remaining AMRTP parent ions were selected for identification using a combination of database searching, spectral matching, elemental composition analysis and in silico fragmentation. For AMRTP identification function 2 MS/MS data was screened in Metlin for MS/MS fragmentation patterns. When available, if MS/MS fragmentation data was present in the database, MS/MS function 2 data in +ve or −ve ionization mode was screened for identification. Elemental composition of the 12 parent compound was determined in MassLynx. 6 of the 12 compounds chosen had % confidence fit of the isotope pattern between 90 and 100%. Function 2 fragmentation data was screened

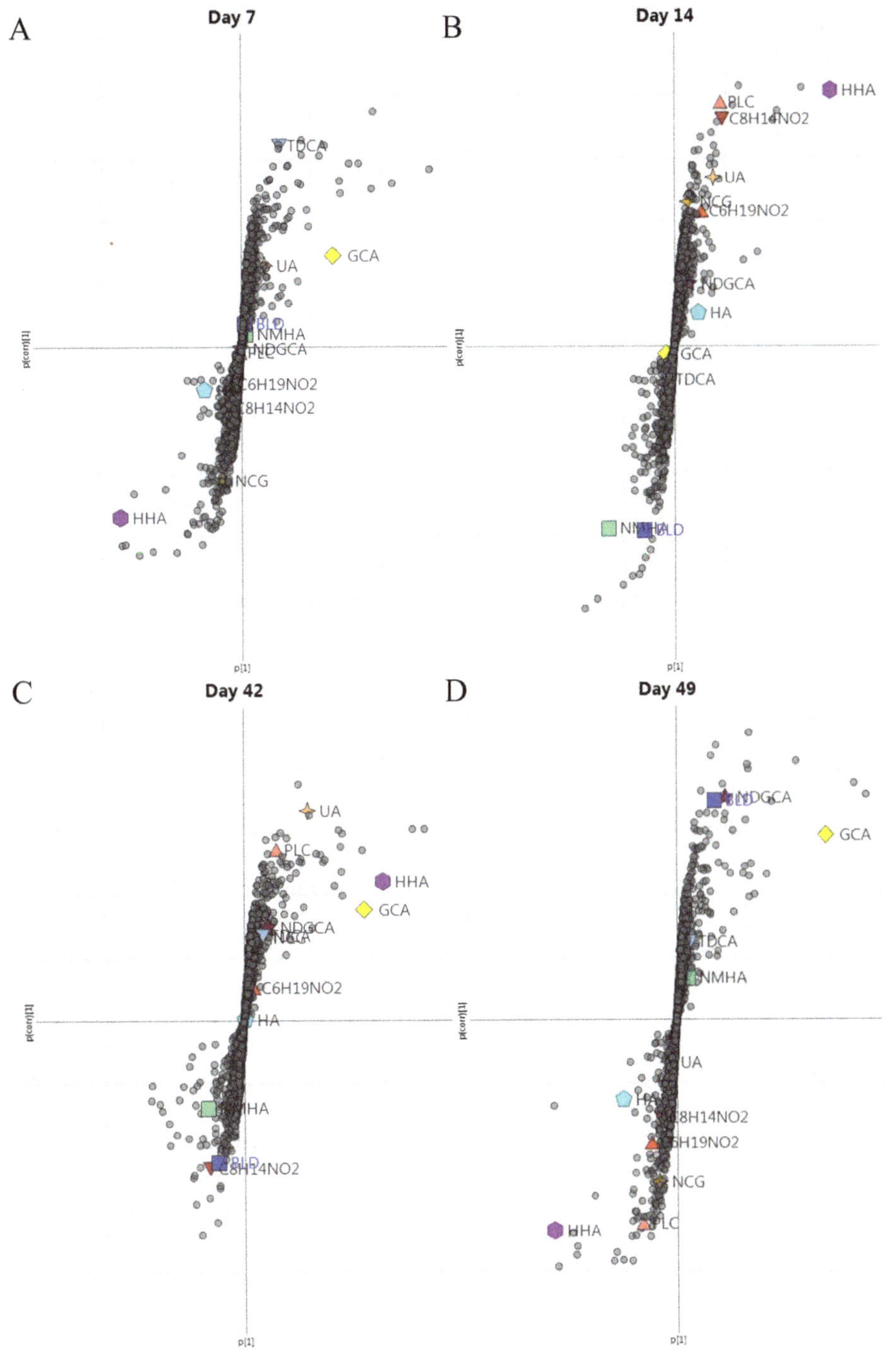

Figure 5 S-plots of supervised OPLS-DA analysis of UPLC-MS profiled plasma from vaccinated and non-vaccinated calves. Supervised OPLS-DA S-plot plots of plasma from vaccinated and non-vaccinated calves at days 7, 14, 42 and 49 are illustrated in Figures 5**A-D** respectively. The location of AMRTPs on the S-Plot is a combination of influence (p [1]) and reliability (p(corr) [1]) on the discrimination of study groups by OPLS-DA. Identified vaccine response markers and AMRPTs selected throughout the study are marked on the S-Plot.

against the Metlin online database. The retention time and accurate mass of identified markers of immune response to vaccination are presented in Table 1 together with the percentage confidence of elemental composition determination in addition to potential database IDs.

Of the 12 potential markers identified to differ significantly between vaccination study groups, 5 had their identities confirmed using pure standards (Uric Acid (UA), Glycocholic Acid (GCA), Taurodeoxycholic Acid (TDCA), Biliverdin (BLD), Hippuric Acid, (HA) and

Table 1 Final AMRPTs selected as metabolomic markers of response to vaccination

AMRTP I.D.	Retention time (mins)	Measured mass (Da)	Elemental composition (M + H)	% Fit confidence	Mass Error (mDa)	PubChem I.D.	Compound
0.4295_151.145	0.4295	151.145	C6H19N2O2	98.17	0.7		Unknown
0.4926_156.105	0.4926	156.105	C8H14NO2	99.66	1.4		Unknown
0.6158_169.039	0.6158	169.039	C5H5N4O3	99.48	−0.4	1175	Uric Acid (UA)[a]
1.4952_218.14	1.4952	218.14	C10H20NO4	95.95	−0.2	107738	Propionylcarnitine (PLC)
4.2427_180.066	4.2427	180.066	C9H10NO3	74.69	1.1	464	Hippuric Acid (HA) [a]
4.5993_194.082	4.5993	194.082	C10H12NO3	54.33	−1.1	97479	N-Methylhippuric Acid (NMHA)
4.8821_184.097	4.8821	184.097	C9H14NO3	34.64	−0.2	149048	N-(Cyclohex-1-en-1-ylcarbonyl)glycine (NCG)
5.006_186.113	5.006	186.113	C9H16NO3	100	0.1	147412	Hexahydrohippuric Acid (HHA)[a]
7.1759_464.3	7.1759	464.3	C26H42NO6	96.92	−0.6	10253857	N-[(3α,5β,12α)-3,12-Dihydroxy-7, 24-dioxocholan-24-yl]glycine (NDGCA)
7.7341_466.317	7.7341	466.317	C26H44NO6	16.22	−0.6	10140	Glycocholic Acid (GCA)[a]
8.2088_500.304	8.2088	500.304	C26H46NO6S	5.8	−0.8	44688	Taurodeoxycholic Acid (TDCA)[a]
8.5105_583.255	8.5105	583.255	C33H35N4O6	18.33	1.4	5280353	Biliverdin (BLD)[a]

Elemental composition of AMPRTs was calculated in MassLynx, with mass error of 3mDa, and elements C, H, O, P, S and N and % fit confidence for 3 isotopic peaks was calculated. Where possible spectral match score against function 2 data in Metlin is indicated. Compounds identified by pure standards are indicated with[a].

Hexahydrohippuric Acid (HHA)). Putative identities based on PubChem database searching and in silico fragmentation using MetFrag were obtained for propionylcarnitine (PLC), N-[(3α,5β,12α)-3,12-dihydroxy-7,24-dioxocholan-24-yl]glycine (NDGCA), N-methylhippuric acid (NMHA) and N-(cyclohex-1-en-1-ylcarbonyl)glycine (NCG) - identities for the AMRTPs 0.4295_151.145 and 0.4926_156.105, could not be assigned. The influence (p[1]) and reliability (p(corr)[1]) of these markers on the OPLS-DA multivariate data analysis can be observed in the S-plots illustrated in Figures 5A-D. AMRTPs with high influence and reliability are indicated in the top right and bottom left corners of the S-plots. The variations in detected marker peak intensities between treatment groups throughout the study are indicated in Figure 6. These findings indicate that fluctuations in metabolite marker levels can occur throughout sampling stages due to environmental factors, as illustrated in the temporal variations apparent in non-vaccinated control animals. Elevated metabolite levels in vaccinated animals, as illustrated at day 14 for 0.4926_156.105, NCG, PLC and HHA, are therefore vaccine induced temporal increases in these markers which contrasts with the normal temporal decrease observed in non-vaccinated controls as a result of environmental factors. HHA and NCG were shown to differ significantly between study groups at day 0. Repeated measures ANOVA with bonferroni post-hoc test revealed significantly different temporal relationships between study groups day 0 to day 7 with HHA and NCG found to decrease significantly ($p < 0.05$) in vaccinated animals only from day 0 to day 7. Peak intensity of HHA and NCG differed significantly between treatment groups at a number of stages, with Pearson correlation showing significant positive correlation ($p < 0.001$, r = 0.982 and r = 0.951 in vaccinated and non-vaccinated animals respectively). Coupled with TDCA these were the only AMRTPs to differ at the earliest post vaccination sampling point (day 7), prior to observable difference in anti-BPI3V IgG titre between study groups. The significant up and down regulation of 0.4926_156.105 and NMHA respectively was limited to primary vaccine dosage, and is likely to be related to the adaptive immune response to vaccination (significant rise in IgG BPI3V antibody titre at day 14). NHMA was found to significantly decrease ($p < 0.05$) from day 0 levels in vaccinated animals at day 14. Significantly higher ($p < 0.05$) 0.4296_156.105 at day 14 in vaccinated animal was a result of vaccine induced deviation from the temporal decrease from day 7 to 14 observed in non-vaccinated control animals. The remaining identified markers were found to differ significantly during the phase of secondary immune response. Peak intensity of UA was significantly higher ($p < 0.05$) in vaccinated calves compared to non-vaccinated calves at day 42 and was significantly higher ($p < 0.05$) than day 0 levels in vaccinated animals at days 7, 14 and 28. GCA was significantly up-regulated in vaccinated calves at days 42 and 49, however, this was a result of booster induced deviation in vaccinated animals which differed from the temporal profile observed in control non-vaccinated animals. Peak intensities of 0.4295_151.145 and HA were found to be significantly lower in vaccinated calves at day 49 and significantly lower ($p < 0.05$ and $p < 0.01$ respectively) than day 0 levels in vaccinated animals. BLD and NDGCA were up-regulated at day 49 in vaccinated animals, significantly higher ($p < 0.05$) than day 0 levels. Furthermore, HHA and NCG levels were found to be significantly correlated with HA throughout the study

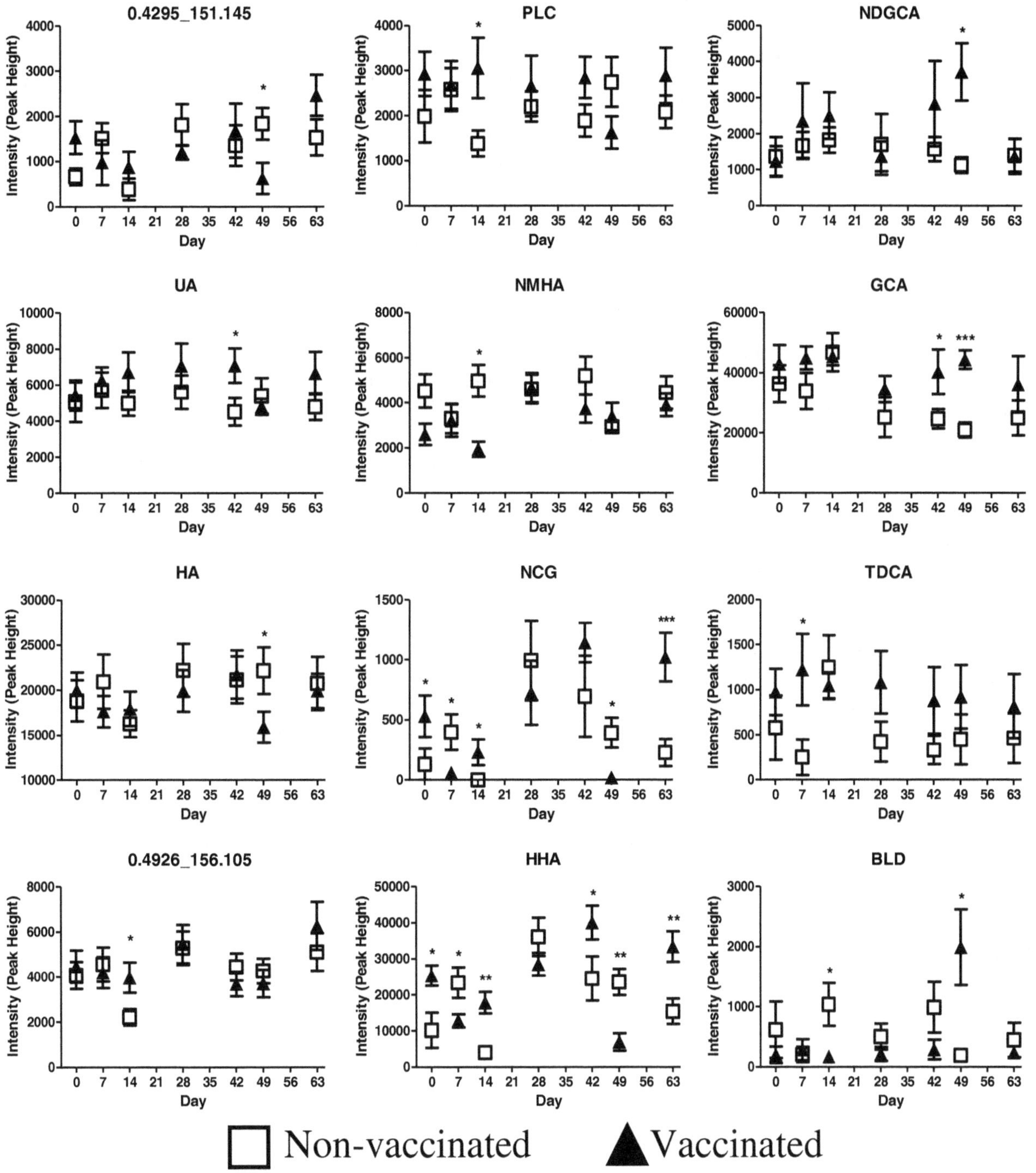

Figure 6 Temporal changes in metabolite peak intensity throughout vaccination program. Raw peak intensity (height) of the selected biomarkers at each sampling stage is indicated ($n = 6$). Significant changes in metabolite peak intensity between vaccinated and non-vaccinated calves at the corresponding study day (height) are indicated *$P < 0.05$, **$p < 0.01$, ***$p < 0.001$. Values represent mean ± S.E.M, $n = 6$.

in vaccinated and non-vaccinated animals (HHA and HA, $p < 0.001$, r = 0.971 in vaccinated animals and $p < 0.01$ and r = 0.894 in non-vaccinated animals; NCG and HA, $p < 0.01$, r = 0.917 in vaccinated animals and $p < 0.05$, r = 0.761 in non-vaccinated animals).

Discussion

Vaccine development strategies have typically focused on the induction of specific antibody responses to antigenic molecules as an indicator of effective immune stimulation (whole virus or viral proteins) with little understanding of how antigens elicit particular immune responses [6]. Whilst this approach has resulted in the majority of vaccines available today, new vaccine development is increasingly costly and it is imperative that the least promising candidates are eliminated from investigation as early as possible. Whilst the identification of immune correlations, in particular proteins such as interleukins and cytokines, has helped to improve the understanding of vaccine mediated immune response mechanisms, emerging metabolomic techniques may offer a novel perspective to vaccine development and selection. This is possible as metabolites are the ultimate end stage products or mediators of biological processes and can provide a holistic view of underlying physiological processes. This study has for the first time employed an untargeted UPLC-MS metabolomic profiling approach to identify plasma components altered by primary and secondary immune responses to an intranasal vaccination containing live modified virus. Vaccination with Pfizer Rispoval® PI3 + RSV resulted in an increase of BPI3V specific IgG antibody titre in vaccinated calves. The IgG responses indicated that the booster immunization was necessary to further increase the titres of BPI3V antibodies. This stimulated IgG response is characteristic of the immune responses typically seen in two dosage vaccination experiments. Furthermore, the high IgG titre maintained in vaccinated animals following experimental challenge with BPI3V indicates a primed immune response to infection. Conversely the non-vaccinated animals showed no significant alterations in BPI3V specific IgG titre during vaccination stages but at post-BPI3V challenge displayed a rise in WCC indicating a stimulated immune response in the absence of prior infection. We can therefore characterize the markers identified in this study which showed altered abundance between vaccinated and non-vaccinated study groups as being related to the immunological responses involved in primary and secondary immune-stimulation. Metabolomic profiling initially revealed a panel of 96 features which differed significantly between calves vaccinated intranasally with Pfizer Rispoval® PI3 + RSV and non-vaccinated calves throughout the study. These features were further refined to identify 12 high confidence parent compounds, 10 of which were identified based on database searching and spectral matching, with 6 further validated using pure standards. Based on the observed stimulated IgG response following two intranasal vaccine dosages (characteristic of the immune response typically seen in two-stage dosage vaccine programs [6]), these markers can be characterized as being related to the responses involved in primary and secondary immune stimulation. All detected markers were shown to be present in plasma prior to vaccine administration, therefore their altered abundance reflects the processes of stimulation of the mucosal immune system following exposure of animals to modified live viral vaccine, and are not associated with vaccine breakdown products.

A significant increase in BLD (10.26 FC) plasma peak intensity in vaccinated calves compared to non-vaccinated calves was observed two weeks after the second Pfizer Rispoval® PI3 + RSV dosage (day 49). BLD is degraded from heme groups by Heme Oxygenases (HO) [25] and rapidly reduced to Bilirubin by Biliverdin Reductase [26]. BLD and the HO isoform HO-1 are involved in promoting anti-inflammatory responses. BLD suppresses IL-2 production and T cell proliferation [27], and activates the aryl hydrocarbon receptor (AHR) [28] regulating T helper cell phenotype towards an anti-inflammatory regulatory T cell, or a pro-inflammatory T helper 17 effector function [29,30]. HO-1, produced from circulating monocytes during acute inflammatory states, has immunomodulatory function by supporting the proliferative capacity and activation of CD4(+) and CD8(+) T cells via CD14(+) monocytes, preventing DC maturation [31-33] and controlling Th1 pro-inflammatory cytokine production [34,35]. The observed increased plasma levels of BLD may be due to either increased HO-1 activity at a rate which cannot be matched by Biliverdin Reductase, or an unknown modulatory effect on Biliverdin Reductase affecting the rate at which it reduces BLD to bilirubin - strongly supporting BLD and HO-1 involvement in the promotion of anti-inflammatory responses as the immune stimulation response following vaccine dosage is deactivated to normal status.

Plasma peak intensities of a number of conjugated Bile Acids (BAs) were found to differ significantly between vaccinated and non-vaccinated calves, with increased TDCA (4.87 FC) after primary vaccine dosage (day 7, prior to observable differences in IgG titre) and increased GCA (1.63 and 2.12 FC) and NDGCA (1.80 and 3.29 FC) after secondary dosage (day 42 and 49 respectively) in vaccinated animals. The up-regulation of different BA conjugates at different stages following vaccination suggests that Cholic acid conjugation may allow for mediation of different immune response pathways, dependent on the amino acid that is conjugated. To date the only other published study assessing metabolomic responses to vaccination reported an up-regulation of serum cholesterol levels at days 5 and 10 in rabbits after primary and secondary immunization (using human red blood cells) respectively [1]. As cholesterol is a precursor to Cholic acid, and hence GCA and TDCA, it's up-regulation could be due to an increased demand for immuno-regulatory BAs. BAs have recently been demonstrated to function as signaling molecules with immunomodulatory effects resulting from their activation of the nuclear receptor Farsenoid X Receptor (FXR) [36,37] and the G-protein coupled receptors Transmembrane G protein coupled receptor 5 (TGR5) [38,39] and the Formyl-peptide receptors (FPR) [40]. TGR5, present in a variety of cells of the immune system including alveolar macrophages and dendritic cells [38,41], can be activated by BAs to stimulate cAMP production which inhibits pro-inflammatory cytokines secretion (TNF-α, IL-1β, IL-1α, IL-6 and IL-8) [38]. This activation favours more hydrophobic BAs [38], with TDCA more likely to activate TGR5 in vivo compared to GCA or NDGCA and its' up-regulation at day 7 in vaccinated calves illustrates a potential role in arresting innate inflammatory response in favour of the progression of adaptive immunity through the activation of TGR5. Dendritic cells demonstrate FXR modulated function following BA treatment, resulting in increased production of IFN-γ producing T-cells and reduced airway eosinophilia and macrophage influx after OVA airway stimulation [42]. Activation of FXR by synthetic bile acid ligands also results in NK T-cell inhibition and reduced pro-inflammatory osteopontin production which indicates FXRs role in maintaining immune homeostasis [43]. Both TDCA and GCA have been shown to activate FXR in vivo, upon transportation into FXR expressing cells [44]. However, the consequences of BA driven FXR modulation would favour an adaptive immune response, which would therefore be associated with secondary booster dosage stages where increased plasma levels of GCA and NDGCA were observed in vaccinated animals. Significant up-regulation of circulating plasma levels of GCA could provide a method by which pro-inflammatory responses at the site of infection are limited after secondary exposure to viral infections. GCA induced activation of FXR at post-booster stages in vaccinated animals may reduce macrophage and neutrophil influx to the site of infection and increase the levels of INF-γ producing CD4+ and CD8+ T-cells, promoting an adaptive immune response.

Significantly higher levels of PLC (2.21 FC) in vaccinated relative to non-vaccinated calves were observed at day 14 post initial vaccine dosage, suggesting a potential role of PLC in either mediating adaptive immune responses following primary immune stimulation, or as an end-stage metabolite produced as a result of these processes. PLC has been demonstrated to modulate innate immune response following transplantation by preventing neutrophil, CD4+, CD8+, ED1+ and MHCII cell infiltration upon transplantation, protecting grafts from oxidative stress injury [45]. In vivo PLC treatment resulted in significant decrease in the release of leukocyte adhesion molecules into plasma (E-selectin, P-selectin, L-selectin ICAM-1 and VCAM-1) [46] suggesting PLC's action in modulating leukocyte function and trafficking, with a potential role in reducing immune cell recruitment to sites of active viral replication with the progression of adaptive immunity associated with increased BPI3V IgG production at day 14 in this study. The immunomodulatory effects of PLC are further demonstrated by its' potential to reduce platelet activating factors when exposed to neutrophils in vitro and in vivo [47]. The significant up-regulation of PLC at day 14 may therefore be due to its' anti-inflammatory effect in arresting pro-inflammatory leukocyte recruitment in favour of adaptive immune response.

UA released from injured cells activates the NALP3 inflammasome leading to IL-1β production [48], but the specific mechanism by which UA promotes its immunosuppressive effects is not fully understood [49,50]. Significantly higher levels of UA (1.57 FC) were observed in vaccinated relative to non-vaccinated calves at day 42 (1 week post second vaccine dosage) and would suggest an increased population of cytotoxic T cells responding to re-exposure to the live attenuated vaccine. Whilst there has been no previously reported evidence of the direct immunosuppressive properties of HA or HHA, significantly lower levels of HA (21.70 FC) were observed in vaccinated animals at day 49 (2 weeks post booster immunization), and significant differences in the plasma peak intensity of HHA in vaccinated animals compared to non-vaccinated at days 7 (−1.82 FC), 14 (4.45 FC) post initial immunization and days 42 (1.63 FC), 49 (− 3.41 FC) and 63 (2.17 FC), 1, 2 and 4 weeks post booster immunization respectively. Reduced plasma HA levels in vaccinated calves compared to non-vaccinated calves, suggests that it does not exert a direct anti-inflammatory effect. HA may instead be involved in the mediation of immune response through its' metabolism to produce compounds which exert a direct immuno-modulatory effect. Hippuric acid is an acyl-glycine, formed through the action of N-acyltransferase involving Acyl-CoA. Circulating HA in mammals is primarily derived from the metabolism and glycine conjugation of phenolic dietary constituents [51]. The metabolites HHA, NMHA and NCG have acyl-glycine like fragmentation patterns, with HHA and NCG levels found to significantly correlate with HA. As dietary composition was consistent between study groups and significant variation in HA occurred only at post-booster stages, the reduced plasma HA levels may result from reduced N-acyltransferase activity (due to increased metabolic demand for acyl-CoA) coinciding with a marked reduction in plasma levels of other metabolites (HHA and NCG).

In conclusion, this study has demonstrated the ability of untargeted UPLC-MS metabolomics to differentiate between vaccinated and non-vaccinated animals via the profiling of metabolite constituents in plasma. A number of plasma constituents were found to be associated with initial and/or booster vaccine dosage events and were therefore characterized as corresponding to primary and/or secondary immune stimulation. The markers associated with primary immune stimulation to vaccine administration, particularly TDCA and HHA which varied in plasma prior to observable variations in BPI3V IgG, may find application as early diagnostic markers to screen for immunogenic candidates during vaccine selection investigations, particularly for vaccines targeting routes of pathogen entry such as through the respiratory tract. The metabolites GCA, NDGCA, UA and BLD, which were altered within plasma at the secondary vaccine dosage stages, may additionally represent key diagnostic markers of established immune protection in animals. A number of the selected markers have demonstrated immunological properties, affecting key cell signaling pathways and receptors located on cells of the immune system. Further validation studies are required to expand upon this initial proof of concept study to discern whether the differences observed in these metabolite marker levels as a result of vaccination are repeatable in a larger external sample set comprising animals of varying ages, genders and breeds coupled with more frequent sampling. However, this study's findings illustrate the potential for untargeted metabolomics to identify key metabolite immune correlates which relate to specific cell signaling pathways involved in immune responses. The assessment of such metabolite markers may provide greater information on the immune pathways stimulated (compared to traditional IgG or IgA serology) by vaccine formulations, and in particular benchmarking early metabolomic responses to highly immunogenic vaccine formulations could provide a means of rapidly assessing new vaccine candidates. Furthermore, a greater understanding of the metabolite pathways altered as a result of vaccination could allow for targeted vaccine design (antigens, adjuvants and nanoparticle carrier systems) to stimulate key immunogenic pathways which can be assessed at the metabolite level. Currently, metabolomics does not lend itself easily to routine vaccine candidate screening, due to the requirement of costly analytical equipment and skilled operators. However, recent advances in portable mass-spectrometers, such as the 908 Devices handheld system (908 Devices, Boston, USA), or the more user friendly Microsaic 4000 MiD® (Microsaic Systems, Surrey, UK), may eventually see the use of metabolites as routine markers for the evaluation of vaccine candidate immune function and immunogenicity. Future research will seek to expand upon the physiological role of these metabolomic markers and focus on establishing the biological pathways in which they may play a role in immuno-modulatory activities.

Additional files

Additional file 1: Rectal temperatures and haematology findings throughout the study. Routine blood haematology was performed on serum samples from vaccinated and non-vaccinated study groups at days 0, 7, 14, 21, 28, 42, 49, 56, 63, 70, 75, 82, 84 and 90 post-initial immunization. Analysis of rectal temperature was performed at days 14, 28, 42 and 63. Values represent mean ± S.E.M.

Additional file 2: Inter-run quality control parameters for UPLC-MS. Retention time deviation and mass accuracy of validated peaks corresponding to L-phenylalanine, L-tryptophan and glycocholic acid analysed in inter-run quality control pools.

Additional file 3: Cross-validation of supervised OPLS-DA analysis. OPLS-DA fitting and predictive statistics generated from cross-validation using 2/3 randomly selected dataset for the generation of predictive models and the remaining 1/3 as a test set.

Additional file 4: Selected AMRTPs of plasma metabolomic markers of response to vaccination. Combined list of markers selected using OPLS-DA at days 7, 14, 42 and 49 and filtered to exclude those with $p < 0.05$, FC < 1.5 and V.I.P. score < 1.

Abbreviations

BRD: Bovine respiratory disease; BPI3V: Bovine Parainfluenza Type3 Virus; UPLC-MS: Ultra Performance liquid chromatography-mass spectrometry; AMRTP: Accurate mass retention time pair; PCAk: Principle component analysis; OPLS-DA: Orthogonal projections to latent structures-discriminant analysis; PC: Principle component; MS/MS: Tandem mass spectrometry; UA: Uric acid; GCA: Glycocholic acid; TDCA: Taurodeoxycholic acid; BLD: Biliverdin; HA: Hippuric acid; HHA: Hexahydrohippuric acid; PLC: Propionylcarnitine; NMHA: N- N-Methylhippuric acid; NCG: N-(cyclohex-1-en-1-ylcarbonyl)glycine; FXR: Farsenoid X Receptor; TGR5: Transmembrane G-Protein Coupled Receptor 5; BA: Bile Acid; NALP3: NACHT, LRR and PYD domains-containing protein 3.

Competing interests

The authors declare that they have no competing interests.

Authors' contributions

DG performed the sample processing, metabolomic analysis, multivariate data analysis and marker identification as well as preparation of the manuscript. FM carried out BPI3V IgG ELISA and preparation of empty-PLGA nanoparticles. MW and SD participated in the design and coordination of the animal study and helped to draft the manuscript. MM, CE and OC participated in the design of metabolomic analysis aspects of the study and helped to draft the manuscript. All authors read and approved the final manuscript.

Acknowledgements

We acknowledge the staff at AFBI Animal Services Unit VSD (Stormont) for their help in the animal study and the staff at the Advanced ASSET Center IGFS QUB for their excellent technical assistance. This research was funded by a Department of Agriculture and Rural Development (DARD) Northern Ireland postgraduate studentship awarded to Darren Gray.

Author details

[1]Institute for Global Food Security (IGFS), School of Biological Sciences, Queen's University Belfast (QUB), Belfast, Northern Ireland, BT9 5AG, UK. [2]Veterinary Sciences Division (VSD), Agri-Food and Biosciences Institute (AFBI), Belfast, Northern Ireland, BT4 3SD, UK.

References

1. Zamani Z, Arjmand M, Tafazzoli M, Gholizadeh A, Pourfallah F, Sadeghi S, Mirzazadeh R, Mirkhani F, Taheri S, Iravani A, Bayat P, Vahabi F (2011) Early detection of immunization: a study based on an animal model using 1H nuclear magnetic resonance spectroscopy. Pak J Biol Sci 14:195–203
2. Light DW, Andrus JK, Warburton RN (2009) Estimated research and development costs of rotavirus vaccines. Vaccine 27:6627–6633
3. Oyston P, Robinson K (2012) The current challenges for vaccine development. J Med Microbiol 61:889–894
4. Agnandji ST, Lell B, Soulanoudjingar SS, Fernandes JF, Abossolo BP, Conzelmann C, Methogo BGNO, Doucka Y, Flamen A, Mordmueller B, Issifou S, Kremsner PG, Sacarlal J, Aide P, Lanaspa M, Aponte JJ, Nhamuave A, Quelhas D, Bassat Q, Mandjate S, Macete E, Alonso P, Abdulla S, Salim N,

Juma O, Shomari M, Shubis K, Machera F, Hamad AS, Minja R, et al. (2011) First results of phase 3 trial of RTS, S/AS01 malaria vaccine in African children. N Engl J Med 365:1863–1875

5. Tameris MD, Hatherill M, Landry BS, Scriba TJ, Snowden MA, Lockhart S, Shea JE, McClain JB, Hussey GD, Hanekom WA, Mahomed H, McShane H (2013) MVA85A 020 Trial Study Team: Safety and efficacy of MVA85A, a new tuberculosis vaccine, in infants previously vaccinated with BCG: a randomised, placebo-controlled phase 2b trial. Lancet 381:1021–1028
5. Tameris MD, Hatherill M, Landry BS, Scriba TJ, Snowden MA, Lockhart S, Shea JE, McClain JB, Hussey GD, Hanekom WA, Mahomed H, McShane H, MVA85A 020 Trial Study Team (2013) Safety and efficacy of MVA85A, a new tuberculosis vaccine, in infants previously vaccinated with BCG: a randomised, placebo-controlled phase 2b trial. Lancet 381:1021–1028
6. Siegrist C (2008) Vaccine immunology, 1st edition. Saunders, Vaccines, pp 17–36
7. Cusack PMV, McMeniman N, Lean IJ (2003) The medicine and epidemiology of bovine respiratory disease in feedlots. Aust Vet J 81:480–487
8. Snowder GD, Van Vleck LD, Cundiff LV, Bennett GL, Koohmaraie M, Dikeman ME (2007) Bovine respiratory disease in feedlot cattle: phenotypic, environmental, and genetic correlations with growth, carcass, and longissimus muscle palatability traits. J Anim Sci 85:1885–1892
9. Fulton RW (2009) Bovine respiratory disease research (1983–2009). Anim Health Res Rev 10:131–139
10. Taylor JD, Fulton RW, Lehenbauer TW, Step DL, Confer AW (2010) The epidemiology of bovine respiratory disease: what is the evidence for preventive measures? Can Vet J 51:1351–1359
11. Kahrs RF (2001) Viral Diseases Of Cattle, 2nd edition. Iowa State University Press, Iowa
12. Ploquin A, Szecsi J, Mathieu C, Guillaume V, Barateau V, Ong KC, Wong KT, Cosset FL, Horvat B, Salvetti A (2013) Protection against henipavirus infection by use of recombinant adeno-associated virus-vector vaccines. J Infect Dis 207:469–478
13. Galli V, Simionatto S, Marchioro SB, Fisch A, Gomes CK, Conceicao PR, Dellagostin OA (2012) Immunisation of mice with Mycoplasma hyopneumoniae antigens P37, P42, P46 and P95 delivered as recombinant subunit or DNA vaccines. Vaccine 31:135–140
14. Skoberne M, Cardin R, Lee A, Kazimirova A, Zielinski V, Garvie D, Lundberg A, Larson S, Bravo FJ, Bernstein DI, Flechtner JB, Long D (2013) An adjuvanted herpes simplex virus 2 subunit vaccine elicits a T cell response in mice and is an effective therapeutic vaccine in Guinea pigs. J Virol 87:3930–3942
15. Martelli P, Ardigo P, Ferrari L, Morganti M, De Angelis E, Bonilauri P, Luppi A, Guazzetti S, Caleffi A, Borghetti P (2013) Concurrent vaccinations against PCV2 and PRRSV: study on the specific immunity and clinical protection in naturally infected pigs. Vet Microbiol 162:558–571
16. Adamczyk-Poplawska M, Markowicz S, Jagusztyn-Krynicka EK (2011) Proteomics for development of vaccine. J Proteomics 74:2596–616
17. DelVecchio VG, Sabato MA, Trichilo J, Dake C, Grewal P, Alefantis T (2010) Proteomics for the development of vaccines and therapeutics. Crit Rev Immunol 30:239–254
18. Zhang T, Wu X, Ke C, Yin M, Li Z, Fan L, Zhang W, Zhang H, Zhao F, Zhou X, Lou G, Li K (2013) Identification of potential biomarkers for ovarian cancer by urinary metabolomic profiling. J Proteome Res 12:505–512
19. Yang J, Zhao X, Liu X, Wang C, Gao P, Wang J, Li L, Gu J, Yang S, Xu G (2006) High performance liquid chromatography-mass spectrometry for metabonomics: potential biomarkers for acute deterioration of liver function in chronic hepatitis B. J Proteome Res 5:554–561
20. Graham SF, Chevallier OP, Roberts D, Hoelscher C, Elliott CT, Green BD (2013) Investigation of the Human brain metabolome to identify potential markers for early diagnosis and therapeutic targets of Alzheimer's disease. Anal Chem 85:1803–1811
21. Xiao JF, Varghese RS, Zhou B, Ranjbar MRN, Zhao Y, Tsai T-H, Di Poto C, Wang J, Goerlitz D, Luo Y, Cheema AK, Sarhan N, Soliman H, Tadesse MG, Ziada DH, Ressom HW (2012) LC-MS based serum metabolomics for Identification of hepatocellular carcinoma biomarkers in Egyptian cohort. J Proteome Res 11:5914–5923
22. Jeffery H, Davis SS, O'Hagan DT (1993) The preparation and characterization of poly(lactide-co-glycolide) microparticles. II. The entrapment of a model protein using a (water-in-oil)-in-water emulsion solvent evaporation technique. Pharm Res 10:362–368
23. Tammen H, Schulte L, Hess R, Menzel C, Kellmann M, Mohring T, Schulz-Knappe P (2005) Peptidomic analysis of human blood specimens: comparison between plasma specimens and serum by differential peptide display. Proteomics 5:3414–3422
24. Brun-Hansen HC, Kampen AH, Lund A (2006) Hematologic values in calves during the first 6 months of life. Vet Clin Pathol 35:182–187
25. Abraham NG, Kappas A (2008) Pharmacological and clinical aspects of heme oxygenase. Pharmacol Rev 60:79–127
26. Ryter SW, Alam J, Choi AMK (2006) Heme oxygenase-1/carbon monoxide: From basic science to therapeutic applications. Physiol Rev 86:583–650
27. Yamashita K, McDaid J, Ollinger R, Tsui TY, Berberat PO, Usheva A, Csizmadia E, Smith RN, Soares MP, Bach FH (2004) Biliverdin, a natural product of heme catabolism, induces tolerance to cardiac allografts. FASEB J 18:765–767
28. Phelan D, Winter GM, Rogers WJ, Lam JC, Denison MS (1998) Activation of the Ah receptor signal transduction pathway by bilirubin and biliverdin. Arch Biochem Biophys 357:155–163
29. Quintana FJ, Basso AS, Iglesias AH, Korn T, Farez MF, Bettelli E, Caccamo M, Oukka M, Weiner HL (2008) Control of T-reg and TH17 cell differentiation by the aryl hydrocarbon receptor. Nature 453:65–71
30. Veldhoen M, Hirota K, Westendorf AM, Buer J, Dumoutier L, Renauld J-C, Stockinger B (2008) The aryl hydrocarbon receptor links T(H)17-cell-mediated autoimmunity to environmental toxins. Nature 453:106–109
31. Yachie A, Toma T, Mizuno I, Okamoto H, Shimura S, Ohta K, Kasahara Y, Koizumi S (2003) Heme oxygenase-1 production by peripheral blood monocytes during acute inflammatory illnesses of children. Exp Biol Med 228:550–556
32. Chauveau C, Remy S, Royer PJ, Hill M, Tanguy-Royer S, Hubert FX, Tesson L, Brion R, Beriou G, Gregoire M, Josien R, Cuturi MC, Anegon I (2005) Heme oxygenase-1 expression inhibits dendritic cell maturation and proinflammatory function but conserves IL-10 expression. Blood 106:1694–1702
33. Burt TD, Seu L, Mold JE, Kappas A, McCune JM (2010) Naive human T cells are activated and proliferate in response to the heme oxygenase-1 inhibitor tin mesoporphyrin. J Immunol 185:5279–5288
34. Poss KD, Tonegawa S (1997) Heme oxygenase 1 is required for mammalian iron reutilization. Proc Natl Acad Sci U S A 94:10919–10924
35. Kapturczak MH, Wasserfall C, Brusko T, Campbell-Thompson M, Ellis TM, Atkinson MA, Agarwal A (2004) Heme oxygenase-1 modulates early inflammatory responses: evidence from the heme oxygenase-1-deficient mouse. Am J Pathol 165:1045–1053
36. Makishima M, Okamoto AY, Repa JJ, Tu H, Learned RM, Luk A, Hull MV, Lustig KD, Mangelsdorf DJ, Shan B (1999) Identification of a nuclear receptor for bile acids. Science 284:1362–1365
37. Parks DJ, Blanchard SG, Bledsoe RK, Chandra G, Consler TG, Kliewer SA, Stimmel JB, Willson TM, Zavacki AM, Moore DD, Lehmann JM (1999) Bile acids: natural ligands for an orphan nuclear receptor. Science 284:1365–1368
38. Kawamata Y, Fujii R, Hosoya M, Harada M, Yoshida H, Miwa M, Fukusumi S, Habata Y, Itoh T, Shintani Y, Hinuma S, Fujisawa Y, Fujino M (2003) A G protein-coupled receptor responsive to bile acids. J Biol Chem 278:9435–9440
39. Hylemon PB, Zhou H, Pandak WM, Ren S, Gil G, Dent P (2009) Bile acids as regulatory molecules. J Lipid Res 50:1509–1520
40. Le YY, Murphy PM, Wang JM (2002) Formyl-peptide receptors revisited. Trends Immunol 23:541–548
41. Ichikawa R, Takayama T, Yoneno K, Kamada N, Kitazume MT, Higuchi H, Matsuoka K, Watanabe M, Itoh H, Kanai T, Hisamatsu T, Hibi T (2012) Bile acids induce monocyte differentiation toward interleukin-12 hypo-producing dendritic cells via a TGR5-dependent pathway. Immunology 136:153–162
42. Willart MAM, van Nimwegen M, Grefhorst A, Hammadt H, Moons L, Hoogsteden HC, Lambrecht BN, KleinJan A (2012) Ursodeoxycholic acid suppresses eosinophilic airway inflammation by inhibiting the function of dendritic cells through the nuclear farnesoid X receptor. Allergy 67:1501–1510
43. Mencarelli A, Renga B, Migliorati M, Cipriani S, Distrutti E, Santucci L, Fiorucci S (2009) The bile acid sensor farnesoid X receptor is a modulator of liver immunity in a rodent model of acute hepatitis. J Immunol 183:6251–6261
44. Wang H, Chen J, Hollister K, Sowers LC, Forman BM (1999) Endogenous bile acids are ligands for the nuclear receptor FXR BAR. Mol Cell 3:543–553
45. Azzollini N, Cugini D, Cassis P, Pezzotta A, Gagliardini E, Abbate M, Arduini A, Peschechera A, Remuzzi G, Noris M (2008) Propionyl-L-carnitine prevents early graft dysfunction in allogeneic rat kidney transplantation. Kidney Int 74:1420–1428
46. Signorelli SS, Malaponte G, Di Pino L, Digrandi D, Pennisi G, Mazzarino MC (2001) Effects of ischaemic stress on leukocyte activation processes in patients with chronic peripheral occlusive arterial disease: role of L-propionyl carnitine administration. Pharmacol Res 44:305–309

47. Triggiani M, Oriente A, Golino P, Gentile M, Battaglia C, Brevetti G, Marone G (1999) Inhibition of platelet-activating factor synthesis in human neutrophils and platelets by propionyl-L-carnitine. Biochem Pharmacol 58:1341–1348
48. Laiakis EC, Morris GAJ, Fornace AJ, Howie SRC (2010) Metabolomic analysis in severe childhood pneumonia in the Gambia, West Africa: findings from a pilot study. PLoS One 5:e12655
49. Kanellis J, Kang DH (2005) Uric acid as a mediator of endothelial dysfunction, inflammation, and vascular disease. Semin Nephrol 25:39–42
50. Kang DH, Park SK, Lee IK, Johnson RJ (2005) Uric acid-induced C-reactive protein expression: Implication on cell proliferation and nitric oxide production of human vascular cells. J Am Soc Nephrol 16:3553–3562
51. Wikoff WR, Anfora AT, Liu J, Schultz PG, Lesley SA, Peters EC, Siuzdak G (2009) Metabolomics analysis reveals large effects of gut microflora on mammalian blood metabolites. Proc Natl Acad Sci U S A 106:3698–3703

9

The immunoglobulin M-degrading enzyme of *Streptococcus suis*, Ide$_{Ssuis}$, is involved in complement evasion

Jana Seele[1], Andreas Beineke[2], Lena-Maria Hillermann[1], Beate Jaschok-Kentner[3], Ulrich von Pawel-Rammingen[4], Peter Valentin-Weigand[1] and Christoph Georg Baums[5*]

Abstract

Streptococcus (*S.*) *suis* is one of the most important pathogens in pigs causing meningitis, arthritis, endocarditis and serositis. Furthermore, it is also an emerging zoonotic agent. In our previous work we identified a highly specific IgM protease in *S. suis*, designated Ide$_{Ssuis}$. The objective of this study was to characterize the function of Ide$_{Ssuis}$ in the host-pathogen interaction. Edman-sequencing revealed that Ide$_{Ssuis}$ cleaves the heavy chain of the IgM molecule between constant domain 2 and 3. As the C1q binding motif is located in the C3 domain, we hypothesized that Ide$_{Ssuis}$ is involved in complement evasion. Complement-mediated hemolysis induced by porcine hyperimmune sera containing erythrocyte-specific IgM was abrogated by treatment of these sera with recombinant Ide$_{Ssuis}$. Furthermore, expression of Ide$_{Ssuis}$ reduced IgM-triggered complement deposition on the bacterial surface. An infection experiment of prime-vaccinated growing piglets suggested attenuation in the virulence of the mutant 10Δ*ide*$_{Ssuis}$. Bactericidal assays confirmed a positive effect of Ide$_{Ssuis}$ expression on bacterial survival in porcine blood in the presence of high titers of specific IgM. In conclusion, this study demonstrates that Ide$_{Ssuis}$ is a novel complement evasion factor, which is important for bacterial survival in porcine blood during the early adaptive (IgM-dominated) immune response.

Introduction

Streptococcus (*S.*) *suis* colonizes different mucosa of pigs, its main host. Virulent strains might, however, cross the mucosal barrier, cause bacteremia and infect various tissues leading to severe pathologies, such as meningitis, arthritis, endocarditis and serositis. Suppurative meningitis caused by *S. suis* is one of the most important diseases in modern swine production as it is associated with severe economic losses. *S. suis* exhibits a high degree of diversity among and within different serotypes. Serotype 2 is worldwide the most important serotype isolated from affected tissues in piglets and also an important zoonotic agent [1-3].

Numerous proteins involved in interaction with the host have been functionally characterized [4,5]. Recently, we identified a 124 kDa large Immunoglobulin M-degrading enzyme of S. suis, designated Ide$_{Ssuis}$ [6]. The N-terminal region of Ide$_{Ssuis}$ is homologous to the 38 kDa IgG specific endoprotease IdeS (also known as Mac-1) expressed by *S. pyogenes* and sufficient for IgM cleavage. Ide$_{Ssuis}$ is a highly specific IgM protease expressed by all investigated *S. suis* strains, which included strains from four different serotypes and clonal complexes. Importantly, it is so far the only known protease cleaving specifically the intact IgM multimer. The specificity of this protease is underscored by several findings: (i) Ide$_{Ssuis}$ does not degrade porcine or human IgG or IgA, (ii) IgM of pigs but not IgM of any other investigated species is cleaved and (iii) incubation of different body liquids with Ide$_{Ssuis}$, including cerebrospinal and joint fluids from diseased piglets, generated only one additional band in SDS-PAGE in accordance with a specific IgM cleavage product [6].

Complement activation leads to formation of C3 convertases (C3Bb or C4b2a) cleaving C3 into the anaphylatoxin C3a and the most important opsonin C3b. In an experimental mouse model the complement system proved to be crucial for protection against

* Correspondence: christoph.baums@vetmed.uni-leipzig.de
[5]Institute for Bacteriology and Mycology, Centre of Infectious Diseases, College of Veterinary Medicine, University Leipzig, An den Tierkliniken 29, 04103 Leipzig, Germany
Full list of author information is available at the end of the article

morbidity and mortality caused by intranasal *S. suis* infection, as recently demonstrated by our group using $C3^{-/-}$ mice [7]. Thus, evasion of complement activation is essential for the survival of *S. suis* in its host and several factors involved in complement evasion have been identified in *S. suis*. Sialic acid moieties of the capsule of serotype 2 strains [8] might interfere with the activation of the alternative complement cascade by increasing the affinity constant of C3b to the complement inhibitor factor H [9,10]. Accordingly, deposition of C3b is increased on the bacterial surface of an unencapsulated mutant [7]. Furthermore, two factor H binding proteins (Fhb and SSU0186) both homologous to PspC (Pneumococcal surface protein C) of *S. pneumoniae* have been identified in *S. suis* [11,12]. FhB was shown to contribute to virulence in experimental infections of piglets and to survival in human blood ex vivo.

The classical complement pathway is activated by immunoglobulins, in particular IgM, and some other host proteins, e. g. choline-binding protein, recognizing bacterial surface structures [13]. Binding of the IgM pentamer to surfaces of pathogens leads to activation of the classical complement (c) cascade, as IgM, including porcine IgM, contains a C1q binding motif [14,15]. The results of this study showed that the cleavage site of Ide_{Ssuis} in porcine IgM is located between the C1q-binding motif and the antigen recognizing part. Thus, we investigated whether IgM protease activity represents a novel complement evasion mechanism protecting the pathogen against classical complement activation.

Materials and methods

Bacterial strains and growth conditions

S. suis strain 10 is a virulent serotype 2 strain that has previously been used for experimental infections of piglets and for generation of isogenic mutants [16-19]. It expresses the virulence-associated muramidase-released protein (MRP), the extracellular factor and suilysin [20]. The capsule deficient isogenic mutant *10cpsΔEF* is attenuated in virulence [19] and shows increased deposition of C3 antigen on its bacterial surface in murine serum [7]. Streptococci were grown on Columbia blood agar plates or in Bacto™ Todd Hewitt broth (THB). *Escherichia (E.) coli* strains were cultured in Luria-Bertani (LB) medium. If appropriate, antibiotics were added at the following concentrations: ampicillin, 100 µg/mL for *E. coli*; chloramphenicol, 3.5 µg/mL for *S. suis*, 8 µg/mL for *E. coli*; spectinomycin 100 µg/mL for *S. suis*.

DNA techniques and primer

Standard DNA manipulations were performed as described [21]. Oligonucleotide primers were designed based on the sequence of SSU0496 in the genome of *S. suis* P1/7 [6]. Chromosomal DNA of strain 10 served as template in all PCRs conducted for generation of inserts. DNA fragments were amplified with Phusion polymerase (Promega, Mannheim, Germany).

Generation of *S. suis* mutants expressing truncated Ide_{Ssuis}

The mutant $10\Delta ide_{Ssuis}$ and its complemented strain $10\Delta ide_{Ssuis}$ pGA14*ideSsuis* were described previously [6]. In frame deletion mutants expressing either the N-terminal part homologous to IdeS ($10\Delta ide_{Ssuis}$_C-terminus) or the large C-terminal part ($10\Delta ide_{Ssuis}$_homologue) were generated within this work using the thermosensitive plasmids pSET5Δide_{Ssuis}_C and pSET5Δide_{Ssuis}_h, respectively, to mutagenize *S. suis* strain 10. The following amplicons were generated with the indicated oligonucleotide primers to generate pSET5Δide_{Ssuis}_C: a 619 bp ide_{Ssuis} 5′-fragment amplified with ide_{Ssuis}delCforPstI and ide_{Ssuis}delCrevBamHI and a 608 bp ide_{Ssuis} 3′-fragment generated with ide_{Ssuis}-delCforBamHI and ide_{Ssuis}delCrevEcoRI (Additional file 1). Both fragments were cut with the restriction enzymes indicated in the name of the primers and inserted into the corresponding sites of pSET5. For the construction of pSET5Δide_{Ssuis}_h a 614 bp 5′-ide_{Ssuis} amplification product was generated with the primer pair preProIde$_{Ssuis}$PstI plus postSSide$_{Ssuis}$BamHI and a 621 bp 3′-ide_{Ssuis} amplification product with the primer pair Ide$_{Ssuis}$delh_for_BamHI and Ide$_{Ssuis}$delh_rev_SacI (Additional file 1). Both fragments were cut with the indicated restriction enzymes and inserted into the corresponding sites in vector pSET5. Restriction analysis and sequencing was performed with pSET5Δide_{Ssuis}_h and pSET5Δide_{Ssuis}_C to verify both constructs.

The allelic exchanges for generation of $10\Delta ide_{Ssuis}$_homologue and $10\Delta ide_{Ssuis}$_C-terminus were performed essentially as described previously [6]. The deletion of the genes was confirmed by PCR and Southern Blot analysis, which included four different probes for each mutant strain.

Generation of an unencapsulated ide_{Ssuis} mutant

In frame deletion mutagenesis of ide_{Ssuis} was conducted in the unencapsulated *S. suis* strain *10cpsΔEF* with the thermosensitive plasmid pSET5Δide_{Ssuis} constructed in our previous study [6]. The unencapsulated double mutant $10cps\Delta EF\Delta ide_{Ssuis}$ was confirmed by comprehensive Southern blot analysis using 4 different probes and two different digestions of DNA (HincII and BamHI).

Expression and purification of recombinant proteins

The expression and the purification of the different recombinant Ide_{Ssuis} constructs, MRP and the fibronectin- and fibrinogen-binding protein of *S. suis* (FBPS) were performed as previously described [6].

Sodium dodecyl sulphate polyacrylamide gel electrophoresis (SDS-PAGE) and Western blot analysis

For αIgM Western blot analysis samples were prepared with reducing or non-reducing sample buffer and separated in 6% or 10% separating gels. For the detection of the Ig light chain the samples were prepared with reducing sample buffer and separated in a 12% separating gel. Western blot analysis was conducted as previously described [6] with antibodies specified together with the final dilution in Additional file 2. Polyclonal antisera were raised against Ide_{Ssuis}, Ide_{Ssuis}_homologue and Ide_{Ssuis}_C-terminus in rabbits within our previous study [6].

Determination of the IgM-cleavage site

The cleavage site of Ide_{Ssuis} in IgM was determined through N-terminal sequencing after Edman degradation of a cleavage product. For this, recombinant Ide_{Ssuis} in a concentration of 0.07 mg/mL was incubated with 0.68 mg/mL purified porcine IgM at 37 °C for 3 h on a rotator. The proteins were then separated under reducing conditions in a 10% separating and 4% stacking gel. The cleavage products were transferred to PVDF-membranes (Merck Millipore, Schwalbach, Germany) and either visualized in an αIgM Western blot or cut out for sequencing via N-terminal Edman degradation performed on an Applied Biosystems Procise Protein Sequencer 494C with reagents supplied by the manufacturer (Life Technologies, Darmstadt, Germany).

Complement hemolysis assay

A hemolysis assay was established to investigate whether Ide_{Ssuis} activity modulates the complement-dependent hemolysis caused by porcine Ig raised against ovine erythrocytes. For generation of sera containing these specific antibodies (αEry sera), two piglets were immunized with purified ovine erythrocytes and 10% Emulsigen (MVP Laboratories Inc., Omaha, NE). Generation of hyperimmune sera in pigs in our institute is registered under 12A226 at the Lower Saxonian State Office for Consumer Protection and Food Safety.

Sera were drawn from these piglets prior and post prime as well as post booster vaccination as indicated. Ovine erythrocytes from defibrinated blood were washed three times with 0.9% sodium chloride solution and were finally diluted to a 2% erythrocyte suspension. Hemolysis experiments were conducted with 1:20 final dilutions of porcine sera. To confirm that the hemolytic activity of the αEry sera depended on complement activity, sera were either inactivated by heat treatment (30 min 56 °C) or by addition of 10 mM EDTA (30 min 25 °C). The classical pathway was specifically inhibited by incubation of the serum with 10 mM EGTA and 15 mM $MgCl_2$ (30 min 25 °C).

For functional analysis of Ide_{Ssuis}, 1.8 μg recombinant protein of either Ide_{Ssuis} or a truncated derivative was incubated with 100 μL of a 1:10 dilution of porcine serum (pre immune or αEry sera) for 1.5 h on a rotator at 37 °C. Erythrocytes were mixed with treated serum (each 100 μL) and incubated for 30 min at 37 °C on a shaker. As control the erythrocytes were incubated in water (defined as complete lysis of erythrocytes) or in a 0.9% sodium chloride solution. Unlysed red blood cells were pelleted by centrifugation (1000 × *g* for 5 min). One hundred μL of the supernatant was transferred into a 96-well flat bottom microplate and the absorbance was measured at 405 nm. For the inhibition assay, 5.2 μg recombinant protein was incubated with 0.4 M iodoacetamide (or as a control PBS) for 30 min. Unbound iodoacetamide was afterwards removed using Amicon Ultra 0.5 mL centrifugal filters with a 10 kDa cut off (Merck Millipore, Schwalbach, Germany). Subsequently, the iodoacetamide-inactivated Ide_{Ssuis} contructs and its controls were investigated for modulation of hemolysis caused by αEry sera as described above but erythrocytes and serum were incubated for 1 h.

Detection of IgM and IgG on the surface of ovine erythrocytes

Porcine sera drawn before and after immunization with ovine erythrocytes (see above) were inactivated by heat treatment (30 min 56 °C). A 2% erythrocyte suspension generated from EDTA-blood was incubated with inactivated pre and post immune serum. Inactivated serum was pretreated with different rIde_{Ssuis} constructs and as control with rMRP as described above to investigate a putative modulation of IgM and IgG binding to erythrocytes. After incubation with porcine sera, erythrocytes were centrifuged, resuspended in 5% goat serum (for the detection of IgM) or 5% rabbit serum (for the detection of IgG) and incubated on a rotator at 8 °C for 1 h. Erythrocytes were washed with PBS and incubated in a 1:250 dilution of a mouse anti-porcine IgM antibody (Serotec, Puchheim, Germany) or in a 1:10 000 dilution of a goat anti-porcine IgG antibody (Serotec) for 1 h at 8 °C. After washing of erythrocytes samples were incubated in a 1:500 dilution of a phycoerythrin-labelled goat anti-mouse IgG antibody (Bio Legend, Fell, Germany) or in a 1:1000 dilution of a Alexa fluor 488–labelled chicken anti-goat IgG antibody (Life Technologies, Darmstadt, Germany), respectively. Erythrocytes were analysed using a BD Accuri™ C6 (Becton Dickinson, Heidelberg, Germany) flow cytometer. For each determination 10 000 events were acquired and analysis of erythrocytes was carried out by dot plot analysis.

C3-deposition assay

For opsonization of *S. suis* with C3b/C3i, 150 μL serum drawn after bacterin prime-vaccination or hyperimmune serum raised against *S. suis* serotype 2 was added to

75 µL of a culture grown to an OD_{600} of 0.8. After 1 h of incubation at 37 °C under rotation, bacteria were centrifuged, washed with PBS and incubated with a polyclonal FITC-labeled rabbit anti-human C3c antibody (Dako, Eching, Germany) (1:150 diluted in PBS) for 1 h at 8 °C. For opsonization of *S. suis* 10*cps*Δ*EF* and 10*cps*Δ*EF*Δ*ideSsuis*, 75 µL serum of colostrum-deprived piglets (SCDP) with or without the addition of purified porcine IgM (0.14 mg/mL) was added to 75 µL of a culture grown to an OD_{600} of 0.8. Porcine IgM were purified as described before (8). Bacteria and serum were incubated for 30 min at 37 °C and labelled with an antibody directed against C3 as described above. Fluorescent bacteria were analysed after washing with PBS and inactivation with 0.375% formaldehyde in flow cytometry as described previously [7].

To deplete serum of complement components, serum was pretreated with zymosan as decribed [22] with the following modifications. A 225 µL aliquot of a zymosan A (Sigma, Taufkirchen, Germany) stock solution (15 mg zymosan A resuspended in 1 mL of a 14 mM sodium chloride solution) was incubated for 30 min at 100 °C. The suspension was centrifuged at 16 000 × *g* for 5 min and the pellet was resuspended in 150 µL of porcine serum, incubated for 30 min at 25 °C and centrifuged at 16 000 × *g* for 5 min. Treatment of bacteria with this supernatant was compared to treatment of bacteria with untreated serum to access the effect of complement depletion by zymosan. All three complement pathways were blocked with 10 mM EDTA (30 min 25 °C) or heat inactivation (30 min 56 °C). To inhibit only the classical complement pathway, sera were incubated with 10 mM EGTA and 15 mM $MgCl_2$ for 30 min at 25 °C. The differently treated serum samples were incubated with the bacteria which were subsequently analyzed for deposition of C3 antigen as described above.

Opsonophagocytosis assay

Opsonophagocytic killing in the presence of 20% (v/v) porcine serum was assessed essentially as described [23]. Porcine neutrophils were purified from freshly drawn blood as outlined previously [24]. To obtain a multiplicity of infection of 0.03, 1.5×10^5 bacteria were added to 400 µL of a neutrophil suspension in RPMI containing 5×10^6 neutrophils and 100 µL serum. The samples were incubated for 1 h at 37 °C on a rotator. Samples incubated with porcine α*S. suis* serotype 2 hyperimmune serum and serum of colostrum-deprived piglets were included as positive and negative control, respectively. The survival factor as defined by the ratio of colony forming units (CFU) at t = 60 min to the respective value at t = 0 min was determined for each strain. The ratio of the survival factors of 10Δide_{Ssuis} and wt was calculated to assess attenuation of the 10Δide_{Ssuis} mutant.

Bactericidal assay

Survival of *S. suis* in porcine blood was determined as described in a previous study [6]. Briefly, 500 µL of heparinized blood (16 I. U. heparin/mL) were infected with 1.5×10^5 CFU using stocks of frozen bacteria with 15% glycerol after thawing. The blood was incubated for 2 h at 37 °C on a rotator. Bactericidal assays were conducted with blood drawn from 5 to 7 week old piglets 6 to 14 days after prime vaccination with a *S. suis* serotype 2 bacterin. These piglets were not included in the experimental infection experiment.

Animal experiment

German Landrace piglets (*n* = 25) free of *sly* + *mrp* + *epf* + *cps*2+ strains were infected experimentally either with strain 10 (*n* = 9) or strain 10Δide_{Ssuis} (*n* = 8) or 10Δide_{Ssuis}_homologue (*n* = 8). Piglets were cared for in accordance with the principles outlined in the European Convention for the Protection of Vertebrate Animals Used for Experimental and Other Scientific Purposes [25]. The animal experiment of this study was approved by the Committee on Animal Experiments of the Lower Saxonian State Office for Consumer Protection and Food Safety (permit no. 33.9-42502-04-12/0965).

All piglets were prime-vaccinated at an age of 5–6 weeks with a bacterin generated with *S. suis* strain 10 grown overnight and inactivated in 0.2% formaldehyde. Emulsigen was added as adjuvant (20% [vol/vol]). Each immunization dose contained approximately 10^9 bacteria.

At an age of 7 to 8 weeks piglets were challenged 12 days after prime vaccination. Piglets were intranasally infected after predisposition through intranasal treatment with 1% acetic acid as described previously [16]. Criteria for morbidity were fever (≥40.2 °C) or specific clinical signs such as convulsions or severe lameness. In the case of high fever (≥40.5 °C), apathy and anorexia persisting over 36 h as well as in all cases of clinical signs of acute polyarthritis or severe meningitis animals were euthanized for reasons of animal welfare. All surviving piglets were sacrificed 15 days post infection (dpi).

After euthanasia every animal went through the same procedure of necropsy including predefined collection of samples for histological and bacteriological investigations. Fibrinous-suppurative inflammations were scored in blinded experiments as described previously [16]. To allow comparison of groups the sum of the highest scores of each animal for any of the investigated organs was divided by the number of animals ($\omega = \Sigma score_{max}/n_{animals}$). Isolation of the challenge strains was confirmed in a PCR for detection of *epf* and *cps*2 [26] and in ide_{Ssuis}-specific PCRs using oligonucleotide primers specified in Additional file 1.

Detection of αMRP IgG as well as α*S. suis* IgM and IgG antibodies

MRP, used as antigen for the IgG ELISA, is a dominant immunogen of this *S. suis* pathotype [17,23,27]. The detection of IgG titers against MRP was performed as described [16]. For the measurement of α*S. suis* IgM or IgG antibody titers Maxisorb® plates (Nunc, Rochester, NY) were coated with 1×10^7 inactivated *S. suis* wt bacteria/well. Every sample and the controls were measured in a duplicate series of four (reference serum: seven) twofold dilutions in PBST starting with a dilution of 1:50. For the detection of *S. suis* specific IgM antibodies the plates were incubated with a dilution of 1:10 000 of a POD-conjugated goat anti-porcine IgM antibody (Thermo Scientific, Schwerte, Germany, catalog number PA1-84625) for 1 h at 37 °C. Blocking, washing and development of ELISA plates as well as calculation of ELISA units was conducted as previously described [17]. Data were only considered if they met the following criteria: a deviation of duplicates of no more than 22%, a slope of the linear portion of the reference standard curve between 0.8 and 1.2, a correlation coefficient between 0.9 and 1.0, and controls within established ranges.

Statistical analysis

Experiments were performed at least three times and if not stated otherwise one-way analysis of variance (ANOVA) using Dunnetts adjustment or Tukeys multiple comparison test was used. ELISA-values were compared using the Mann–Whitney U-Test. Statistical analysis of Kaplan-Meier diagrams was conducted with the log-rank test. Means and standard deviation of the results are shown. Probabilities lower than 0.05 were considered significant ($p < 0.05$ *, $p < 0.01$ ** and $p < 0.001$ ***).

Results

Ide$_{Ssuis}$ cleaves the heavy chain of IgM at the N-terminus of the C3 domain

Cleavage of IgM by Ide$_{Ssuis}$ was previously identified and characterized in Western blot analysis under non-reducing conditions [6]. In this study we used a different αIgM antibody recognizing only the reduced heavy chain of IgM to detect IgM cleavage products after Ide$_{Ssuis}$ incubation (Figure 1). This allowed us to successfully determine the N-terminal sequence of the 32 kDa cleavage product as SPITVFAIAP via Edman sequencing (Figure 1). Based on the N-terminal sequence, Ide$_{Ssuis}$ cleaves the heavy chain of IgM at the N-terminus of the C3 domain. In accordance with this result, reducing αIgM Western blot analysis revealed two cleavage products of 41 kDa and 32 kDa, which putatively included V1-C1-C2 and C3-C4 domains of the heavy IgM chain, respectively (Noteworthy, this αIgM antibody does not recognize the light chain of IgM).

Cysteines involved in disulphide bonds are conserved between human and porcine IgM. Assuming that constitution of disulfide bonds is also conserved between the two species, the cysteines of C1 and C2 domains of porcine IgM should form intradomain and interchain disulphide bonds but not link monomers to the multimer. The Western blot in Figure 1 and further analysis with antibodies recognizing unreduced IgM [6] and the light chain of IgM only (Figure 1A), suggested that IgM is cleaved by Ide$_{Ssuis}$ only at the indicated site. IgM bound to the bacterial surface is also cleaved by Ide$_{Ssuis}$ and results in release of Fcμ cleavage products [6], which most likely include the C3 and C4 domain of the heavy chain of porcine IgM. This cleavage pattern is likely to affect IgM effector functions, in particular reduced activation of the classical complement pathway, as the C3 domain includes the C1q binding motif of porcine IgM [28,29].

Ide$_{Ssuis}$ abrogates activation of the classical complement pathway

The classical complement activation pathway can be studied in hemolysis assays using sera containing antibodies directed against erythrocytes. We investigated the impact of Ide$_{Ssuis}$ on complement activation in a hemolysis assay including sera drawn from piglets vaccinated with erythrocytes (αEry sera). In accordance with complement activation, treatment of αEry sera with heat, EDTA or EGTA plus $MgCl_2$ completely abolished the hemolytic activity of the αEry sera (Figure 2A). For functional analysis of Ide$_{Ssuis}$, αEry sera drawn after prime and booster vaccination were treated with different rIde$_{Ssuis}$ constructs (Figure 2B) prior incubation with erythrocytes. Incubation of the post-prime αEry serum with rIde$_{Ssuis}$ and rIde$_{Ssuis}$_homologue (the domain containing the IgM protease), almost completely abolished this hemolysis (Figure 2C). Noteworthy, treatment of the post-prime αEry serum with two recombinant control proteins (MRP and FBPS), did not result in abrogation of hemolysis (Figure 2C). Interestingly, treatment of αEry sera with proteolytic inactive construct rIde$_{Ssuis}$_C_terminus led also to a significant reduction of hemolysis indicating a separate role of the C-terminus in complement evasion. However, significant differences between inhibition of complement activation through αEry sera drawn after prime and booster vaccination were only observed for the Ide$_{Ssuis}$ constructs with IgM protease activity (Figure 2C).

The different recombinant Ide$_{Ssuis}$ constructs were treated with the protease inhibitor iodoacetamide prior to incubation with αEry serum to assess the impact of proteolytic activity on complement inhibition. Preincubation of rIde$_{Ssuis}$ and rIde$_{Ssuis}$_homologue with iodoacetamide completely abrogated the complement inhibiting activity of these proteins (Figure 2D).

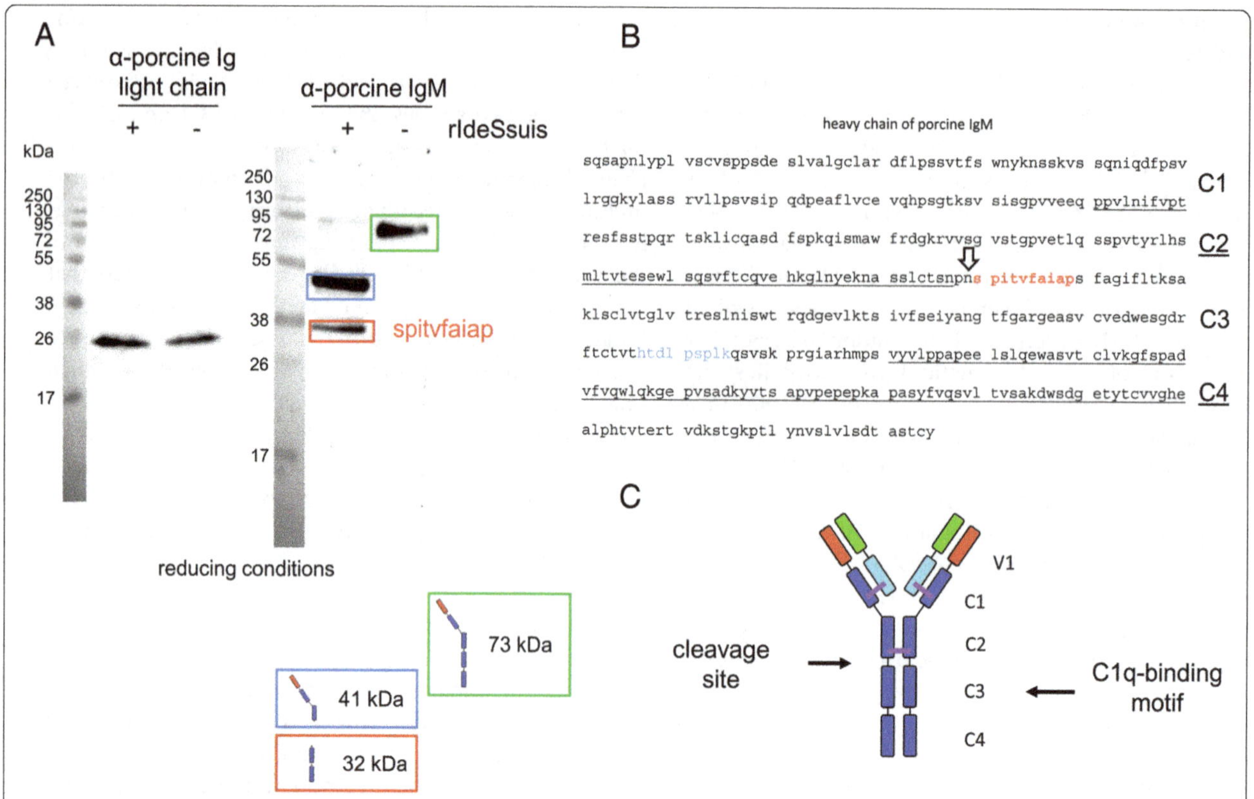

Figure 1 Ide$_{Ssuis}$ cleaves the heavy chain of porcine IgM. (A) αIg light chain and αIgM Western blot analysis of purified porcine IgM after incubation +/− rIde$_{Ssuis}$. Samples were separated in an SDS-gel under reducing conditions. The marker bands are shown on the left side (sizes in kDa). **(B)** The IgM-cleavage product highlighted in red was characterized by N-terminal Edman-sequencing. The identified sequence is shown in red and corresponds to the constant domain 3 of the IgM heavy chain. The putative C1q binding motif is marked in blue. Domains C2 and C4 are underlined. The obtained sequence was taken directly from the NCBI database. **(C)** Illustration of an IgM-monomer with the indicated cleavage site and the location of the putative C1q-binding motif.

Furthermore, flow cytometry analysis was conducted with erythrocytes after incubation with inactivated post prime and post booster αEry sera to differentiate binding of specific IgM and IgG in these sera. Both sera contained erythrocyte-specific IgG and IgM in contrast to the pre immune serum. Incubation with the post prime serum led to significantly higher percentage of IgM-labelled erythrocytes and respective mean fluorescence intensity (MFI) in comparison to the post booster serum. Vice versa, IgG staining on erythrocytes resulted in a much higher MFI after incubation in post booster serum (Figures 3A and B). We investigated modulation of IgM and IgG antigen binding to erythrocytes by treatment of the post prime αEry serum with the different recombinant Ide$_{Ssuis}$ constructs. Treatment of this serum with proteolytic active rIde$_{Ssuis}$ and rIde$_{Ssuis}$_homologue led to a significant reduction of the percentage of erythrocytes labelled with IgM and the respective MFI (Figures 3C and D) in contrast to the treatment with the non-proteolytic constructs. Binding of IgG to the erythrocytes was not modulated by incubation of the αEry serum with any of the recombinant Ide$_{Ssuis}$ constructs.

In conclusion, Ide$_{Ssuis}$ interferes with the classical complement activation pathway. The results of the hemolysis assay suggest that Ide$_{Ssuis}$ interferes with complement activation by two mechanisms, firstly, by its IgM protease activity and, secondly, by some yet unknown function of the large non-proteolytic C-terminal domain.

Expression of Ide$_{Ssuis}$ reduces IgM-triggered complement deposition on the bacterial surface of an unencapsulated mutant

We investigated deposition of C3 on the surface of opsonized *S. suis* strains by flow cytometry to further investigate the hypothesis that Ide$_{Ssuis}$ is involved in complement evasion. After opsonization of *S. suis* wt and 10Δ*ide*$_{Ssuis}$ with different porcine sera with moderate to high specific IgM titers the percentage of bacteria with stained C3 antigen (most likely C3b/C3i) was slightly increased in the mutant 10Δ*ide*$_{Ssuis}$ (Additional file 3). Specifically, 39.2% of wt (SD = 11.0%) and 42.8% of 10Δ*ide*$_{Ssuis}$ (SD = 10.2%) bacteria were C3-labelled after opsonization in sera of bacterin-primed piglets (Additional file 3). The sera of these bacterin-primed

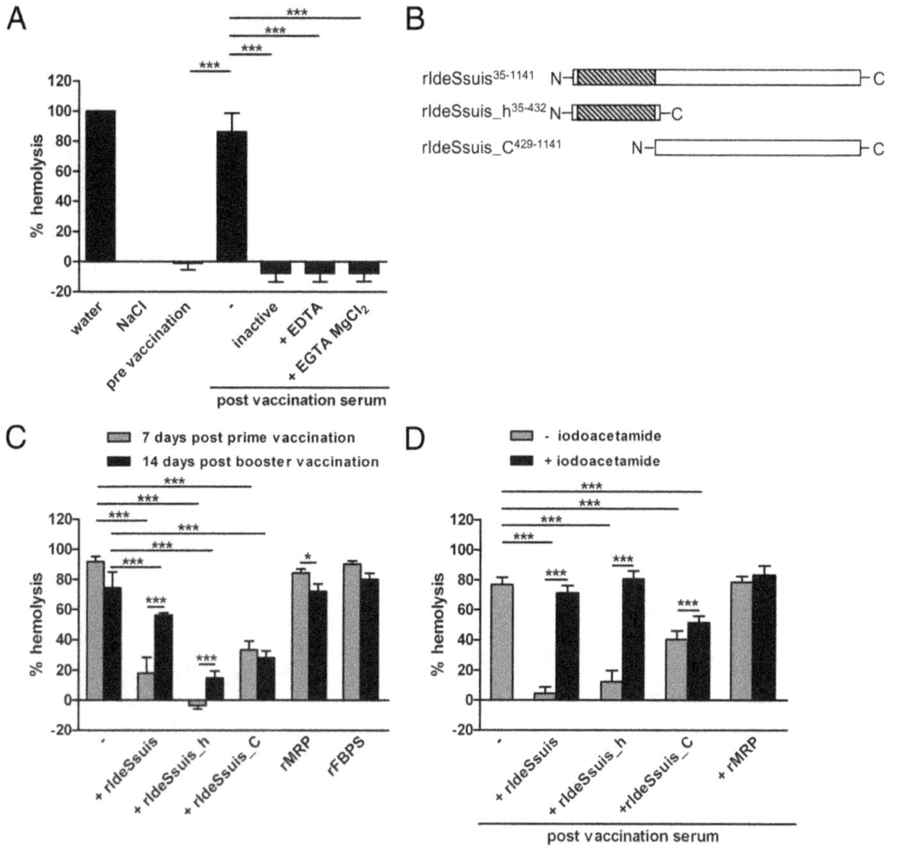

Figure 2 Hemolysis caused by the classical complement activation pathway is abrogated by Ide$_{Ssuis}$ in dependence of the protease activity. (A) Purified sheep erythrocytes were incubated with water (defined as 100% hemolysis), physiological sodium chloride solution (NaCl), sera of a piglet drawn before (pre vaccination serum) and 7 days after prime vaccination (post vaccination αEry serum) with ovine erythrocytes. The αEry serum was heat inactivated or treated with EDTA to access the impact of complement activation. To specifically inhibit the classical complement pathway 10 mM EGTA plus 15 mM $MgCl_2$ was used. **(B)** Illustration of rIde$_{Ssuis}$ and its truncated derivatives. The amino acids of Ide$_{Ssuis}$ included in these constructs are superscribed. The region homologous to IdeS is shaded. **(C)** Complement dependent hemolysis is reduced by pretreatment of the indicated different αEry sera with rIde$_{Ssuis}$, rIde$_{Ssuis}$_homologue (rIdeSsuis_h) and rIde$_{Ssuis}$_C_terminus (rIdeSsuis_C) but not with rMRP and rFBPS. **(D)** Proteolytic activity of rIde$_{Ssuis}$ and rIde$_{Ssuis}$_homologue is crucial for complement inhibition. The Ide$_{Ssuis}$ constructs were incubated with the cysteine-protease inhibitor iodoacetamide prior to incubation with the αEry sera as indicated. The final dilutions of porcine sera in the hemolysis assay were 1:20 in all cases. Bars and error bars represent mean values and standard deviations, respectively. Significant differences are indicated (* $p < 0.05$; ** $p < 0.01$; *** $p < 0.001$).

piglets had moderate to high titers of α*S. suis* IgM (34 – 103 ELISA units) and α*S. suis* IgG (69 – 161 ELISA units) but low αMRP titers (below 15 ELISA units). After addition of EGTA and $MgCl_2$ to these sera only 7.1% (SD = 4.8%) and 7.7% (SD = 6.8%) of wt and 10Δ*ide*$_{Ssuis}$ bacteria, respectively, were labelled with the αC3 antibody indicating that complement is mainly activated by the classical activation pathway during early adaptive immune responses (Additional file 3).

We hypothesized that activation of the classical complement pathway in this assay was determined by specific IgM and IgG and that redundant complement evasion mechanisms in *S. suis* serotype 2 might limit detection of phenotypic differences between wt and 10Δ*ide*$_{Ssuis}$. Thus, we deleted *ide*$_{Ssuis}$ in an unencapsulated isogenic strain (10*cps*Δ*EF*Δ*ide*$_{Ssuis}$) to avoid complement inhibition through the sialylated capsule of *S. suis* serotype 2. Furthermore, effects of specific IgG were excluded using serum from colostrum-deprived piglets (SCDP). As shown in Figure 4A approximately 10% of either 10*cps*Δ*EF* or 10*cps*Δ*EF*Δ*ide*$_{Ssuis}$ bacteria were stained with C3 after opsonization with SCDP. Importantly, the percentages of C3-stained 10*cps*Δ*EF* increased to about 20% after addition of purified porcine IgM to SCDP prior to opsonization, but fourfold (to 40%) for 10*cps*Δ*EF*Δ*ide*$_{Ssuis}$ bacteria lacking IgM protease activity (Figure 4). Differences in C3 deposition between 10*cps*Δ*EF* and 10*cps*Δ*EF*Δ*ide*$_{Ssuis}$ were highly significant for the percentage of labelled bacteria and the MFI (Figure 4). Addition of the classical complement pathway inhibitor (EGTA plus $MgCl_2$) reduced the percentage of C3 labelled bacteria to 4.7% (10*cps*Δ*EF*) and 4.9% (10*cps*Δ*EF*Δ*ide*$_{Ssuis}$)

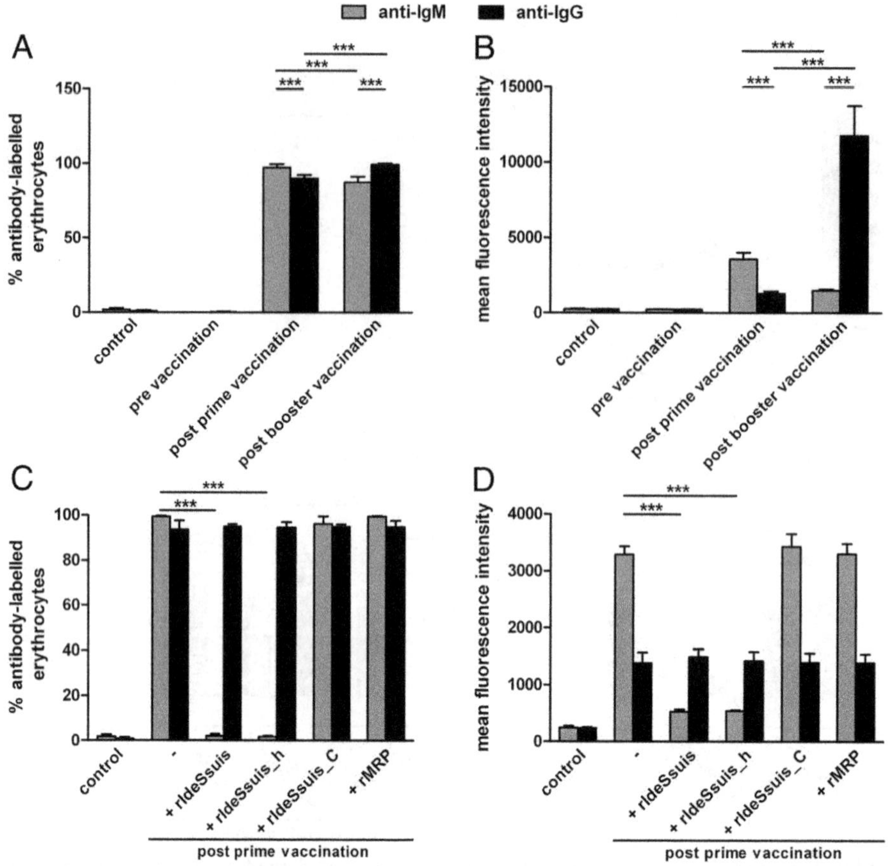

Figure 3 The proteolytic rIde$_{Ssuis}$ constructs modulate IgM binding to the surface of erythrocytes after incubation in αEry sera. (A, B) Flow cytometry analysis of IgM and IgG binding to ovine erythrocytes after incubation with porcine sera drawn pre, post prime or post booster vaccination with ovine erythrocytes (generation of αEry sera). **(C, D)** Binding of specific IgM antigen to the surface of ovine erythrocytes is significantly reduced after pretreatment of a post prime αEry serum with rIde$_{Ssuis}$ and rIde$_{Ssuis}$_homologue. The post prime αEry serum was preincubated with the indicated Ide$_{Ssuis}$ constructs and as a control with MRP. **(A, C)** The percentage of erythrocytes labelled with IgM or IgG and **(B, D)** the mean fluorescence intensities are shown. αEry sera were inactivated in these assays to allow flow cytometric analysis of erythrocytes. Bars and error bars represent mean values and standard deviations, respectively. Significant differences are indicated (***p < 0.001) except for differences between pre and post vaccination sera.

and diminished the phenotype of the double mutant. These results confirm that C3 deposition on the surface of *S. suis* might be determined by IgM-mediated activation of the classical complement pathway and show that *S. suis* reduces this IgM-mediated C3 deposition by expression of Ide$_{Ssuis}$.

The mutant 10Δ*ide*$_{Ssuis}$ is attenuated in survival in opsonophagocytosis assays in the presence of specific IgM

As rIde$_{Ssuis}$ interfered with complement activation using sera with specific antibodies, we hypothesized that expression of the IgM protease Ide$_{Ssuis}$ contributes to survival in opsonophagocytosis assays including a porcine serum with specific IgM and comparatively low specific IgG titers (α*S. suis* IgM: 29.2 ELISA-units and for comparison: αMRP IgG: 12.8 ELISA-units). Phenotypic analysis of *S. suis* was conducted in this study using the mutant 10Δ*ide*$_{Ssuis}$ [6] and two new in frame deletion mutants expressing truncated Ide$_{Ssuis}$ constructs. These new mutants, designated 10Δ*ide*$_{Ssuis}$_C-terminus and 10Δ*ide*$_{Ssuis}$_homologue, expressed the N-terminal part homologous to IdeS and the large C-terminal part lacking homologies, respectively (Additional file 4). Noteworthy, 10Δ*ide*$_{Ssuis}$ _C-terminus released IgM protease activity in the supernatant in contrast to 10Δ*ide*$_{Ssuis}$ and 10Δ*ide*$_{Ssuis}$_homologue (Additional file 4). As shown in Figure 5A 10Δ*ide*$_{Ssuis}$ and 10Δ*ide*$_{Ssuis}$_homologue had a significant lower survival factor compared to the wt strain and the survival factor for 10Δ*ide*$_{Ssuis}$_C-terminus was also found to be lower compared to the wt strain. The extent of attenuation of 10Δ*ide*$_{Ssuis}$ was significantly lower in opsonophagocytosis assays including serum from a colostrum-deprived piglet in comparison to assays including specific IgM. Inhibition of complement reduced the attenuation of the mutant 10Δ*ide*$_{Ssuis}$ significantly (Figure 5B).

Experimental infection of prime-vaccinated growing piglets suggests attenuation of the mutant 10Δide_{Ssuis}

Based on the in vitro results we considered Ide_{Ssuis} to be a putative virulence factor of *S. suis* in piglets with high titers of specific IgM. Thus, we conducted experimental infection of piglets prime vaccinated with a bacterin. Immunological screening of these piglets confirmed that these piglets had high specific IgM titers and low IgG titers against MRP, a main immunogen of this invasive *S. suis* pathotype (Additional file 5). We infected piglets with the wt and the 10Δide_{Ssuis} mutant as well as with the partial mutant 10Δide_{Ssuis}_homologue, which expressed only the C-terminus and showed no IgM proteolysis (Additional file 4). The complemented mutant was not included in the experimental infection because it showed attenuation in growth in medium (unpublished results). Sixty three percent of the piglets infected with the mutant 10Δide_{Ssuis} survived this experiment, whereas only 33% did so in the wt infected group ($p = 0.125$) (Figure 6A). Furthermore, 50% and 11% of 10Δide_{Ssuis} and wt infected piglets, respectively, were free of clinical signs throughout the observation period ($p = 0.076$; Figure 6B). Furthermore, 10Δide_{Ssuis} infected piglets had a lower pathohistological score ($\omega = 2.2$) in comparison to wt infected animals ($\omega = 3.7$; Table 1). In general, detection of fibrinosuppurative lesions was associated with detection of the infection strain. The mutant 10Δide_{Ssuis} was not detectable in any inner organ in 5 of 8 infected piglets (Table 2). However, the group infected with the deletion mutant 10Δide_{Ssuis}_homologue showed mortality and morbidity as well as a high rate of infection of inner organs very similar to the wt infected group (Figure 6; Table 2).

In summary, the results of the experimental infection suggested an attenuation of the mutant 10Δide_{Ssuis} in prime-vaccinated growing piglets with high titers of specific IgM.

Ide_{Ssuis} positively affects survival of *S. suis* in blood of piglets with high specific IgM titers ex vivo

As bacteremia is considered to be a critical step in the pathogenesis of invasive *S. suis* diseases, we further investigated survival of the different ide_{Ssuis} mutants and the wt in porcine blood with high IgM titers ex vivo. Thus, we evaluated Ide_{Ssuis}-dependent survival in blood from bacterin prime-vaccinated piglets. These piglets had significantly higher IgM titers against *S. suis* than unvaccinated weaning piglets investigated for comparison ($p < 0.01$; Additional file 6). As shown in Figure 7, the two mutants deficient in IgM proteolysis (10Δide_{Ssuis} and 10Δide_{Ssuis}_homologue) are significantly attenuated in survival in blood drawn from piglets prime-vaccinated with a bacterin. In contrast, the mutant expressing the truncated N-terminal domain with IgM protease activity (10Δide_{Ssuis}_C-terminus) was not attenuated in growth in porcine blood ex vivo.

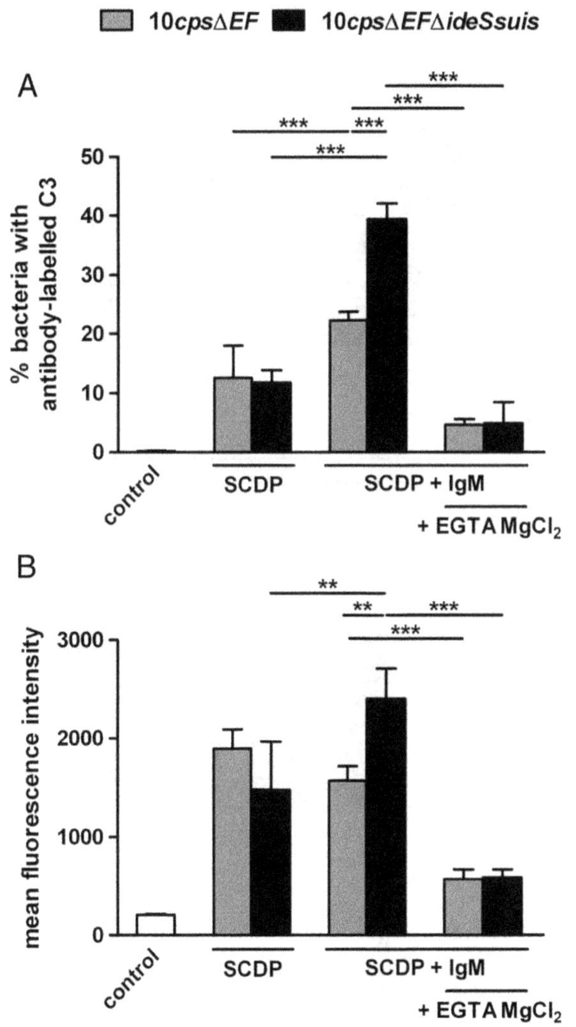

Figure 4 Expression of Ide_{Ssuis} reduces C3 deposition on the surface of an unencapsulated mutant triggered by IgM-mediated activation of the classical complement pathway. C3 antigen bound to the surface of the unencapsulated mutant 10*cps*Δ*EF* and the double mutant 10*cps*Δ*EF*Δide_{Ssuis} was detected through flow cytometry analysis. Bacteria were opsonized with sera from colostrum-deprived piglets (SCDP) or SCDP spiked with purified porcine IgM (SCDP plus IgM). To inactivate the classical complement activation pathway SCDP plus IgM was pretreated with EGTA $MgCl_2$. As control non-opsonized bacteria (incubated in PBS) were incubated with the C3 specific antibody. **(A)** The percentage of bacteria with antibody-labelled C3 and **(B)** the mean fluorescence intensity of the samples are shown. Bars and error bars represent mean values and standard deviations, respectively. Significant differences are indicated (*, $p < 0.05$; **, $p < 0.01$; ***, $p < 0.001$).

In conclusion, expression of the IgM protease Ide_{Ssuis} promotes increased survival of *S. suis* in porcine blood ex vivo, at least in the presence of specific IgM.

Discussion

The IgM pentamer is a very important activator of the classical complement pathway. It has been estimated

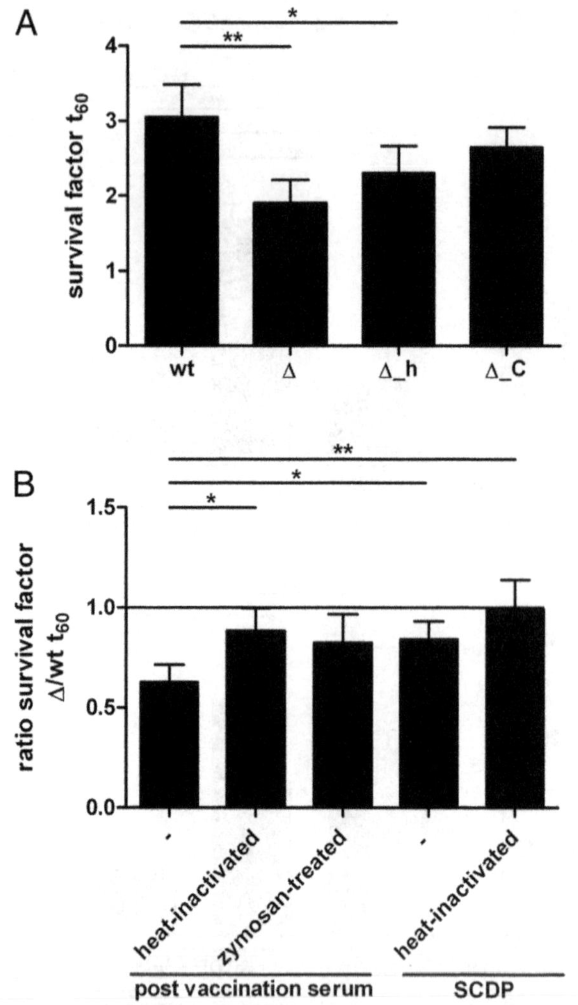

Figure 5 Ide$_{Ssuis}$ promotes survival in opsonophagocytosis assays including purified porcine neutrophilic granulocytes and serum with specific IgM titers. (A) Survival of strain 10 (wt), 10Δ*ide*$_{Ssuis}$ (Δ), 10Δ*ide*$_{Ssuis}$_homologue (Δ_h) and 10Δ*ide*$_{Ssuis}$_C-terminus (Δ_C) in opsonophagocytosis assays with serum from a piglet with specific IgM. **(B)** Attenuation of 10Δ*ide*$_{Ssuis}$ in opsonophagocytosis assays depends on active complement and adaptive immunity. The ratios of the survival factors of 10Δ*ide*$_{Ssuis}$ to the respective survival factors of wt are shown. A ratio of 1 is depicted by the horizontal line and refers to a lack of attenuation. To access the impact of complement, the post immune serum with specific IgM used for experiments shown in **(A)** was heat-inactivated or treated with zymosan. Samples with active and heat-inactivated serum from a colostrum-deprived pig were included to investigate whether this Ide$_{Ssuis}$-mediated phenotype depends on adaptive immunity. Bars and error bars represent mean values and standard deviations, respectively. Significant differences between strains and ratios of survival factors in **(A)** and **(B)**, respectively, are indicated (* $p < 0.05$, ** $p < 0.01$).

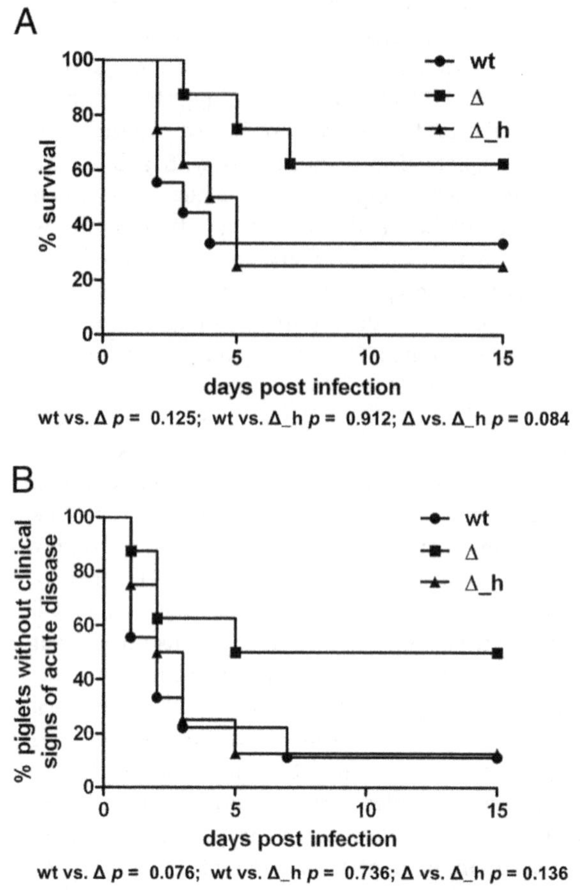

Figure 6 Mortality (A) and morbidity (B) of prime-vaccinated growing piglets intranasally challenged with the indicated *S. suis* strains. Growing piglets were infected with wild type strain 10 (wt), 10Δ*ide*$_{Ssuis}$ (Δ) and 10Δ*ide*$_{Ssuis}$ _homologue (Δ_h) 12 days after prime vaccination with a homologous *S. suis* serotype 2 bacterin. A piglet was determined as morbid in the case of elevated body temperature (≥40.2 °C) or specific clinical signs (signs of central nervous dysfunction or severe lameness). Statistical analysis of the Kaplan-Meier diagrams was conducted with the log-rank test (all *p*-values are shown below the diagrams).

that the efficiency of one pentameric IgM molecule to activate complement is equivalent to the respective efficiency of 1000 IgG molecules [29]. As cleavage of IgM by Ide$_{Ssuis}$ occurs at a site located between the antigen-recognizing part and the Fc-part containing the putative C1q binding motif, it was reasonable to hypothesize that IgM cleavage by Ide$_{Ssuis}$ is an important complement evasion mechanism of *S. suis*. In this study we obtained in vitro data supporting the hypothesis that Ide$_{Ssuis}$ is involved in complement evasion: (i) different recombinant Ide$_{Ssuis}$ constructs abolished the hemolysis induced by activation of the classical complement pathway in serum with specific IgM directed against erythrocytes; (ii) attenuation of the mutant 10Δ*ide*$_{Ssuis}$ in opsonophagocytosis assays was complement-dependent; (iii) IgM-triggered deposition of C3 on the bacterial surface is reduced by Ide$_{Ssuis}$ expression and (iv) attenuation of 10Δ*ide*$_{Ssuis}$ in survival in porcine blood ex vivo was observed in blood from piglets with high specific IgM titers.

Table 1 Scoring of fibrinosuppurative lesions of growing piglets intranasally infected with the indicated *S. suis* strains after prime-vaccination with a *S. suis* serotype 2 bacterin

Infection strain[a]	Piglets without lesions	Piglets with lesions in three or more locations	Brain			Serosae			Joint			Spleen and liver			Lung			Heart			
			Meningitis, chorioiditis			Pleuritis or peritonitis			Synovialitis			Splenitis[b] or hepatitis			Pneumonia			Endocarditis			
			5[c]	3[d]	1[e]	4[c]	2[d]	1[e]	4[c]	2[d]	1[e]	4[c]	2[d]	1[e]	4[c]	2[d]	1[e]	4[c]	2[d]	1[e]	ω[f]
wt	1/9	5/9	1/9	0/9	0/9	4/9	0/9	0/9	2/9	0/9	0/9	3/9	3/9	0/9	6/9	0/9	0/9	0/9	0/9	0/9	3.7
Δ	3/8	3/8	3/8	0/8	0/8	0/8	1/8	0/8	1/8	2/8	0/8	1/8	1/8	3/8	1/8	2/8	0/8	0/8	0/8	0/8	2.2
Δ_h	2/8	4/8	2/8	0/8	0/8	3/8	0/8	0/8	0/8	0/8	0/8	0/8	4/8	2/8	3/8	1/8	0/8	2/8	0/8	0/8	2.9

[a]Infection strains were strain 10 (wt), 10Δide_{Ssuis} (Δ) and 10Δide_{Ssuis}_homologue (Δ_h).
[b]Neutrophilic accumulation of the splenic red pulp.
[c]Scoring of 4 and 5 indicates moderate to severe diffuse or multifocal fibrinosuppurative inflammations.
[d]Scoring of 2 and 3 indicates mild focal fibrinosuppurative inflammation.
[e]Individual single perivascular neutrophils received a score of 1.
[f]$\omega = \Sigma score_{max}/n_{animals}$ [15].

The hemolysis assays of this study showed that Ide_{Ssuis} interferes substantially with activation of the classical complement pathway. Importantly, Ide_{Ssuis} mediated inhibition of complement activation by erythrocyte specific IgM was abrogated by pretreatment of Ide_{Ssuis} and Ide_{Ssuis}_homologue with the protease inhibitor iodoacetamide. As IgM is the only known substrate of this protease [6] and inhibition of IgM proteolysis by iodoacetamide was confirmed in this assay, we conclude that IgM proteolysis is involved in interference of Ide_{Ssuis} with complement activation. Accordingly, C3 deposition on *10cpsΔEFΔ*ide_{Ssuis} bacteria in serum from colostrum-deprived piglets spiked with specific IgM is significantly higher compared to C3 deposition on the Ide_{Ssuis} expressing strain *10cpsΔEF*.

Though IgM is much more powerful in activation of the classical complement pathway than IgG, immune evasion mechanism of bacteria counteracting the classical complement pathway have so far only been described for factors interacting with IgG. Specifically, protein H expressed by group A streptococci (GAS) reduces C3 deposition on IgG-coated beads and inhibits immune hemolysis of IgG-sensitized erythrocytes [30]. Furthermore, protection against opsonophagocytic killing of GAS in the presence of specific IgG is mediated by M-proteins and M-like proteins acting as Fc-receptors [31] and by the IgG protease IdeS [32]. In light of the different virulence factors counteracting IgG-mediated activation of the classical complement pathway, it is very much surprising that a bacterial evasion mechanism counteracting IgM-mediated complement activation has to the best of our knowledge not been described. The interference of Ide_{Ssuis} with IgM-mediated complement activation is important for pathogenesis, since survival of *S. suis* in porcine blood of prime-vaccinated piglets is significantly increased by Ide_{Ssuis} expression and clinical as well as pathological findings after experimental infection of respective piglets suggested attenuation of the isogenic mutant 10Δide_{Ssuis}.

Deposition of C3b on the surface of the encapsulated *S. suis* serotype 2 strains was only slightly determined by Ide_{Ssuis} expression under the chosen experimental conditions. The percentage of bacteria with detectable C3b deposition was below 16% after incubation of *S. suis* strains 10 and 10Δide_{Ssuis} in serum of colostrum-deprived piglets supplemented with purified porcine IgM (results not

Table 2 Reisolation of the infection strain from pigs primed with a bacterin and then infected with the indicated strains

Infection strain[a]	Number of pigs with an isolate of the infection strain in at least one inner organ[b]	Number of pigs with indicated site of infection strain[a] isolation/total number of pigs							
		Tonsils	Lung[c]	Serosa[d]	Spleen	Liver	Brain, CSF[e]	Joint fluid[f]	Endocard
wt	6/9	5/9	5/9	5/9	5/9	6/9	1/9	3/9	3/9
Δ	3/8	2/8	1/8	0/8	3/8	2/8	3/8	1/8	1/8
Δ_h	7/8	3/8	6/8	5/8	6/8	5/8	3/8	5/8	6/8

[a]Infection strains were strain 10 (wt), 10Δide_{Ssuis} (Δ) and 10Δide_{Ssuis}_homologue (Δ_h). Identification was conducted through PCR as described in Materials and methods.
[b]Piglets with isolates of the challenge strain exclusively from the tonsil were not considered.
[c]One cranial lobe was investigated.
[d]Pleural, peritoneal or pericardial cavity.
[e]Cerebrospinal fluid.
[f]Punctures of both tarsal and carpal joints were investigated in each animal. In cases of lameness additional joint punctures of the respective limb were screened.

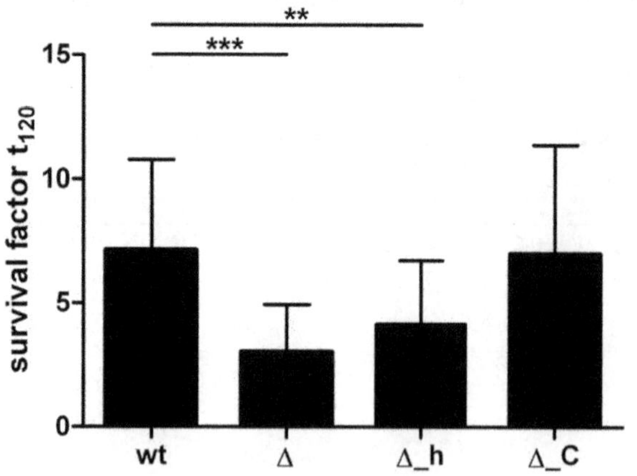

Figure 7 The mutants 10Δ*ide*$_{Ssuis}$ (Δ) and 10Δ*ide*$_{Ssuis}$ _homologue (Δ_h) are attenuated in survival in porcine blood ex vivo. The blood was drawn from 7 different growing piglets with an age of 5–7 weeks 6–14 days after prime vaccination with a *S. suis* bacterin. The mutant 10Δ*ide*$_{Ssuis}$ _C-terminus (Δ_C) not deficient in IgM proteolysis was also included. The bars and error bars represent mean values and standard deviations, respectively. Significant differences are indicated (** $p < 0.01$; *** $p < 0.001$).

shown) in contrast to the results shown for the unencapsulated mutants (Figure 4). This indicates in accordance with published results [7] that the capsule of serotype 2 is a main inhibitor of C3b deposition. Thus, we speculate that Ide$_{Ssuis}$ expression might be crucial for bacterial survival (i) during reduced capsule expression, (ii) in the presence of very high IgM titers against the polysaccharide capsule and (iii) in strains of serotypes that lack capsular sialic acid [8].

Two factor H binding proteins, have recently been identified in *S. suis* [12,13]. Factor H bound to the surface of *S. suis* serves as a cofactor for the factor-I mediated cleavage of C3b [12]. Deletion of the gene *fhb* encoding one of the factor H binding proteins led to a significant increase in C3b/iC3b deposition after opsonization with human serum. Activation of human complement was elicited by *S. suis* mainly via the alternative pathway under the chosen experimental conditions. However, in this work we demonstrate that in growing piglets with high titers of specific IgM the percentage of bacteria with antibody-labelled C3 is mainly determined by the classical pathway. This is important, because piglets with early adaptive immune responses are often affected by *S. suis* diseases and development of vaccines eliciting protection during this early immune response stage would substantially improve animal health.

Cleavage of IgM might have important biological consequences in addition to prevention of C3b deposition on the bacterial surface. Based on the identified cleavage site in the IgM heavy chain, Ide$_{Ssuis}$ activity should lead to release of a pentameric Fc-molecule including only C3 and C4 domains of the heavy IgM chains. We speculate that the cleavage product detected above the 250 kDa marker lane in Western blot analysis under non-reducing conditions [6] constitutes this pentameric molecule. Future studies should consider whether this putative C3-C4-pentamer modulates functions of the immune system. It is known that ½Fc IgG fragments released upon cleavage of IgG by IdeS prime neutrophils to respond to a second stimulus with an enhanced rate of reactive oxygen species production [33]. This might lead to activation of immune cells at sites remote from the pathogen. Similarly, the putative C3-C4 pentamer might also activate immune cells, e.g. by binding to the Fcμ receptor [34].

The results of the experimental infection suggested attenuation of the mutant 10Δide$_{Ssuis}$. However, the mutant expressing only the C-terminus of Ide$_{Ssuis}$ (10Δ*ide*$_{Ssuis}$_homologue) caused morbidity in prime-vaccinated piglets comparable to the wt and unlike the mutant 10Δ*ide*$_{Ssuis}$, which suggests that IgM proteolysis as such was not crucial for the outcome of the animal experiment and that the C-terminus of Ide$_{Ssuis}$ carries out important, yet unknown functions. Accordingly, the recombinant truncated protein consisting only of the C-terminus of Ide$_{Ssuis}$ showed also a significant interference with complement activation in the hemolysis assay suggesting an additional function of Ide$_{Ssuis}$ in complement inhibition but IgM proteolysis. Interestingly, the interference of this non-proteolytic construct did not seem to depend on the ratio of erythrocyte-specific IgM and IgG titers, in contrast to the interference by the IgM protease domain (as estimated by comparative analysis of post prime and post booster αEry sera). Further studies are certainly needed to decipher further functions of Ide$_{Ssuis}$ in complement evasion and their role in host-pathogen interaction.

Host-pathogen interaction of *S. suis* was investigated during early adaptive immune responses in this study. Survival in porcine blood with high specific IgM titers is significantly determined by expression of the IgM protease Ide$_{Ssuis}$. Accordingly, the in vitro results of this study demonstrate that Ide$_{Ssuis}$ abrogates activation of the classical complement system. As Ide$_{Ssuis}$ is expressed by all investigated *S. suis* strains [6], this unique virulence mechanism appears to be crucial for the evolutionary success of this pathogen.

Additional files

Additional file 1: Sequences of oligonucleotide primers. Name, sequence and position of target sequence of primers used in this study.

Additional file 2: Antibodies used in Western blot analysis. Specificity, source, conjugation and used dilution of antibodies.

Additional file 3: Flow cytometry analysis of C3 antigen (C3b/C3i) bound to opsonized *S. suis* strain 10 (wt) and 10Δide_{Ssuis} (Δ). Mean values and standard deviations (S. D.) for the percentage of C3-labelled bacteria and respective mean fluorescence intensity after opsonization of bacteria with sera including specific immunoglobulins as indicated.

Additional file 4: 10Δide_{Ssuis}_homologue (Δ_h) and 10Δide_{Ssuis}_C-terminus (Δ_C) release stabile fragments of Ide_{Ssuis} into the supernatant in accordance with IgM cleavage activity in the case of Δ_C. (A) αIde_{Ssuis}_C-terminus and αIde_{Ssuis}_homologue Western blot analysis of culture supernatants of 10Δide_{Ssuis} _homologue (Δ_h), 10Δide_{Ssuis}_C-terminus (Δ_C), 10Δide_{Ssuis} (Δ) and wild type strain 10 (wt). (B) 10Δide_{Ssuis}_C-terminus but not 10Δide_{Ssuis}_homologue exhibits IgM-cleaving activity. αIgM Western blot analysis of diluted porcine serum incubated with concentrated culture supernatants of 10Δide_{Ssuis}_homologue (Δ _h), 10Δide_{Ssuis} _C-terminus (Δ_C), 10Δide_{Ssuis} (Δ) and wild type strain 10 (wt) or with PBS.

Additional file 5: Immunological analysis of piglets used in the experimental infection (see Figure 6). (A) α-*S. suis* serotype 2 (ST2) IgM, (B) α-ST2 IgG titers and (C) α-MRP IgG titers were determined in serum samples of piglets after prime vaccination with a *S. suis* ST2 bacterin (before experimental infection) and as a control in unvaccinated piglets. Significant differences are indicated. Mean values are shown by horizontal lines.

Additional file 6: Immunological analysis of piglets used for the bactericidal assay (see Figure 7). (A) α-*S. suis* serotype 2 (ST2) IgM and (B) α-MRP IgG titers were determined in serum samples of these 7 growing piglets (prime-vaccinated) and for comparison in unvaccinated piglets. Prime vaccination was conducted with a *S. suis* serotype 2 bacterin. Significant differences are indicated (** $p < 0.01$). Horizontal lines represent mean values.

Abbreviations

S.: *Streptococcus*; Ide_{Ssuis}: Immunoglobulin M-degrading enzyme of *S. suis*; Ig: Immunglobulin; *E.*: *Escherichia*; MRP: Muramidase-released protein; FBPS: Fibronectin-and fibrinogen-binding protein of *S. suis*; TBST: Tris-buffered saline plus 0.1% Tween 20; PBST: PBS plus 0.1% Tween 20; SCDP: Serum of colostrum-deprived piglets; MFI: Mean fluorescence intensity; CFU: Colony forming units; Dpi: Days post infection; GAS: Group A streptococci; Fhb: Factor H binding protein; ST: Serotype; CSF: Cerebrospinal fluid.

Competing interests

The authors declare that they have no competing interests.

Authors' contributions

JS conducted mutagenesis, all complement assays and phenotyping of the mutants in vitro. Furthermore, she supported experimental infections, conducted statistical analysis and participated in experimental design and drafting the manuscript. AB conducted histopathological analysis. Immunological analysis of the piglets was performed by LMH. BJK conducted N-terminal sequencing of the cleavage products. UvPR and PVW participated in study design and manuscript revision. CGB conceived of the study, designed experiments, conducted experimental infections and drafted the manuscript. All authors read and approved the final manuscript.

Acknowledgements

We thank H. Smith (DLO-Lelystad, Netherlands) for *S. suis* strains 10 and 10*cps*Δ*EF*. Daisuke Takamatsu (National Institute of Animal Health, Japan) kindly provided the plasmid pSET5s. This study was supported by a grant of the Deutsche Forschungsgemeinschaft (DFG), Bonn, Germany (SFB587), IDT Biologika GmbH and by the German Federal Ministry for Research and Education (BMBF) within the Helmholtz – CAS – Joint Research Group ZooStrep (HCJRG-116). UvPR is supported by the Carl Tryggers foundation, Sweden. We acknowledge support from the German Research Foundation (DFG) and Universität Leipzig within the program of Open Access Publishing.

Author details

[1]Institute for Microbiology, Centre for Infection Medicine, University of Veterinary Medicine Hannover, 30173 Hannover, Germany. [2]Department of Pathology, University of Veterinary Medicine Hannover, 30559 Hannover, Germany. [3]Department of Structure and Function of Proteins, Helmholtz Centre for Infection Research, 38124 Braunschweig, Germany. [4]Department of Molecular Biology and Umeå Centre for Microbial Research, Umeå University, 90187 Umeå, Sweden. [5]Institute for Bacteriology and Mycology, Centre of Infectious Diseases, College of Veterinary Medicine, University Leipzig, An den Tierkliniken 29, 04103 Leipzig, Germany.

References

1. Wangkaew S, Chaiwarith R, Tharavichitkul P, Supparatpinyo K (2006) Streptococcus suis infection: a series of 41 cases from Chiang Mai University Hospital. J Infect 52:455–460
2. Mai NT, Hoa NT, Nga TV, le Linh D, Chau TT, Sinh DX, Phu NH, Chuong LV, Diep TS, Campbell J, Nghia HD, Minh TN, Chau NV, de Jong MD, Chinh NT, Hien TT, Farrar J, Schultsz C (2008) Streptococcus suis meningitis in adults in Vietnam. Clin Infect Dis 46:659–667
3. Tang J, Wang C, Feng Y, Yang W, Song H, Chen Z, Yu H, Pan X, Zhou X, Wang H, Wu B, Wang H, Zhao H, Lin Y, Yue J, Wu Z, He X, Gao F, Khan AH, Wang J, Zhao GP, Wang Y, Wang X, Chen Z, Gao GF (2006) Streptococcal toxic shock syndrome caused by Streptococcus suis serotype 2. PLoS Med 3:e151
4. Baums CG, Valentin-Weigand P (2009) Surface-associated and secreted factors of Streptococcus suis in epidemiology, pathogenesis and vaccine development. Anim Health Res Rev 10:65–83
5. Fittipaldi N, Segura M, Grenier D, Gottschalk M (2012) Virulence factors involved in the pathogenesis of the infection caused by the swine pathogen and zoonotic agent Streptococcus suis. Future Microbiol 7:259–279
6. Seele J, Singpiel A, Spoerry C, Pawel-Rammingen U, Valentin-Weigand P, Baums CG (2013) Identification of a novel host-specific IgM protease in Streptococcus suis. J Bacteriol 195:930–940
7. Seitz M, Beineke A, Singpiel A, Willenborg J, Dutow P, Goethe R, Valentin-Weigand P, Klos A, Baums CG (2014) Role of capsule and suilysin in mucosal infection of complement-deficient mice with Streptococcus suis. Infect Immun 82:2460–2471
8. Smith HE, de Vries R, van't Slot R, Smits MA (2000) The cps locus of Streptococcus suis serotype 2: genetic determinant for the synthesis of sialic acid. Microb Pathog 29:127–134
9. Marques MB, Kasper DL, Pangburn MK, Wessels MR (1992) Prevention of C3 deposition by capsular polysaccharide is a virulence mechanism of type III group B streptococci. Infect Immun 60:3986–3993
10. Lewis LA, Carter M, Ram S (2012) The relative roles of factor H binding protein, neisserial surface protein A, and lipooligosaccharide sialylation in regulation of the alternative pathway of complement on meningococci. J Immunol 188:5063–5072
11. Pian Y, Gan S, Wang S, Guo J, Wang P, Zheng Y, Cai X, Jiang Y, Yuan Y (2012) Fhb, a novel factor H-binding surface protein, contributes to the antiphagocytic ability and virulence of Streptococcus suis. Infect Immun 80:2402–2413
12. Vaillancourt K, Bonifait L, Grignon L, Frenette M, Gottschalk M, Grenier D (2013) Identification and characterization of a new cell surface protein possessing factor H-binding activity in the swine pathogen and zoonotic agent Streptococcus suis. J Med Microbiol 62:1073–1080
13. Volanakis JE (2001) Human C-reactive protein: expression, structure, and function. Mol Immunol 38:189–197
14. Butler JE, Zhao Y, Sinkora M, Wertz N, Kacskovics I (2009) Immunoglobulins, antibody repertoire and B cell development. Dev Comp Immunol 33:321–333
15. Czajkowsky DM, Shao Z (2009) The human IgM pentamer is a mushroom-shaped molecule with a flexural bias. Proc Natl Acad Sci U S A 106:14960–14965
16. Baums CG, Kaim U, Fulde M, Ramachandran G, Goethe R, Valentin-Weigand P (2006) Identification of a novel virulence determinant with serum opacification activity in Streptococcus suis. Infect Immun 74:6154–6162
17. Baums CG, Kock C, Beineke A, Bennecke K, Goethe R, Schröder C, Waldmann KH, Valentin-Weigand P (2009) Streptococcus suis bacterin and subunit vaccine immunogenicities and protective efficacies against serotypes 2 and 9. Clin Vaccine Immunol 16:200–208
18. de Greeff A, Buys H, Verhaar R, Dijkstra J, van Alphen L, Smith HE (2002) Contribution of fibronectin-binding protein to pathogenesis of Streptococcus suis serotype 2. Infect Immun 70:1319–1325

19. Smith HE, Damman M, van der Velde J, Wagenaar F, Wisselink HJ, Stockhofe-Zurwieden N, Smits MA (1999) Identification and characterization of the cps locus of Streptococcus suis serotype 2: the capsule protects against phagocytosis and is an important virulence factor. Infect Immun 67:1750–1756
20. Smith HE, Vecht U, Wisselink HJ, Stockhofe-Zurwieden N, Biermann Y, Smits MA (1996) Mutants of Streptococcus suis types 1 and 2 impaired in expression of muramidase-released protein and extracellular protein induce disease in newborn germfree pigs. Infect Immun 64:4409–4412
21. Sambrook J, Fritsch EF, Maniatis T (1989) Molecular cloning: a laboratory manual, 2nd edition. Cold Spring Harbor Laboratory Press, Cold Spring Harbor, N.Y
22. Wang Z, Zhang S, Wang G, An Y (2008) Complement activity in the egg cytosol of zebrafish Danio rerio: evidence for the defense role of maternal complement components. PLoS One 3:e1463
23. Kock C, Beineke A, Seitz M, Ganter M, Waldmann KH, Valentin-Weigand P, Baums CG (2009) Intranasal immunization with a live Streptococcus suis isogenic ofs mutant elicited suilysin-neutralization titers but failed to induce opsonizing antibodies and protection. Vet Immunol Immunopathol 132:135–145
24. Benga L, Fulde M, Neis C, Goethe R, Valentin-Weigand P (2008) Polysaccharide capsule and suilysin contribute to extracellular survival of Streptococcus suis co-cultivated with primary porcine phagocytes. Vet Microbiol 132:211–219
25. European Convention for the Protection of Vertebrate Animals Used for Experimental and Other Scientific Purposes. [http://www.conventions.coe.int/Treaty/en/Treaties/Html/123.htm]
26. Silva LM, Baums CG, Rehm T, Wisselink HJ, Goethe R, Valentin-Weigand P (2006) Virulence-associated gene profiling of Streptococcus suis isolates by PCR. Vet Microbiol 115:117–127
27. Wisselink HJ, Stockhofe-Zurwieden N, Hilgers LA, Smith HE (2002) Assessment of protective efficacy of live and killed vaccines based on a non-encapsulated mutant of Streptococcus suis serotype 2. Vet Microbiol 84:155–168
28. Arya S, Chen F, Spycher S, Isenman DE, Shulman MJ, Painter RH (1994) Mapping of amino acid residues in the C mu 3 domain of mouse IgM important in macromolecular assembly and complement-dependent cytolysis. J Immunol 152:1206–1212
29. Klimovich VB (2011) IgM and its receptors: structural and functional aspects. Biochemistry (Mosc) 76:534–549
30. Berge A, Kihlberg BM, Sjoholm AG, Bjorck L (1997) Streptococcal protein H forms soluble complement-activating complexes with IgG, but inhibits complement activation by IgG-coated targets. J Biol Chem 272:20774–20781
31. Nordenfelt P, Waldemarson S, Linder A, Mörgelin M, Karlsson C, Malmström J, Björck L (2012) Antibody orientation at bacterial surfaces is related to invasive infection. J Exp Med 209:2367–2381
32. Pawel-Rammingen U, Johansson BP, Bjorck L (2002) IdeS, a novel streptococcal cysteine proteinase with unique specificity for immunoglobulin G. EMBO J 21:1607–1615
33. Soderberg JJ, Pawel-Rammingen U (2008) The streptococcal protease IdeS modulates bacterial IgGFc binding and generates 1/2Fc fragments with the ability to prime polymorphonuclear leucocytes. Mol Immunol 45:3347–3353
34. Kubagawa H, Oka S, Kubagawa Y, Torii I, Takayama E, Kang DW, Gartland GL, Bertoli LF, Mori H, Takatsu H, Kitamura T, Ohno H, Wang JY (2009) Identity of the elusive IgM Fc receptor (FcmuR) in humans. J Exp Med 206:2779–2793

10

PCV2 vaccination induces IFN-γ/TNF-α co-producing T cells with a potential role in protection

Hanna C Koinig[1,2], Stephanie C Talker[2], Maria Stadler[2], Andrea Ladinig[1], Robert Graage[1,3], Mathias Ritzmann[1,4], Isabel Hennig-Pauka[1], Wilhelm Gerner[2†] and Armin Saalmüller[2*†]

Abstract

Porcine circovirus type 2 (PCV2) is one of the economically most important pathogens for swine production worldwide. Vaccination is a powerful tool to control porcine circovirus diseases (PCVD). However, it is not fully understood how PCV2 vaccination interacts with the porcine immune system. Especially knowledge on the cellular immune response against PCV2 is sparse. In this study we analysed antigen-specific T cell responses against PCV2 in a controlled vaccination and infection experiment. We focused on the ability of $CD4^+$ T cells to produce cytokines using multicolour flow cytometry (FCM). Vaccination with a PCV2 subunit vaccine (Ingelvac CircoFLEX®) induced PCV2-specific antibodies only in five out of 12 animals. Conversely, vaccine-antigen specific $CD4^+$ T cells which simultaneously produced IFN-γ and TNF-α and had a phenotype of central and effector memory T cells were detected in all vaccinated piglets. After challenge, seroconversion occurred earlier in vaccinated and infected pigs compared to the non-vaccinated, infected group. Vaccinated pigs were fully protected against viremia after subsequent challenge. Therefore, our data suggests that the induction of IFN-γ/TNF-α co-producing T cells by PCV2 vaccination may serve as a potential correlate of protection for this type of vaccine.

Introduction

Since the first description of porcine circovirus by Tischer et al. in 1982 [1], porcine circovirus type 2 (PCV2) has become one of the most important pathogens affecting the swine industry worldwide [2]. PCV2 is the causative agent of a number of disease syndromes summarized as porcine circovirus diseases (PCVD) among which postweaning multisystemic wasting syndrome (PMWS) is the economically most important [3,4]. Single PCV2 infection rarely results in clinical disease [5]. In the majority of cases pigs are subclinically infected [4]. However, coinfections with porcine reproductive and respiratory syndrome virus (PRRSV), porcine parvovirus (PPV) or *Mycoplasma hyopneumoniae* (*M. hyo*) are common and lead to more severe clinical symptoms [6,7].

In 2006 the first commercial PCV2 vaccines were introduced to the market [8]. Open reading frame 2 (ORF2) encoded capsid proteins were found to be immunogenic which made them suitable for vaccine development [9,10]. Indeed, two of four commercial PCV2 vaccines are based on recombinant ORF2 capsid proteins. Currently, PCV2 vaccination is widely used to combat PCVD. Different vaccines are commercially available and have successfully contributed to a decrease in mortality and an increase in growth parameters [11], probably via a reduction of PMWS severity [12]. Therefore, they are considered as an efficient tool to control PMWS [13].

The majority of domestic pigs are seropositive for PCV2-specific antibodies [12,14]. Of note, viremia is frequently detected in seropositive pigs. This led to the assumption that antibodies against PCV2 are not fully protective [15,16]. Furthermore, previous studies indicated that the analysis of antibody titres is often not sufficient to evaluate a protective immune response against PCV2 [17]. Other findings underline the importance of neutralizing antibodies. PMWS-affected pigs have lower titres of neutralizing antibodies than subclinically infected animals [18] and high titres of neutralizing antibodies are inversely

* Correspondence: armin.saalmueller@vetmeduni.ac.at
†Equal contributors
[2]Institute of Immunology, Department of Pathobiology, University of Veterinary Medicine, Vienna, Austria
Full list of author information is available at the end of the article

correlated with PCV2 load [19]. The role of cellular immune responses for protection against PCV2 is less well studied. It was shown that cellular immune responses are directed against capsid proteins as well as against the ORF1 encoded replicase protein [20]. Apparently, CD4$^+$ and CD8$^+$ T cells are involved in this response [21]. In addition, one study showed that virus clearance coincides with the appearance of PCV2-specific IFN-γ secreting cells (SC) [22].

The aim of the present study was to elucidate the role of antigen-specific cellular immune responses after PCV2 vaccination with a commercially available PCV2 subunit vaccine (Ingelvac CircoFLEX®). Since the analysis of PCV2-specific antibodies is not sufficient to predict protection against PCVD, antigen-specific cellular immune responses might play an important role. During a controlled vaccination and infection experiment we monitored clinical signs and analysed PCV2 viral load in serum samples by quantitative polymerase chain reaction (qPCR). Additionally, we investigated the humoral immune response by determination of PCV2-specific antibodies using a commercially available ELISA kit. The main interest was the determination of antigen-specific T cell responses. We analysed in detail the ability of CD4$^+$ T cells to produce IFN-γ and TNF-α by intracellular cytokine staining using multicolour flow cytometry (FCM). Our results provide first indications that the induction of IFN-γ/TNF-α co-producing CD4$^+$ T cells by PCV2 vaccination is associated with a reduction of viremia and therefore, might contribute to a protection against PCVD.

Materials and methods

Animals and study design

24 crossbred three week-old piglets (Large White X Landrace X Pietrain) were obtained from a conventional farm in Lower Austria and housed in the isolation unit of the Vetmeduni Vienna. On arrival, the piglets were weighed and divided into two groups according to their bodyweight. Half of the animals were vaccinated with a PCV2 subunit vaccine (Ingelvac CircoFLEX®, Boehringer Ingelheim Vetmedica, Ingelheim, Germany) according to the manufacturer's instructions on study day 0. Twenty-four days post vaccination (dpv) half of the vaccinated and non-vaccinated pigs were intranasally infected with a PCV2a field isolate (93965, origin Poland, provided by Boehringer Ingelheim). One mL of a virus suspension containing 10^5 $TCID_{50}$ of PCV2/mL was administered into each nostril. During the entire experiment the pigs were kept under ordinary husbandry conditions. Infected and non-infected animals were kept in separate compartments. Clinical signs were monitored daily. Blood samples were taken by puncture of the *V. cava cranialis* or *V. jugularis* as indicated in the timeline (Figure 1). Sera were obtained for the detection of PCV2-specific antibodies and for the determination of PCV2 viremia. Whole blood samples were taken to isolate PBMCs at 0 dpv, 24 dpv, 42 dpv and 56 dpv. For calculation of the average daily weight gain, piglets were weighed three times (Figure 1). The animal experiment was approved by the institutional ethics committee, the Advisory Committee for Animal Experiments (§12 of Law for Animal Experiments, Tierversuchsgesetz – TVG) and the Federal Ministry for Science and Research (reference number BMWF 68.205/0109-II/3b/2011).

Determination of viral load

Viremia was analysed by qPCR specific for ORF1 PCV2 DNA. The protocol for the qPCR was established at the University Clinic for Swine in cooperation with Dr Ingrid Huber (Bavarian Health and Food Safety Authority, Oberschleißheim, Germany). Both PCV2 primers and the probe attached within ORF1. Forward primer 5′-GGT ACT CCT CAA CTG CTG TCC-3′, reverse primer 5′-GGG AAA GGG TGA CGA ACT GG-3′ and the probe 5′-ACA GAA CAA TCC ACG GAG GAA GGG-3′ were purchased from TIB MOLBIOL (TIB MOLBIOL GmbH, Berlin, Germany). 6-carboxyfluorescein was used as fluorochrome and tetramethylrhodamine as quencher (TIB MOLBIOL GmbH). To create a standard curve for quantification of PCV2 DNA in the samples, a PCV2 PCR product was cloned into the PCR Cloning Vector pSC-A-amp/kan according to the manufacturer's instructions (StrataClone™ PCR Cloning Kit, Stratagene, Amsterdam,

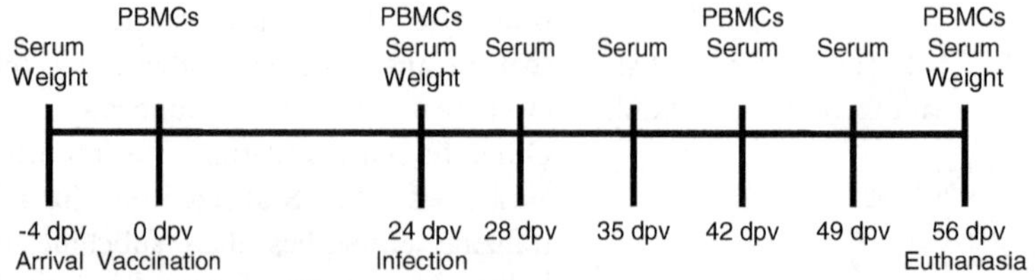

Figure 1 Time schedule of the animal experiment. Piglets were weighed after arrival and subsequently two more times in the course of the experiment. PCV2 vaccination was performed on study day 0. Piglets were inoculated with a PCV2a isolate 24 days post vaccination (dpv). Serum samples were taken twice before challenge (−4, 24 dpv) and 5 times thereafter (28, 35, 42, 49, 56 dpv). Heparinized blood samples for the isolation of PBMCs were taken on the day of vaccination, on day 24 post vaccination, 42 dpv and at the end of the study (56 dpv).

Netherlands). The insert was located in ORF1 and was produced by PCV2-specific PCR. After accumulation in *Escherichia coli* the obtained plasmid DNA was purified using Plasmid Midi Kit (Qiagen, Hilden, Germany) as recommended by the manufacturer. Different dilutions (10^2-10^9 copies/mL) of the purified plasmid DNA were used to establish a standard curve. As internal PCR control system a 125 bp fragment of *Nicotiana tabacum* (provided by I. Huber, Bavarian Health and Food Safety Authority) was used to avoid false negative results due to inhibitory effects of the sample matrix. Viral DNA was extracted from serum samples using High Pure PCR Template Preparation Kit (Roche, Mannheim, Germany) as recommended by the manufacturer. Thereafter DNA samples were diluted 1:10 with diethylpyrocarbonate-treated water (DEPC-treated water, Thermo Fisher Scientific, Waltham, MA, USA). A mastermix was prepared which contained Brilliant II QPCR MasterMix (Stratagene), PCV2 primers and PCV2 probe (TIB MOLBIOL GmbH) as well as primers and probe for the internal PCR control (provided by I. Huber, Bavarian Health and Food Safety Authority). The internal PCR control was added and the mastermix was pipetted to the DNA samples. A known positive serum was used as positive control. Additionally, a negative control containing DEPC-treated water (Thermo Fisher Scientific) was included in the qPCR assay. Finally, DNA fragments were amplified using Mx3005P Real Time Cycler (Stratagene). Thermocycling conditions involved an initial activation step of 95 °C for 10 min followed by 45 cycles of 95 °C for 15 s and 60 °C for 1 min. The PCR raw data was analysed using MxPro Software (Stratagene). The detection limit of the PCR was 25 virus copies/mL serum. Samples below this detection level were regarded as negative.

Determination of PCV2-specific antibody titres

Sera were analysed for PCV2-specific antibodies by a commercially available ELISA kit (INGEZIM Circovirus IgG/IgM, Ingenasa, Madrid, Spain) according to manufacturer's instructions. The ELISA was performed using an automated ELISA processing system (Dynex DS2®, Dynex Technologies, Chantilly, VA, USA).

Isolation of peripheral blood mononuclear cells (PBMCs)

PBMCs were isolated from heparinized blood samples by gradient centrifugation using lymphocyte separation medium (PAA, Pasching, Austria). The isolation procedure was performed as previously described [23]. After isolation, $3–6 \times 10^7$ PBMCs per cryo tube were frozen in freezing medium (50% RPMI 1640, PAN Biotech, Aidenbach, Germany, 40% fetal calf serum (FCS), PAA, 10% Dimethylsulfoxide, Sigma, Vienna, Austria) and stored at −150 °C.

In vitro re-stimulation of PBMCs and intracellular cytokine staining (ICS)

Defrosted PBMCs were counted and 5×10^5 cells per well were plated (U-bottomed 96-well microtitreplates, Greiner Bio One, Frickenhausen, Germany) in 150 μL culture medium (RPMI 1640, 10% FCS, 100 IU/mL penicillin, PAA). Cells were cultured at 37 °C and 5% CO_2 for four hours. Subsequently, PBMCs were stimulated with 4 μg/mL baculovirus-expressed capsid protein (PCV2-ORF2, provided by Boehringer Ingelheim). Cells cultured in medium only served as negative control. Stimulation with supernatant of baculovirus infected cell cultures was performed in separate experiments and did not show any difference to the medium control. After overnight incubation, 1 μg/mL Brefeldin A (BD GolgiPlug™, BD Biosciences, San Jose, CA, USA) was added and cells were incubated for another four hours. Afterwards, 12 wells per stimulation group were pooled and PBMCs were washed twice using phosphate buffered saline (PBS, PAN Biotech) containing 3% FCS (PAA). Six-colour FCM staining was performed in U-bottomed 96-well microtitreplates (Greiner Bio One). Table 1 provides information on antibodies used for FCM staining. Prior to use, all antibodies had been titrated and optimal working dilutions were determined according to the maximal staining index. Mastermixes of antibodies were prepared for each incubation step; incubations were performed for

Table 1 Antibodies for FCM staining

Antigen	Clone	Isotype	Fluorochrome	Labelling strategy	Source of primary Ab
CD4	74-12-4	IgG2b	Alexa488[a]	Secondary antibody	In house
CD8α	76-2-11	IgG2a	PE-Cy7[b]	Secondary antibody	In house
CD27	b30c7	IgG1	Alexa647[c]	Directly conjugated	In house
IFN-γ	P2G10	IgG1	PE[d]	Directly conjugated	BD Biosciences
TNF-α	MAb11	IgG1	BV605[e]	Directly conjugated	BioLegend

[a]Alexa488: Goat anti-Mouse IgG2b-Alexa488, Life Technologies, Carlsbad, CA, USA.
[b]PE-Cy7: Goat anti-Mouse IgG2a-PE-Cy7, Southern Biotech, Birmingham, AL, USA.
[c]Alexa647: Protein Labelling Kit Alexa 647, Life Technologies, Carlsbad, CA, USA.
[d]PE, BD Biosciences, San Jose, CA, USA.
[e]Brilliant Violet605, BioLegend, San Diego, CA, USA.

20 min at 4 °C in the fridge. Each incubation was followed by two washing steps with 200 μL of FCM buffer (PBS containing 3% FCS) and centrifugation. The cells were re-suspended using a plate shaker after each washing step. Cell surface markers were labelled by monoclonal antibodies (mAbs) against CD4, CD8α and CD27 (see Table 1 for details), followed by incubation with isotype-specific fluorochrome-labelled secondary antibodies. Fixable Near-IR Dead Cell Stain Kit (Life Technologies, Carlsbad, CA, USA) was included in the mastermix of secondary antibodies to discriminate live from dead cells. Mastermixes for primary antibodies were prepared in PBS containing 3% FCS; secondary antibodies were prepared in PBS only. After labelling of cell surface markers, cells were fixed and permeabilized by BD Cytofix/Cytoperm (BD Biosciences) according to manufacturer's instructions. Finally, mAbs against IFN-γ and TNF-α were added. Single stain samples for each fluorochrome were prepared as compensation controls.

Flow cytometry analysis

Samples were analysed using a FACSCanto II (BD Biosciences) flow cytometer equipped with three lasers (405, 488 and 633 nm). After measurement of compensation controls, compensation was calculated by FACSDiva software Version 6.1.3 (BD Biosciences). Flow cytometric data was analysed with the same version of FACSDiva software.

Statistics and preparation of diagrams

Statistics were calculated using IBM SPSS® Statistics 20 (IBM Corp., Armonk, NY, USA). Data was tested for normal distribution using Kolmogorov-Smirnov test. Analysis of variance (ANOVA) was performed to compare the four study groups. Tukey's range test was used for post-hoc analysis. For not normally distributed data Kruskal-Wallis test and consequently Mann–Whitney tests were executed to evaluate differences between the treatment groups. To analyse differences within one study group, paired t-tests were conducted for normally distributed data and Wilcoxon tests were used for not normally distributed data. Bar charts and scatter diagrams were created in Excel 2010 (Microsoft, Redmond, WA, USA).

Results

To evaluate the influence of vaccination against PCV2 with the recombinant baculovirus PCV2-ORF2 vaccine (Ingelvac CircoFLEX®) and subsequent challenge on the generation of antigen-specific T cells, 24 piglets were divided into four groups. Six piglets were immunized intramuscularly with the Ingelvac CircoFLEX® vaccine and represented the vaccinated group (VA). Another six piglets were vaccinated and intranasally infected (VI) at 24 dpv with a PCV2a isolate. An additional group of six animals was non-vaccinated and infected with the same virus strain at day 24 and represented the infection group (IN). Six non-vaccinated and non-infected animals served as controls (CO). The time course of the experiment is presented in Figure 1.

Clinical signs

On arrival, all piglets included in the study were clinically healthy. Vaccination did not induce any clinical signs. Likewise, no signs of disease were detected after PCV2 inoculation. None of the piglets showed any signs of PCVD throughout the entire study, despite the fact that PCV2 DNA could be detected in serum of five out of six animals in the IN group starting from day 35 (see below). No significant difference was found in average daily weight gain before and after PCV2 inoculation between the four study groups (data not shown).

PCV2 viral load in serum samples

Sera of all animals were investigated by qPCR for ORF1 DNA. No PCV2 nucleic acids were found in the serum samples taken on study day −4 and 24 dpv, i.e. prior to infection, and also four days after infection (28 dpv). The earliest time point for the detection of PCV2 DNA in the sera was 35 dpv (11 days after infection), and only one animal in the IN group was positive (Figure 2, IN, animal #3, IN3). In IN animals viremia could be detected at 42 dpv (18 days after infection) in four out of six animals. A viral load of $> 10^4$ PCV2 copies/mL serum was found in four of the positive pigs (IN3, IN4, IN5, IN6). One animal (IN1) had a viral load of $>10^6$ PCV2 copies/mL on two consecutive examination time points (42 dpv, 49 dpv) (Figure 2, IN). Another animal (IN2) did not show any detectable viremia at all investigated time points after infection. At 56 dpv (32 days after infection) no viral DNA could be detected in any sera of the IN group. All animals in the VI group (Figure 2) stayed negative for PCV2 DNA during the entire experiment. Likewise, sera of the CO and VA group remained free of PCV2 nucleic acids (Figure 2 and summarized in Figure 3A).

Serology

For a determination of the humoral immune response after PCV2 vaccination and infection, we analysed serum samples by a commercial ELISA (INGEZIM Circovirus IgG/IgM, Ingenasa, Madrid, Spain) which differentiates between PCV2-specific IgM and IgG antibodies. Results are displayed in a heat map, indicating the presence of PCV2-specific IgM and IgG antibodies, or both (Figure 3A). In addition, OD-values derived from this ELISA are shown in Figure 3B to allow a semi-quantitative evaluation of the titres in individual animals.

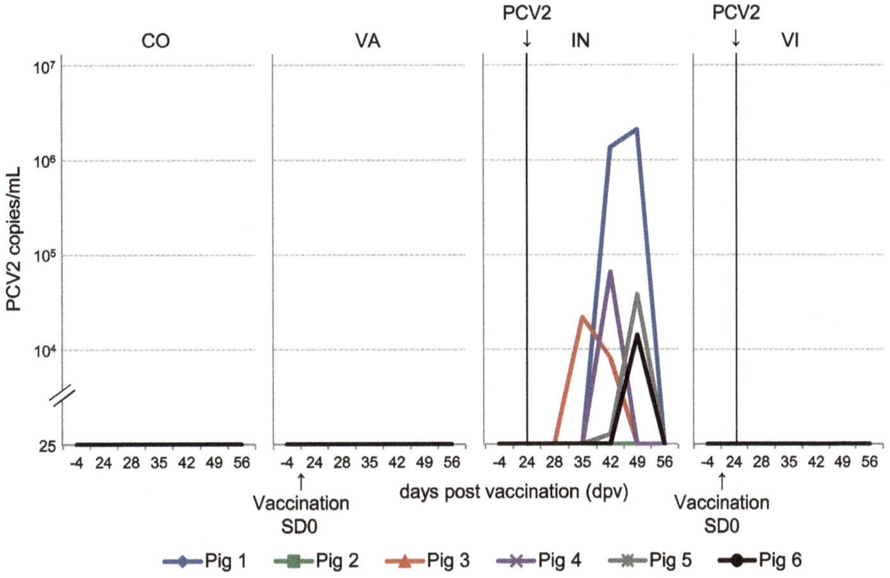

Figure 2 Viral load in animals of the different treatment groups. Sera were analysed for PCV2 DNA by quantitative PCR specific for ORF1. Line charts represent levels of virus titres in serum samples of individual animals within the four study groups (CO = control, VA = vaccinated, IN = infected, VI = vaccinated & infected) at all investigated time points before and after PCV2 infection. The detection level of the qPCR was 25 virus copies/mL serum. Samples below this level were regarded as negative. The arrows indicate PCV2 vaccination on study day 0 (SD0) and experimental PCV2 infection on day 24 post vaccination, respectively.

Due to the parallel IgM/ IgG detection, early after birth the test potentially discriminates between maternal PCV2-specific IgG antibodies and PCV2-specific IgM antibodies produced by the piglet. At the beginning of the experiment at day −4, twelve out of 24 piglets had PCV2-specific IgG antibodies, which were most likely maternally derived antibodies (Figures 3A and B). However, at 24 dpv only two animals were positive for IgG, indicating a decline of maternal antibodies. At this time point (24 dpv), within vaccinated animals (VA, VI), four were positive for IgM which most probably were induced by vaccination and one was positive for IgG. Of note, although titres remained below the cut-off value, in tendency all vaccinated animals showed an increase in OD-values for IgM from −4 dpv to 24 dpv (Figure 3B, VA, VI). After PCV2 inoculation (day 24), piglets from the vaccinated group (Figures 3A and B, VI) showed an earlier seroconversion than piglets from the IN group. Four days after infection (28 dpv), three out of six VI piglets had PCV2-specific antibodies. One animal (Figures 3A and B, VI1) showed IgG and IgM antibodies, whereas two other animals (VI5 and VI6) had IgG only. At 35 dpv four out of six animals in the VI group had seroconverted; 18 days after infection (42 dpv) all animals of the VI group showed a detectable antibody titre, with IgG antibodies being present in five of out of six animals. Only one animal (VI2) had IgM antibodies which could still be detected seven days later (49 dpv) together with IgG molecules. Another seven days later (56 dpv) only IgG could be identified in piglet VI2. PCV2-specific antibodies developed later in IN animals (Figures 3A and B, IN). Four days after infection (28 dpv), all piglets were negative. Seven days later (35 dpv) two out of six animals showed PCV2-specific antibodies, IN2 IgG and IN3 IgM. The IgM antibodies in IN3 coincided with viremia (Figure 3A, IN, black crosses). Another seven days later (18 days after infection, 42 dpv) IgM antibodies were present in three animals, all with a detectable viremia (IN1, IN3, IN4). One animal with detectable virus DNA (IN5) had not yet seroconverted and one animal without detectable viral DNA showed seroconversion to IgG antibodies (IN2). At 49 dpv individual animals of the IN group had either IgG, IgM or both types of antibodies and 56 dpv all IN animals were seropositive. Unlike VI animals, which were predominantly IgG positive, antibodies of both investigated isotypes were found across animals of the IN group. In contrast to the infected groups (IN, VI), pigs of the VA and CO group were seronegative at the three time points at the end of the experiment (42 dpv, 49 dpv, and 56 dpv), with the exception of one VA animal (Figure 3, VA5). Nevertheless, although titres remained below the cut-off value, in tendency all VA animals showed an increase in OD-values for IgG from 35 dpv to 56 dpv (Figure 3B).

Cytokine production of CD4$^+$ T cells and phenotype of cytokine-producing cells

The main focus of this study was the analysis of PCV2-specific CD4$^+$ T cell responses in regard to IFN-γ/TNF-α

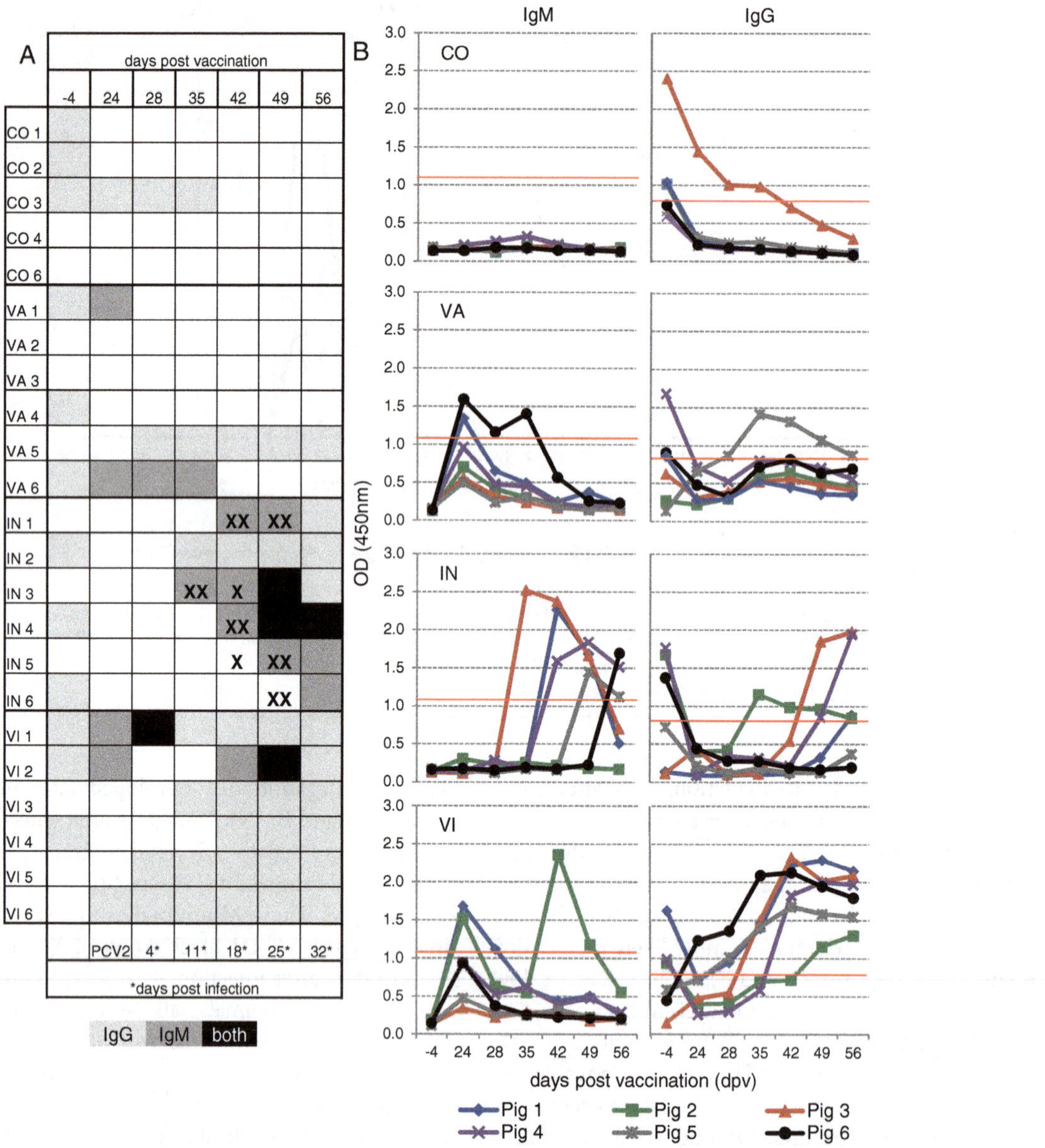

Figure 3 PCV2-specific IgM/IgG antibodies and coincidence with viremia. Serum samples were analysed for PCV2-specific antibodies by a commercially available ELISA kit (INGEZIM Circovirus IgG/IgM, Ingenasa, Madrid, Spain). **A)** The heatmap shows the detection of PCV2-specific IgM and IgG antibodies for all animals of the different study groups (CO = control, VA = vaccinated, IN = infected, VI = vaccinated & infected). Light grey fields represent samples positive for IgG. Dark grey fields indicate the detection of IgM antibodies. Black fields illustrate samples containing both IgM and IgG antibodies. PCV2 infection was performed 24 days post vaccination. Corresponding days post infection are indicated at the bottom of the table. Occurrence of PCV2 DNA in individual samples is marked by X. X indicates serum samples with < 10^4 PCV2 copies/mL, XX stands for > 10^4 PCV2 copies/mL. **B)** Raw data of the INGEZIM Circovirus IgG/IgM ELISA is depicted. OD-values, measured at 450 nm, of IgM (left) and IgG antibodies (right) for individual animals and all sampling points are shown. The red lines indicate the cut-off OD = 1.108 for IgM and OD = 0.821 for IgG, respectively.

production and phenotyping of responding cells. PBMCs were re-stimulated with the vaccine antigen (PCV2-ORF2) in vitro and analysed by multicolour FCM. Cells cultured in medium alone served as controls. In order to identify rare subsets of cytokine-producing T cells, at least 8×10^5 lymphocytes per sample, identified by light scatter properties, were acquired during FCM analyses. Total CD4$^+$ T cells were gated (Figure 4A) and analysed for IFN-γ and TNF-α production. To evaluate the memory phenotype of cytokine-producing T cells we further analysed the expression of the surface markers CD8α and CD27. The gating strategy and the cytokine analysis are displayed from representative experiments with PBMCs isolated from a control (CO, left) and a vaccinated (VA, right) animal in Figure 4A. Hardly any IFN-γ and IFN-γ/TNF-α co-producing T cells were detected in pigs belonging

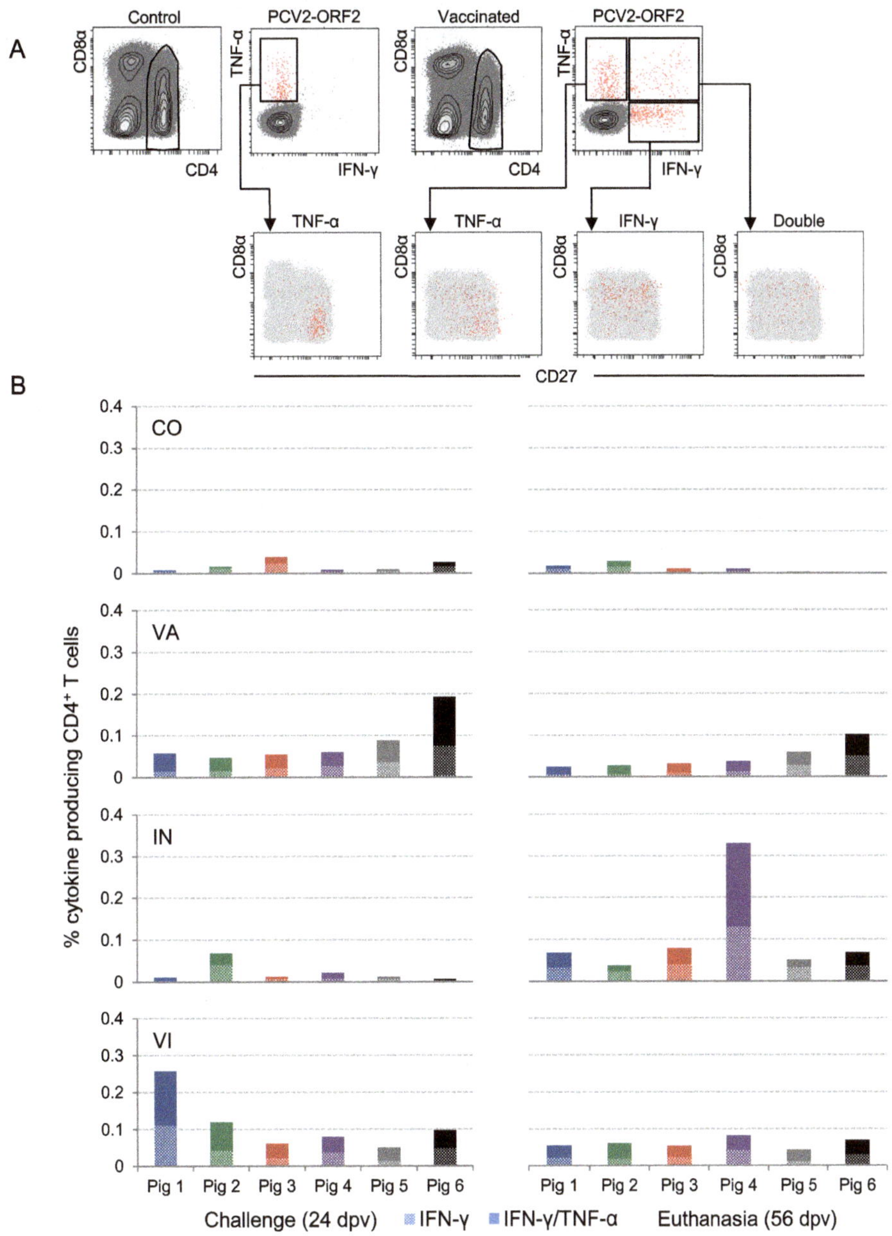

Figure 4 Frequency of PCV2-ORF2-specific cytokine-producing CD4$^+$ T cells. A) Porcine PBMCs were stimulated with PCV2-ORF2 over night or were cultured in medium as negative control. CD4$^+$ T cells were gated and analysed for production of IFN-γ and TNF-α by intracellular cytokine staining (top panel). Cytokine-producing CD4$^+$ T cell subsets were further sub-gated for the analysis of CD8α and CD27 expression (bottom panel). Red dots indicate cytokine-producing CD4$^+$ T cells; grey dots represent total CD4$^+$ T cells. FCM data is shown for one representative animal of the control (CO) and vaccinated group (VA) at 24 dpv. **B)** Stacked bar charts indicate percentages of cytokine-producing CD4$^+$ T cells within total CD4$^+$ T cells from individual animals of the treatment groups (CO = control, VA = vaccinated, IN = infected, VI = vaccinated & infected) prior to infection (24 dpv) and at the end of the study (56 dpv). Hatched bars represent percentages of IFN-γ single-producing CD4$^+$ T cells and filled bars illustrate percentages of IFN-γ/TNF-α co-producing CD4$^+$ T cells within total CD4$^+$ T cells.

to the CO group. In contrast, TNF-α single production in response to PCV2-ORF2 was also found in CO animals. These TNF-α single-producing T cells from CO animals were CD4$^+$ and mostly had a naïve phenotype (CD8α$^-$), indicating that this subpopulation does not represent PCV2-specific memory cells. Therefore, TNF-α single-producing T cells were excluded from further analyses. In contrast, in the vaccinated groups (VA, VI) IFN-γ single-producing as well as IFN-γ/TNF-α co-producing T cells were induced after vaccination. These cells were mainly CD8α$^+$ and therefore, considered as antigen experienced. CD27$^+$ central memory T cells (T_{CM}) and CD27$^-$

effector memory T cells (T_{EM}) were present in this population of cytokine-producing T cells (Figure 4A).

Percentages of CD4$^+$ IFN-γ single and IFN-γ/TNF-α co-producing T cells at two investigated time points, prior to challenge (24 dpv) and at the end of the study (56 dpv), for the individual animals within respective groups are shown in Figure 4B. Moreover, the mean values of these two subpopulations for each treatment group were calculated and subjected to statistical analyses (Additional file 1). Background levels of about 0.02% IFN-γ single-producing cells within total CD4$^+$ T cells were identified in PBMCs isolated from CO animals at 24 dpv and at the end of the study (56 dpv) and the frequencies of IFN-γ/TNF-α co-producing T cells were even lower (≤0.014%). Cytokine production prior to vaccination was tested for three animals belonging to either the VI or the VA group. At 0 dpv CD4$^+$ T cells of all animals showed minimal IFN-γ/TNF-α production (IFN-γ$^+$TNF-α$^-$ ≤ 0.014%, IFN-γ$^+$TNF-α$^+$ ≤ 0.0098%; Additional file 2). Also, cytokine production in samples incubated with cell culture medium only was close to zero for all animals and time points (data not shown).

Compared to the CO group the frequency of IFN-γ producing T cells isolated from animals of the VA group was higher at 24 dpv. By this time, all animals of the VA group had higher levels of IFN-γ/TNF-α co-producing T cells than the controls ($p = 0.044$). Animal VA6 showed the most prominent response to vaccination, especially regarding the development of double cytokine-producing T cells. The frequency of IFN-γ single as well as IFN-γ/TNF-α co-producing T cells declined in all VA animals ($p = 0.004$ for IFN-γ and $p = 0.028$ for IFN-γ/TNF-α co-producing T cells, respectively) towards the end of the study (56 dpv).

Before challenge, the IN pigs had similar low frequencies of IFN-γ$^+$ and IFN-γ$^+$TNF-α$^+$ T cells as animals from the CO group. After experimental PCV2 infection, we observed a strong increase of IFN-γ single-producing T cells in this group. IN4 had the strongest response to PCV2 infection with a 15-fold enhancement of IFN-γ$^+$CD4$^+$ T cells by the end of the study. Similar results were obtained for IFN-γ/TNF-α co-producing T cells ($p = 0.046$). We found a strong increase of double cytokine-producing T cells after PCV2 infection in five IN pigs, among which IN4 was outstanding (0.1996%). IN2 had low levels (0.03%) of double cytokine-producing T cells before challenge which did not further increase after PCV2 infection.

Similar to VA animals, VI pigs had elevated frequencies of IFN-γ producing CD4$^+$ T cells compared to their non-vaccinated counterparts at 24 dpv. Furthermore, a clear induction of bi-functional T cells in response to vaccination was detected in all VI animals 24 dpv. In contrast to IN pigs, no further increase of single or double cytokine-producing CD4$^+$ T cells was observed after PCV2 infection. Instead, the frequency of cytokine-producing T cells slightly declined towards the end of the study.

Results from the VI group had indicated that an increase in IFN-γ single and IFN-γ/TNF-α double-producing CD4$^+$ T cells led to an accelerated occurrence of PCV2-specific IgG antibodies following PCV2 infection. This raised the question if the IgG antibodies seen at 32 days post infection (dpi) in four out six animals of the IN group were also preceded by an increase of PCV2-specific cytokine-producing CD4$^+$ T cells. Therefore, PBMCs isolated from the IN group were tested also 18 dpi and data is displayed in a time course (Figure 5). Indeed, three of the four animals with PCV2-specific IgG antibodies at

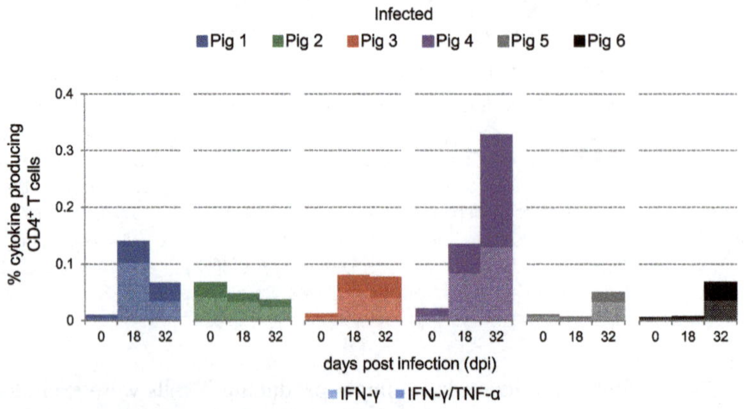

Figure 5 Kinetics of PCV2-specific cytokine-producing CD4$^+$ T cells following PCV2 infection. PBMCs isolated from PCV2 infected animals (not vaccinated, IN-group) before infection and 18 or 32 days post infection (dpi) were stimulated with PCV2-ORF2. CD4$^+$ T cells were gated as described before and analysed for IFN-γ and TNF-α production. Stacked bar charts indicate percentages of cytokine-producing CD4$^+$ T cells from individual animals. Hatched bars represent percentages of IFN-γ single-producing CD4$^+$ T cells and filled bars illustrate percentages of IFN-γ/TNF-α co-producing CD4$^+$ T cells within total CD4$^+$ T cells.

32 dpi (IN1, IN3, IN4) showed a strong increase of IFN-γ single and IFN-γ/TNF-α double-producing $CD4^+$ T cells at 18 dpi. IN5 and IN6 who lacked single and double cytokine-producing T cells 18 dpi were only positive for IgM by the end of the study and did not perform a class switch to IgG.

Lastly, having observed the marked induction of IFN-γ/TNF-α co-producing $CD4^+$ T cells following PCV2 vaccination and also PCV2 infection, we compared the CD27 expression in PCV2-specific IFN-γ^+TNF-$\alpha^+$$CD4^+$ T cells from VA animals at 24 dpv (day of experimental infection), IN animals at the day of euthanasia and VI animals at both time points (Figure 6). Regardless of the treatment group and the time point, $CD27^+$ central memory T cells (T_{CM}) were present in higher frequencies than $CD27^-$ effector memory T cells (T_{EM}) in the vast majority of samples.

Discussion

PCV2 continues to be a highly relevant pathogen for modern swine production which needs to be controlled by vaccination [2]. The role of the humoral immune response after PCV2 vaccination has been extensively studied

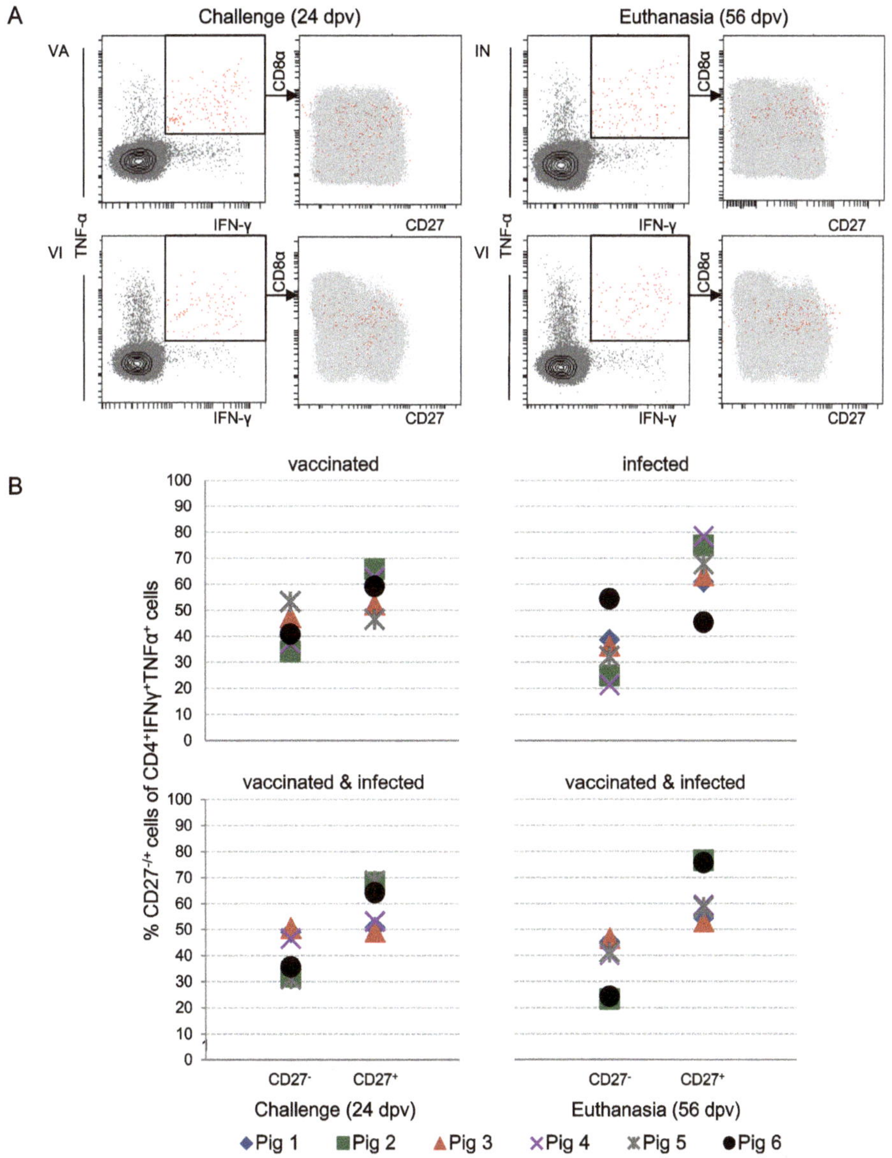

Figure 6 Memory phenotype of IFN-γ/TNF-α co-producing $CD4^+$ T cells. A) $CD4^+$ T cells were gated (not shown) and analysed for IFN-γ and TNF-α production following PCV2-ORF2 restimulation. IFN-γ/TNF-α double cytokine-producing $CD4^+$ T cells were sub-gated and investigated for CD8α and CD27 expression. Representative data of animals VA6 (24 dpv), IN3 (56 dpv) and VI6 (challenge and euthanasia) are shown. **B)** Symbols in the scatter diagrams represent percentages of $CD27^-$ effector memory T cells (T_{EM}) and $CD27^+$ central memory T cells (T_{CM}) within the subpopulation of IFN-γ/TNF-α co-producing T cells. Data is shown for individual animals of the vaccinated (VA), infected (IN) and vaccinated & infected (VI) group. The investigated time points correspond to 24 dpv (challenge) and 56 dpv (euthanasia).

but knowledge on cellular immune responses is sparse. Based on a controlled PCV2 vaccination-infection experiment, the present study puts a strong focus on the role of $CD4^+$ T cells and their potential role following vaccination and/ or infection.

Clinical signs

Clinical manifestation of PCV2 infection varies and can result in distinct diseases. Most pigs are subclinically infected. In other cases lung disease, enteric disease, reproductive failure or porcine dermatitis and nephropathy syndrome (PDNS) may occur. PMWS is the economically most important manifestation of PCV2 infection [3,4]. It is generally accepted, that PCV2 alone is not sufficient to induce PCVD. Coinfections with other viral or bacterial pathogens are needed to provoke more severe clinical symptoms [5]. Accordingly, we did not observe any signs of PCVD after singular PCV2 infection in our animal experiment.

PCV2 viral load in serum samples

Detection of PCV2 antigen within characteristic microscopic lesions is one of the key requirements for PCVD diagnosis [24,25]. In addition, determination of high viral loads (> $10^{4.7}$ PCV2 copies/mL) in serum samples by qPCR is an indicator for PCVD [4]. Hence, we analysed serum samples collected at regular intervals throughout the vaccination-infection experiment for the amount of PCV2 DNA. In our study, viremia occurred in the IN group only. Interestingly, piglets vaccinated with the PCV2 subunit vaccine seemed to be protected and did not develop viremia after PCV2 inoculation (Figure 2). This is in accordance with other studies: in field studies, the same PCV2 subunit vaccine significantly reduced PCV2 viral load and duration of viremia in sera of pigs suffering from PMWS and porcine respiratory disease complex (PRDC), respectively [26,27]. Under experimental conditions, four commercially available PCV2 vaccines, including the subunit vaccine used in our study, significantly decreased PCV2 DNA in the blood after PCV2 challenge [28]. However, in all these studies viremia was not completely prevented by PCV2 vaccination. Nevertheless, we assume that our experimental infection was successful because similar levels of viremia were achieved after singular PCV2 infection elsewhere [28].

Serology

Serum antibodies against PCV2 are wide spread in pig populations all over the world [12,14]. However, the analysis of PCV2-specific antibody titres is challenging from a technical perspective. Several studies revealed that vast differences among laboratories and various ELISA test systems exist [29,30]. Despite these issues, we decided to use a qualitative ELISA capable of distinguishing IgM from IgG antibodies. This enabled us to differentiate between maternally derived and vaccine induced antibodies. 24 dpv PCV2-specific antibodies, which were considered to be induced by vaccination, were detected in five out of 12 vaccinated piglets. After experimental infection, all infected animals seroconverted independent of vaccination status. Of note, seroconversion occurred earlier in VI pigs than in IN pigs. These results are comparable to previous data. Several recent studies described that pigs vaccinated with PCV2 subunit vaccines showed a prompt seroconversion and had increased antibody titres compared to their non-vaccinated counterparts under experimental conditions as well as after natural PCV2 infection [28,31].

Although all animals of the VI group had detectable PCV2-specific IgG titres at the end of the study, for some individuals this was not preceded by a clear IgM response. However, although titres remained below the cut-off value, in tendency also VI animals 3, 4, 5 and 6 showed an increase in OD-values for IgM from –4 dpv to 24 dpv. In addition, it is conceivable that these animals with IgM titres below the cut-off had higher titres before day 24 post vaccination. Nevertheless, antibodies of the IgG isotype were predominant in samples of VI pigs, whereas a mixture of IgM and IgG antibodies was found in IN pigs (Figure 3). The early occurrence of IgG antibodies is most probably a beneficial effect of the vaccination which may be related to the presence of vaccine-specific $CD4^+$ T cells with a helper function (see also below).

Cytokine production of $CD4^+$ T cells and phenotype of cytokine-producing cells

It is likely that a sufficient protection against PCV2 infection is achieved by a response of both the humoral and the cellular immune system following vaccination. So far, little is known about the cellular immune response and knowledge on the development of antigen-specific T memory cells after PCV2 vaccination is sparse. Therefore, a detailed examination of vaccine induced antigen-specific $CD4^+$ T cells and their IFN-γ/TNF-α production was the main focus of our study. To evaluate the memory phenotype of cytokine-producing cells, we further analysed the expression of CD8α and CD27. As mentioned above, CD8α can be found on activated, antigen experienced T cells and memory T cells whereas naïve T helper cells are considered CD8α negative [32]. Similar to humans CD27 distinguishes between porcine central and effector memory T cells [33]. IFN-γ single and IFN-γ/TNF-α co-producing $CD4^+$ T cells induced after vaccination were mainly activated $CD8\alpha^+$ T cells. We detected a homogenous distribution of $CD27^+$ central memory T cells (T_{CM}) and $CD27^-$ effector memory T cells (T_{EM}) within IFN-γ/TNF-α co-producing T cells in VA, IN and VI pigs. Apparently, all memory phenotypes were addressed equally by PCV2 vaccination and/ or infection (Figure 4A and Figure 6). With these findings we expand previous knowledge that PCV2 vaccination elicits $CD4^{+}CD8\alpha^{+}$ memory T cells [34].

So far, it is known that the development of IFN-γ secreting cells (SC) is a key event in cell-mediated PCV2 immunity [35]. A good example for that is the inverse correlation of IFN-γ SC and numbers of PCV2 copies in serum samples [28,36]. In the present study, we additionally investigated the phenotype of the IFN-γ producing T cells by ICS after in vitro re-stimulation with PCV2-ORF2. We detected a higher frequency of IFN-γ single-producing $CD4^{+}$ T cells in vaccinated animals compared to their non-vaccinated counterparts at 24 dpv. Similarly, the frequency of IFN-γ producing $CD4^{+}$ T cells increased in the IN group after experimental PCV2 infection (Figure 4B, Figure 5). Obviously, this increase of antigen-specific IFN-γ producing cells is a response to vaccination and infection. Similar results were obtained in studies investigating cell-mediated immune responses against PCV2 based on determination of IFN-γ SC by ELISpot assay. In accordance with our data, IFN-γ SC in response to capsid protein were induced in vaccinated as well as in vaccinated and challenged pigs [37]. Amounts of PCV2-specific IFN-γ SC increased also in vaccinated and naturally PCV2 infected pigs [38]. Unlike others, we did not detect a further enhancement of cytokine-producing cells after experimental infection in vaccinated and infected pigs [39].

Evidence exists that the magnitude of IFN-γ production by $CD4^{+}$ T cells alone is not always sufficient to predict protection [40] and that multi-functional T cells, which simultaneously produce IFN-γ, interleukin-2 (IL-2) and TNF-α, are strongly correlated with protection [41]. Hence, in addition to IFN-γ, we investigated TNF-α expression by $CD4^{+}$ T cells and consequently evaluated the appearance of IFN-γ/TNF-α co-producing T cells. 24 dpv we found elevated levels of $IFN\text{-}\gamma^{+}TNF\text{-}\alpha^{+}CD4^{+}$ T cells in all vaccinated animals (VA, VI). The frequency of these cells declined in the VA group towards the end of the study (56 dpv). In the IN group we also observed these double cytokine-producing T cells following PCV2 inoculation. Similar to IFN-γ single-producing cells, no further increase of co-producing T cells was observed in the VI group after PCV2 challenge (Figure 4B). Nevertheless, it is conceivable that the induction of PCV2-specific IFN-γ/ TNF-α co-producing $CD4^{+}$ T cells by a non-replicative agent, i.e. the ORF2 subunit vaccine, is sufficient to control a subsequent PCV2 infection. Another important finding of this study is that the occurrence of cytokine-producing $CD4^{+}$ T cells 18 dpi was associated with a subsequent isotype-switch from IgM to IgG in the IN group. This phenomenon may be interpreted as a helper function of $CD4^{+}$ T cells for antibody production and antibody class switch and support the hypothesis that these double cytokine-producing T cells play a role in protection against PCV2.

In conclusion, our data shows that PCV2 vaccination did not induce stable titres of PCV2-specific IgG antibodies in all vaccinated animals. Nevertheless, the PCV2 subunit vaccine was highly efficacious and prevented viremia in all vaccinated and infected pigs. Moreover, the amount of IFN-γ producing $CD4^{+}$ T cells increased after PCV2 vaccination and/ or infection. Contrary to PCV2-specific antibodies, antigen-specific $IFN\text{-}\gamma^{+}TNF\text{-}\alpha^{+}CD4^{+}$ T cells were induced in all vaccinated pigs. The appearance of these cells seems to be linked to a switch from IgM to IgG indicating their relevance for protection after PCV2 infection. Therefore, IFN-γ/TNF-α co-producing T cells might represent a new correlate of an immune reaction after PCV2 vaccination and their existence after vaccination might correlate with protection. This finding needs further investigation.

Additional files

Additional file 1: Mean cytokine production of PCV2-ORF2 specific $CD4^{+}$ T cells. Stacked bar charts indicate mean percentages of cytokine-producing $CD4^{+}$ T cells of the respective groups (CO = control, VA = vaccinated, IN = infected, VI = vaccinated & infected) at the investigated time points prior to challenge (C, 24 days post vaccination) and at the day of euthanasia (E, 56 days post vaccination). Hatched bars represent percentages of IFN-γ single-producing $CD4^{+}$ T cells and filled bars illustrate percentages of IFN-γ/TNF-α co-producing $CD4^{+}$ T cells. Minuscules indicate significant differences ($p < 0.05$) between treatment groups and investigated time points, respectively. For IFN-γ single-producing $CD4^{+}$ T cells significant differences were detected between CO and IN at the end of the study (E) (a:b $p = 0.035$) and within the VA group between 24 dpv (C) and 56 dpv (E) (c:d $p = 0.004$). For IFN-γ/TNF-α co-producing $CD4^{+}$ T cells differences were significant on day 24 post vaccination between CO and VA (e:f $p = 0.044$), CO and VI (e:g $p = 0.006$) and IN and VI (g:h $p = 0.011$). On study day 56 post vaccination differences were significant between CO and VA, IN and VI, respectively (i:j $p = 0.006$). Within the IN group more IFN-γ/TNF-α co-producing $CD4^{+}$ T cells were detected after experimental infection (h:j $p = 0.046$) and in both vaccinated groups (VA and VI) frequency of double cytokine-producing cells declined towards the end of the study (56 dpv) (f:j; g:j $p = 0.028$).

Additional file 2: Cytokine production of $CD4^{+}$ T cells in the time course before and after PCV2 vaccination. The frequency of PCV2-ORF2-specific cytokine-producing $CD4^{+}$ T cells in the time course before and after vaccination for three animals of the vaccinated (VA, top panel) and three animals of the vaccinated and infected group (VI, bottom panel) was analysed. Contour plots display data from one representative animal (VI1) before vaccination and 24 days post vaccination (dpv). PBMCs were stimulated with PCV2-ORF2 and $CD4^{+}$ T cells were gated as described above. Stacked bar charts indicate percentages of cytokine-producing $CD4^{+}$ T cells before vaccination as well as 24 and 56 dpv from individual animals. Hatched bars represent percentages of IFN-γ single-producing $CD4^{+}$ T cells and filled bars illustrate percentages of IFN-γ/ TNF-α co-producing $CD4^{+}$ T cells within total $CD4^{+}$ T cells.

Abbreviations

BV: Brilliant violet; CD: Cluster of differentiation; CO: Control group; DMSO: Dimethyl sulfoxide; dpi: Days post infection; dpv: Days post vaccination; ELISA: Enzyme linked immunosorbent assay; ELISpot: Enzyme linked immunosorbent spot; FCM: Flow cytometry; FCS: Fetal calf serum; ICS: Intracellular cytokine staining; IFN-γ: Interferon gamma; IL-2: Interleukin 2;

IN: Infection group; IU: International unit; mAB: Monoclonal antibody; *M. hyo*: *Mycoplasma hyopneumoniae*; ORF: Open reading frame; PBMCs: Peripheral blood mononuclear cells; PBS: Phosphate buffered saline; PCV2: Porcine circovirus type 2; PCVD: Porcine circovirus diseases; PDNS: Porcine dermatitis and nephropathy syndrome; PE: Phycoerythrin; PMWS: Postweaning multisystemic wasting syndrome; PPV: Porcine parvovirus; PRRSV: Porcine reproductive and respiratory syndrome virus; qPCR: Quantitative polymerase chain reaction; SC: Secreting cells; T_{CM}: Central memory T cells; T_{EM}: Effector memory T cells; TNF-α: Tumor necrosis factor alpha; VA: Vaccination group; VI: Vaccinated and infected group.

Competing interests

The authors declare that they received funding for this project from the company Boehringer Ingelheim Animal Health GmbH.

Authors' contributions

HK participated in practical work during the animal experiment, performed the FCM analysis and wrote the manuscript. ST established the protocol for the intracellular cytokine staining. MS participated in the practical work during FCM experiments. WG was involved in the planning and establishment of the experiments and preparation of the manuscript. AL organized and guided the animal experiment. RG helped to conduct the animal experiment. IH assisted to edit the manuscript. MR and AS conceived the study. MR further contributed to the organization of the animal experiment and AS helped to set up the FCM experiments and draft the manuscript. All authors read and approved the final manuscript.

Acknowledgements

The authors thank Pamela Lakits, Heidelore Arbinger and Christiane Weissenbacher-Lang for the generation of the qPCR results and for performing the INGEZIM Circovirus IgM/IgG ELISA. The authors acknowledge Boehringer Ingelheim for the supply of the challenge virus and the baculovirus-expressed capsid protein as well as for funding. Hanna Koinig was funded by the Comet program "Preventive veterinary medicine: Improving pig health for safe pork production" sponsored by BMVIT, BMWFJ and the government of Lower Austria.

Author details

[1]University Clinic for Swine, Department for Farm Animals and Veterinary Public Health, University of Veterinary Medicine, Vienna, Austria. [2]Institute of Immunology, Department of Pathobiology, University of Veterinary Medicine, Vienna, Austria. [3]Current address: Institute of Veterinary Pathology, Vetsuisse-Faculty, University of Zurich, Zurich, Switzerland. [4]Current address: Clinic for Swine, Ludwig-Maximilians-University, Munich, Germany.

References

1. Tischer I, Gelderblom H, Vettermann W, Koch MA (1982) A very small porcine virus with circular single-stranded DNA. Nature 295:64–66
2. Segalés J, Kekarainen T, Cortey M (2013) The natural history of porcine circovirus type 2: From an inoffensive virus to a devastating swine disease? Vet Microbiol 165:13–20
3. Chae C (2005) A review of porcine circovirus 2-associated syndromes and diseases. Vet J 169:326–336
4. Segalés J (2012) Porcine circovirus type 2 (PCV2) infections: clinical signs, pathology and laboratory diagnosis. Virus Res 164:10–19
5. Opriessnig T, Halbur PG (2012) Concurrent infections are important for expression of porcine circovirus associated disease. Virus Res 164:20–32
6. Opriessnig T, O'Neill K, Gerber PF, de Castro AMMG, Gimenéz-Lirola LG, Beach NM, Zhou L, Meng X, Wang C, Halbur PG (2013) A PCV2 vaccine based on genotype 2b is more effective than a 2a-based vaccine to protect against PCV2b or combined PCV2a/2b viremia in pigs with concurrent PCV2, PRRSV and PPV infection. Vaccine 31:487–494
7. Seo HW, Park SJ, Park C, Chae C (2014) Interaction of porcine circovirus type 2 and *Mycoplasma hyopneumoniae* vaccines on dually infected pigs. Vaccine 32:2480–2486
8. Opriessnig T, Meng X, Halbur PG (2007) Porcine circovirus type 2-associated disease: Update on current terminology, clinical manifestations, pathogenesis, diagnosis and intervention strategies. J Vet Diagn Invest 19:591–615
9. Mahé D, Blanchard P, Truong C, Arnauld C, Le Cann P, Cariolet R, Madec F, Albina E, Jestin A (2000) Differential recognition of ORF2 protein from type 1 and type 2 porcine circoviruses and identification of immunorelevant epitopes. J Gen Virol 81:1815–1824
10. Blanchard P, Mahé D, Cariolet R, Keranflec'h A, Baudouard MA, Cordioli P, Albina E, Jestin A (2003) Protection of swine against post-weaning multisystemic wasting syndrome (PMWS) by porcine circovirus type 2 (PCV2) proteins. Vaccine 21:4565–4575
11. Beach NM, Meng X (2012) Efficacy and future prospects of commercially available and experimental vaccines against porcine circovirus type 2 (PCV2). Virus Res 164:33–42
12. Velasova M, Alarcon P, Werling D, Nevel A, Wieland B (2013) Effectiveness of porcine circovirus type 2 vaccination in reducing the severity of post-weaning multisystemic wasting syndrome. Vet J 197:842–847
13. Alarcon P, Rushton J, Nathues H, Wieland B (2013) Economic efficiency analysis of different strategies to control post-weaning multi-systemic wasting syndrome and porcine circovirus type 2 subclinical infection in 3-weekly batch system farms. Prev Vet Med 110:103–118
14. Puvanendiran S, Stone S, Yu W, Johnson CR, Abrahante J, Jimenez LG, Griggs T, Haley C, Wagner B, Murtaugh M (2011) Absence of porcine circovirus type 1 (PCV1) and high prevalence of PCV2 exposure and infection in swine finisher herds. Virus Res 157:92–98
15. Rodríguez-Arrioja GM, Segalés J, Calsamiglia M, Resendes AR, Balasch M, Plana-Durán J, Casal J, Domingo M (2002) Dynamics of porcine circovirus type 2 infection in a herd of pigs with postweaning multisystemic wasting syndrome. Am J Vet Res 63:354–357
16. Sibila M, Calsamiglia M, Segalés J, Blanchard P, Badiella L, Le Dimna M, Jestin A, Domingo M (2004) Use of polymerase chain reaction assay and an ELISA to monitor porcine circovirus type 2 infection in pigs from farms with and without postweaning multisystemic wasting syndrome. Am J Vet Res 65:88–92
17. Trible BR, Ramirez A, Suddith A, Fuller A, Kerrigan M, Hesse R, Nietfeld J, Guo B, Thacker E, Rowland RRR (2012) Antibody responses following vaccination versus infection in a porcine circovirus-type 2 (PCV2) disease model show distinct differences in virus neutralization and epitope recognition. Vaccine 30:4079–4085
18. Meerts P, Misinzo G, Lefebvre D, Nielsen J, Bøtner A, Kristensen CS, Nauwynck HJ (2006) Correlation between the presence of neutralizing antibodies against porcine circovirus 2 (PCV2) and protection against replication of the virus and development of PCV2-associated disease. BMC Vet Res 2:6
19. Fort M, Olvera A, Sibila M, Segalés J, Mateu E (2007) Detection of neutralizing antibodies in postweaning multisystemic wasting syndrome (PMWS)-affected and non-PMWS-affected pigs. Vet Microbiol 125:244–255
20. Fort M, Sibila M, Nofrarías M, Pérez-Martín E, Olvera A, Mateu E, Segalés J (2010) Porcine circovirus type 2 (PCV2) Cap and Rep proteins are involved in the development of cell-mediated immunity upon PCV2 infection. Vet Immunol Immunopathol 137:226–234
21. Steiner E, Balmelli C, Gerber H, Summerfield A, McCullough K (2009) Cellular adaptive immune response against porcine circovirus type 2 in subclinically infected pigs. BMC Vet Res 5:45
22. Fort M, Fernandes LT, Nofrarías M, Díaz I, Sibila M, Pujols J, Mateu E, Segalés J (2009) Development of cell-mediated immunity to porcine circovirus type 2 (PCV2) in caesarean-derived, colostrum-deprived piglets. Vet Immunol Immunopathol 129:101–107
23. Saalmüller A, Reddehase MJ, Bühring HJ, Jonjic S, Koszinowski UH (1987) Simultaneous expression of CD4 and CD8 antigens by a substantial proportion of resting porcine T lymphocytes. Eur J Immunol 17:1297–1301
24. Chae C (2004) Postweaning multisystemic wasting syndrome: A review of aetiology, diagnosis and pathology. Vet J 168:41–49
25. Meng X (2013) Porcine circovirus type 2 (PCV2): Pathogenesis and interaction with the immune system. Annu Rev Anim Biosci 1:43–64
26. Kixmöller M, Ritzmann M, Eddicks M, Saalmüller A, Elbers K, Fachinger V (2008) Reduction of PMWS-associated clinical signs and co-infections by vaccination against PCV2. Vaccine 26:3443–3451
27. Fachinger V, Bischoff R, Jedidia SB, Saalmüller A, Elbers K (2008) The effect of vaccination against porcine circovirus type 2 in pigs suffering from porcine respiratory disease complex. Vaccine 26:1488–1499

28. Seo HW, Han K, Park C, Chae C (2014) Clinical, virological, immunological and pathological evaluation of four porcine circovirus type 2 vaccines. Vet J 200:65–70
29. Patterson AR, Johnson J, Ramamoorthy S, Meng X, Halbur PG, Opriessnig T (2008) Comparison of three enzyme-linked immunosorbent assays to detect porcine circovirus-2 (PCV-2)-specific antibodies after vaccination or inoculation of pigs with distinct PCV-1 or PCV-2 isolates. J Vet Diagn Invest 20:744–751
30. Patterson AR, Johnson JK, Ramamoorthy S, Hesse RA, Murtaugh MP, Puvanendiran S, Pogranichniy RM, Erickson GA, Carman S, Hause B, Meng X, Opriessnig T (2011) Interlaboratory comparison of porcine circovirus-2 indirect immunofluorescent antibody test and enzyme-linked immunosorbent assay results on experimentally infected pigs. J Vet Diagn Invest 23:206–212
31. Martelli P, Ardigò P, Ferrari L, Morganti M, De Angelis E, Bonilauri P, Luppi A, Guazzetti S, Caleffi A, Borghetti P (2013) Concurrent vaccination against PCV2 and PRRSV: Study on specific immunity and clinical protection in naturally infected pigs. Vet Microbiol 162:558–571
32. Saalmüller A, Werner T, Fachinger V (2002) T-helper cells from naive to committed. Vet Immunol Immunopathol 87:137–145
33. Reutner K, Leitner J, Müllebner A, Ladinig A, Essler SE, Duvigneau JC, Ritzmann M, Steinberger P, Saalmüller A, Gerner W (2013) CD27 expression discriminates porcine T helper cells with functionally distinct properties. Vet Res 44:18
34. Ferrari L, Borghetti P, De Angelis E, Martelli P (2014) Memory T cell proliferative responses and IFN-γ productivity sustain a long-lasting efficacy of a Cap-based PCV2 vaccine upon PCV2 natural infection and associated disease. Vet Res 45:44
35. Kekarainen T, McCullough K, Fort M, Fossum C, Segalés J, Allan GM (2010) Immune responses and vaccine-induced immunity against porcine circovirus type 2. Vet Immunol Immunopathol 136:185–193
36. Seo HW, Oh Y, Han K, Park C, Chae C (2012) Reduction of porcine circovirus type 2 (PCV2) viremia by a reformulated inactivated chimeric PCV1-2 vaccine-induced humoral and cellular immunity after experimental PCV2 challenge. BMC Vet Res 8:194
37. Fort M, Sibila M, Nofrarías M, Pérez-Martín E, Olvera A, Mateu E, Segalés J (2012) Evaluation of cell-mediated immune responses against porcine circovirus type 2 (PCV2) Cap and Rep proteins after vaccination with a commercial PCV2 sub-unit vaccine. Vet Immunol Immunopathol 150:128–132
38. Martelli P, Ferrari L, Morganti M, De Angelis E, Bonilauri P, Guazzetti S, Caleffi A, Borghetti P (2011) One dose of a porcine circovirus 2 subunit vaccine induces humoral and cell-mediated immunity and protects against porcine circovirus-associated disease under field conditions. Vet Microbiol 149:339–351
39. Fort M, Sibila M, Pérez-Martín E, Nofrarías M, Mateu E, Segalés J (2009) One dose of a porcine circovirus 2 (PCV2) sub-unit vaccine administered to 3-week-old conventional piglets elicits cell-mediated immunity and significantly reduces PCV2 viremia in an experimental model. Vaccine 27:4031–4037
40. Seder RA, Darrah PA, Roederer M (2008) T-cell quality in memory and protection: implications for vaccine design. Nat Rev Immunol 8:247–258
41. Darrah PA, Patel DT, De Luca PM, Lindsay RWB, Davey DF, Flynn BJ, Hoff ST, Andersen P, Reed SG, Morris SL, Roederer M, Seder RA (2007) Multi-functional T_H1 cells define a correlate of vaccine-mediated protection against *Leishmania major*. Nat Med 13:843–850

Functional analysis of bovine TLR5 and association with IgA responses of cattle following systemic immunisation with H7 flagella

Amin Tahoun[1,2], Kirsty Jensen[1], Yolanda Corripio-Miyar[1], Sean P McAteer[1], Alexander Corbishley[1,3], Arvind Mahajan[1], Helen Brown[1], David Frew[3], Aude Aumeunier[4], David GE Smith[3,4], Tom N McNeilly[3], Elizabeth J Glass[1] and David L Gally[1*]

Abstract

Flagellin subunits are important inducers of host immune responses through activation of TLR5 when extracellular and the inflammasome if cytosolic. Our previous work demonstrated that systemic immunization of cattle with flagella generates systemic and mucosal IgA responses. The IgA response in mice is TLR5-dependent and TLR5 can impact on the general magnitude of the adaptive response. However, due to sequence differences between bovine and human/murine TLR5 sequences, it is not clear whether bovine TLR5 (bTLR5) is able to stimulate an inflammatory response following interaction with flagellin. To address this we have examined the innate responses of both human and bovine cells containing bTLR5 to H7 flagellin from *E. coli* O157:H7. Both HEK293 (human origin) and embryonic bovine lung (EBL) cells transfected with bTLR5 responded to addition of H7 flagellin compared to non-transfected controls. Responses were significantly reduced when mutations were introduced into the TLR5-binding regions of H7 flagellin, including an R90T substitution. In bovine primary macrophages, flagellin-stimulated CXCL8 mRNA and secreted protein levels were significantly reduced when TLR5 transcript levels were suppressed by specific siRNAs and stimulation was reduced with the R90T-H7 variant. While these results indicate that the bTLR5 sequence produces a functional flagellin-recognition receptor, cattle immunized with R90T-H7 flagella also demonstrated systemic IgA responses to the flagellin in comparison to adjuvant only controls. This presumably either reflects our findings that R90T-H7 still activates bTLR5, albeit with reduced efficiency compared to WT H7 flagellin, or that other flagellin recognition pathways may play a role in this mucosal response.

Introduction

Flagella have been shown to play a significant role in bacterial pathogenesis, primarily through their function as motility organelles, but also as adhesins and as pro-inflammatory agonists. As a consequence, flagella have been trialled as vaccine antigens in a number of species [1-5] and it is evident that flagellins promote specific immune responses and may increase the magnitude of the response, functioning as an adjuvant for the presentation of heterologous antigens [6,7]. It has been demonstrated in cattle that systemic vaccination with H7 flagella leads to the production of IgA and IgG1 against $\mathrm{FliC_{H7}}$ with both IgA and IgG1 detected at the mucosal surface [3,8,9]. Toll like receptors (TLRs) are crucial components that allow recognition of microbial associated molecular patterns (MAMPs), including Lipid A of LPS, lipoteichoic acid, peptidoglycan, certain nucleic acids and flagellin [10,11]. TLRs are a family of transmembrane proteins, each consisting of a Leucine-rich extracellular domain (ectodomain) that recognizes distinct MAMPs and hence is variable between different TLRs. Most TLRs form dimers following MAMP binding and some TLRs can function as heterodimers, for example TLR2 makes a heterodimer with TLR6 to sense lipoteichoic acid and a heterodimer with TLR1 to sense lipid-protein combination [12].

TLR5 recognises the flagellin monomer [13,14] and they are considered to form a TLR5:flagellin complex

* Correspondence: dgally@ed.ac.uk
[1]Division of Immunity and Infection, The Roslin Institute and R(D)SVS, The University of Edinburgh, Easter Bush, Midlothian EH25 9RG, UK
Full list of author information is available at the end of the article

with a 2:2 stoichiometry [15]. TLRs have an intracellular domain (endodomain) that is relatively conserved between the different TLRs including the presence of a toll/interleukin-1 (TIR) region that contains specific amino acids that are phosphorylated upon MAMP binding and can then interact with different adaptor proteins leading to signalling cascades resulting in pro-inflammatory cytokine release [16,11]. In terms of flagellin, it is evident that specific residues within the more conserved D1 domains are required for binding to the TLR5 ectodomain, with the more variable D2 and D3 regions responsible for the antigenic variability of flagellins [17]. While the D0 and D1 domains of flagellin are relatively conserved, variation in these regions has been shown to limit innate responses to flagellin expressed by α and ε Proteobacteria, including *Helicobacter pylori* [18,19].

Recent research in mice has indicated that induction of IgA following systemic immunization with flagellin from *Salmonella enterica serovar* Typhimurium is considered to be dependent on the capacity of monomeric flagellin to stimulate toll-like receptor 5 (TLR5) signalling in specific intestinal dendritic cells [20]. Another study in mice has also shown that the magnitude of the response to flagellin as an antigen is also TLR5-dependent [21]. There is 79% amino acid homology between the bovine (NP_001035591.1) and human (NP_003259.2) TLR5 sequences. In cattle (*Bos taurus*), there are specific changes in both the extracellular domain and the TIR domain in TLR5 in comparison to other mammalian sequences [22]. For example, codon S268 has been positively selected in the artiodactyl clade [22] and is within the LRR9 loop region identified by Yoon et al. [17] as being particularly important in the TLR5 interaction with the N- and C-terminal helices of the flagellin D1 domain. Variation in the human and murine amino acids at this site (TLR5 268) has also been shown to at least partially account for differences between these species in their interactions with flagellins [23]. With the addition of further artiodactyla TLR5 sequences we have identified a further potentially functional change in bovine TLR5 at position 798 in the TIR region, which in most species including humans and mice is a tyrosine, but in cattle and other ruminants is a Phenylalanine. It has been suggested that Tyr798 plays an important role in TLR5 signaling as mutation of murine TLR5 Tyr798 to Leu798 resulted in negligible capacity to signal in response to flagellin [23]. Very recent work demonstrated that bovine TLR5 transfected into HEK293T cells did not appear to signal. However there was some indication of P38 phosphorylation in bovine macrophages following addition of flagella although there was no indication as to whether this was TLR5-dependent [24]. Taken together, it is unclear whether TLR5 is functionally important in the recognition of flagellin in cattle.

Nonetheless, systemic immunization in cattle with H7 flagellin induces IgA responses [3,8] in line with similar murine responses to flagellin that were dependent on TLR5 [20,21,23]. This might indicate that these bovine IgA responses are also TLR5-dependent and that bovine TLR5 is functional despite variation in the ectodomain and the TIR domain. To test this we have transfected bovine TLR5 (bTLR5) clones into both human HEK293 and bovine EBL cells and analysed responses following stimulation with wild type H7 and with flagellins engineered to contain site-specific mutations in the TLR5-binding domains. We also investigated gene expression and CXCL8 secretion from bovine peripheral blood monocyte-derived macrophages following addition of H7 flagellin, with and without siRNA knock-down of bovine TLR5 expression. Finally, immunization studies were carried out in cattle comparing stimulation of mucosal humoral responses following systemic delivery of H7 flagella and a variant with reduced capacity to stimulate TLR5.

Materials and methods

Flagella expression and purification

H7 flagella or engineered variants were expressed from *E. coli* O157 TUV93-0 Δ*fliC* transformed with pEW7 (wild type $fliC_{H7}$) or plasmid-encoded site-directed mutants (Table 1). Flagella were purified by shearing for all the in vitro experiments according to published procedures and by acid de- and re-naturation for the calf immunization trials [3,8,25]. In brief, one colony was grown overnight on motility agar at 30 °C. 10 μL agar plugs from the edge of the motility circle were then inoculated overnight in LB broth with ampicillin (100 μg/mL). The next day this was diluted 1:100 into LB with ampicillin and 1 mM IPTG added when the culture reached $OD_{600} = 0.5$, and the cultures left to grow at 30 °C for 4-5 h ($OD_{600} > 2$). The bacteria were harvested at 4100 × *g* at 4 °C for 30 min. The supernatants were discarded and the pellets suspended overnight at 4 °C in 0.9% NaCl at 4% of the initial culture volume. For acid preparations the pellets were suspended in PBS at 2% of the initial culture volume.

Table 1 Bacterial strains used in the study

Strain	Source
TUV93-0 Δ*fliC*	Lab stock
TUV93-0 Δ*fliC* transformed with pEW7 ($fliC_{H7}$)	Lab stock
TUV93-0 Δ*fliC fliC* transformed with pAT12	This study
TUV93-0 Δ*fliC fliC* transformed with pAT13	This study
TUV93-0 Δ*fliC fliC* transformed with pAT14	This study
TUV93-0 Δ*fliC fliC* transformed with pAT15	This study
TUV93-0 Δ*fliC fliC* transformed with pAT16	This study

For acid preparation 1 M HCl was added on a stirring platform until a pH ~ 2 was reached and stirred for 30 min. The preparations were centrifuged at 5000 × *g* for 30 min. The supernatants were transferred and neutralised with 1 M NaOH. The volume of supernatants was measured and $(NH_4)_2SO_4$ added to 2.67 M (35.2 g/100 mL) and left overnight at 4 °C. Then the preparations were centrifuged at 15 000 × *g* at 4 °C for 15 min. The supernatants were discarded and pellets suspended in PBS (2 mL for an original litre of culture). Flagella preparations were dialysed overnight three times at 4 °C in at 500-1000 volumes of PBS and stored at −20 °C.

For sheared flagella preparations, the cultures suspended in a 2% volume of PBS bacterial cultures were made up to 20 mL in PBS. The cultures were sheared for 2 min on ice with an IKA T-10 homogeniser (Ultra-Turrax). The cultures were then centrifuged at 4100 × *g* for 15 min. The supernatants were collected and re-centrifuged. This step was repeated 4 to 5 times until the supernatants were clear. The cleared supernatants were centrifuged at 15 000 × *g* for 10 min to remove any remaining bacteria. The supernatant from this step were transferred into fresh tubes and centrifuged at 145 000 × *g* at 4 °C for 90 min to pellet the flagella. Flagella pellets were suspended in 500 μL PBS and stored at −20 °C.

Flagellin concentrations were determined by BCA and purity by coomassie staining following separation on SDS-polyacrylamide gels.

LPS removal and monomerization of flagella

The first step to remove LPS involved repeated extraction in 1% TritonX114. This was added to flagella (1 in 500) in an Eppendorf and rotated overnight at 4 °C. The mixture was then incubated at 37 °C for 10 min and centrifuged for 15 min at 13 000 rpm in desktop centrifuge at RT. The aqueous phase was collected from clearly visible Tx114 at bottom of tube. This extraction was repeated 4 times and the collected flagellin filter-sterilized and dialyzed to remove any remaining of detergent. The second step was a column clean up using Pierce® High-Capacity Endotoxin binding resin following manufacturer's instructions (Thermo Scientific). Endotoxin levels were measured using an EndoLISA kit according to manufacturer's instructions (Hyglos GmbH) and expressed as endotoxin units (EU) per μg protein.

When required, monomerisation of flagellins was carried out by heating flagella at 70 °C for 15 min followed by filtration by centrifugation at 5000 × *g* at 4 °C for 30 min using 100 kDa 4 mL filter units (Millipore) [13].

Site-directed mutagenesis of H7 flagella

L500A/I505A, Q89A, and R90A mutations were selected based on effects previously demonstrated for *Salmonella* FliC [13,18] and Q89D and R90T mutations were selected based on naturally-acquired alleles demonstrated to reduce activation of TLR5 in *Helicobacter pylori* [18]. Site directed mutants were made following the manufacturer's protocols (QuikChange, Agilent technologies). The primers used for these reactions are in Table 2. Amplified and treated constructs were transformed into *E. coli* XL10-Gold Ultra competent bacteria and plated on LB–ampicillin plates and incubated overnight on 37 °C. Plasmids were extracted and sequenced (DNA Sequencing and Bioinformatics - GATC Biotech, Germany). Selection of required alleles followed sequence analysis using Lazergene software.

Motility assay

TUV93-0 Δ*fliC* transformed with pEW7 (*fliC*$_{H7}$) and altered alleles: pAT12 (Q89A), pAT13 (Q89D), pAT14 (R90A), pAT15 (R90T) and pAT16 (L500A/I504A) (Table 1) were stab inoculated into the centre of motility agar plates [18] (0.3% agar, with ampicillin and 1 mM final concentration of IPTG). The plates were incubated at 30 °C overnight and then examined for the extent of spread.

Cell lines

Embryonic bovine lung (EBL) cells were from laboratory stocks. The cells were grown at 37 °C in a 5% CO_2 and 80% humidity in Dulbecco's modified Eagle's medium (DMEM) supplemented with 10% (v/v) (FBS, Sigma), 1 U of penicillin (Invitrogen), 1 μg/mL of streptomycin (Invitrogen) and 2 mM L-glutamine (Invitrogen). HEK293 and HEK blue (PDRIVE5s-mIFN-ß) cells were grown in the above medium with additions when required zeocin 100 μg/mL (InvivoGen), pUNo1 selection blasticidin 30 μg/mL (InvivoGen) and Normocin (100 μg/mL) (InvivoGen) was used as antifungal and mycoplasma agent.

Table 2 Primers used for H7-FliC mutagenesis

SDM	Orientation	Oligonucleotide sequence (5′ – 3′)
L500A/I504A	F	CCCGCTTGCTGCCGCGGACGACGCAGCC AGCTCCATCGAC
	R	GTCGATGGAGCTGGCTGCGTCGTCCGCGG CAGCAAGCGGG
Q89A	F	CAACAACAACTTAGCGCGTATTCGTGAAC
	R	GTTCACGAATACGCGCTAAGTTGTTGTTG
Q89D	F	CAACAACAACTTAGACCGTATTCGTGAAC
	R	GTTCACGAATACGGTCTAAGTTGTTGTTG
R90A	F	CAACAACTTACAGGCTATTCGTGAACTGAC
	R	GTCAGTTCACGAATAGCCTGTAAGTTGTTG
R90A	F	CAACAACTTACAGACTATTCGTGAACTGAC
	R	GTCAGTTCACGAATAGTCTGTAAGTTGTTG

TLR5 clones and transfections

The human and bovine TLR5 clones were obtained from InvivoGen. The human clone was supplied in embryonic kidney cells (HEK293) transfected with pUNo1-hTLR05 (InvivoGen) under control of a hEF1-HTLV promoter. These cells were also transfected with PDRIVE5s-mIFN-ß containing SEAP as a reporter for NF-κB transcriptional activation as the mIFNß promoter has four binding sites for NF-κB. Cells containing the two plasmids are referred to as "hHEK blue cells" while those just the SEAP construct are referred to as "Null cells". Confluent cultured (HEK blue cells) were used to study the capacity of H7 flagellin to activate hTLR5. The bovine clone was supplied by InvivoGen in *E. coli*, and so was purified and transfected into the HEK Null cells. Permanent transfection was selected by addition of zeocin for the SEAP reporter plasmid and Blasticidin for the bTLR5 clone.

For transfection of the bovine EBLs, the bTLR5 clone was sub-cloned into a modified ptGFP1 vector [26]. Briefly, the full-length bTLR5 was amplified using specific primers encoding bovine TLR5 alongside restriction enzymes sites XhoI and SacII (bTLR5xsFW: CTCGAG CAC CATGGGAGACTGCCTTG, bTLR5xsRV: CCGCG GCTAGGAGATGGTGG). Invivogen bTLR5 plasmid was used as a template in a 25 μL reaction containing 1 μL of plasmid, 5 μL of GoTaq colourless reaction buffer, 0.5 μL of each of the primers at 10 mM, 0.5 μL dNTP (10 mM each), 0.25 μL of a mix of 10:1 GoTaq DNA polymerase (5 U/μL) and Pfu DNA polymerase (5 U/mL) (both Promega, Madison, USA). The PCR product was then gel extracted using QIAquick Gel Extraction Kit (Qiagen Inc., Netherlands) and ligated into pGEM®-T Easy Cloning Vector (Promega, Madison, USA).

Following transformation into competent XL1-Blue Competent Cells (Stratagene, Agilent Technologies Division, USA), cells were grown on LB agar (Sigma Aldrich, USA) supplemented with X-Gal and 10 mM IPTG. White colonies were grown overnight in 5 mL of LB medium with ampicillin (100 μg/mL), in a shaking incubator at 37 °C. Plasmid DNA from 4 independent colonies was then purified using a QIAprep Plasmid DNA Miniprep kit (Qiagen Inc., Netherlands) following the manufacturer's instructions and sent for sequencing to confirm correct sequence. The confirmed bTLR5 plasmid and modified vector ptGFP1 were then digested with XhoI and SacII at 37 °C for 3 h in a 50 μL reaction. Digestion was then purified with a QIAquick PCR Purification kit (Qiagen Inc., Netherlands) and ligated at 4 °C overnight using T4 DNA ligase (Promega, Madison, USA). Ligated products were then transformed into competent JM109 cells (Promega, Madison, USA), and seeded into LB agar + kanamycin (50 μg/mL). Positive colonies were grown overnight in 5 mL of LB medium with kanamycin in a shaking incubator at 37 °C. Plasmid DNA was purified as above and concentrations determined by spectrophotometry (Nanodrop, Labtech International, UK).

EBL cells were incubated in DMEM media supplemented with 10% foetal calf serum (FCS, Labtech International, UK), 100 U/mL penicillin and 100 mg/mL streptomycin (P/S, Invitrogen Life Technologies, BV, Netherlands) and 1% L-Glutamine. Cells were passaged 48 h prior to transfection by electroporation in a Nucleofector™ 2d Device (Lonza Group Ltd., USA) as described elsewhere [27]. Briefly approximately 2 μg of bTLR5-ptGFP1 construct or empty ptGFP1 vector (control) were used to transfect 10^6 cells alongside 100 μL Amaxa Nucleofactor solution V, by running program T-030. 500 μl of DMEM, 10% FCS, 1% L-Glutamine and P/S was added to the electrophoresis cuvette and then transferred into tissue culture flasks or plates. After 24 h, all media was replaced with fresh media supplemented with 500 μg/mL of neomycin (G418, Sigma Aldrich, UK). This was replenished every day to remove dead cells, and the concentration of neomycin reduced to 250 μg/mL a week after transfection. Once around 25-50% of the cells were GFP positive, they were cell sorted using a FACSAria™ III which generated a culture with >95% GFP+ cells.

In order to further confirm the presence of bTLR5 in the transfected cells, a PCR was carried out using cDNA obtained from EBL cells transfected with bTLR5-ptGFP1 and empty ptGFP1 vector as template. Forward primer was specific for bTLR5 (bTLR5FW: GTGCCTCGAAGC CTTCAGTTAT) and reverse primer (bTLR5-ptGFP1-RV: CTAGCCGCGGCTCTAGATCAT AATCAG) was designed spanning both bTLR5 and ptGFP1 to ascertain that the amplified fragment was the transfected bTLR5 and not any endogenous TLR5 which could be naturally produced by EBL cells. The reactions for the amplification of the vector/bTLR5 and the endogenous control GAPDH (GAPDH-FW: GATGCTGGTGCTGAGTATG TAGTG and GAPDH-RV: ATCCACAACAGACACGT TGGGAG) was subjected to an initial denaturation of 2 min at 95 °C, followed by 35 cycles of 95 °C for 30 s, 60 °C for 30 s and 72 °C for 45 s using a 25 μL reaction as detailed previously. All PCR products were visualised on a 1% agarose gel containing SYBR® Safe DNA Gel Stain (Life Technologies, BV, Netherlands).

Bovine monocyte-derived macrophages

Bovine monocyte-derived macrophages (MDM) were generated as described previously [28,29], except that the MDM were differentiated for 14 days. In brief, PBMC were initially cultured for 2 h in RPMI-1640 medium without serum at 5×10^6 cells/mL, before the medium was replaced with MDM medium (RPMI-1640 supplemented with 20% FBS, 4 mM L-glutamine and 50 μM β-mercaptoethanol) with 100 U/mL Penicillin-Streptomycin. The MDM medium was replaced on days 4 and 11. On day 14 the adherent cells were rigorously washed with phosphate buffered saline (PBS) and detached with TrypLE Express (Invitrogen). Flow cytometry, using a mouse anti-bovine SIRPα antibody directly conjugated with RPE-Cy5 (AbD Serotec: Cat. No. MCA2041C), confirmed that the MDM purity exceeded 90% (data not shown). Purified MDM were resuspended at 3×10^5 cells/mL in MDM medium without Penicillin-Streptomycin, dispensed into 12 well plates and cultured for 24 h before transfection of siRNA.

Analysis of NfκB activation using a secreted alkaline phosphatase reporter

Cells were treated with trypsin and diluted to be 5×10^5 cell per mL. 180 μL/well of the cells were added to 96 well plate and 20 μL of the required flagella concentration added and incubated with the cells overnight at 37 °C in a 5% CO_2 and 80% humidity. Next day 20 μL of the culture media was added to 200 μL of a ready-to-use substrate (Quanti blue) in a 96 well plate format (p7998, Sigma, St. Louis, MI, USA) for 10 min at RT and the readings made at 650 nm using Promega plate reader.

CXCL8/IL8 determination by ELISA

Cells were treated as above and CXCL8/IL8 levels in the cell culture supernatants was assessed following capture with mouse anti-sheep IL-8 and detection with rabbit anti-sheep IL-8 (AbD Serotec, Raleigh, N.C.) followed by goat anti-rabbit IgG conjugated to HRP (DAKO) according to manufacturer's instructions. Briefly, ELISA plates (Thermoelectron 3455) were coated with mouse anti-sheep CXCL8/IL8 antibody (MCA1660) diluted in carbonate coating buffer (50 μL per well). The plates were sealed and incubated at 4 °C overnight. The plates were washed 6 times in wash buffer (0.05% Triton in PBS) and 100 μL/well blocking buffer (3% bovine serum albumen in wash buffer) was added and incubated at RT for 1 h. Samples and standards were prepared as appropriate in dilution buffer (wash buffer + 1% BSA). Plates were washed 5 times in wash buffer and 50 μL of sample and standard were added in duplicate to the plates. The plates were incubated at RT for 1 h. The plates were then washed 6 times and 50 μL/well of the rabbit anti-sheep IL-8 antibody (AHP425) diluted in dilution buffer was added. The plates were then incubated at RT for 1 h. The plates washed 6 times and 50 μL/well of goat anti-rabbit-HRP (Dako P0448) diluted 1:1000 in RDB was added and incubated at RT for 1 h. The plates were wash 6 times and 100 μL OPD substrate (Sigmafast OPD P9187 Sigma-Aldrich) was added per well and incubated for 5-10 min depending on reaction time of the controls and this varied depending on the room temperature. The reactions were stopped by addition of 50 μL 2.5 M H_2SO_4 and plates were read at 492 nm using a BMG FLUORstar ELISA reader. The concentration of CXCL8 was determined according to manufacturer's instructions using recombinant bovine CXCL8 (Kingfisher Biotech, Inc.) to make the standard curve.

We note that sets of experiments were performed with EBL cells at different densities and transfection efficiencies which, in combination with different flagellin preparations may account for variation in CXCL8 levels measured at specific flagellin concentrations between experiments.

Real time PCR analysis of TLR5 and CXCL8 transcripts

Total RNA was extracted from all MDM samples using the RNeasy mini kit (Qiagen), including a DNase digestion step, according to the manufacturer's instructions. The quality and quantity of the resulting RNA was determined by a Nanodrop spectrophotometer. First strand cDNA was reverse transcribed from 0.2 μg total RNA using an oligo(dT) primer and GoScript reverse transcriptase (Promega) according to the manufacturer's protocols. The resulting cDNA was diluted 1:20 for RT-qPCR analysis.

Oligonucleotides were designed for bovine TLR5, IL1β and CXCL8/IL8 using Primer3 [30] and Netprimer (Biosoft International) software (Table 3). The mRNA levels of each transcript were quantified by qPCR using the

Table 3 Additional primers used in the study

Gene	Accession no.	Orientation	Oligonucleotide sequence (5′ – 3′)
Toll-like receptor 5 (TLR5)	NM_001040501	F	CGATGCCTATTTGTGCTTCA
		R	CACCACCCGTCTCTAAGGAA
Interleukin 1B (IL1B)	NM_174093	F	TCCGACGAGTTTCTGTGTGA
		R	TGTGAGAGGAGGTGGAGAGC
Interleukin/CXCL 8 (IL8/CXCL8)	NM_173925	F	CACATTCCACACCTTTCCAC
		R	GGCAGACCTCGTTTCCATT
Chromosome alignment	NM_001205506	F	AGCAGTGACCAAGAGCAGGT
Maintaining phosphoprotein 1		R	TCATAGCACGACAGCAACAA

F and R denote forward and reverse primers respectively.

Brilliant III ultra-fast SYBR Green Mastermix kit (Agilent) as described previously [28]. The relative quantities of mRNA were calculated using the method described by Pfaffl [31]. The RT-qPCR results for chromosome alignment maintaining phosphoprotein 1 (CHAMP1) were used to calculate differences in the template RNA levels and thereby standardize the results for the genes of interest. CHAMP1 was previously selected from microarray and RT-qPCR analyses as a constitutively and moderately expressed gene in activated bovine monocytes and macrophages [28,29].

siRNA knock-down of TLR5

Prior to the experiments reported here, three siRNA duplexes specific for bovine TLR5 (RefSeq Accession No. NM_001040501) were obtained from Sigma-Aldrich and assessed for their ability to knockdown TLR5 mRNA levels. The siRNAs TLR5#2 (target sequence CAATTTC ATCCAATTATCA) and TLR5#3(target sequence CGT ACAAATACGATGCCUA) were found to consistently knock-down TLR5 mRNA levels between 24 and 96 h. The third siRNA TLR5#1 (target sequence GTCTGA ACCCATTCAGAAA) failed to modulate TLR5 mRNA levels. In addition, the AllStars negative control siRNA, which does not share homology with any known mammalian gene (Qiagen), was used as a non-target siRNA control.

The transfection reagent Lipofectamine RNAiMAX (Invitrogen) has previously been shown to be suitable for transfecting siRNA into bovine MDM [28]. The MDM were transfected with siRNA following the manufacturer's protocol, initially generating a mix of 3 μL Lipofectamine RNAiMAX and 3 μL 20μM siRNA in 200 μL Opti-MEM I reduced serum medium (Invitrogen). After 20 min incubation at RT the siRNA/Lipofectamine RNAiMAX mix was added to MDM in 1 mL MDM medium, giving a final concentration of 50 μM siRNA. Additional controls included in each experiment were MDM treated with Lipofectamine RNAiMAX only (transfection control) and untreated MDM (negative control). After 24 h the medium was replaced with fresh MDM medium to remove the residual siRNA/Lipofectamine RNAiMAX mix.

Immunization of cattle

Immunizations were performed at Moredun Research Institute (MRI) under Home Office licence 60/3179. Ethical approval was obtained from the MRI Animal Experiments Committee. Two groups of conventionally reared male Holstein–Friesian calves ($n = 6$) were immunized on two separate occasions two weeks apart with either 60 μg of WT-H7 + 5mg Quil A adjuvant (Brenntag Biosector, Frederikssund, Denmark) or 60 μg R90T-H7 + 5 mg Quil A adjuvant via the intra-muscular route. A control group ($n = 3$) was immunized in an identical manner with adjuvant only. Serum samples were collected at days -1, 7, 21 and 28 relative to the first immunization. The average age of calves at the time of the first immunization was 14 ± 3 weeks. Faecal samples obtained from each calf prior to immunization were confirmed to be negative for *E. coli* O157:H7 by immunomagnetic separation, performed according to the manufacturer's instructions (Dynabeads® anti-*E. coli* O157, Invitrogen).

Measurement of serum immunoglobulin levels

WT-H7 and R90T-H7 specific IgA antibodies were quantified by indirect ELISA as previously described [8] using LPS-free antigen preparations. Antibody titres were calculated as follows: the $\log_{10}$ optical density (OD) was plotted against the $\log_{10}$ sample dilution and regression analysis of the linear part of the curve allowed the calculation of the endpoint titre with an OD of 0.1 above the average negative control value. Inter-plate variation was normalised to a known positive control sample.

Statistical analyses

Mixed models were used to analyse each experiment. These models are an extension to ANOVA and take account of variation occurring both between- and within-experiments, and of correlations between measurements repeated over time-points or concentrations. Treatment, concentration (or time) and the treatment by concentration (or time) interaction were fitted as fixed effects, and experiment as a random effect, in each model. Pairwise comparisons between treatment effects at individual concentration (or time) levels were made within each model using t-tests. The variance for these comparisons was determined by the mixed model, taking into account the between- and within- experiment variation. Adjustments were made for multiple testing in the statistical tests. When measurements were not repeated over concentration or time, only treatment was fitted as a fixed effect in the mixed model. Log transformations of the data were used when necessary to ensure that normality requirements for the model were satisfied. The analyses were carried out using the MIXED procedure in the SAS/STAT(r) software. Further information on mixed models may be found in Brown and Prescott [32].

Results

Signalling from HEK293 cells transfected with human and bovine TLR5 clones

The bovine TLR5 (bTLR5) and human TLR5 (hTLR5) clones were obtained from InvivoGen. As a read-out for activity of HEK293 cells transfected with these constructs, the cells also contained a plasmid encoding an NF-κB/AP-1-inducible secreted alkaline phosphatase (SEAP) reporter

(Materials and methods, InvivoGen). HEK293 cells stably transfected with just the reporter construct but no TLR5 clones were used as a control (Null cells). Both the bTLR5 and hTLR5 clones activated the NF-kB reporter at levels significantly higher ($p < 0.005$) than the Null cells over a range of H7 flagellin concentrations (0.5-5000 ng/mL, Figure 1A). There was evidence that hTLR5 was more sensitive than bTLR5 to activation by flagellin at lower concentrations (0.05 and 0.5 ng/mL, $p = 0.027$ and $p < 0.001$ respectively), but differences in expression levels between the two constructs cannot be ruled out. There was no significant difference in their maximum levels of induction above a concentration of 5 ng/mL flagellin. This indicated that the bTLR5 was capable of signalling through NF-kB in this human-derived cell background.

Mutational analysis of H7 flagellin

Previous mutational analyses of *Salmonella enterica* serovar Typhimurium Phase 1 FliC flagellin has helped define key amino acids required for TLR5 recognition and signalling within the TLR5 binding domains in the D1 regions of the flagellin monomer (Figure 2A) [13]. We mutated amino acid residues based on this previous work as well as analysis of *Helicobacter* FlaA and FlaB

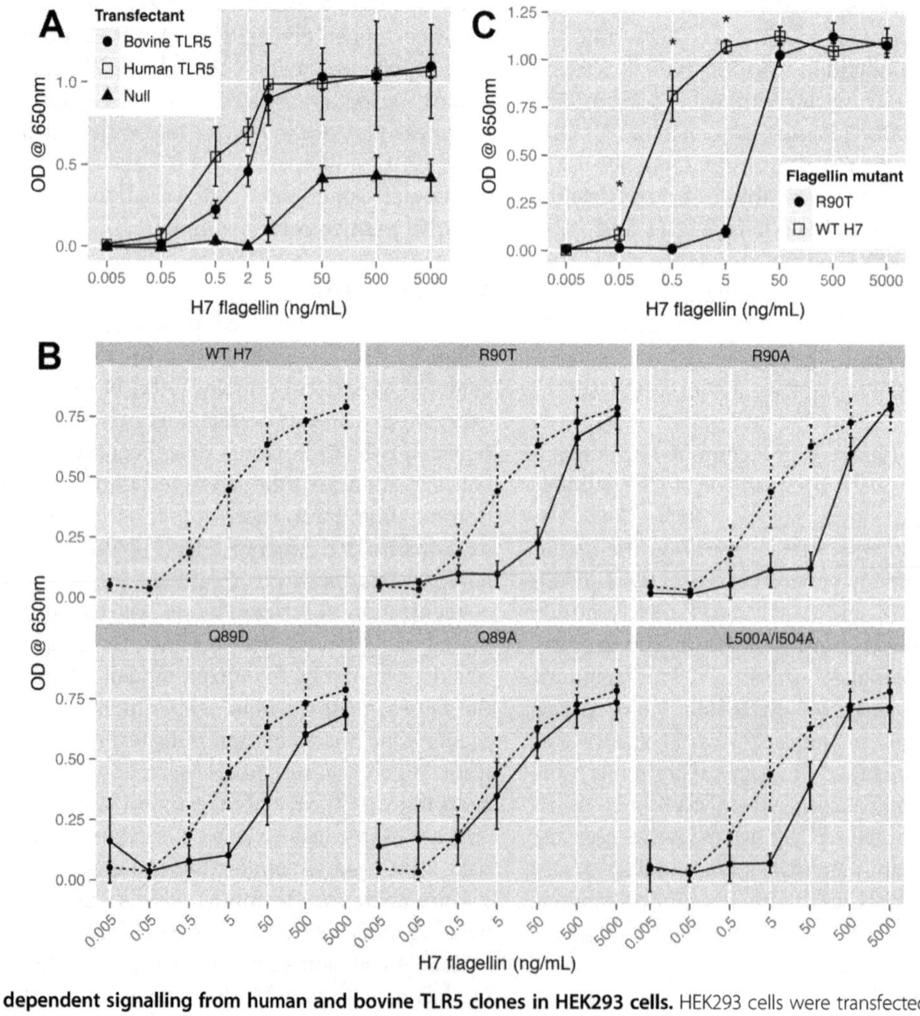

Figure 1 NF-kB dependent signalling from human and bovine TLR5 clones in HEK293 cells. HEK293 cells were transfected with an NF-κB-dependent secreted alkaline phosphatase (SEAP) reporter plasmid alone (Null cells) or with the reporter in combination with either a human TLR5 (hTLR5) or bovine (bTLR5) expression plasmid. SEAP levels were determined following addition of different concentrations of WT-H7 flagellin or site-directed flagellin mutants. **(A)** NF-kB dependent SEAP production from bTLR5 and hTLR5 following overnight stimulation with a range of H7 flagellin concentrations. SEAP activity from cells transfected with either TLR5 construct was significantly higher than the non-transfected control at levels of 0.5 ng/mL flagellin or greater ($p < 0.005$). hTLR5 produced higher SEAP activity compared to bTLR5 at two concentrations of flagellin, 0.05 and 0.5 ng/mL ($p = 0.027$ and $p < 0.001$ respectively). **(B)** NF-kB dependent SEAP production from bTLR5 in HEK293 cells stimulated overnight with different concentrations of WT-H7 and the indicated flagellin mutants. The dashed line indicates the response to WT-H7. **(C)** NF-kB dependent SEAP production from hTLR5 in HEK293 cells following addition of WT H7 and an R90T variant. Differences of $p < 0.001$ are indicated by an asterisk. All experiments in this figure were performed a minimum of three times with at least three technical repeats. The data shown are the means and 95% confidence intervals.

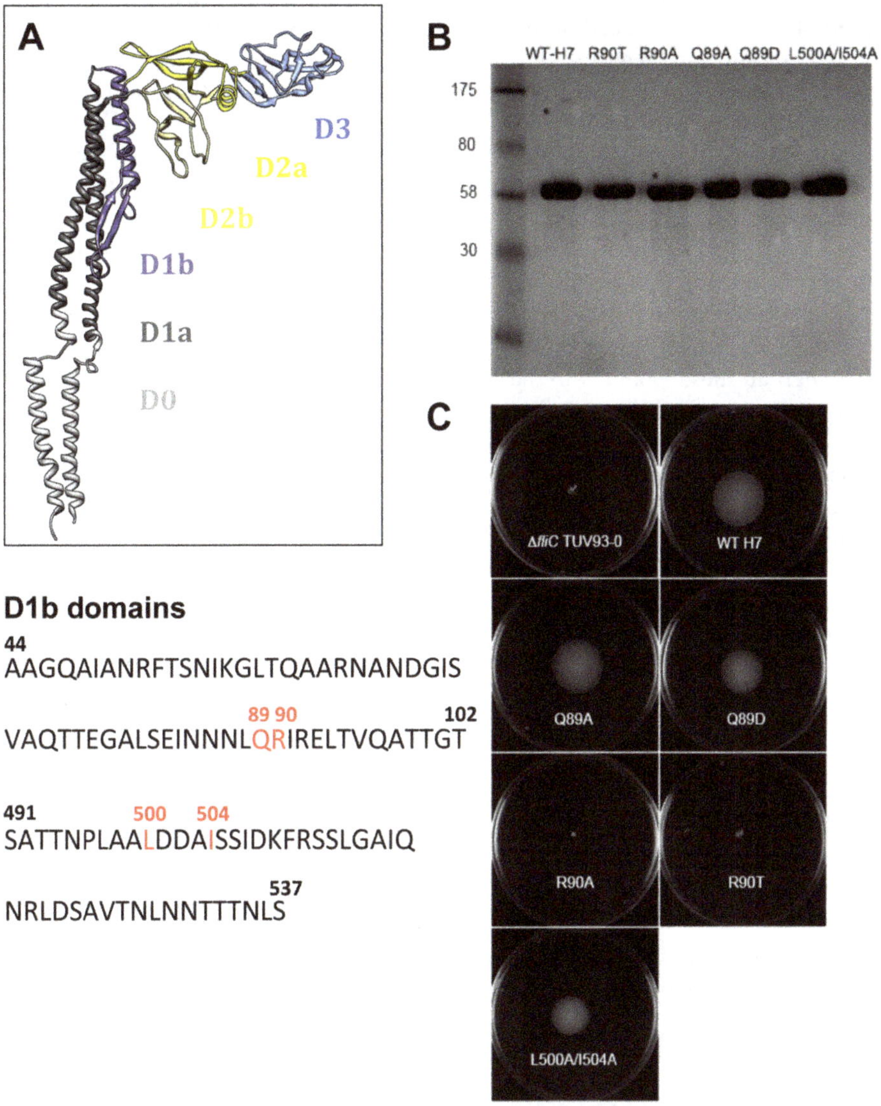

Figure 2 Site-directed mutagenesis of H7 flagellin to reduce TLR5 signalling. (A) Predicted TLR5-binding regions of H7 flagellin (FliC). Top panel shows the structure of FliC (*Salmonella* Typhimurium) from PDB entry 1UCU (R-type straight flagellar filament) and is coloured in UCSF Chimera according to structural domains as indicated. TLR5 binding residues have been mapped within the D1b regions (dark grey). The bottom panel shows the FliC-H7 D1b regions which are homologous to those from *S.* Typhimurium and the 4 residues that have been mutated in this study are shown in red. Q89 and R90 in the D1b amino terminal regions have the same position in *S.* Typhimurium, whereas the L500 and I504 in FliC-H7 are equivalent to I411 and L415 (leucine and isoleucine are interchanged) respectively in *S.* Typhimurium phase 1 FliC (13). **(B)** Coomassie-stained SDS-PAGE of WT-H7 and variants. Flagella were purified from *E. coli* O157 TUV93-0 Δ*fliC* and total protein concentration adjusted following a BCA assay to 2.5 µg per lane. The left margin shows the approximate molecular size (kDa). **(C)** Motility of *E. coli* O157 expressing altered flagellins. Motility was assessed following inoculation of *E. coli* O157 (TUV93-0) Δ*fliC* containing WT $fliC_{H7}$ clone (pEW7) and site-directed mutants as indicated. Motility was assessed after overnight incubation.

which have been shown to have a reduced capacity to stimulate TLR5 [18] as part of a proposed immune evasion strategy. Five mutations (Figure 2A) were introduced successfully into a clone of $fliC_{H7}$ on plasmid pEW7 (Materials and methods). Flagella expression was analysed in *E. coli* O157 (TUV93-0) Δ*fliC* transformed with the WT $fliC_{H7}$ or the site-directed mutants. Flagella were purified from all the mutants by shearing and concentrations were adjusted based on bicinchoninic acid assays and then analysed by gel electrophoresis for purity and relative concentration (Figure 2B). The Q89A, Q89D, L500A/I504A demonstrated motility on 0.3% agar following overnight culture, whereas R90A-H7 and R90T-H7 were non motile (Figure 2C). The different flagellins were tested over a range of concentrations for their capacity to stimulate NF-kB activity in HEK293 cells containing the bTLR5 clone (Figure 1B). All variants with the exception of Q89A showed reduced SEAP levels at flagellin concentrations of 5 ng/mL and 50 ng/mL ($p < 0.001$). R90T was selected for further work as this could easily be purified at high levels and showed a markedly reduced signalling capacity compared to WT-H7. R90T was then compared against the WT-H7 using the hTLR5 clone in HEK293 cells and analysis demonstrated significantly reduced NF-kB dependent SEAP production over a range of flagellin concentrations (0.005-5 ng/mL, $p < 0.001$), with approximately 100-fold more mutated flagellin (R90T) required to induce equivalent levels of response to the WT monomer at these points on the response curves (Figure 1C).

Analysis of bovine TLR5 activity in bovine epithelial cells

There are possible complications with using the HEK293 cell background to read out for functionality of bTLR5. These include that the adaptor signalling pathways are human not bovine and the possibility of some complementing activity from residual TLR5 activity in the HEK293 cells [17,33], as our non-transfected cells did show a level of activation, especially at high flagellin concentrations (Figure 1A). It was important therefore to test the activity of the bTLR5 clone in a bovine cell context. To our knowledge there are two main immortalized bovine epithelial cell lines that are currently used by research community: Mac-T, a bovine mammary epithelial cell line [34] and EBLs, an embryonic bovine epithelial cell line (supplied by the Leibniz Institute DSMZ-German Collection of Microorganisms and Cell Cultures). We use EBLs routinely for bacterial infections studies so we investigated whether these cells were able to produce CXCL8 following addition of H7 flagellin. There was no detectable endogenous TLR5 activity in these cells as determined by CXCL8 assays 16 h after addition of up to 10 μg of flagellin (data not shown) and so they were considered an appropriate background in which to study the bTLR5 clone. In order to aid detection and selection of transfected EBLs, the bTLR5 region was sub-cloned into ptGFP1 (Material and Methods) allowing detection of transfected cells through expression of GFP.

EBL cells with and without sub-cloned bTLR5 were then tested for CXCL8 secretion following addition of flagellin (0.5 ng/mL - 50 μg/mL). The results indicated that transfecting these cells with the bTLR5 clone enabled them to respond to the addition of flagellin by releasing CXCL8 over a range of flagellin concentrations (Figure 3A, $p < 0.001$ compared to control cells). Induction of CXCL8 by LPS was ruled out in two ways; (1) the majority of LPS was removed from an H7 flagellin preparation (Materials and methods) leaving less that 0.05 endotoxin units/μg protein (EU) and this still was able to promote CXCL8 production to a level equivalent to the original (LPS high) preparation (Figure 3B). Secondly, addition of purified LPS (1 EU) alone failed to induce any CXCL8 production from EBLs transfected with bTLR5 (data not shown).

The site-directed mutations in the TLR5 binding domain of $FliC_{H7}$ were tested at 50 ng/mL on EBL cells transfected with bTLR5 (Figure 3C). The R90T, R90A and L500A/I504A constructs all showed significantly reduced levels of CXCL8 secretion compared to stimulation with WT-H7 ($p < 0.001$). At this flagellin concentration R90T produced lower levels of CXCL8 than the R90A construct (Figure 3C, $p < 0.001$). Of note was the finding that neither Q89A nor Q89D had any impact on levels of CXCL8 produced compared to WT-H7 at this flagellin concentration while this was not the case when these were tested on the hTLR5 in the HEK293 cells, indicative of different recognition or signalling between the clones and cell types. The R90T flagellin was compared with WT-H7 over a range of concentrations on the bTLR5-EBL cells and shown to induce significantly lower levels of CXCL8 when 50 ng/mL and 500 ng/mL flagellin was added (Figure 3D, $p < 0.001$). At these concentrations approximately 10-fold more R90T than WT was required to induce an equivalent level of CXCL8 release (Figure 3D).

Analysis of TLR5 responses in bovine primary macrophages derived from PBMCs

We wanted to determine if CXCL8 responses from bovine peripheral blood monocyte-derived macrophages (MDMs) exposed to flagellin were TLR5-dependent. MDMs were derived as described previously ([28,29] and Materials and methods). To determine the initial response of the bMDMs to flagellin, TLR5 and CXCL8 transcript levels were determined at 4 and 24 h by RT-PCR following addition of 26.5 ng/mL H7 flagellin (Figure 4A). CXCL8 mRNA levels increased at both time points relative to the T0 value ($p < 0.001$) while TLR5 levels were significantly reduced at 4 h ($p < 0.001$) while there was no significant difference at 24 h ($p = 0.073$, Figure 4A).

In order to assess the requirement of TLR5 for CXCL8 production following flagellin stimulation, three different siRNAs were tested to try and reduce TLR5 transcript levels in the bovine MDMs using established methods [28]. The bovine MDMs were cultured for 48 h following siRNA transfection. TLR5 and CXCL8 mRNA levels are shown at 0 and 24 h following addition of 26.5 ng/mL flagellin (Figures 4B and 4C). It was evident that two of the TLR5 siRNAs, #2 & #3, had significantly reduced levels of TLR5 mRNA at 24 h post flagellin stimulation relative to both non-transfected and scrambled siRNA controls ($p < 0.001$, Figure 4B). The third siRNA had no

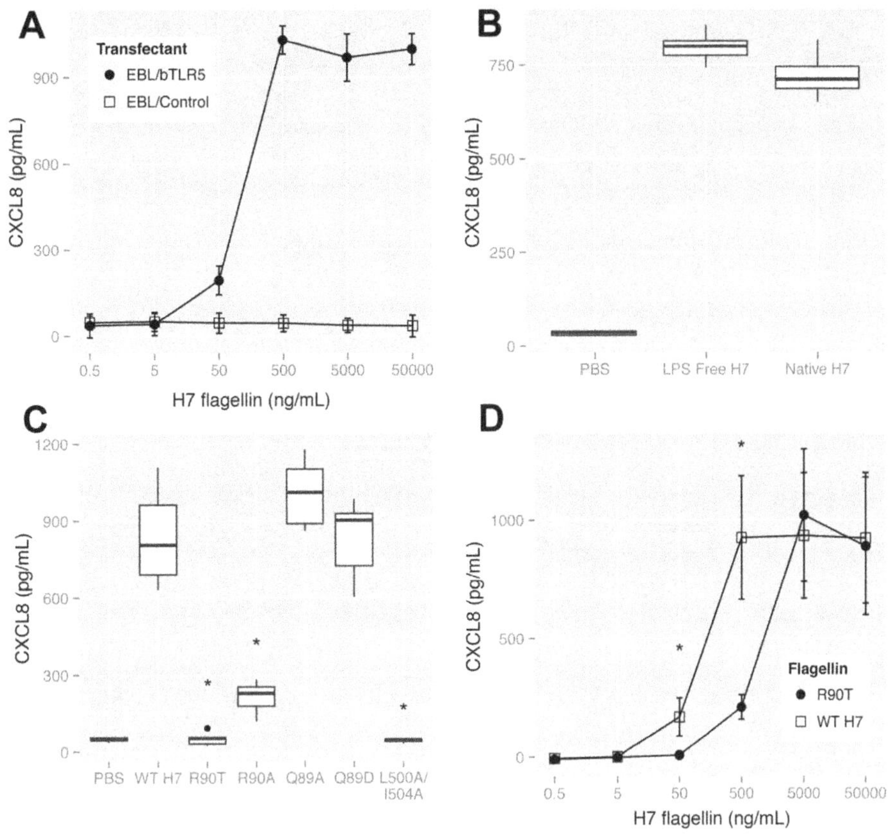

Figure 3 Analysis of bovine TLR5 activity in bovine epithelial cells. The bovine EBL cell line was stably transfected with a bTLR5 clone and CXCL8 secretion assayed following challenge with flagellin. **(A)** CXCL8 levels from EBLs with and without transfection of bTLR5. H7 flagellin at a range of concentrations was added to the cells and CXCL8 levels were measured by ELISA following overnight incubation. Transfection with bTLR5 resulted in significantly higher levels of CXCL8 being produced by the bTLR5+ cells with addition of 50-50 000 ng/mL of H7 flagellin ($p < 0.001$). The data shown are the means and 95% confidence intervals. **(B)** Analysis of CXCL8 production from EBL-TLR5 in response to addition of native H7 or an H7 flagellin preparation from which the majority of LPS has been removed. Medians and interquartile ranges are shown. **(C)** Secreted CXCL8 following addition of WT and mutated H7 flagellins to EBLs with transfected bTLR5. 50 ng/mL of WT-H7 and mutated flagellins were added to the EBLs transfected with bTLR5 and incubated overnight. CXCL8 was measured by ELISA. Addition of the R90T, R90A and L500A/I504A variants led to significantly lower levels of cytokine release ($p < 0.001$) relative to WT-H7 stimulation (asterisks). R90T showed a significantly lower induction than R90A ($p < 0.001$). Medians and interquartile ranges are shown. **(D)** Secreted CXCL8 following addition of WT H7 and the R90T flagellin mutant to EBL cells. A range of flagellin concentrations was incubated overnight with the cells and CXCL8 measured by ELISA. R90T flagellin demonstrated significantly reduced levels of CXCL8 activation at 50 ng/mL and 500 ng/mL ($p < 0.001$), marked by asterisks. The data shown are the means and 95% confidence intervals. All CXCL8 data shown is from a minimum of three biological replicates.

effect and is not shown. CXCL8 mRNA levels (Figure 4C) were reduced at 24 h post flagellin addition for the cells transfected with siRNAs #2 & #3 relative to the controls ($p < 0.05$) and this correlated with a significant reduction in secreted CXCL8 for siRNA #2 at 24 h ($p = 0.012$) and for siRNA #3 at 24 h ($p < 0.001$) relative to controls (Figure 4D). Bovine MDMs treated with siRNA #3 produced less CXCL8 in response to crude LPS activation than measured in siRNA #2-treated and control MDMs (data not shown), suggesting another effect of this siRNA on bovine MDM function or viability. This may explain the enhanced effect of siRNA #3 compared to siRNA #2 with respect to CXCL8 mRNA expression and protein secretion. Taken together, these data indicate a positive association of TLR5 expression in bovine MDMs with both CXCL8 mRNA expression and CXCL8 secreted cytokine production in response to addition of H7 flagellin.

To determine if a variant flagellin with reduced TLR5 activation (relative to WT-H7) also had a reduced capacity to stimulate CXCL8 when added to the bovine MDMs, the R90T flagellin was tested. While addition of 50 ng/mL R90T produced significantly lower levels of secreted CXCL8 compared to addition of WT H7 ($p = 0.02$, Figure 4E), this reduction in secreted CXCL8 levels was only 50% compared to the >10 fold difference demonstrated for the same variant on EBLs expressing bTLR5 (Figure 3C).

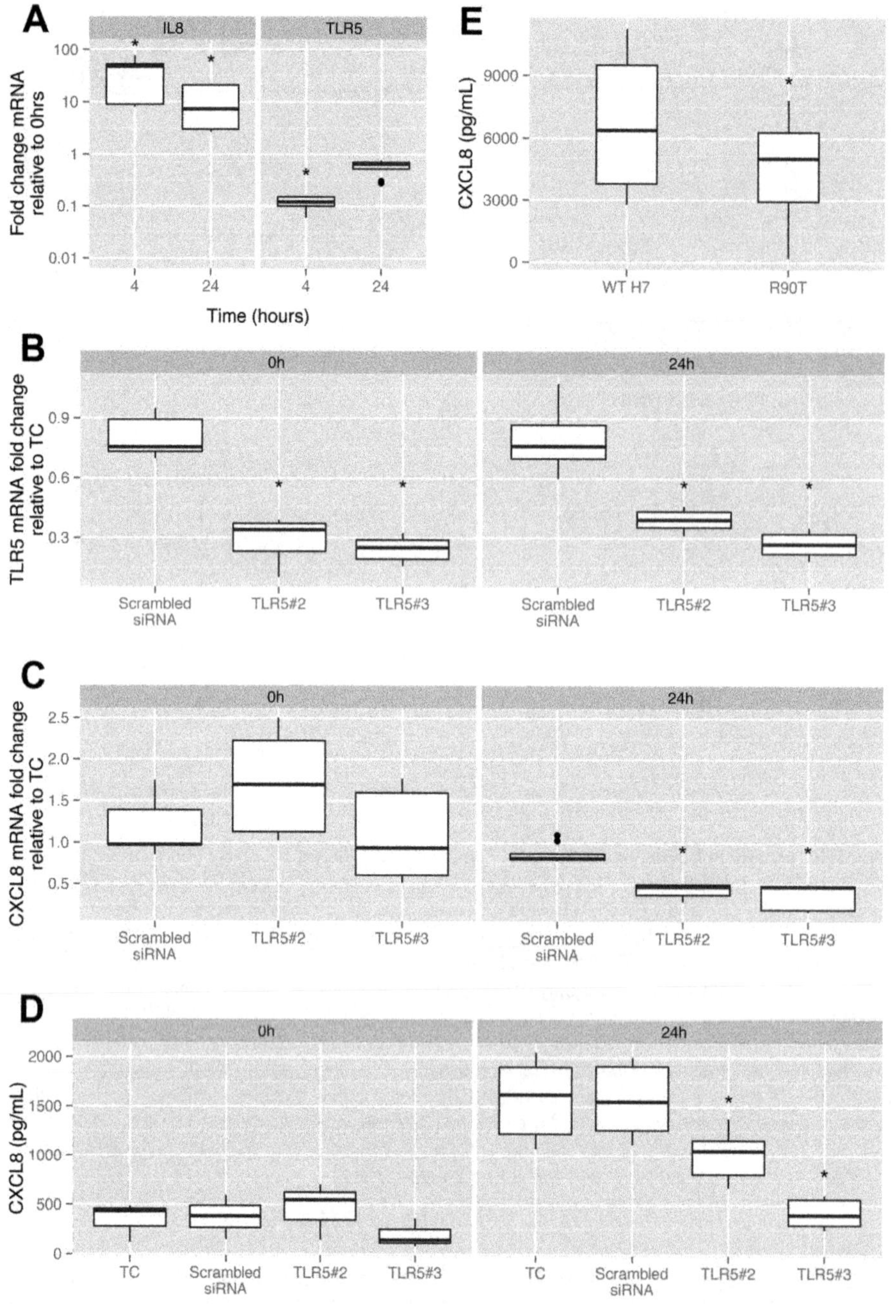

Figure 4 Responses of bovine monocyte-derived macrophages (bMDMs) to flagellin. (A) mRNA levels of CXCL8 and TLR5 following addition of flagellin to bMDMs. Transcript levels are plotted relative to time 0 and increase significantly at 4 h and 24 h ($p < 0.001$), while TLR5 transcript levels are lower ($p < 0.001$) 4 h after addition of flagellin but not significantly different ($p = 0.073$) at 24 h, significance marked by asterisks. **(B)** Assessment of TLR5 transcript levels in bMDMs. Transfected cells were pre-incubated with siRNAs for 48 h then WT H7 flagellin (26.5 ng/mL) added (time 0). TLR5 transcripts were reduced by treatment with both TLR5#2 and TLR5#3 relative to controls at both time 0 and 24 h ($p < 0.001$), marked by asterisks. **(C)** Assessment of CXCL8 transcript levels in bMDMs. CXCL8 mRNA levels were measured in cells challenged with WT H7 flagellin as above. CXCL8 transcript levels were significantly reduced in the cells treated with the TLR5#2 and TLR5#3 siRNAs relative to the controls at 24 h ($p < 0.001$), indicated by asterisks. Data is from three biological repeats with a minimum of three technical replicates. **(D)** Determination of released CXCL8 from bMDMs with reduced TLR5 expression. bMDMs were treated as above and supernatant CXCL8 determined by ELISA. TLR5 #3 siRNA significantly reduced secreted levels of CXCL8 relative to un-transfected controls at 24 h ($p < 0.001$), while a significant reduction was evident for TLR5 #2 at 24 h ($p = 0.012$), marked with asterisks. **(E)** CXCL8 release from bMDMs challenged with WT and altered H7 flagellin. CXCL8 was measured in the supernatants of the bMDMs 24 h after stimulation with WT or R90T H7 flagellin. The CXCL8 levels released were significantly lower for R90T compared with WT flagellin ($p = 0.022$, asterisk). All plots show medians with upper and lower quartiles; outliers as dark circles.

Analysis of bovine humoral responses to systemic immunization with WT-H7 flagella and R90T derivative

Two groups of male Holstein-Friesian calves ($n = 6$) were immunized twice with an interval of two weeks (day 0 and day 14) with either WT-H7 plus Quil A adjuvant or R90T-H7 plus Quil A adjuvant. A further group of three calves were immunized with adjuvant only. The LPS levels in the two flagellin preparations were equivalent (Materials and Methods). Serum IgA titres against both LPS-free (<0.05 EU per μg protein) WT-H7 and R90T-H7 were determined by end-point ELISA until two weeks after the second immunization (Figure 5). Immunization with both WT-H7 and R90T-H7 resulted in significant increases in serum IgA antibodies against WT-H7 from 7 days after the first immunization and these remained elevated until two weeks after the second immunization by comparison to serum from animals immunized with adjuvant only (Figure 5, $p < 0.01$). The same pattern was observed when IgA responses were analysed with plates coated with R90T-H7 indicating that the amino acid change was unlikely to have altered overall presentation of the flagellin and epitopes (data not shown). There was no significant difference in IgA levels produced between the groups immunized with WT-H7 and R90T-H7, although median levels of IgA from the animals immunized with WT-H7 were consistently higher than those receiving R90T-H7 (Figure 5A). The variation between samples and low animal numbers means that the study was underpowered to detect relatively subtle differences in IgA titres. Combining the T2-T4 IgA responses for the two groups approaches significance ($p = 0.07$) in terms of a reduced IgA response for the animals immunized with R90T.

Discussion

There is considerable interest in using factors that stimulate pattern recognition receptors (PRRs) as adjuvants. MAMPs are a logical inclusion in vaccine formulations as they stimulate the natural recognition systems allied to host innate and adaptive responses [35,36]. Flagellin monomers are powerful agonists through TLR5 activation as demonstrated in mice and humans [20,37] but their potency to activate TLR5 in cattle is unclear. Our work is focused on responses stimulated by H7 flagellin in cattle for two reasons: (1) generically, as an adjuvant that can stimulate mucosal responses in ruminants; (2) as an antigen to limit EHEC O157:H7 colonisation following vaccination in the reservoir host. Our previous research has demonstrated that systemic immunization with H7 flagella can limit EHEC O157:H7 colonisation possibly by eliciting specific IgA response and high IgG titres [3,8]. The nature of this response was in line with recent findings in mice that have shown the importance of TLR5 in mediating an IgA response to flagellins following systemic injection [20]. However, the responses in cattle were counter to a recent report that indicated minimal activity of cells containing a bovine TLR5 clone [24]. The purpose of the current study was therefore to investigate the functionality of bovine TLR5 using a combination of in vitro and in vivo approaches.

The research presented provides evidence that bovine TLR5 (EMBL ABC68311.1) is functional in terms of flagellin recognition and signalling. The TLR5 clone signalled through an NFkB reporter when transfected into HEK293 cells; the signalling was reduced when specific mutations were introduced into the H7 flagellin TLR5-

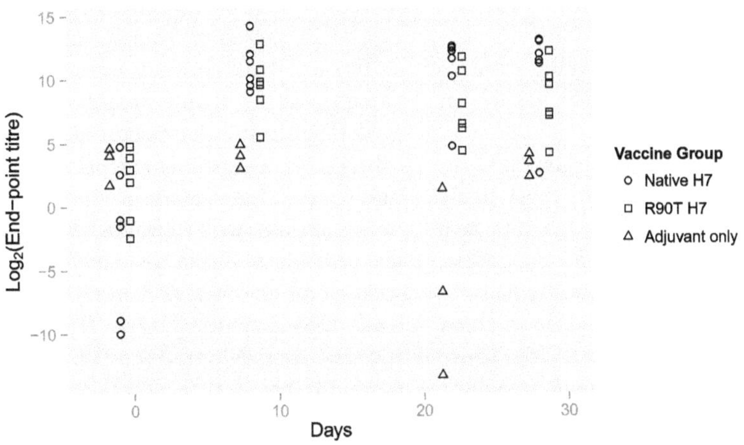

Figure 5 IgA responses of cattle immunized with WT and R90T H7 flagellin. Three groups of calves were immunized twice via the intramuscular route 2 weeks apart with either 60 μg of WT H7 flagellin + 5mg Quil A ($n = 6$), 60 μg of R90T H7 flagellin + 5mg Quil A ($n = 6$) or 5mg Quil A alone ($n = 3$) as described in the Materials and methods. Levels of anti WT-H7 specific IgA were determined by end-point ELISA from serum sampled at the times indicated. Animals were immunized at day 0 and day 14. Plots show the $\log_2$ transformed endpoint titre values for each animal sample for each of the three groups. The sampling times were a day before immunization, and days, 8, 22 and 28 post-immunization; the groups have been separated to ease visualization.

binding domain. It was apparent that the human clone used in our study did activate the NK-kB reporter to higher levels than the bovine clone in the HEK293 background, at least at when the cells were challenged with lower levels of H7 flagellin. We do not know whether this is due to differences in expression levels of the different TLR5s, and/or signalling activity. Recently reported research on bovine TLR5 by Metcalfe et al. [24] provided no evidence of bTLR signalling in HEK293T cells and we reasoned that this may be due to: (1) either very low levels of transfection and a different reporter system in their study; (2) differences in signalling in the HEK293 and HEK293T cells based on residual human TLR activity. We have found positively selected codons in the bovine TIR domain which may alter its interactions with MyD88 and other signalling molecules and impact on signalling in cells of different animal origin [22]. To ensure compatibility, we tested the bovine TLR5 clone in a bovine cell line. Prior to transfection, the bovine epithelial cell line, EBL, showed no production of IL8/CXCL8 when flagellin was added. This cell line was then transfected with a bTLR5 sub-clone generated in this study and this resulted in cells that secreted CXCL8 in response to addition of flagella in a dose-dependent manner. This secretion was reduced when the mutated H7 flagellin R90T was added. While this data indicated that the bTLR5 clone is active in response to flagellin in a bovine cell background, further work is required to assess which cells and tissues express TLR5 in cattle. It was interesting that un-transfected EBL cells did not express a TLR5 transcript (data not shown) and were not activated by addition of H7 flagellin; this is in line with reports that udder tissue does not express TLR5 [38] and both bovine primary colonocyte cultures and bovine neutrophils were negative for TLR5 expression [39,40]. A key restriction for future work on cell- and tissue-specific expression is the development of reagents that recognise ruminant TLR5, particularly in its native conformation.

Based on current research, the key cells involved in stimulating host responses to flagellins are most likely specific subsets of dendritic cells and/or macrophages [20,21]. We therefore wanted to analyse TLR5-dependent responses to H7 flagellin by bovine macrophages. Macrophages were derived from blood monocytes [29] for which RNA silencing methods have been developed [28]. These cells showed detectable expression of TLR5 mRNA which could be knocked down by various TLR5 specific siRNAs. These cells produced CXCL8 mRNA and cytokine in response to flagella and this response was restricted by the anti-TLR5 siRNAs. It was interesting that the level of TLR5 mRNA reduced significantly 4 h following addition of flagellin, indicating that recognition of the agonist leads to a regulatory shift in the sensing cells. However, this immediate repression appeared to be temporary as the TLR5 transcript levels were similar to the initial levels at 24 h, perhaps indicating some type of homeostatic response to continuous flagellin activation. While this study did demonstrate functional TLR5-dependent signalling by bovine macrophages it was evident from the TLR5 knockdowns and studies with the mutated flagellins that other TLR5-independent responses to the flagellins were occurring which did not appear to be the case for the transfected EBL cells. It has been shown that flagellin recognition can also be mediated through cytosolic NAIP and NLRC4-dependent inflammasomes [41,42]. Thus bovine macrophages, unlike bovine EBLs, presumably internalise flagellin into the cytosol, leading to activation of inflammasomes, but further research is required to confirm if this is the case and the consequences of this activation.

To test whether the reduced capacity to stimulate bTLR5 in vitro might alter the humoral IgA response to flagellin, cattle were immunized with either WT-H7 or R90T-H7 flagellin preparations. IgA responses in cattle serum to both flagellins were determined by end-point titration ELISAs. Immunization with the R90T led to levels of serum IgA that were consistently lower than those detected for the WT-H7 irrespective of the coated flagellin antigen used in the ELISA (WT or R90T). However, these differences were not significant ($P > 0.05$) as a consequence of high titre variation between animals and the relatively small numbers of calves in each group ($n = 6$). The finding that the variant R90T-H7 was also able to stimulate IgA responses was perhaps not surprising given that this variant was still able to activate bTLR5 signalling, although at a reduced level compared to WT-H7. Differences in vitro were dependent on the amount of flagellin used and how these levels translate to the sensitivity in vivo is unknown. Furthermore the difference in terms of CXCL8 secretion from bovine MDMs stimulated with WT-H7 vs R90T-H7, while significantly reduced for the variant, was less than two-fold at the concentration examined (Figure 4E). As discussed above, it is possible that other TLR5-independent signalling pathways may contribute to the IgA response in cattle following systemic immunization with flagellin. Another consideration for the cattle immunizations experiments is that QuilA was used as an adjuvant and immune stimulating complexes (ISCOMS) containing Quil A can help induce IgA responses when delivered mucosally. However, we are aware from our previous work examining systemic delivery of antigens other than flagellin that Quil A does not usually induce IgA responses to these [8,9]. So while we appreciate there may well be synergy between the adjuvants, QuilA and flagellin, flagellin is required for overt IgA responses.

Proof of TLR5-dependent IgA production in cattle would ideally require cattle that do not express functional

TLR5. Recent work has shown that TLR5 alleles are present in cattle with stop codons in the ectodomain which are likely to impair function [22]. However their frequencies would indicate that where present, they would probably be heterozygous. Nonetheless a different stop codon mutation in human TLR5 is a dominant negative mutation and its presence as a heterozygote in humans leads to significantly lower natural levels of flagellin-specific IgG and IgA [43]. Thus it may be possible to investigate whether cattle carrying the STOP codon mutants respond less well to systemic immunisation with H7 flagellin. It may also be possible to identify bovine sires carrying these STOP codons and select homozygotes which would be TLR5 negative, allowing more definitive experiments on the role of bovine TLR5 in vivo.

The TIR domain is important for signal transduction for TLR5, although less is known about the TLR5 signaling motifs and pathways for other TLRs. It is intriguing that the bTLR5 is functional given that it possesses a Y798P change compared to other mammalian TLR5 sequences and that Y798L has been shown to negate TLR5 signalling activity in mice [23]. However, the serine at position 805 may also be critical for signalling [44], and this is present in the WT bovine TLR5. Evidence suggests that ruminant TLR5 has undergone adaptive evolution which is still ongoing as SNPs were co-localised with predicted adaptive codons [22]. This would suggest that the interactions between flagellins and bovine TLR5 are drivers of evolutionary changes which may have functional consequences in terms of both infectious disease susceptibility and/or inflammatory disorders as described for humans [43,45]. On-going work is investigating the critical residues required for bTLR5 responses and the pathways induced by flagellin recognition. Potentially polymorphisms might account for variation seen in the responses in the flagellin immunisation experiments carried out in the present animal study.

Flores-Langarica et al. [20] have shown in mice that CD103+ TLR5+ dendritic cell numbers drop in the lamina propria following systemic immunization with flagellins, and that this reduction is associated with an increase in these cells within the local mesenteric lymph nodes. They conclude that this subset of cells traffics to the local node following TLR5-dependent flagellin stimulation to present flagellin peptides to T cells and promote class switching of flagellin-specific B cells to IgA. It has been also been shown that humoral immunity in response to flagellin can depend on other TLR5 independent pathways which involve NAIPs and NLRC4 inflammasome activation [27] and/or a novel MyD88 independent pathway [46]. Their relevance for cattle is unknown at present. A logical progression of the work in this area is to obtain similar mucosal responses to systemically delivered heterologous antigens expressed either within or conjugated to flagellins. Future work will test immune responses in cattle induced by heterologous flagellin-antigen constructs, as well as defining the specificity of bovine TLR5 stimulation by different flagellin sequences to determine the most appropriate flagellin constructs for use as an adjuvant in this species.

Competing interests

The authors declare that they have no competing interests.

Authors' contributions

Conceived and designed the experiments: DLG, DGES, EJG, KJ, AM, AT, TM. Performed the experiments: AT, KJ, YC-M, SM, DF, AA, TM. Analyzed the data: KJ, AT, AC, TM, DLG, HB. Contributed reagents/materials/analysis tools: HB, AC, SM. Wrote and approved the final manuscript: DLG, AT, KJ, TM, DGES, AA, EJG.

Acknowledgements

We thank Dr. Jun Zou from the Scottish Fish Immunology Centre, University of Aberdeen for supplying the modified ptGFP1. We thank Dr. Eliza Wolfson for helping with Figure 2. AA, AM, DGES, TM and DLG were supported by grant BB/I011625/1 from the BBSRC; EG and YCM acknowledge BBSRC Industrial Partnership Awards with Bio-Rad AbD Serotec, BB/I020519/1 and BB/I019863/1. DLG, EG, SM, KJ acknowledge support of an Institute Strategic Programme Grant to the Roslin Institute from the BBSRC. TM and DGES receive funding from the Scottish Government.

Author details

[1]Division of Immunity and Infection, The Roslin Institute and R(D)SVS, The University of Edinburgh, Easter Bush, Midlothian EH25 9RG, UK. [2]Faculty of Veterinary Medicine, Kafrelsheikh University, 33516 Kafr el-Sheikh, Egypt. [3]Moredun Research Institute, Pentlands Science Park, Bush Loan, Penicuik, Edinburgh EH26 0PZ, UK. [4]Institute of Infection, Immunity & Inflammation, Glasgow Biomedical Research Centre, University of Glasgow, Glasgow G12 8TA, UK.

References

1. Döring G, Meisner C, Stern M, Flagella Vaccine Trial Study Group (2007) Double-blind randomized placebo-controlled phase III study of a *Pseudomonas aeruginosa* flagella vaccine in cystic fibrosis patients. Proc Natl Acad Sci U S A 104:11020–11025
2. Roy K, Hamilton D, Ostmann MM, Fleckenstein JM (2009) Vaccination with EtpA glycoprotein or flagellin protects against colonization with enterotoxigenic *Escherichia coli* in a murine model. Vaccine 27:4601–4608
3. McNeilly TN, Naylor SW, Mahajan A, Mitchell MC, McAteer S, Deane D, Smith DG, Low JC, Gally DL, Huntley JF (2008) *Escherichia coli* O157:H7 colonization in cattle following systemic and mucosal immunization with purified H7 flagellin. Infect Immun 76:2594–2602
4. Ricci ML, Torosantucci A, Scaturro M, Chiani P, Baldassarri L, Pastoris MC (2005) Induction of protective immunity by *Legionella pneumophila* flagellum in an A/J mouse model. Vaccine 23:4811–4820
5. Mori J, Vranac T, Smrekar B, Cernilec M, Serbec VČ, Horvat S, Ihan A, Benčina M, Jerala R (2012) Chimeric flagellin as the self-adjuvanting antigen for the activation of immune response against *Helicobacter pylori*. Vaccine 30:5856–5863
6. Stocker BA, Newton SM (1994) Immune responses to epitopes inserted in Salmonella flagellin. Int Rev Immunol 11:167–178
7. Westerlund-Wikström B (2000) Peptide display on bacterial flagella: principles and applications. Int J Med Microbiol 290:223–230
8. McNeilly TN, Mitchell MC, Nisbet AJ, McAteer S, Erridge C, Inglis NF, Smith DG, Low JC, Gally DL, Huntley JF (2010) IgA and IgG antibody responses following systemic immunization of cattle with native H7 flagellin differ in epitope recognition and capacity to neutralise TLR5 signalling. Vaccine 28:1412–1421
9. McNeilly TN, Mitchell MC, Rosser T, McAteer S, Low JC, Smith DG, Huntley JF, Mahajan A, Gally DL (2010) Immunization of cattle with a combination of purified intimin-531, EspA and Tir significantly reduces shedding of *Escherichia coli* O157:H7 following oral challenge. Vaccine 28:1422–1428
10. Medzhitov R (2001) Toll-like receptors and innate immunity. Nat Rev Immunol 1:135–145

11. Song DH, Lee J-O (2012) Sensing of microbial molecular patterns by Toll-like receptors. Immunol Rev 250:216–229
12. Farhat K, Riekenberg S, Heine H, Debarry J, Lang R, Mages J, Buwitt-Beckmann U, Röschmann K, Jung G, Wiesmüller KH, Ulmer AJ (2008) Heterodimerization of TLR2 with TLR1 or TLR6 expands the ligand spectrum but does not lead to differential signaling. J Leukoc Biol 83:692–701
13. Smith KD, Andersen-Nissen E, Hayashi F, Strobe K, Bergman MA, Barrett SLR, Cookson BT, Aderem A (2003) Toll-like receptor 5 recognizes a conserved site on flagellin required for protofilament formation and bacterial motility. Nat Immunol 4:1247–1253
14. Andersen-Nissen E, Smith KD, Bonneau R, Strong RK, Aderem A (2007) A conserved surface on toll-like receptor 5 recognizes bacterial flagellin. J Exp Med 204:393–403
15. Ivicak-Kocjan K, Panter G, Bencina M, Jerala R (2013) Determination of the physiological 2:2 TLR5:flagellin activation stoichiometry revealed by the activity of a fusion receptor. Biochem Biophys Res Commun 435:40–45
16. Yamamoto M, Takeda K, Akira S (2004) TIR domain-containing adaptors define the specificity of TLR signaling. Mol Immunol 40:861–868
17. Yoon SI, Kurnasov O, Natarajan V, Hong M, Gudkov AV, Osterman AL, Wilson IA (2012) Structural basis of TLR5-flagellin recognition and signaling. Science 335:859–864
18. Andersen-Nissen E, Smith KD, Strobe KL, Barrett SL, Cookson BT, Logan SM, Aderem A (2005) Evasion of Toll-like receptor 5 by flagellated bacteria. Proc Natl Acad Sci U S A 102:9247–9252
19. Lee SK, Stack A, Katzowitsch E, Aizawa SI, Suerbaum S, Josenhans C (2003) *Helicobacter pylori* flagellins have very low intrinsic activity to stimulate human gastric epithelial cells via TLR5. Microbes Infect 5:1345–1356
20. Flores-Langarica A, Marshall JL, Hitchcock J, Cook C, Jobanputra J, Bobat S, Ross EA, Coughlan RE, Henderson IR, Uematsu S, Akira S, Cunningham AF (2012) Systemic flagellin immunization stimulates mucosal CD103+ dendritic cells and drives Foxp3+ regulatory T cell and IgA responses in the mesenteric lymph node. J Immunol 189:5745–5754
21. Atif SM, Uematsu S, Akira S, McSorley SJ (2014) CD103-CD11b + dendritic cells regulate the sensitivity of CD4 T-cell responses to bacterial flagellin. Mucosal Immunol 7:68–77
22. Smith SA, Jann OC, Haig D, Russell GC, Werling D, Glass EJ, Emes RD (2012) Adaptive evolution of Toll-like receptor 5 in domesticated mammals. BMC Evol Biol 12:122
23. Ivison SM, Khan MA, Graham NR, Bernales CQ, Kaleem A, Tirling CO, Cherkasov A, Steiner TS (2007) A phosphorylation site in the Toll-like receptor 5 TIR domain is required for inflammatory signalling in response to flagellin. Biochem Biophys Res Commun 352:936–941
24. Metcalfe HJ, La Ragione RM, Smith DG, Werling D (2014) Functional characterisation of bovine TLR5 indicates species-specific recognition of flagellin. Vet Immunol Immunopathol 157:197–205
25. Ibrahim GF, Fleet GH, Lyons MJ, Walker RA (1985) Method for the isolation of highly purified Salmonella flagellins. J Clin Microbiol 22:1040–1044
26. Corripio-Miyar Y, Secombes CJ, Zou J (2012) Long-term stimulation of trout head kidney cells with the cytokines MCSF, IL-2 and IL-6: Gene expression dynamics. Fish Shellfish Immunol 32:35–44
27. Vijay-Kumar M, Carvalho FA, Aitken JD, Fifadara NH, Gewirtz AT (2010) TLR5 or NLRC4 is necessary and sufficient for promotion of humoral immunity by flagellin. Eur J Immunol 40:3528–3534
28. Jensen K, Anderson JA, Glass EJ (2014) Comparison of small interfering RNA (siRNA) delivery into bovine monocyte-derived macrophages by transfection and electroporation. Vet Immunol Immunopathol 158:224–232
29. Jensen K, Talbot R, Paxton E, Waddington D, Glass EJ (2006) Development and validation of a bovine macrophage specific cDNA microarray. BMC Genomics 7:224
30. Rozen S, Skaletsky H (2000) Primer3 on the WWW for general users and for biologist programmers. Methods Mol Biol 132:365–386
31. Pfaffl MW (2001) A new mathematical model for relative quantification in real-time RT–PCR. Nucleic Acids Res 29:e45
32. Brown HK, Prescott RP (2006) Applied Mixed Models in Medicine, 2nd edition. John Wiley, Chichester
33. Smith MF, Mitchell A, Li G, Ding S, Fitzmaurice AM, Ryan K, Crowe S, Goldberg JB (2003) Toll-like receptor (TLR) 2 and TLR5, but not TLR4, are required for Helicobacter pylori-induced NF-κB activation and chemokine expression by epithelial cells. J Biol Chem 278:32552–32560
34. Huynh HT, Robitaille G, Turner JD (1991) Establishment of bovine mammary epithelial cells (MAC-T): an *in vitro* model for bovine lactation. Exp Cell Res 197:191–199
35. Van Duin D, Medzhitov R, Shaw AC (2006) Triggering TLR signaling in vaccination. Trends Immunol 27:49–55
36. Reed SG, Bertholet S, Coler RN, Friede M (2009) New horizons in adjuvants for vaccine development. Trends Immunol 30:23–32
37. Szabó C (2003) Role of flagellin in the pathogenesis of shock and acute respiratory distress syndrome: therapeutic opportunities. Crit Care Med 31:S39–S45
38. Porcherie A, Cunha P, Trotereau A, Roussel P, Gilbert FB, Rainard P, Germon P (2012) Repertoire of *Escherichia coli* agonists sensed by innate immunity receptors of the bovine udder and mammary epithelial cells. Vet Res 43:14
39. Bridger P, Mohr M, Stamm I, Fröhlich J, Föllmann W, Birkner S, Metcalfe H, Werling D, Baljer G, Menge C (2010) Primary bovine colonic cells: a model to study strain-specific responses to *Escherichia coli*. Vet Immunol Immunopathol 137:54–63
40. Conejeros I, Patterson R, Burgos RA, Hermosilla C, Werling D (2011) Induction of reactive oxygen species in bovine neutrophils is CD11b, but not dectin-1-dependent. Vet Immunol Immunopathol 139:308–312
41. Miao EA, Alpuche-Aranda CM, Dors M, Clark AE, Bader MW, Miller SI, Aderem A (2006) Cytoplasmic flagellin activates caspase-1 and secretion of interleukin 1beta via Ipaf. Nat Immunol 7:569–575
42. Franchi L, Amer A, Body-Malapel M, Kanneganti TD, Ozören N, Jagirdar R, Inohara N, Vandenabeele P, Bertin J, Coyle A, Grant EP, Núñez G (2006) Cytosolic flagellin requires Ipaf for activation of caspase-1 and interleukin 1beta in salmonella-infected macrophages. Nat Immunol 7:576–582
43. Gewirtz AT, Vijay-Kumar M, Brant SR, Duerr RH, Nicolae DL, Cho JH (2006) Dominant-negative TLR5 polymorphism reduces adaptive immune response to flagellin and negatively associates with Crohn's disease. Am J Physiol Gastrointest Liver Physiol 290:G1157–G1163
44. Ivison SM, Graham NR, Bernales CQ, Kifayet A, Ng N, Shobab LA, Steiner TS (2007) Protein kinase D interaction with TLR5 is required for inflammatory signaling in response to bacterial flagellin. J Immunol 178:5735–5743
45. Chantratita N, Tandhavanant S, Myers ND, Chierakul W, Robertson JD, Mahavanakul W, Singhasivanon P, Emond MJ, Peacock SJ, West TE (2014) Screen of whole blood responses to flagellin identifies TLR5 variation associated with outcome in melioidosis. Genes Immun 15:63–71
46. López-Yglesias AH, Zhao X, Quarles EK, Lai MA, VandenBos T, Strong RK, Smith KD (2014) Flagellin induces antibody responses through a TLR5- and inflammasome-independent pathway. J Immunol 192:1587–1596

12

Incubation of ovine scrapie with environmental matrix results in biological and biochemical changes of PrP^{Sc} over time

Ben C Maddison[1], John Spiropoulos[2], Christopher M Vickery[2], Richard Lockey[2,3], Jonathan P Owen[1], Keith Bishop[1], Claire A Baker[1] and Kevin C Gough[4*]

Abstract

Ovine scrapie can be transmitted via environmental reservoirs. A pool of ovine scrapie isolates were incubated on soil for one day or thirteen months and eluted prion was used to challenge tg338 mice transgenic for ovine PrP. After one-day incubation on soil, two PrP^{Sc} phenotypes were present: G_{338} or $Apl_{338}ii$. Thirteen months later some divergent PrP^{Sc} phenotypes were seen: a mixture of $Apl_{338}ii$ with either G_{338} or P_{338}, and a completely novel PrP^{Sc} deposition, designated Cag_{338}. The data show that prolonged ageing of scrapie prions within an environmental matrix may result in changes in the dominant PrP^{Sc} biological/biochemical properties.

Introduction, methods and results

Prion diseases (or transmissible spongiform encephalopathies, TSEs) are fatal, progressive neurological disorders that have no effective treatment or cure. Prion diseases include human Creutzfeldt-Jakob disease (CJD), bovine spongiform encephalopathy (BSE), scrapie in sheep and goats, and chronic wasting disease (CWD) in deer and elk. The prion hypothesis states that the causal agent is a misfolded version of the cellular prion protein (PrP^C), termed PrP^{Sc} [1].

It is known that particular prion diseases can include strains that display distinct and reproducible disease phenotypes. It is most likely that the prion agent is not a single entity but is made up of a plethora of different conformers of PrP^{Sc} and the dominant PrP^{Sc} conformation causes the specific disease characteristics for a particular infection including pathology, clinical signs and PrP^{Sc} molecular signatures [2]. The identification of prion strains is in fact therefore a description of the dominant disease characteristics. The "gold standard" method employed to define scrapie strains is mouse bioassay using either wild type or preferably transgenic mice such as the tg338 line [3]. These transgenic mice overexpress an ovine PrP transgene and display high sensitivity and specificity to ovine scrapie prions. Of the several phenotypic parameters exhibited in a host species which are used to discriminate TSEs, PrP^{Sc} distribution in the brain detected by immunohistochemistry (IHC) or PET/Histo-blot offers the highest discriminatory power and it can be applied on an individual mouse basis [4-8]. This biological property of prions in conjunction with analysis of the biochemical properties of the agent recovered from the same host species offer a powerful means to identify TSE strains even when they are applied at primary passage as they remain essentially unchanged through serial passages [4,6,9,10].

Scrapie is effectively transmitted between susceptible sheep and goats by animal-to-animal contact and via environmental reservoirs, a disease trait that is shared with CWD in deer/elk. For both diseases, the agent is disseminated widely in vivo and excreted/secreted via multiple routes (reviewed in [11]). The likely location of environmental reservoirs are water, soil, metal surfaces, wood surfaces and concrete surfaces ([12,13] reviewed in [14]). Furthermore, environmental prion is stable and remains infectious for years [15].

The purpose of the present study was to assess the viability of scrapie prions in a soil matrix over time. Pools of hindbrain from nine scrapie-infected sheep with VRQ/VRQ (amino acid positions 136, 156 and 171

* Correspondence: kevin.gough@nottingham.ac.uk
[4]School of Veterinary Medicine and Science, The University of Nottingham, Sutton Bonington Campus, College Road, Sutton Bonington, Leicestershire, UK
Full list of author information is available at the end of the article

respectively) *PRNP* genotypes and twenty genotype matched scrapie-free controls were made into homogenates and applied to soil columns containing a sandy loam soil as previously described [16]. Soil columns were kept at 16–20 °C and constant water content and sampled 1 day and 13 months after the addition of the prion sample. Equivalent samples were taken for soil incubated with the prion-free control sample, and soil unexposed to brain material was used as a further control. All soil was removed from a column and homogenised by mixing. Prion protein was then extracted from soil [15]: 100 mg of soil was re-suspended for 1 h in 500 μL PBS prior to centrifugation at 800 *g* for 10 min. The soil pellet was re-suspended in 100 μL of 1% (w/v) SDS in PBS and shaken vigorously for 1 h. After centrifugation at 800 *g* for 10 min prion protein in the supernatant was removed. Extracted prion was then precipitated for 30 min at 37 °C by the addition of 15 μL of 4% (w/v) sodium phosphotungstic acid (Napta) and 170 mM magnesium chloride, and recovered by centrifugation at 12 100 *g* for 30 min. The pellet was air-dried and re-suspended in 20 μL sterile saline. Each inoculum (20 μL) was used to challenge intracranially 5–10 week old tg338 mice ($n = 10$) as described previously [9]. After inoculation the mice were monitored for signs of neurological disease and were euthanized after exhibiting clinical signs. All animal work was approved by the Animal and Plant Health Agency local ethics committee and was carried out in accordance with the Animals (Scientific Procedures) Act 1986 under Home Office project license 70/6310. In combination with clinical signs, immunohistochemical (IHC) analysis was used to diagnose prion infection for all mice in the study. After euthanasia the brain of each mouse was removed and processed as described previously [9]. TSE diagnosis was based on PrP^{Sc} detection in brain sections with polyclonal antibody Rb486 following a standard protocol [17]. Identification of different PrP^{Sc} types and their distribution in the murine brain was used to identify defined PrP^{Sc} distribution patterns as described previously for wild type and transgenic mice [4-7]. Slides were analysed blind by two independent observers (J.S. and C.V.); the agreement between the two observers regarding PrP^{Sc} deposition pattern identification was 100%.

With inoculum extracted from soil incubated with the scrapie sample for 1 day, eight out of the 10 challenged mice succumbed to TSE with incubation periods <170 days post inoculation (dpi) (Figure 1A). IHC analysis of the mice revealed granular PrP^{Sc} deposits distributed mainly along the brainstem, thalamus and basal ganglia with little involvement of the cerebral or cerebellar cortex; this pattern has been previously designated as G_{338} (Figure 2A) [4]. One further mouse died 483 dpi (Figure 1A) and the main PrP^{Sc} pattern feature was plaques and large aggregates of PrP^{Sc} in the brain parenchyma and perivascular plaques in round meningeal vessels (Figure 2B), a distribution pattern previously recorded as $Apl_{338}ii$. One mouse that died 243 dpi was TSE negative and was treated as an intercurrent death. No mice displayed signs of TSE between 170–483 dpi.

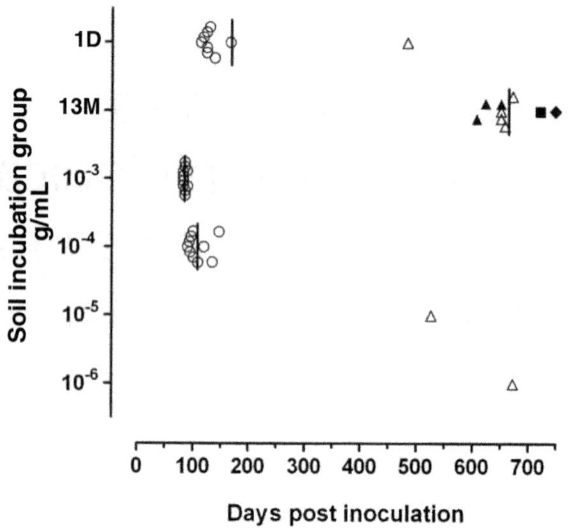

Figure 1 Incubation periods of mice after challenge with scrapie. Mice were inoculated with extracts of soil incubated with a pool of classical scrapie isolates or with a dilution series of the same scrapie pool without soil incubation g/mL of brain inoculum are shown). Open circles: the PrP^{Sc} distribution phenotype G_{338}; open triangles: $Apl_{338}ii$; square: Cag_{338}; solid triangles: $G_{338}/Apl_{338}ii$ mix; diamond: $P_{338}/Apl_{338}ii$ mix. Each vertical line indicates the mean incubation period of a group of mice irrespective of their PrP^{Sc} distribution phenotype. 1D and 13 M are the prion eluted from soil after a 1 day or 13 month incubation respectively.

After 13 months incubation of the scrapie sample on soil, prions were extracted and inoculated into tg338 mice. One mouse was diagnosed TSE negative (intercurrent death) and the remaining nine were TSE positive. The incubation period of the TSE positive mice was 606–748 dpi (Figure 1A). With one exception all mice showed a pattern that was compatible with $Apl_{338}ii$. This was the only pattern observed in four mice, while in another three it was observed in conjunction with G_{338} (Figures 2D-F) and in a single mouse signs of $Apl_{338}ii$ and P_{338} were observed concomitantly (Figure 2G). P_{338} is a pattern characterised by punctate deposits in the neuropil and prominent well-defined intraneuronal PrP^{Sc} accumulations as described previously [4]. One mouse also showed a previously unrecognised PrP^{Sc} pattern designated Cag_{338} characterised by granular PrP^{Sc} deposits, which increased in intensity multifocally, to give rise to coalescing aggregates in the neuropil (Figure 2C). The areas affected more extensively were the midbrain and the medulla.

Previous studies have shown that the P_{338} IHC presentation of PrP^{Sc} is accompanied by a relatively low

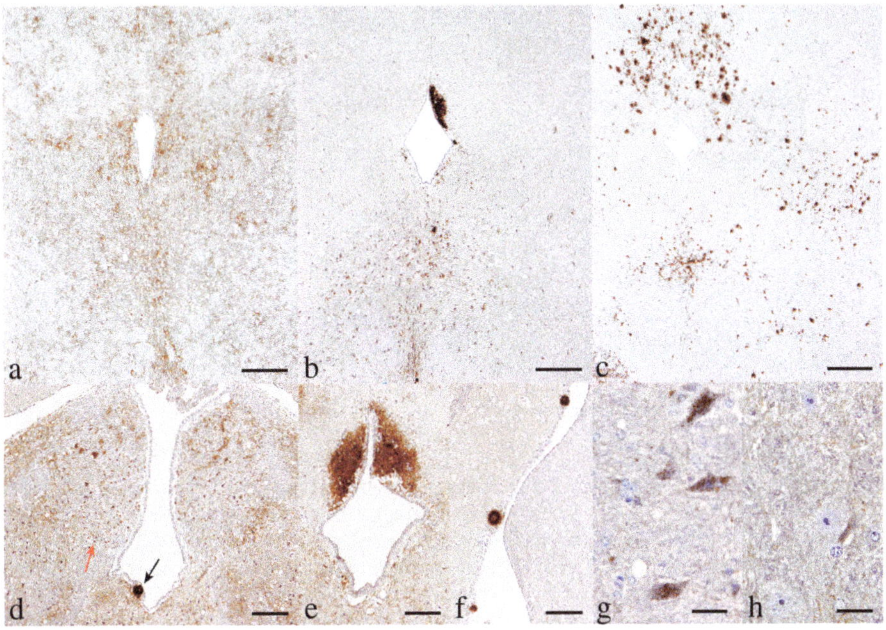

Figure 2 Representative images of PrP^{Sc} deposition in the midbrain of tg338 mice after challenge with scrapie. The deposition patterns observed were characteristic of strains G_{338} **(a)**, $Apl_{338}ii$ **(b)** and Cag_{338} **(c)**. Three mice showed phenotypic characteristics typical of both G_{338} and $Apl_{338}ii$ patterns; photos d-f are all from a single mouse showing small discrete aggregates (**d**, red arrow) in the habenular bodies which is a G_{338} characteristic feature in addition to plaques and large aggregates in subpial areas (**d**, black arrow; **e**, periaqueductal grey matter; **f**, lateral ventricle) which are associated with $Apl_{338}ii$. In a single mouse with $Apl_{338}ii$ phenotype, punctate and prominent intraneuronal labelling **(g)** which are features associated with the P_{338} pattern were also observed; the $Apl_{338}ii$ phenotype is not usually associated with intraneuronal labelling **(h)**. The neurons in **g** and **h** are located in the olive nucleus. Scale bar in **a-c** represents 250 μm; **d-f** 100 μm; **g** and **h** 25 μm.

molecular weight for the PK-resistant PrP^{Sc} compared to both $Apl_{338}ii$ and G_{338} [4,6]. We looked to investigate whether the distinct IHC presentations described here were accompanied by distinct PrP^{Sc} properties. Both the original sheep samples and the murine samples were digested with PK, analyzed on western blots and the prion detected with the antibody SHa31 as previously described [18] (Figures 3A and B). The results show that all ovine samples had indistinguishable PrP^{Sc} profiles with an unglycosylated PrP^{Sc} size of 19.0 +/− 0.3 kDa. The G_{338}, $Apl_{338}ii$ and $G_{338}/Apl_{338}ii$ mixed IHC phenotypes had a similar size of 19.1 +/− 0.3 kDa. However, the $Apl_{338}ii/P_{338}$ mixed phenotype had a relatively low molecular mass by comparison of 17.1 kDa, consistent with previously published data for P_{338} [4,6]. Also, the unglycosylated PrP^{Sc} of Cag_{338} had a relatively high molecular mass of 20.6 kDa (Figure 3B). In addition, we determined that the G_{338} and $Apl_{338}ii$ IHC phenotypes could be readily distinguished by the stability of their PrP^{Sc} (Figures 3C and D). The assay was carried out as described previously [19]. Briefly, aliquots of each murine brain homogenate were incubated with increasing molar concentrations of GdnHCl (final concentrations of 0.5, 2.5, 3.0, 3.5, and 4 M) 1 h at 37 °C. Subsequently all samples were adjusted to a final GdnHCl concentration of 0.4 M, proteinase K was added to a final concentration of 50 μg/mL and the samples incubated for 1 h at 37 °C. Reactions were stopped with 5 mM PMSF. Samples were analysed by western blot using antibody SHa31. The level of signal for each PrP triplet treated with 2.5, 3.0, 3.5 or 4 M GdnHCl was expressed as a percentage of the signal for the same sample treated with 0.5 M. G_{338} was more susceptible to GdnHCl treatment becoming PK sensitive after treatment with 3 M of the denaturant. In contrast, $Apl_{338}ii$ was relatively stable to denaturation with readily detectable PK-resistant PrP^{Sc} after treatment with 4 M GdnHCl (Figures 3C and D). Overall, the PrP^{Sc} biochemical characteristics were distinct for each of $Apl_{338}ii$, G_{338}, $Apl_{338}ii/P_{338}$ mixed and Cag_{338} IHC phenotypes.

Extracts from soil unexposed to brain material and soil treated with scrapie-free brain homogenate were bioassayed in tg338 mice and were TSE negative.

For comparison, the original scrapie sample without any incubation with soil was also titrated in tg338 mice over a range of 10-fold dilutions ($n = 10$ mice for each dilution; Figure 1B). All mice challenged with 20 μg and 2 μg scrapie brain succumbed to scrapie with a G_{338} IHC phenotype. Only one of the 10 mice challenged with either 200 or 20 ng of brain pool was diagnosed with scrapie and in each case this produced an $Apl_{338}ii$ IHC phenotype. Challenge with lower amounts of brain

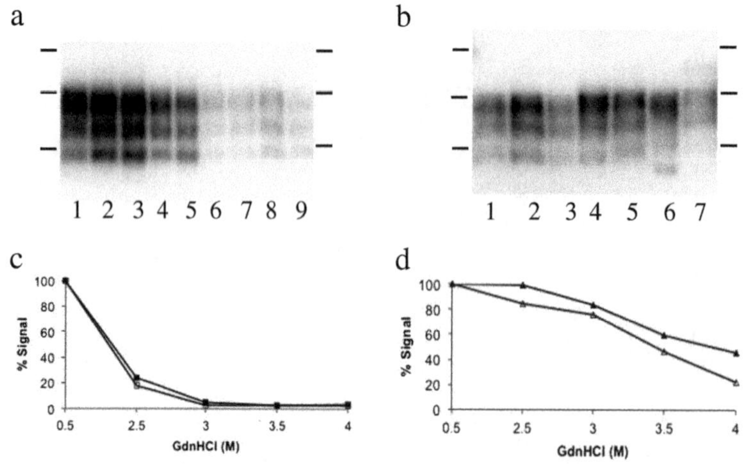

Figure 3 PrP^{Sc} characteristics of the scrapie isolates. Nine ovine hindbrain samples that were pooled and incubated with soil **(a)** were analysed by western blot. Murine isolates **(b)** designated G_{338} (lanes 1, 2 and 3), $Apl_{338}ii$ (lane 4), $Apl_{338}ii/G_{338}$ mixed phenotype (lane 5), $Apl_{338}ii/P_{338}$ mixed phenotype (Lane 6) and Cag_{338} (Lane 7) are also shown. Blots were probed with anti-PrP antibody SHa31 and molecular mass markers of 20, 30 and 40 kDa are indicated. All samples were analysed twice to determine the molecular mass of unglycosylated PrP^{Sc} and gave consistent results. The strains G_{338} **(c)** and $Apl_{338}ii$ **(d)** were further analysed by the conformational stability assay and gave distinct profiles. These molecular traits were consistent both before (closed symbols) and after (open symbols) treatment with SDS and Napta. Analysis was carried out on 3 murine isolates of G_{338} and 2 murine isolates of $Apl_{338}ii$ and the presented data is representative of these isolates.

pool did not cause disease. Prion desorbed from soil after 1 day displayed the same IHC and PrP^{Sc} phenotypes as the original scrapie pool, that is $Apl_{338}ii$ and G_{338}. However, it is possible that the extraction and precipitation treatments have an effect on PrP^{Sc} phenotype or recovery. To test this, murine brain homogenates for G_{338} and $Apl_{338}ii$ phenotypes (10% w/v; 100 μL) were diluted to 200 μL with 2% (w/v) SDS and shaken vigorously for 1 h. After centrifugation at 800 *g* for 10 min prion in the supernatant was precipitated with Napta and brain homogenate and Napta precipitate were analyzed by western blot as detailed above and the total signal for the PrP triplet was determined by densitometry. The percentage recovery after SDS treatment/Napta precipitation for each isolate was determined and comparison of the recoveries of G_{338} and $Apl_{338}ii$ was carried out using a two-tailed students *t*-test. The percentage recoveries for 3 isolates of murine G_{338} and 2 isolates of murine $Apl_{338}ii$ were determined and the mean recoveries were 57 and 56% respectively, differences in the recoveries of the two PrP^{Sc} phenotypes were not significant ($p = 0.97$). In addition, the molecular phenotypes were maintained before and after SDS/Napta treatment (Figures 3C and D).

Discussion

The bioassay data show that the hit rate was equivalent for sheep scrapie extracted from soil after 1 day or 13 months incubation indicating ovine scrapie infection was retained on soil over a prolonged time period. The data also clearly suggest that between day 1 and month 13 the biological and biochemical properties of the prion that is desorbed from soil change considerably. In our view, this concomitant change of biological and biochemical properties as described here is indicative of strain variation. Indeed many of these phenotypic characteristics have been attributed to characterised strains isolated and studied in tg338 mice (Table 1) [4,6]. Some

Table 1 Main features of characterised strains identified in this study [4,6]

		Main PrP^{Sc} characteristics	
Strain	**Incubation period (IP)***	**Immunohistochemistry (IHC)**	**Western blot#**
G_{338}	78 ± 6	Granular deposits mainly in brain stem and thalamus	21 KDa
P_{338}	153 ± 8	Punctate and intraneuronal deposits mainly in brain stem and thalamus	19 KDa
$Apl_{338}ii$	249 ± 59	Aggregates and plaques. Midbrain is most affected area	21 KDa

*Incubation period (IP) values denote mean ± SD and indicate days post inoculation (dpi) after three serial passages. At first passage IP values of certain strains such as Apl_{338} may be prolonged [6]. G_{338} is an exceptional strain as shorter IP values can be observed at primary passage [21] with serial passages resulting in IP prolongation by approximately 12 dpi.

#Western blot values refer to the molecular mass of the unglycosylated band. Absolute values may differ depending on the western blot conditions. However, the P_{338} unglycosylated band always migrates further indicating a 2 KDa lower molecular mass compared to G_{338} and $Apl_{338}ii$.

of the strain phenotypes identified after a 13 month incubation are highly novel. Both G_{338} and P_{338} strains are relatively fast incubation strains and have not been reported before in a mixed phenotype with $Apl_{338}ii$ or at these prolonged incubation times. The identification particularly of G_{338} IHC characteristics, in conjunction with $Apl_{338}ii$, in the brains of mice showing incubation period >600 dpi is intriguing as the maximum incubation period associated with G_{338} is known to be <200 dpi [20]. Therefore the possibility that G_{338} was existing as an independent entity in the inoculum used to challenge the mice is unlikely even if we accept that in the presence of a significantly slower strain, such as $Apl_{338}ii$, the propagation of G_{338} was delayed. Another possible explanation would be that agents with G_{338} or P_{338} properties could emerge from $Apl_{338}ii$ at a later stage of the incubation period. Alternatively the G_{338} and P_{338} phenotypic characteristics that were observed in conjunction with $Apl_{338}ii$ indicate phenotypes that have some G_{338} or P_{338} properties associated with unusually prolonged incubation periods. Without isolating each of these agents in a pure state to study their properties it is not possible to draw definitive conclusions regarding their exact strain characteristics. However, their existence at this stage, particularly of the P_{338} IHC phenotype, which is also accompanied with biochemical properties that are attributed to the P_{338} strain, cannot be ignored and adds valuable information regarding the diversity of scrapie phenotypes that can emerge after prolonged incubation period with soil. The Cag_{338} strain phenotype is reported here for the first time. Collectively, therefore, these data suggest that the ageing of prions within an environmental matrix can affect their biological and biochemical properties suggesting strain alterations. The three novel phenotypes of desorbed prion strains observed after 13 months incubation on soil were not detected in a range of 10-fold dilutions of the original scrapie sample and the SDS/Napta treatment of samples to desorb them from soil had no apparent effect on G_{338} or $Apl_{338}ii$ recovery or PrP^{Sc} phenotype. Therefore, these novel PrP^{Sc} presentations must be a consequence of their interaction with soil or ageing or both. It is not known whether this emergence of novel phenotypes seen here during ageing on soil reflects the selection of existing conformers present in the original sample or *de novo* mutation to produce novel conformations of the prion. The study compared PrP^{Sc} phenotypes that are recovered from soil after 1 day and 13 month periods and the effects of soil interaction and incubation time alone are not considered separately. Therefore it is also not known whether the observed changes in dominant prion strains are dictated by incubation time at ambient temperature alone or by interaction with soil over a prolonged period. However, regardless of the mechanisms of the observed ageing, the unequivocal finding is that when a mixture of prion phenotypes are added to a soil environment the dominant pathologies change over time. Whether analogous ageing of prions occurs in other natural environments that may harbour prion reservoirs remains to be established. The presence of "dynamic" reservoirs of environmental scrapie infectivity could possibly lead to the emergence of novel strains of scrapie in natural infections. Such events may have contributed to the significant (and unusual) diversity of the scrapie disease agent.

Abbreviations
TSE: Transmissible spongiform encephalopathy; CWD: Chronic wasting disease; PrP/PrP^C: Cellular prion protein; PrP^{Sc}: Disease-associated prion protein; IHC: Immunohistochemistry; Napta: Sodium phosphotungstic acid.

Competing interests
The authors declare that they have no competing interests.

Authors' contributions
KCG and BCM conceived this study and participated in its design and coordination. JS, RL and CMV carried out the bioassay JS and CMV conducted IHC analysis of the samples and the interpretation of the findings. JO, KB and CB carried out the soil experiments and prepared the inoculums, analysed samples by western blot and conformational stability assay. KCG and BCM have written the manuscript with inputs from all authors. All authors read and approved the final manuscript.

Acknowledgements
This work was supported by the Department for Environment, Food and Rural Affairs, UK (Defra project SE1858). The authors would like to thank colleagues in Pathology and Animal Science Unit at APHA for their skilled technical expertise and support. We thank the Biological-archive, APHA (Addlestone, Surrey, UK) for the provision of sheep brain material.

Author details
[1]ADAS UK, School of Veterinary Medicine and Science, The University of Nottingham, Sutton Bonington Campus, College Road, Sutton Bonington, Leicestershire, UK. [2]Animal and Plant Health Agency, Woodham Lane, New Haw, Addlestone, Surrey, UK. [3]Current address: University of Southampton, Southampton SO17 1BJ, UK. [4]School of Veterinary Medicine and Science, The University of Nottingham, Sutton Bonington Campus, College Road, Sutton Bonington, Leicestershire, UK.

References
1. Prusiner SB (1998) Prions. Proc Natl Acad Sci U S A 95:13363–13383
2. Collinge J, Clarke AR (2007) A general model of prion strains and their pathogenicity. Science 318:930–936
3. Vilotte JL, Soulier S, Essalmani R, Stinnakre MG, Vaiman D, Lepourry L, Da Silva JC, Besnard N, Dawson M, Buschmann A, Groschup M, Petit S, Madelaine MF, Rakatobe S, Le Dur A, Vilette D, Laude H (2001) Markedly increased susceptibility to natural sheep scrapie of transgenic mice expressing ovine PrP. J Virol 75:5977–5984
4. Thackray AM, Hopkins L, Lockey R, Spiropoulos J, Bujdoso R (2011) Emergence of multiple prion strains from single isolates of ovine scrapie. J Gen Virol 92:1482–1491
5. Beck KE, Vickery CM, Lockey R, Holder T, Thorne L, Terry LA, Denyer M, Webb P, Simmons MM, Spiropoulos J (2012) The interpretation of disease phenotypes to identify TSE strains following murine bioassay: characterisation of classical scrapie. Vet Res 43:77
6. Thackray AM, Hopkins L, Lockey R, Spiropoulos J, Bujdoso R (2012) Propagation of ovine prions from "poor" transmitter scrapie isolates in ovine PrP transgenic mice. Exp Mol Pathol 92:167–174
7. Beck KE, Sallis RE, Lockey R, Vickery CM, Beringue V, Laude H, Holder TM, Thorne L, Terry LA, Tout AC, Jayasena D, Griffiths PC, Cawthraw S, Ellis R, Balkema-Buschmann A, Groschup MH, Simmons MM, Spiropoulos J (2012) Use of murine bioassay to resolve ovine transmissible spongiform

encephalopathy cases showing a bovine spongiform encephalopathy molecular profile. Brain Pathol 22:265–279

8. van Keulen LJ, Langeveld JP, Dolstra CH, Jacobs J, Bossers A, van Zijderveld FG: TSE strain differentiation in mice by immunohistochemical PrP profiles and triplex Western blot. Neuropathol Appl Neurobiol, in press
9. Corda E, Beck KE, Sallis RE, Vickery CM, Denyer M, Webb PR, Bellworthy SJ, Spencer YI, Simmons MM, Spiropoulos J (2012) The interpretation of disease phenotypes to identify TSE strains in mice: characterisation of BSE using PrP^{Sc} distribution patterns in the brain. Vet Res 43:86
10. Le Dur A, Beringue V, Andreoletti O, Reine F, Lai TL, Baron T, Bratberg B, Vilotte J-L, Sarradin P, Benestad SL, Laude H (2005) A newly identified type of scrapie agent can naturally infect sheep with resistant PrP genotypes. Proc Natl Acad Sci U S A 102:16031–16036
11. Gough KC, Maddison BC (2010) Prion transmission: prion excretion and occurrence in the environment. Prion 4:275–282
12. Maddison BC, Baker CA, Terry LA, Bellworthy SJ, Thorne L, Rees HC, Gough KC (2010) Environmental sources of scrapie prions. J Virol 84:11560–11562
13. Nichols TA, Pulford B, Wyckoff AC, Meyerett C, Michel B, Gertig K, Hoover EA, Jewell JE, Telling GC, Zabel MD (2009) Detection of protease-resistant cervid prion protein in water from a CWD-endemic area. Prion 3:171–183
14. Bartelt-Hunt SL, Bartz JC (2013) Behavior of prions in the environment: implications for prion biology. PLoS Pathog 9:e1003113
15. Seidel B, Thomzig A, Buschmann A, Groschup MH, Peters R, Beekes M, Terytze K (2007) Scrapie agent (strain 263 k) can transmit disease via the oral route after persistence in soil over years. PLoS One 2:e435
16. Maddison BC, Owen JP, Bishop K, Shaw G, Rees HC, Gough KC (2010) The interaction of ruminant PrP^{Sc} with soils is influenced by prion source and soil type. Environ Sci Technol 44:8503–8508
17. Vickery CM, Beck KE, Simmons MM, Hawkins SA, Spiropoulos J (2013) Disease characteristics of bovine spongiform encephalopathy following inoculation into mice via three different routes. Int J Exp Pathol 94:320–328
18. Owen JP, Maddison BC, Whitelam GC, Gough KC (2007) Use of thermolysin in the diagnosis of prion diseases. Mol Biotechnol 35:161–170
19. Peretz D, Scott MR, Groth D, Williamson RA, Burton DR, Cohen FE, Prusiner SB (2001) Strain-specified relative conformational stability of the scrapie prion protein. Protein Sci 10:854–863
20. Andréoletti O, Orge L, Benestad SL, Beringue V, Litaise C, Simon S, Le Dur A, Laude H, Simmons H, Lugan S, Corbière F, Costes P, Morel N, Schelcher S, Lacroux C (2011) Atypical/Nor98 Scrapie Infectivity in Sheep Peripheral Tissues. PLoS Pathog 7:e1001285
21. Thackray AM, Hopkins L, Spiropoulos J, Budjoso R (2008) Molecular and transmission characteristics of primary-passaged ovine scrapie isolates in conventional and transgenic mice. J Virol 82:11197–11207

13

Vaccination of pigs with the S48 strain of *Toxoplasma gondii* – safer meat for human consumption

Alison Burrells[1], Julio Benavides[1,2], German Cantón[1,3], João L Garcia[1,4], Paul M Bartley[1], Mintu Nath[5], Jackie Thomson[1], Francesca Chianini[1], Elisabeth A Innes[1] and Frank Katzer[1*]

Abstract

As clinical toxoplasmosis is not considered a problem in pigs, the main reason to implement a control strategy against *Toxoplasma gondii* (*T. gondii*) in this species is to reduce the establishment of *T. gondii* tissue cysts in pork, consequently reducing the risk of the parasite entering the human food chain. Consumption of *T. gondii* tissue cysts from raw or undercooked meat is one of the main sources of human infection, with infected pork being considered a high risk. This study incorporates a mouse bioassay with molecular detection of *T. gondii* DNA to study the effectiveness of vaccination (incomplete S48 strain) in its ability to reduce tissue cyst burden in pigs, following oocyst (M4 strain) challenge. Results from the mouse bioassay show that 100% of mice which had received porcine tissues from vaccinated and challenged pigs survived compared with 51.1% of mice which received tissues from non-vaccinated and challenged pigs. The presence (or absence) of *T. gondii* DNA from individual mouse brains also confirmed these results. This indicates a reduction in viable *T. gondii* tissue cysts within tissues from pigs which have been previously vaccinated with the S48 strain. In addition, the study demonstrated that the main predilection sites for the parasite were found to be brain and highly vascular muscles (such as tongue, diaphragm, heart and masseter) of pigs, while meat cuts used as human food such as chop, loin, left tricep and left semitendinosus, had a lower burden of *T. gondii* tissue cysts. These promising results highlight the potential of S48 strain tachyzoites for reducing the number of *T. gondii* tissues cysts in pork and thus improving food safety.

Introduction

The protozoan parasite *Toxoplasma gondii* (*T. gondii*) has the ability to infect all warm blooded mammals, including humans and livestock. Livestock are known intermediate hosts of *T. gondii*. Food animals such as pigs, sheep, goats and cattle become infected with the parasite, either from consumption of oocysts shed in the environment by the definitive host (felids), or in the case of pigs, from consuming other infected intermediate hosts such as rodents [1]. Following *T. gondii* infection, cysts form in the tissues of the animal (tissue cysts), these cysts contain the bradyzoite stage of the parasite and can survive for the lifetime of the host. The ability of tissue cysts to establish within food producing animals varies; cattle rarely have detectable tissue cysts, even in animals which have been experimentally challenged [2,3], whilst in sheep, pigs and goats, tissue cysts are more commonly identified [4]. Tissue cysts have a preference to establish in specific tissues of the host, such as liver, heart, brain, tongue, diaphragm, and skeletal muscle [5,6]. Viable parasites and tissue cysts have also been isolated from cuts of meat and meat products destined for human consumption from naturally and experimentally infected animals [7-11]. Consumption of raw or undercooked meat from animals containing tissue cysts is a main source of *T. gondii* infection in humans, with infected pork considered to be the major source of infection [12,13].

Outdoor reared pigs are more likely to become infected with the parasite compared with those reared indoors [14,15], with the main source of infection thought to be from consumption of oocyst contaminated feed, water and/or soil [16]. In addition, outdoor housing

* Correspondence: frank.katzer@moredun.ac.uk
[1]Moredun Research Institute, Pentlands Science Park, Bush Loan, Midlothian EH26 0PZ, Scotland, UK
Full list of author information is available at the end of the article

systems also allow pigs to come into contact with rodents and other wildlife species. Due to their omnivorous nature pigs will consume rodents or rodent cadavers as well as other small mammals and birds, which may be infected with *T. gondii* and several studies have demonstrated how rodent control programs can reduce *T. gondii* seropositivity in pigs [1,17].

Although clinical toxoplasmosis in pigs is rare, and certainly not a common enough problem to warrant the commercial use of a vaccine against the parasite, the formation of tissue cysts in the muscles of infected animals can pose a significant risk for food safety and is thought to be one of the most important sources of *T. gondii* infection for humans, particularly when pork is eaten undercooked or raw [18,19].

A vaccine which can reduce or eliminate the formation of infective tissues cysts in pigs would be beneficial for pork products intended for human consumption, reducing the potential public health risk from *T. gondii* infection. Previous research into the reduction of the formation of tissue cysts in pigs has included work using live and killed vaccine approaches [20-25]. It is currently unknown whether the commercially available vaccine Toxovax® (comprised of the S48 strain of *T. gondii* and used to protect against ovine abortion caused by the parasite), offers any protection against tissue cyst formation in livestock species. This lack of knowledge regarding the ability of S48 to protect against tissue cyst formation was highlighted, as a key knowledge gap, in a recent document produced for the Food Standards Agency [26]. The document stated that one of the gaps in the current knowledge relevant to a UK risk assessment was: "*Vaccines based on live attenuated strains of tachyzoites are effective in reducing morbidity in sheep but it is not known whether vaccination has any effect on the formation of tissue cysts*". Therefore, to address this knowledge gap and potentially improve food safety, this study focused on the effect of vaccination of pigs with the S48 strain of *T. gondii* in order to reduce tissue cyst formation. The S48 strain was originally isolated from a case of ovine abortion in New Zealand, which after approximately 3000 passages in mice lost its ability to develop into tissue cysts (bradyzoites) in mice and oocysts in cats [27,28].

The objective of this research was to evaluate the effectiveness of this live attenuated strain of *T. gondii* (S48) in its ability to reduce viable tissue cysts within porcine tissues. A reduction, or indeed elimination, of viable tissue cysts in pork would make this food source safer for human consumption. In addition, another objective was to ensure that the S48 strain used for vaccination did not persist in the pig tissues. Finally, the research aimed to provide an insight into the predilection sites for the parasite within specific porcine tissues, including tissues used within the human food chain.

Materials and methods

Pig vaccination and challenge

A total of 18 pigs, six week old Large White/Landrace cross bred pigs (*Sus scrofa*) of mixed gender, were divided into four groups (G) depending on experimental challenge; G1 ($n = 5$) non-vaccinated and oocyst challenged animals, G2 ($n = 5$) vaccinated and oocyst challenged animals, G3 ($n = 5$) vaccinated non-challenged animals, G4 ($n = 3$) non-vaccinated and non-challenged animals. The five animals in G2 and G3 were vaccinated subcutaneously (SC) with 1.2×10^5 S48 tachyzoites 4 weeks prior to experimental challenge (day 0) (see Table 1). Four weeks following vaccination (day 28) animals in G1 and G2 were orally challenged with 10^3 *T. gondii* oocysts of the M4 strain. During the experiment all animals were fed using a commercial pig feed and water was available *ad libitum*. All animal procedures complied with the Animals (Scientific Procedures) Act 1986 and were approved by the Moredun Research Institute ethics committee.

Sampling and measurements

Rectal temperatures of all pigs were monitored daily for 14 days post vaccination. At day 28 all animals were micro-chipped, iDENTICHIP® with Bio-Thermo (Animalcare Ltd., York, UK), and temperature monitored for 14 days post challenge. Blood sampling was carried out weekly from days 0 to 70 of the experiment. Blood was collected from the anterior vena cava using a 2.7 mL S-monovette serum tube with an S-monovette 20G × 1.5" safety needle (Sarstedt, Leicester, UK). Blood was left to clot overnight at 4 °C, tubes centrifuged for 10 min at 2000 *g* and serum transferred to a sterile 1.5 mL tube. Serum samples were stored at −20 °C until required. All 18 pigs were euthanised six weeks post challenge (day 70 of the experiment), by electrical stunning followed by severing of the jugular vein and exsanguination. Tissues (brain, chop, loin, left tricep, left semitedinosus, heart, masseter, tongue and diaphragm) were collected at *post mortem* for DNA extraction, pathology and mouse bioassay.

Table 1 Animal groupings for vaccination and *T. gondii* challenge

Group	Vaccination and/or challenge		Number of animals
	Day 0	Day 28	
1	n/a	1000 M4 oocysts	5
2	1.2×10^5 S48 tachyzoites	1000 M4 oocysts	5
3	1.2×10^5 S48 tachyzoites	n/a	5
4	n/a	n/a	3

Mouse bioassay

Mouse bioassay is considered the gold standard for determining the viability of *T. gondii* tissue cysts [29]. Ninety Porton mice (a minimally inbred stain), were used for the mouse bioassay. Food and water was supplied *ad libitum* and animals clinically monitored twice daily. Tissues from pigs in G1 (unvaccinated and oocyst challenged) and G2 (vaccinated and oocyst challenged pigs) were used for the mouse bioassay. Tissues were separated into three different 50 g groups, each group was based on the tissue type and divided into the following; "Brain" (50 g of brain), "Food" (a 50 g pooled sample which included 12.5 g each of chop, loin, left tricep and left semitendinosus), and "Other" (a 50 g pooled sample which included 12.5 g each of diaphragm, heart, tongue and masseter). These tissues were digested with acid/pepsin using a method previously described [30]. The tissue homogenate was centrifuged for 10 min at 1200 *g*, the supernatant was poured off gently and the final pellet was resuspended in 3 mL sterile saline (which contained 400 μg/mL penicillin and 400 units/mL streptomycin). Three mice were intraperitoneally injected with 400 μL of each inocula. An additional 400 μL of the inocula was stored at −20 °C for subsequent DNA extraction.

Tissues from pigs in G3 (vaccinated and non-challenged) and G4 (negative control group animals) were not included in the mouse bioassay.

Mice that showed either signs of infection, or which survived until the end of the six week bioassay, were euthanised by cervical dislocation. Blood samples were taken and brain tissue collected from each mouse. Half of each brain was stored separately in a sterile vial containing 1 mL PBS for DNA extraction, whist the remaining half was placed in 1 mL 10% buffered formalin for pathological examination.

Detection of *T. gondii* DNA from mouse brains following bioassay

DNA extraction followed by a *T. gondii* specific nested ITS1 PCR (n-PCR) was completed for all mice used in the bioassay ($n = 90$). DNA extraction (adapted from [31]) initially required the homogenisation of each brain sample, which was achieved by passing the material through an increasing gradient of fine gauge needles (18G, 21G and 25G needles). 900 μL of Nuclei Lysis Solution (Promega, UK). Each 400 μL of mouse brain homogenate was incubated overnight at 55 °C, then once cooled, 300 μL of Protein Precipitation Solution (Promega) was added, mixed and incubated on ice for 5 min. The mixture was then centrifuged at 13 000 *g* for 5 min and the resulting supernatant transferred to a 2 mL tube containing 900 μL of isopropanol. Each tube was mixed by inversion and incubated at −20 °C overnight. The DNA was pelleted by centrifugation at 13 000 *g* for 5 min, supernatant removed and DNA pellet washed with 600 μL 70% ethanol. To avoid contamination, a DNA extraction control was included within each batch of extractions. The DNA pellet was centrifuged a second time and any residual ethanol removed and the pellet briefly air dried, with final re-suspension in 200 μL sterile H_2O. To identify the presence of *T. gondii* DNA, a *T. gondii* specific ITS1 PCR was used, as previously described [32]. The ITS1 PCR was completed in triplicate for each mouse brain DNA sample. A positive control (*T. gondii* RH DNA) and multiple negative controls as well as the DNA extraction control were included within each PCR run.

Detection of *T. gondii* DNA from mouse bioassay inocula

DNA was extracted from a 400 μL aliquot of the acid/pepsin porcine tissue homogenate (as previously described within this paper for DNA extraction from homogenised mouse brains). The DNA generated was tested for the presence of *T. gondii* by two different molecular methods; a qPCR targeting the *T. gondii* 529 bp repeat element [10], and the *T. gondii* ITS1 n-PCR [32] which is described throughout this study. By using both of these methodologies, the molecular detection of the parasite can be compared between the different techniques. In addition, this also allows the results from the molecular detection of the parasite, using DNA from the inocula, to be compared to detection of the parasite within individual mouse brains from the bioassay (mouse bioassay vs. molecular detection from bioassay inocula).

Molecular detection of *T. gondii* DNA from pig tissues

DNA was extracted and tested for the presence of *T. gondii* from the following porcine tissues: brain, chop, loin, left tricep, left semitendinosus, diaphragm, heart, tongue and masseter. Aliquots of 1 g of each tissue for all pigs ($n = 18$) were tested individually. DNA was extracted using Precellys tubes containing ceramic beads (Peqlab, UK), followed by the *T. gondii* n-ITS1 specific PCR (used to detect *T. gondii* DNA), using the methodology previously described [31,32]. Each PCR was carried out in triplicate, with a positive control (*T. gondii* RH DNA), multiple negative controls and DNA extraction controls included within each PCR run.

Porcine *T. gondii* IgG enzyme linked immunosorbent assay (ELISA)

The porcine *T. gondii* IgG ELISA was adapted from a similar methodology described for detection of *T. gondii* IgG in sheep [33]. Flat-bottom 96 well polystyrene microtitration plates (MICROLON, 96K, F-form, medium binding, Greiner Bio-one, Germany) were coated with 0.1 mL (2.5 μg/mL) of *T. gondii* tachyzoite antigens prepared as previously described [34], diluted in 0.1 M carbonate buffer (pH 9.6) and incubated overnight at 6 °C. The plates were washed 3 times with PBS-Tween 20 (0.07 M PBS/ 0.05% Tween 20 (PBS-T)) and non-specific immune sites blocked by incubation for 1 h at 37 °C with 125 μL of PBS-1% bovine serum albumin (BSA). Control and test sera were diluted 1:100 in PBS-T-1% BSA and added to the microtitre plates in duplicate, 0.1 mL in each well, and incubated for 1 h at 37 °C. Positive and negative control sera (pool of three animals) were included in each plate. After washing, peroxidase-labeled anti-pig IgG antibody (Sigma A5670, diluted 1:10 000 in PBS-T-1% BSA) was added 0.1 mL in each well and incubated for 1 h at 37 °C. After washing, the peroxidase activity was revealed by adding 0.1 mL of substrate solution (SureBlue TMB Microwell Peroxidase Substrate, KPL, Gaithersburg, MD, USA), and the reaction was stopped by adding 0.1 mL of 2 M H_2SO_4, and the optical density (OD) was read at 450 nm in an ELISA microplate reader (MRXII, thermo Labsystems). The average OD-value for the blank controls on a plate was subtracted from the OD-values of the sera on each plate. For control of plate-to-plate variation, the same positive and negative control sera were included on every plate and a corrected OD value was calculated for each sample as described previously [35]. A serum sample was considered to be positive when OD-value of the serum sample is greater than OD mean (from negative sera obtained from all plates, $n = 64$ – negative sera from the current experiment) plus 2 standard deviation (SD from negative serum from all plates).

Quantification of histopathological lesions and imunohistochemistry labelling of porcine tissues

Methodology was carried out as described by [11]. Briefly, during histopathological examination, the numbers of glial foci and perivascular cuffs were counted for each tissue. IHC labelled slides were examined for labelled *T. gondii*-like structures (tachyzoites and tissue cysts). An animal was considered positive by IHC when positive labelling of tissue cysts or tachyzoites were found in at least one of its tissue sections.

Murine *T. gondii* IgG ELISA

The ID Screen Toxoplasmosis Indirect Multi-species ELISA kit (ID.vet, Montpellier, France) was used to detect IgG against *T. gondii* from mouse serum. The supplied manufacturer's instructions were followed and plates were read at 450 nm using the same ELISA reader as previously described. An ELISA was valid if the mean value of the positive control OD (OD_{pc}) was greater than 0.035 ($OD_{pc} > 0.035$), and if the ratio of the mean OD values for the positive and negative controls (OD_{pc} and OD_{nc}), were greater than 3.5 ($OD_{pc}/OD_{nc} > 3.5$).

The interpretation of the result was classed as percent seropositivity (SP). A sample with an SP value of 50% or higher was positive, a negative result was an SP of 40% or less, and the result classed as doubtful if the SP was between 40% - 50%.

Statistical analysis

To account for the increased variability with the mean, the weekly data on OD-value obtained from ELISA of serum samples of pigs post-vaccination were transformed using square root transformation. A repeated measures model was fitted to the transformed data incorporating treatment group, time (week post-vaccination as a categorical variable) and interaction between treatment group and time as fixed effects. The model considered a first-order autoregressive correlation structure between observations for each pig. The data on weekly rectal temperature of pigs were also analysed using a similar repeated measures model. Possible biologically interesting comparisons of differences in mean values between treatment groups were obtained using two-sided probabilities for each comparison. These probabilities were then adjusted using a False Discovery Rate (FDR) approach [36] to take into account the multiple comparisons of means so that the overall FDR was less than 5%. All *p*-values in this paper refer to FDR-adjusted probabilities unless they are specified to be global *p*-values.

For the mouse bioassay, all 45 mice, that received tissues (15 mice each fed with brain, food and other tissues) from the pigs of the G2 group (vaccinated and oocyst challenged), survived until the end of the experiment (day 42), and therefore, all data in this group were censored. A total of 22 mice, inoculated with tissues from the pigs of the G1 group (unvaccinated and oocyst challenged), died at different intervals. A Kaplan-Meir survival curve was plotted to present the mean survival proportions of mice between the two groups and the equality between two survival curves was tested using G-rho family of test [37]. Similarly, the equality of survival distributions between a pair of tissues within G1 group was also tested considering pig as a stratum variable. To account for multiple comparisons, these probabilities were then adjusted using a False Discovery Rate (FDR) approach as discussed earlier.

To test the agreement of each of the two molecular tests used for detection of parasite DNA from bioassay inocula (*T. gondii* 529 bp qPCR and conventional PCR incorporating the *T. gondii* specific ITS1 region) with gold standard test (the detection of *T. gondii* DNA directly from mouse brains following bioassay), the data on discordant cells were tested using an exact test of a null hypothesis about the equal probability of success ($p = 0.5$) in a Bernoulli distribution. Additionally, the data from the contingency table were used to estimate the sensitivity and specificity of both molecular tests and corresponding exact binomial confidence intervals.

All statistical analyses were carried out using R software version 3.0.1 with appropriate R packages (stats, nlme, multcomp, survival, ggplot) [38].

Results

Clinical observations in pigs

Rectal temperatures of all animals were recorded from days –5 to 14 of the experiment. Estimates of mean rectal temperature and 95% confidence intervals for four treatment groups along with observed temperature on each individual pig at each day post-vaccination (until day 14) are presented in Figure 1, although this can be noted in absence of oocyst challenge (which occurred on day 28), G1 & G4 and G2 & G3 are identical. Due to the increasing size of the animals, the technique used for recording the temperature from days 28 – 42 (daily for 14 days following oocyst challenge) was an implanted Thermochip®. However, this technique did provide accurate recording of the rectal temperature, probably due to the location of the chip. Temperatures fluctuated greatly resulting in vast variations of temperature readings. These readings were not reliable or informative, and therefore, were not used for further statistical analysis. On day 7 post-challenge (i.e. on day 35 of the experiment), all five animals in G2 appeared subdued/depressed for approximately 24 h, although they remained interested in food and movement was unaffected. All other animals remained clinically normal throughout the experiment.

Molecular detection of *T. gondii* from individual pig tissues

DNA extracted from individual tissues (brain, chop, loin, left tricep, left semitendinosus, diaphragm, heart, tongue and masseter) from all pigs in G1, G2, G3 and G4 was tested for the presence of *T. gondii* DNA using the ITS1 n-PCR. Parasite DNA was not detected from any of these tissues, despite each DNA sample being tested in triplicate.

Porcine *T. gondii* IgG ELISA

Estimates of the mean transformed OD values (square root transformation) and corresponding 95% confidence

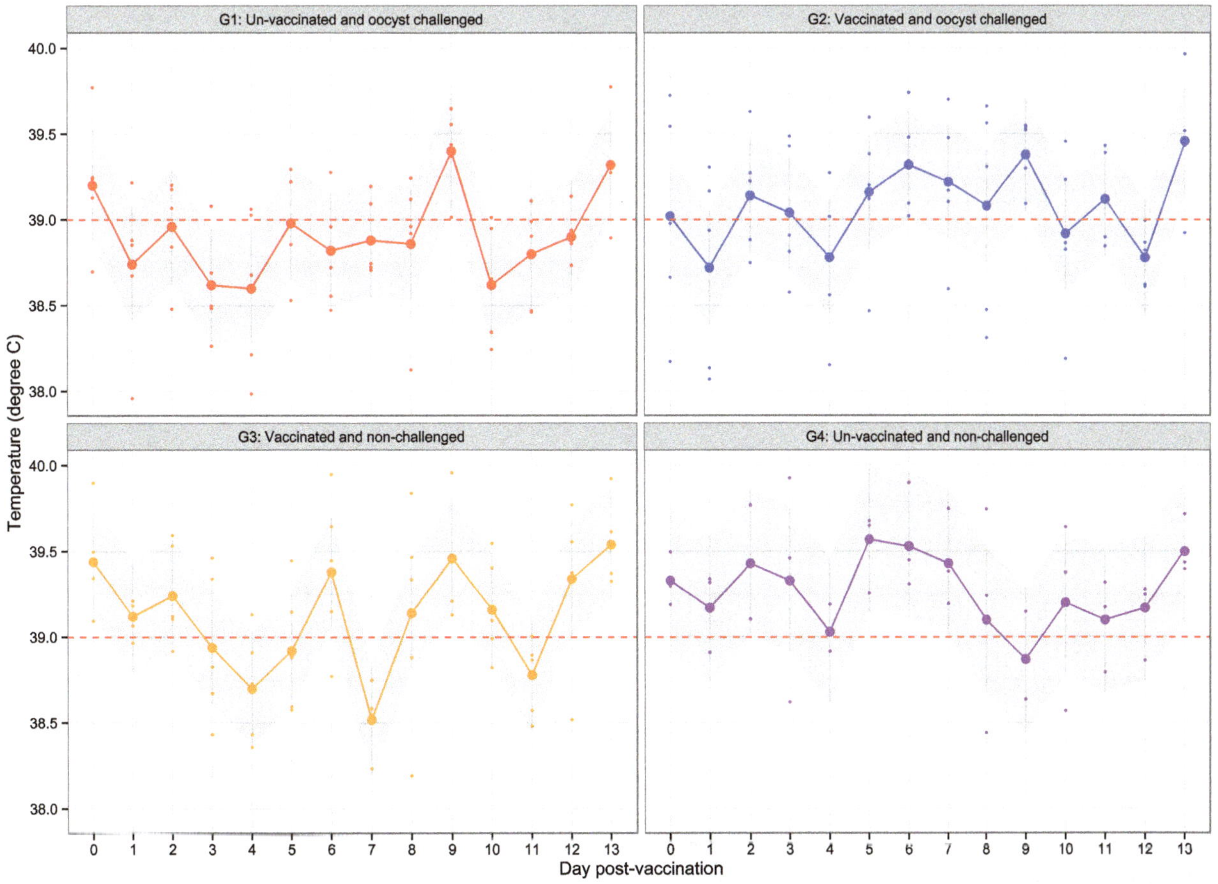

Figure 1 Average porcine temperature per experimental group following vaccination with S48 tachyzoites. Rectal temperatures of each pig was recorded daily prior to challenge. Between days 0 – 14 post vaccination, treatment groups G1 and G4, and G2 and G3 are identical. The red cut off line indicates the normal rectal temperature for pigs. G1 = Oocyst (M4) challenged pigs, G2 = Vaccinated (S48) and oocyst (M4) challenged pigs, G3 = Vaccinated (S48) pigs, G4 = Negative control pigs.

intervals for four treatment groups along with observed OD values on each individual pig at each week post-vaccination are presented in Figure 2. Briefly, all pigs tested negative by ELISA for *T. gondii* IgG at the beginning of the experiment (day 0 post-vaccination), however, by day 42 post-vaccination (or 2 weeks after challenge with *T. gondii* oocysts for G1 and G2), most of the pigs (apart from the pigs in G4 – negative control animals) were *T. gondii* IgG positive (OD-value greater or equal to 0.34, or equivalently, square root of OD-value greater or equal to 0.58; see Figure 2). The interaction effect of treatment group and time had a statistically significant (global $p < 0.001$) effect on the mean OD. The results showed that the mean OD value of pigs from G2 (pigs which were vaccinated with S48 and then challenged four weeks later with 10^3 M4 *T. gondii* oocysts) were statistically significantly higher compared with G3 animals (pigs which were vaccinated and not challenged) at day 49 ($p = 0.019$), 63 ($p < 0.001$) and 70 ($p = 0.017$) post-vaccination (Figure 2). Mean OD values were higher in magnitude for the G2 group compared with G3 on day 42 and 70, but the mean differences were not statistically significant ($p > 0.05$). The negative control animals (G4) remained seronegative throughout the experiment as OD values were below the threshold during the entire experimental period (see Figure 2).

Quantification of histopathological lesions and immunohistochemistry labelling of porcine tissues

Histological examination of the brain from the infected pigs showed mild non purulent perivascular infiltration, randomly distributed, in four animals from G1 and one animal from G2, mainly formed by CD3 positive lymphocytes. Besides these lesions, mild, focal, non-specific infiltration of few mononuclear inflammatory cells, mainly lymphocytes in the lungs and the different muscles studied were found in the all the animals studied. No differences were found between the studied groups regarding these non specific changes. Immunohistochemical labelling showed few intracellular *T. gondii*

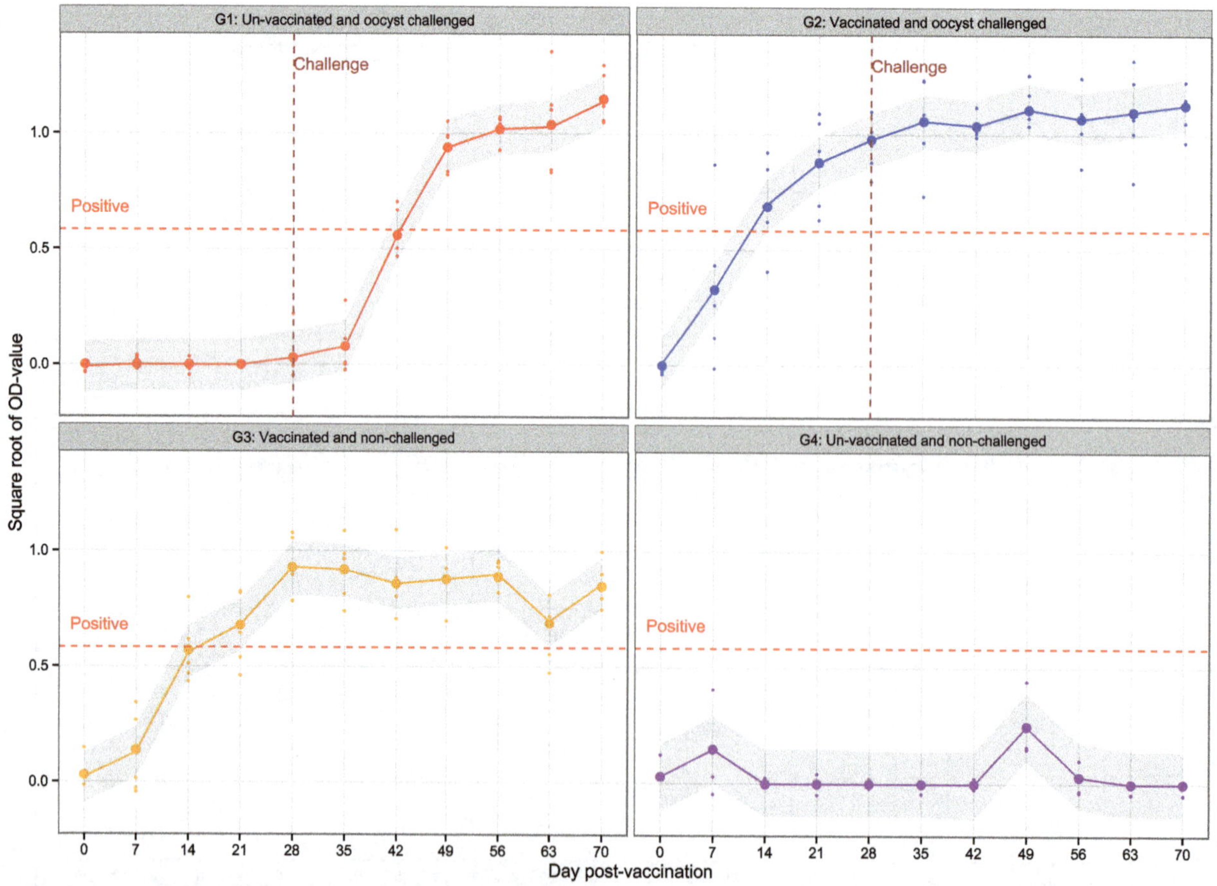

Figure 2 *T. gondii* IgG ELISA. *T. gondii* IgG ELISA results for all pigs from week 0 to 70 post vaccination. Plots show observed ELISA value of each pig (small dots), estimated mean ELISA value of each group (large solid dots joined by solid line) and corresponding 95% confidence intervals (shaded region). The vertical dashed line indicates the point at which pigs were challenged with 1000 M4 *T. gondii* oocysts. The horizontal dashed line indicates when animals were classed as seropositive for *T. gondii*.G1 = Oocyst (M4) challenged pigs, G2 = Vaccinated (S48) and oocyst (M4) challenged pigs, G3 = Vaccinated (S48) pigs, G4 = Negative control pigs.

tachyzoites-like structures in the jejunal lymph node from one animal from G1 and in the retromandibular lymph node of another animal from G2.

Mouse bioassay

During the 6 week mouse bioassay 75.6% (68/90) of mice survived until the end of the experiment. Twenty two of 90 mice (24.4%) had to be euthanised due to the manifestations of clinical signs of *T. gondii* infection (ruffled coat, reluctance to move). All of these mice had received tissues from G1 pigs (unvaccinated and challenged with M4 *T. gondii* oocysts). From G1 mice, four animals were euthanised on day 11 of the experiment, and a further18 mice were euthanised on day 12, which left a total of 51.1% (23/45) of mice surviving until the end of the experiment (day 42) (see Figure 3A). In contrast, all mice, which received tissues from G2 pigs (vaccinated with S48 and challenged with M4 *T. gondii* oocysts), survived to the end of the experiment, resulting in 100% (45/45) survival of mice (Figure 3A). It was therefore not surprising that the independent two-sample log-rank test of the censored survival data until day 42 of the experiment showed strong evidence ($p < 0.001$), that mice which received porcine tissues from G2 pigs had a higher probability of survival across the entire range of the experimental period compared with mice which received G1 porcine tissues.

For mice that received tissues from G1 pigs, there was evidence that the mean proportion of mice that survived, differed between the porcine tissues (brain, food and other) that they were inoculated with (Figure 3B). Among them, 40% (6/15), 26.7% (4/15) and 86.7% (13/15) of mice survived when they were inoculated with "brain", "other" and "food" tissues, respectively. Mice that received "food" tissues had a statistically significantly higher chance of surviving during the entire study period compared with mice that received "brain" ($p = 0.018$) and "other" ($p < 0.001$) tissues. The probability of survival between the mice that received "brain" and "other" tissues did not differ significantly ($p = 0.340$).

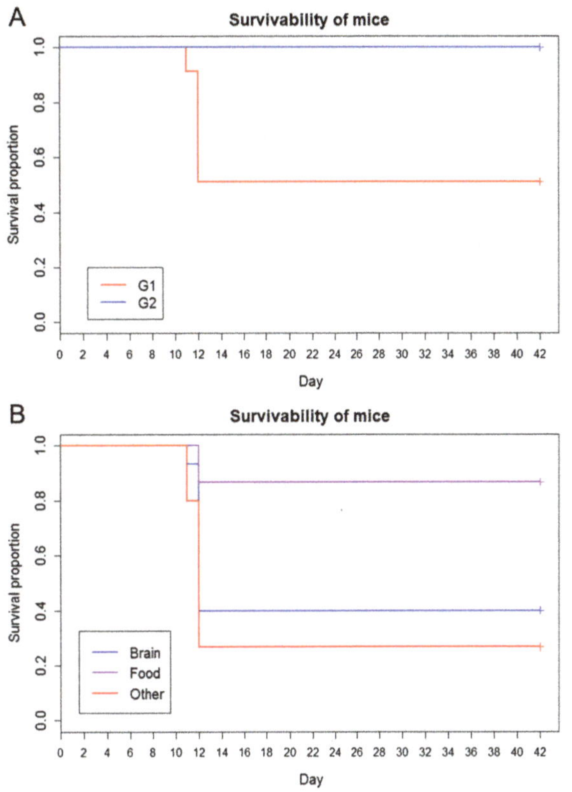

Figure 3 Kaplan-Meir survival curves. Kaplan-Meir survival curve in relation to vaccination highlighting proportion of mice that survived when fed tissues from G1 and G2 pigs **(A)**. All mice which received tissues from vaccinated and challenged pigs (G2) survived (blue line) until the end of the bioassay (day 42). Only 51.1% of mice which received tissues from unvaccinated and challenged pigs (G1) survived until the end of the bioassay (day 42). G1 = Mice inoculated with porcine tissues from pigs which were vaccinated (S48) and oocyst (M4) challenged. G2 = Mice which were inoculated with porcine tissues from pigs which were oocyst (M4) challenge. Kaplan-Meir survival curve from mice fed different tissues from pigs in G1 highlighting proportion of mice that survived when fed different tissue types (brain, food and other) **(B)**. Brain = brain tissue, Food = pooled sample of chop, loin, left tricep and left semitendinosus, Other = pooled sample of diaphragm, heart, tongue and masseter.

Detection of *T. gondii* DNA from mouse brains following bioassay

Brains from the 22 mice which were euthanised prior to the end of the six week mouse bioassay (all fed with G1 pig tissues – as shown in Figure 4), were positive by ITS1 n-PCR and *T. gondii* DNA was detected within the brains of all 22 mice. When DNA was extracted from the brains of the remaining 66 mice (which did not show any signs of *T. gondii* infection and were euthanised on day 42 of the bioassay), an additional two mice, which had been inoculated with brain tissue from G1 pigs, were identified as ITS1 positive. Therefore, *T. gondii* DNA was detected in 53.3% (24/45) of mouse brains which had been inoculated with tissues from G1 pigs (see Table 2). In contrast, 100% (45/45) of mice, which had been inoculated with tissues from G2 pigs, tested negative for *T. gondii* by ITS1 PCR (see Table 2).

Detection of *T. gondii* DNA from bioassay inocula

Homogenised and acid/pepsin digested pig tissues used as inocula to challenge the mice were tested for the presence of *T. gondii* DNA. All inocula ($n = 30$) were tested ("food", "brain" and "other" per pig, giving 15 inocula per experimental group), using both the *T. gondii* ITS1 PCR and the *T. gondii* 529 bp qPCR. *T. gondii* DNA could not be detected in any of the inocula (0/15) generated from G2 pigs by either of conventional *T.*

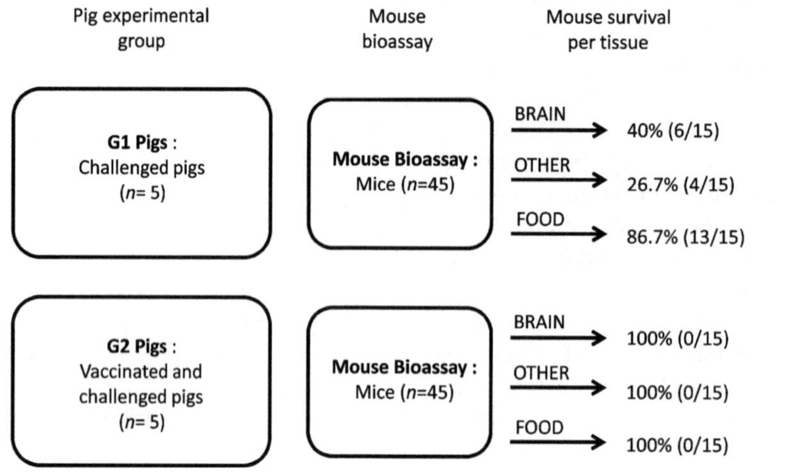

Figure 4 Mouse survival rate related to specific porcine tissues (experimental groups G1 and G2). All mice which received homogenised tissue from G2 pigs survived. Not all mice which received porcine tissues from G1 pigs survived, with only 40% of mice which received brain tissue surviving, followed by 26.7% which received food and 86.7% receiving other.

gondii ITS1 n-PCR, or 529 bp qPCR (Table 3). The results from the ITS1 n-PCR showed that 7/15 (46.7%) of inocula comprised of tissues from pigs in G1 were positive for *T. gondii* DNA (Table 4). Of the seven positives, four were from the inocula containing "brain" tissue, two from the inocula comprised of the "other" tissues and one from the inocula comprised of the "food" tissues (Table 4). However, among inocula generated with tissues from G1 pigs, detection of *T. gondii* DNA using the qPCR was slightly lower compared with detection using the ITS1 n-PCR, with 6/15 (40.0%) of inocula testing positive by qPCR (compared to 7/15 (46.7%) by ITS1 PCR) (see Table 4). Inocula, which were used for bioassay in mice, with subsequent detection of *T. gondii* DNA directly from mouse brain, detects the greatest number of *T. gondii* positive tissue samples, resulting in 9/15 (60%) of pig tissue inocula testing positive. Four of these positives were detected in inocula comprised of "brain", four from "other" and one from "food" tissues. Considering the data on bioassay results, there was however no evidence that mean proportions of detectable infected and non-infected samples differed between tissues (global $p = 0.201$).

Comparison of molecular detection methods for detection of *T. gondii* DNA using bioassay inocula

Two molecular tests (*T. gondii* 529 bp qPCR and the *T. gondii* specific n-ITS1 PCR) were compared for their detection of parasite DNA from bioassay inocula using a gold standard test. The detection of *T. gondii* DNA directly from mouse brains following bioassay was considered as the "gold standard" as parasite DNA was detected in 9 out of 15 samples (60%) (see Table 4). The qPCR detected 6 out of 15 samples (40%), compared with 7 out of 15 samples (46.7%) by ITS1-PCR. Results showed that both qPCR ($p = 0.250$) and ITS1-PCR ($p = 0.500$) are in agreement with the gold standard test. However, the estimate of sensitivity of the ITS1 PCR (0.78 with 95% confidence interval: 0.40, 0.97) was higher compared with the 529pb qPCR (0.67 with 95% confidence interval: 0.30, 0.93). The estimates of specificity and 95% confidence interval for both tests were identical for both methods (1.00; 0.77, 1.00).

Mouse serology and pathology

Serum samples from all mice ($n = 90$) were collected at *post mortem* and tested for the presence *T. gondii* IgG

Table 2 Summary of *T. gondii* DNA detected by ITS1 PCR in mouse brains following bioassay with porcine tissues

Mouse Group	ITS1 positive mice (n)	% ITS1 positive	ITS1 negative mice (n)	% ITS1 negative
1	24[a]	53.3	21	46.7
2	0	0	45	100
TOTAL	24	26.7	66	73.3

[a] = including two mice which survived until the end of the end of the experiment (42 dpi).
1 = mice inoculated with porcine tissues from oocyst challenged pigs.
2 = mice inoculated with porcine tissues from vaccinated and oocyst challenged pigs.

Table 3 Detection of *T. gondii* DNA from bioassay inocula (homogenised tissues) compared to detection of *T. gondii* DNA from mouse brain (bioassay) from vaccinated and oocyst challenged pigs (G2)

Pig No.	Brain			Other			Food		
	qPCR	ITS1	Bio	qPCR	ITS1	Bio	qPCR	ITS1	Bio
820	–	–	–	–	–	–	–	–	–
821	–	–	–	–	–	–	–	–	–
822	–	–	–	–	–	–	–	–	–
823	–	–	–	–	–	–	–	–	–
824	–	–	–	–	–	–	–	–	–
Positives	0/5	0/5	0/5	0/5	0/5	0/5	0/5	0/5	0/5

Results from the 529 bp *T. gondii* qPCR (qPCR), conventional *T. gondii* ITS1 PCR (ITS1) and ITS1 PCR from mouse brain - bioassay result (Bio), from vaccinated and oocyst challenged pigs (G2).

antibodies using the commercially available ID vet ELISA. The majority of mice (98.9%, 89/90) tested seronegative (with seropositivity (SP) ≤ 3%), which included all 22 mice euthanised due to signs of *T. gondii* infection. One mouse (C11-1), which was inoculated with brain tissue from a pig G1 pig, tested positive by ITS1 PCR and survived until the end of the experiment (day 42), was classified as seronegative (23% SP). However, the percentage seropositivity of this mouse was much higher than that of the remaining 89 seronegative mice. Only one mouse (C11-2), which was also inoculated with brain tissue from a pig in G1, tested positive for *T. gondii* IgG (189% SP, this mouse was euthanised at the end of the experiment (day 42) and tested positive by ITS1 PCR.

The pathological results completed on half of each mouse brain ($n = 90$) could not identify any differences between mice inoculated with different porcine tissues (brain, food and other), with the exception of three animals, where tissue cysts were observed (C11-2, C14-3 and C18-2), which had been inoculated with tissues from pigs in G1.

Table 4 Detection of *T. gondii* DNA from bioassay inocula (homogenised tissues) compared to detection of *T. gondii* DNA from mouse brain (bioassay) from oocyst challenged pigs (G1)

Pig No.	Brain			Other			Food		
	qPCR	ITS1	Bio	qPCR	ITS1	Bio	qPCR	ITS1	Bio
825	+	+	+	–	–	–	–	–	–
826	+	+	+	+	–	+	–	–	–
827	+	+	+	–	–	+	–	–	–
828	+	+	+	–	+	+	–	–	–
829	–	–	–	–	+	+	+	+	+
Positives	4/5	4/5	4/5	1/5	2/5	4/5	1/5	1/5	1/5

Results from the 529 bp *T. gondii* qPCR (qPCR), conventional *T. gondii* ITS1 PCR (ITS1) and ITS1 PCR from mouse brain - bioassay result (Bio), from oocyst challenged pigs (G1).

Discussion

The results from this work clearly show that vaccination with a live attenuated strain of the parasite (S48) and subsequent challenge with *T. gondii* oocysts (M4) in pigs is successful in significantly reducing infective tissue cysts from establishing within porcine tissues, as shown by the mouse bioassay. Mouse survival rates from the bioassay at day 42 pi show a clear difference between those mice inoculated with tissues from pigs in G1 (unvaccinated and oocyst challenged pigs), compared with mice inoculated with tissues from pigs in G2 (vaccinated and oocyst challenged pigs) (Figure 3A). In our experience, infection with the M4 strain (type II) of *T. gondii* is likely to cause clinical signs in Porton mice, where viable tissue cysts present in the inocula (homogenised porcine tissue), generally results in severe clinical signs in mice and euthanasia is required. Therefore, in this study, reporting of mouse survival was important as it was a good indicator of the presence or absence of viable tissue cysts. It has previously been reported that as little as one tissue cyst (containing possibly thousands of infective bradyzoites) is enough to cause infection [39]. Other research, which has studied the vaccination of pigs to reduce tissue cyst burden, has mainly focused on microscopic identification of tissue cysts and/or detection of parasite DNA from mice used in the bioassay [21,23-25,35,40,41]. In these studies there is no detailed information about mouse survival and clinical signs of *T. gondii* during the bioassay itself. In fact, very few *T. gondii* studies, which incorporate mouse bioassays to assess the viability of tissue cysts, describe mouse survival rates in any detail. However, this might also be related to the strain of mouse used, as Swiss Webster mice (although susceptible to *T. gondii*) are generally thought to be more resistant to the parasite and are less likely to show clinical signs of infection. Research by Pena et al. [42], have reported mouse mortality rates following bioassay of cat tissues in relation to the genotype of *T. gondii* present. Our current research describes mouse survival rates using a Kaplan-Meir survival curve. Mouse survival provides an indication of the viability of *T. gondii* tissue cysts, however, this data is lacking in the majority of studies which incorporate mouse bioassay.

In addition to mouse survival rates, *T. gondii* DNA was not detected in any mice (0/45) following challenge with inocula comprised of porcine tissues from G2 pigs (vaccinated and oocysts challenged pigs) (Table 3), whilst parasite DNA was detected in 53.3% (24/45) of mice following challenge with inocula from G1 pigs (non-vaccinated oocyst challenged) (Table 4). Other research, investigating vaccination and *T. gondii* challenge of pigs and subsequent mouse bioassay, have focused only on the microscopic detection of tissues cysts from mouse brain following bioassay [18,21,25,41], rather than detection of

T. gondii DNA from the mouse brain. Therefore, as the pathology results from the current research provide limited information, it is difficult to draw direct comparisons between these vaccination and challenge experiments and the current research. However, as 100% of mice from the bioassay survived following inoculation with tissues from pigs vaccinated and oocyst challenge, vaccination with S48 tachyzoites appears to be a very promising approach for reducing parasite burden in porcine tissues. Previous research into vaccination of pigs against *T. gondii*, which have incorporated mouse bioassay, have not shown such a protective response against tissue cyst formation in mouse brains. For example, following immunisation of pigs with crude *T. gondii* rhoptry proteins with Quil-A as an adjuvant, da Cunha et al. [41] found only partial protection from formation of tissue cysts in mouse brains following bioassay with porcine tissues, with the parasite detected in 5/11 (45.4%) mice in the vaccinated and challenged group. In a similar experiment, partial protection was observed by Garcia et al. [21], who used *T. gondii* rhoptry proteins and immunostimulating complexes (ISCOMS) as an adjuvant to vaccinate pigs. Dubey et al. [25] tested a vaccine incorporating a low dose of irradiated *T. gondii* oocysts, and although fewer tissue cysts were observed in mice, cysts were detected in 45/110 (40.9%) of mice which had received porcine tissues from vaccinated pigs. In other work by Dubey et al. [18] using tachyzoites of a non-persistent strain of *T. gondii* (RH) to vaccinate pigs, only partial protection was described, with fewer tissues cysts in mice inoculated with porcine tissues. Similar results were also reported using the *T. gondii* TS-4 mutant to vaccinate pigs [43,44], where the vaccine alone did not persist, however only partial protection was observed following challenge with GT-1 oocysts. In summary, apart for the research described within this manuscript, none of the literature currently available can describe 100% protection against tissue cyst formation in mice, following bioassay of porcine tissues.

From the current results, it appears that vaccination with S48 alone does not induce tissue cyst formation in porcine tissues, as results from the mouse bioassay, which included inocula with porcine tissues from the vaccinated and challenged animals, were all PCR negative for *T. gondii*. If a positive had been obtained from this group, the experiment had been designed to verify whether infection was due to vaccination (S48) or oocyst challenge (M4), as previously shown in lambs [11] (both S48 and M4 are different *T. gondii* genotypes; S48 = type I, M4 = type II). However, a bioassay using porcine tissues from animals that were vaccinated alone (which was not included in this study), could further support this result.

The results also show that there were differences in survival rates within groups of mice which were inoculated using tissues from G1 pigs, depending on which type of tissue they had been inoculated with (Figure 4). A greater proportion of mice survived which had received porcine inocula from the "food" tissue group (chop, loin, left triceps and left semitendinosus), compared with mice which had received tissues from the "brain" and "other" tissue groups (diaphragm, heart, tongue and masseter). This suggests that there are a greater number of viable parasites within tissues from the "brain" and "other" groups in comparison to tissues that are used routinely for human consumption ("food"). To further confirm this result, *T. gondii* DNA was detected in the brains of all mice which were euthanised due to clinical signs of *T. gondii* infection, with parasite DNA being detected in fewer bioassay mice which had received porcine tissues from the "food" group using tissues from G1 pigs (oocysts challenged pigs), compared with mice which received brain or tissues from the "other" group (Table 4).

In addition, two mice (C11-1 and C11-2), which had been inoculated with tissues from G1 pigs that survived until the end of the experiment (day 42) but also tested positive for *T. gondii* by detection of parasite DNA in their brains. Accordingly, they were the only two mice which gave a seropositivity of greater than 3% with the *T. gondii* IgG ELISA. It is likely that mice, which were euthanised within the first 14 days of the bioassay, which also tested positive for the presence of *T. gondii* DNA in their brains, may only just have started to mount a humoral immune response against the parasite, however, the levels of IgG present were possibly too low to be detected by the ELISA.

Although the *T. gondii* specific ITS1 PCR was carried out using DNA from individual porcine tissues (brain, chop, loin, left tricep, left semitendinosus, diaphragm, heart, tongue and masseter), parasite DNA could not be detected from any tissues. When comparing this result with a similar study carried out in lambs [11], where *T. gondii* DNA was detected from individual tissues by ITS1 PCR, it is likely that the challenge dose of 1000 oocysts may be too low to be detected by this method. Although 1000 M4 oocysts is more likely to reflect that of a natural infection, it appears that a higher challenge dose (500 000 M4 oocysts as used by [11]), may result in a greater chance of detecting parasite DNA directly from the hosts tissue, without the need for mouse bioassay or detection of parasite DNA from bioassay inocula. In addition, direct detection of parasite DNA from porcine tissues used only 1 g of starting material, compared with 50 g of tissue which was prepared for mouse bioassay, therefore, due to the inhomogeneous distribution of parasite tissue cysts there was less chance of detecting the parasite from a smaller 1 g sample. In the current study, detection of parasite DNA from bioassay inocula was tested by two different molecular techniques; the

529 bp *T. gondii* qPCR and the *T. gondii* ITS1 PCR, to determine which test was more sensitive and whether either technique was as sensitive as mouse bioassay (the "gold standard" assay for detection of viable tissue cysts). Although detection of parasite DNA from mouse brains, following bioassay by ITS1 PCR, detected the greatest number of positive samples there was no evidence of a difference between two molecular tests. However, the sensitivity of the ITS1 PCR was slightly higher than the 529 bp qPCR (0.78 and 0.67 respectively). It should also be noted that although these two molecular techniques successfully detect parasite DNA, it is still currently only the mouse bioassay which has the ability to detect viable tissue cysts, and their potential to infect another host. However, perhaps future methodology could employ both molecular detection of the parasite from bioassay inocula in conjunction with mouse bioassay, with a view to reducing the number of mice used within the bioassay, such as magnetic capture qPCR (MC-qPCR) of *T. gondii* DNA as described by [10]. Histological examination of porcine samples was of limited use to detect the parasite in the porcine tissue or to show differences between the groups of infected mice. However, it showed how vaccination protected against the occurrence of lesions in the brain (perivascular foci) after infection. Immmunohistochemical labelling was also ineffective when trying to localize the parasite, as only in two animals tachyzoites-like structures were detected. These results from pathological studies suggest that these techniques are not adequate when studying parasite distribution in studies where no (porcine experiment) or very similar (murine bioassay) lesions are originated.

Overall, in terms of vaccination to reduce viable tissue cysts in meat, these results are promising, as this is the first description of 100% protection against tissue cyst formation in mice following mouse bioassay of tissues from pigs. The results also provide an answer to the question raised by the Food Standards Agency, in a recent report published by the Advisory Committee on the Microbiological Safety of Food (ACMSF), the document states that one of the knowledge gaps relevant to a risk assessment in the UK is: "*vaccines based on live attenuated strains of tachyzoites are effective in reducing morbidity in sheep but it is not known whether vaccination has any effect on the formation of tissue cysts*" [26]. From the current research it is now clear that S48 does have a significant effect in reducing the formation of tissue cysts in pigs. Vaccination of other "high risk" livestock species should be addressed and it has recently been demonstrated that vaccination of sheep with S48 also results in a reduction in the number of ovine tissue samples in which parasite DNA can be detected [11].

Competing interests
The authors declare that they have no competing interests.

Authors' contributions
FK, EAI, AB, JLG conceived and designed the experiment; AB and FK conducted the experiment; AB, FK, GC, PMB, JB, FC, JL and JT completed pig *post mortem* examinations, mouse bioassays, serology and molecular analysis; FK, AB and MN carried out statistical analysis and contributed to the interpretation of data; AB, FK, MN wrote the paper and provided important intellectual content; all authors read and approved the final version.

Acknowledgements
This project was partially funded by a transnational access project funded through the European Union Seventh Framework Network of Animal Disease Infectiology Research Facilities (NADIR; reference number FP7-228394). AB was funded by the Moredun Foundation. FK, PMB, MN, JT, FC, EAI were supported by the Scottish Government, Rural and Environmental Sciences and Analytical Services (RESAS). JB was supported by CSIC and financed in part by European Social Fund (ESF). JLG was financed by Coordenação de Aperfeiçoamento de Pessoal de Nível Superior (CAPES, BEX 10259-/12-0), Brazil and GC by the Instituto Nacional de Tecnologia Agropecuaria (INATA), Argentina.

Author details
[1]Moredun Research Institute, Pentlands Science Park, Bush Loan, Midlothian EH26 0PZ, Scotland, UK. [2]Instituto de Ganadería de Montaña (CSIC-ULE), León, Spain. [3]Instituto Nacional de Tecnología Agropecuaria (INATA), EEA Balcarce, Argentina. [4]Departamento de Medicina Veterinária Preventiva, Universidade Estadual de Londrina, Londrina, Brazil. [5]Biomathematics & Statistics Scotland, The King's Buildings, Edinburgh EH9 3JZ, Scotland, UK.

References

1. Kijlstra A, Meerburg B, Cornelissen J, De Craeye S, Vereijken P, Jongert E (2008) The role of rodents and shrews in the transmission of *Toxoplasma gondii* to pigs. Vet Parasitol 156:183–190
2. Esteban-Redondo I, Maley SW, Thomson K, Nicoll S, Wright S, Buxton D, Innes EA (1999) Detection of *T. gondii* in tissues of sheep and cattle following oral infection. Vet Parasitol 86:155–171
3. Garcia JL, Innes EA, Katzer F (2014) Current progress toward vaccines against *Toxoplasma gondii*. Vaccine (Auckl) 4:23–37
4. Tenter AM, Heckeroth AR, Weiss LM (2000) *Toxoplasma gondii*: from animals to humans. Int J Parasitol 30:1217–1258
5. Swierzy IJ, Muhammad M, Kroll J, Abelmann A, Tenter AM, Luder CG (2014) *Toxoplasma gondii* within skeletal muscle cells: a critical interplay for food-borne parasite transmission. Int J Parasitol 44:91–98
6. Dubey JP (1988) Long-term persistence of *Toxoplasma gondii* in tissues of pigs inoculated with T gondii oocysts and effect of freezing on viability of tissue cysts in pork. Am J Vet Res 49:910–913
7. Kijlstra A, Jongert E (2009) Toxoplasma-safe meat: close to reality? Trends Parasitol 25:18–22
8. Dubey JP, Murrell KD, Fayer R, Schad GA (1986) Distribution of *Toxoplasma gondii* tissue cysts in commercial cuts of pork. J Am Vet Med Assoc 188:1035–1037
9. Aspinall TV, Marlee D, Hyde JE, Sims PFG (2002) Prevalence of *Toxoplasma gondii* in commercial meat products as monitored by polymerase chain reaction - food for thought? Int J Parasitol 32:1193–1199
10. Opsteegh M, Langelaar M, Sprong H, den Hartog L, De Craeye S, Bokken G, Ajzenberg D, Kijlstra A, van der Giessen J (2010) Direct detection and genotyping of *Toxoplasma gondii* in meat samples using magnetic capture and PCR. Int J Food Microbiol 139:193–201
11. Katzer F, Canton G, Burrells A, Palarea-Albaladejo J, Horton B, Bartley PM, Pang Y, Chianini F, Innes EA, Benavides J (2014) Immunization of lambs with the S48 strain of *Toxoplasma gondii* reduces tissue cyst burden following oral challenge with a complete strain of the parasite. Vet Parasitol 205:46–56
12. Cook AJ, Gilbert RE, Buffolano W, Zufferey J, Petersen E, Jenum PA, Foulon W, Semprini AE, Dunn DT (2000) Sources of toxoplasma infection in pregnant women: European multicentre case-control study. European Research Network on Congenital Toxoplasmosis. BMJ 321:142–147

13. Dubey JP (2008) The history of Toxoplasma gondii–the first 100 years. J Eukaryot Microbiol 55:467–475
14. Kijlstra A, Eissen OA, Cornelissen J, Munniksma K, Eijck I, Kortbeek T (2004) *Toxoplasma gondii* infection in animal-friendly pig production systems. Invest Ophthalmol Vis Sci 45:3165–3169
15. van der Giessen J, Fonville M, Bouwknegt M, Langelaar M, Vollema A (2007) Seroprevalence of Trichinella spiralis and *Toxoplasma gondii* in pigs from different housing systems in The Netherlands. Vet Parasitol 148:371–374
16. Lehmann T, Graham DH, Dahl E, Sreekumar C, Launer F, Corn JL, Gamble HR, Dubey JP (2003) Transmission dynamics of *Toxoplasma gondii* on a pig farm. Infect Genet Evol 3:135–141
17. Hill DE, Haley C, Wagner B, Gamble HR, Dubey JP (2010) Seroprevalence of and risk factors for *Toxoplasma gondii* in the US swine herd using sera collected during the National Animal Health Monitoring Survey (Swine 2006). Zoonoses Public Health 57:53–59
18. Dubey JP, Urban JF, Jr, Davis SW (1991) Protective immunity to toxoplasmosis in pigs vaccinated with a nonpersistent strain of *Toxoplasma gondii*. Am J Vet Res 52:1316–1319
19. Djurković-Djaković O, Bobić B, Nikolić A, Klun I, Dupouy-Camet J (2013) Pork as a source of human parasitic infection. Clin Microbiol Infect 19:586–594
20. Innes EA, Bartley PM, Rocchi M, Benavidas-Silvan J, Burrells A, Hotchkiss E, Chianini F, Canton G, Katzer F (2011) Developing vaccines to control protozoan parasites in ruminants: dead or alive? Vet Parasitol 180:155–163
21. Garcia JL, Gennari SM, Navarro IT, Machado RZ, Sinhorini IL, Freire RL, Marana ER, Tsutsui V, Contente AP, Begale LP (2005) Partial protection against tissue cysts formation in pigs vaccinated with crude rhoptry proteins of *Toxoplasma gondii*. Vet Parasitol 129:209–217
22. Jongert E, Melkebeek V, De Craeye S, Dewit J, Verhelst D, Cox E (2008) An enhanced GRA1-GRA7 cocktail DNA vaccine primes anti-Toxoplasma immune responses in pigs. Vaccine 26:1025–1031
23. Kringel H, Dubey JP, Beshah E, Hecker R, Urban JF, Jr (2004) CpG-oligodeoxynucleotides enhance porcine immunity to *Toxoplasma gondii*. Vet Parasitol 123:55–66
24. Dubey JP, Baker DG, Davis SW, Urban JF, Jr, Shen SK (1994) Persistence of immunity to toxoplasmosis in pigs vaccinated with a nonpersistent strain of *Toxoplasma gondii*. Am J Vet Res 55:982–987
25. Dubey JP, Lunney JK, Shen SK, Kwok OC (1998) Immunity to toxoplasmosis in pigs fed irradiated *Toxoplasma gondii* oocysts. J Parasitol 84:749–752
26. AMCSF (2012) *Ad Hoc* Group on Vulnerable Groups: Risk profile in relation to toxoplasma in the food chain. Advisory Committee on the Microbiological Safety of Food. http://www.food.gov.uk/sites/default/files/multimedia/pdfs/committee/acmsfrtaxopasm.pdf
27. Buxton D, Innes EA (1995) A commercial vaccine for ovine toxoplasmosis. Parasitology 110:S11–S16
28. Innes EA, Bartley PM, Maley S, Katzer F, Buxton D (2009) Veterinary vaccines against *Toxoplasma gondii*. Mem Inst Oswaldo Cruz 104:246–251
29. Jacobs L, Remington JS, Melton ML (1960) A survey of meat samples from swine, cattle, and sheep for the presence of encysted Toxoplasma. J Parasitol 46:23–28
30. Dubey JP (1998) Refinement of pepsin digestion method for isolation of *Toxoplasma gondii* from infected tissues. Vet Parasitol 74:75–77
31. Bartley PM, Wright SE, Zimmer IA, Roy S, Kitchener AC, Meredith A, Innes EA, Katzer F (2013) Detection of Neospora caninum in wild carnivorans in Great Britain. Vet Parasitol 192:279–283
32. Burrells A, Bartley PM, Zimmer IA, Roy S, Kitchener AC, Meredith A, Wright SE, Innes EA, Katzer F (2013) Evidence of the three main clonal *Toxoplasma gondii* lineages from wild mammalian carnivores in the UK. Parasitology 140:1768–1776
33. Katzer F, Brulisauer F, Collantes-Fernandez E, Bartley PM, Burrells A, Gunn G, Maley SW, Cousens C, Innes EA (2011) Increased *Toxoplasma gondii* positivity relative to age in 125 Scottish sheep flocks; evidence of frequent acquired infection. Vet Res 42:121
34. Opsteegh M, Swart A, Fonville M, Dekkers L, van der Giessen J (2011) Age-related *Toxoplasma gondii* seroprevalence in Dutch wild boar inconsistent with lifelong persistence of antibodies. PLoS One 6:e16240
35. Garcia JL, Gennari SM, Machado RZ, Navarro IT (2006) *Toxoplasma gondii*: Detection by mouse bioassay, histopathology, and polymerase chain reaction in tissues from experimentally infected pigs. Exp Parasitol 113:267–271
36. Benjamini Y, Hochberg Y (1995) Controlling the false discovery rate: a practical and powerful approach to multiple testing. J R Stat Soc Ser B Stat Methodol 7:289–300
37. Harrington DP, Fleming TR (1982) A class of rank test procedures for censored survival data. Biometrika 69:553–566
38. R-Core-Team (2014) A language and environment for statistical computing. Foundation for Statistical Computing, Vienna, Austria. http://www.R-project.org/
39. Dubey JP, Lindsay DS, Speer CA (1998) Structures of *Toxoplasma gondii* tachyzoites, bradyzoites, and sporozoites and biology and development of tissue cysts. Clin Microbiol Rev 11:267–299
40. Freire RL, Navarro IT, Bracarense APFRL, Gennari SM (2003) Vaccination of pigs with *Toxoplasma gondii* antigens incorporated in immunostimulating complexes (iscoms). Arq Bras Med Vet Zootec 55:388–396
41. da Cunha IA, Zulpo DL, Bogado AL, de Barros LD, Taroda A, Igarashi M, Navarro IT, Garcia JL (2012) Humoral and cellular immune responses in pigs immunized intranasally with crude rhoptry proteins of *Toxoplasma gondii* plus Quil-A. Vet Parasitol 186:216–221
42. Pena HF, Soares RM, Amaku M, Dubey JP, Gennari SM (2006) *Toxoplasma gondii* infection in cats from Sao Paulo state, Brazil: seroprevalence, oocyst shedding, isolation in mice, and biologic and molecular characterization. Res Vet Sci 81:58–67
43. Lindsay DS, Blagburn BL, Dubey JP (1993) Safety and results of challenge of weaned pigs given a temperature-sensitive mutant of *Toxoplasma gondii*. J Parasitol 79:71–76
44. Pinckney RD, Lindsay DS, Blagburn BL, Boosinger TR, McLaughlin SA, Dubey JP (1994) Evaluation of the safety and efficacy of vaccination of nursing pigs with living tachyzoites of two strains of *Toxoplasma gondii*. J Parasitol 80:438–448

14

Evaluation of biological safety in vitro and immunogenicity in vivo of recombinant *Escherichia coli* Shiga toxoids as candidate vaccines in cattle

Katharina Kerner[1], Philip S Bridger[1], Gabriele Köpf[1], Julia Fröhlich[1], Stefanie Barth[1,2], Hermann Willems[3], Rolf Bauerfeind[1], Georg Baljer[1] and Christian Menge[1,2*]

Abstract

Cattle are the most important reservoir for enterohemorrhagic *Escherichia coli* (EHEC), a subset of shigatoxigenic *E. coli* (STEC) capable of causing life-threatening infectious diseases in humans. In cattle, Shiga toxins (Stx) suppress the immune system thereby promoting long-term STEC shedding. First infections of animals at calves' age coincide with the lack of Stx-specific antibodies. We hypothesize that vaccination of calves against Shiga toxins prior to STEC infection may help to prevent the establishment of a persistent type of infection. The objectives of this study were to generate recombinant Shiga toxoids ($rStx1_{mut}$ & $rStx2_{mut}$) by site-directed mutagenesis and to assess their immunomodulatory, antigenic, and immunogenic properties. Cultures of bovine primary immune cells were used as test systems. In ileal intraepithelial lymphocytes both, recombinant wild type Stx1 ($rStx1_{WT}$) and $rStx2_{WT}$ significantly induced transcription of IL-4 mRNA. $rStx1_{WT}$ and $rStx2_{WT}$ reduced the expression of Stx-receptor CD77 (syn. Globotriaosylceramide, Gb3) on B and T cells from peripheral blood and of CD14 on monocyte-derived macrophages. At the same concentrations, $rStx1_{mut}$ and $rStx2_{mut}$ exhibited neither of these effects. Antibodies in sera of cattle naturally infected with STEC recognized the $rStx_{mut}$ toxoids equally well as the recombinant wild type toxins. Immunization of calves with $rStx1_{mut}$ plus $rStx2_{mut}$ led to induction of antibodies neutralizing Stx1 and Stx2. While keeping their antigenicity and immunogenicity recombinant Shiga toxoids are devoid of the immunosuppressive properties of the corresponding wild type toxins in cattle and candidate vaccines to mitigate long-term STEC shedding by the reservoir host.

Introduction

Enterohemorrhagic *Escherichia coli* (EHEC), a subset of Shiga toxin-producing *E. coli* (STEC), are food-borne pathogens which can evoke life-threatening diseases, such as hemorrhagic colitis and hemolytic-uremic syndrome, in humans. Cattle and other ruminants are primary reservoirs for EHEC serotypes that are frequently associated with human disease, e.g., EHEC O157:H7. Calves become infected with a plethora of different STEC strains early in life via horizontal or vertical transmission. Although calves rarely develop clinical signs of STEC infection they may shed these bacteria for several months and shed STEC quantities may be considerably high at some sampling points [1-4].

To prevent humans from EHEC infection, interventions must be applied at several stages of the food chain, starting in the animal itself and continuing in slaughterhouses, processing plants, distributors, and households [5]. A systematic review of vaccinations to reduce the shedding of *E. coli* O157 in the faeces of domestic ruminants revealed that vaccination may be a sensible control option [6]. Current vaccination strategies are promising but only succeed partially in reducing *E. coli* O157:H7 excretion (as reviewed by [5]). In some instances, e.g., when vaccinating cattle against H7 flagellin, an important adhesion factor to

* Correspondence: christian.menge@fli.bund.de
[1]Institute of Hygiene and Infectious Diseases of Animals, Justus Liebig University, Frankfurter Str. 85-89, 35392 Giessen, Germany
[2]Current Address: Friedrich-Loeffler-Institut, Institute of Molecular Pathogenesis, Naumburger Str. 96a, 07743 Jena, Germany
Full list of author information is available at the end of the article

bovine intestinal epithelium during early stages of colonization [7], systemically induced H7-specific IgG may even impair innate immune responses to *E. coli* O157:H7 when getting into contact with the epithelium via neutralisation of TLR5-mediated activation of epithelial cells [5].

Shiga toxins (Stx) are potent protein cytotoxins and represent the principal STEC virulence factor in the pathogenesis of human infections. Cumulating evidence exist that Stx act as immunomodulating agents during STEC infections in cattle. Stx1 alters the cytokine expression pattern in mucosal macrophages [8] and intraepithelial lymphocytes [9] and suppresses the activation and proliferation of mucosal [10] and peripheral lymphocytes in vitro [11]. The development of an adaptive cellular immune response is significantly delayed following experimental infection of calves with $Stx2^{+}$ STEC O157:H7 compared to that in animals inoculated with Stx-negative *E. coli* O157:H7 [12]. In vitro and in vivo studies revealed that Stx operate during the early phases of immune activation rather than depressing an established immunity [11-14]. Consequently, Stx likely acts as immunomodulator only upon first STEC infection of hitherto immunologically naïve calves. Of note, a significant portion of calves lacks anti-Stx antibodies at the time of first encountering STEC [2]. We hypothesize that passive (maternal) and active vaccination against Stx1 and Stx2 confers a protection against the toxins' immunosuppressive effects and subsequently enables the calves to actively mount a rapid immune response against STEC strains circulating in the respective cohort. Kuribayashi et al. showed that immunization of pregnant cows with Stxs led to an enrichment of colostra with anti-Stx1 and anti-Stx2 antibodies [15]. Subsequent application of bovine colostral anti-Stx2 to experimentally infected dogs indeed reduced STEC shedding [16].

Development of anti-Stx antibodies is remarkably delayed after natural [2] and experimental STEC infection of cattle [17]. Although Stx primarily targets $CD8^{+}$ cells [11], the immunomodulating capacity of Stx may also impair the humoral anti-Stx response. A strategy to circumvent this obstacle is the use of toxoid vaccines. Chemically inactivated Stx2e, however, was only partially effective in protecting piglets against oedema disease [18]. A more promising approach is the inactivation of Stx by genetic modification. Replacement of amino acids E167 and R170, located within the enzymatically active cleft of Stx2e [19,20] and vaccination of piglets with the recombinant protein fully protected piglets during challenge with native Stx2e [21]. Similar results have been reported for mice [22,23].

In order to follow a novel approach to add on or to improve current vaccination strategies to mitigate STEC shedding by cattle, the objectives of this proof-of-concept study were to generate recombinant Shiga toxoids ($rStx1_{mut}$ & $rStx2_{mut}$) by site-directed mutagenesis and to assess the immunomodulatory, antigenic, and immunogenic properties of the resulting proteins in cattle.

Material and methods

Generation of recombinant toxins and toxoids for in vitro and in vivo applications

For generating recombinant Stx ($rStx_{WT}$) and Stx mutants ($rStx_{mut}$), *stx1* and *stx2* genes from the *E. coli* reference strain EDL 933 (ATCC 43895) were PCR amplified (primers [5′→3′], Stx1_for: GGAGTATTGTGTCATA TGAAAAT, Stx1_rev: TATTCGAATTCAACGAAAAA TAA, Stx2_for: TATATGCATATGAAGTGTATATTAT TTAAA, Stx2_rev: AACCGTGAATTCAGTCATTATTA AACTGCACT). After restriction of PCR products with *Nde*I and *Eco*RI, resulting fragments were ligated into a compatible pET-24(b) + plasmid vector (Novagen, Merck KGaA, Darmstadt, Germany). Recombinant plasmids were transformed into *E. coli* BLR(DE3) and plasmid DNA bearing the *stx1* and *stx2* inserts, respectively, was prepared for site-directed mutagenesis. To replace E167 and R170 with glutamine (Q) and leucine (L), respectively, we used the QuickChange® Site-Directed Mutagenesis Kit (Stratagene, Amsterdam, The Netherlands). Sequencing of recombinant plasmids revealed, that the gene sequences of the wild type toxins $rStx1_{WT}$ and $rStx2_{WT}$ were identical with the original sequences (Acc.No. AE005174 for Stx1, NC_000924 for Stx2) and those of the mutant toxins $rStx1_{mut}$ and $rStx2_{mut}$ contained the desired mutations (E167Q, R170L; Table 1). Both, $rStx_{WT}$ and $rStx_{mut}$ were expressed in *E. coli* BLR(DE3). Control preparations were obtained from *E. coli* BLR(DE3) transformed with an empty vector (vector control). After incubation of the bacterial pellet with Polymyxin B (1 mg/mL) expressed toxin was collected from the periplasmic space and depleted from endotoxin (Detoxi-Gel™ Endotoxin Removing Gel, Thermo Scientific, Nidderau, Germany).

Quantification of $rStx_{WT}$ was done by VCA and Stx ELISA (see below), quantification of $rStx_{mut}$ only by Stx ELISA. For adjustment of the vector control, the lowest dilution determined for $rStx_{WT}$/$rStx_{mut}$ preparations to be applied in functional assays was also used for the vector control. The content of endotoxin was 51 fg/mL or less in $rStx_{WT}$, $rStx_{mut}$, and vector control preparations at working dilutions.

Vero cell cytotoxicity assay (VCA) and Vero cell cytotoxicity neutralization assay (VNA)

The VCA was performed in 96-well microtiter plates (Nunc, Wiesbaden, Germany) using Vero cells (ATCC CRL 1587, LGC-Promochem GmbH, Wesel, Germany) as previously described [24] to determine the cytotoxicity (verocytotoxic doses 50%, CD_{50}/mL) of the

Table 1 Comparison of the gene sequences of Stx1 and Stx2 before and after mutagenesis

Gene	Relevant nucleotide sequence (codon triplets for amino acids 164 to 174 in 5′ to 3′ direction)*	Compared to wild type amino acid replacements on position†
stx1$_{WT}$	-gtg aca gct **g**aa gct tta c**g**t ttt cgg caa ata-	none
stx1$_{mut}$	-gtg aca gct **C**aa gct tta c**T**t ttt cgg caa ata-	E167Q, R170L
stx2$_{WT}$	-gtc aca gca **g**aa gcc tta c**g**c ttc agg cag ata-	none
stx2$_{mut}$	-gtc aca gca **C**aa gcc tta c**T**c ttc agg cag ata-	E167Q, R170L

*Bold letters indicate positions of replaced nucleotides, with small letters marking the nucleotides in wild type toxin sequences and capital letters marking replaced nucleotides in mutant toxin sequences.
†E = glutamine acid, Q = glutamine; R = arginine; L = leucine.

$rStx_{WT}$ preparations and for adjustment of stock solutions (20 000 CD_{50}/mL).

The VNA was used for the determination of the neutralization activity in serum of vaccinated calves and was done as previously described [2] in order to determine the titre of neutralizing antibodies [nAb titre] against either wild type Stx1 or wild type Stx2 (Sigma-Aldrich Chemie GmbH, Taufkirchen, Germany).

Enzyme-linked immunosorbent assay (ELISA)

To quantify rStx protein in the preparations, a commercial Stx ELISA was used (Novitec® Verotoxin ELISA-Test, HISS Diagnostics, Freiburg, Germany) following the manufactures instructions. $rStx_{mut}$ concentrations used for the functional assays were adjusted to reach an OD equivalent to the OD of $rStx_{WT}$ stock solutions containing 20 000 CD_{50}/mL. Stock solutions were further diluted accordingly to reach a final concentration of 200 CD_{50}/mL or equivalent doses.

Stx-specific antibodies in sera from naturally exposed calves collected during a proceeding study [2] were analysed in a modified form of the ELISA. Briefly, 19 serum samples with Stx1 nAb titres between 60 and 2000 (as determined by VNA) were pre-diluted to achieve an approx. 50% reduction of the relative optical density [OD_{rel}]. Four serum samples with a Stx2 nAb titre of 30 were used un-diluted. Serum samples were incubated with either $rStx_{WT}$ or $rStx_{mut}$ preparations for 30 min at 37 °C. Subsequently, pre-incubated rStx was used as sample in the ELISA assay and subsequent steps were performed as described by the manufacturer. OD_{rel} was calculated by the following formula: OD_{rel} [%] = ($OD_{rStx + serum\ sample}$ - $OD_{vector\ control + serum\ sample}$)/($OD_{rStx + negative\ serum}$ - $OD_{vector\ control + serum\ sample}$) × 100.

Primary cell cultures

Peripheral blood mononuclear cells (PBMC) were isolated as previously described [11]. Cells were diluted in cell culture medium 1 (RPMI 1640, 10% fetal calf sera, 1% Penicillin/Streptomycin, 0.03% 1 mM 2-β-mercaptoethanol) to 1.5×10^6/mL and aliquoted into a 96-well flat-bottom plate (Greiner Bio-One, Frickenhausen, Germany) at 150 µL per well (2.25×10^5/well). Challenge material ($rStx_{WT}$, $rStx_{mut}$ or vector control, respectively) was added to reach a final concentration of 200 CD_{50}/mL or equivalent doses, respectively. For proliferation the mitogen phytohemagglutinin P [PHA-P] was added in a final concentration of 5 µg/mL. Plates were incubated for 96 h in 5% CO_2 at 37 °C.

Ileal intraepithelial lymphocytes (iIEL) were isolated as described elsewhere [25]. Cells were harvested and diluted in cell culture medium 2 (RPMI 1640, 20% fetal calf sera, 1% Penicillin/Streptomycin, 1% Amphotericin B, 0.01% Gentamicin) to 2×10^7/mL. Nine millilitre of this cell suspension were pipetted into a well of a 6-well plate and challenge material ($rStx_{WT}$, $rStx_{mut}$ or vector control) was added to a final concentration of 200 CD_{50}/mL or equivalent doses. Additionally, PHA-P was added to a final concentration of 2.5 µg/mL. Plates were incubated for 6 h in 5% CO_2 at 37 °C.

Monocyte-derived macrophages (MDM) were isolated as described elsewhere [26,27]. Briefly, a whole blood sample was centrifuged (2380 × *g*, 20 min) and the buffy coat was collected. After several washing and lysis steps, buffy coat was layered onto Ficoll for density centrifugation (800 × *g*, 45 min). Cells were collected by taking the interphase and washed three times with PBS buffer. Cells were adjusted to 4×10^6/mL in cell culture medium 3 (Iscove's Modified Dulbecco's Medium (IMDM) without Phenol Red, 20% fetal calf sera, 1% Penicillin/Streptomycin, 1% Amphotericin B, 0.05% 100 mM 2-β-mercaptoethanol) and 25 mL of this cell suspension were transferred to Teflon bags (VueLife Bags, American Fluoroseal Corp., Gaithersburg, USA) and incubated for 8 days (37 °C, 5% CO_2). At the end of the incubation period, cells were harvested and diluted to 2×10^6/mL in cell culture medium 4 (IMDM without phenol red, 2% fetal calf sera, 1% Penicillin/Streptomycin, 1% Amphotericin B, 0.05% 100 mM 2-β-mercaptoethanol). Five millilitre of the cell suspension was cultured in petri dishes (Greiner Bio-One, Frickenhausen, Germany) for 18 h. Lymphocytes were removed by careful washing and adherent MDMs were left within the dishes in cell culture medium 4. Challenge material was added in cell culture medium 4 to reach a final concentration of 200 CD_{50}/mL or equivalent doses and incubated for 6 h.

Immunophenotyping

At the end of the respective incubation times (see above), cells were resuspended and transferred to V-shape microtitre plates (Greiner Bio-One, Frickenhausen, Germany). After centrifugation (300 × *g*, 3 min, 4 °C) supernatants were flicked out. Pellets were resuspended in washing buffer (PBS supplemented with 1% bovine serum albumin, 0.01% sodium azide, and 0.5% goat serum) as negative control or with 50 μL of primary antibody dilution (diluted 1:50 through 1:500 in washing buffer). Antibodies were purchased from VMRD (Labor Diagnostik Leipzig, Leipzig, Germany; CD4 clone IL-A11, CD8β clone BAT82A, CD14 clone CAM36A, CD21 clone GB25A, γδT/N24 clone GB21A), AbDSerotech (Puchheim, Germany; CD77 clone 38–13) or kindly provided by Dirk Werling (The Royal Veterinary College, London, United Kingdom; CD80 clone N32/52-3, CD86 clone IL-A190). Cells were incubated for 20 min on ice, washed with washing buffer and resuspended in 50 μL of washing buffer with secondary antibodies (fluorescein isothiocyanate (FITC)-labelled α-rat IgM (Dianova GmbH, Hamburg, Germany); allophycocyanin (APC)-labelled α-mouse IgG_1, APC-labelled α-mouse IgG_{2a}, APC-labelled α-mouse IgG_{2b} (Jackson ImmunoResearch Europe Ltd., Suffolk, United Kingdom)) supplemented with 7-amino actinomycin D (7-AAD; final concentration 2 μg/mL; Sigma-Aldrich, Taufkirchen, Germany). After 20 min on ice, cells were washed with washing buffer and analysed with BD FACSCalibur™ Analyzer (Becton-Dickinson, Heidelberg, Germany). For analysis of PBMC, following the last incubation step, cells were incubated with 50 μL of Annexin V-phycoerythrin [PE]-Dilution (1:500; Dianova GmbH, Hamburg, Germany), washed with Annexin V binding buffer (10 mM HEPES pH 7.4, 140 mM NaCl, 2.5 mM $CaCl_2$), diluted in Annexin V binding buffer and analysed. Cells were gated according to their size and granularity. Only morphologically intact cells were used for further analysis. Cells positive for 7-AAD uptake or Annexin-V-PE binding were excluded and defined as early apoptotic (positive for Annexin-V-PE), late apoptotic (positive for Annexin-V-PE and 7-AAD), and necrotic (positive for 7-AAD), respectively. Data analysis was performed with FCSExpress (Version 2, De Novo-Software, Thornhill, Ontario, Canada).

RNA isolation

At the end of the incubation period, iIEL were resuspended, transferred to 50 mL tubes, washed with PBS (200 × *g*, 7 min), lysed in 600 μL RLT buffer (RNeasy MiniKit, Qiagen, Hilden, Germany) supplemented with 1% β-mercaptoethanol, and stored at –70 °C.

All samples were thawed at 37 °C for 5 min, and then homogenized by passing through a 20 G needle. RNA isolation was performed with the RNeasy MiniKit following the manufacturers' instruction with modifications described by Moussay et al. [9]. Reverse transcription and real-time PCR using primers and probes labelled at the 5′-end with the reporter dye FAM (6-carboxyfluorescein) and at the 3′-end with the quencher dye TAMRA (6-carboxytetramethyl-rhodamine) was conducted as described [9]. PCR amplification was performed on an automated fluorometer (ABI PRISM™ 5700 Sequence Detection System, Applied Biosystems) using 96-well optical plates. Each sample was analysed in duplicates. For analysis of the data, the comparative C_t method ($\Delta\Delta C_t$ method) was applied with first, normalization of the C_t values referring to the housekeeping gene GAPDH and second, comparing the C_t values for the quantitation of IL-4-specific mRNA in cultures treated with challenge material ($rStx_{WT}$, $rStx_{mut}$) and in cultures treated with vector control (control cultures) [9].

Immunization study

The experiment was carried out in strict accordance with European and German laws for the care and use of animals, approved by Thüringer Landesamt für Lebensmittelsicherheit und Verbraucherschutz, Bad Langensalza, Germany (permit no. 22-268-04-04-105/11).

Prior to the experiment, two conventionally raised bull calves aged 11 months tested negative for Stx-specific antibodies (16 and 4 weeks before the trial by VNA). Calves were tested for STEC shedding 16 weeks before the trial and immediately prior to the 1st and the 2nd vaccination. For this purpose coliform bacteria from fecal samples were enriched by growth on Gassner agar (3 plates per sample) [28]. Subsequently, the enriched bacterial culture material was tested with a *stx1/stx2*-duplex-PCR modified from Nguyen et al. [29]. While all fecal samples were *stx*-negative at the first and last sampling, in both calves genes encoding Stx1 and Stx2 were present in the fecal sample taken prior to the 1st vaccination at low frequencies (only 1 of 3 enrichment cultures from these fecal samples tested positive). Calves were double-vaccinated i.m. with both, a $rStx1_{mut}$ vaccine and a $rStx2_{mut}$ vaccine on trial days 0 and 21. Immediately prior to application, vaccines had been freshly prepared as follows: $rStx1_{mut}$ and $rStx2_{mut}$ preparations were diluted separately with NaCl solution (0.89%) to 1 000 000 CD_{50} equivalents in 1.4 mL and then supplemented with 0.6 mL of aluminium hydroxide (Alu-Gel-S, Serva Electrophoresis GmbH, Heidelberg, Germany). Blood samples were taken weekly, centrifuged, and sera were frozen at –20 °C. Nine weeks after first immunization, last samples were drawn. Detection of specific antibodies in the sera was done by VNA. Titres below the detection limit were given an arbitrary value of 30.

Statistical analysis

Unless otherwise indicated, data obtained after applying $rStx_{WT}$ and $rStx_{mut}$ preparations in biological assays were normalized relative to data obtained after application of vector control.

Statistical analysis was done with "SPSS for windows" (Version 15, SPSS Inc., Chicago, Illinois, USA). Single factor variance analyses with repeated measurements were carried out applying Greenhouse Geisser Test for all data from in vitro testing of the preparations. Pearsons's correlation analysis was used to compare quantitative values from the VNA. Two-tailed p-values with $p \leq 0.05$ were considered significant. The following description was used: n.s. = not significant ($p > 0.05$); * = $p \leq 0.05$; ** = $p \leq 0.01$; *** = $p \leq 0.001$.

Results

Generation of Shiga toxins and toxoids

Lysates from *E. coli* BLR(DE3) transformed with plasmids coding for either of the $rStx_{WT}$ possessed a considerable Vero cytotoxicity (2.7×10^6 and 0.8×10^6 CD_{50}/mL for $rStx1_{WT}$ and $rStx2_{WT}$, respectively; geometric mean of n = 4 determinations; Figure 1). Lysates containing $rStx_{mut}$ only had low cytotoxic activities (40 and < 20 CD_{50}/mL for $rStx1_{mut}$ and $rStx2_{mut}$, respectively) not different from lysates of *E. coli* BLR(DE3) transformed with the empty expression vector (<20 CD_{50}/mL). In order to functionally test $rStx_{WT}$ and $rStx_{mut}$ at comparable yet biologically relevant concentrations, a concentration of 200 CD_{50}/mL was chosen and $rStx_{mut}$ containing lysates were adjusted to their $rStx_{WT}$ containing counterparts according to the results of an ELISA test (resulting working dilutions indicated in Figure 1).

Viability and phenotype of bovine PBMC upon in vitro challenge with $rStx_{WT}$ and $rStx_{mut}$

Purified wild type Stx1 from *E. coli* blocks activation and proliferation of bovine lymphocyte subpopulations in vitro without inducing cellular death [11]. Neither incubation of PHA-P (phytohemagglutinin-P) stimulated PBMC with $rStx_{WT}$ nor incubation with $rStx_{mut}$ led to a significant increase in the percentage of late apoptotic/necrotic cells and the percentage of early apoptotic cells as compared to PHA-P stimulated bovine PBMC cultures incubated in the presence of the vector control (referred to as "control cultures" throughout; data not shown).

Control cultures phenotyped after four days of in vitro maintenance consisted of 13.2 ± 6.4%, 9.8 ± 4.9%, 30.0 ± 8.4%, and 18.9 ± 6.0% (mean ± standard deviation; n = 3–6) of $CD4^+$, $CD8\beta^+$, $\gamma\delta T^+$, and B cells ($CD21^+$), respectively (data not shown). Addition of $rStx1_{WT}$ or $rStx2_{WT}$ preparations to the culture medium both significantly reduced the portion of $CD8\beta^+$ PBMC while incubation with $rStx_{mut}$

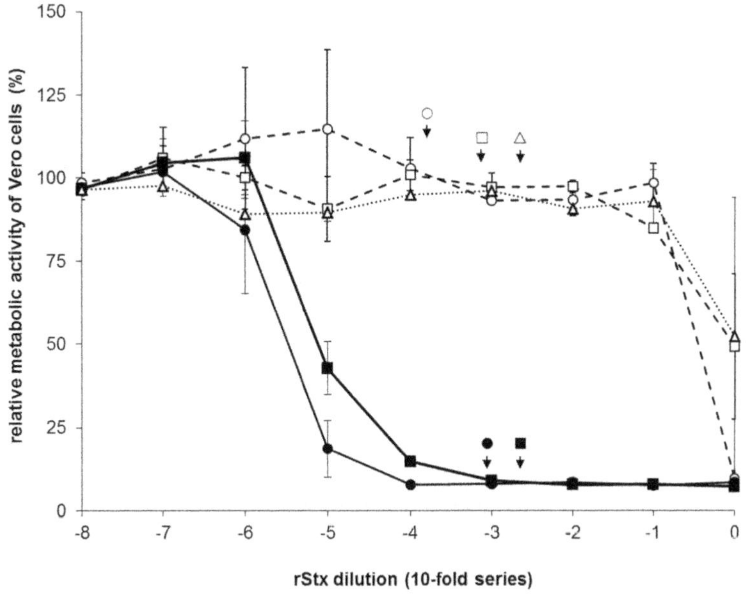

Figure 1 Effect of recombinant Shiga toxins and toxoids on the cellular metabolic activity of Vero cells. Cells were incubated for 96 h at 37 °C with 10-fold dilutions of endotoxin-deprived lysates prepared from *E. coli* BLR(DE3) transformed with plasmids encoding for $rStx1_{WT}$ (filled circle, solid line), $rStx1_{mut}$ (open circle, dashed line), $rStx2_{WT}$ (filled square, solid line), $rStx2_{mut}$ (open square, dashed line) or vector control (open triangle, dashed line). Results of VCA are presented relative to data obtained with cells incubated with plain medium as negative control (set to 100%) and data from cells treated with 1% SDS as positive control (set to 0%). Data is depicted as means ± standard deviations from duplicate determinations in one representative out of four independent experiments. Missing error bars are within symbols. For functional assays with bovine primary cell cultures, lysates containing $rStx_{WT}$ were adjusted to reach a final concentration of 200 verocytotoxic doses 50% per mL. Lysates containing $rStx_{mut}$ were diluted to yield the same OD as the corresponding $rStx_{WT}$–containing lysate in an ELISA assay (for details see Material and methods). To visualize the verocytotoxic activities of the respective rStx working dilutions, the calculated dilution factors are depicted by arrows and a corresponding symbol in the diagram.

left the proportion of CD8β$^+$ cells unaffected (Figure 2). Similarly, incubation with rStx1$_{WT}$ and rStx2$_{WT}$ reduced the portion of CD21$^+$ PBMC in the cultures compared to rStx$_{mut}$ treated cells. In turn, the portion of CD4$^+$ cells increased after incubation with rStx$_{WT}$ (significant for rStx2$_{WT}$ only). Incubation with rStx$_{mut}$ did not result in significant changes in PBMC composition except a slight but significant increase of CD21$^+$ PBMC after challenge with rStx1$_{mut}$ (Figure 2).

CD77 acts as the Stx receptor on a variety of cells from different species including bovine lymphocytes [14] and is up-regulated by bovine lymphocytes upon activation in vitro and in vivo [13]. Sustained down-regulation of CD77 by bovine PBMC is a hallmark of the activity purified wild type Stx1 exerts in bovine PBMC cultures [30]. Incubation with rStx1$_{WT}$ and rStx2$_{WT}$ also caused a significant reduction of the percentage of PBMC expressing CD77 to about half the values detected in control cultures (Figure 3) while incubation with rStx1$_{mut}$ and rStx2$_{mut}$ had no effect. In control cultures, 10.7 ± 1.4% (mean ± standard deviation; $n = 6$) of all PBMC expressed CD77 but the portion of CD77-expressing cells varied between the PBMC subsets analysed. Four days after initiation of cultures, 12.3 ± 9.6%, 23.5 ± 11.5%, 22.9 ± 12.6%, and 29.4 ± 9.6% of CD4$^+$, CD8β$^+$, γδT$^+$, and B cells (CD21$^+$), respectively, co-expressed CD77. Effects of rStx1$_{WT}$ and rStx2$_{WT}$ on CD77$^+$ cells differed between subsets and showed no correlation with the percentage of cells co-expressing CD77 in that subset. While a comparably high proportion of CD8β$^+$ cells (Figure 4) and γδT cells co-expressed CD77 and the portion of CD77$^+$ cells was significantly reduced by exposure to rStx$_{WT}$ (Figures 3 and 4), toxins exhibited minor effects on CD21$^+$ B cells also expressing CD77 in high numbers in control cultures (Figure 3). CD4$^+$ cells showed little CD77 expression which was clearly albeit not significantly reduced in the

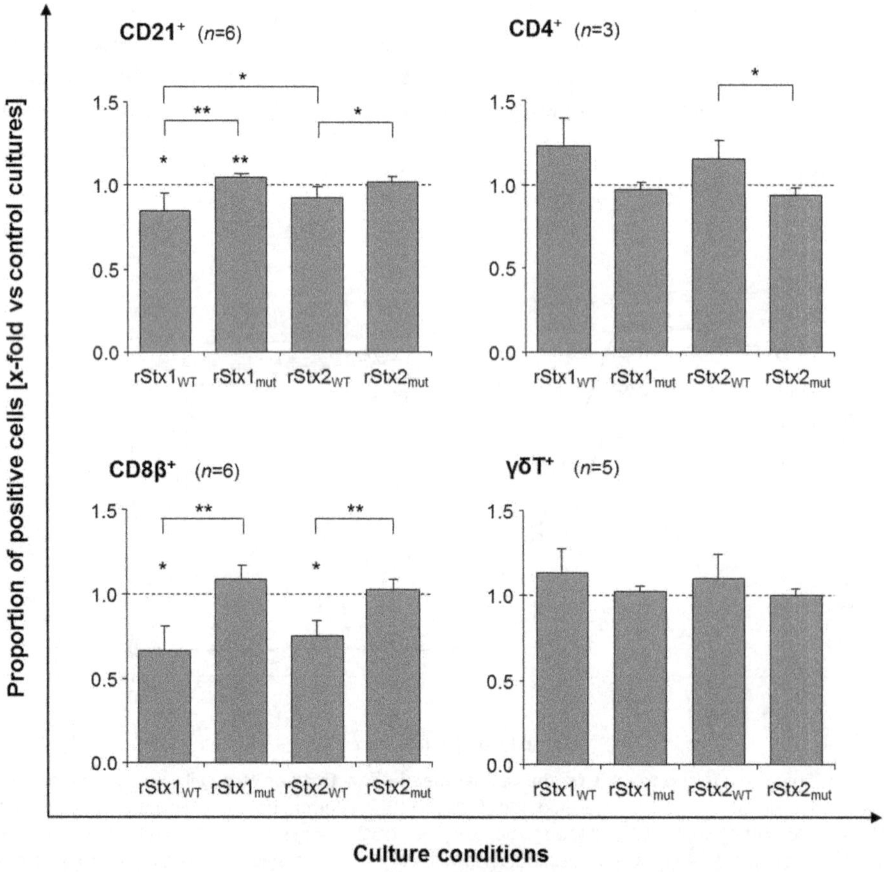

Figure 2 Proportion of CD21$^+$, CD4$^+$, CD8β$^+$, and γδT$^+$ cells in cultures of PHA-P stimulated bovine PBMC after incubation with recombinant Shiga toxins and toxoids. Results are shown relative to data obtained from cultures incubated in the presence of the vector control (control cultures; defined as 1.0, indicated by the dashed line). Data is depicted as means ± standard deviations of 3 to 6 repetitive experiments as indicated. ANOVA was performed (1) comparing non-normalized data with the values from control cultures (asterisks above bars) and (2) comparing values of normalized data obtained after incubation with rStx1$_{WT}$ versus rStx1$_{mut}$, rStx2$_{WT}$ versus rStx2$_{mut}$, rStx1$_{WT}$ versus rStx2$_{WT}$, and rStx1$_{mut}$ versus rStx2$_{mut}$ (asterisks above brackets). Significance levels were defined as $p \leq 0.001$ [***], $p \leq 0.01$ [**], and $p \leq 0.05$ [*].

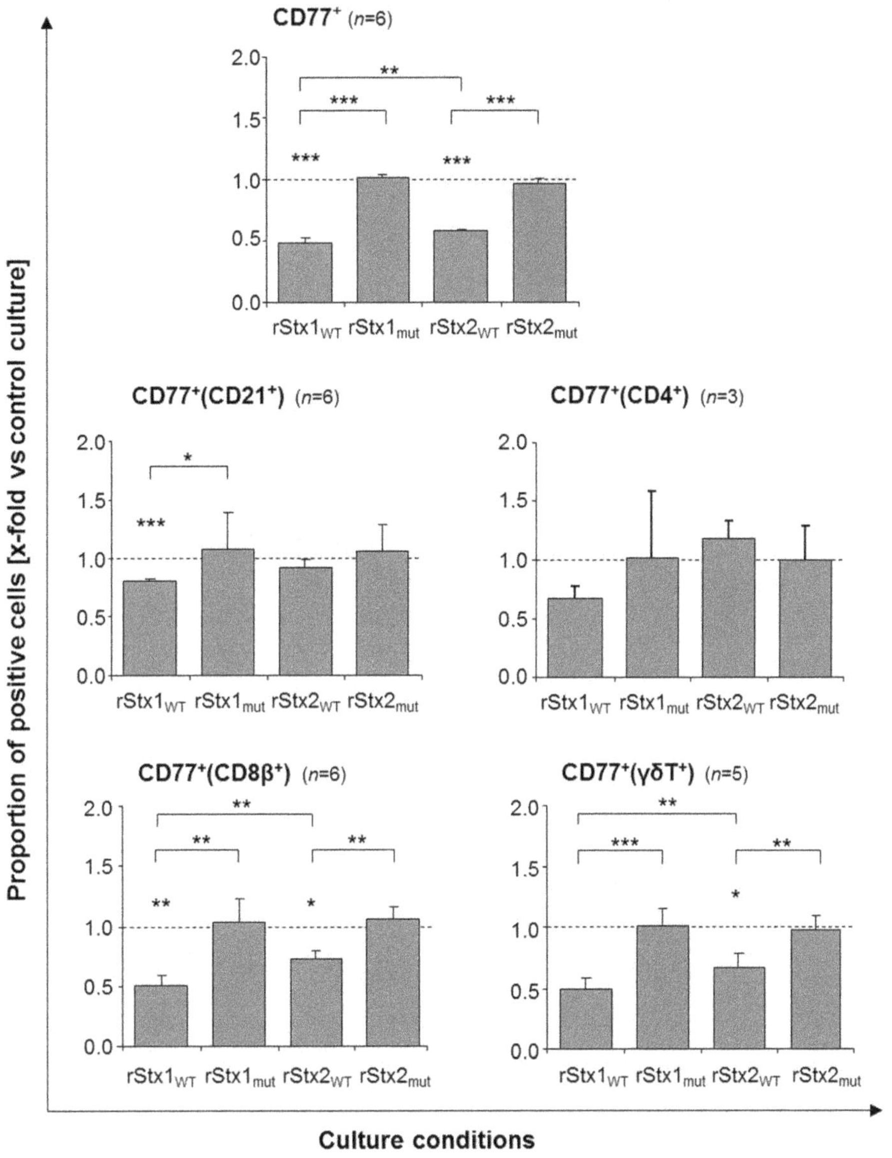

Figure 3 Bovine PBMC subsets co-expressing CD77 after in vitro challenge with recombinant Shiga toxins and toxoids. Proportions of bovine PBMC and of PBMC subsets co-expressing CD77 in PHA-P stimulated cultures are shown relative to data obtained from PHA-P stimulated cultures incubated in the presence of the vector control (control cultures; defined as 1.0, indicated by the dashed line). Data is depicted as means ± standard deviations of 3 to 6 repetitive experiments as indicated. Statistical analysis was performed as described in legend to Figure 2. Significance levels were defined as $p \le 0.001$ [***], $p \le 0.01$ [**], and $p \le 0.05$ [*].

presence of $rStx1_{WT}$ only (analysis of variance [ANOVA], $p = 0.378$). Incubation with $rStx1_{mut}$ and $rStx2_{mut}$ did not reduce CD77 expression by any of the PBMC subsets.

Changes in PBMC culture composition induced by $rStx_{WT}$ were partially reflected by alterations in the proportion of non-viable cells. The overall portions of early apoptotic cells within lymphocyte populations were not affected by the presence of $rStx_{WT}$ and $rStx_{mut}$ except a decrease in early apoptotic $CD8\beta^+$ PBMC after incubation with $rStx2_{mut}$ (ANOVA; $p = 0.009$; data not shown). However, wild type toxins induced a significant increase of late apoptotic/necrotic cells within the $CD21^+$ population (ANOVA; $rStx1_{WT}$: $p = 0.004$; $rStx2_{WT}$: $p = 0.036$; data not shown) and within the $CD4^+$ population (ANOVA; $rStx1_{WT}$: $p = 0.004$; data not shown). Effects became more apparent when analysing the percentage of late apoptotic/necrotic cells in the $CD77^+$ and $CD77^-$ subsets of the lymphocyte populations separately (Figure 5). Incubation with wild type toxins increased the portion of $CD77^+$ late apoptotic/necrotic cells in the $CD21^+$, $CD4^+$, $CD8\beta^+$, and $\gamma\delta T^+$ subsets even though differences did not always statistically significant levels. $CD77^-$ cells within

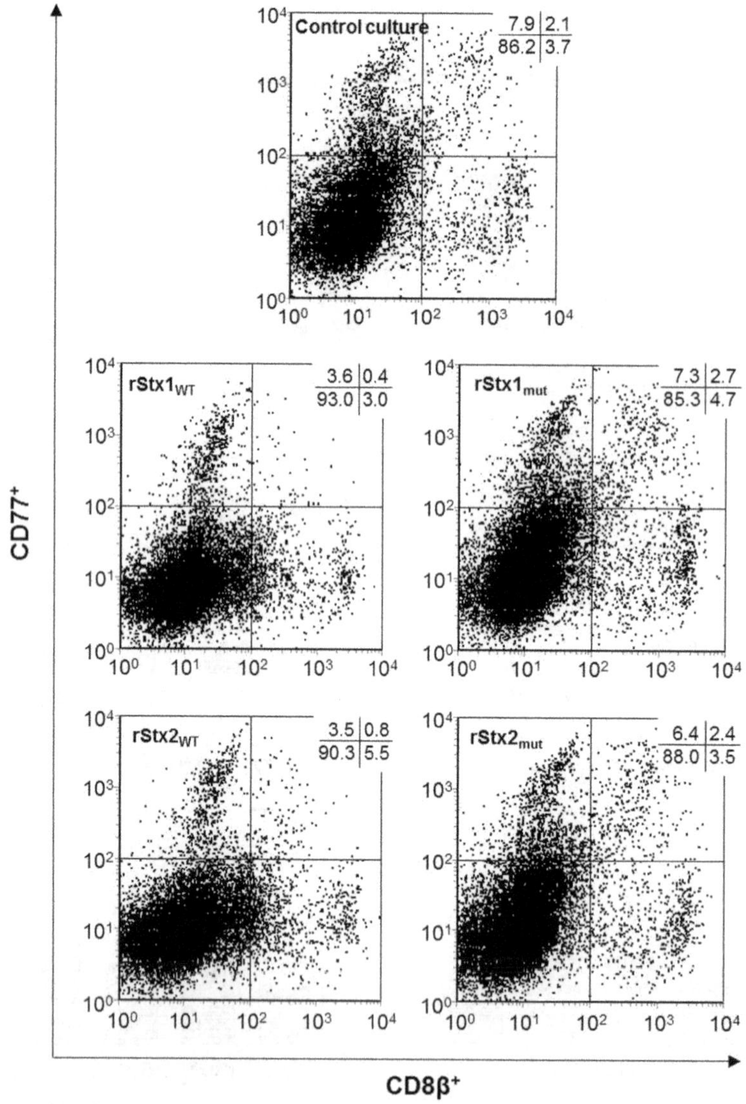

Figure 4 Effect of recombinant Shiga toxins and toxoids on CD77 expression by bovine CD8β⁺ PBMC. Cells were incubated in culture medium containing 5 μg/mL PHA-P and $rStx_{WT}$ or $rStx_{mut}$ as indicated. After four days of incubation cells were submitted to immunolabelling and flow cytometry analysis. Percentages of CD8β⁺ PBMC co-expressing CD77 (events in the upper right quadrant) are given in the upper right corner of the dot plots. PBMC incubated in the presence of PHA-P and vector control were used as control (upper graph).

the subsets were less or not affected. Incubation with toxoids neither resulted in proportions of early apoptotic nor of late apoptotic/necrotic cells that were significantly elevated compared to control cultures for any of the subpopulations tested irrespective of CD77 co-expression.

IL-4 transcription in bovine iIEL upon in vitro challenge with $rStx_{WT}$ and $rStx_{mut}$

Ileal intraepithelial lymphocytes (iIEL) are also sensitive to purified wild type Stx1 with a strong induction of IL-4 transcription being the most prominent and reproducible functional implication [9,25]. In corroboration of these findings, incubation of bovine iIEL for 6 h with $rStx1_{WT}$ or $rStx2_{WT}$ both led to a dramatic increase in the amounts of IL-4-specific mRNA (Figure 6A). Again, incubation with comparable amounts of $rStx1_{mut}$ and $rStx2_{mut}$ had no detectable biological effect.

CD14 expression by bovine MDM upon in vitro challenge with $rStx_{WT}$ and $rStx_{mut}$

Monocyte-derived macrophages (MDM) have recently been discovered as yet another Stx-sensitive cell type in cattle [31]. Incubation with $rStx_{WT}$ or $rStx_{mut}$ for 6 h did not significantly alter the percentage of early apoptotic cells as compared control cultures (data not shown). However, MDM responded to the exposure to $rStx1_{WT}$

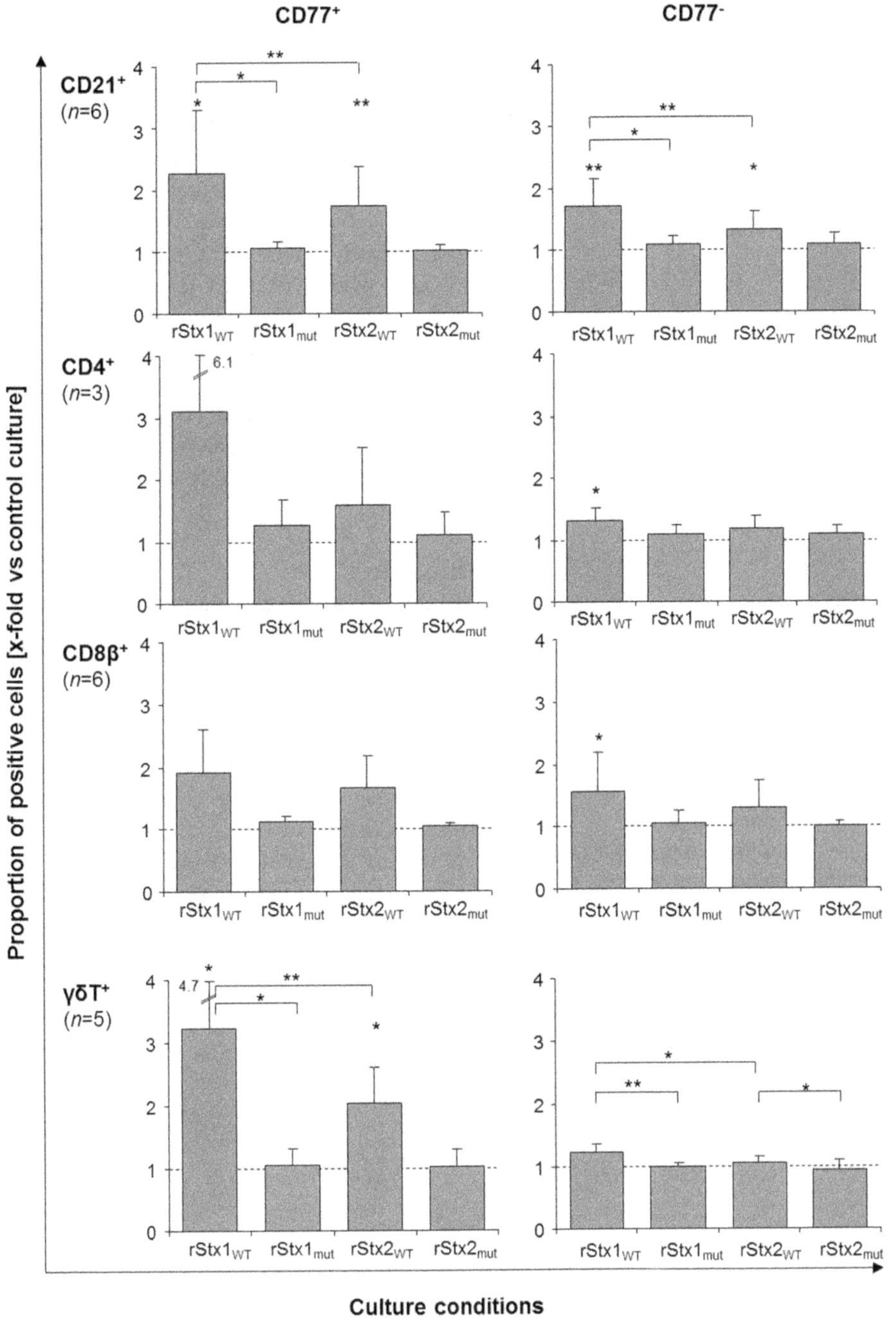

Figure 5 Late-apoptotic/necrotic cells within PBMC subsets after in vitro challenge with recombinant Shiga toxins and toxoids. Proportions of 7AAD positive cells expressing (left row) or not expressing CD77 (right row) within PBMC subsets in PHA-P stimulated cultures are shown relative to data obtained from PHA-P stimulated cultures incubated in the presence of the vector control (control cultures; defined as 1.0, indicated by the dashed line). Data is depicted as means ± standard deviations of 3 to 6 repetitive experiments as indicated. Statistical analysis was performed as described in legend to Figure 2. Significance levels were defined as $p \leq 0.001$ [***], $p \leq 0.01$ [**], and $p \leq 0.05$ [*].

or rStx2$_{WT}$ with a clear decrease in the number of CD14 molecules on the cellular surface (as deduced from quantitation of fluorescence intensities (MFI) for the detection of this antigen). The effect was most prominent in the CD77 co-expressing subset of MDM (Figure 6B, data not shown for CD77$^-$ MDM). The recombinant toxins had no influence on the number of surface-expressed CD80 and CD86 molecules on CD77$^+$ bovine MDM (data not shown). Incubation with comparable amounts of rStx1$_{mut}$ and rStx2$_{mut}$ had no significant effect on CD14, CD80, and CD86 expression by CD77$^+$ bovine MDM (Figure 6B; data not shown for CD80 and CD86).

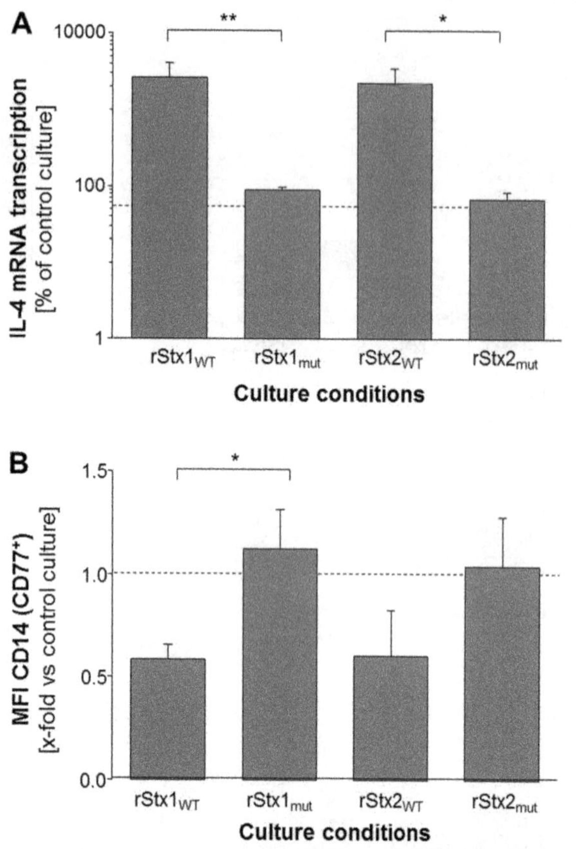

Figure 6 Gene transcription in bovine iIEL and surface marker expression on bovine MDM incubated for 6 h with $rStx_{WT}$ or $rStx_{mut}$. (A) Relative amounts of gene transcripts for IL-4 harboured by PHA-P-stimulated (2.5 mg/mL) bovine iIEL normalized to the transcription of the housekeeping gene GAPDH. Vector control cultures were used as reference and set to 100% (dashed line). **(B)** Expression (i.e., mean fluorescence intensity; MFI) of CD14 on bovine $CD77^+$ MDM relative to vector control cultures defined as 1.0 (dashed line). Data is depicted as means ± standard deviations from 5 independent experiments each. Statistical analysis was performed as described in legend to Figure 2. Significance levels were defined as $p \leq 0.01$ [**], and $p \leq 0.05$ [*].

Recognition of $rStx_{WT}$ and $rStx_{mut}$ by sera from calves naturally exposed to wild type toxins

Sera with known specific amounts of Stx antibodies, as defined by VNA and western blotting in a previous study [2], were used to occupy epitopes on $rStx_{WT}$ and $rStx_{mut}$ antigens that were afterwards subjected to the ELISA assay. As the titers of the different sera to Stx1 and Stx2 substantially differed with anti-Stx2 titers being just above the detection limit of the VNA, anti-Stx1 containing sera were pre-diluted to achieve an approx. 50% reduction of the rStx binding to the ELISA plate. Subsequently, pairs of values ($rStx_{WT}$ and $rStx_{mut}$) obtained for the individual sera at a given dilution were analysed by correlation analysis. The competitive ELISA revealed that naturally induced antibodies recognized the corresponding $rStx_{WT}$ and $rStx_{mut}$ equally well (Pearson's $r = 0.886$; $p < 0.001$; Figure 7).

Immunization of calves with $rStx1_{mut}$ and $rStx2_{mut}$

Until trial day 21, the day of the second immunization with both toxoids, serum samples of both calves tested negative for Stx1 neutralizing antibodies [nAbs] (Figure 8). Beginning one week later, anti-Stx1 nAbs were detectable in both calves. Stx1 nAb titres peaked on trial day 35 and remained on high levels through the end of the trial. Stx2 nAb titres were detectable as early as trial day 14. Titres of calf 1 fell below the detection limit of 60 on trial day 21 and started to rise again beginning on trial day 28. Calf 2 developed a Stx2 nAb titre beginning with trial day 14, one week before the second vaccination. Titre rose constantly until the end of the sampling period.

Discussion

The immunomodulatory and -suppressive effects of Shiga toxins (Stx) disturb the development of an adaptive immune response against STEC-specific antigens in the course of the initial infection of that far naïve calves [11,12]. In order to develop an effective but biologically safe antigen to vaccinate cattle against the immunologically distinct types 1 and 2 of Stx the objectives of this study were to prove that recombinant Shiga toxoids devoid of the enzymatic activity of the wild type toxins have lost their activity against all types of bovine immune cells identified as potential Stx targets thus far. For functional

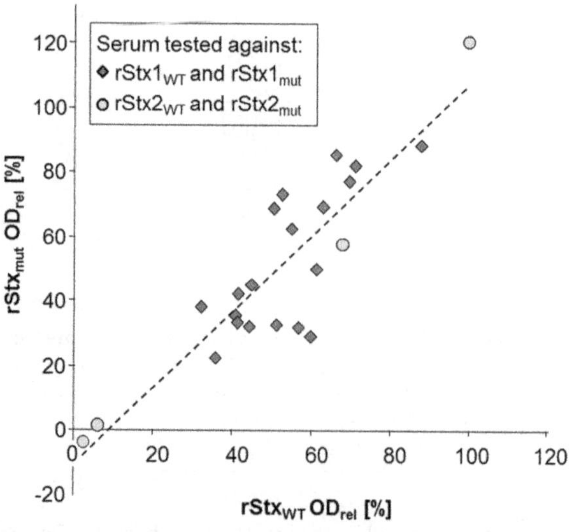

Figure 7 Antigenicity of recombinant Shiga toxins and toxoids as assessed with calf sera harbouring naturally induced Stx-specific antibodies. Results obtained with 23 sera in the competitive ELISA are presented. Figure represents OD_{rel} values of defined $rStx_{WT}$ and $rStx_{mut}$ samples, respectively, after pre-incubation with serum (dashed line: trend line [$y = 1.179x - 10.702$]).

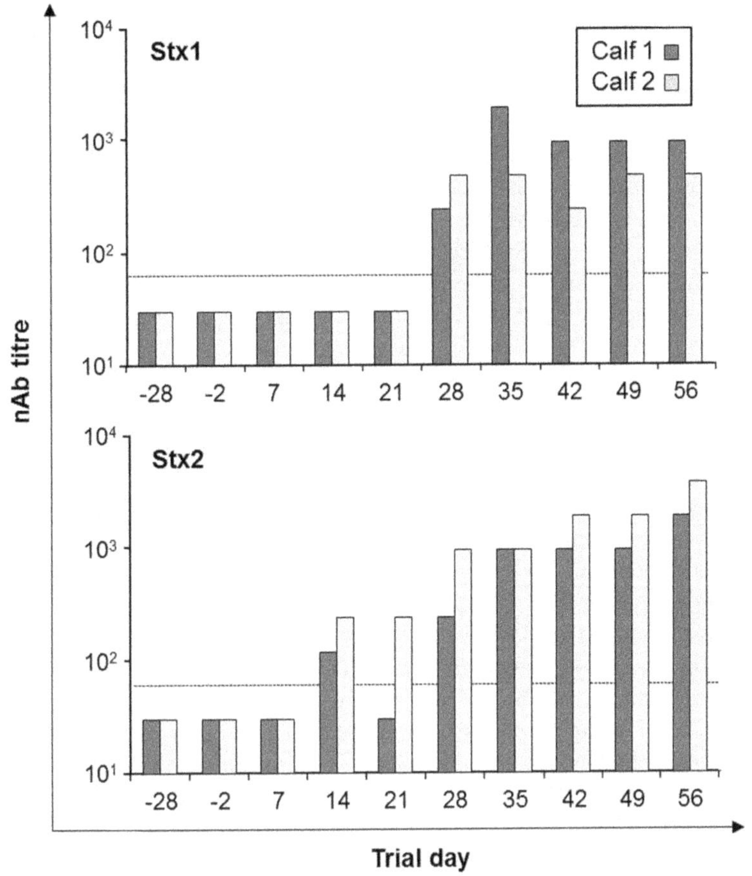

Figure 8 Detection of Stx1 and Stx2 neutralizing antibodies (nAb) in sera from two calves vaccinated with $rStx1_{mut}$ and $rStx2_{mut}$. Results from the Vero cell neutralization assay (VNA). Dashed line indicates the detection limit. Calves were vaccinated on days 0 and 21 of the trial. A titre of 30 was attributed to all those samples that gave negative test results in the highest concentration tested.

studies, a concentration of rStx of 200 CD_{50}/mL was chosen. Extensive previous studies had shown that purified Stx1 reliably induces maximum modulating effects on bovine immune cells in vitro at this concentration [9]. Concentrations of 2000 CD_{50}/mL may induce effects that cannot be fully neutralized by anti-StxB1 and therefore not clearly ascribed to Stx1 even when purified toxin is used [11]. Partially purified (i.e., endotoxin-deprived) preparations were used in the current study causing some depression of the metabolic activity of the robust Vero cells when applied undiluted. As the aim of this study was to provide a broad proof of loss of immunomodulating function of $rStx_{mut}$ in bovines and experiments were exclusively conducted with primary cells availability of which was limited, we refrained from conducting dose–response assays for any of the parameters under study. Consequently, we cannot rule out the possibility that the toxoids may cause adverse effects when applied in significantly higher concentrations. However, efficient induction of a humoral immune response in two calves locally exposed to 1 000 000 CD_{50} equivalents upon vaccination points against such assumptions. Having accomplished this proof-of-principle study presented herein, an extensive experiment is currently under way assessing the immunomodulating, immunogenic, and protective capacity of $rStx_{mut}$-based vaccines under field conditions.

Wild type Stx1 purified from a STEC field isolate blocks the proliferation of bovine peripheral blood T cells, with $CD8^+$ T cells in particular, and induces a down-regulation of the Stx receptor CD77 on several lymphocyte subsets without inducing significant cell death by apoptosis or necrosis [11,13]. Results of the present study show that non-purified endotoxin-deprived periplasmic preparations containing recombinant $rStx_{WT}$ induce comparable biological effects in bovine PBMC cultures. Similar to studies with purified Stx1, addition of recombinant $rStx_{WT}$ containing periplasmic preparations did not significantly affect the overall percentage of early or late apoptotic/necrotic cells within major PBMC subsets. In-depth analysis of multicolour flow cytometry data, applied here for the first time, provided evidence, however, that $rStx_{WT}$ treatment has led to an increase in the portion of late apoptotic cells in all lymphocyte populations. Notably, this effect (1) predominantly affected the respective $CD77^+$

expressing cells of the subsets and (2) could not be confirmed when analysing for early apoptotic cells. Further studies will be needed to dissect whether this effect can also be induced by purified toxins or is augmented by auxiliary factors present in the periplasmic preparations. Nevertheless, results presented here strongly imply that – despite several reports linking differences in the virulence of EHEC strains for humans to the Stx type or even subtype encoded for by the strains [32] - Stx1 and Stx2 do not differ significantly in their biological activities in bovines, the STEC/EHEC reservoir host, a finding that has direct implications for vaccine development.

Incubation of PBMC with $rStx1_{mut}$ and $rStx2_{mut}$ neither influenced the percentage of lymphocytes expressing $CD77^{+}$ nor the overall subset composition. Toxoids did not induce a down-regulation of CD14 in MDM cultures and did not lead to an up-regulation of IL-4 transcription in iIEL cultures, effects that occurred in the presence of wild type toxins. Even though the molecular mechanism by which Stx induce cell death in a variety of cell lines and primary cells is well understood [33-35], the molecular basis of the immunomodulatory effects of wild type Stx to bovine immune cells is not entirely clear. In most cells, Stx primarily inhibit protein synthesis by acting on the 23S rRNA incorporated in ribosomes [36]. THP-1 cells show an up-regulation of TNF-α upon treatment with Stx1 [37], an effect traced back to the ribotoxic stress response triggered by the enzymatic activity of Stx towards ribosomes. It would also be plausible that cross-linking of CD77 molecules on the cellular surfaces by the multivalent 5B plus 1A structured Stx has initiated cellular responses independent from the enzymatic activity as toxin binding induces apoptosis in sensitive cell lines [14]. We previously showed that incubation of bovine iIEL neither with Stx1 holotoxin nor with purified Stx1B subunit or with anti-CD77 antibody induces IL-4 transcription [9]. By contrast, binding of rStxB1 to CD77 on bovine PBMC induced a holotoxin like activity, e.g., an inhibition of lymphocyte proliferation [14]. The results presented here using genetically modified Stx devoid of verocytotoxic activity as well as lacking any detectable biological activities of $rStx1_{mut}$ and $rStx2_{mut}$ in all in vitro systems applied strongly suggest that the enzymatic activity is essentially required for the immunomodulating effect of Stx in cattle and underscore that the toxoids may represent biologically safe vaccines.

Final prove of biological safety can only come from immunization trials in vivo. Of note, the interferon-α receptor (IFNAR) harbours potential binding sites for CD77 in its extracellular domains, structurally related to CD77 binding sites of StxB subunits [38] raising the possibility that Stx immunization may induce auto-antibodies. The detrimental potential of vaccine-induced auto-antibodies has become dramatically apparent by the occurrence of bovine neonatal panleucocytopenia (BNP). In this clinical entity, prevalent in several European countries in recent years, anti-leukocytic antibodies induced by vaccination of dams are transmitted to their offspring causing severe bleedings and bone marrow depletion [39]. Anti-Stx1 antibodies can frequently be found in adult cattle [2,40] and anti-Stx2 antibodies, although with strikingly lower frequencies and titres, can also be detected. Two calves could be successfully vaccinated by two shots of vaccines containing $rStx1_{mut}$ and $rStx2_{mut}$, and immunization did not exert adverse effects indicative of auto-antibodies.

Antigenicity of $rStx_{mut}$ was evaluated in comparison to $rStx_{WT}$ in a competitive ELISA format using sera obtained from naturally exposed calves with known anti-Stx1 and anti-Stx2 titres [2]. Pre-incubation of the sera with $rStx_{mut}$ and $rStx_{WT}$ equally well reduced binding of the toxins to the capture antibodies. We take this as a strong hint that the structure of important epitopes being the target of a significant portion of naturally induced antibodies are conserved irrespective of the amino acid exchanges in the toxoids introduced by genetic modification.

To be used as vaccine component, inactivated Stx molecules must remain immunogenic. Chemical inactivation of Stx2e by formaldehyde treatment abolishes the cytotoxic effect in vitro but application of the toxoid failed to prevent piglets from developing edema disease upon intravenous challenge with wild type Stx2e [21]. By contrast, inactivation of Stx2e by means of genetic amino acid exchange in the enzymatic cleft of the A subunit resulted in a vaccine able to induce protective antibodies in piglets [41]. Similarly, the survival rate of mice after Stx1 challenge could be raised to 100% when animals had been immunized with mutagenized Stx1 (E167Q, R170L) [23]. It remains unclear whether the poor induction of an anti-Stx response in cattle after natural STEC infection [2] is due to an active immunosuppression by Stx, due to an insufficient antigen exposure by small amounts of toxins produced in vivo or due to poor immunogenicity of the toxins. The latter may result from the structural similarity of StxB subunit with bovine IFNAR and be the consequence of a centrally induced immunological tolerance. Nevertheless, i.m. application to calves of the toxoids generated and characterized in this study led to the induction of substantial anti-Stx1 as well as anti-Stx2 titres, presumably protective in that they at least are able to neutralize the biological activity of Stx holotoxin in vitro. The study design applied here does not allow for concluding on the specificity of the antibodies to each of the toxoids. Kinetics of shedding of Stx1- and Stx2-producing STEC strains as well as kinetics and magnitude of maternal and endogenous anti-Stx antibodies in calves substantially differ [2]. Further studies are worthwhile to separately optimize the immunogenic capacity of the two toxoids and to assess their relative protective efficacy, e.g., by modifications of the vaccine formulation and application scheme.

The STEC/EHEC pathovar consists of a plethora of different *E. coli* strains varying in serotype and virulence gene pattern. By definition, Stx's are the only virulence factors harboured by all STEC strains. Up to now, success of attempts to vaccinate cattle was mostly restricted to single subpopulations of STEC, e.g. strains positive for O157 [42], harbouring the genes for Tir (translocated intimin receptor) [42], for adhesion factor intimin [43], Esp's (*E. coli* secreted proteins) A and B [44,45] or flagellin H7 [46]. Stx rather act as immunomodulating agents during bovine STEC infections [8-12] by affecting the early phases of immune activation than by depressing an established immunity [13,14]. Consequently, Stx may principally be effective upon first STEC infection of hitherto immunologically naïve animals at the time they first encounter STEC antigens. In the absence of Stx, animals may be able to mount an efficient adaptive immune response with the potential to prevent persistent STEC colonization of the intestinal mucosa. However, Stx always co-occurs with STEC antigens in spatial and temporal terms during infection. In this particular situation, Stx apparently hinders calves from properly responding, creating an immunologically privileged niche and thereby paving the way for persistent colonization. Application of Stx toxoid-based vaccines may enable calves to actively mount a primary immune response to antigens other than Stx that are harboured by STEC strains circulating in the respective cohort. In case future studies show that this does not suffice, subsequent application of aforementioned vaccines as booster shall be evaluated as to their ability to eventually induce a robust anti-STEC adaptive immune response mitigating long-term STEC shedding by cattle.

Competing interests

The authors declare that they have no competing interests.

Authors' contributions

Design of study and experiments: CM, GB. Production of $rStx_{WT}$ and $rStx_{mut}$: HW, GK, SB and RB. Vero cell assays: KK, JF, SB. Primary cell assays: KK, PSB. Statistical analysis: PSB, SB. Drafting of the manuscript: CM, SB, KK. All authors read and approved the final manuscript.

Acknowledgements

KK was in part financially supported by the German Research Foundation (Deutsche Forschungsgemeinschaft, DFG) as part of the SFB535. The authors would like to thank U. Leidner (Institute of Hygiene and Infectious Diseases of Animals, Giessen, Germany) for her excellent technical assistance and the staff of the experimental animal facility (Friedrich-Loeffler-Institut, Jena, Germany) for their support during the animal trial.

Author details

[1]Institute of Hygiene and Infectious Diseases of Animals, Justus Liebig University, Frankfurter Str. 85-89, 35392 Giessen, Germany. [2]Current Address: Friedrich-Loeffler-Institut, Institute of Molecular Pathogenesis, Naumburger Str. 96a, 07743 Jena, Germany. [3]Clinic for Ruminants and Swine (Internal Medicine & Surgery), Justus Liebig University, Giessen, Germany.

References

1. Caprioli A, Morabito S, Brugere H, Oswald E (2005) Enterohaemorrhagic *Escherichia coli*: emerging issues on virulence and modes of transmission. Vet Res 36:289–311
2. Fröhlich J, Baljer G, Menge C (2009) Maternally and naturally acquired antibodies to Shiga toxins in a cohort of calves shedding Shiga-toxigenic *Escherichia coli*. Appl Environ Microbiol 75:3695–3704
3. Naylor SW, Gally DL, Low JC (2005) Enterohaemorrhagic *E. coli* in veterinary medicine. Int J Med Microbiol 295:419–441
4. Geue L, Segura-Alvarez M, Conraths FJ, Kuczius T, Bockemühl J, Karch H, Gallien P (2002) A long-term study on the prevalence of shiga toxin-producing *Escherichia coli* (STEC) on four German cattle farms. Epidemiol Infect 129:173–185
5. Vande Walle K, Vanrompay D, Cox E (2013) Bovine innate and adaptive immune responses against *Escherichia coli* O157:H7 and vaccination strategies to reduce faecal shedding in ruminants. Vet Immunol Immunopathol 152:109–120
6. Snedeker KG, Campbell M, Sargeant JM (2012) A systematic review of vaccinations to reduce the shedding of *Escherichia coli* O157 in the faeces of domestic ruminants. Zoonoses Public Health 59:126–138
7. Mahajan A, Currie CG, Mackie S, Tree J, McAteer S, McKendrick I, McNeilly TN, Roe A, La Ragione RM, Woodward MJ, Gally DL, Smith DG (2009) An investigation of the expression and adhesin function of H7 flagella in the interaction of *Escherichia coli* O157:H7 with bovine intestinal epithelium. Cell Microbiol 11:121–137
8. Stamm I, Mohr M, Bridger PS, Schröpfer E, König M, Stoffregen WC, Dean-Nystrom EA, Baljer G, Menge C (2008) Epithelial and mesenchymal cells in the bovine colonic mucosa differ in their responsiveness to *Escherichia coli* Shiga toxin 1. Infect Immun 76:5381–5391
9. Moussay E, Stamm I, Taubert A, Baljer G, Menge C (2006) *Escherichia coli* Shiga toxin 1 enhances *il-4* transcripts in bovine ileal intraepithelial lymphocytes. Vet Immunol Immunopathol 113:367–382
10. Menge C, Stamm I, Van Diemen PM, Sopp P, Baljer G, Wallis TS, Stevens MP (2004) Phenotypic and functional characterization of intraepithelial lymphocytes in a bovine ligated intestinal loop model of enterohaemorrhagic *Escherichia coli* infection. J Med Microbiol 53:573–579
11. Menge C, Wieler LH, Schlapp T, Baljer G (1999) Shiga toxin 1 from *Escherichia coli* blocks activation and proliferation of bovine lymphocyte subpopulations in vitro. Infect Immun 67:2209–2017
12. Hoffman MA, Menge C, Casey TA, Laegreid W, Bosworth BT, Dean-Nystrom EA (2006) Bovine immune response to shiga-toxigenic *Escherichia coli* O157: H7. Clin Vaccine Immunol 13:1322–1327
13. Menge C, Stamm I, Wuhrer M, Geyer R, Wieler LH, Baljer G (2001) Globotriaosylceramide (Gb_3/CD77) is synthesized and surface expressed by bovine lymphocytes upon activation in vitro. Vet Immunol Immunopathol 83:19–36
14. Stamm I, Wuhrer M, Geyer R, Baljer G, Menge C (2002) Bovine lymphocytes express functional receptors for *Escherichia coli* Shiga toxin 1. Microb Pathog 33:251–264
15. Kuribayashi T, Seita T, Fukuyama M, Furuhata K, Honda M, Matsumoto M, Seguchi H, Yamamoto S (2006) Neutralizing activity of bovine colostral antibody against verotoxin derived from enterohemorrhagic *Escherichia coli* O157:H7 in mice. J Infect Chemother 12:251–256
16. Kuribayashi T, Seita T, Matsumoto M, Furuhata K, Tagata K, Yamamoto S (2009) Bovine colostral antibody against verotoxin 2 derived from *Escherichia coli* O157:H7: resistance to proteases and effects in beagle dogs. Comp Med 59:163–167
17. Johnson RP, Cray WC, Jr, Johnson ST (1996) Serum antibody responses of cattle following experimental infection with *Escherichia coli* O157:H7. Infect Immun 64:1879–1883
18. MacLeod DL, Gyles CL (1991) Immunization of pigs with a purified Shiga-like toxin II variant toxoid. Vet Microbiol 29:309–318
19. Hovde CJ, Calderwood SB, Mekalanos JJ, Collier RJ (1988) Evidence that glutamic acid 167 is an active-site residue of Shiga-like toxin I. Proc Natl Acad Sci U S A 85:2568–2572
20. Yamasaki S, Furutani M, Ito K, Igarashi K, Nishibuchi M, Takeda Y (1991) Importance of arginine at position 170 of the A subunit of Vero toxin 1 produced by enterohemorrhagic *Escherichia coli* for toxin activity. Microb Pathog 11:1–9

21. Makino S, Watarai M, Tabuchi H, Shirahata T, Furuoka H, Kobayashi Y, Takeda Y (2001) Genetically modified Shiga toxin 2e (Stx2e) producing *Escherichia coli* is a vaccine candidate for porcine edema disease. Microb Pathog 31:1–8
22. Ohmura-Hoshino M, Yamamoto M, Yuki Y, Takeda Y, Kiyono H (2004) Non-toxic Stx derivatives from *Escherichia coli* possess adjuvant activity for mucosal immunity. Vaccine 22:3751–3761
23. Ishikawa S, Kawahara K, Kagami Y, Isshiki Y, Kaneko A, Matsui H, Okada N, Danbara H (2003) Protection against Shiga toxin 1 challenge by immunization of mice with purified mutant Shiga toxin 1. Infect Immun 71:3235–3239
24. Gentry MK, Dalrymple JM (1980) Quantitative microtiter cytotoxicity assay for *Shigella* toxin. J Clin Microbiol 12:361–366
25. Menge C, Blessenohl M, Eisenberg T, Stamm I, Baljer G (2004) Bovine ileal intraepithelial lymphocytes represent target cells for Shiga toxin 1 from *Escherichia coli*. Infect Immun 72:1896–1905
26. Adler H, Peterhans E, Jungi TW (1994) Generation and functional characterization of bovine bone marrow-derived macrophages. Vet Immunol Immunopathol 41:211–227
27. Werling D, Howard CJ, Niederer E, Straub OC, Saalmüller A, Langhans W (1998) Analysis of the phenotype and phagocytic activity of monocytes/macrophages from cattle infected with the bovine leukaemia virus. Vet Immunol Immunopathol 62:185–195
28. Barth S, Duncker S, Hempe J, Breves G, Baljer G, Bauerfeind R (2009) *Escherichia coli* Nissle 1917 for probiotic use in piglets: evidence for intestinal colonization. J Appl Microbiol 107:1697–1710
29. Nguyen TV, Le Van P, Le Huy C, Gia KN, Weintraub A (2005) Detection and characterization of diarrheagenic *Escherichia coli* from young children in Hanoi, Vietnam. J Clin Microbiol 43:755–760
30. Menge C, Stamm I, Blessenohl M, Wieler LH, Baljer G (2003) Verotoxin 1 from *Escherichia coli* affects $Gb_3/CD77^+$ bovine lymphocytes independent of interleukin-2, tumor necrosis factor-alpha, and interferon-alpha. Exp Biol Med 228:377–386
31. Loos D (2012) Untersuchungen zum Einfluss von Shigatoxin auf Makrophagen und dendritische Zellen des Rindes. Doctoral thesis, Justus Liebig University Gießen, Institute of Hygiene and Infectious Diseases of Animals.
32. Friedrich AW, Bielaszewska M, Zhang WL, Pulz M, Kuczius T, Ammon A, Karch H (2002) *Escherichia coli* harboring Shiga toxin 2 gene variants: frequency and association with clinical symptoms. J Infect Dis 185:74–84
33. O'Loughlin EV, Robins-Browne RM (2001) Effect of Shiga toxin and Shiga-like toxins on eukaryotic cells. Microbes Infect 3:493–507
34. Karmali MA (2004) Infection by Shiga toxin-producing *Escherichia coli*: an overview. Mol Biotechnol 26:117–122
35. Foster GH, Tesh VL (2002) Shiga toxin 1-induced activation of c-Jun NH (2)-terminal kinase and p38 in the human monocytic cell line THP-1: possible involvement in the production of TNF-alpha. J Leukoc Biol 71:107–114
36. Obrig TG, Moran TP, Brown JE (1987) The mode of action of Shiga toxin on peptide elongation of eukaryotic protein synthesis. Biochem J 244:287–294
37. Harrison LM, van Haaften WC, Tesh VL (2004) Regulation of proinflammatory cytokine expression by Shiga toxin 1 and/or lipopolysaccharides in the human monocytic cell line THP-1. Infect Immun 72:2618–2627
38. Maloney MD, Binnington-Boyd B, Lingwood CA (1999) Globotriaosyl ceramide modulates interferon-alpha-induced growth inhibition and CD19 expression in Burkitt's lymphoma cells. Glycoconj J 16:821–828
39. Bridger PS, Bauerfeind R, Wenzel L, Bauer N, Menge C, Thiel HJ, Reinacher M, Doll K (2011) Detection of colostrum-derived alloantibodies in calves with bovine neonatal pancytopenia. Vet Immunol Immunopathol 141:1–10
40. Pirro F, Wieler LH, Failing K, Bauerfeind R, Baljer G (1995) Neutralizing antibodies against Shiga-like toxins from *Escherichia coli* in colostra and sera of cattle. Vet Microbiol 43:131–141
41. Gordon VM, Whipp SC, Moon HW, O'Brien AD, Samuel JE (1992) An enzymatic mutant of Shiga-like toxin II variant is a vaccine candidate for edema disease of swine. Infect Immun 60:485–490
42. Potter AA, Klashinsky S, Li Y, Frey E, Townsend H, Rogan D, Erickson G, Hinkley S, Klopfenstein T, Moxley RA, Smith DR, Finlay BB (2004) Decreased shedding of *Escherichia coli* O157:H7 by cattle following vaccination with type III secreted proteins. Vaccine 22:362–369
43. van Diemen PM, Dziva F, Abu-Median A, Wallis TS, van den Bosch H, Dougan G, Chanter N, Frankel G, Stevens MP (2007) Subunit vaccines based on intimin and Efa-1 polypeptides induce humoral immunity in cattle but do not protect against intestinal colonisation by enterohaemorrhagic *Escherichia coli* O157:H7 or O26:H. Vet Immunol Immunopathol 116:47–58
44. Dziva F, Vlisidou I, Crepin VF, Wallis TS, Frankel G, Stevens MP (2007) Vaccination of calves with EspA, a key colonisation factor of *Escherichia coli* O157:H7, induces antigen-specific humoral responses but does not confer protection against intestinal colonisation. Vet Microbiol 123:254–261
45. Bretschneider G, Berberov EM, Moxley RA (2007) Isotype-specific antibody responses against *Escherichia coli* O157:H7 locus of enterocyte effacement proteins in adult beef cattle following experimental infection. Vet Immunol Immunopathol 118:229–238
46. McNeilly TN, Naylor SW, Mahajan A, Mitchell MC, McAteer S, Deane D, Smith DG, Low JC, Gally DL, Huntley JF (2008) *Escherichia coli* O157:H7 colonization in cattle following systemic and mucosal immunization with purified H7 flagellin. Infect Immun 76:2594–2602

Gene expression profiling of porcine mammary epithelial cells after challenge with *Escherichia coli* and *Staphylococcus aureus* in vitro

Alexandra Jaeger[1], Danilo Bardehle[2], Michael Oster[1], Juliane Günther[1], Eduard Muráni[1], Siriluck Ponsuksili[1], Klaus Wimmers[1*] and Nicole Kemper[3]

Abstract

Postpartum Dysgalactia Syndrome (PDS) represents a considerable health problem of postpartum sows, primarily indicated by mastitis and lactation failure. The poorly understood etiology of this multifactorial disease necessitates the use of the porcine mammary epithelial cell (PMEC) model to identify how and to what extent molecular pathogen defense mechanisms prevent bacterial infections at the first cellular barrier of the gland. PMEC were isolated from three lactating sows and challenged with heat-inactivated potential mastitis-causing pathogens *Escherichia coli* (*E. coli*) and *Staphylococcus aureus* (*S. aureus*) for 3 h and 24 h, in vitro. We focused on differential gene expression patterns of PMEC after pathogen challenge in comparison with the untreated control by performing microarray analysis. Our results show that a core innate immune response of PMEC is partly shared by *E. coli* and *S. aureus*. But *E. coli* infection induces much faster and stronger inflammatory response than *S. aureus* infection. An immediate and strong up-regulation of genes encoding cytokines (IL1A and IL8), chemokines (CCL2, CXCL1, CXCL2, CXCL3, and CXCL6) and cell adhesion molecules (VCAM1, ICAM1, and ITGB3) was explicitly obvious post-challenge with *E. coli* inducing a rapid recruitment and activation of cells of host defense mediated by IL1B and TNF signaling. In contrast, *S. aureus* infection rather induces the expression of genes encoding monooxygenases (CYP1A1, CYP3A4, and CYP1B1) initiating processes of detoxification and pathogen elimination. The results indicate that the course of PDS depends on the host recognition of different structural and pathogenic profiles first, which critically determines the extent and effectiveness of cellular immune defense after infection.

Introduction

Postpartum Dysgalactia Syndrome (PDS), with Coliform Mastitis (CM) as cardinal symptom, is known as a multifactorial infectious disease in postpartum sows and a serious problem with high economic relevance in modern piglet production worldwide [1]. Significant milk production failure and other clinical signs including increased rectal temperature (>39.3 °C) postpartum, loss of appetite or low water intake, redness and inflammation of teats, pain, failure to expose teats and nurse, and sometimes vaginal discharge are typical indicators of affected animals [2]. While initial research focused on husbandry- and management-influenced occurrence of PDS, current studies rather concentrate on the role of causative pathogens, immune defense mechanisms, infection pressure and genetic predisposition. Gram-negative pathogens, e.g. *Escherichia coli* (*E. coli*) and gram-positive pathogens, e.g. *Staphylococcus aureus* (*S. aureus*) were most commonly isolated from milk of PDS-positive, but also from non-affected sows [3,4]. The major question is why only some sows develop subclinical or clinical signs of infection within 12 h to 48 h postpartum after contact with ubiquitous bacteria while others remain clinically healthy. Frequency and severity of this complex disease appear to depend on immune competence including resistance to infection of the sow. While the heritability of CM resistance has been estimated in a range from 0.02 up to 0.20 [5], further genetic studies on mastitis susceptibility are lacking. Extremely low infectious dose for colonization of

* Correspondence: wimmers@fbn-dummerstorf.de
[1]Institute for Genome Biology, Leibniz-Institute for Farm Animal Biology, Wilhelm-Stahl-Allee 2, D-18196 Dummerstorf, Germany
Full list of author information is available at the end of the article

mammary gland of sows of less than 100 coliform microorganisms [6] abet microbial mammary tissue invasion. In sows as well as in other animal species *E. coli* pathogenesis has been associated with lipopolysaccharide (LPS) endotoxin release inducing acute and severe inflammation [7]. In contrast, mastitis induced by *S. aureus* infection is mostly characterized as subclinical, mild and persistent [8]. Pathogenesis of both infections may proceed to pathogen clearance or to chronic infection depending on the effectiveness of host defense mechanisms especially at early stages of cellular response [8]. When pathogens have overcome physical barriers and entered the lumen of the mammary gland through the teat canal, macrophages and mammary epithelial cells (MEC) are important for initiating and driving the immediate non-specific innate immune response [9]. Inflammation response of periparturient sows after inoculation of porcine mammary gland with different potential mastitis-causing *E. coli* strains specified a dominant role of that pathogen species in CM [10]. The development of clinical symptoms of CM in the sow was suggested to be associated with a locally increased production of pro-inflammatory cytokines such as interleukin 1-beta (IL1-beta), IL6, IL8, and tumor necrosis factor-alpha (TNF-alpha) in response to intramammary *E. coli* infection [10,11]. Additionally, the time of infection of the mammary gland relative to parturition and the number of circulating neutrophils at the time of infection were shown to influence the development of clinical CM in the sow [12]. No published study was found regarding the inflammatory response of periparturient sows after inoculation of mammary gland with *S. aureus*. But it was commonly shown that *E. coli* and *S. aureus* are also the main causative agents of bovine mastitis, the most economically important disease of dairy ruminants. Comparative kinetic studies on infected udder of cows and inoculation of primary bovine mammary epithelial cells (pbMEC) with *E. coli* and *S. aureus* showed that *E. coli* swiftly and strongly induced the expression of cytokines and bactericidal factors, while *S. aureus* elicited a retarded response and failed to quickly induce the expression of bactericidal factors [8]. Both pathogens induced similar patterns of immune response genes, but the host response to *E. coli* was observed to be much faster and stronger than that to *S. aureus* infection [8]. Also different expression profiles of upstream as well as downstream regulators of early responses of pbMEC to *E. coli* and *S. aureus* may contribute to the different clinical manifestations and outcome of mastitis caused by these two pathogens [13]. Except for few referred studies on pathogen defense mechanisms of porcine mammary glands, the role of porcine mammary epithelial cells (PMEC) in the initiation of the innate immune response remains largely unknown. Our study focused on inflammatory response mechanisms of PMEC, isolated from lactating sows, after challenge with potential mastitis-causing pathogens such as *E. coli* and *S. aureus*. Strains from both pathogens used in our study were isolated from milk of PDS-positive sows. The molecular characterization of affected signaling pathways and involved signaling molecules in PMEC dependent on challenge time was performed by microarray analysis. Similarities and differences in the response of PMEC to both heat-inactivated pathogen species were determined by comparing the expression profile between the pathogen-challenged PMEC groups and unchallenged control as well as among the challenged groups. Selective analysis of most and strongest affected molecular and cellular functions, canonical pathways, upstream regulators and signaling networks were performed to throw light on the role of PMEC in pathogen clearance after bacterial invasion. Our results may especially improve the understanding of the specific reaction of PMEC to pathogen challenge and may help to get insight in how and to what extent environmental bacteria trigger inflammatory and immune responses in porcine mammary gland in general. To our knowledge, this is the first microarray-based study investigating genetic factors that determine the initial immune response of PMEC in vitro, at 3 h and at 24 h post-challenge (hpc) with heat-inactivated *E. coli* and *S. aureus* strains, potentially causing mastitis of sows.

Materials and methods

Cell culture and pathogen challenge

Primary cell cultures were established from mammary glands of three lactating sows of commercial herds. Animal care and tissue collection was performed in compliance with the German Law of Animal Protection. The experimental protocol was approved by the Animal Care Committee of the Leibniz-Institute for Farm Animal Biology, Dummerstorf, Germany. Tissues from eight mammary complexes cranial of the navel were collected aseptically immediately after slaughter from each individual. Subsequently, tissue samples were washed in Hank's Balanced Salt Solution (HBSS, PAN Biotech, Aidenbach, Germany) containing 17 mM 4-(2-hydroxyethyl)-1-piperazineethanesulfonic acid (HEPES, PAN Biotech) and 2% Antibiotic/Antimycotic Solution (APS, 10 000 U/mL penicillin, 10 mg/mL streptomycin sulphate, 25 µg/mL amphotericin B, PAA, Cölbe, Germany). After a second washing step, tissue samples were finely minced using sharp blades and placed in 15 mL falcon tubes. Washing steps were repeated until the supernatant was clear. Tissue digestion steps were performed in collagenase solution (Type III, 200 U/mL, Biochrom, Berlin, Germany) at 37 °C for 45 min. Occasionally, digested tissue was mixed with washing buffer and filtered through stainless steel meshes (100–380 μm pore size, Sigma-Aldrich, Steinheim, Germany) to remove undissociated tissue and debris. Cells were collected by centrifugation at 1000 rpm and 15 °C for 10 min and pellets were resuspended in washing buffer without APS. This step was repeated until the supernatant was clear (3–4 digestion steps in total). At the end, cell pellets were resuspended in complete medium consisting of Dulbecco's Modified Eagle Medium/Nutrient Mixture F-12 (DMEM/F12, PAN Biotech), 10% fetal bovine serum (FBS, PAA), 1% APS, 10 μg/mL insulin (Sigma-Aldrich) and 1 μg/mL hydrocortisone (Sigma-Aldrich). Primary cells were cryopreserved in 90% FBS and 10% dimethyl sulfoxide (DMSO, Carl Roth, Karlsruhe, Germany). Before starting the experiments, cells were thawn, plated onto collagen-coated (1:10 collagen R in destilled water, Menal, Emmendingen, Germany) 10 cm petri dishes and cultured in complete medium for several days at 37 °C and 5% CO_2 in a humidified atmosphere. Fibroblasts, adipocytes and other cell types were removed by selective trypsinization (Trypsin/EDTA (0.25%/0.02%, Sigma-Aldrich) during the following days. These cell types detach more rapidly from plastic after trypsinization than do the epithelial cell islands. The culture was quickly rinsed with growth medium to stop the enzymatic dispersion and to remove the fibroblastic cell areas. The relatively undisturbed epithelial cell islands were further incubated with growth medium. This procedure was repeated several times until a uniform and confluent monolayer of epithelial cells was formed.

Staphylococcus aureus (not characterized) and *E. coli* (gMEc240, sequence type 101, phylogroup B1, C+) strains used for this experiment were isolates from milk of PDS-positive sows. Both strains were grown in brain-heart-infusion-broth (BHB, Oxoid, Wesel, Germany) at 37 °C to the logarithmic phase of culture growth (Optical Density at 600 nm [OD_{600}] 0.5, ~ 5×10^7/mL). Dilution series were plated to calibrate cell counts from the OD readings. Heat-inactivation of bacteria was performed at 80 °C for 1 h and verified by control plating. Afterwards, bacteria were spun down at 3000 rpm for 15 min, washed twice with DMEM/F12 medium and resuspended herein at a density of 1×10^8/mL. Aliquots were stored at −20 °C.

Approximately 4.4×10^5 of the isolated PMEC from each individual (three biological replicates) were seeded and cultured in collagen-coated 6-well plates in complete medium without APS (three technical replicates per individual and treatment condition). On the next day, medium was changed. Forty eight hours after seeding, cells reached 90% confluency. PMEC were challenged with 10^7/mL heat-inactivated *S. aureus* and *E. coli*, respectively, for 3 h and for 24 h (Figure 1A). Equivalent challenge treatments have been considered as robust cell stimulation based on previously published reports. After incubation periods, pathogen-challenged and unchallenged cells (control) were washed three times with phosphate buffered saline (PBS, PAA) to remove the bacteria. Cells were collected for total RNA isolation.

Immunocytochemistry/microscopy

PMEC were seeded on 12 mm coverslips (Carl Roth) in 24-well plate (Biochrom) at a density of 10 000 cells/well. After two days of culturing, medium was discarded, and coverslips were washed twice with PBS and fixed with ice-cold methanol (−20 °C, Carl Roth) for 20 min. Cells were permeabilized with 0.2% Triton X-100 (Carl Roth), diluted with PBS for 5 min and washed twice with PBS. Non-specific binding sites were blocked by incubating the coverslips with 10% FBS in PBS for 30 min at room temperature. Coverslips were washed twice with PBS and incubated with mouse anti-cytokeratin 18-fluorescein isothiocyanate (anti-Cy18-FITC, Sigma-Aldrich) and mouse anti-alpha-smooth muscle actin antibodies (clone 1A4, Sigma-Aldrich), respectively in a humidified chamber for 1 h. Coverslips were washed three times with PBS. Bound anti-alpha-smooth muscle actin antibody was visualized by 1 h incubation of the coverslips with goat anti-mouse FITC-labeled secondary antibody (Sigma-Aldrich). Nuclei of the cells were stained with 4',6-diamidino-2-phenylindole (DAPI, Carl Roth) for 15 min. Coverslips were washed twice with PBS, air dried and mounted with 1,4-diazabicyclo[2.2.2]octane (DABCO) on glass slides (both from Carl Roth). Coverslips were analyzed by immunofluorescence microscopy (Microphot-FXA, Nikon, Düsseldorf, Germany).

RNA extraction, target preparation, and hybridization

Total RNA was isolated using the TRI® reagent (Sigma-Aldrich) according to the manufacturer's instructions. Isolated RNA was purified using RNeasy Mini Kit (Qiagen, Hilden, Germany), and contaminating DNA was removed by DNase I digestion (Qiagen). RNA integrity and quantity were checked by agarose gel electrophoresis and by spectrometry with a NanoDrop ND1000 spectrophotometer (PEQLAB, Erlangen, Germany). Absence of DNA contamination was verified by PCR of the porcine beta-actin gene (forward primer, GAGAAG CTCTGCTACGTCGC, reverse primer, CCTGATGTC CACGTCGCACT, Promega, Mannheim, Germany) with isolated RNA as templates. For the microarray analysis individual biotin-labeled cRNA was synthesized by the Gene Chip 3' Express Kit (Affymetrix, Santa Clara, CA, USA). cRNA was fragmented (~100 bp) and hybridized for 16 h at 45 °C to Affymetrix Gene Chip® Porcine Genome Arrays. The microarrays were scanned using GeneChip Scanner 3000 (Affymetrix). Raw data was

A

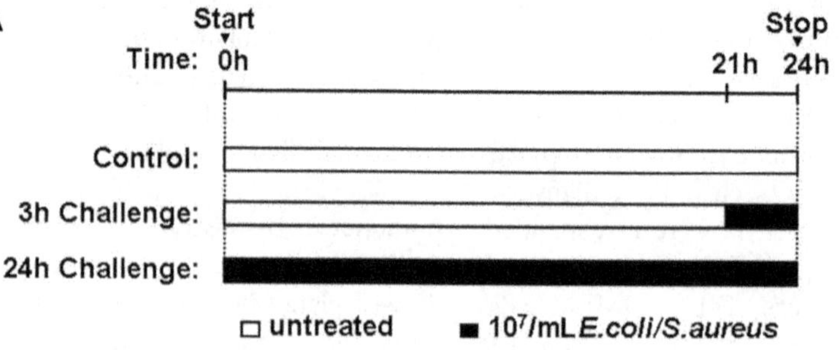

B

Microarray calculation	treatment				
	untreated	*E. coli*		*S. aureus*	
PMEC	controls	3 h	24 h	3 h	24 h
sow I	3x	3x	3x	3x	3x
sow II	3x	3x	3x	3x	3x
sow III	3x	3x	3x	3x	3x
					Σ 45 arrays

Figure 1 Schema of experimental setting. (A) Confluent PMEC cultures were challenged with 10^7/mL heat-inactivated *S. aureus* and *E. coli*, respectively, for 3 h and 24 h. In parallel unchallenged control cells were cultivated. After incubation periods, cells were collected and total RNA was isolated. **(B)** PMEC isolated from three lactating sows represent three biological replicates. Three technical replicates were analysed of each challenge (*S. aureus*, *E. coli*), unchallenged control and the two challenge times (3 h, 24 h), respectively. A total of 45 microarrays were obtained.

deposited in a MIAME-compliant database [14,15] (accession number: GSE64246).

Microarray data analysis

A microarray experiment was conducted in triplicate; three biological replicates were performed for each bacterial strain and experimental condition (3 h, 24 h, and control). A total of 45 microarrays were analysed (Figure 1B). Five experimental groups were built, including cells challenged with *E. coli* (3 hpc and 24 hpc), cells challenged with *S. aureus* (3 hpc and 24 hpc) and unchallenged control cells. Data pre-processing was done using Bioconductor/ R packages. After quality control [16], background correction and data normalization were performed using GC-RMA (Log2). To improve statistical power [17], inappropriate probe sets were excluded from further analysis due to three criteria: (i) probe sets absent in >50% of PMEC culture within each experimental group (MAS5 filtering); (ii) probe sets with a small standard deviation (SD < 0.2); (iii) probe sets with a small mean value (M < 2.5). A mixed-model analysis was performed using statistical analysis software (SAS, SAS Institute, Cary, NC, USA) to determine relative changes in mRNA levels, including effects mediated by experimental group and individual animal [$V_{ij} = \mu + \text{experimental group}_i + \text{animal}_j + e_{ij}$]. Corresponding q-values were calculated to estimate the proportion of false positives among all significant hypotheses and thus to correct for multiple testing [18]. Alterations in transcript abundances were considered to be statistically significant at $p < 0.05$ and $q < 0.05$. Subsequently, data was filtered by fold change (FC < −1.5; FC > 1.5). The Ensembl gene annotation (Sus scrofa 9) was used as previously described [19]. A principal component analysis (PCA) was performed in R to assess an overall trend about the gene expression data and inspection about outliers. Gene lists from microarray results (Additional files 1, 2, 3 and 4) were evaluated with Ingenuity Pathway Analysis (IPA, Ingenuity Systems, Redwood City, CA, USA) to identify most affected molecular and cellular functions, canonical pathways, upstream regulators, and functional networks ($p \leq 0.05$, Fisher's exact test).

Real-time quantitative PCR

First strand cDNA synthesis was performed with the same RNA samples used for the microarray analysis applying SuperScript III MMLV reverse transcriptase (Invitrogen, Karlsruhe, Germany) in a reaction containing 1 μg RNA, 500 ng oligo (dT)13VN primer and 500 ng random hexamer primers (Promega) according to the manufacturer's protocol. Real-time quantitative PCR (RT-qPCR) was performed in duplicate to validate the differential expression results. Quantification of mRNA copy numbers was performed on a LightCycler 480 System using the LightCycler 480 SYBR Green I Master (all Roche Applied Science). Sequences of the oligonucleotide primers used (Sigma-Aldrich) and amplicons are given in Additional file 5. The reaction conditions for PCR were as follows: initial denaturation step at 95 °C for 5 min and 45 cycles consisting of denaturation at 95 °C for 10 s, annealing at 60 °C for 15 s and extension/ fluorescence acquisition at 72 °C for 25 s. Melting curve analysis and agarose gel electrophoresis were performed after completion of the qPCR run to confirm specificity of the amplification and absence of primer dimers. Threshold cycles were converted to copy numbers using a standard curve generated by amplifying serial dilutions of an external PCR-generated standard (10^8–10^2 copies). The calculated copy numbers were normalized with a factor derived from expression of the reference genes *HPRT1* and *RN7SK* according to the method described by Vandesompele et al. [20]. Significance of differences was assessed with ANOVA. The results were declared to be statistically significant at $p < 0.05$. Spearman's Rank Correlation was used to compare microarray and RT-qPCR measurements using the SAS 9.3 software (SAS Institute, Inc., Cary, NC, USA).

Results

Morphological characterization of PMEC cultures

Heterogeneous population of epithelial, fibroblast-like, and adipose cells isolated from mammary glands of lactating sows were purified by continuous removal of non-epithelial cells by trypsin/EDTA treatment. Fibroblastic cells detached from their substratum, while epithelial cells were found to be more resistant. Most of the PMEC had a typical cobblestone shape and were connected tightly, visualized by phase contrast microscopy (Figure 2A). The purity of PMEC cultures was determined by immunocytochemistry. Cytokeratin elements of the PMEC cytoskeleton were stained with specific anti-cytokeratin-18 antibody. Almost all of the cells in our primary cell cultures were positive for cytokeratin-18 staining (~97%) confirming high purity of luminal epithelial cells (Figure 2B). Some cells were found negative for cytokeratin-18 staining, but positive for alpha-smooth muscle actin staining (~3%) with a specific antibody showing that only few myoepithelial cells were present in our PMEC cultures (Figure 2C). The homogeneity of our established PMEC cultures ensures clarity and reproducibility of the subsequent experimental results.

PMEC respond more prominently and earlier to challenge with E. coli than to challenge with S. aureus

Gene expression profiling of PMEC from three lactating sows was performed at 3 hpc and at 24 hpc with *E. coli* and *S. aureus*, respectively, in comparison with unchallenged control cells using Affymetrix Gene Chip® Porcine Genome Arrays. Filtering of raw data based on MAS5 algorithm and variability of expression of probe sets revealed 8494 probe sets for further analysis. A principal component analysis (PCA) showed that PMEC biological replicates were distantly clustered indicating individual differences, but had some similarity and reproducibility within the five experimental groups (Additional file 6). These were clustered into three distinct coloured groups (green dots: control; red dots: *E. coli*-challenge; blue dots: *S. aureus*-challenge) according to the density and consisting of three technical replicates, respectively. It was also shown that gene expression diverged most significantly with increasing challenge time (3 h to 24 h). No outliers were detected. Further data analysis showed that more genes were differentially expressed at 24 h compared to 3 h after pathogen challenge, and following challenge with *E. coli* compared to challenge with *S. aureus* (Figures 3A-D). Significant expression changes of 156 and 1250 genes were observed at 3 hpc and at 24 hpc with *E. coli*, respectively. The expressions of 73 and 1073 genes were altered at 3 hpc and at 24 hpc with *S. aureus*, respectively. Approximately 50% of the genes which were differentially expressed at 3 hpc with *S. aureus* also differed at 3 hpc with *E. coli* (Figure 3E). But 85% of the genes which were

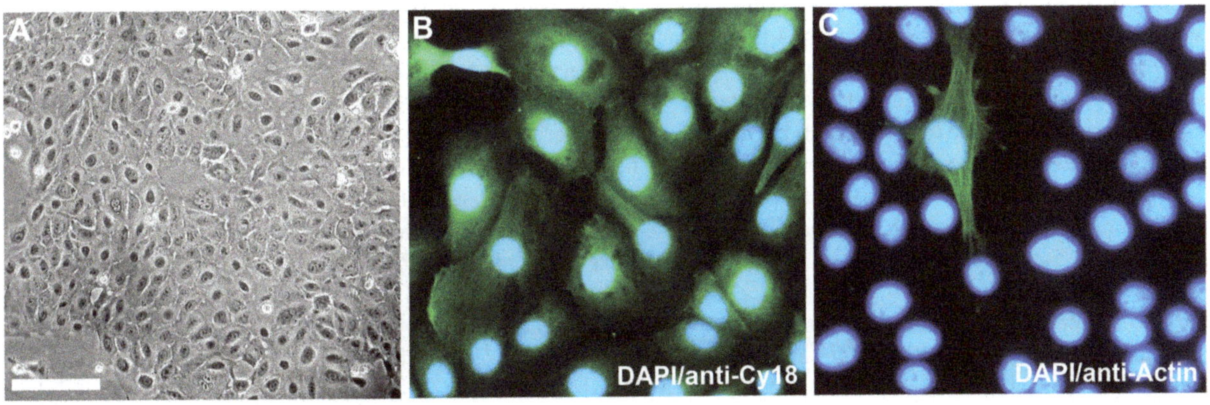

Figure 2 Validation of cell types in PMEC cultures. **(A)** Phase contrast micrograph of a confluent PMEC monolayer grown on collagen-coated tissue culture dishes demonstrating typical epithelial cobblestone morphology (bar = 100 μm). **(B)** Dominant luminal mammary epithelial cells were stained with anti-cytokeratin-18 antibody (anti-Cy18, green fluorescence; nuclei, DAPI, blue fluorescence). **(C)** Sporadically found myoepithelial cells were stained with anti-smooth muscle actin antibody (anti-Actin, green fluorescence; nuclei, DAPI, blue fluorescence).

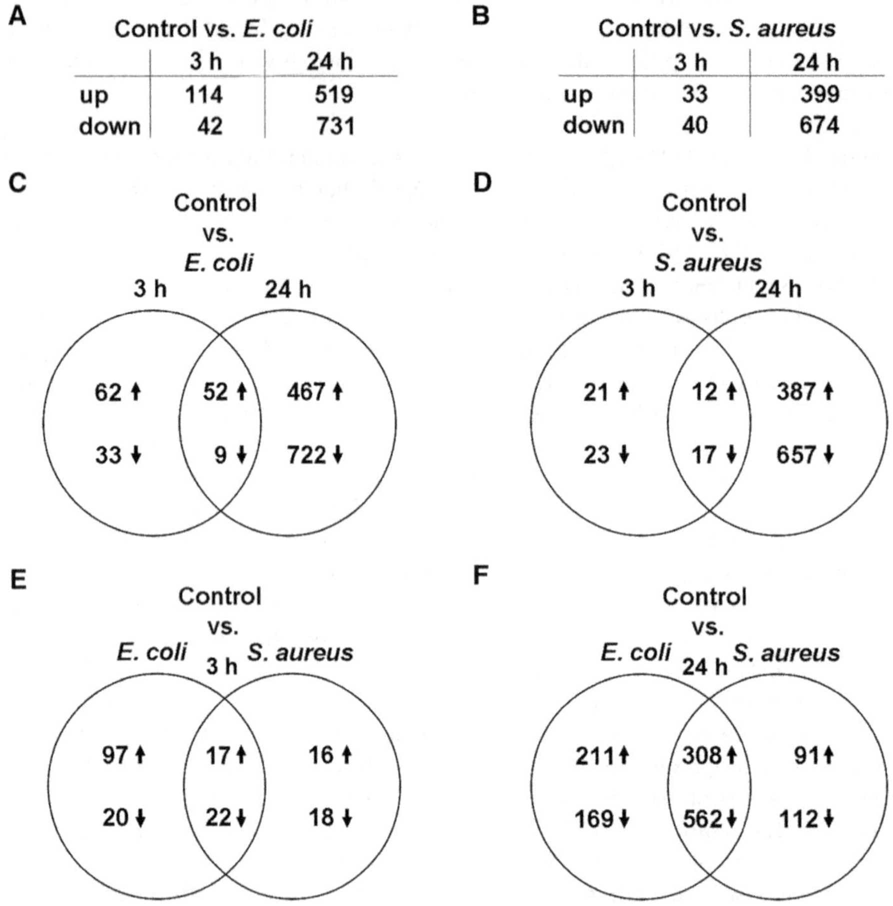

Figure 3 Significantly differentially expressed genes comparing *E. coli*-challenged and *S. aureus*-challenged PMEC. (A, B) More genes were differentially expressed at 24 h than at 3 h after pathogen challenge, and following challenge with *E. coli* than challenge with *S. aureus*. **(C-F)** Venn diagrams showing numbers of differentially expressed genes as a function of time and pathogen stimulus vs. untreated PMEC (control) of three independent biological replicates; $p < 0.05$, $q < 0.05$, $-1.5 > FC > 1.5$. The numbers in the intersections represent the genes differentially expressed in the two groups. The early response of PMEC to both pathogen species (3 hpc, **E**) was followed by a late, more intensive host response (24 hpc, **F**).

up-regulated at 3 hpc with *E. coli* were not found up-regulated at 3 hpc with *S. aureus* (Figure 3E). The early response of PMEC to both pathogen species (3 hpc) was followed by a late more intensive host response (24 hpc) as indicated by an 8-fold and 14-fold increase of differentially expressed genes at 24 hpc with *E. coli* and *S. aureus*, respectively (Figures 3A-D). However, the number of shared up- and down-regulated genes was increased up to a maximum of 80% at 24 hpc with both pathogen species (Figure 3F).

Molecular and cellular functions predominantly affected in PMEC by *E. coli* and *S. aureus* are different at 3 h, but similar at 24 h post-challenge

Top five categories of molecular and cellular functions which were affected in PMEC at 3 hpc and at 24 hpc with *E. coli* or *S. aureus* were identified using Ingenuity Pathway Analysis (IPA) software (Table 1). At 3 hpc with *E. coli*, most of the differentially expressed genes in PMEC were categorized by functions comprising "gene expression", "cellular movement", "cellular growth and proliferation", "cellular development", and "cell death and survival". Except for the two first named categories, all other molecular and cellular functions are also affected in cells at 24 hpc with *E. coli*. Additionally, at the same time, differentially expressed genes associated with "RNA post-transcriptional modification" and "cell cycle" were affected by challenge with *E. coli*. In contrast, at 3 hpc of PMEC with *S. aureus*, most differentially expressed genes were categorized by functions comprising "small molecule biochemistry", "drug metabolism", "lipid metabolism", "vitamin and mineral metabolism", and "energy production". Genes belonging to these functional categories were also affected at 3 hpc with *E. coli*, but were not predominantly involved in the early response of PMEC to this pathogen as well as

Table 1 Molecular and cellular functions affected in PMEC by pathogen challenge

3 h *E. coli*-challenged vs. unchallenged control cells	*p*-value	#Molecules
Gene Expression	1.72E-14 - 1.71E-04	46
Cellular Growth and Proliferation	3.56E-14 - 3.13E-04	55
Cellular Development	1.46E-13 - 3.95E-04	52
Cell Death and Survival	1.29E-11 - 3.95E-04	50
Cellular movement	4.13E-11 - 3.95E-04	40
3 h *S. aureus*-challenged vs. unchallenged control cells	***p*-value**	**#Molecules**
Small Molecule Biochemistry	4.30E-08 - 4.53E-03	14
Drug Metabolism	2.15E-07 - 4.53E-03	8
Lipid Metabolism	2.15E-07 - 4.53E-03	11
Vitamin and Mineral Metabolism	2.15E-07 - 3.39E-03	4
Energy Production	8.97E-07 - 2.27E-03	4
24 h *E. coli*-challenged vs. unchallenged control cells	***p*-value**	**#Molecules**
Cellular Growth and Proliferation	1.46E-15 - 5.35E-03	255
RNA Post-Transcriptional Modification	3.21E-14 - 4.88E-03	53
Cell Cycle	1.46E-12 - 4.88E-03	115
Cell Death and Survival	7.44E-10 - 5.09E-03	226
Cellular Development	4.90E-08 - 5.35E-03	219
24 h *S. aureus*-challenged vs. unchallenged control cells	***p*-value**	**#Molecules**
RNA Post-Transcriptional Modification	9.24E-15 - 1.62E-02	42
Cell Cycle	8.61E-10 - 1.62E-02	95
Cellular Growth and Proliferation	8.88E-10 - 1.37E-02	202
Cell Death and Survival	4.29E-08 - 1.62E-02	187
Gene Expression	3.25E-07 - 6.69E-03	156

Top five categories of molecular and cellular functions affected in PMEC at 3 h and at 24 h post-challenge with *E. coli* and *S. aureus*, respectively, compared with unchallenged control cells with their respective *p*-value and number of molecules included in each class obtained from IPA software.

in the late response of cells (24 hpc) to both *E. coli* and *S. aureus*.

Similar late response effects in terms of most affected with molecular and cellular functions comprising "RNA post-transcriptional modification", "cell cycle", "cellular growth and proliferation" and "cell death and survival" were apparent in PMEC at 24 hpc with *E. coli* and *S. aureus*, respectively, compared with unchallenged control cells. In contrast, differentially expressed genes associated with "cellular development" or "gene expression" were most affected by long-term challenge (24 h) with *E. coli* and *S. aureus*, respectively. Overall, PMEC are more responsive to the challenge with *E. coli* than *S. aureus* as early as 3 hpc and as late as 24 hpc in term of the number of differentially expressed genes involved in molecular and cellular functions (243 vs 41 at 3 hpc; 868 vs 682 at 24 hpc, see also Table 1).

Genes of different canonical pathways are involved in response of PMEC to pathogen challenge dependent on pathogen species and incubation time

At 3 hpc, IPA analysis identified 250 canonical pathways affected by the challenge with *E. coli* compared to 170 pathways by *S. aureus*. After long-term challenge (24 h) of PMEC with *E. coli* or *S. aureus* 295 and 267 canonical pathways were affected, respectively.

The most prominent genes which were significantly up-regulated in PMEC at 3 hpc with *E. coli* encode pro-inflammatory cytokines and chemokines (chemokine (C-C motif) ligand 2, CCL2; chemokine (C-X-C motif) ligands CXCL1, CXCL2, CXCL3, and CXCL6; interleukin 1 alpha, IL1A), cell adhesion proteins (vascular cell adhesion molecule 1, VCAM1; intercellular adhesion molecule, ICAM1; integrin beta 3, ITGB3), and interferon signaling proteins (interferon-induced protein with tetratricopeptide repeats, IFIT1 and IFIT3; interferon receptors, IFNAR1 and IFNAR2) responsible for pathogen recognition by granulocytes and the first line of host defense against bacterial infection (Table 2).

Consistent with the up-regulation of the metabolism and degradation of various substrates (bupropion, acetone, nicotine, and melatonin) and estrogen biosynthesis in PMEC at 3 hpc with *S. aureus*, the most represented up-regulated genes involved in these canonical pathways are *cytochrome P450, family 1, subfamily A, polypeptide 1*

Table 2 Up-regulated canonical pathways in PMEC at 3 hpc

***E. coli*-challenged vs. unchallenged control cells**	
Canonical pathway (Genes involved in pathway)	***p*-value**
Granulocyte Adhesion and Diapedesis (*CXCL3,IL1A,VCAM1,ICAM1,CCL2,CLDN1,CXCL1,CXCL2,IL1RAP, CXCL6,ITGB3*)	8.52E-11
Interferon Signaling (*IFIT3,IFIT1,JAK2,IFNAR2,IFNAR1,IRF1*)	4.11E-09
Agranulocyte Adhesion and Diapedesis (*CXCL3,IL1A,VCAM1,ICAM1,CCL2,CLDN1,CXCL1,CXCL2,CXCL6*)	4.92E-08
Hepatic Fibrosis/Hepatic Stellate Cell Activation (*CXCL3,IL1A,VCAM1,ICAM1,CCL2,IFNAR2,IL1RAP,IFNAR1*)	8.20E-08
Role of IL-17A in arthritis (*CXCL3,NFKBIA,CCL2,CXCL1,CXCL6*)	2.43E-06
***S. aureus*-challenged vs. unchallenged control cells**	
Canonical pathway (Genes involved in pathway)	***p*-value**
Bupropion Degradation	3.44E-06
Acetone Degradation I (to Methylglyoxal)	3.86E-06
Estrogen Biosynthesis	1.11E-05
Nicotine Degradation III	2.87E-05
Melatonin Degradation I (*CYP1A1,CYP3A4,CYP1B1 are involved in all five canonical pathways*)	3.39E 05

Top five categories of up-regulated canonical pathways in PMEC at 3 hpc with *E. coli* and *S. aureus*, respectively, compared with unchallenged control cells with their respective *p*-value and genes involved in each pathway obtained from IPA software.

(*CYP1A1*), *CYP3A4* and *CYP1B1* encoding monooxygenases (Table 2).

Furthermore, most of the significantly up-regulated canonical pathways, which were identified in PMEC at 3 hpc with *E. coli* were also up-regulated at 24 hpc with *E. coli* (Tables 2 and 3). For example, "interferon signalling" was also one of the top up-regulated canonical pathways in PMEC at 24 hpc with *S. aureus* (Table 3).

In addition, at 24 hpc of PMEC with *E. coli* genes involved in inflammatory response signaling pathways such as "HMGB1 signaling" were significantly up-regulated, and at 24 hpc with *S. aureus* genes regulating cell growth, proliferation, apoptosis and activation of natural killer cells were significantly up-regulated (Table 3).

Genes encoding growth factors (bone morphogenic protein 2, BMP2 and BMP4) as well as different transcription factors (FBJ murine osteosarcoma viral oncogene homolog, FOS; jun proto-oncogene, JUN; vav3 guanine nucleotide exchange factor, VAV3; early growth response 1, EGR1) involved in BMP, IL-2 and TGF-beta signaling pathways are significantly down-regulated at 3 hpc with *E. coli* (Table 4). "Differential regulation of cytokine production in macrophages and T helper cells by IL-17A and IL-17 F" and "MIF regulation of innate immunity" are some of the top five significantly down-regulated canonical pathways, critically involved in early response (3 hpc) of PMEC to challenge with *S. aureus* and which are different from early response (3 hpc) of the cells to *E. coli* (Table 4). The most prominent down-regulated genes, which are involved in almost all of these pathways, encode transcription factor FOS and the cytokines colony stimulating factor 2 (CSF2) and CXCL1.

Canonical pathways regulating cell cycle and protein ubiquitination are some of the top five significantly down-regulated canonical pathways, which were mostly affected in PMEC at 24 hpc with *E. coli* as well as at 24 hpc with *S. aureus* (Table 5). Genes involved in these pathways encode heat shock proteins (DnaJ (Hsp40) homolog, subfamily C, member 9, DNAJC9; DNAJC11; DnaJ (Hsp40) homolog, subfamily A, member 1,

Table 3 Up-regulated canonical pathways in PMEC at 24 hpc

Canonical pathway (Genes involved in pathway)	*p*-value
***E. coli*-challenged vs. unchallenged control cells**	
Interferon Signaling (*IFIT3,IFIT1,PTPN2,MX1,TYK2,JAK2,STAT1,TAP1,IRF1*)	1.31E-06
Hepatic Fibrosis/Hepatic Stellate Cell Activation (*CXCL3,VCAM1,IL1A,CTGF,CCL2,ICAM1,FGF2,IGFBP3,TGFA, IGF1R,FGFR2,STAT1,FAS,COL3A1*)	4.17E-06
Granulocyte Adhesion and Diapedesis (*HRH1,CXCL3,VCAM1,IL1A,MMP7,ICAM1,SDC1,CLDN8, CCL2,CLDN1,CCL28,CXCL1,CXCL2,CXCL6,ITGB3*)	7.71E-06
Agranulocyte Adhesion and Diapedesis (*CXCL3,HRH1,VCAM1,IL1A,MMP7,ICAM1,CLDN8,CCL2, CLDN1,CCL28,CXCL1,CXCL2,CXCL6*)	6.97E-05
HMGB1 Signaling (*MAP2K6,PIK3R3,FOS,IL1A,VCAM1,ICAM1, RHOQ,CCL2,DIRAS3,FNBP1,KAT6B*)	1.75E-04
***S. aureus*-challenged vs. unchallenged control cells**	
Canonical pathway (Genes involved in pathway)	***p*-value**
Interferon Signaling (*IFIT3,IFIT1,PTPN2,TYK2,JAK2,BCL2*)	8.94E-04
Growth Hormone Signaling (*PIK3R3,FOS,SOCS6,IGF1R,IGFBP3,RPS6KA5,SOCS4,JAK2, PRKCZ,PRKD1*)	1.89E-03
Hepatic Fibrosis/Hepatic Stellate Cell Activation (*VCAM1,CTGF,IGF1R,IGFBP3,FGFR2,SERPINE1,COL3A1,BCL2*)	2.09E-03
Thrombopoietin Signaling (*PIK3R3,FOS,IRS2,JAK2,PRKCZ,PRKD1*)	5.34E-03
IGF-1 Signaling (*PIK3R3,FOS,YWHAG,CTGF,SOCS6,IGF1R,IGFBP3,IRS2,SOCS4, JAK2,PRKCZ*)	7.80E-03

Top five categories of up-regulated canonical pathways in PMEC at 24 hpc with *E. coli* and *S. aureus*, respectively, compared with unchallenged control cells with their respective *p*-value and genes involved in each pathway obtained from IPA software.

Table 4 Down-regulated canonical pathways in PMEC at 3 hpc

Canonical pathway (Genes involved in pathway)	*p*-value
***E. coli*-challenged vs. unchallenged control cells**	
BMP signaling pathway (*SOSTDC1,JUN,BMP4,BMP2*)	1.27E-04
Regulation of IL-2 Expression in Activated and Anergic T Lymphocytes (*FOS,JUN,NFKBIA,VAV3*)	1.55E-04
TGF-b Signaling (*FOS,JUN,BMP4,BMP2*)	1.79E-04
T Cell Receptor Signaling (*FOS,JUN,NFKBIA,VAV3*)	2.84E-04
PKCq Signaling in T Lymphocytes (*FOS,JUN,NFKBIA,VAV3,MAP3K8*)	4.80E-04
***S. aureus*-challenged vs. unchallenged control cells**	
Canonical pathway (Genes involved in pathway)	***p*-value**
Differential Regulation of Cytokine Production in Macrophages and T Helper Cells by IL-17A and IL-17 F (*CXCL1,CSF2*)	1.75E-04
Role of Tissue Factor in Cancer (*EGR1,CXCL1,JAK2,CSF2*)	2.35E-04
Differential Regulation of Cytokine Production in Intestinal Epithelial Cells by IL-17A and IL-17 F (*CXCL1,CSF2*)	2.88E-04
IL-17A Signaling in Gastric Cells (*FOS,CXCL1*)	3.42E-04
MIF Regulation of Innate Immunity (*FOS,PTGS2*)	9.24E-04

Top five categories of down-regulated canonical pathways in PMEC at 3 hpc with *E. coli* and *S. aureus*, respectively, compared with unchallenged control cells with their respective p-value and genes involved in each pathway obtained from IPA software.

Table 5 Down-regulated canonical pathways in PMEC at 24 hpc

E. coli-challenged vs. unchallenged control cells	
Canonical pathway (Genes involved in pathway)	***p*-value**
Estrogen-mediated S-phase Entry (*CCNA2,E2F4,CCNE1,TFDP1,E2F1,CDK2*)	1.84E-05
Protein Ubiquitination Pathway (*USP28,PSMB9,DNAJC9,MED20,HSPA1A/HSPA1B,HSPH1, UBE2N,UBE2R2,HSPA6,CDC23,UBE2S,DNAJA1,HSPA5,TAP1, DNAJC11,USP31,USP3,PSMD12,USP46,USP34,BIRC*)	5.29E-04
Adenine and Adenosine Salvage I (*PNP*)	5.89E-04
Phosphatidylglycerol Biosynthesis II (Non-plastidic) (*GPAM,ABHD5,PTPMT1,MBOAT2*)	6.36E-04
Cell Cycle: G1/S Checkpoint Regulation (*E2F4,CCNE1,CCND2,TFDP1,E2F1,GNL3,CDK2*)	7.40E-04
***S. aureus*-challenged vs. unchallenged control cells**	
Canonical pathway (Genes involved in pathway)	***p*-value**
Phosphatidylglycerol Biosynthesis II (Non-plastidic) (*GPAM,ABHD5,PTPMT1,MBOAT2*)	4.27E-04
Protein Ubiquitination Pathway (*DNAJC9,HSPA1A/HSPA1B,HSPH1,UBE2N,UBE2R2,HSPA6, DNAJC25,CDC23,UBE2S,DNAJA1,HSPA5,DNAJC11, PSMD12,USP46,USP34*)	5.14E-04
Aldosterone Signaling in Epithelial Cells (*ICMT,DNAJC9,HSPA1A/HSPA1B,HSPH1,HSPA6,DNAJC25, DNAJA1,HSPA5,PRKCZ,DNAJC11,PIK3R3,SCNN1G,PRKD1*)	5.21E-04
Estrogen-mediated S-phase Entry (*E2F4,CCNE1,TFDP1,E2F1*)	1.69E-03
Vitamin-C Transport (*SLC2A1,TXN,TXNRD1*)	3.15E-03

Top five categories of down-regulated canonical pathways in PMEC at 24 hpc with *E. coli* and *S. aureus*, respectively, compared with unchallenged control cells with their respective *p*-value and genes involved in each pathway obtained from IPA software.

DNAJA1; heat shock 70 kDa protein 1A/1B, HSPA1A/HSPA1B; heat shock 70 kDa protein 6, HSPA6; heat shock 105 kDa/110 kDa protein 1, HSPH1), cell cycle and cell growth regulating proteins (cell division cycle 23, CDC23; ubiquitin-conjugating enzyme E2S, UBE2S; ubiquitin-conjugating enzyme E2R2, UBE2R2) and ubiquitin specific peptidases (USP34, USP46) (Table 5).

"iNOS signalling" is one of the top five shared canonical pathways, which was affected at 3 hpc with *E. coli* and *S. aureus*, respectively (data not shown), indicating the production of radical effectors of the innate immune system to eliminate invading pathogens. The top five shared canonical pathways, which were affected at 24 hpc with the respective pathogens, include Janus kinase 2 (JAK2), insulin-like growth factor 1 (IGF-1) and signal transducer and activator of transcription 3 (STAT3) signaling indicating the activation of cytokine-mediated immune response and regulatory effects on cell proliferation, apoptosis and migration (data not shown).

Different upstream regulators are involved in response of PMEC to the challenge with *E. coli* or *S. aureus*

Using IPA, we considered the top five upstream regulators when comparing pathogen challenged vs. unchallenged PMEC. We found considerable overlap in the identity and direction of activation of these upstream regulators between the compared data sets.

"IL1B" (interleukin-1 beta), "lipopolysaccharide", "IRAK4" (interleukin-1 receptor-associated kinase 4), "TNF" (tumor necrosis factor) and "cycloheximide" are the top five upstream regulators during the early response (3 hpc) of cells to *E. coli* (Table 6). In contrast, at 3 hpc of cells with *S. aureus*, "beta-estradiol", "ESR1" (estrogen receptor 1), "U0126" (1,4-diamino-2,3-dicyano-1,4-bis[2-aminophenylthio] butadiene), "3-methylcholanthrene" and "paclitaxel" are the top five upstream regulators associated with host-pathogen interaction (Table 6). While upstream regulators of the early response (3 hpc) of PMEC to *E. coli* and *S. aureus* are completely different from another, at 24 hpc with the respective pathogen species, "RAF1" (proto-oncogene serine/threonine-protein kinase 1) and "PD98059" (2'-Amino-3'-methoxyflavone) were involved in both host-pathogen interactions. Furthermore, "IKBKB" (inhibitor of kappa light polypeptide gene enhancer in B-cells, kinase beta), "TGFB1" (transforming growth factor beta 1), "HGF" (hepatocyte growth factor) and "E2F1" (E2F transcription factor 1), "TP53" (tumor protein p53), "INSR" (insulin receptor) were considered as the top upstream regulators in PMEC at 24 hpc with *E. coli* and *S. aureus*, respectively (Table 6). The identified transcriptional upstream regulators affect the observed gene expression patterns after pathogen stimulation and control the complex cellular response mechanisms e.g. proliferation, apoptosis, migration and cell cycle progression to fine-tune the innate immune response of PMEC (Table 6).

Different genes are involved in "inflammatory response" of PMEC challenged with *E. coli* or *S. aureus*

With particular focus on differentially expressed genes annotated by IPA as signaling molecules involved in "inflammatory response", heatmaps were generated to illustrate the details of the defense mechanisms of PMEC to challenge with *E. coli* or *S. aureus*.

Our data show that more inflammatory response genes were up- and down-regulated at 24 h than at 3 h after pathogen challenge, and following challenge with *E. coli* than challenge with *S. aureus* (Figures 4A and B). In the early inflammatory response (3 hpc) of the cells to *E. coli* 40 genes were involved, mainly encoding cytokines, enzymes, transcription regulators and transmembrane receptors (Figure 4A). Most of these genes were up-regulated (maximum FC 6.68) rather than down-regulated (minimum FC −1.84). Only nine inflammatory response genes were affected at 3 hpc of the cells with

Table 6 Upstream regulators and their biological functions

3 h *E. coli*-challenged vs. unchallenged control cells	*p*-value of overlap
IL1B (proinflammatory; proliferation; differentiation; apoptosis)	6.80E-23
lipopolysaccharide (increase of TLR4 expression; innate immune response)	8.75E-22
IRAK4 (activation of NF-kB; innate immune response)	6.93E-21
TNF (proinflammat.; proliferation; differentiation; apoptosis; lipid metabolism; coagulation)	1.17E-20
cycloheximide (inhibitor of protein synthesis; apoptosis, cell death)	3.04E-20
3 h *S. aureus*-challenged vs. unchallenged control cells	***p*-value of overlap**
beta-estradiol (proliferation; growth; apoptosis; breast cancer signaling)	1.20E-10
ESR1 (growth; proliferation; transcription; transactivation)	2.00E-09
U0126 (inhibitor of MAP kinase kinase; apoptosis; proliferation; migration)	3.74E-09
3-methylcholanthrene (carcinogen; transformation; proliferation)	1.59E-08
paclitaxel (antimitotic; apoptosis; growth; survival; cell viability)	2.55E-08
24 h *E. coli*-challenged vs. unchallenged control cells	***p*-value of overlap**
PD98059 (inhibitor of MAP kinase kinase; apoptosis; proliferation; migration)	1.98E-11
IKBKB (activation of NF-kB; apoptosis; proliferation)	8.45E-11
TGFB1 (proliferation; differentiation; adhesion; migration; apoptosis; growth)	1.47E-10
RAF1 (activation of MEK1/2; apoptosis; proliferation; differentiation; cell cycle; migration)	1.90E-10
HGF (activation of tyrosine kinases; migration; proliferation; scattering; apoptosis; growth)	9.20E-10
24 h *S. aureus*-challenged vs. unchallenged control cells	***p*-value of overlap**
RAF1 (activation of MEK1/2; apoptosis; proliferation; differentiation; cell cycle; migration)	2.30E-09
E2F1 (apoptosis; proliferation; cell cycle)	3.32E-08
TP53 (tumor suppressor; apoptosis; cell cycle; growth; proliferation)	3.45E-07
INSR (proliferation; growth; differentiation; migration; mitogenesis)	9.61E-07
PD98059 (inhibitor of MAP kinase kinase; apoptosis; proliferation; migration)	1.24E-06

Top five categories of upstream regulators and their functions in PMEC at 3 hpc and at 24 hpc with *E. coli* and *S. aureus*, respectively, compared with unchallenged control cells with their respective *p*-value of overlap in each class obtained from IPA software.

S. aureus (Figure 4A). Equal amounts of these genes were up- and down-regulated (maximum FC 3.38; minimum FC −2.17) and most of them encode enzymes, cytokines and transcription regulators. Four out of the nine genes affected by challenge with *S. aureus* were also affected by challenge with *E. coli*.

In the late inflammatory response (24 hpc) of the cells to *E. coli* 70 genes were involved, mainly encoding enzymes, cytokines, transmembrane receptors, transcription regulators and kinases (Figure 4B). Equal amounts of these genes were up- and down-regulated (maximum FC 7.87; minimum FC −2.51). In contrast, only 17 inflammatory response genes were affected at 24 hpc of the cells with *S. aureus*, mainly encoding enzymes, kinases, transmembrane receptors, transcription regulators and G-protein coupled receptors (Figure 4B). Moreover, equal amounts of these genes were up- and down-regulated (maximum FC 2.38; minimum FC -4.28). Eleven of the 17 genes involved in late inflammatory response of the cells to *S. aureus* were also affected by challenge with *E. coli*.

Gene network analysis revealed different key molecules regulating defense mechanisms of PMEC against *E. coli* and *S. aureus*

Gene interactions were examined using IPA based on the known contributions of genes to regulatory networks in order to identify key regulators of the specific immune response of PMEC to pathogen challenge. The analysis was focused on the top 50 up-regulated and the top 50 down-regulated genes at 3 hpc and at 24 hpc with *E. coli* and *S. aureus*. Figure 5 shows that the networks of key regulatory genes associated with host response to challenge with *E. coli* are more complex than that of challenge with *S. aureus*. Especially at 3 hpc with *E. coli* a wider range of cytokines and growth factors were induced (Figure 5A) compared to 3 h challenge with *S. aureus* (Figure 5B). Our results indicated key regulatory functions of *IL1A*, *CXCL2*, *NFKBIA*, *mitogen-activated protein kinase kinase kinase 8* (*MAP3K8*), *JUN*, *FOS* and *EGR1* within a network consisting of 32 response genes of PMEC at 3 hpc with *E. coli*. In contrast, a network consisting of 14 response genes at 3 hpc with *S. aureus* was created with *CSF2*, *prostaglandin-endoperoxide synthase 2* (*PTGS2*), *FOS* and *EGR1* as key regulators. Furthermore, *CXCL1*, *CYP1B1*, *dual specificity phosphatase 6* (*DUSP6*), *FOS* and *EGR1* were affected in PMEC at 3 hpc with both pathogens.

Tumor necrosis factor (ligand) superfamily, member 10 (*TNFSF10*), *NFKBIA*, and *FOS* were found to be key regulators within a network consisting of 22 response genes at 24 hpc of PMEC with *E. coli* (Figure 5C). In contrast, a network consisting of 17 response genes at 24 hpc with *S. aureus* was created with *CSF2*, *FOS* and *proliferating cell nuclear antigen* (*PCNA*) as key regulators (Figure 5D). *VCAM1*, *MAP2K6*, *CYP1B1*, *leucyl-tRNA synthetase* (*LARS*), *proteasome activator subunit 3* (*PSME3*), *CDC6* and *FOS* were affected in PMEC at 24 hpc with both pathogens. Almost all of the named key regulatory genes, which were involved in defense mechanisms of PMEC against *E. coli* and *S. aureus* are categorized by IPA as genes of "inflammatory response".

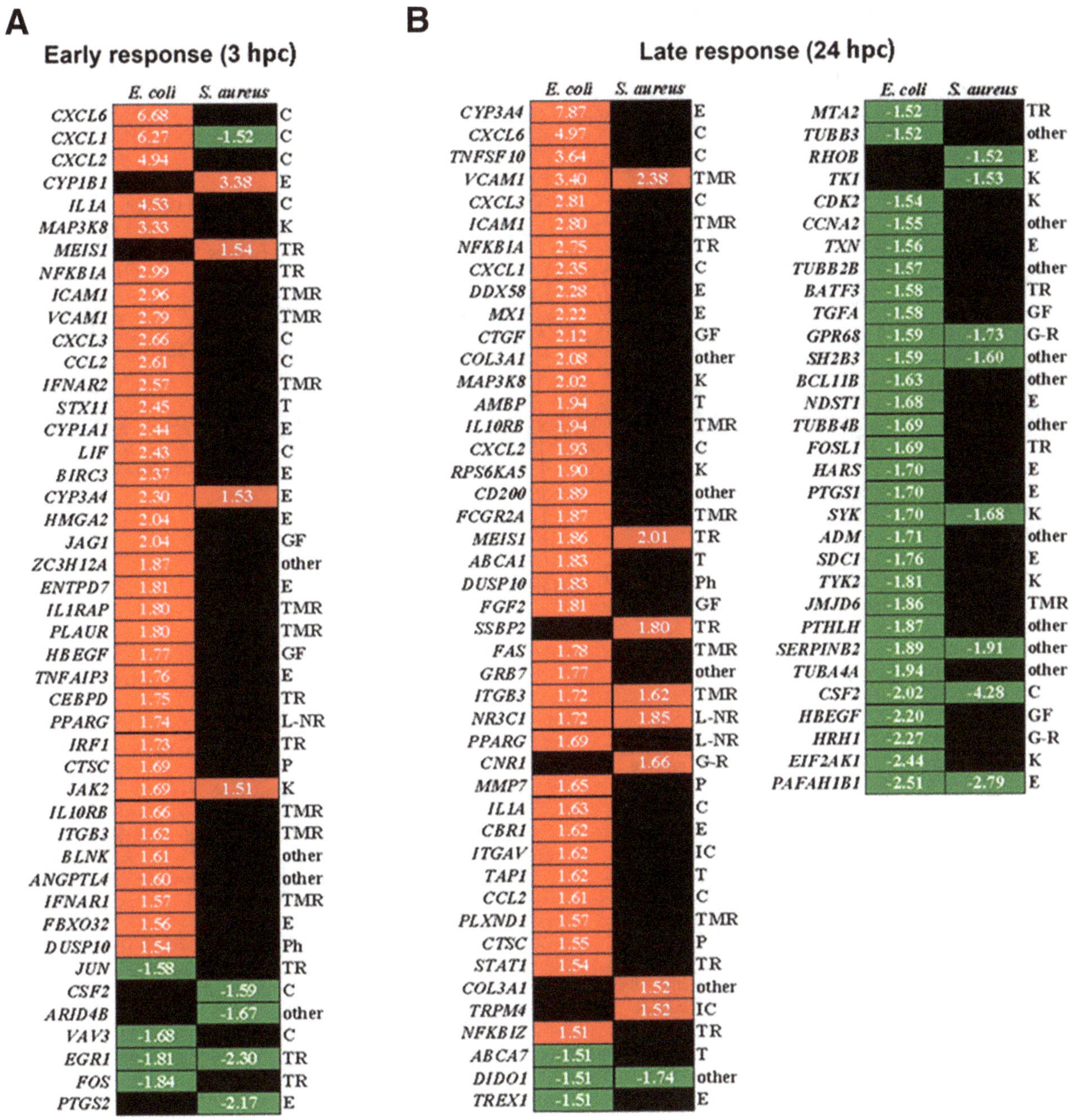

A
Early response (3 hpc)
E. coli S. aureus
CXCL6 6.68 C
CXCL1 6.27 -1.52 C
CXCL2 4.94 C
CYP1B1 3.38 E
IL1A 4.53 C
MAP3K8 3.33 K
MEIS1 1.54 TR
NFKBIA 2.99 TR
ICAM1 2.96 TMR
VCAM1 2.79 TMR
CXCL3 2.66 C
CCL2 2.61 C
IFNAR2 2.57 TMR
STX11 2.45 T
CYP1A1 2.44 E
LIF 2.43 C
BIRC3 2.37 E
CYP3A4 2.30 1.53 E
HMGA2 2.04 E
JAG1 2.04 GF
ZC3H12A 1.87 other
ENTPD7 1.81 E
IL1RAP 1.80 TMR
PLAUR 1.80 TMR
HBEGF 1.77 GF
TNFAIP3 1.76 E
CEBPD 1.75 TR
PPARG 1.74 L-NR
IRF1 1.73 TR
CTSC 1.69 P
JAK2 1.69 1.51 K
IL10RB 1.66 TMR
ITGB3 1.62 TMR
BLNK 1.61 other
ANGPTL4 1.60 other
IFNAR1 1.57 TMR
FBXO32 1.56 E
DUSP10 1.54 Ph
JUN -1.58 TR
CSF2 -1.59 C
ARID4B -1.67 other
VAV3 -1.68 C
EGR1 -1.81 -2.30 TR
FOS -1.84 TR
PTGS2 -2.17 E
B
Late response (24 hpc)
E. coli S. aureus
CYP3A4 7.87 E
CXCL6 4.97 C
TNFSF10 3.64 C
VCAM1 3.40 2.38 TMR
CXCL3 2.81 C
ICAM1 2.80 TMR
NFKBIA 2.75 TR
CXCL1 2.35 C
DDX58 2.28 E
MX1 2.22 E
CTGF 2.12 GF
COL3A1 2.08 other
MAP3K8 2.02 K
AMBP 1.94 T
IL10RB 1.94 TMR
CXCL2 1.93 C
RPS6KA5 1.90 K
CD200 1.89 other
FCGR2A 1.87 TMR
MEIS1 1.86 2.01 TR
ABCA1 1.83 T
DUSP10 1.83 Ph
FGF2 1.81 GF
SSBP2 1.80 TR
FAS 1.78 TMR
GRB7 1.77 other
ITGB3 1.72 1.62 TMR
NR3C1 1.72 1.85 L-NR
PPARG 1.69 L-NR
CNR1 1.66 G-R
MMP7 1.65 P
IL1A 1.63 C
CBR1 1.62 E
ITGAV 1.62 IC
TAP1 1.62 T
CCL2 1.61 C
PLXND1 1.57 TMR
CTSC 1.55 P
STAT1 1.54 TR
COL3A1 1.52 other
TRPM4 1.52 IC
NFKBIZ 1.51 TR
ABCA7 -1.51 T
DIDO1 -1.51 -1.74 other
TREX1 -1.51 E
E. coli S. aureus
MTA2 -1.52 TR
TUBB3 -1.52 other
RHOB -1.52 E
TK1 -1.53 K
CDK2 -1.54 K
CCNA2 -1.55 other
TXN -1.56 E
TUBB2B -1.57 other
BATF3 -1.58 TR
TGFA -1.58 GF
GPR68 -1.59 -1.73 G-R
SH2B3 -1.59 -1.60 other
BCL11B -1.63 other
NDST1 -1.68 E
TUBB4B -1.69 other
FOSL1 -1.69 TR
HARS -1.70 E
PTGS1 -1.70 E
SYK -1.70 -1.68 K
ADM -1.71 other
SDC1 -1.76 E
TYK2 -1.81 K
JMJD6 -1.86 TMR
PTHLH -1.87 other
SERPINB2 -1.89 -1.91 other
TUBA4A -1.94 other
CSF2 -2.02 -4.28 C
HBEGF -2.20 GF
HRH1 -2.27 G-R
EIF2AK1 -2.44 K
PAFAH1B1 -2.51 -2.79 E

Figure 4 Differentially expressed genes associated with "inflammatory response" in PMEC after pathogen challenge. Heat maps show differentially expressed genes annotated by IPA and grouped according to their maximal altered mRNA concentrations as well as a function of challenge time (red, up-regulated; green, down-regulated; fold changes are given inside the boxes). **(A)** More genes were affected at 3 hpc (early response) with *E. coli* (40 genes) than with *S. aureus* (9 genes). **(B)** The majority of differentially expressed genes of PMEC was also involved in late response (24 hpc) to challenge with *E. coli* (70 genes) than to challenge with *S. aureus* (17 genes). Gene functions according to the IPA annotation are given to the right. The affected inflammatory response genes encoding cytokines (C), enzymes (E), kinases (K), transcription regulators (TR), transmembrane receptors (TMR), transporter (T), growth factors (GF), ligand-dependent nuclear receptors (L-NR), peptidases (P), phosphatases (Ph), G-protein coupled receptors (G-R) and ion channel proteins (IC).

Validation of selected key transcripts by RT-qPCR

In order to validate the microarray experiment, eight selected key transcripts encoding cytokines (IL1A, CXCL2, CCL2, TNFSF10, and CSF2), kinase (MAP3K8), transcription regulator (NFKBIA) and transmembrane receptor (VCAM1) associated with "inflammatory response" were analysed by RT-qPCR (Additional file 7). Between microarray and RT-qPCR data the correlation coefficients were highly significant and ranged between 0.84 and 0.98 for the selected genes. The RT-qPCR data

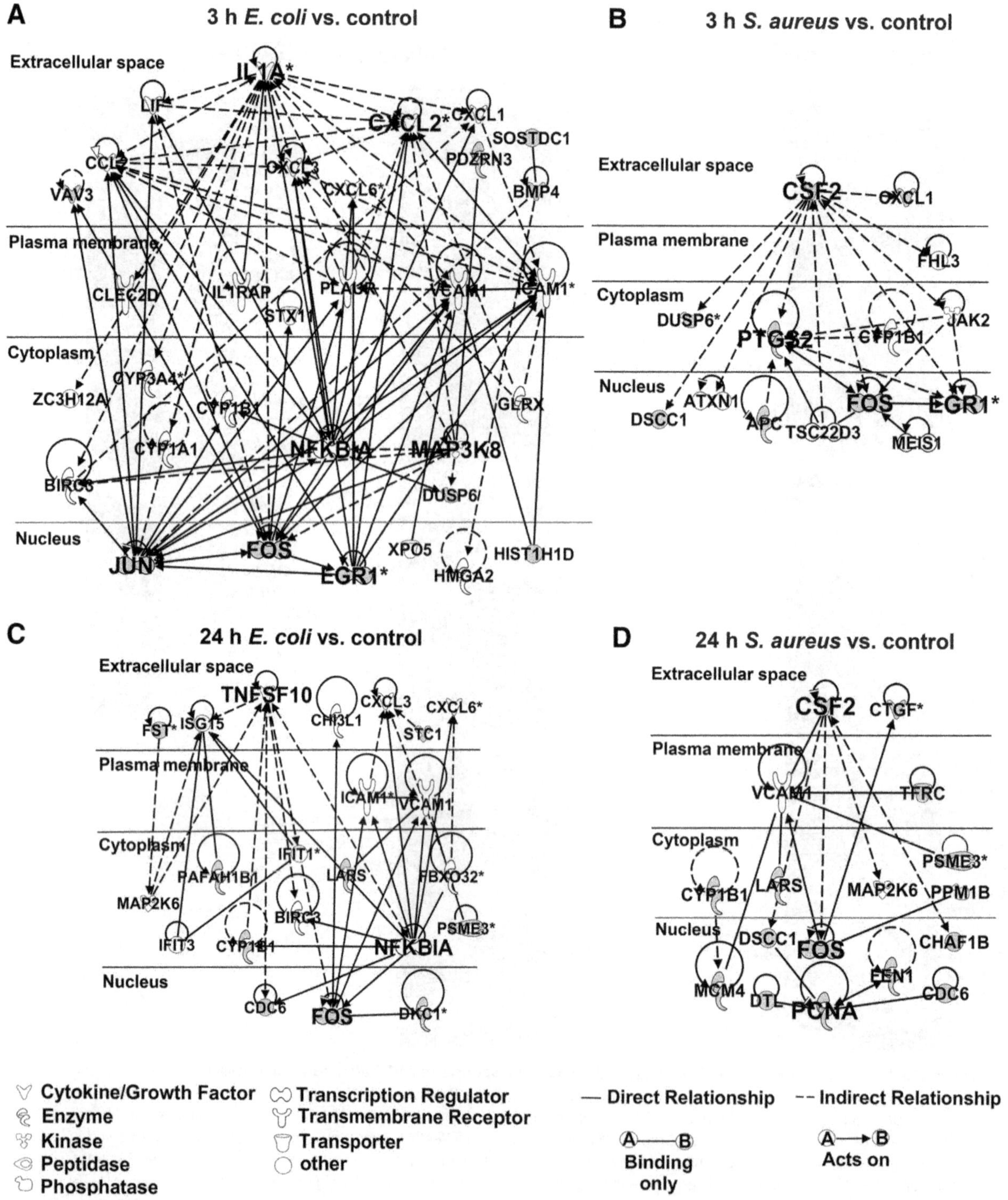

Figure 5 Most highly rated networks of genes triggered in PMEC after pathogen challenge. Network analysis was performed with top 50 up-regulated and top 50 down-regulated genes at 3 hpc and at 24 hpc with *E. coli* and *S. aureus*, respectively, and calculated by IPA. The down-regulated genes are in grey. **(A)** The gene interaction network of the early response (3 hpc) to *E. coli* was dominated by *IL1A*, *NFKBIA*, *MAP3K8*, *JUN*, *FOS* and *EGR1*. **(B)** *CSF2*, *PTGS2*, *FOS* and *EGR1* are the key regulatory genes of the early response (3 hpc) to *S. aureus*. **(C)** The gene interaction network of the late response (24 hpc) to *E. coli* was dominated by *TNFSF10*, *NFKBIA* and *FOS*. **(D)** *CSF2*, *FOS* and *PCNA* are the key regulatory genes of the late response (24 hpc) to *S. aureus*.

confirmed the selected results of microarray analysis with a good reproducibility.

Discussion

This study aimed to examine details about signaling pathways and key signaling molecules involved in PMEC defense mechanisms against pathogen infection which can help to elucidate the contribution of PMEC in pathogenesis of PDS in postpartum sows. To our knowledge, this is the first report describing the transcriptional response of PMEC at 3 hpc and at 24 hpc with heat-inactivated *E. coli* and *S. aureus*, in vitro.

However, it is difficult to compare the infection pressure of in vitro to in vivo situations. Therefore, we performed our experiments with heat-inactivated bacteria to provide standardized experimental conditions. In the PMEC model, the time course of the pathogen-specific immune response is well-defined and bacteria concentrations are constant throughout the entire experiments. This is to avoid bacterial overgrowth and depletion of nutrients during experiments. Since in vivo different cell types contribute to the immune response of the porcine mammary gland and the individual variation is high, PMEC model is less complex and therefore useful to describe molecular mechanisms of host-pathogen interactions with good reproducibility. We keep in mind that the PMEC model does not properly reflect the mastitis-induced regulation of chemokines and the complement system in the gland. Also the function of heat-labile proteins during inflammatory response may not be displayed in the PMEC model. Our study consists of a small number of biological replica, which might limit the statistical power, but the variability of pathogen-induced gene expression between biological cell culture replicates seems to be much less than that between pigs itself.

It is known that gram-negative (*E. coli*) and gram-positive (*S. aureus*) bacteria have relatively different structural and pathogenic profiles causing a similar, but time-delayed pattern of shock in the host [21]. The major pathogenic protein of gram-negative bacteria is the cell wall component LPS [22]. In contrast, gram-positive bacteria express cell wall-associated and secreted proteins (e.g., protein A, hemolysins, and phenol-soluble modulin) and cell wall components (e.g., peptidoglycan and alanylated lipoteichoic acid) which have been shown to be inflammatory [23]. While intramammary infection by *E. coli* is acute in nature and generally clears within a few days [24], infection by *S. aureus* is often less severe but results in a chronic infection that can persist for a life time of an animal [8]. The reasons for these pathogen-related differences in the host immune defense might reside in factors contributing to the innate immune system [25]. Innate recognition of pathogen-associated molecular patterns (PAMP) is mediated by evolutionary conserved pattern recognition receptors (PRR) [26]. For example, TLR2 recognizes cell wall components of gram-positive bacteria [27], whereas TLR4 recognizes LPS from gram-negative bacteria [28]. A simultaneous recognition of different pathogens is also possible, although the type of signal and co-receptor may differ. TLR2 mRNA expression was shown to be higher in porcine mammary glands after inoculation with *E. coli* as well as in sows that developed clinical signs of mastitis than in the non-inoculated mammary glands of sows that remained clinically healthy [9]. However, in our study, we did not observe significant changes in TLR expression of PMEC after both pathogen challenges.

Main effects on molecular and cellular functions of PMEC after pathogen challenge depend on different initial host defense mechanisms

The initial response of PMEC to the challenge with *E. coli* was more prominent than with *S. aureus*. During the long infection procedure (24 hpc), a more intense host response with a maximum increase of shared up- and down-regulated genes was identified after challenge with both pathogens. This is in accordance with observations by Günther et al. [8], who described that *S. aureus* elicits a much weaker and slower immune response in primary bovine mammary epithelial cells (pbMEC) than *E. coli*. To explain these, we focused on affected molecular and cellular functions in PMEC after pathogen challenge. While short-term as well as long-term challenge of PMEC with *E. coli* affected genes which are mostly involved in cellular processes such as growth, proliferation, development, death, survival, movement, and gene expression, short-term challenge with *S. aureus* rather induced metabolism of small molecules, lipids, vitamins and minerals. This is in line with the studies by Foster [29], who described that *S. aureus* cytotoxicity mainly depends on proteases, hyaluronidases, lipases, and nucleases which facilitate tissue destruction, membrane-damaging toxins that cause cytolytic effects in host cells, and superantigens which contribute to symptoms of septic shock. At 24 hpc of PMEC with the respective pathogens, the most affected molecular and cellular functions are more analog, for example the post-transcriptional modification of RNA, cell cycle, growth, proliferation, death, and survival. This is in agreement with other transcriptional profiling studies which have demonstrated that immune competent cells respond to bacterial stimuli with common transcriptional activation program which can be interpreted as generic "alarm signals" for infection [30,31]. Both, cell death and lipid metabolism were found to be among the most significant molecular functions altered in proteins of cows infected with either *E. coli* or *S. aureus* [32].

Pathogen defense mechanisms of PMEC are driven by different canonical pathway mediators

Our analysis of most affected canonical pathways and genes involved in that pathways in PMEC after pathogen challenge revealed that *E. coli* induced an early innate immune response at 3 hpc indicated by a strong up-regulation of genes encoding pro-inflammatory cytokines and chemokines such as CCL2, CXCL1, CXCL2, CXCL3, CXCL6, IL1A, and IL8 as well as cell adhesion proteins such as VCAM1, ICAM1, and ITGB3. The up-regulation of cytokine production by epithelial cells is a key component of the host innate immune response [33]. Cronin et al. [34] reported that TLR4 on cells of the immune system of cow bind to LPS which in turn stimulates the secretion of the pro-inflammatory cytokines IL1B and IL6, and the chemokine IL8. The monokine IL1A was first appreciated as an endogenous pyrogen and lymphocyte-activating factor [35]. The NF-kappaB-mediated secretion of the chemotactic factor IL8 and TLR-induced expression of vascular endothelial adhesion molecules promote the rapid recruitment and activation of immune cells including neutrophils, macrophages, lymphocytes and monocytes at the site of inflammation which kill invading bacteria [36-38]. These correlate well with our findings that the induced adhesion and activation of granulocytes, agranulocytes and stellate cells by PMEC at 3 hpc and at 24 hpc with *E. coli* were significant. In contrast, only stellate cell activation is one of the top five canonical pathways, which was affected at 24 hpc of PMEC with *S. aureus*. Therefore, we suggest the early activation of cytokines and of cells of the innate immune system as critical factors driving the different downstream cascades of host defense mechanisms. Interferons play also an important role in the first line of defense of PMEC against *E. coli* indicated by the up-regulation of IFN signaling genes *IFIT1* and *IFIT3* as well as type I IFN receptor genes such as *IFNAR1* and *IFNAR2*, which are expressed by leukocytes. An up-regulation of this gene cluster was also present at 24 hpc with *E. coli* as well as at 24 hpc with *S. aureus*. The higher up-regulation of chemokines that target mononuclear leukocytes by LPS than by *S. aureus* culture supernatant is likely to be related to the differential activation of the type I IFN pathway, and could induce a different profile of the initial recruitment of leukocytes [13].

The enhanced gene expression of *IL-17A* in PMEC at 3 hpc with *E. coli* is a sign for antibacterial activity of the cells as well, mediated by indirect enhancement of neutrophil migration and secretion of cytokines and chemokines to infected tissue. With regard to the innate immune response to infection, *IL-17A* was found in milk cell RNA extracts in the early phase (8 hpc) of the inflammatory response [39] as well as in milk leukocytes from cows suffering from *S. aureus* mastitis [40,41]. In contrast, IL-17A signaling pathways were down-regulated in PMEC at 3 hpc with *S. aureus*. Genini et al. [31] stated that the comparison of *E. coli* and *S. aureus* infections in cattle in vivo reveals affected genes showing opposite regulation with the same altered biological functions and this provides evidence that *E. coli* can cause a stronger host response. Gilbert et al. [13] suggested that *E. coli* induces a more intense response associated with strong NF-kappaB stimulation and the recruitment of a wider repertoire of immune cells, whereas *S. aureus* interferes with cell DNA integrity and may induce a more restricted immune response involving the IL-17A pathway. In contrast to the short-term challenge of PMEC with *E. coli*, at 3 hpc with *S. aureus* we observed a strong up-regulation of *CYP1A1*, *CYP3A4* and *CYP1B1* encoding monooxygenases, which have pivotal roles in primary and secondary metabolic pathways and are involved in the detoxification and elimination of reactive oxygen species and other poisonous compounds [42,43]. Thus, as expected canonical pathways including different metabolic degradation processes as well as estrogen biosynthesis were mostly affected in PMEC at 3 hpc with *S. aureus*. Genes encoding the cell adhesion molecules VCAM1 and ITGB3 were also up-regulated in PMEC at 3 hpc and at 24 hpc with *S. aureus*. This can lead to an induction of infiltration of immune cells to the site of infection to act there as key factors in the host defense against invading pathogens [44]. These differences in the initial innate immune response of PMEC to *E. coli* or *S. aureus* are consistent with studies in mammary epithelial cells from cows and sheep where it was argued that the response of mammary epithelial cells (MEC) to *S. aureus* was not the result of an overwhelming cytotoxicity, because the early response was an increase of the reduction activity [8,45]. This may also explain a very rapid increase in somatic cell count (SCC) in bovine milk during *E. coli* infection compared to a slower but longer increase in *S. aureus* infections [46]. In general, most of the canonical pathways such as interferon signaling and the activation of immune competent cells, which were up-regulated in PMEC at 3 hpc with *E. coli* were also up-regulated at 24 hpc with *E. coli* and, to a lesser extent, at 24 hpc with *S. aureus*. Additionally, at the same challenge time High-Mobility-Group-Protein B1 (HMGB1) signaling is induced by *E. coli* suggesting an activation of antigen-presenting dendritic cells [47]. Insulin-like growth factor 1 (IGF-1) signaling was induced in PMEC at 24 hpc with *S. aureus* indicating an induction of SCC. It was reported that the concentration of IGF-1 and the numbers of SCC in milk of cows were greatly elevated in secretions of quarters affected by acute clinical as well as subclinical mastitis compared with the corresponding clinically healthy quarters [48]. The pathogen *E. coli* can also induce apoptosis in vivo and thereby properly contribute to a decrease of milk production in mastitis [49]. In our probe sets the expressions of both, pro- and anti-apoptotic genes, were modulated in PMEC, especially at 24 hpc with both pathogens.

Fine-tuning of host defense mechanisms is important for preventing host cell damage

While a robust and rapid initiation of the host defense mechanism is essential for a successful pathogen clearance during the acute phase, on the other hand an excessive but ineffective immune defense can produce temporary or permanent damage of the host. Therefore, a restriction of an exuberant innate immune response is necessary to limit host defense. We observed an increased expression of genes encoding immune dampening factors such as NF-kappaB pathway suppressors IkappaB-alpha (NFKBIA) which function in the cytoplasm to sequester NF-kappaB, and the kinase MAP3K8 [30,50] at 3 hpc and at 24 hpc of PMEC with *E. coli*, but not with *S. aureus*. Both, NF-kappaB and MAPK cascades are induced by myeloid differentiation primary response 88 (MyD88) which is activated by LPS [51]. In agreement with our results, an increased expression of *NFKBIA* was also reported at 4 h after infusion of LPS into mouse mammary glands [52]. The panel of immune suppressors in PMEC was extended by increased expression of *TNFAIP8* at 24 hpc with *E. coli* which functions in a negative feedback loop regulating TLR-ligand and TNF-induced responses [53]. Besides, the up-regulation of anti-inflammatory genes as well as the down-regulation of pro-inflammatory genes balances the host immune response. For example, at 3 hpc with *S. aureus*, we observed a down-regulation of *CXCL1* and the cytokine *CSF2* (also known as *GM-CSF*) in PMEC, which is contrary to challenge with *E. coli*. Proteins encoded by both genes are known to control the production, differentiation and recruitment of neutrophils and macrophages [54,55]. Neutrophils from cows affected by subclinical mastitis demonstrated a significant delay of apoptosis as compared with neutrophils obtained from healthy cows and were unresponsive to GM-CSF [56]. Gilbert et al. [13] observed an induction of *CXCL1* and *CSF2* at 3 hpc and at 6 hpc of bovine mammary epithelial cells (bMEC) with *E. coli* crude LPS, but not with *S. aureus* culture supernatant. Down-regulation of these genes could be a result of steroid hormones (e.g. glucocorticoid), which orchestrate physiological processes such as metabolism, immunity and development and suppress cytokines, adhesion molecules and inflammatory response proteins as well as the recruitment of leukocytes to allow a systemic response to external stresses and resources [57]. This is in congruence with our transcriptome analysis of PMEC highlighting steroid hormone (estrogen) biosynthesis as one of the most enriched canonical pathways at 3 hpc with *S. aureus*.

Networks of specific pathogen-affected upstream and downstream regulators associated with inflammatory response emphasize the complexity of the innate immune response of PMEC

The activation of downstream signal transduction pathways via phosphorylation, ubiquitination, or protein-protein interactions, ultimately culminate in activation of transcription factors regulating the expression of genes involved in inflammation and antimicrobial host defenses [58]. Our results are in agreement with that, showing a down-regulation of genes encoding heat-shock proteins which are involved in protein ubiquitination pathways in PMEC at 24 hpc with *E. coli* as well as with *S. aureus*, and contributing to a decreasing receptor-mediated activation of the innate immune response.

Nevertheless, the common transcriptional response of PMEC to both pathogens is characterized by expression changes of genes interacting in activation, regulation and limitation of the innate immune response. Upstream analysis of genes mostly affected in PMEC at 3 hpc with *E. coli* are associated with TLR4-mediated recognition of LPS and downstream signaling cascades involving *IL1B*, *interleukin-1 receptor-associated kinase 4* (*IRAK4*) and *TNF* to initiate local and systemic inflammatory response. This is in accordance with the study of Günther et al. [8], who reported that genes that are exclusively and most strongly up-regulated by *E. coli* may be clustered into a regulatory network with TNF-alpha and IL1. An association between clinical mastitis and local production of IL1-beta, IL6 and TNF-alpha is suggested in mammary glands of sows [26]. IL1-beta is found in greater concentration in milk of *E. coli* mastitis than in milk of *S. aureus* mastitis, and TNF-alpha is found in bovine milk in case of *E. coli* but not *S. aureus* mastitis [40,59]. In contrast, upstream regulation of the innate immune response of PMEC at 3 hpc with *S. aureus* is mediated for example by beta-estradiol, known to regulate the innate immunity by suppressing the secretion and/or expression of pro-inflammatory mediators by human uterine epithelial cells, but also stimulates the production of antimicrobials [60]. Different upstream regulators affected in PMEC at 24 hpc with *E. coli* and with *S. aureus* have similar functions by controlling gene expressions involved in the cell division cycle, apoptosis, cell differentiation, cell adhesion, cell migration and metabolism. This reflects the complexity of the innate immune response of PMEC to the respective pathogens. The networks of key regulatory genes associated with host response of PMEC challenged with *E. coli* are more complex than that challenged with *S. aureus*. Almost all of the key regulatory genes involved in the defense mechanisms against *E. coli* and *S. aureus* are categorized by IPA as genes of "inflammatory response". *IL1A, CXCL2, TNFSF10, NFKBIA* and *MAP3K8* are the main key regulatory genes of the innate immune response of PMEC challenged with *E. coli*, which act on gene expression of *JUN, FOS* and *EGR1*, while challenge with *S. aureus* mostly affected gene expression of *FOS, EGR1* and *PCNA* via CSF2 and PTGS2 signaling. Apart from the different mostly affected genes encoding proteins which act in several cell-to-cell communications or cytoplasmic protein interactions, their effects on regulation of transcription centered to the active down-regulation of some immediate early genes (*EGR1, JUN, FOS*) executing distinct biological functions.

Our results show that PMEC do not only pose a physical barrier against extracellular pathogens, but are immune competent as well. They are capable of recognizing invading pathogens and initiate local and systemic immune responses. The extent and the course of the infection depend on: (i) pathogen stimuli; (ii) pathogen recognition and (iii) immune status of the animal. Individual differences in one of these objects critically influence the innate host immune response and PDS pathogenesis. The much faster and stronger inflammatory response of PMEC to challenge with *E. coli* results from immediately induced IL1B and TNF signaling initiating the rapid mobilization of immune cells mediated by various cytokines and chemokines. In contrast, such strong and rapid effects on expressions of immune relevant genes are not elicited by challenge with *S. aureus*, which rather affected metabolic pathway signaling resulting in a more moderate innate immune response.

Overall, our results suggest PMEC as a suitable mechanistic model, which especially contributes the understanding of pathogenesis of porcine mastitis induced by *E. coli* or *S. aureus*, and generally confirm comprehensive expression patterns of innate immune response in other cell types as well as animal species. Further comparative investigations on these gene expression patterns of the innate immune response of PDS-negative and PDS-positive sows may aid elucidation of the PDS etiology.

Additional files

Additional file 1: Overview of differentially expressed genes at 3 h post-challenge with *E. coli* compared to unchallenged control. Table giving Affymetrix probe set numbers, fold changes (control vs. treatment), *p*-values and corresponding q-values, gene symbols and gene names.

Additional file 2: Overview of differentially expressed genes at 3 h post-challenge with *S. aureus* compared to unchallenged control. Table giving Affymetrix probe set numbers, fold changes (control vs. treatment), *p*-values and corresponding q-values, gene symbols and gene names.

Additional file 3: Overview of differentially expressed genes at 24 h post-challenge with *E. coli* compared to unchallenged control. Table giving Affymetrix probe set numbers, fold changes (control vs. treatment), *p*-values and corresponding q-values, gene symbols and gene names.

Additional file 4: Overview of differentially expressed genes at 24 h post-challenge with *S. aureus* compared to unchallenged control. Table giving Affymetrix probe set numbers, fold changes (control vs. treatment), *p*-values and corresponding q-values, gene symbols and gene names.

Additional file 5: Sequences of oligonucleotide primers used for real-time PCR quantification. Table providing primer sequences, length of PCR products, annealing temperatures and GenBank accession number of respective nucleotide sequences.

Additional file 6: Principle component analysis. The 2D condition scatter plot view clustering of gene expressions in PMEC after challenge with *E. coli* (red dots) or *S. aureus* (blue dots) for 3 h and 24 h compared to unchallenged control (green dots). The two main principal components of the expression of the most significant genes show significant separation of the three biological replicates by location (PC1 and PC2). It is also shown that gene expression diverges most significantly with increasing treatment time. In contrast, the technical replicates show more consistent gene expression clusters. No outliers were detected.

Additional file 7: Comparison of microarray and RT-qPCR results for selected transcripts associated with "inflammatory response". Table giving fold changes, *p*-values and corresponding q-values detailed for various comparisons obtained with microarrays and RT-qPCR and correlation coefficient for the two methods.

Competing interests
The authors declare that they have no competing interests.

Authors' contributions
KW and NK designed the study. AJ and KW sampled the tissue probes during the slaughter process. DB and NK collected and classified the bacteria samples. AJ, DB, JG and KW designed and carried out the cell culture experiments and microscopy. EM coordinated the RNA sampling and RT-qPCR analyses. SP participated in the microarray analyses. MO performed the statistical and bioinformatic analyses of microarray data and RT-qPCR data. AJ and JG analysed and interpreted the data. AJ drafted the manuscript and prepared figures and tables. MO, EM, KW and NK critically revised the manuscript. All authors read and approved the final manuscript.

Acknowledgements
The authors are grateful for the excellent technical support from Angelika Deike, Hannelore Tychsen and Anette Jugert. This research project was funded by the German Federal Ministry of Education and Research (BMBF) in the research program "FUGATO - Functional Genome Analysis in Animal Organisms", project "geMMA - structural and functional analysis of the genetic variation of the MMA syndrome" (FKZ0315138).

Author details
[1]Institute for Genome Biology, Leibniz-Institute for Farm Animal Biology, Wilhelm-Stahl-Allee 2, D-18196 Dummerstorf, Germany. [2]Institute of Agricultural and Nutritional Sciences, Martin-Luther-University Halle-Wittenberg, Theodor-Lieser-Straße 11, D-06120 Halle (Saale), Germany. [3]Institute for Animal Hygiene, Animal Welfare and Livestock Ethology, University of Veterinary Medicine Hannover, Foundation, Bischofsholer Damm 15, D-30173 Hannover, Germany.

References
1. Gerjets I, Kemper N (2009) Coliform mastitis in sows: a review. J Swine Health Prod 17:97–105
2. López J, Ubiergo A (2005) Pig Progress. Reed Business Information, Doetinchem, Netherlands 21:12–14

3. Kemper N, Bardehle D, Lehmann J, Gerjets I, Looft H, Preissler R (2013) The role of bacterial pathogens in coliform mastitis in sows. Berl Munch Tierarztl Wochenschr 126:130–136
4. Gerjets I, Traulsen I, Reiners K, Kemper N (2011) Comparison of virulence gene profiles of Escherichia coli isolates from sows with coliform mastitis and healthy sows. Vet Microbiol 152:361–367
5. Preissler R, Hinrichs D, Reiners K, Looft H, Kemper N (2012) Estimation of variance components for postpartum dysgalactia syndrome in sows. J Anim Breed Genet 129:98–102
6. Bertschinger HU, Bühlmann A (2001) Absence of protective immunity in mammary glands after experimentally induced coliform mastitis. In: Congress, Swiss Association of Swine Medicine (ed) International Pig Veterinary Society. Proceedings of the 11th International Pig Veterinary Society Congress: 1–5 July 2001, Lausanne, Switzerland, p 175
7. Elmore RG, Martin CE, Berg P (1978) Absorption of Escherichia coli endotoxin from the mammmary glands and uteri of early postpartum sows and gilts. Theriogenol 10:439–445
8. Günther J, Esch K, Poschadel N, Petzl W, Zerbe H, Mitterhuemer S, Blum H, Seyfert HM (2011) Comparative kinetics of Escherichia coli- and Staphylococcus aureus-specific activation of key immune pathways in mammary epithelial cells demonstrates that S. aureus elicits a delayed response dominated by interleukin-6 (IL-6) but not by IL-1A or tumor necrosis factor alpha. Infect Immun 79:695–707
9. Zhu Y (2007) Early inflammatory response in periparturient sows to experimentally induced Escherichia coli mastitis. PhD thesis. Swedish University of Agricultural Sciences, Division of Reproduction, Department of Clinical Sciences, Faculty of Veterinary Medicine and Animal Science, Uppsala, Sweden
10. Zhu Y, Berg M, Fossum C, Magnusson U (2007) Proinflammatory cytokine mRNA expression in mammary tissue of sows following intramammary inoculation with Escherichia coli. Vet Immunol Immunopathol 116:98–103
11. Zhu Y, Fossum C, Berg M, Magnusson U (2007) Morphometric analysis of proinflammatory cytokines in mammary glands of sows suggests an association between clinical mastitis and local production of IL-1beta, IL-6 and TNF-alpha. Vet Res 38:871–882
12. Magnusson U, Pedersen Mörner A, Persson A, Karlstam E, Sternberg S, Kindahl H (2001) Sows intramammarily inoculated with Escherichia coli influence of time of infection, hormone concentrations and leucocyte numbers on development of disease. J Vet Med B Infect Dis Vet Public Health 48:501–512
13. Gilbert FB, Cunha P, Jensen K, Glass EJ, Foucras G, Robert-Granié C, Rupp R, Rainard P (2013) Differential response of bovine mammary epithelial cells to Staphylococcus aureus or Escherichia coli agonists of the innate immune system. Vet Res 44:40
14. Edgar R, Domrachev M, Lash A (2002) Gene expression omnibus: Ncbi gene expression and hybridization array data repository. Nucleic Acids Res 30:207–210
15. The National Center for Biotechnology Information Gene Expression Omnibus. www.ncbi.nlm.nih.gov/geo Accessed 16 December 2014
16. Kauffmann A, Gentleman R, Huber W (2009) arrayQualityMetrics–a bioconductor package for quality assessment of microarray data. Bioinformatics 25:415–416
17. Bourgon R, Gentleman R, Huber W (2010) Independent filtering increases detection power for high-throughput experiments. Proc Natl Acad Sci U S A 107:9546–9551
18. Storey JD, Tibshirani R (2003) Statistical significance for genomewide studies. Proc Natl Acad Sci U S A 100:9440–9445
19. Naraballobh W, Chomdej S, Muráni E, Wimmers K, Ponsuksili S (2010) Annotation and in silico localization of the Affymetrix GeneChip Porcine Genome Array. Arch Anim Breed 53:230–238
20. Vandesompele J, De Preter K, Pattyn F, Poppe B, Van Roy N, De Paepe A, Speleman F (2002) Accurate normalization of real-time quantitative RT-PCR data by geometric averaging of multiple internal control genes. Genome Biol 3:RESEARCH0034
21. Sriskandan S, Cohen J (1999) Gram-positive sepsis. Mechanisms and differences from gram-negative sepsis. Infect Dis Clin North Am 13:397–412
22. Wellnitz O, Reith P, Haas SC, Meyer HHD (2006) Immune relevant gene expression of mammary epithelial cells and their influence on leukocyte chemotaxis in response to different mastitis pathogens. Vet Med 51:125–132
23. Fournier B, Philpott DJ (2005) Recognition of Staphylococcus aureus by the innate immune system. Clin Microbiol Rev 18:521–540
24. Smith KL, Hogan JS (1993) Environmental mastitis. Vet Clin N Am Food Anim Pract 9:489–498
25. Miller SI, Ernst RK, Bader MW (2005) LPS, TLR4 and infectious disease diversity. Nat Rev Microbiol 3:36–46
26. Aderem A, Ulevitch RJ (2000) Toll-like receptors in the induction of the innate immune response. Nature 406:782–787
27. Yoshimura A, Lien E, Ingalls RR, Tuomanen E, Dziarski R, Golenbock D (1999) Cutting edge: recognition of Gram-positive bacterial cell wall components by the innate immune system occurs via Toll-like receptor 2. J Immunol 163:1–5
28. Hirschfeld M, Ma Y, Weis JH, Vogel SN, Weis JJ (2000) Cutting edge: repurification of lipopolysaccharide eliminates signaling through both human and murine toll-like receptor 2. J Immunol 165:618–622
29. Foster TJ (2005) Immune evasion by Staphylococci. Nat Rev Microbiol 3:948–958
30. Jenner RG, Young RA (2005) Insights into host responses against pathogens from transcriptional profiling. Nat Rev Microbiol 3:281–294
31. Genini S, Badaoui B, Sclep G, Bishop SC, Waddington D, Pinard van der Laan MH, Klopp C, Cabau C, Seyfert HM, Petzl W, Jensen K, Glass EJ, de Greeff A, Smith HE, Smits MA, Olsaker I, Boman GM, Pisoni G, Moroni P, Castiglioni B, Cremonesi P, Del Corvo M, Foulon E, Foucras G, Rupp R, Giuffra E (2011) Strengthening insights into host responses to mastitis infection in ruminants by combining heterogeneous microarray data sources. BMC Genomics 12:225
32. Ibeagha-Awemu EM, Ibeagha AE, Messier S, Zhao X (2010) Proteomics, genomics, and pathway analyses of Escherichia coli and Staphylococcus aureus infected milk whey reveal molecular pathways and networks involved in mastitis. J Proteome Res 9:4604–4619
33. Kolls JK, McCray PB, Jr, Chan YR (2008) Cytokine-mediated regulation of antimicrobial proteins. Nat Rev Immunol 8:829–835
34. Cronin JG, Turner ML, Goetze L, Bryant CE, Sheldon IM (2012) Toll-like receptor 4 and MYD88-dependent signaling mechanisms of the innate immune system are essential for the response to lipopolysaccharide by epithelial and stromal cells of the bovine endometrium. Biol Reprod 86:51
35. Dinarello CA (1991) Interleukin-1 and interleukin-1 antagonism. Blood 77:1627–1652
36. Harada A, Sekido N, Akahoshi T, Wada T, Mukaida N, Matsushima K (1994) Essential involvement of interleukin-8 (IL-8) in acute inflammation. J Leukoc Biol 56:559–564
37. Paape MJ, Shafer-Weaver K, Capuco AV, Van Oostveldt K, Burvenich C (2000) Immune surveillance of mammary tissue by phagocytic cells. Adv Exp Med Biol 480:259–277
38. Leitner G, Eligulashvily R, Krifucks O, Perl S, Saran A (2003) Immune cell differentiation in mammary gland tissues and milk of cows chronically infected with Staphylococcus aureus. J Vet Med B Infect Dis Vet Public Health 50:45–52
39. Rainard P, Cunha P, Bougarn S, Fromageau A, Rossignol C, Gilbert FB, Berthon P (2013) T helper 17-associated cytokines are produced during antigen-specific inflammation in the mammary gland. PLoS One 8:e63471
40. Riollet C, Mutuel D, Duonor-Cerutti M, Rainard P (2006) Determination and characterization of bovine interleukin-17 cDNA. J Interferon Cytokine Res 44:141–149
41. Tao W, Mallard B (2007) Differentially expressed genes associated with Staphylococcus aureus mastitis of Canadian Holstein cows. Vet Immunol Immunopathol 44:201–211
42. Barouki R, Morel Y (2001) Repression of cytochrome P450 1A1 gene expression by oxidative stress: mechanisms and biological implications. Biochem Pharmacol 61:511–516
43. Murray GI, Melvin WT, Greenlee WF, Burke MD (2001) Regulation, function, and tissue-specific expression of cytochrome P450 CYP1B1. Annu Rev Pharmacol Toxicol 41:297–316
44. Paape M, Mehrzad J, Zhao X, Detilleux J, Burvenich C (2002) Defense of the bovine mammary gland by polymorphonuclear neutrophil leukocytes. J Mammary Gland Biol Neoplasia 7.109–121
45. Bonnefont CM, Rainard P, Cunha P, Gilbert FB, Toufeer M, Aurel MR, Rupp R, Foucras G (2012) Genetic susceptibility to S. aureus mastitis in sheep: differential expression of mammary epithelial cells in response to live bacteria or supernatant. Physiol Genomics 44:403–416
46. De Haas Y, Veerkamp RF, Barkema HW, Gröhn YT, Schukken YH (2004) Associations between pathogen-specific cases of clinical mastitis and somatic cell count patterns. J Dairy Sci 87:95–105

47. Dumitriu IE, Baruah P, Bianchi ME, Manfredi AA, Rovere-Querini P (2005) Requirement of HMGB1 and RAGE for the maturation of human plasmacytoid dendritic cells. Eur J Immunol 35:2184–2190
48. Liebe A, Schams D (1998) Growth factors in milk: interrelationships with somatic cell count. J Dairy Res 65:93–100
49. Long E, Capuco AV, Wood DL, Sonstegard T, Tomita G, Paape MJ, Zhao X (2001) Escherichia coli induces apoptosis and proliferation of mammary cells. Cell Death Differ 8:808–816
50. Bottero V, Imbert V, Frelin C, Formento JL, Peyron JF (2003) Monitoring NF-kappa B transactivation potential via real-time PCR quantification of I kappa B-alpha gene expression. Mol Diagn 44:187–194
51. Fujihara M, Muroi M, Tanamoto K, Suzuki T, Azuma H, Ikeda H (2003) Molecular mechanisms of macrophage activation and deactivation by lipopolysaccharide: roles of the receptor complex. Pharmacol Ther 100:171–194
52. Zheng J, Watson AD, Kerr DE (2006) Genome-wide expression analysis of lipopolysaccharide-induced mastitis in a mouse model. Infect Immun 44:1907–1915
53. Dixit VM, Green S, Sarma V, Holzman LB, Wolf FW, O'Rourke K, Ward PA, Prochownik EV, Marks RM (1990) Tumor necrosis factor-alpha induction of novel gene products in human endothelial cells including a macrophage-specific chemotaxin. J Biol Chem 265:2973–2978
54. Mantovani A, Cassatella MA, Costantini C, Jaillon S (2011) Neutrophils in the activation and regulation of innate and adaptive immunity. Nat Rev Immunol 11:519–531
55. De Filippo K, Dudeck A, Hasenberg M, Nye E, van Rooijen N, Hartmann K, Gunzer M, Roers A, Hogg N (2013) Mast cell and macrophage chemokines CXCL1/CXCL2 control the early stage of neutrophil recruitment during tissue inflammation. Blood 121:4930–4937
56. Boutet P, Boulanger D, Gillet L, Vanderplasschen A, Closset R, Bureau F, Lekeux P (2004) Delayed neutrophil apoptosis in bovine subclinical mastitis. J Dairy Sci 87:4104–4114
57. Regan JC, Brandão AS, Leitão AB, Mantas Dias AR, Sucena E, Jacinto A, Zaidman-Rémy A (2013) Steroid hormone signaling is essential to regulate innate immune cells and fight bacterial infection in Drosophila. PLoS Pathog 9:e1003720
58. Akira S, Uematsu S, Takeuchi O (2006) Pathogen recognition and innate immunity. Cell 124:783–801
59. Bannerman DD, Paape MJ, Lee JW, Zhao X, Hope JC, Rainard P (2004) Escherichia coli and Staphylococcus aureus elicit differential innate immune responses following intramammary infection. Clin Diagn Lab Immunol 11:463–472
60. Fahey JV, Wright JA, Shen L, Smith JM, Ghosh M, Rossoll RM, Wira CR (2008) Estradiol selectively regulates innate immune function by polarized human uterine epithelial cells in culture. Mucosal Immunol 1:317–325

Effects of bovine leukemia virus infection on milk neutrophil function and the milk lymphocyte profile

Alice Maria Melville Paiva Della Libera[1*], Fernando Nogueira de Souza[2], Camila Freitas Batista[1], Bruna Parapinski Santos[1], Luis Fernando Fernandes de Azevedo[1], Eduardo Milton Ramos Sanchez[3], Soraia Araújo Diniz[2], Marcos Xavier Silva[2], João Paulo Haddad[2] and Maiara Garcia Blagitz[1]

Abstract

The effects of bovine leukemia virus (BLV) on the immune response have been extensively investigated; however, its effects on mammary gland immunity are only speculative. Although BLV has a tropism for B cells, it can affect both adaptive and innate immunities because these systems share many effector mechanisms. This scenario is the basis of this investigation of the effects of BLV on mammary gland immunity, which is largely dependent upon neutrophilic functions. Thus, the present study sought to examine neutrophilic functions and the lymphocyte profile in the milk of naturally BLV-infected cows. The viability of the milk neutrophils and the percentage of milk neutrophils that produced reactive oxygen species (ROS) or phagocytosed *Staphylococcus aureus* were similar between BLV-infected and BLV-uninfected dairy cows. Furthermore, the expression of CD62L and CD11b by the milk neutrophils and the percentage of milk neutrophils ($CH138^+$ cells) that were obtained from the udder quarters of the BLV-infected cows were not altered. Conversely, the median fluorescence intensity (MFI) representing intracellular ROS production and the phagocytosis of *S. aureus*, the expression of CD44 by the milk neutrophils and the percentage of apoptotic B cells were lower in the milk cells from BLV-infected dairy cows, particularly those from animals with persistent lymphocytosis (PL). The lymphocyte subsets were not different among the groups, with the exception of the percentage of $CD5^-/CD11b^-$ B cells, which was higher in the milk cells from BLV-infected cows, particularly those with PL. Thus, the present study provides novel insight into the implications of BLV infection for mammary gland immunity.

Introduction

Bovine leukemia virus (BLV) is a member of the Retroviridae family and the *Deltaretrovirus* genus that is genetically and structurally similar to the primate T-lymphotropic viruses types 1–5 (i.e., HTLV-1 to 4). Although BLV has been successfully eradicated in some regions of Europe, it is among the most widespread livestock pathogens in many countries, particularly in dairy herds. BLV infections in cattle may remain clinically silent or present as persistent lymphocytosis (PL); more rarely, BLV infection may result in B cell lymphoma. PL is characterized by a chronic elevation in the number of circulating B lymphocytes and is found in approximately 20-30% of BLV-infected cattle [1].

Various studies have investigated the effects of BLV infection on lymphocyte subsets [1-8], neutrophil functions [9-14] and B cell viability [15-22]. All of these studies evaluated these parameters in the blood, and therefore, the effects of BLV infection on the lymphocyte subsets, neutrophil functions and B cell viability in milk are only speculative. However, mastitis [23-30] and decreased milk production [31-35] have been associated with BLV infection, particularly in BLV-infected cows with PL [31] and high-performing infected dairy herds [35]. These findings prompted an investigation into the effects of BLV, which is a B cell tropic virus [1,6,15], on mammary gland immunity, which is largely dependent upon neutrophil functions and recruitment. Notably, the impact of some chronic diseases with low lethality, such

* Correspondence: dellalibera@usp.br
[1]Departamento de Clínica Médica, Faculdade de Medicina Veterinária e Zootecnia, Universidade de São Paulo, Av. Prof. Dr. Orlando Marques de Paiva, 87, Cidade Universitária, São Paulo 05508-270, Brazil
Full list of author information is available at the end of the article

as BLV infection, may be underestimated because they may be associated with comorbidities, such as mastitis, which is the most costly dairy cattle disease. This disease threatens the image of the dairy sector because of animal welfare issues and issues related to milk quality and public health due to increased risks of antimicrobial residues and the emergence of resistant bacteria. A better understanding of the implications of BLV infection on mammary gland immunity is critical for controlling mastitis and facilitating the strict control of these infections to improve dairy cattle productivity. Thus, the present study sought to explore milk lymphocyte subsets, neutrophil functions and B cell viability from naturally BLV-infected cows.

Materials and methods

Experimental design and collection of samples

The present study used 57 quarters of the mammary glands of 19 dairy cows in a commercial herd, at different lactation stages. Due to the effects of bacterial mastitis pathogens on neutrophil function [36-40], the following exclusion criteria were applied: 1) bacteriologically positive quarters; 2) quarters with abnormal secretions in the strip cup test; and 3) quarters with high somatic cell counts (SCCs) based on the previously proposed threshold for SCC [41,42].

The sera of all of the animals were tested for BLV using an agar gel immunodiffusion (AGID) assay (Tecpar®, Curitiba, Brazil) and an ELISA (VMRD Pullman Inc., Pullman, WA, USA, cat. number 284–5), using gp51 as the antigen. These animals were divided uniformly into the following three groups according to the sera test results: negative for BLV infection according to the AGID and ELISA assays and lacking hematological alterations [43] (healthy; $n = 8$; 24 quarters); positive for BLV according to both tests and lacking hematological alterations [43], which is commonly referred to as aleukemic (AL; $n = 6$; 16 quarters); and positive for BLV according to both tests and exhibiting PL ($n = 5$; 17 quarters). The BLV-infected cattle were classified as having PL when their lymphocyte counts exceeded 1×10^4 mL^{-1} and their leukocyte counts exceeded 1.5×10^4 mL^{-1} as established by Thurmond et al. [44]. One hundred ten days after the first sampling for the serodiagnosis of BLV, additional blood samples for the hematological procedures and serodiagnoses of BLV were collected to confirm the persistence of lymphocytosis. At this time (110 days after the first sampling), milk cells for the SCC, bacteriological analysis and flow cytometry analysis to determine neutrophil function and lymphocyte profile were also collected.

First, the strip cup test was performed to determine the presence of clots or flakes or otherwise obviously abnormal secretions. Then, predipping was performed, using one towel for each teat. After discarding the first three milk streams, the ends of the teats were scrubbed with 70% ethanol using a piece of cotton, and single milk samples from the individual mammary quarters were aseptically collected in sterile vials for the bacteriological analysis. Finally, milk samples for the SCC and the evaluation of neutrophilic function and lymphocyte profile were collected. The samples were maintained at 4 °C until they arrived at the laboratory. The milk samples for the bacteriological analysis were stored at −20 °C for a maximum of 30 days until the analysis.

Subsequently, each sample was codified and randomized, and further analyses were performed in which the researcher was blinded to the BLV status of the animal from which the sample was drawn. This research complied with the Ethical Principles for Animal Research and was approved by the Bioethics Commission.

Hematological procedures

The total leukocyte counts were determined using an automated cell counter (ABX VET ABC, Horiba ABX Diagnostic®, Montpellier, France). The differential leukocyte counts were performed using routine smears.

Bacteriological analysis

The bacteriological analysis was performed by culturing 0.01 mL of each milk sample on 5% sheep blood agar plates. The plates were incubated for 72 h at 37 °C, followed by Gram staining, observation of colony morphologies and biochemical testing [45]. A milk sample was considered to be culture-positive when the growth of ≥ 3 colonies was detected, with the exception of animals with *Staphylococcus aureus* or *Streptococcus agalactiae* infections in their quarters, which were considered to be culture-positive when the growth of ≥ 1 colony was detected [46,47].

Determination of SCC

The milk samples for SCC determination were collected in 40-mL vials containing microtablets of the preservant agent bronopol (2-bromo-2-nitropane-1,3-diol). Subsequently, the SCC were performed using the Somacount 300 automated somatic cell counter (Bentley Instruments, Chaska, MN, USA).

Separation of milk cells

The separation of the milk cells was performed as described by Koess and Hamann [48]. Briefly, 1 L of milk was diluted with 1 L of phosphate-buffered saline (PBS; pH 7.4; 1.06 mM Na_2HPO_4, 155.17 mM NaCl and 2.97 mM $Na_2HPO_4.7H_2O$). After centrifugation at $1000 \times g$ for 15 min, the cream layer and supernatant were discarded. The cell pellet was then washed once using 30 mL of PBS and centrifuged at $400 \times g$ for 10 min. The cells were resuspended in 1 mL of RPMI-1640 nutritional medium (R7638, Sigma Aldrich, USA) supplemented with 10% fetal bovine serum (Cultilab, Brazil) and counted using a Neubauer chamber. Cell viability was first evaluated by trypan blue exclusion. The milk cells were then diluted with nutritional medium containing 10% fetal bovine serum to a concentration of 2×10^6 viable cells mL^{-1}.

Enumeration of lymphocyte subpopulations

The cells were washed with PBS and stained to detect the combination of CD3, CD4 and CD8, the combination of CD3, CD4 and CD25 and the combination of CD21, CD5 and CD11b following incubation with the primary antibodies (Abs) for 30 min at room temperature. The identification of lymphocyte subsets was based on their cytoplasmic granularities and mean fluorescence intensities following a two-step fluorescent immunolabeling protocol using primary anti-bovine monoclonal Abs and secondary Abs coupled to long-wavelength fluorescent probes. Thus, the following primary monoclonal antibodies (mAbs) directed against bovine lymphocytes were used: mouse IgG1 anti-bovine CD3 (T lymphocytes, MM1A, VMRD Pullman Inc. Corp®), mouse IgG2a anti-bovine CD4 (IL-A11, VMRD Pullman Inc. Corp®), mouse IgM anti-bovine CD8α (BAQ111A, VMRD Pullman Inc. Corp®), mouse IgG3 anti-bovine CD25 (LCTB2A; VMRD Pullman Inc. Corp®), mouse IgM anti-bovine CD21 (B lymphocytes, BAQ15A, VMRD Pullman Inc. Corp®), mouse IgG2a anti-bovine CD5 (B29A, VMRD Pullman Inc. Corp®) and mouse IgG1 anti-bovine CD11b (MM12A, VMRD Pullman Inc. Corp®). After washing with PBS, the cells were incubated for 30 min at room temperature with the following secondary Abs: goat anti-mouse IgG1 conjugated to phycoerythrin-Cy5 (PE-Cy5) (M32018; Invitrogen, Carlsbad, CA, USA), goat anti-mouse IgM conjugated to fluorescein isothiocyanate (FITC) (M31501, Invitrogen), goat anti-mouse IgG2a conjugated to phycoerythrin (PE) (M32204, Invitrogen) and goat anti-mouse IgG3 conjugated to FITC (M32701, Invitrogen). The cells were then washed with PBS and immediately analyzed using flow cytometry. A total of 20 000 milk cells, excluding most of the cellular debris, was examined per sample. The FlowJo software (TreeStar Inc., Ashland, OR, USA) was used to analyze the data. The results were corrected for autofluorescence content, which was defined as the fluorescence that was associated with the non-labeled freshly isolated milk cells from the same cow.

Identification of neutrophils

Milk neutrophils were differentiated from other cells by indirect fluorescent labeling. The cells were incubated with an unlabeled primary monoclonal anti-bovine granulocyte antibody (anti-CH138A, VMRD Pullman Inc. Corp®) for 30 min at room temperature. Next, 1 mL of PBS was added to the cell suspension, which was centrifuged at 400 × *g* for 8 min. Finally, a labeled secondary Ab was added, and the sample was incubated for 30 min at room temperature in the dark to visualize the bound CH138A. The neutrophils were identified using flow cytometry based on the cells' cytoplasmic granularities and CH138A positivities as previously described [40,49]. The labeled secondary mAbs included allophycocyanin- (APC; M31505, Invitrogen), FITC- (M31501, Invitrogen) or PE-conjugated (M31504, Invitrogen) goat anti-mouse IgM mAb. A total of 20 000 milk cells, excluding most of the cellular debris, was examined per sample. The FlowJo software (TreeStar Inc., Ashland, OR, USA) was used to analyze the data. The results were corrected for autofluorescence content, which was defined as the fluorescence that was associated with the non-labeled freshly isolated milk cells from the same cow.

Detection of apoptosis by flow cytometry

The death of neutrophils ($CH138^+$) and B cells ($CD21^+$) was assessed using dual labeling with an annexin V antibody and propidium iodide (PI; K2350, APOPTEST-FITC, Dako Cytomation, The Netherlands) and flow cytometric analyses as previously described [40,49]. Briefly, 2×10^5 viable milk cells were suspended in 100 μL of binding buffer (10 mM HEPES, 150 mM NaCl, 1 mM $MgCl_2$ and 1.8 mM $CaCl_2$) containing anti-annexin V-FITC antibody and incubated at room temperature for 20 min in the dark. Immediately before flow cytometry analysis, 5 μL of a 250 μg/mL PI solution was added. Next, the neutrophils were labeled using mAbs as described above.

To analyze the data, scatter plots were generated for the gated neutrophils or B cells. The living, nonapoptotic cells were negative for both FITC-labeled anti-annexin V and PI. The cells that were positive for FITC-labeled anti-annexin V but negative for PI were classified as apoptotic cells [40,49]. The necrotic subpopulation was excluded from the analysis [49]. A total of 20 000 milk cells, excluding most of the cellular debris, was examined per sample. The FlowJo software (TreeStar Inc., Ashland, OR, USA) was used to analyze the data.

Intracellular reactive oxygen species production

Intracellular reactive oxygen species (ROS) production was assessed by flow cytometry using 2′,7′-dichlorofluorescein diacetate (DCFH-DA) as a probe [50]. Briefly, 2×10^5 viable milk cells from each quarter that were previously assessed by trypan blue exclusion were incubated at 37 °C for 30 min with 0.3 μM DCFH-DA (D6883, Sigma Aldrich, St. Louis, MO, USA).

The intracellular 2′,7′-dichlorofluorescein (DCF) fluorescence of the neutrophils was determined by flow cytometry using an excitation wavelength of 488 nm. DCFH-DA, which is a cell-permeable, nonfluorescent probe, is converted to DCF by ROS in a dose-dependent manner, resulting in fluorescence emission. The green fluorescence of DCF was detected at 500–530 nm.

The percentage of neutrophils producing ROS was calculated as the number of fluorescent neutrophils divided by the total neutrophil count and multiplied by 100. The median fluorescence intensity (MFI) of ROS production was estimated from the median of DCF fluorescence divided by the number of neutrophil that produced ROS [40]. For this assay, 10 000 gated neutrophils were examined per sample. The FlowJo software (TreeStar Inc., Ashland, USA) was used to analyze the data. The results were corrected for autofluorescence content, which was defined as the fluorescence that was associated with the non-labeled freshly isolated milk cells from the same cow.

Preparation of PI-labeled bacteria

PI-labeled *Staphylococcus aureus* (ATCC 25923) was prepared as proposed by Hasui et al. [50] with some modifications. Briefly, *S. aureus* was cultured for 18 h at 37 °C on brain-heart infusion agar. Subsequently, the bacteria were heat-killed by incubation at 60 °C for 30 min, after which they were washed three times using a sterile saline solution (0.9% NaCl). The bacterial density was adjusted to an absorbance of 2.50 at 620 nm, yielding approximately 2.4×10^9 bacteria mL^{-1}, as previously described [50]. The bacteria were then labeled using a 5% PI (P4170, Sigma Aldrich, St. Louis, MO, USA) solution for 30 min at room temperature. The fluorescent bacteria were washed three times and suspended in PBS containing 5 mM glucose and 0.1% gelatin, and aliquots were stored at −80 °C. Thereafter, the PI labeling of the bacteria was confirmed by flow cytometry.

Phagocytosis assay

The phagocytosis assay was performed using flow cytometry of PI-labeled *S. aureus* as previously described by Hasui et al. [50]. Briefly, 2×10^5 viable milk cells were incubated with 100 μL of heat-killed, PI-labeled *S. aureus* and 900 μL of PBS for 30 min at 37 °C. Subsequently, 2 mL of 3 mM EDTA was added, and after centrifugation at $400 \times g$ for 10 min, the leukocytes were resuspended in 300 μL of PBS and analyzed by flow cytometry.

The percentage of neutrophils that phagocytized the bacteria was equal to the number of fluorescent neutrophils divided by the total neutrophil count and multiplied by 100. The MFI of *S. aureus* phagocytosis was estimated from the median value of PI fluorescence divided by the number of neutrophils that phagocytized *S. aureus* [40]. At least 20 000 cells were examined per sample. The Flow Jo Tree Star Software (TreeStar Inc., Ashland, OR, USA) was used to analyze the data.

Expression of L-selectin, β_2-integrin and CD44

The identification of neutrophils expressing L-selectin (CD62L), the β-chain of β_2-integrin (CD11b) and one of the three endothelial-selectin (E-selectin) ligands (CD44) was performed by flow cytometry using the following mAbs: a FITC-conjugated mouse anti-bovine CD62L (MCA1649F, AbDSerotec, Oxford, England), a primary mouse IgG1 anti-CD11b mAb (MM12A, Pullman Inc. Corp®), a phycoerythrin-Cy5 (PE-Cy5)-conjugated goat anti-mouse IgG1 Ab (M32018, Invitrogen), a primary mouse IgG3 anti-CD44 mAb (BAG40A, Pullman Inc. Corp®) and an FITC-conjugated goat anti-mouse IgG3 Ab (M32701, Invitrogen). First, dot plots of gated neutrophils ($CH138A^+$) were generated as previously described. The neutrophils were identified as previously described. Then, unlabeled primary mAbs that were directed against CD11b and CD44 were added to the cell suspension and incubated for 30 min at room temperature. The isolated milk cell suspension was centrifuged at $400 \times g$ for 8 min, and a labeled CD62L mAb and secondary labeled mAbs for the detection of the anti-CD11b and -CD44 Abs were added. Finally, the isolated milk cells were incubated for 30 min at room temperature in the dark to allow for the visualization of cells expressing CD62L, CD11b and CD44. We chose the relative MFI because this parameter was much more discriminating compared with the percentage of positive cells. The MFI provides an accurate measurement of the brightness of the stained cells and is thus an indicator of the number of receptors per cell [51]. For this assay, 10 000 gated neutrophil cells were examined per sample. The Flow Jo Tree Star Software (TreeStar Inc., Ashland, OR, USA) was used to analyze the data.

Statistical analyses

First, the distributions of all of the variables were examined using normal probability plots obtained using the Shapiro and Wilk tests. The data were analyzed using a multivariate analysis of variance. Then, the Kruskal-Wallis and Mann–Whitney tests were applied. The model considered the quarters and the cows to be nested within the cows. The statistical analyses were performed using the STATA statistical software version 12 (Stata Corp., College Station, Texas, USA). The results are reported as the mean ± standard deviation. Significance was set at $P \leq 0.05$.

Results

The results are summarized in Tables 1, 2 and 3. The SCC, lactational status and parity (data not shown) values did not differ among the groups. Here, we found that BLV infection detrimentally affected some important milk neutrophilic functions. For instance, the MFI that represented the amount of intracellular ROS production by the milk

Table 1 Characteristics of neutrophils in the milk of healthy and bovine leukemia virus (BLV)-infected cows

Group/Variable	Negative ($n = 24$)	AL ($n = 16$)	PL ($n = 17$)
CH138$^+$ (%)	13.72 ± 14.91^a	8.89 ± 9.72^a	11.88 ± 15.34^a
Annexin V$^-$/PI$^-$ (%)	30.74 ± 12.92^a	39.05 ± 16.06^a	24.97 ± 16.01^a
Annexin V$^+$/PI$^-$(%)	39.50 ± 14.48^a	37.03 ± 21.92^a	39.27 ± 19.64^a
ROS production (%)	54.91 ± 22.92^a	68.20 ± 21.85^a	69.98 ± 15.39^a
Intensity of ROS production (MFI)	2069 ± 1008^a	1603 ± 585.7^b	865.6 ± 447.3^c
S. aureus phagocytosis (%)	63.23 ± 17.80^a	55.11 ± 20.88^a	58.84 ± 15.21^a
Intensity of *S. aureus*phagocytosis (MFI)	219.8 ± 100.3^a	211.2 ± 80.77^a	104.2 ± 39.11^b
CD44 expression (MFI)	22.03 ± 22.65^a	1.07 ± 0.18^b	1.03 ± 0.09^b
CD62L expression (MFI)	13.45 ± 15.41^a	1.01 ± 0.00^a	1.01 ± 0.00^a
CD11b expression (MFI)	755.8 ± 344.6^a	633.3 ± 555.0^a	843.7 ± 334.9^a

Different superscripted letters[a,b,c] within a row indicate significant differences ($P \leq 0.05$) between the values. The results are shown as the mean ± SD.
AL: aleukemic BLV-infected cows; PL: BLV-infected cows with persistent lymphocytosis; PI: propidium iodide; *S. aureus*: *Staphylococcus aureus*; ROS: reactive oxygen species; MFI: median fluorescence intensity.

neutrophils was lower for the BLV-infected cows, particularly those with PL, than for the uninfected cows. Furthermore, the MFI that represented the amount of *S. aureus* phagocytosis by the milk neutrophils was also the lowest for the PL group. Moreover, the level of CD44 expression by milk neutrophils from the BLV-infected dairy cows was lower than that of milk neutrophils collected from the uninfected cows (Table 1).

The lymphocyte subsets did not differ among the groups, with the exception of the percentage of CD5$^-$/CD11b$^-$ B cells, which was higher in the BLV-infected cows, particularly those with PL (Table 2). Furthermore, the percentage of apoptotic B cells was lower in the BLV-infected dairy cows (Table 3), particularly those with PL, than in the uninfected cows.

Discussion

It is not easy to precisely delineate innate immunity because it is intricately enmeshed with adaptive immunity, and the two systems share many effector mechanisms [37]. Thus, various viruses can affect the general functions of both innate and adaptive immunities. This phenomenon predisposes animals to different coinfections or superinfections and can increase the severity of infections [25,28,30,52-55]. As previously mentioned, the impact of some chronic diseases with low lethalities may be underestimated because of their associations with comorbidities. This scenario prompted an investigation into the effects of BLV, which is a B cell tropic virus [1,6,15], on mammary gland immunity, which is largely dependent on neutrophil function and recruitment [36-40].

Table 2 Percentage of lymphocyte subsets in the milk from healthy and bovine leukemia virus (BLV)-infected cows

Group/Variables	Negative ($n = 25$)	AL ($n = 16$)	PL ($n = 17$)
CD3$^+$ (T cells) (%)	7.13 ± 5.04^a	10.46 ± 9.30^a	11.66 ± 7.27^a
CD4$^+$/CD8$^-$ T cells (%)	1.32 ± 1.19^a	1.83 ± 1.73^a	2.55 ± 2.48^a
CD4$^-$/CD8$^+$ T cells (%)	3.15 ± 2.57^a	4.45 ± 2.02^a	4.51 ± 3.86^a
CD4$^+$/CD8$^+$ T cells (%)	0.41 ± 0.36^a	0.33 ± 0.30^a	0.23 ± 0.19^a
CD4$^-$/CD8$^-$ T cells (%)	$2..24 \pm 2.33^a$	3.84 ± 5.74^a	4.38 ± 3.87^a
CD3$^+$ (T cells) (%)	6.31 ± 4.99^a	10.28 ± 10.44^a	11.06 ± 6.81^a
CD4$^+$/CD25$^-$ T cells (%)	1.38 ± 1.32^a	1.84 ± 1.67^a	2.70 ± 2.46^a
CD4$^-$/CD25$^+$ T cells (%)	0.06 ± 0.04^a	0.13 ± 0.18^a	0.15 ± 0.14^a
CD4$^+$/CD25$^+$ T cells (%)	0.24 ± 0.23^a	0.21 ± 0.29^a	0.29 ± 0.36^a
CD4$^-$/CD25$^-$ T cells (%)	4.63 ± 4.11^a	8.11 ± 8.58^a	7.92 ± 4.62^a
CD21$^+$(B cells) (%)	7.90 ± 5.53^a	13.02 ± 8.14^a	17.44 ± 7.20^a
CD5$^+$/CD11$^-$ B cells (%)	0.87 ± 0.88^a	0.71 ± 0.45^a	0.72 ± 0.47^a
CD5$^-$/CD11$^+$ B cells (%)	3.84 ± 4.01^a	6.80 ± 6.97^a	8.59 ± 5.15^a
CD5$^+$/CD11$^+$ B cells (%)	0.85 ± 0.78^a	0.85 ± 0.51^a	1.01 ± 0.66^a
CD5$^-$/CD11$^-$ B cells (%)	2.35 ± 1.73^a	4.67 ± 3.26^b	7.11 ± 3.89^c

Different superscripted letters[a,b,c] within a row indicate significant differences ($P \leq 0.05$) between the values. The results are shown as the mean ± SD.
AL: aleukemic BLV-infected cows; PL: BLV-infected cows with persistent lymphocytosis.

Table 3 Viability of B cells in milk from healthy and bovine leukemia virus (BLV)-infected cows.

Group/Variables	Negative ($n = 25$)	AL ($n = 16$)	PL ($n = 17$)
Annexin V^-/PI^-(%)	37.13 ± 17.99^a	51.15 ± 16.73^a	71.31 ± 13.02^a
Annexin V^+/PI^-(%)	55.72 ± 17.59^a	31.22 ± 18.43^b	12.35 ± 6.44^c

Different superscripted letters[a,b,c] within a row indicate significant differences ($P \leq 0.05$) between the values. The results are shown as the mean ± SD.
AL: aleukemic BLV-infected cows; PL: BLV-infected cows with persistent lymphocytosis; PI: propidium iodide.

Neutrophils form the first line of cellular defense against invading pathogens [36-40] and are essential for the innate host defense against invading microorganisms. These cells eliminate pathogens by a process known as phagocytosis. During phagocytosis, neutrophils produce ROS to kill invading pathogens [36-40,56].

Apoptosis of bovine neutrophils implies impaired phagocytic and oxidative burst activities [47,57,58]. Neutrophil viability is closely related to neutrophil phagocytosis and oxidative burst activities [56,58]. Thus, the non-significant difference that was observed in neutrophil viability rates among the groups in this study may be related to the results for the percentage of neutrophils that produced ROS or phagocytosed *S. aureus*.

While the study size is limited, we observed a lower MFI representing the phagocytosis of *S. aureus* and the intracellular production of ROS by the milk neutrophils from the BLV-infected cows, particularly those with PL. BLV-infected cows with PL have higher proviral loads [59,60] that are linked to lower levels of interferon (IFN)-γ expression by peripheral blood mononuclear cells [7,61-63], which is regulated by many factors, such as the PD-1 [7,62] and Tim-3/Gal-9 pathways [63]. IFN-γ has a positive effect on bovine neutrophil phagocytosis and ROS production [64], and this characteristic together with the altered production of IFN-γ by the peripheral blood mononuclear cells of BLV-infected cattle may explain our results regarding the deficient functions of the milk neutrophils. Consistent with our findings, Takamatsu et al. [11] found that most sera from leukemic cattle inhibit the phagocytosis of blood neutrophils.

In this study, no significant differences were observed in the levels of CD62L and CD11b expression by the milk neutrophils of BLV-infected cows. CD62L mediates the initial transient attachment of circulating granulocytes to the activated endothelium. The surface expression and rapid functional activation of Mac-1 (CD11b/CD18) is essential for the subsequent granulocyte migration to the site of inflammation. Following activation, CD62L is shed from the cell surface by proteolysis, whereas the surface expression of Mac-1 is up-regulated [51]. Therefore, the migration of neutrophils across endothelial cells is almost completely dependent upon CD18, the β-chain of β_2 integrins and to a lesser extent on CD11b, which is one of the α-chains of β_2 integrins [36].

Further, we found decreased levels of CD44 expression in the milk neutrophils from the BLV-infected dairy cows. CD44 was identified as one of the three endothelial-selectin ligands that are present on neutrophils, which are responsible for hindering their movement and activating their rolling. However, CD44 is required, but not essential, for neutrophil extravasation during inflammation [65]. CD44 is also regarded as a competent phagocytic receptor that efficiently mediates pathogen recognition and phagocytosis by neutrophils [66,67].

Together, these findings indicate that BLV infection, particularly BLV-infected cows with PL, may impact the outcome of intramammary infections because the resident milk neutrophils have an enormous impact on the elimination of bacteria by phagocytosis and the intracellular production of ROS [36,56]. Thus, we believe that BLV can affect mastitis control programs.

A feasible alternative to reduce the transmission of BLV infection could be achieved by eliminating animals with high proviral loads, which mainly exhibit PL instead of AL [59,60]. Thus, our findings regarding the milk neutrophil function in BLV-infected cows, particularly those with PL, indicated that the elimination of PL animals may also lead to a lower probability of comorbidities, such as mastitis, which is regarded as the most costly dairy cattle disease and is thus associated with important economic and public health implications.

No perturbations in the percentages of T lymphocyte subsets among the milk cells from the BLV-infected cows were found, as was previously described for the peripheral blood of BLV-infected cows [4,6], although no consensus exists [2,3,8]. It is generally accepted that the infected cells (mainly B cells) frequently co-express CD5 and CD11b molecules [1,6]. Conversely, the present study shows an increase in the percentage of $CD5^-$/$CD11b^-$ $CD21^+$ cells (mainly B-1b cells) in the milk of BLV-infected cows, particularly those with PL. Although this observation is puzzling, it may lend insight into the roles of CD5 [68] and CD11b [69] on B cells in mammary gland immunity.

BLV infection is correlated with the inhibition of the apoptotic process, leading to the generation of a reservoir of apparently latent cells [1]. This phenomenon, together with the B cell tropism of BLV, may explain the lower percentage of milk B cells that was observed in the BLV-infected cows, particularly those with PL, that were undergoing apoptosis, which has been previously described for B cells that were obtained from blood [1,16,18,19,21,22].

In conclusion, the present study provides novel insight into the implications of BLV infections for mammary gland immunity, which is mainly supported here by the dysfunction of the milk neutrophils. Thus, this study highlights the importance of controlling BLV infections due to their indirect effects, such as the higher susceptibilities of BLV-infected cows to secondary diseases, such as mastitis, which is the most costly disease affecting cattle.

Abbreviations

BLV: Bovine leukemia virus; ROS: Reactive oxygen species; MFI: Median fluorescence intensity; PL: Persistent lymphocytosis; SCC: Somatic cell count; AGID: Agar gel immunodiffusion; AL: Aleukemic; PBS: Phosphate-buffered saline; PE-Cy5: Phycoerythrin-Cy5; FITC: Fluorescein isothiocyanate; PE: Phycoerythrin; APC: Allophycocyanin; mAb: Monoclonal antibody; Ab: Antibody; PI: Propidium iodide; DCFH-DA: 2′,7′-dichlorofluorescein diacetate; DCFH: 2′,7′-dichlorofluorescein; CD62L: L-selectin; CD11b: β-chain of β_2-integrin; IFN-γ: Interferon-γ.

Competing interests

The authors declare that they have no competing interests.

Authors' contributions

AMMPDL designed the experiments, supervised the studies and drafted and edited the manuscript. MGB designed the experiments, performed all of the analyses and edited the manuscript. FNS designed the experiments, performed all of the analyses and drafted the paper. BPS and CFB participated in the flow cytometric analysis. EMRS provided technical help, supervised the studies and edited the manuscript. LFFA collected all of the samples and provided technical help. SAD, JPH and MXS performed the statistical analyses and edited the manuscript. All authors read and approved the final manuscript.

Authors' information

Alice MMP Della Libera and Fernando N Souza should be considered co-first authors.

Acknowledgments

The authors are grateful for the financial support of the São Paulo State Research Foundation (Project number 2009/50672-0). We thank Claudia Regina Stricagnolo for her technical support.

Author details

[1]Departamento de Clínica Médica, Faculdade de Medicina Veterinária e Zootecnia, Universidade de São Paulo, Av. Prof. Dr. Orlando Marques de Paiva, 87, Cidade Universitária, São Paulo 05508-270, Brazil. [2]Departamento de Medicina Veterinária Preventiva, Escola de Veterinária, Universidade Federal de Minas Gerais, Belo Horizonte 31270-010, Brazil. [3]Laboratório de Sorologia e Imunobiologia, Instituto de Medicina Tropical, Universidade de São Paulo, São Paulo 05403-000, Brazil.

References

1. Gillet N, Florins A, Boxus M, Burteau C, Nigro A, Vandermeers F, Balon H, Bouzar AB, Defoiche J, Burny A, Reichert M, Kettman R, Willems L: **Mechanisms of leukomogenesis induced by bovine leukemia virus: prospects for novel anti-retroviral therapies in human.** *Retrovirology* 2007, **4:**18.
2. Williams DL, Amborski GF, Davis WC: **Enumeration of T and B cells lymphocytes in bovine leukemia virus-infected cattle, using monoclonal antibodies.** *Am J Vet Res* 1988, **49:**1098–1103.
3. Gatei MH, Brandon RB, Naif HM, Mclennan MW, Daniel RCW, Lavin MF: **Changes in B cell and T cell subsets in bovine leukaemia virus-infected cattle.** *Vet Immunol Immunopath* 1989, **23:**139–147.
4. Taylor BC, Stott JL, Thurmond MA, Picanso JP: **Alteration in lymphocyte subpopulations in bovine leukosis virus-infected cattle.** *Vet Immunol Immunopath* 1992, **31:**35–47.
5. Wu D, Takahashi K, Liu N, Koguchi A, Makara M, Sasaki J, Goryo M, Okada K: **Distribution of T-lymphocyte subpopulation in blood and spleen of normal cattle and cattle with enzootic bovine leukosis.** *J Comp Pathol* 1999, **120:**117–127.
6. Della Libera AMMP, Blagitz MG, Batista CF, Latorre AO, Stricagnolo CR, Souza FN: **Quantification of B cells and T lymphocytes subsets in bovine leukemia virus infected dairy cows.** *Semin-Cienc Agrar* 2012, **33:**1487–1494.
7. Ikebuchi R, Konnai S, Okagawa T, Yokoyama K, Nakajima C, Suzuki Y, Murata S, Ohashi K: **Blockade of bovine PD-1 increases T cell function and inhibits bovine leukemia virus expression in B cells in vitro.** *Vet Res* 2013, **44:**59.
8. Suzuki S, Konnai S, Okagawa T, Ikebuchi R, Shirai T, Sunden Y, Mingala CN, Murata S, Ohashi K: **Expression analysis of Foxp3 in T cells from bovine leukemia virus infected cattle.** *Microbiol Immunol* 2013, **57:**600–604.
9. Rademacher R, Sodomkova D, Vanasek J: **Alkaline phosphatase in neutrophil granulocytes of the peripheral blood of healthy and leukotic cattle.** *Vet Med (Praha)* 1977, **22:**673–677 (in German).
10. Walker AF, Lumsden JH, Stirtzinger T: **Neutrophil function in sheep experimentally infected with bovine leukemia virus.** *Vet Immunol Immunopathol* 1987, **14:**67–76.
11. Takamatsu H, Inumaru S, Nakajima H: **Inhibition of in vitro immunocyte function by sera from cattle with bovine leukosis.** *Vet Immunol Immunopathol* 1988, **18:**349–359.
12. Flaming KP, Frank DE, Carpenter S, Roth JA: **Longitudinal studies of immune function in cattle experimentally infected with bovine immunodeficiency virus and/or bovine leukemia virus.** *Vet Immunol Immunopathol* 1997, **56:**27–38.
13. Kaczmarczyk E, Bojarojc-Nosowicz B, Fiedorowicz A: **Leukocyte acid phosphatase and metabolic efficiency of phagocytes in the first lactation trimester of cows from a leukaemic herd.** *J Appl Genet* 2005, **46:**59–67.
14. Souza FN, Blagitz MG, Latorre AO, Ramos Sanchez EM, Batista CF, Weigel RA, Rennó FP, Sucupira MCA, Della Libera AMMP: **Intracellular reactive oxygen production by polymorphonuclear leukocytes in bovine leukemia virus-infected dairy cows.** *J Vet Med Sci* 2012, **74:**221–225.
15. Schwartz-Cornil I, Chevallier N, Belloc C, Rhun DL, Lainé V, Berthelemy M, Mateo A, Levy D: **Bovine leukaemia virus-induced lymphocytosis in sheep is associated with reduction of spontaneous B cell apoptosis.** *J Gen Virol* 1997, **78:**153–162.
16. Cantor GL, Pritchard SM, Dequiet F, Willems L, Kettman R, Davis WC: **CD5 is associated from the B-cell receptor in B cells from bovine leukemia virus-infected, persistently lymphocytotic cattle: consequences to B-cell receptor-mediated-apoptosis.** *J Virol* 2001, **75:**1689–1696.
17. Debacq C, Asquith B, Reichert M, Burny A, Kettmann R, Willems L: **Reduced cell turnover in bovine leukemia virus-infected persistently lymphocytotic cattle.** *J Virol* 2003, **77:**13073–13083.
18. Takahashi M, Tajima S, Takeshima S-N, Konnai S, Yin SA, Okada K, Davis WC, Aida Y: **Ex vivo survival of pheripheral blood mononuclear cells in sheep induced by bovine leukemia vírus (BLV) mainly occurs in CD5$^-$ B cells that express BLV.** *Microb Infect* 2004, **6:**584–595.
19. Florins A, Gillet N, Asquith B, Boxus M, Burtheau C, Twizere J-C, Urbain P, Vandermeers F, Debacq C, Sanchez-Alcaraz MT, Schwartz-Cornil I, Kerkhofs P, Jean G, Thewis A, Hay J, Mortheux F, Wattel E, Reichert M, Burny A, Kettmann R, Bangham C, Willems L: **Cell dynamics and immune response to BLV infection: an unifying model.** *Front Biosci* 2007, **12:**1520–1531.
20. Florins A, Boxus M, Vandermeers F, Verlaeten O, Bouzar A-B, Defoiche J, Hubaux R, Burny A, Kettmann R, Willems L: **Emphasis on cell turnover in two hosts infected by bovine leukemia virus: a rationale for host susceptibility to disease.** *Vet Immunol Immunopathol* 2008, **125:**01–07.
21. Erskine RJ, Corl CM, Gandy JC, Sordillo LM: **Effect of infection with bovine leucosis virus on lymphocyte proliferation and apoptosis in dairy cattle.** *Am J Vet Res* 2011, **72:**1059–1064.
22. Souza FN, Latorre AO, Caniceiro BD, Sakai M, Kieling K, Blagitz MG, Della Libera AMMP: **Apoptosis of CD5$^+$ cells and lymphocyte proliferation in bovine leukemia virus-infected dairy cows.** *Arq Bras Med Vet Zoot* 2011, **63:**1124–1130.
23. Emanuelson U, Scherling K, Pettersson H: **Relationship between herd bovine leukemia virus infection status and reproduction, disease incidence, and productivity in Swedish dairy herds.** *Prev Vet Med* 1992, **12:**121–131.
24. Rusov V, Milojevic Z, Stojanovic L: **Occurence of mastitis and sanitary-hygienic quality of milk of cows infected with enzootic leukosis.** *Vet Glasnik* 1994, **48:**303–308.
25. Sandev N, Koleva M, Binev R, Ilieva D: **Influence of enzootic bovine leukosis virus upon the incidence of subclinical mastitis in cows at a different stage of lactation.** *Vet Arch* 2004, **74:**411–416.

26. Jacobs RM, Pollari FL, McNab B, Jefferson B: **A serological survey of bovine syncytial in Otario: Associations with bovine leukemia and immunodeficiency-like viruses, production records, and management practices.** *Can J Vet Res* 1995, **59:**271–278.
27. Yoshikawa H, Xie B, Otamada T, Hiraga A, Yoshikawa T: **Detection of bovine leukemia viruses (BLV) in mammary tissues of BLV antibody-positive cows affected by subclinical mastitis.** *J Vet Med Sci* 1997, **59:**301–302.
28. Wellenberg GJ, Van der Poel WHM, Van Oirschot JT: **Viral infections and bovine mastitis: a review.** *Vet Microbiol* 2002, **88:**27–45.
29. Bojarojc-Nosowicz B, Kaczmarczyk E: **Somatic cell count and chemical composition of milk in naturally BLV-infected cows with different phenotypes of blood leukocyte acid phosphatase.** *Arch Tierz* 2006, **49:**17–28.
30. Rinaldi M, Li RW, Capuco AV: **Mastitis associated transcriptomic disruptions in cattle.** *Vet Immunol Immunopathol* 2010, **138:**267–279.
31. Da Y, Shanks RD, Stewart JA, Lewin HA: **Milk and fat yields decline in bovine leukemia virus-infected Holstein cattle with persistent lymphocytosis.** *Proc Natl Acad Sci U S A* 1993, **90:**6538–6541.
32. Sargeant JM, Kelton DF, Martin SW, Mann ED: **Associations between farm management practices, productivity, and bovine leukemia virus infection in Ontario dairy herds.** *Prev Vet Med* 1997, **31:**211–221.
33. D'Angelino JL, Garcia M, Birgel EH: **Productive and reproductive performance in cattle infected with bovine leukosis virus.** *J Dairy Res* 1998, **65:**693–695.
34. Ott SL, Johnson R, Wells SJ: **Association between bovine-leukosis virus seroprevalence and herd-level productivity on US dairy farms.** *Prev Vet Med* 2003, **61:**249–262.
35. Erskine RJ, Bartlett PC, Byrem TM, Render CL, Febvay C, Houseman JT: **Association between bovine leukemia virus, production, and population age in Michigan dairy herds.** *J Dairy Sci* 2012, **95:**727–734.
36. Paape MJ, Bannerman DD, Zhao X, Lee JW: **The bovine neutrophil: structure and function in blood and milk.** *Vet Res* 2003, **34:**597–627.
37. Rainard P, Riollet C: **Innate immunity of bovine mammary gland.** *Vet Res* 2006, **37:**369–400.
38. Elazar S, Gone E, Livneh-Kol I, Rosenshine I, Sphigel NY: **Essential role of neutrophils but not mammary gland alveolar macrophages in a murine model of acute *Escherichia coli* mastitis.** *Vet Res* 2010, **41:**53.
39. Souza FN, Ramos Sanchez EM, Heinemann MB, Gidlund MA, Reis LC, Blagitz MG, Della Libera AMMP, Cerqueira MMOP: **The innate immunity in bovine mastitis: the role of pattern-recognition receptors.** *Am J Immunol* 2012, **8:**166–178.
40. Blagitz MG, Souza FN, Santos BP, Batista CF, Parra AC, Azevedo LFF, Melville PA, Benites NR, Della Libera AMMP: **Function of milk polymorphonuclear neutrophils leukocytes in bovine mammary glands infected with *Corynebacterium bovis*.** *J Dairy Sci* 2013, **96:**3750–3757.
41. Schepers AJ, Lam TJGM, Schukken YH, Wilmink JBM, Hanekamp WJA: **Estimation of variance components for somatic cell counts to determine threshold for uninfected quarters.** *J Dairy Sci* 1997, **80:**1833–1840.
42. Schukken YH, Wilson DJ, Welcome F, Garrison-Tikofsky L, Gonzales RN: **Monitoring udder health and milk quality using somatic cell counts.** *Vet Res* 2003, **34:**579–596.
43. Divers TJ, Peek SF: *Rebhunn's diseases of dairy cattle.* St. Louis: Saunders Elsevier; 2008.
44. Thurmond MC, Carter RL, Picanso JP, Stralka K: **Upper-normal prediction limits of lymphocyte count for cattle not infected with bovine leukemia virus.** *Am J Vet Res* 1990, **51:**466–470.
45. Oliver SP, González RN, Hogan JS, Jayarao BM, Owens WE: *Microbiological procedures for the diagnosis of bovine udder infection and determination of milk quality.* Verona: National Mastitis Council; 2004.
46. Piepers S, De Meulemeester L, de Kruif A, Opsomer G, Barkema HW, De Vliegher S: **Prevalence and distribution of mastitis pathogens in subclinically infected dairy cows in Flanders, Belgium.** *J Dairy Res* 2007, **74:**478–483.
47. Piepers S, De Vliegher S: **Oral supplementation of medium-chain fatty acids during the dry period supports the neutrophil viability of peripartum dairy cows.** *J Dairy Res* 2013, **80:**309–318.
48. Koess C, Hamann J: **Detection of mastitis in the bovine mammary gland by flow cytometry at early stages.** *J Dairy Res* 2008, **75:**225–232.
49. Piepers S, De Vliegher S, Demeyere K, Lamrecht BN, de Kruif A, Meyer E, Opsomer G: **Technical note: flow cytometric identification of bovine milk neutrophils and simultaneous quantification of their viability.** *J Dairy Sci* 2009, **92:**626–631.
50. Hasui M, Hirabayashi Y, Kobayashi Y: **Simultaneous measurement by flow cytometry of phagocytosis and hydrogen peroxide production of neutrophils in whole blood.** *J Immunol Methods* 1989, **117:**53–58.
51. Diez-Fraile A, Meyer E, Paape MJ, Burvenich C: **Analysis of the selective mobilization of L-selectin and Mac-1 reservoirs in bovine neutrophils and eosinophils.** *Vet Res* 2003, **34:**57–70.
52. Trainin Z, Brenner J, Meirom R, Ungar-Waron H: **Detrimental effect of bovine leukemia virus (BLV) on immunological state of cattle.** *Vet Immunol Immunopathol* 1996, **56:**39–51.
53. Marinho J, Galvão-Castro B, Rodrigues LC, Barreto ML: **Increased risk of tuberculosis with human T-lymphotropic virus-1 infection.** *J Acquir Defic Syndr* 2005, **40:**625–628.
54. Verdonck K, González E, Schrooten W, Vanham G, Gotuzzo E: **HTLV-1 is associated with history of active tuberculosis among family members of HTLV-1 infected patients in Peru.** *Epidemiol Infect* 2008, **136:**1076–1083.
55. Vanleeuwen JA, Haddad JP, Dohoo IR, Keefe GP, Tiwari A, Scott HM: **Risk factors associated with *Neospora caninum* seropositivity in randomly samples Canadian dairy cows and herds.** *Prev Vet Med* 2010, **93:**129–138.
56. Mehrzad J, Duchateau L, Burvenich C: **Viability of milk neutrophils and severity of bovine coliform mastitis.** *J Dairy Sci* 2004, **87:**4150–4162.
57. Van Oostveldt K, Paape MJ, Dosogne H, Burvenich C: **Effect of apoptosis on phagocytosis, respiratory burst and CD18 adhesion receptor expression of bovine neutrophils.** *Domest Anim Endocrinol* 2002, **22:**37–50.
58. Mehrzad J, Duchateau L, Burvenich C: **High milk neutrophil chemiluminescence limits the severity of bovine coliform mastitis.** *Vet Res* 2005, **36:**101–116.
59. Juliarena MA, Gutierrez SE, Ceriani C: **Determinationof proviral load in bovine leukemia virus-infected cattle with and without lymphocytosis.** *Am J Vet Res* 2007, **68:**1220–1225.
60. Alvarez I, Gutiérrez G, Gammella M, Martinez C, Politzki R, González C, Caviglia L, Carignano H, Fondevila N, Poli M, Trono K: **Evaluation of total white blood cell count as a marker for proviral load of bovine leukemia virus in dairy cattle from herds with a high seroprevalence of antibodies against bovine leukemia virus.** *Am J Vet Res* 2013, **74:**744–749.
61. Yakobson B, Brenner J, Ungar-Waron H, Trainin Z: **Cellular immune response cytokine expression during initial stage of bovine leukemia virus (BLV) infection determines the disease progression to persistent lymphocytosis.** *Comp Immunol Microbiol Infect Dis* 2000, **23:**197–208.
62. Ikebuchi R, Konnai S, Shirai T, Sunden Y, Murata S, Onuma M, Ohashi K: **Increase of cells expressing PD-L1 in bovine leukemia virus infection and enhancement of anti-viral immune responses in vitro via PD-L1 blockade.** *Vet Res* 2011, **42:**103.
63. Okagawa T, Konnai S, Ikebuchi R, Suzuki S, Shirai T, Sunden Y, Onuma M, Murata S, Ohashi K: **Increased bovine Tim-3 and its ligand expressions during bovine leukemia virus infection.** *Vet Res* 2012, **43:**45.
64. Sordillo LM, Babiuk LA: **Modulation of bovine mammary gland function during the periparturient period following in vitro exposure to recombinant bovine intereferon gamma.** *Vet Immunol Immunopathol* 1991, **27:**393–402.
65. Gonen E, Nedvetzki S, Naor D, Shpigel NY: **CD44 is highly expressed on milk neutrophils in bovine mastitis and plays a role in their adhesion to matrix and mammary epithelium.** *Vet Res* 2008, **39:**29.
66. Vachon E, Martin R, Plumb J, Kwok V, Vandivier W, Glogauer M, Kapus A, Wang X, Chow C-W, Grinstein S, Downey GP: **CD44 is a phagocytic receptor.** *Blood* 2006, **107:**4149–4158.
67. Sladek Z, Rysanek D: **Expression of macrophage CD44 receptor in the course of experimental inflamammatory response of bovine mammary gland induced by lipopolysaccharide and muramyl dipeptide.** *Res Vet Sci* 2009, **89:**235–240.
68. Berland R, Wortis HH: **Origins and functions of B-1 cells with notes of the role of CD5.** *Annu Rev Immunol* 2002, **20:**253–300.
69. Kawai K, Tsuno NH, Matsuhashi M, Kitayama J, Osada T, Yamada J, Tsuchiya T, Yoneyama S, Watanabe T, Takahashi K, Nagawa H: **CD11b-mediated migratory property of peripheral blood B cells.** *J Allergy Clin Immunol* 2005, **16:**192–197.

Permissions

All chapters in this book were first published in VR, by BioMed Central; hereby published with permission under the Creative Commons Attribution License or equivalent. Every chapter published in this book has been scrutinized by our experts. Their significance has been extensively debated. The topics covered herein carry significant findings which will fuel the growth of the discipline. They may even be implemented as practical applications or may be referred to as a beginning point for another development.

The contributors of this book come from diverse backgrounds, making this book a truly international effort. This book will bring forth new frontiers with its revolutionizing research information and detailed analysis of the nascent developments around the world.

We would like to thank all the contributing authors for lending their expertise to make the book truly unique. They have played a crucial role in the development of this book. Without their invaluable contributions this book wouldn't have been possible. They have made vital efforts to compile up to date information on the varied aspects of this subject to make this book a valuable addition to the collection of many professionals and students.

This book was conceptualized with the vision of imparting up-to-date information and advanced data in this field. To ensure the same, a matchless editorial board was set up. Every individual on the board went through rigorous rounds of assessment to prove their worth. After which they invested a large part of their time researching and compiling the most relevant data for our readers.

The editorial board has been involved in producing this book since its inception. They have spent rigorous hours researching and exploring the diverse topics which have resulted in the successful publishing of this book. They have passed on their knowledge of decades through this book. To expedite this challenging task, the publisher supported the team at every step. A small team of assistant editors was also appointed to further simplify the editing procedure and attain best results for the readers.

Apart from the editorial board, the designing team has also invested a significant amount of their time in understanding the subject and creating the most relevant covers. They scrutinized every image to scout for the most suitable representation of the subject and create an appropriate cover for the book.

The publishing team has been an ardent support to the editorial, designing and production team. Their endless efforts to recruit the best for this project, has resulted in the accomplishment of this book. They are a veteran in the field of academics and their pool of knowledge is as vast as their experience in printing. Their expertise and guidance has proved useful at every step. Their uncompromising quality standards have made this book an exceptional effort. Their encouragement from time to time has been an inspiration for everyone.

The publisher and the editorial board hope that this book will prove to be a valuable piece of knowledge for researchers, students, practitioners and scholars across the globe.

List of Contributors

Igor Kolotilin
Department of Biology, University of Western Ontario, 1151 Richmond St, London, ON, Canada

Ed Topp
AAFC, Southern Crop Protection and Food Research Centre, 1391 Sandford St, London, ON, Canada

Eric Cox
Laboratory of Immunology, Faculty of Veterinary Medicine, Ghent University, Salisburylaan 133, 9820 Merelbeke, Belgium

Bert Devriendt
Laboratory of Immunology, Faculty of Veterinary Medicine, Ghent University, Salisburylaan 133, 9820 Merelbeke, Belgium

Udo Conrad
Leibniz Institute of Plant Genetics and Crop Plant Research, Gatersleben, Germany

Jussi Joensuu
VTT Technical Research Centre of Finland, Espoo, Finland

Eva Stöger
Department for Applied Genetics and Cell Biology, University of Natural Resources and Life Sciences, Vienna, Austria

Heribert Warzecha
Technische Universität Darmstadt, FB Biologie, Schnittspahnstr. 5, D-64287 Darmstadt, Germany

Tim McAllister
AAFC, Lethbridge Research Centre, 5403, 1 Avenue South, Lethbridge, Alberta, Canada

Andrew Potter
Vaccine and Infectious Disease Organization (VIDO), University of Saskatchewan, 120 Veterinary Road, Saskatoon, Saskatchewan, Canada
Department of Veterinary Microbiology, University of Saskatchewan, 120 Veterinary Road, Saskatoon, Saskatchewan, Canada

Michael D McLean
PlantForm Corp., c/o Room 2218, E.C. Bovey Bldg, University of Guelph, Guelph, Ontario N1G 2 W1, Canada

J Christopher Hall
School of Environmental Sciences, University of Guelph, 50 Stone Road East, Guelph, Ontario N1G 2 W1, Canada

Rima Menassa
Department of Biology, University of Western Ontario, 1151 Richmond St, London, ON, Canada
AAFC, Southern Crop Protection and Food Research Centre, 1391 Sandford St, London, ON, Canada

Chandrika Senthilkumaran
Department of Pathobiology, University of Guelph, Guelph, ON, N1G 2W1, Canada

Joanne Hewson
Department of Clinical Studies, University of Guelph, Guelph, ON, N1G 2W1, Canada

Theresa L Ollivett
Department of Population Medicine, University of Guelph, Guelph, ON, N1G 2W1, Canada

Dorothee Bienzle
Department of Pathobiology, University of Guelph, Guelph, ON, N1G 2W1, Canada

Brandon N Lillie
Department of Pathobiology, University of Guelph, Guelph, ON, N1G 2W1, Canada

Mary Ellen Clark
Department of Pathobiology, University of Guelph, Guelph, ON, N1G 2W1, Canada

Jeff L Caswell
Department of Pathobiology, University of Guelph, Guelph, ON, N1G 2W1, Canada

Line Olsen
Department of Basic Sciences and Aquatic Medicine, Faculty of Veterinary Medicine and Biosciences, Norwegian University of Life Sciences, Oslo, Norway

Caroline Piercey Åkesson
Department of Basic Sciences and Aquatic Medicine, Faculty of Veterinary Medicine and Biosciences, Norwegian University of Life Sciences, Oslo, Norway

Anne K Storset
Department of Food Safety & Infection Biology, Faculty of Veterinary Medicine and iosciences, Norwegian University of Life Sciences, Oslo, Norway

Sonia Lacroix-Lamandé
Institut National de la Recherche Agronomique, UMR1282, Infectiologie et Santé Publique, Laboratoire Apicomplexes et Immunité Muqueuse, Nouzilly, France

Preben Boysen
Department of Food Safety & Infection Biology, Faculty of Veterinary Medicine and iosciences, Norwegian University of Life Sciences, Oslo, Norway

CoralieMetton
Institut National de la Recherche Agronomique, UMR1282, Infectiologie et Santé Publique, Laboratoire Apicomplexes et Immunité Muqueuse, Nouzilly, France

Timothy Connelley
The Roslin Institute, Royal (Dick) School of Veterinary Studies, University of Edinburgh, Edinburgh, UK

Arild Espenes
Department of Basic Sciences and Aquatic Medicine, Faculty of Veterinary Medicine and Biosciences, Norwegian University of Life Sciences, Oslo, Norway

Fabrice Laurent
Institut National de la Recherche Agronomique, UMR1282, Infectiologie et Santé Publique, Laboratoire Apicomplexes et Immunité Muqueuse, Nouzilly, France

Françoise Drouet
Institut National de la Recherche Agronomique, UMR1282, Infectiologie et Santé Publique, Laboratoire Apicomplexes et Immunité Muqueuse, Nouzilly, France

Jean-Rémy Sadeyen
Avian Infectious Diseases Programme, The Pirbright Institute, Compton, Berkshire, RG20 7NN, UK

Zhiguang Wu
The Roslin Institute and Royal (Dick) School of Veterinary Studies, University of Edinburgh, Easter Bush, Midlothian EH25 9RG, UK

Holly Davies
Avian Infectious Diseases Programme, The Pirbright Institute, Compton, Berkshire, RG20 7NN, UK

Pauline M van Diemen
The Jenner Institute, University of Oxford, Oxford OX3 7DQ, UK

Anita Milicic
The Jenner Institute, University of Oxford, Oxford OX3 7DQ, UK

Roberto M La Ragione
School of Veterinary Medicine, University of Surrey, Guildford, GU2 7TE, UK
Department of Bacteriology, AHVLA, Weybridge, Surrey, KT15 3NB, UK

Pete Kaiser
The Roslin Institute and Royal (Dick) School of Veterinary Studies, University of Edinburgh, Easter Bush, Midlothian EH25 9RG, UK

Mark P Stevens
The Roslin Institute and Royal (Dick) School of Veterinary Studies, University of Edinburgh, Easter Bush, Midlothian EH25 9RG, UK

Francis Dziva
Avian Infectious Diseases Programme, The Pirbright Institute, Compton, Berkshire, RG20 7NN, UK
Present address: School of Veterinary Medicine, The University of the West Indies, St Augustine, Trinidad and Tobago

Ornampai Japa
School of Veterinary Medicine and Science, University of Nottingham, Sutton Bonington, Nottingham LE12 5RD, UK

Jane E Hodgkinson
Department of Infection Biology, Institute of Infection and Global Health, University of Liverpool, Liverpool L3 5RF, UK

Richard D Emes
School of Veterinary Medicine and Science, University of Nottingham, Sutton Bonington, Nottingham LE12 5RD, UK
Advanced Data AnalysisCentre, University of Nottingham, Sutton Bonington, Nottingham LE12 5RD, UK

Robin J Flynn
School of Veterinary Medicine and Science, University of Nottingham, Sutton Bonington, Nottingham LE12 5RD, UK

Jin Ju Lee
Animal and Plant Quarantine Agency, Anyang, Gyeonggi-do 430-757, Republic of Korea

Hannah Leah Simborio
Institute of Animal Medicine, College of Veterinary Medicine, Gyeongsang National University, Jinju, 660-701, Republic of Korea

Alisha Wehdnesday Bernardo Reyes
Institute of Animal Medicine, College of Veterinary Medicine, Gyeongsang National University, Jinju, 660-701, Republic of Korea

Dae Geun Kim
Institute of Animal Medicine, College of Veterinary Medicine, Gyeongsang National University, Jinju, 660-701, Republic of Korea

Huynh Tan Hop
Institute of Animal Medicine, College of Veterinary Medicine, Gyeongsang National University, Jinju, 660-701, Republic of Korea

Wongi Min
Institute of Animal Medicine, College of Veterinary Medicine, Gyeongsang National University, Jinju, 660-701, Republic of Korea

Moon Her
Animal and Plant Quarantine Agency, Anyang, Gyeonggi-do 430-757, Republic of Korea

Suk Chan Jung
Animal and Plant Quarantine Agency, Anyang, Gyeonggi-do 430-757, Republic of Korea

Han Sang Yoo
Department of Infectious Diseases, College of Veterinary Medicine, Seoul National University, Seoul 151-742, Republic of Korea

Suk Kim
Institute of Animal Medicine, College of Veterinary Medicine, Gyeongsang National University, Jinju, 660-701, Republic of Korea
Institute of Agriculture and Life Science, Gyeongsang National University, Jinju, 660-701, Republic of Korea

Fernando Núñez-Hernández
Centre de Recerca en Sanitat Animal (CReSA), UAB-IRTA, Campus de la Universitat Autònoma de Barcelona, Bellaterra, Cerdanyola del Vallès, Spain

Lester J Pérez
Centro Nacional de Sanidad Agropecuaria (CENSA), La Habana, Cuba

Marta Muñoz
Centre de Recerca en Sanitat Animal (CReSA), UAB-IRTA, Campus de la Universitat Autònoma de Barcelona, Bellaterra, Cerdanyola del Vallès, Spain

Gonzalo Vera
Departament de Genètica Animal, Centre de Recerca en AgriGenòmica (CRAG), CSIC- IRTA-UAB-UB, Universitat Autònoma de Barcelona, Bellaterra, Barcelona, Spain

Anna Tomás
Programa Infección e Inmunidad, Fundació d́ Investigació Sanitària de les illes Balears, 07110 Buynola, Spain

Raquel Egea
Departament de Genètica Animal, Centre de Recerca en AgriGenòmica (CRAG), CSIC- IRTA-UAB-UB, Universitat Autònoma de Barcelona, Bellaterra, Barcelona, Spain

Sarai Córdoba
Departament de Genètica Animal, Centre de Recerca en AgriGenòmica (CRAG), CSIC- IRTA-UAB-UB, Universitat Autònoma de Barcelona, Bellaterra, Barcelona, Spain

Joaquim Segalés
Centre de Recerca en Sanitat Animal (CReSA), UAB-IRTA, Campus de la Universitat Autònoma de Barcelona, Bellaterra, Cerdanyola del Vallès, Spain
Departament de Sanitat I Anatomia Animals, Universitat Autònoma de Barcelona, Bellaterra, Barcelona, Spain

Armand Sánchez
Departament de Genètica Animal, Centre de Recerca en AgriGenòmica (CRAG), CSIC- IRTA-UAB-UB, Universitat Autònoma de Barcelona, Bellaterra, Barcelona, Spain
Departament de Ciència Animal i dels Aliments, Universitat Autònoma de Barcelona (UAB), Bellaterra, Barcelona, Spain

José I Núñez
Centre de Recerca en Sanitat Animal (CReSA), UAB-IRTA, Campus de la Universitat Autònoma de Barcelona, Bellaterra, Cerdanyola del Vallès, Spain

Darren W Gray
Institute for Global Food Security (IGFS), School of Biological Sciences, Queen's University Belfast (QUB), Belfast, Northern Ireland, BT9 5AG, UK

Michael D Welsh
Veterinary Sciences Division (VSD), Agri-Food and Biosciences Institute (AFBI), Belfast, Northern Ireland, BT4 3SD, UK

Simon Doherty
Veterinary Sciences Division (VSD), Agri-Food and Biosciences Institute (AFBI), Belfast, Northern Ireland, BT4 3SD, UK

Fawad Mansoor
Veterinary Sciences Division (VSD), Agri-Food and Biosciences Institute (AFBI), Belfast, Northern Ireland, BT4 3SD, UK

Olivier P Chevallier
Institute for Global Food Security (IGFS), School of Biological Sciences, Queen's University Belfast (QUB), Belfast, Northern Ireland, BT9 5AG, UK

Christopher T Elliott
Institute for Global Food Security (IGFS), School of Biological Sciences, Queen's University Belfast (QUB), Belfast, Northern Ireland, BT9 5AG, UK

Mark H Mooney
Institute for Global Food Security (IGFS), School of Biological Sciences, Queen's University Belfast (QUB), Belfast, Northern Ireland, BT9 5AG, UK

Jana Seele
Institute for Microbiology, Centre for Infection Medicine, University of Veterinary Medicine Hannover, 30173 Hannover, Germany

Andreas Beineke
Department of Pathology, University of Veterinary Medicine Hannover, 30559 Hannover, Germany

Lena-Maria Hillermann
Institute for Microbiology, Centre for Infection Medicine, University of Veterinary Medicine Hannover, 30173 Hannover, Germany

Beate Jaschok-Kentner
Department of Structure and Function of Proteins, Helmholtz Centre for Infection Research, 38124 Braunschweig, Germany

Ulrich von Pawel-Rammingen
Department of Molecular Biology and Umeå Centre for Microbial Research, Umeå University, 90187 Umeå, Sweden

Peter Valentin-Weigand
Institute for Microbiology, Centre for Infection Medicine, University of Veterinary Medicine Hannover, 30173 Hannover, Germany

Christoph Georg Baums
Institute for Bacteriology and Mycology, Centre of Infectious Diseases, College of Veterinary Medicine, University Leipzig, An den Tierkliniken 29, 04103 Leipzig, Germany

Hanna C Koinig
University Clinic for Swine, Department for Farm Animals and Veterinary Public Health, University of Veterinary Medicine, Vienna, Austria
Institute of Immunology, Department of Pathobiology, University of Veterinary Medicine, Vienna, Austria

Stephanie C Talker
Institute of Immunology, Department of Pathobiology, University of Veterinary Medicine, Vienna, Austria

Maria Stadler
Institute of Immunology, Department of Pathobiology, University of Veterinary Medicine, Vienna, Austria

Andrea Ladinig
University Clinic for Swine, Department for Farm Animals and Veterinary Public Health, University of Veterinary Medicine, Vienna, Austria

Robert Graage
University Clinic for Swine, Department for Farm Animals and Veterinary Public Health, University of Veterinary Medicine, Vienna, Austria
Current address: Institute of Veterinary Pathology, Vetsuisse-Faculty, University of Zurich, Zurich, Switzerland

Mathias Ritzmann
University Clinic for Swine, Department for Farm Animals and Veterinary Public Health, University of Veterinary Medicine, Vienna, Austria
Current address:Clinic for Swine, Ludwig-Maximilians-University, Munich, Germany

Isabel Hennig-Pauka
University Clinic for Swine, Department for Farm Animals and Veterinary Public Health, University of Veterinary Medicine, Vienna, Austria

Wilhelm Gerner
Institute of Immunology, Department of Pathobiology, University of Veterinary Medicine, Vienna, Austria

Armin Saalmüller
Institute of Immunology, Department of Pathobiology, University of Veterinary Medicine, Vienna, Austria

Amin Tahoun
Division of Immunity and Infection, The Roslin Institute and R(D)SVS, The University of Edinburgh, Easter Bush, Midlothian EH25 9RG, UK
Faculty of Veterinary Medicine, Kafrelsheikh University, 33516 Kafr el-Sheikh, Egypt

Kirsty Jensen
Division of Immunity and Infection, The Roslin Institute and R(D)SVS, The University of Edinburgh, Easter Bush, Midlothian EH25 9RG, UK

Yolanda Corripio-Miyar
Division of Immunity and Infection, The Roslin Institute and R(D)SVS, The University of Edinburgh, Easter Bush, Midlothian EH25 9RG, UK

Sean P McAteer
Division of Immunity and Infection, The Roslin Institute and R(D)SVS, The University of Edinburgh, Easter Bush, Midlothian EH25 9RG, UK

Alexander Corbishley
Division of Immunity and Infection, The Roslin Institute and R(D)SVS, The University of Edinburgh, Easter Bush, Midlothian EH25 9RG, UK
Moredun Research Institute, Pentlands Science Park, Bush Loan, Penicuik, Edinburgh EH26 OPZ, UK

Arvind Mahajan
Division of Immunity and Infection, The Roslin Institute and R(D)SVS, The University of Edinburgh, Easter Bush, Midlothian EH25 9RG, UK

Helen Brown
Division of Immunity and Infection, The Roslin Institute and R(D)SVS, The University of Edinburgh, Easter Bush, Midlothian EH25 9RG, UK

David Frew
Moredun Research Institute, Pentlands Science Park, Bush Loan, Penicuik, Edinburgh EH26 OPZ, UK

Aude Aumeunier
Institute of Infection, Immunity & Inflammation, Glasgow Biomedical Research Centre, University of Glasgow, Glasgow G12 8TA, UK

David GE Smith
Moredun Research Institute, Pentlands Science Park, Bush Loan, Penicuik, Edinburgh EH26 OPZ, UK
Institute of Infection, Immunity & Inflammation, Glasgow Biomedical Research Centre, University of Glasgow, Glasgow G12 8TA, UK

Tom N McNeilly
Moredun Research Institute, Pentlands Science Park, Bush Loan, Penicuik, Edinburgh EH26 OPZ, UK

Elizabeth J Glass
Division of Immunity and Infection, The Roslin Institute and R(D)SVS, The University of Edinburgh, Easter Bush, Midlothian EH25 9RG, UK

David L Gally
Division of Immunity and Infection, The Roslin Institute and R(D)SVS, The University of Edinburgh, Easter Bush, Midlothian EH25 9RG, UK

Ben C Maddison
ADAS UK, School of Veterinary Medicine and Science, The University of Nottingham, Sutton Bonington Campus, College Road, Sutton Bonington, Leicestershire, UK

John Spiropoulos
Animal and Plant Health Agency, Woodham Lane, New Haw, Addlestone, Surrey, UK

Christopher M Vickery
Animal and Plant Health Agency, Woodham Lane, New Haw, Addlestone, Surrey, UK

Richard Lockey
Animal and Plant Health Agency, Woodham Lane, New Haw, Addlestone, Surrey, UK
Current address: University of Southampton, Southampton SO17 1BJ, UK

Jonathan P Owen
ADAS UK, School of Veterinary Medicine and Science, The University of Nottingham, Sutton Bonington Campus, College Road, Sutton Bonington, Leicestershire, UK

Keith Bishop
ADAS UK, School of Veterinary Medicine and Science, The University of Nottingham, Sutton Bonington Campus, College Road, Sutton Bonington, Leicestershire, UK

Claire A Baker
ADAS UK, School of Veterinary Medicine and Science, The University of Nottingham, Sutton Bonington Campus, College Road, Sutton Bonington, Leicestershire, UK

Kevin C Gough
School of Veterinary Medicine and Science, The University of Nottingham, Sutton Bonington Campus, College Road, Sutton Bonington, Leicestershire, UK

Alison Burrells
Moredun Research Institute, Pentlands Science Park, Bush Loan, Midlothian EH26 0PZ, Scotland, UK

Julio Benavides
Moredun Research Institute, Pentlands Science Park, Bush Loan, Midlothian EH26 0PZ, Scotland, UK
Instituto de Ganadería de Montaña (CSIC-ULE), León, Spain

German Cantón
Moredun Research Institute, Pentlands Science Park, Bush Loan, Midlothian EH26 0PZ, Scotland, UK
Instituto Nacional de Tecnología Agropecuaria (INATA), EEA Balcarce, Argentina

João L Garcia
Moredun Research Institute, Pentlands Science Park, Bush Loan, Midlothian EH26 0PZ, Scotland, UK
Departamento de Medicina Veterinária Preventiva, Universidade Estadual de Londrina, Londrina, Brazil

Paul M Bartley
Moredun Research Institute, Pentlands Science Park, Bush Loan, Midlothian EH26 0PZ, Scotland, UK

Mintu Nath
Biomathematics & Statistics Scotland, The King's Buildings, Edinburgh EH9 3JZ, Scotland, UK

Jackie Thomson
Moredun Research Institute, Pentlands Science Park, Bush Loan, Midlothian EH26 0PZ, Scotland, UK

Francesca Chianini
Moredun Research Institute, Pentlands Science Park, Bush Loan, Midlothian EH26 0PZ, Scotland, UK

Elisabeth A Innes
Moredun Research Institute, Pentlands Science Park, Bush Loan, Midlothian EH26 0PZ, Scotland, UK

Frank Katzer
Moredun Research Institute, Pentlands Science Park, Bush Loan, Midlothian EH26 0PZ, Scotland, UK

Katharina Kerner
Institute of Hygiene and Infectious Diseases of Animals, Justus Liebig University, Frankfurter Str. 85-89, 35392 Giessen, Germany

Philip S Bridger
Institute of Hygiene and Infectious Diseases of Animals, Justus Liebig University, Frankfurter Str. 85-89, 35392 Giessen, Germany

Gabriele Köpf
Institute of Hygiene and Infectious Diseases of Animals, Justus Liebig University, Frankfurter Str. 85-89, 35392 Giessen, Germany

Julia Fröhlich
Institute of Hygiene and Infectious Diseases of Animals, Justus Liebig University, Frankfurter Str. 85-89, 35392 Giessen, Germany

Stefanie Barth
Institute of Hygiene and Infectious Diseases of Animals, Justus Liebig University, Frankfurter Str. 85-89, 35392 Giessen, Germany
Current Address: Friedrich-Loeffler-Institut, Institute of Molecular Pathogenesis, Naumburger Str. 96a, 07743 Jena, Germany

Hermann Willems
Clinic for Ruminants and Swine (Internal Medicine & Surgery), Justus Liebig University, Giessen, Germany

Rolf Bauerfeind
Institute of Hygiene and Infectious Diseases of Animals, Justus Liebig University, Frankfurter Str. 85-89, 35392 Giessen, Germany

Georg Baljer
Institute of Hygiene and Infectious Diseases of Animals, Justus Liebig University, Frankfurter Str. 85-89, 35392 Giessen, Germany

Christian Menge
Institute of Hygiene and Infectious Diseases of Animals, Justus Liebig University, Frankfurter Str. 85-89, 35392 Giessen, Germany
Current Address: Friedrich-Loeffler-Institut, Institute of Molecular Pathogenesis, Naumburger Str. 96a, 07743 Jena, Germany

Alexandra Jaeger
Institute for Genome Biology, Leibniz-Institute for Farm Animal Biology, Wilhelm-Stahl-Allee 2, D-18196 Dummerstorf, Germany

Danilo Bardehle
Institute of Agricultural and Nutritional Sciences, Martin-Luther-University Halle-Wittenberg, Theodor-Lieser-Straße 11, D-06120 Halle (Saale), Germany

Michael Oster
Institute for Genome Biology, Leibniz-Institute for Farm Animal Biology, Wilhelm-Stahl-Allee 2, D-18196 Dummerstorf, Germany

Juliane Günther
Institute for Genome Biology, Leibniz-Institute for Farm Animal Biology, Wilhelm-Stahl-Allee 2, D-18196 Dummerstorf, Germany

Eduard Muráni
Institute for Genome Biology, Leibniz-Institute for Farm Animal Biology, Wilhelm-Stahl-Allee 2, D-18196 Dummerstorf, Germany

Siriluck Ponsuksili
Institute for Genome Biology, Leibniz-Institute for Farm Animal Biology, Wilhelm-Stahl-Allee 2, D-18196 Dummerstorf, Germany

Klaus Wimmers
Institute for Genome Biology, Leibniz-Institute for Farm Animal Biology, Wilhelm-Stahl-Allee 2, D-18196 Dummerstorf, Germany

Nicole Kemper
Institute for Animal Hygiene, Animal Welfare and Livestock Ethology, University of Veterinary Medicine Hannover, Foundation, Bischofsholer Damm 15, D-30173 Hannover, Germany

Alice Maria Melville Paiva Della Liber
Departamento de Clínica Médica, Faculdade de Medicina Veterinária e Zootecnia, Universidade de São Paulo, Av. Prof. Dr. Orlando Marques de Paiva, 87, Cidade Universitária, São Paulo 05508-270, Brazil

Fernando Nogueira de Souza
Departamento de Medicina Veterinária Preventiva, Escola de Veterinária, Universidade
Federal de Minas Gerais, Belo Horizonte 31270-010, Brazil

Camila Freitas Batista
Departamento de Clínica Médica, Faculdade de Medicina Veterinária e Zootecnia, Universidade de São Paulo, Av. Prof. Dr. Orlando Marques de Paiva, 87, Cidade Universitária, São Paulo 05508-270, Brazil

Bruna Parapinski Santos
Departamento de Clínica Médica, Faculdade de Medicina Veterinária e Zootecnia, Universidade de São Paulo, Av. Prof. Dr. Orlando Marques de Paiva, 87, Cidade Universitária, São Paulo 05508-270, Brazil

Luis Fernando Fernandes de Azevedo
Departamento de Clínica Médica, Faculdade de Medicina Veterinária e Zootecnia, Universidade de São Paulo, Av. Prof. Dr. Orlando Marques de Paiva, 87, Cidade Universitária, São Paulo 05508-270, Brazil

Eduardo Milton Ramos Sanchez
Laboratório de Sorologia e Imunobiologia, Instituto de Medicina Tropical, Universidade de São Paulo, São Paulo 05403-000, Brazil

Soraia Araújo Diniz
Departamento de Medicina Veterinária Preventiva, Escola de Veterinária, Universidade Federal de Minas Gerais, Belo Horizonte 31270-010, Brazil

Marcos Xavier Silva
Departamento de Medicina Veterinária Preventiva, Escola de Veterinária, Universidade Federal de Minas Gerais, Belo Horizonte 31270-010, Brazil

João Paulo Haddad
Departamento de Medicina Veterinária Preventiva, Escola de Veterinária, Universidade Federal de Minas Gerais, Belo Horizonte 31270-010, Brazil

Maiara Garcia Blagitz
Departamento de Clínica Médica, Faculdade de Medicina Veterinária e Zootecnia, Universidade de São Paulo, Av. Prof. Dr. Orlando Marques de Paiva, 87, Cidade Universitária, São Paulo 05508-270, Brazil

Lightning Source UK Ltd.
Milton Keynes UK
UKHW052052080922
408534UK00002B/57

9 781682 860656

ORIGINAL
PONTIAC FIREBIRD
AND
TRANS AM

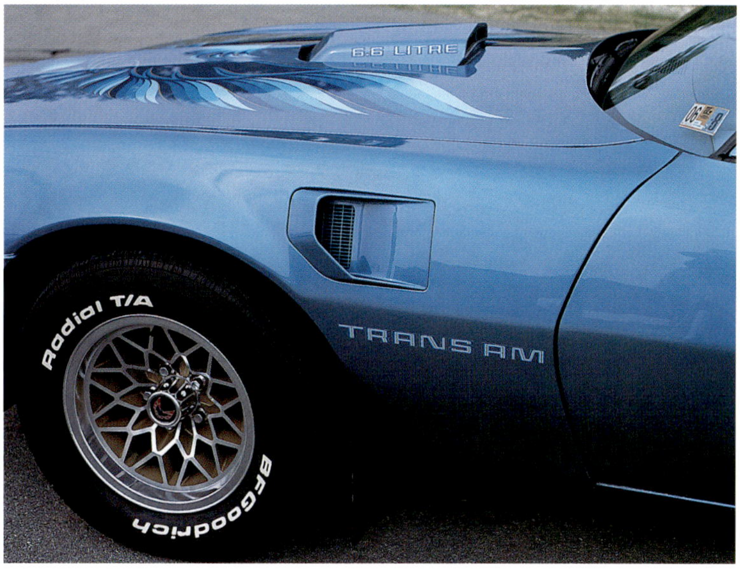

Other titles available in the *Original* series are:

Original Alfa Romeo Spider
by Chris Rees
Original Allis-Chalmers
by Guy Fay
Original Austin-Healey (100 & 3000)
by Anders Ditlev Clausager
Original BMW M-Series
by James Taylor
Original BMW Air-Cooled Boxer Twins
by Ian Falloon
Original Camaro 1967–1969
by Jason Scott
Original Challenger & Barracuda 1970–1974
by Jim Schild
Original Chevelle 1964–1972
by Jim Schild
Original Chevrolet 1955–1957
by Robert Genat
Original Citroën DS
by John Reynolds with Jan de Lange
Original Corvette 1953–1962
by Tom Falconer
Original Corvette 1968–1982
by Tom Falconer
Original Dodge & Plymouth 1966–1970
by Jim Schild
Original Ducati Sport & Super Sport 1972–1986
by Ian Falloon
Original Farmall Cub and Cub Cadet
by Kenneth Updike
Original Farmall Hundred Sereis, 1954–1958
by Guy Fay
Original Ferrari V8
by Keith Bluemel
Original Ferrari V12 1965–1973
by Keith Bluemel
Original Ford Model A
by Jim Schild
Original Harley-Davidson Knucklehead
by Greg Field
Original Harley-Davidson Panhead
by Gregg Field
Original Jaguar E-Type
by Philip Porter
Original Jaguar XJ
by Nigel Thorley
Original Jaguar XK
by Philip Porter
Original John Deere Letter Series Tractors
by Brian Rukes
Original John Deere Model A
by Brian Rukes
Original Mercedes-Benz
Coupes, Cabriolets and V8 Sedans
1960–1972
by Tim Slade
Original Mercedes SL
by Laurence Meredith
Original MGA
by Anders Ditlev Clausager
Original MGB, C & V8
by Anders Ditlev Clausager
Original Mini Cooper and Cooper S
by John Parnell
Original Morgan
by John Worrall and Liz Turner
Original Mustang 1964½–1966
by Colin Date
Original Mustang, 1967–1970
by Colin Date
Original Pontiac GTO 1964–1974
by Tom de Mauro
Original Porsche 356
by Laurence Meredith
Original Porsche 356: The Restorer's Guide
by Laurence Meredith
Original Porsche 911
by Peter Morgan
Original Porsche 924/944/968
by Peter Morgan
Original Rolls-Royce & Bentley 1946–65
by James Taylor
Original Sprite & Midget
by Terry Horler
Original Triumph Bonneville
by Gerard Kane
Original Triumph TR4/4A/5/6
by Bill Piggott
Original Triumph TR7 & TR8
by Bill Piggott

ORIGINAL
PONTIAC FIREBIRD
AND
TRANS AM
1967–2002

by Jim Schild

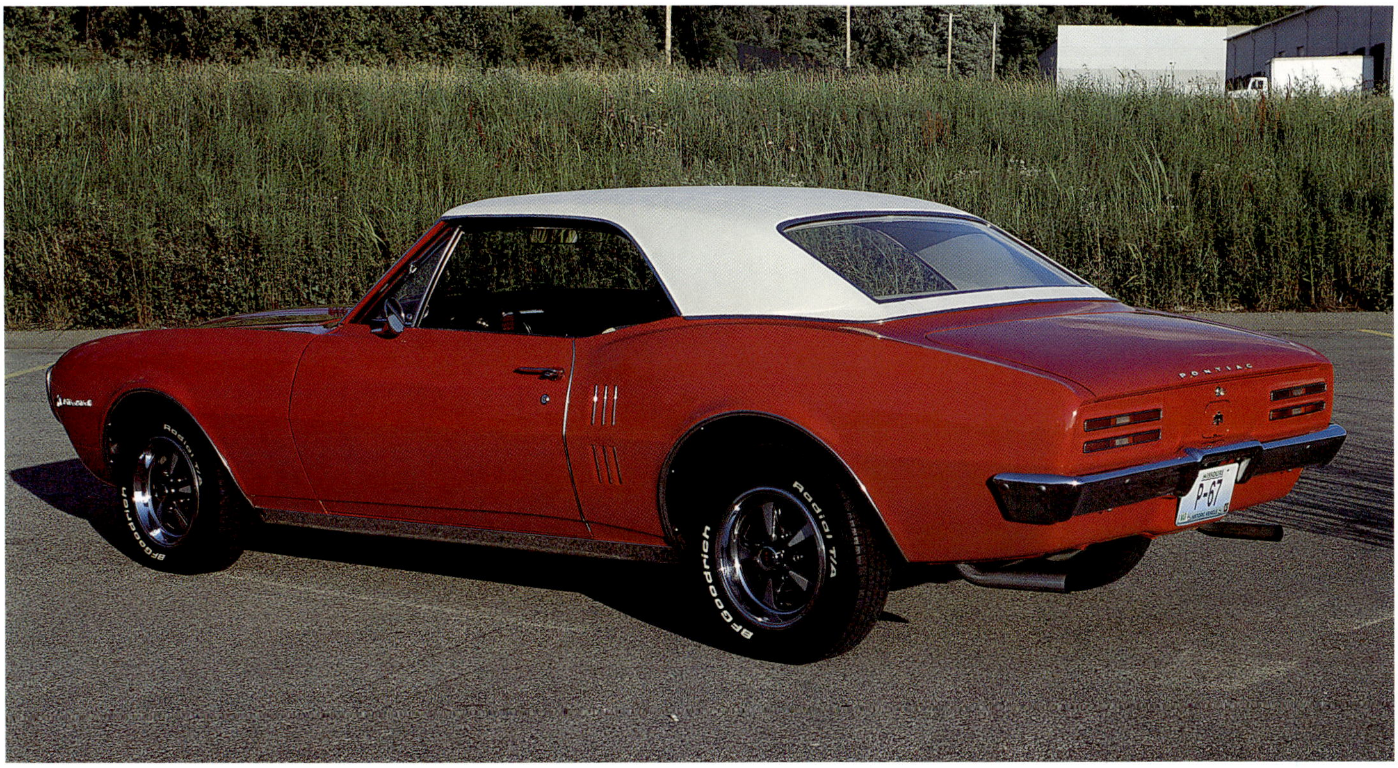

MOTORBOOKS

First published in 2007 by Motorbooks, an imprint of MBI Publishing Company, Galtier Plaza, Suite 200, 380 Jackson Street, St. Paul, MN 55101 USA

The information in this book is true and complete to the best of our knowledge. All recommendations are made without any guarantee on the part of the author or Publisher, who also disclaim any liability incurred in connection with the use of this data or specific details.

This publication has not been prepared, approved, or licensed by General Motors.

We recognize, further, that some words, model names, and designations mentioned herein are the property of the trademark holder. We use them for identification purposes only. This is not an official publication.

Motorbooks titles are also available at discounts in bulk quantity for industrial or sales-promotional use. For details write to Special Sales Manager at MBI Publishing Company, Galtier Plaza, Suite 200, 380 Jackson Street, St. Paul, MN 55101 USA.

To find out more about our books, join us online at www.motorbooks.com.

Editor: Lindsay Hitch
Designer: Christopher Fayers

Printed in China

Library of Congress Cataloging-in-Publication Data

Schild, James J., 1947-
Original Pontiac Firebird and Trans Am 1967–2002 : the restorer's guide / by Jim Schild.
p. cm.
Includes index.
ISBN-13: 978-0-7603-2839-2 (hardbound w/ jacket)
ISBN-10: 0-7603-2839-0 (hardbound w/ jacket)
1. Firebird automobile—Conservation and restoration. 2. Firebird automobile—History. I. Title.
TL215.F57S348 2007
629.222'2—dc22

2006101680

On the front cover: Don Bennett owns this original 1973 Trans Am 455 Super Duty.

On the back cover: The left side view of this Brentwood Brown 1977 Trans Am sport coupe shows the smooth, flowing lines of the popular second-generation body. This Trans Am has Rally II wheels with trim rings and an accessory rear window louver.

Frontispiece: This is a detail view of the left front fender and hood on a Bright Blue 1979 Trans Am equipped with the 6.6-liter V-8. Note the distinctive extractor vent on the rear of the fender.

Title: This red 1967 Firebird 326 coupe is equipped with an optional white vinyl Cordova roof. This left rear quarter view shows the optional Rally II wheels and bright door edge moldings.

Contents: The left front view shows the front fender on a Bright Red 1996 Trans Am coupe with optional T-top hatch roof. This view shows the lines of the fourth-generation Firebird composite body structure.

Contents

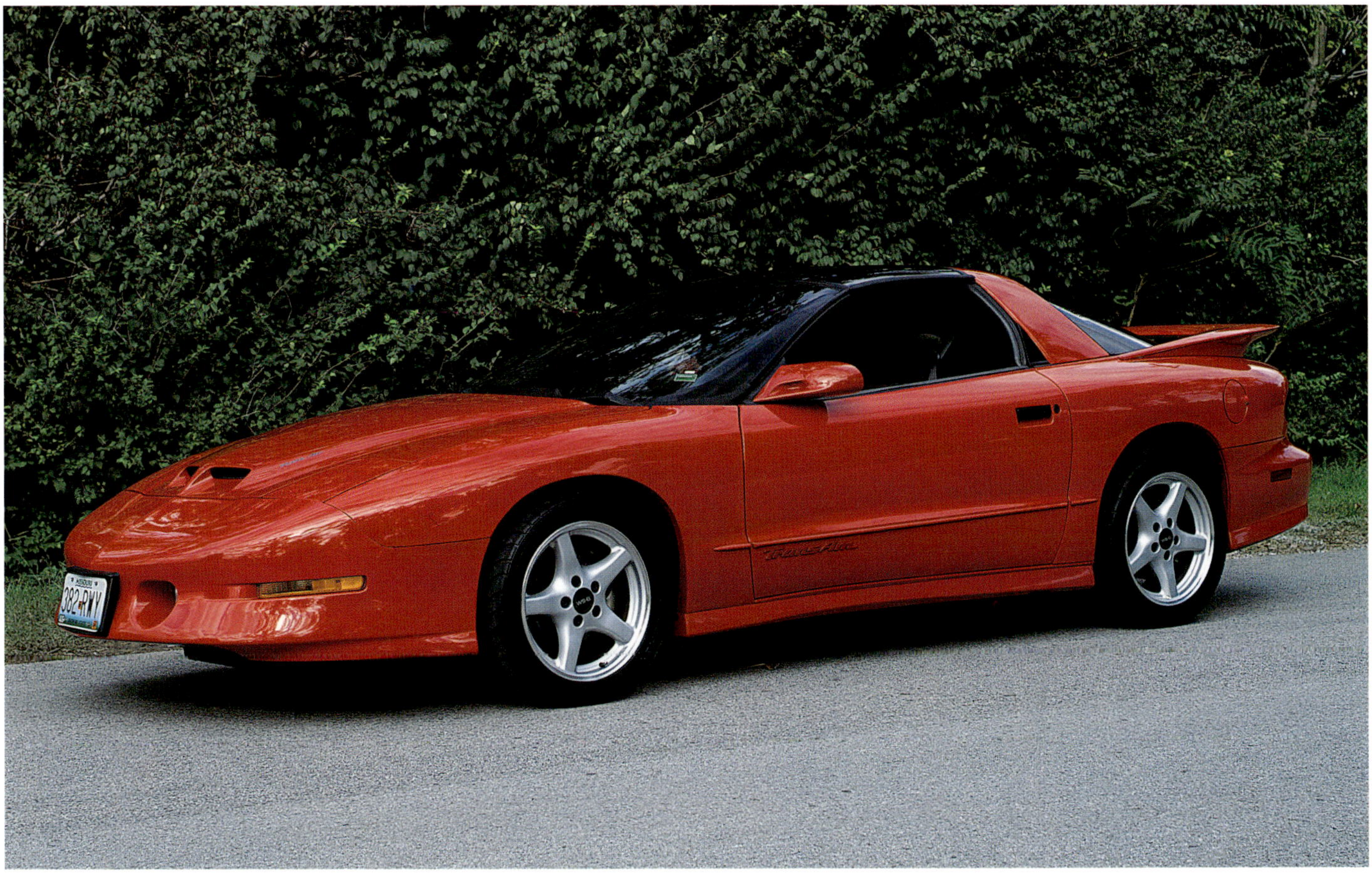

Acknowledgments

Any book of this type cannot be completed successfully without the cooperation, knowledge, and experience of many people. Although I have more than 40 years of experience working on, researching, and writing about automobiles of all kinds, the value of this work has been greatly enhanced by the contributions of a number of knowledgeable Firebird enthusiasts and owners. This is my fifth Original Series book for MBI, and I have to note that Firebird owners and enthusiasts have been the most enthusiastic, generous, and helpful of any I have met.

I must first thank the members of the St. Louis Area Pontiac Oakland Club International and especially John Folluo for providing contacts for research information and cars to photograph. I appreciate the efforts of local POCI members Tony Becker, Paul Epperson, and Paul Carmi for generously offering to read and review the entire text of this book to help ensure its accuracy and completeness. I appreciate the efforts of Christine Schnee for additional proofreading of Chapter 2. Much thanks must also go to my friend and Firebird owner and enthusiast Noel Wilson for providing original documents, loaning his entire collection of original Firebird showroom brochures, and for reading and reviewing the entire text.

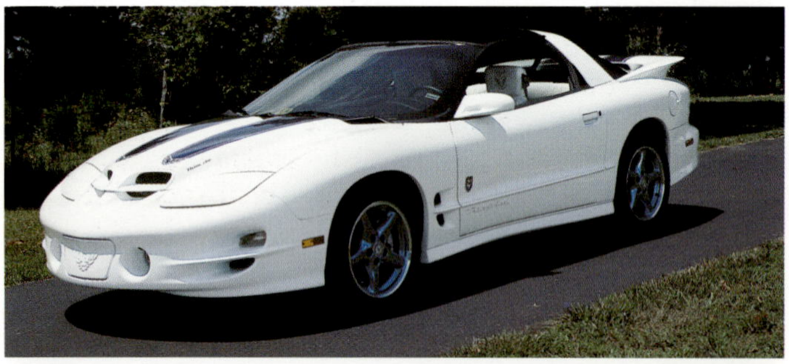

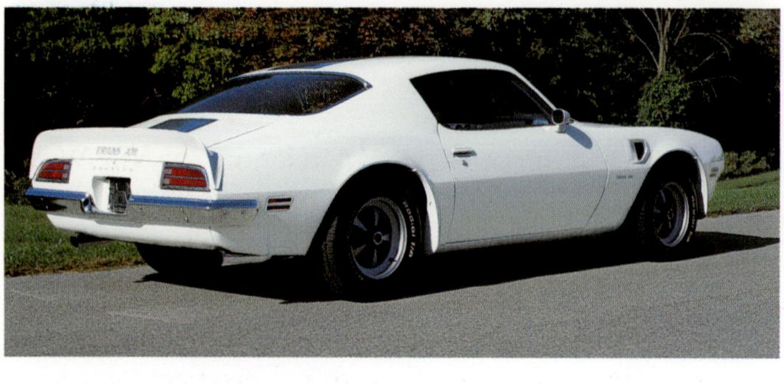

Top: 1999 Trans Am 30th Anniversary Edition coupe with new Ram Air hood scoop design. ***Above:*** 1970 Trans Am sport coupe.

My gratitude also goes to very knowledgeable Firebird enthusiasts and collectors Don Bennett and Steve Hamilton for reviewing significant portions of the text and providing a wealth of technical information. Thanks also to Joe Genera of the Firebird and Trans Am Club for providing a copy of the 1993–2002 Firebird parts catalog and reviewing the text. Firebird owner Cliff Mathus generously loaned his books, literature, and showroom brochures on the first- and second-generation Firebirds. The completeness and quality of the photography could not have been accomplished without the participation of the many owners attending the 2006 Trans Am Club of America Trans Am Nationals in Dayton, Ohio.

In addition to the original Pontiac Firebird parts manuals, owner's manuals, and showroom brochures, any book on Firebirds could not be completed without referencing the superb work of fellow Society of Automotive Historians member Michael Lamm in his book, *The Fabulous Firebird* (Lamm-Morada Publishing Company, 1979). Although now out of print, this excellent book should be in every Firebird owner's library, as it is a reliable source of historical and technical details. John Gunnell's books *Standard Catalog of Firebird 1967–2002* (KP Books, 2002) and *Firebird Illustrated Buyer's Guide* (MBI Publishing, 1998) were also helpful in verifying production details and codes. Thanks to Paul Herd and PAH Publishing for providing a copy of the book, *Trans Am and Firebird Formula 1970–1981* by Joe Moore.

Owners of the cars featured in this book are Noel Wilson, Jeff and Angela Davis, Paul and Kelly Carmi, Tony Becker, Ron and Betsy Thomas, Glenn Meyer, Cliff Mathus, Rick and Mary Kay Murray, Mark Kiefer, Eric Stambaugh, Dave and Yvonne Rose, Tom Gaines, Dan Turner, John Uleski, Nathan Marion, Jack Rhoades, Andy Ryner, Roxann Halsey, Ken Mosier, Ron Hutchens, Rick Shaver, Anson Adams, Frank Ciampi, Steve Coyle, George Berg, Jeff Berry, David Collins, Rebecca Robbins, Kim Hoover, Greg Bleamer, and Scott Biancardi. Thanks must also go to Dean Fait of Rock Island, Illinois, for providing information and photos of his 1995 Comp T/A.

I cannot ignore the extraordinary efforts of Steve Hamilton of Oaklandon, Indiana, and Don Bennett of Vienna, Missouri, whose time, knowledge, and energy were generously donated while allowing me to photograph a significant number of Firebirds (a total of 14 cars) from their extensive and interesting collections.

I must also thank my wife, Myrna, who diligently proofread and edited the entire text.

Chapter 1

Basic 1967–2002 Identification

Model Years

American manufacturers started a system in the 1950s where the model year and the introduction of new models did not coincide with the calendar year. The 1967–2002 Firebird was included in this system, and the new models were generally introduced in September of the previous year. The initial introduction of the new 1967 Firebird and the second-generation 1970 1/2 models were exceptions to this rule, and they were introduced later in the model year. The identification numbers, available models, and significant equipment usually reflect the model year of the vehicle rather than the year it was built.

Vehicle Identification Number

All American automobiles are required by law to have a vehicle identification number (VIN). All 1967 VIN plates were stamped bright metal tags riveted to the left front door hinge (A) pillar and were readable from outside the car with the door open. The 1967 VIN consisted of 13 digits that identified the series, year, body type, assembly plant, and production sequence.

The first character of the 1967 VIN was a number that represented the General Motors division, in this case a 2 for Pontiac. The second and third characters were numbers that identified the series, which was 23 for Firebird. The fourth and fifth numbers represent the body type, such as 37 for a two-door sport coupe and 67 for a two-door convertible. The sixth character represented the year, which was 7 for 1967. The seventh character was a letter that identified the assembly plant. All 1967 Firebirds were built at Lordstown, Ohio, (U). The last six digits represent the production sequence numbers, which were 100001 and up for the V-8 and 600001 and up for the six-cylinder.

In 1968, the VIN plate was moved by government mandate to the left front edge of the instrument panel and was readable through the windshield. This location required removal of the windshield to alter or remove the plate, which was attached with special tamper-proof rivets. The 1968–1971 VIN consisted of 13 characters that identified the series, year, body type, assembly plant, and production sequence.

The 1968–1971 VIN system was similar to that used in 1967 with a few variations. Beginning in 1968, Firebirds were also built at the Los Angeles/Van Nuys, California, plant, adding an L to the assembly plant codes. In 1969, a new plant in Norwood, Ohio, was added with a code of N. In 1970 and 1971, all Firebirds were built at either the Norwood or Los Angeles/Van Nuys plants. Another change was made in 1970 and 1971 when separate model or series codes were created for the base Firebird (23), Firebird Esprit (24), Firebird Formula (26), and Trans Am (28).

In 1972, an entirely new VIN system was introduced and used for 1972–1980. The first character was a number that represented the division, as it had in the previous design, with 2 for Pontiac. The second character was a single letter that identified the series: S for base Firebird, T for Esprit, U for Formula 400, and V or W for Trans Am. There was a special X code for the 1979 10th Anniversary Trans Am. The third and fourth character identified the body type, and since all were two-door sport coupes, the code will always be 87. The fifth character was a letter that identified the engine: D for the 250 six-cylinder; A or C for the 231 V-6; E, L, M, N, P, R for the 350 V-8; P, R, S, T, or Z for the 400 V-8; and W, Y, and X for the 455 V-8. Engine codes varied according to the year and model. The sixth character was a number that identified the year: 2 for 1972, 3 for 1973, etc. The seventh character identified the assembly plant: N for Norwood and L for Van Nuys. The last six digits are the sequence numbers, which were 500001 and up in 1972, and 100001 and up for 1973 and 1974. In 1975 and 1976, the VIN sequence numbers were again 500001 and up. For 1977–1980, the numbers were 100001 and up. The 1980 model year VIN was similar to that used in 1979, but the model year was identified by the letter A for 1980.

For the 1981 model year, the VIN system changed significantly and consisted of 17 characters. The first character was the number 1 for United States and represented the country of origin. The second character was the manufacturer code, which was G for General Motors. The third character was 2, which identified the Pontiac division. The fourth character identified the restraint system type and was A for nonpassive, manual seatbelts. The fifth character identified the series: S for the base Firebird, T for Esprit, V for Formula, and W for Trans Am. The six and seventh characters identified the body type, with 87 representing the two-door sport coupe. The eighth character identified the engine: A for the V-6, S for the 265 V-8, W and T for the 301 V-8, and H for the 305 V-8. The ninth character was a check digit and was X. The tenth character was the model year, with B representing 1981. The assembly plant was identified by the eleventh character, with N for Norwood and L for Van Nuys as before. The last six digits were the sequence number beginning with 100001 and up. This system was maintained much the same from 1982 to 1984 except for the model year and engines codes. The series code also changed with the dropping of the Formula and Esprit and the addition of the S/E with an X code.

The 17-character VIN was modified again for 1985 and 1986. The first three characters were the same as the previous model year, but the fourth character now identified the car line, with F representing Firebird. The remaining 13 characters were the same as those used in 1982–1984, except for the model year code and engine codes. For 1987–1989, the VIN was modified again. There were still 17 characters, but there were a number of changes from the previous system. The first five characters were the same as those used in 1986, but the sixth character representing the body type was now a 2 for sport coupe and the S/E line was dropped. The seventh character was a 1, representing the restraint system as manual seatbelts. The Norwood assembly plant code was dropped for 1988 because all Firebirds were being built at Van Nuys only. The remaining 10 characters identified the same features as the 1986 number with obvious updates in model year and engine codes.

The VIN system remained the same for 1990 and1991, except that the restraint system code changed from 1 to 3 to represent the manual belts and driver-side air bag. For 1991, an additional body type code, 3, was used to represent the two-door convertible and a 2 represented the two-door hatchback. In 1992, the restraint system code could have been either a 1 (manual seatbelts) or 2 (driver-side air bag). For the 1993–2002 model years, the VIN system remained the same except the restraint system code 2 now represented driver and passenger air bags. Beginning in 1993, a new plant code of 2 represented the St. Therese, Ontario, plant, and for 1994 and later, all Firebirds were built at the Canadian facility. The 1993 model year code was P, and the letter codes advanced for each year.

Body Number Plate

The Fisher Body number plate, or trim tag, was located on the upper left engine side of the firewall or cowl on the 1967–1970 Firebird and was attached with two rivets. The 1973–1981 body number plates were attached with two special screws with a hex head and an X or + in the center. The rectangular metal plate was attached before the body was painted so it would be the same semigloss black finish as the firewall. The body number plate identified the model year, interior trim type and color, build date, body style and series, and body sequence number. The 1979–1985 plate also identified the paint type.

There were a number of different design body number plates and labels used on Firebirds. The first design was used in 1967, but a new design plate was adopted for 1968–1985. The 1967 plate featured General Motors Corporation at the top of the plate and placed the build date code at top right of the plate (with nothing else on that line). The alphanumeric build date identified the month and week of scheduled production. The second line is read from right to left starting with (ST) the model year (67) and a code representing the car division, series, and body type. In the center was a one- to three-letter code identifying the assembly plant location with N for Norwood or LOR for Lordstown. The six-digit body sequence number was next.

At the left of the third line (TR) was the three-digit trim code that identified the interior trim color. After 1971, there was a three-digit code identifying the seat type to the right of the trim code. A51 was the code for bucket seats, standard in the Firebird. To the right was a letter (1967 and 1968) or two-digit number (1969–1985) that identified the body color followed by PNT. The next line had a three-character build date under the trim code. Body by Fisher was embossed at the bottom center of the plate. The 1968–1985 plate was similar to the 1967 version, but a federal safety compliance legend was added to the bottom.

Beginning in 1985, the build and identifying information was printed in black on a white Service Parts Identification (Option) Label attached to the inside rear wall of the glove box. This label had much of the same information previously

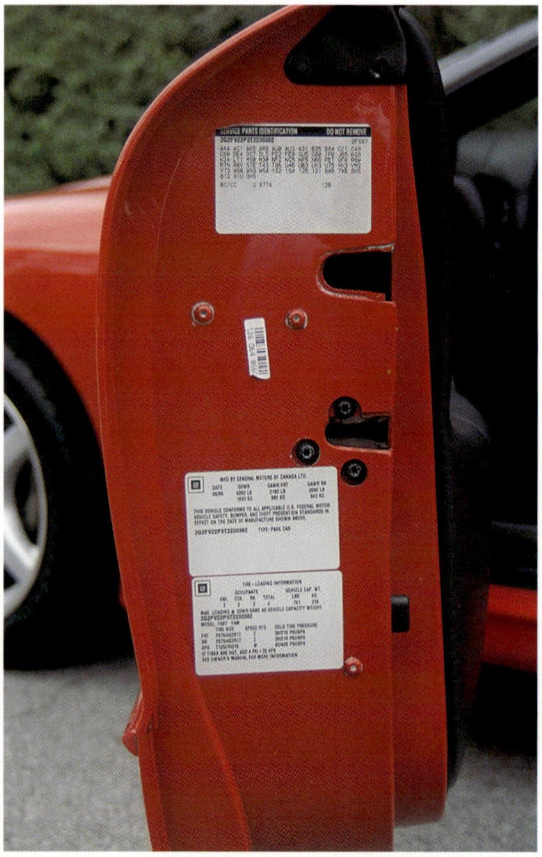

This is the left door pillar on a Bright Red 1996 Trans Am WS6 Ram Air hatchback coupe. The three white decals on the door provide identification numbers, options codes, and tire inflation information.

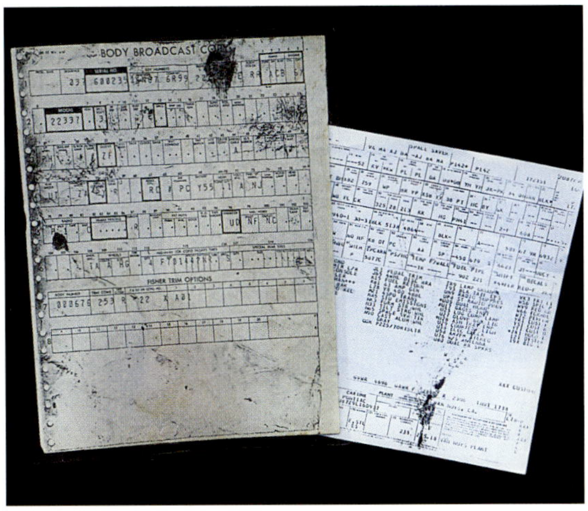

It is always important to locate and preserve the original build sheet for the car. The build sheet will identify the correct options and equipment. Many owners make copies of their original build sheet to display at shows or assist with appraisals.

provided on the body number plate, but the VIN was printed on top of the label in place of the old body sequence number. Beginning in 1998, the Service Parts Identification Label was attached to the upper rear surface of the driver's door and included all of the important option codes.

Additional Numbers

In addition to the identification and option numbers and codes found on the VIN plate and body number plate, there are other locations where numbers might be found. All engines, beginning with the 1968 models, were stamped with the number 2 followed by the last eight digits of the VIN. For example: 23N145623.

In addition to the year, plant, and VIN, the engine also had head and manifold casting numbers and casting date codes cast in the engine components. These numbers should always be dated prior to the build date of the car, as shown on the body number plate. The factory service and parts manuals provide specific details about the location and identification of all engine numbers.

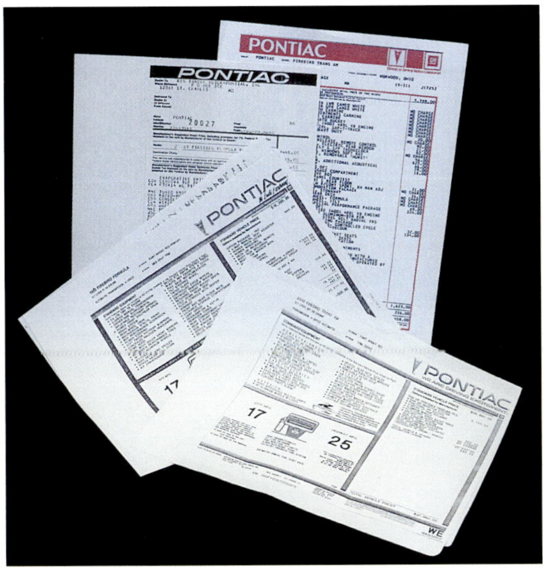

Copies of the original retail price label help to identify the correct equipment and options on the car when it was delivered. These documents, also called "window stickers," are often displayed at car shows. Their design and information varies by year and model.

Documentation

In addition to the serial and identification numbers stamped on various components of the car, there are a number of other methods to identify, date, and authenticate the vehicle. When a car was assembled and delivered, there were a number of documents to direct the assembly line workers in building the car, and there were other documents for the dealer and buyer noting the model, options, and price for the car. These documents included the factory build sheet, factory build card, dealer order form, and retail price label.

Build Sheet

The build sheet is a rectangular form with a number of small blocks coded with information for each assembly line worker to identify parts or operations that went on each car. A different design form might be used depending upon the assembly plant and model year. The form was used in the metal department to detail the various panels, holes or welding required, depending on the model and options. A build sheet in the trim department at Fisher Body detailed the body paint, moldings, interior trim panels, and materials required to finish the body. The build sheet was attached to the body or chassis at various locations as necessary so that workers would immediately find the needed information. When the car was completed, the build sheet was no longer needed and it was either left somewhere in the car or thrown away. Sometimes, the build sheet may be found above the fuel tank. The trim department build sheet may also be found under the rear seat springs, behind the rear seat back or in the front seat springs. Although it is not necessarily the final word, the build sheet is a very accurate record of the correct parts used to build a particular car. If you have an original build sheet it should be preserved as one of the most important items of documentation to prove the authenticity of the car. Some owners make a color copy of the original build sheet and use that copy for show and keep the original in a safe place.

Manufacturer's Suggested Retail Price Label

Commonly called the window sticker, this document was sometimes saved by the original owner. This document, a Monroney label, was originally named for the Oklahoma senator who was chairman of the U.S. Senate subcommittee on automobile marketing practices in 1958. Senator Mike Monroney proposed this label as a means to assure consumers that they were paying the correct prices for their new cars. This label was attached to every car and disclosed details of the retail price.

The label provided the name of the selling dealer, make, VIN, and order number in the upper section of the early versions. The VIN was printed at the lower border of the later labels. The lower section identified the model and sales codes in the early versions, but the sales codes were omitted in the later versions. This section also listed the basic standard equipment, color, trim, and all extra-cost options and packages on the car when it was delivered. Early versions of the form also included the option or sales codes. As its name implies, the form also listed the suggested retail price of the basic vehicle and all options, plus the destination and delivery charges. Later forms noted the fuel economy information in a box at the lower left of the form. Some later cars may have been delivered with an additional form listing dealer- or aftermarket-installed options or special services. Many owners like to display a copy of the window sticker or original dealer sales invoice with their car as a conversation piece at car shows.

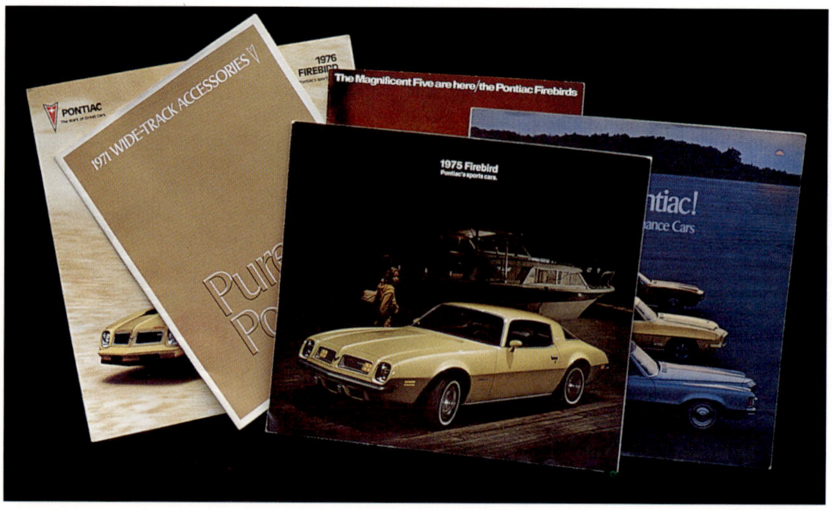

These original Firebird sales and showroom brochures and catalogs from the 1960s and 1970s are excellent sources for identifying the correct equipment and colors of the car when new. They may be found at swap meets and from literature dealers. These copies were preserved by an original Firebird owner.

Sales Catalogs and Dealer Publications

A great deal of important restoration and historical information may be acquired from original and reproduction sales catalogs and dealer data books. Sales catalogs are not always totally accurate because they may have been published prior to the car's actual release, and option availability and prices often changed during the model year, but they provide a wealth of data on the options and equipment offered. The illustrations may be helpful with trim details and colors of the various components and models. Some special edition and collector edition Firebirds may have had their own catalogs and were not shown in the standard line catalogs. These catalogs are available from parts-and-literature vendors. They may also be found at swap meets and car shows.

Dealer color and upholstery selector books are an excellent source to see the exact colors and materials used in the car's construction. These heavy, quality-bound publications can be expensive, but they are available from automobile literature dealers and are sometimes found at swap meets. This is the best source to accurately identify the precise colors and trim materials for any model or year.

The original owner's manual is a valuable source of technical information, such as oil and fuel quantities, lamp model numbers, maintenance schedules, and lubrication requirements. The owner's manual also shows the location and operation of instruments and accessories. Reproduction owner's manuals are sometimes available

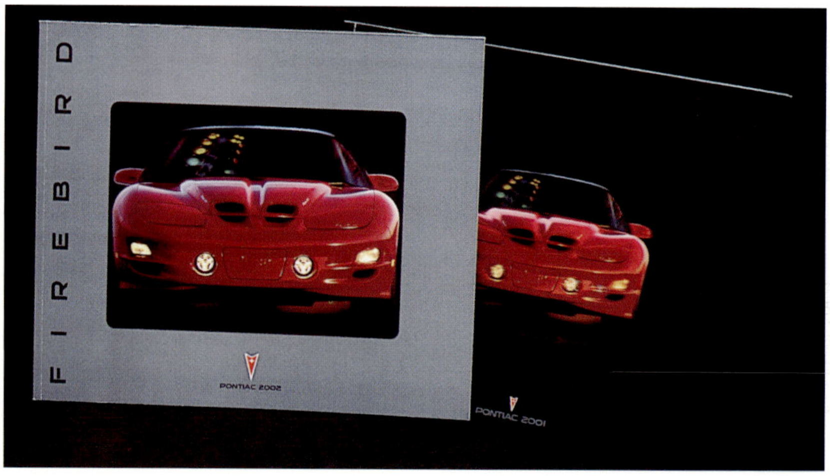

These original, full-color, Firebird catalogs and brochures from 2001 and 2002 provide a great deal of detailed information on the equipment and options available each year. Most options are listed by RPO number and description.

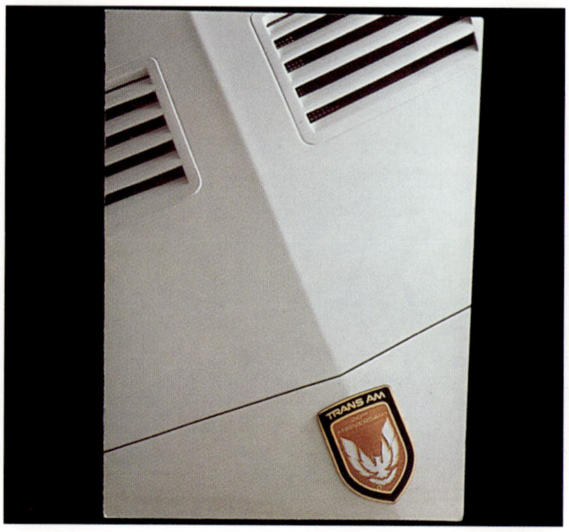

Sometimes, smaller specialized factory brochures have more emphasis on certain models, as is the case with this original publication from 1989. The cover and information inside feature the limited-production 1989 Turbo Trans Am 20th Anniversary Edition.

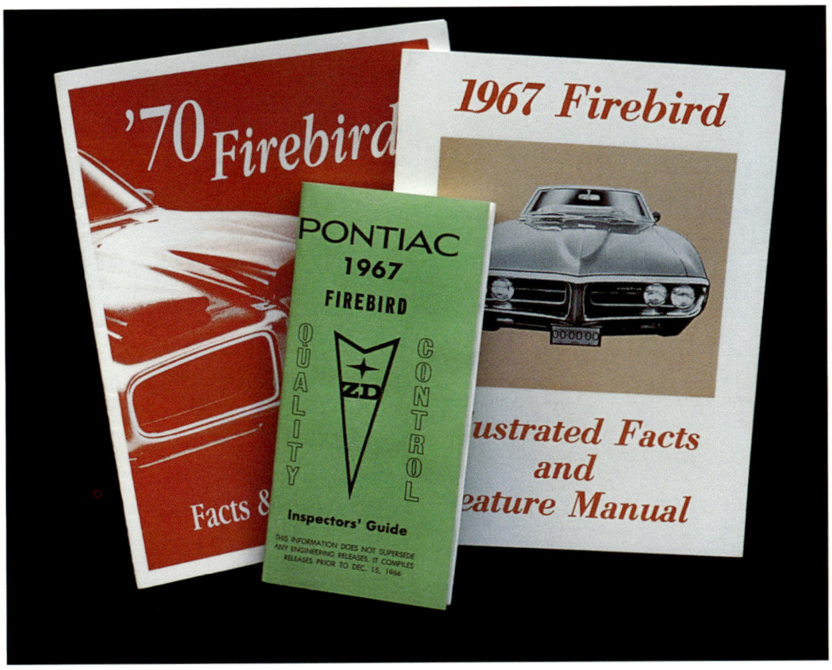

There are also a limited number of reproduction sales catalogs and facts-and-features publications available from parts dealers. These books provide detailed information on options and sales codes in addition to original illustrations of the various models.

from Firebird parts suppliers, or originals may be found at shows and swap meets.

Many owners like to display these catalogs, manuals, and color publications with their cars at car shows. These publications are usually very interesting to the public and indicate that the owner has followed factory specifications in the vehicle's restoration.

Parts-and-Illustration Catalogs

One of the most important sources of correct information for any restoration or authentication is the factory parts-and-illustration catalog. These publications list each component for the car and detail the application and model. Catalogs are generally dependable, but they were usually produced ahead of the production cars and there may be production or assembly changes not reflected in the parts catalog. Parts catalogs or service manuals, service bulletins, and change notices sent to dealers are helpful for research.

A caution regarding the parts catalogs: GM often superseded parts with newer revisions that, while functionally equal, may not look the same. The original part number may also be changed, so a parts catalog published in September 1980 may list many revised part numbers for earlier model years. It is best to obtain a parts catalog that was published as close to the model year of your car as possible.

Sometimes, these catalogs are the only way to determine the correct parts used with each year, model, and body type. These catalogs are available from parts and literature dealers and also may be found on Internet auction sites. Some are available in bound or unbound paper form, and others are only available on CD in Adobe PDF format. There are also product assembly drawings (PADs), but very few were ever available outside of the assembly plants.

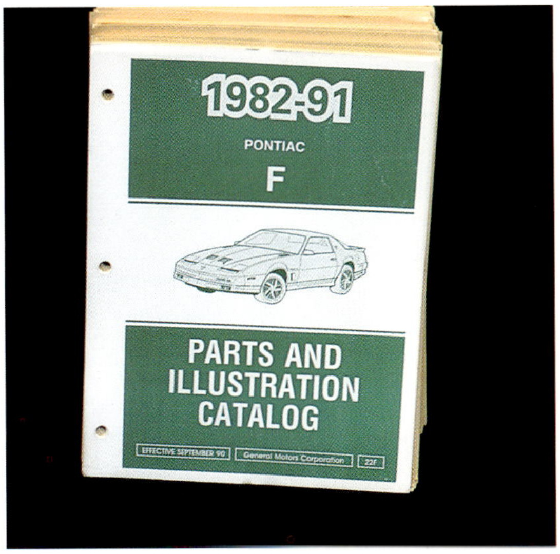

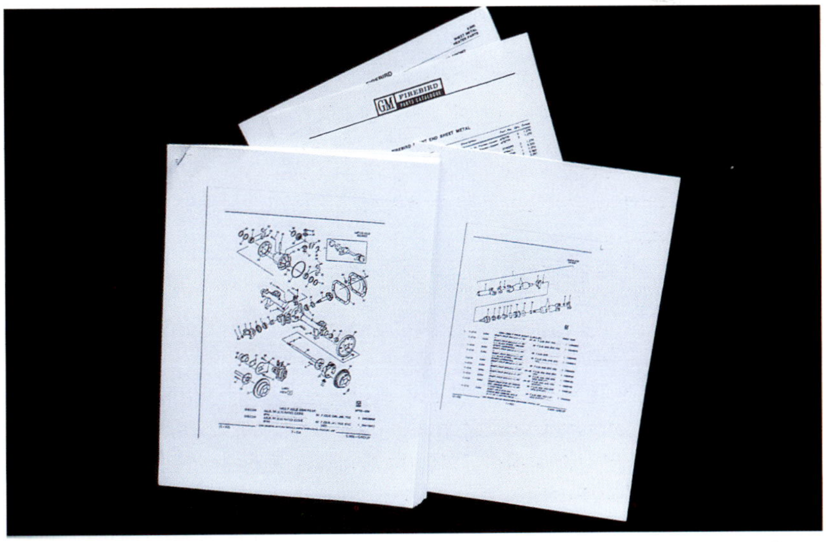

Above left: The most important publication for any owner is the factory parts-and-illustration catalog. Original copies are sometimes difficult to locate, but reproduction copies in paper or digital files are available for most years. Firebird parts catalogs are available in series containing a number of years in each book. ***Above right:*** In addition to identifying the correct parts and numbers, the parts-and-illustration catalog provides valuable assembly details. These publications are usually the definitive source for correct information for restoration or maintenance. These are pages printed from a digital file on compact disc. The 1992–2002 Firebird parts catalog information is only available as a digital file, as no paper publication was produced after 1991.

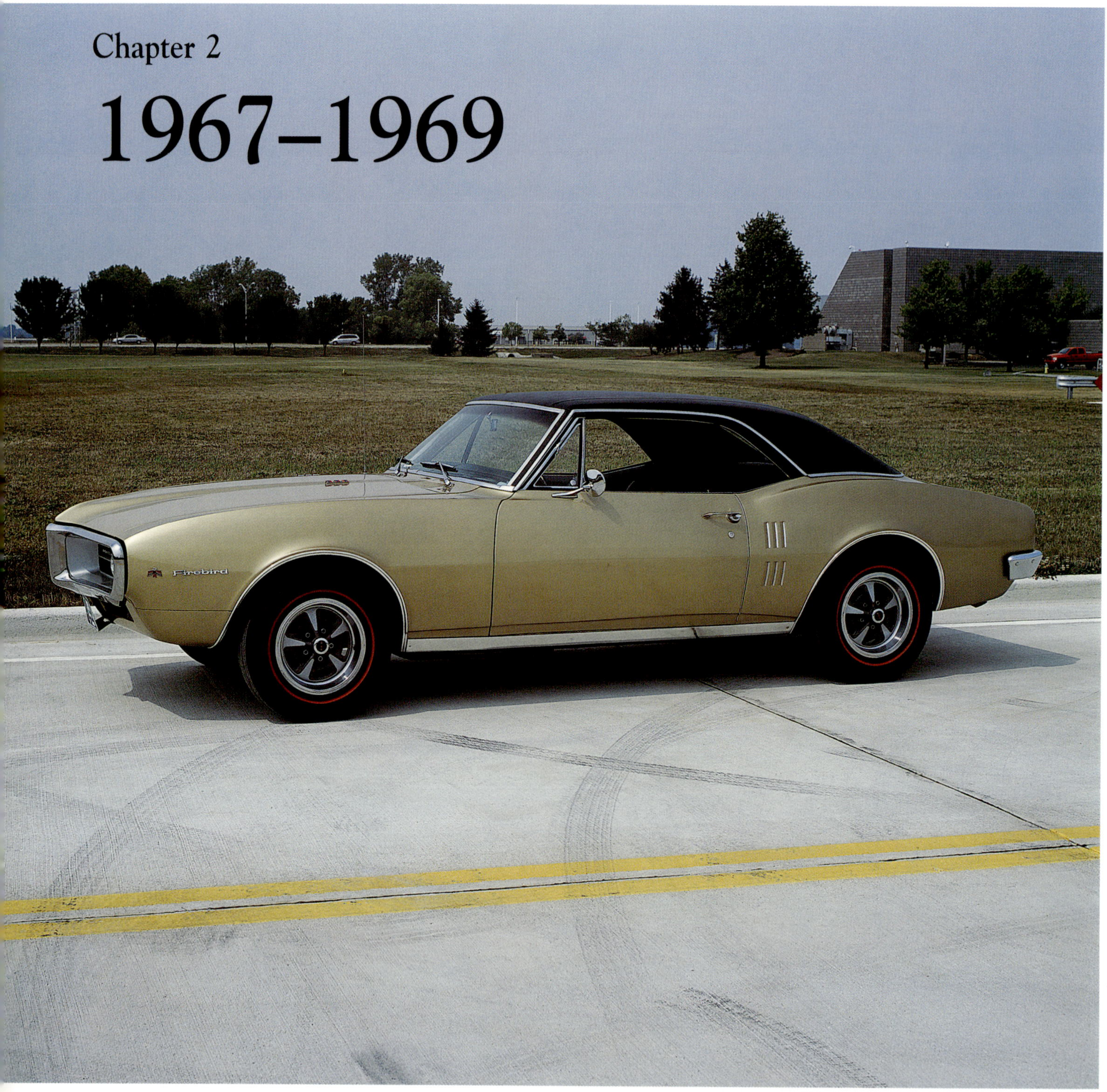

Chapter 2

1967–1969

General Motors arrived late to the pony car market created by Ford's 1964 Mustang. GM's first entry was the 1967 Chevrolet Camaro, introduced in the fall of 1966. Although the Camaro was the first commercial offering to the General Motors pony car line, the Pontiac Division was not idle. John Z. DeLorean of Pontiac wasted no time in creating the two-seater XP-833 concept cars that convinced GM management that Pontiac was adept at design. The XP-833 concept may have been too good, however, as it looked too much like competition for the Corvette and that was clearly unacceptable.

There was actually another, lesser-known John DeLorean-directed concept car called the Banshee, or XP-798, that was slated to appear at the 1966 New York auto show. This first Banshee had some of the styling features that were included in the 1967½ Firebird, but the car was pulled from the Pontiac display at the last minute by General Motors President James M. Roche because he apparently felt it did not comply with Pontiac's

This Signet Gold 1967 Firebird coupe with an optional black vinyl Cordova roof is equipped with optional 14-inch Rally II wheels and the correct redline tires.

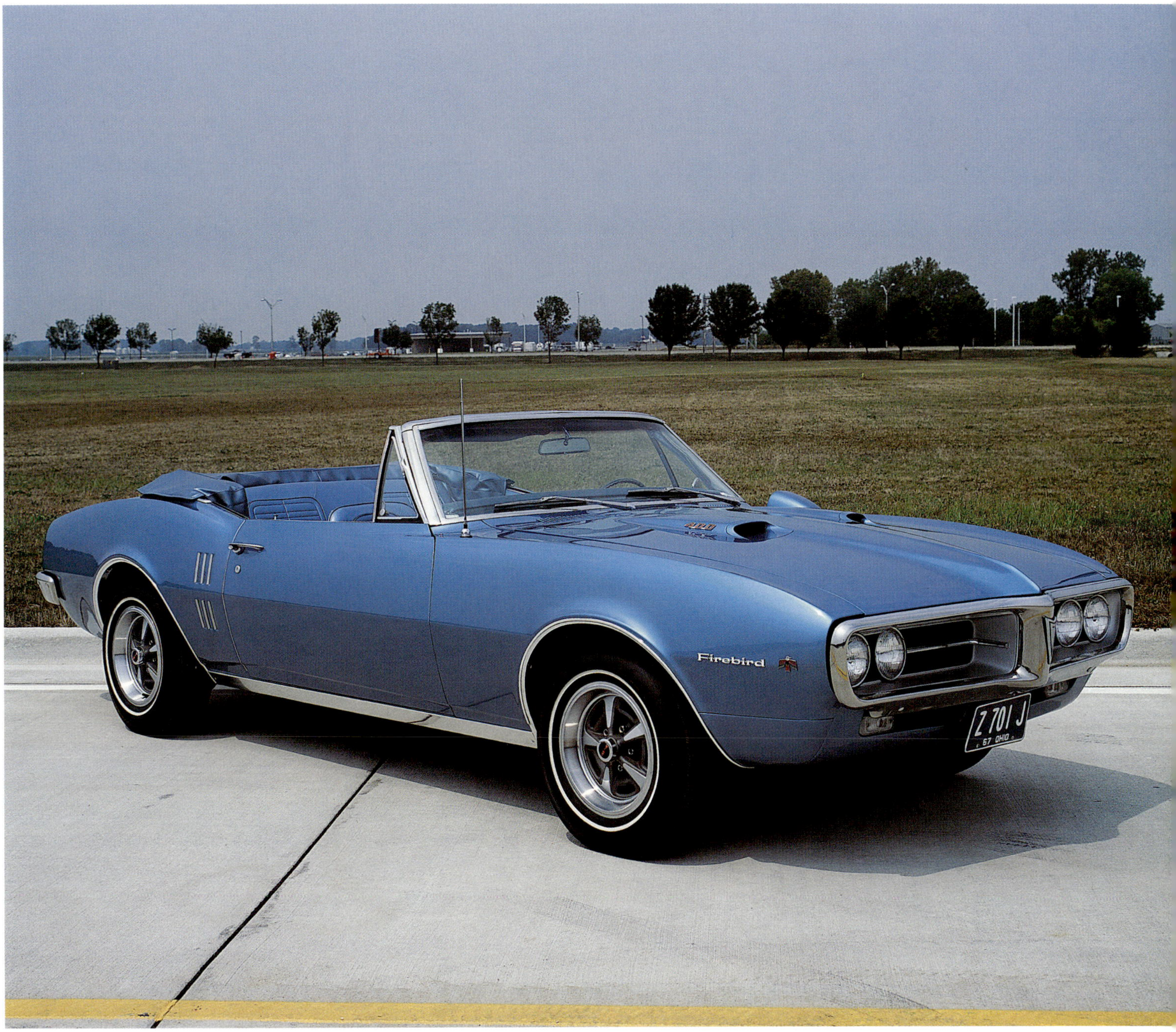

Above: A 3/4 right front view of a Tyrol Blue (E) 1967 Firebird convertible with a medium blue vinyl (255) interior trim. This Firebird has an optional hood-mounted tachometer and Rally II wheels with white-sidewall tires. Note the 400 engine badge on the hood scoops and the arrowhead medallion on the center of the grille surround.

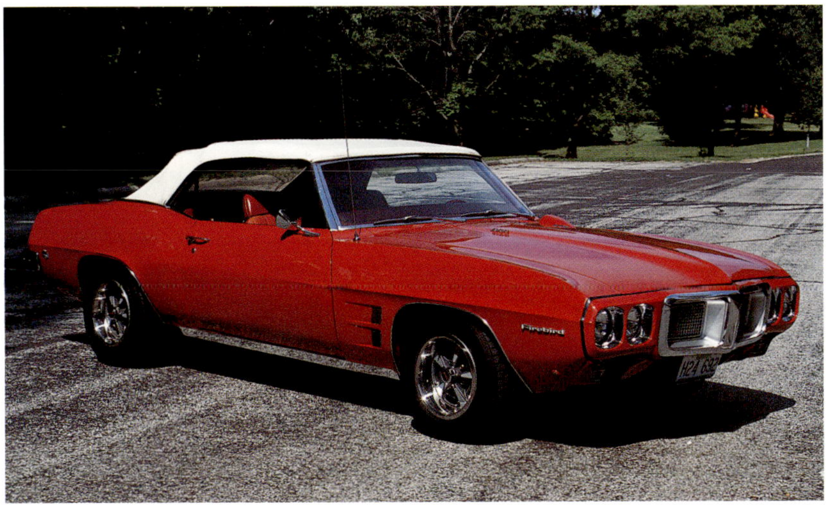

Left: This is a right front quarter view of a red 1969 Firebird convertible equipped with the optional Rally II wheels and simulated extractor vents on the rear of the front fender. The convertible top was available in four colors, including the white ivory shown here.

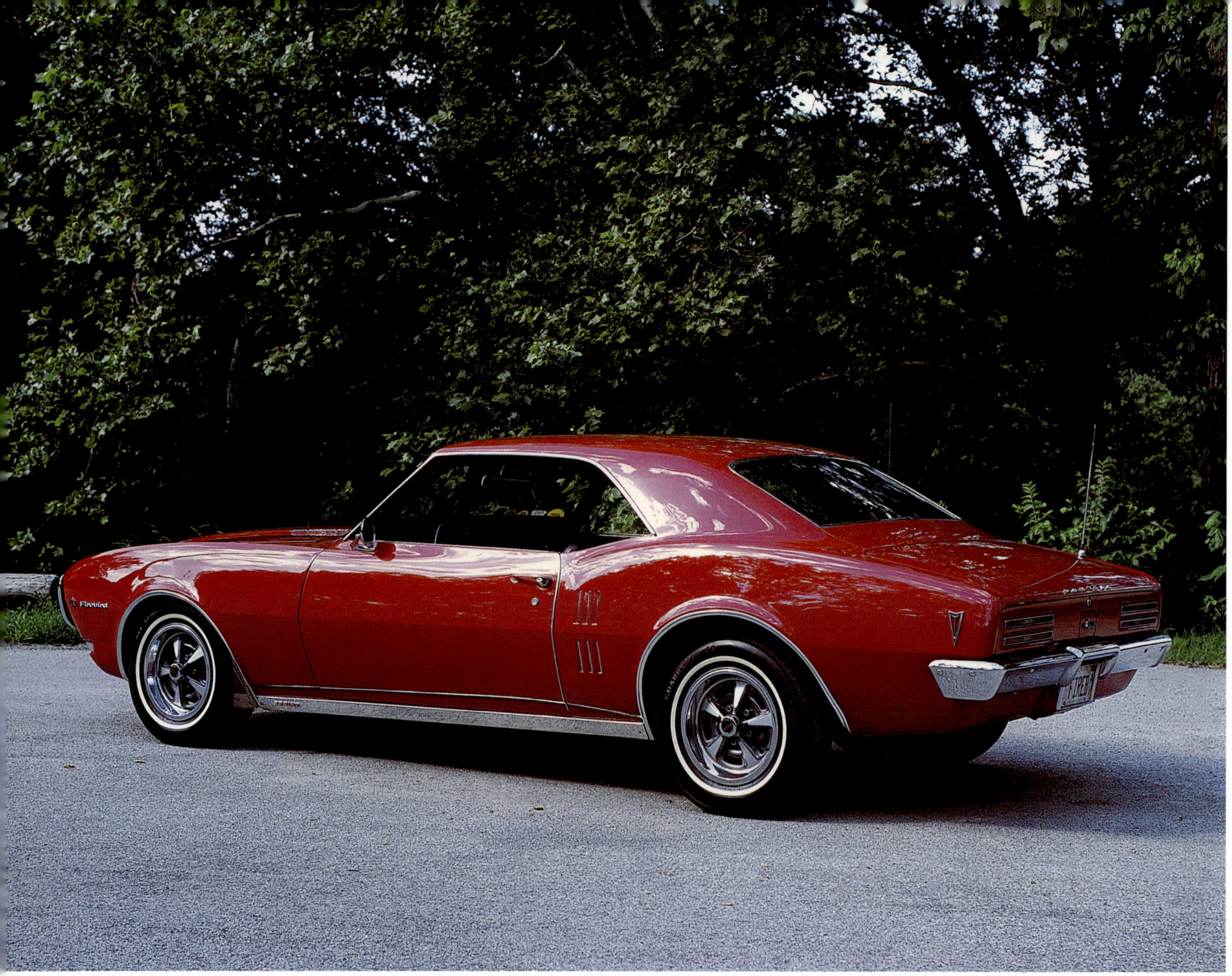

image of safety. The XP-798 Banshee was never shown to the public and was probably destroyed.

As development of the new F-body Camaro advanced, General Motors' management decided that Pontiac would offer a comparable model, although the body shell and basic platform would be shared with the Camaro. It is a credit to Pontiac designers that they were able to bring a unique appearance to the new Firebird. Pontiac styling created a split-nose front-end design that was clearly derived from the popular GTO but had an identity of its own. This identity included a sporty, performance-oriented image that was a step above the Camaro in trim level.

Performance was always a key component of the Firebird image. The new model was available with engine and transmission options ranging from the economy and performance versions of the six-cylinder with three-speed or four-speed manual transmissions to the high-performance 400 with four-speed manual or three-speed automatic transmissions. This new player in Pontiac performance was introduced February 23, 1967, as a mid-year model. Total Firebird production for 1967 was 82,560. Production increased to 107,112 in 1968, but the total production for 1969 dropped to 87,708.

The 1967 Firebird was introduced with a 108.1-inch wheelbase and was advertised as the "Magnificent Five," referring to the five different engine and model configurations offered. There is some confusion about the usage of the model codes as the factory build sheet and broadcast sheet often showed a series 223 code for all models, but the data plate on the firewall showed a specific series code for each model such as 224, 225, or 226. The unitized-construction body shell was based on the long-front, short-rear Camaro. The Firebird used the previously mentioned unique front-end design with a split nose incorporating a separate grille opening on each side with quad round headlights and a full one-piece chrome bumper surround. The Firebird rear fascia included distinctive twin horizontal-slot taillights on each side with a rectangular fuel filler door in the center. The chrome rear bumper was relatively straight and incorporated the license plate mounting in its lower center.

The base Firebird was equipped with the standard Pontiac-built overhead-cam (OHC) inline

Left rear view of a Solar Red (R) 1968 Firebird Sprint coupe (2437) equipped with a 4.1-liter overhead-cam six-cylinder engine. This Sprint is equipped with optional 14-inch Rally II wheels and white-sidewall tires. Note the Sprint badge on the bright front rocker molding.

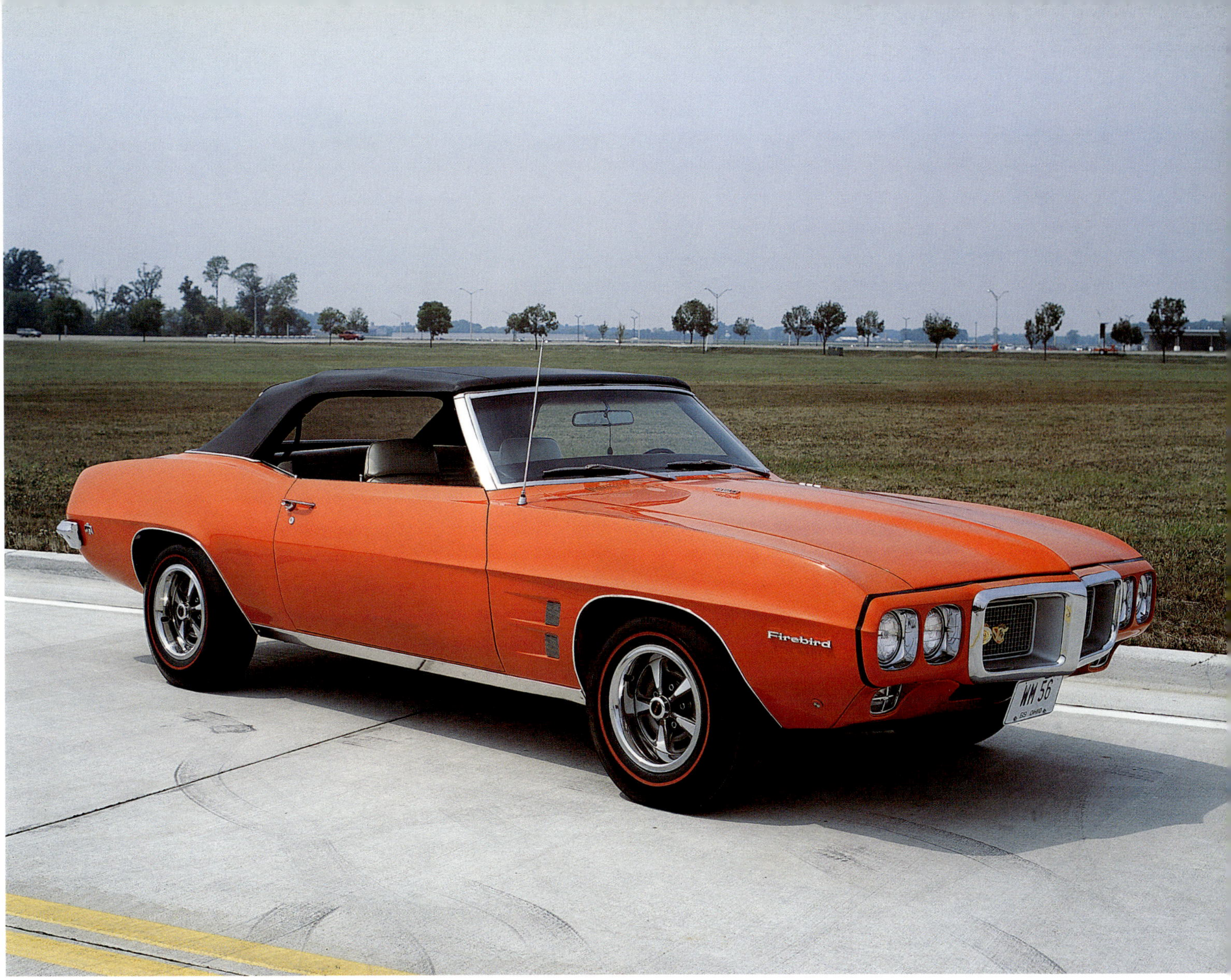

Above: This Carousel Red (72) 1969 Firebird convertible with 350 V-8 engine has optional 14-inch Rally II wheels and redline tires. The interior trim is parchment, and the convertible roof is black (B). *Right:* The Firebird Trans Am coupe was introduced in the 1969 model year and was available only in Cameo Ivory with twin longitudinal Nassau Blue stripes. This Trans Am has the UPC L74 400 Ram Air engine, black vinyl interior, and Rally II wheels. The tires are aftermarket replacements.

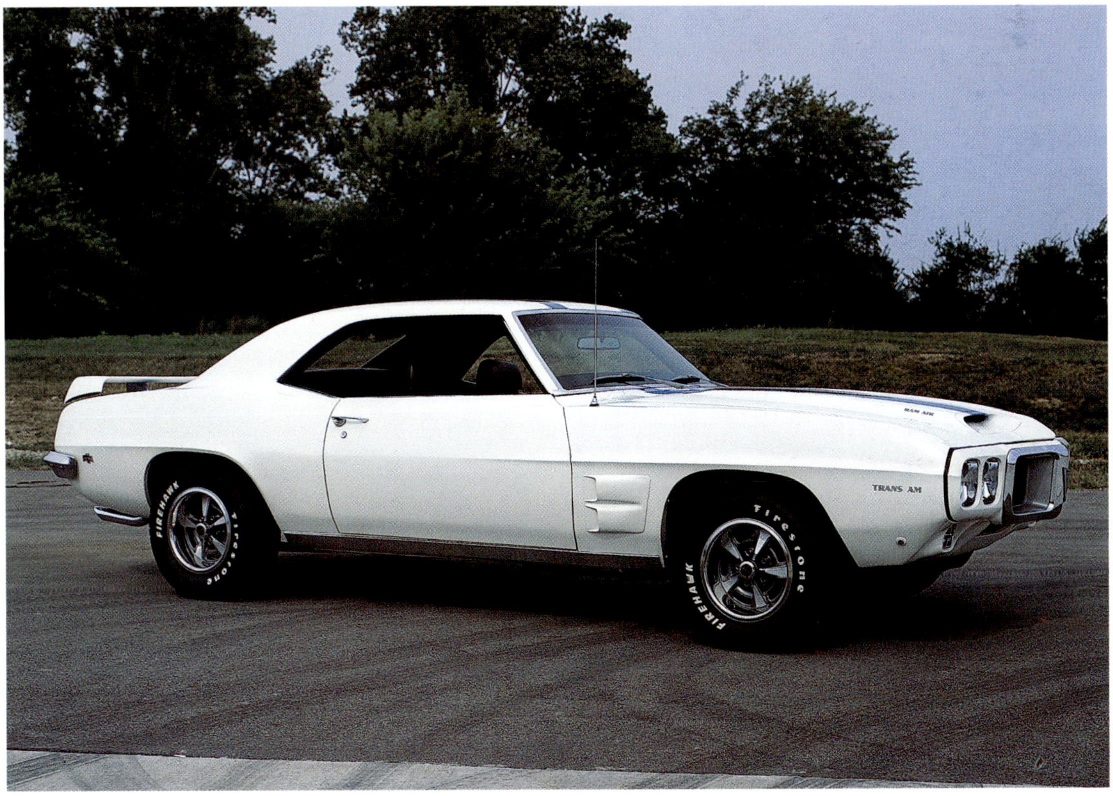

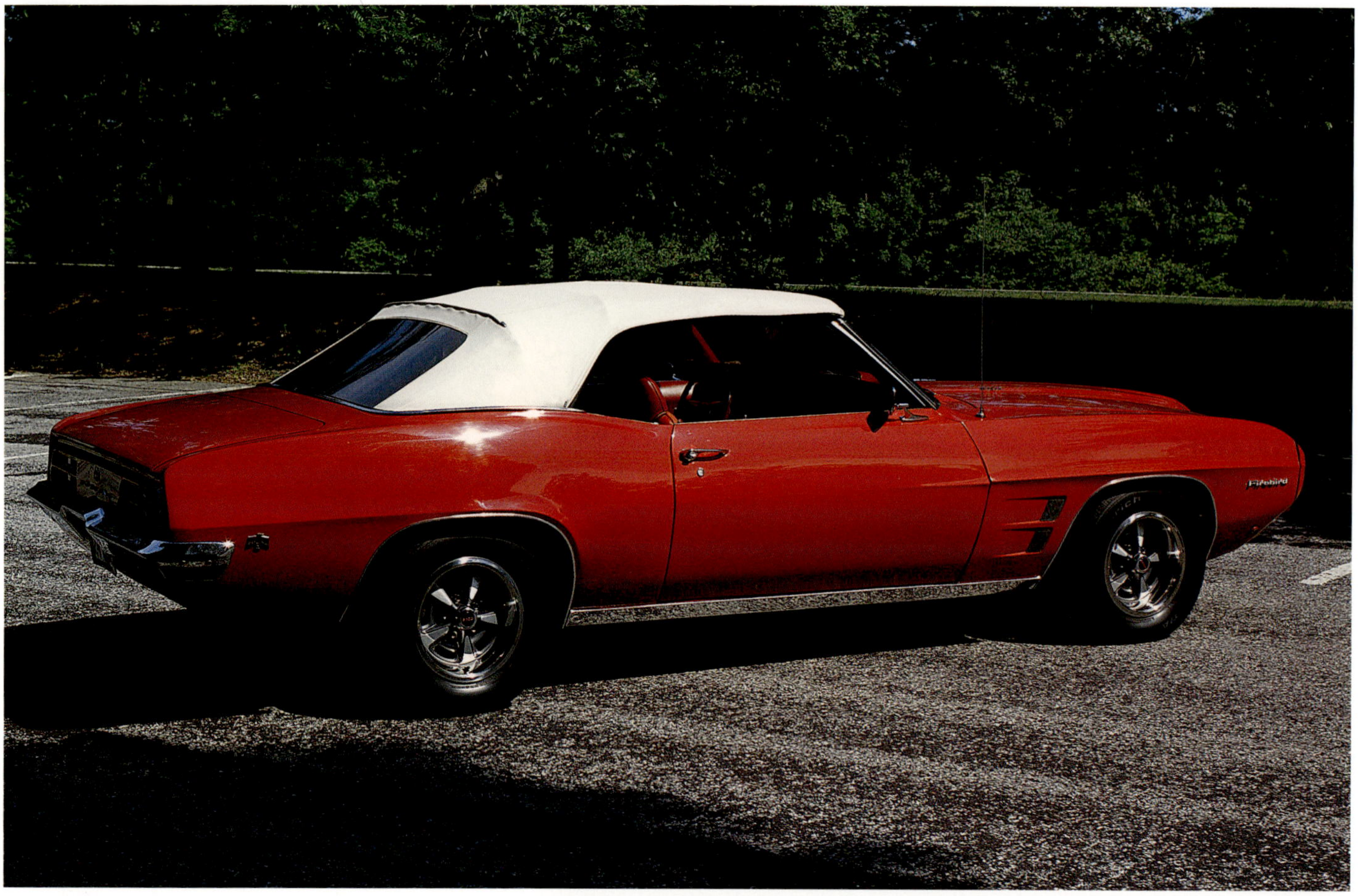

six-cylinder engine with the 326-ci V-8 optional. The Firebird Sprint (Uniform Production Code W53) included a standard slightly-higher-performance (215 horsepower) version of the 230-ci OHC six. The Firebird was available with V-8 engine options as the Firebird 326 (UPC L30), 326 HO (UPC L76), and Firebird 400 (UPC W66). The Firebird 400 and UPC L67 400 Ram Air versions were identified by their distinctive twin simulated hood scoops. All models were available in sport coupe (37) or convertible (67) versions.

The 1967 Firebird was available with five transmission choices. The standard OHC six-cylinder was available with the three-speed manual or air-cooled two-speed automatic transmissions. The Sprint six and V-8 engine options were available with a three-speed manual, four-speed manual, and water-cooled ST-300 two-speed automatic. A water-cooled three-speed Turbo Hydra-Matic was available with the 400 V-8 only.

The 1967 Firebird was available in 15 body color choices. Three vinyl top colors, five convertible top colors, and eleven vinyl interior trim combinations complemented the body color choices.

For 1968, the Firebird was changed little, but the industry-wide adaptation of side markers on the rear quarters, wrap-around front signals, and the loss of the previous year's door vent windows

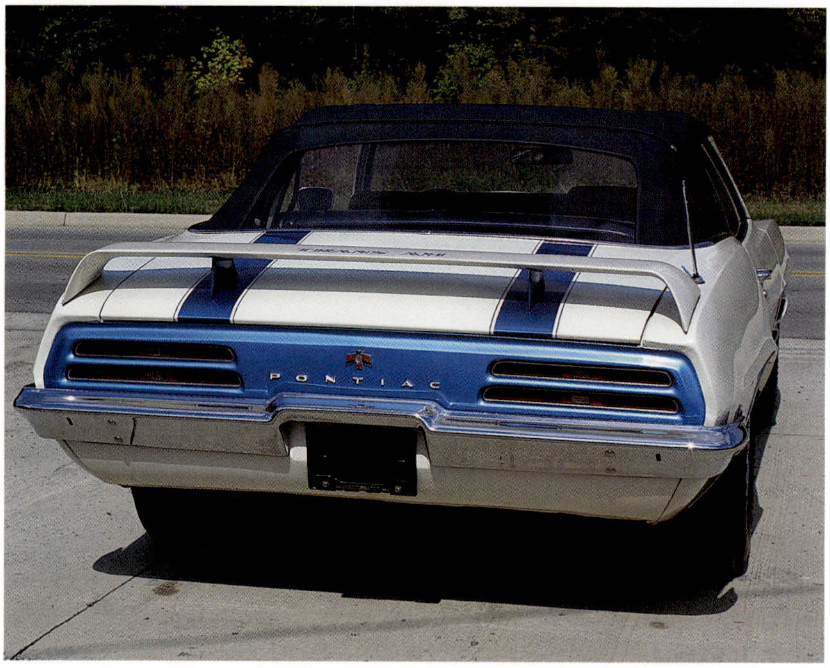

Top: This Matador Red 1969 Firebird convertible (2267) with the optional 350 HO engine has a custom red vinyl interior trim and white convertible roof (A). Note the optional Rally II wheels (UPC N98) and trim rings. ***Above:*** This is a rear view of a replica 1969 Trans Am convertible. The standard Trans Am colors for 1969 were Cameo Ivory with blue stripes. The convertible top is dark blue (C), one of four optional convertible-top colors.

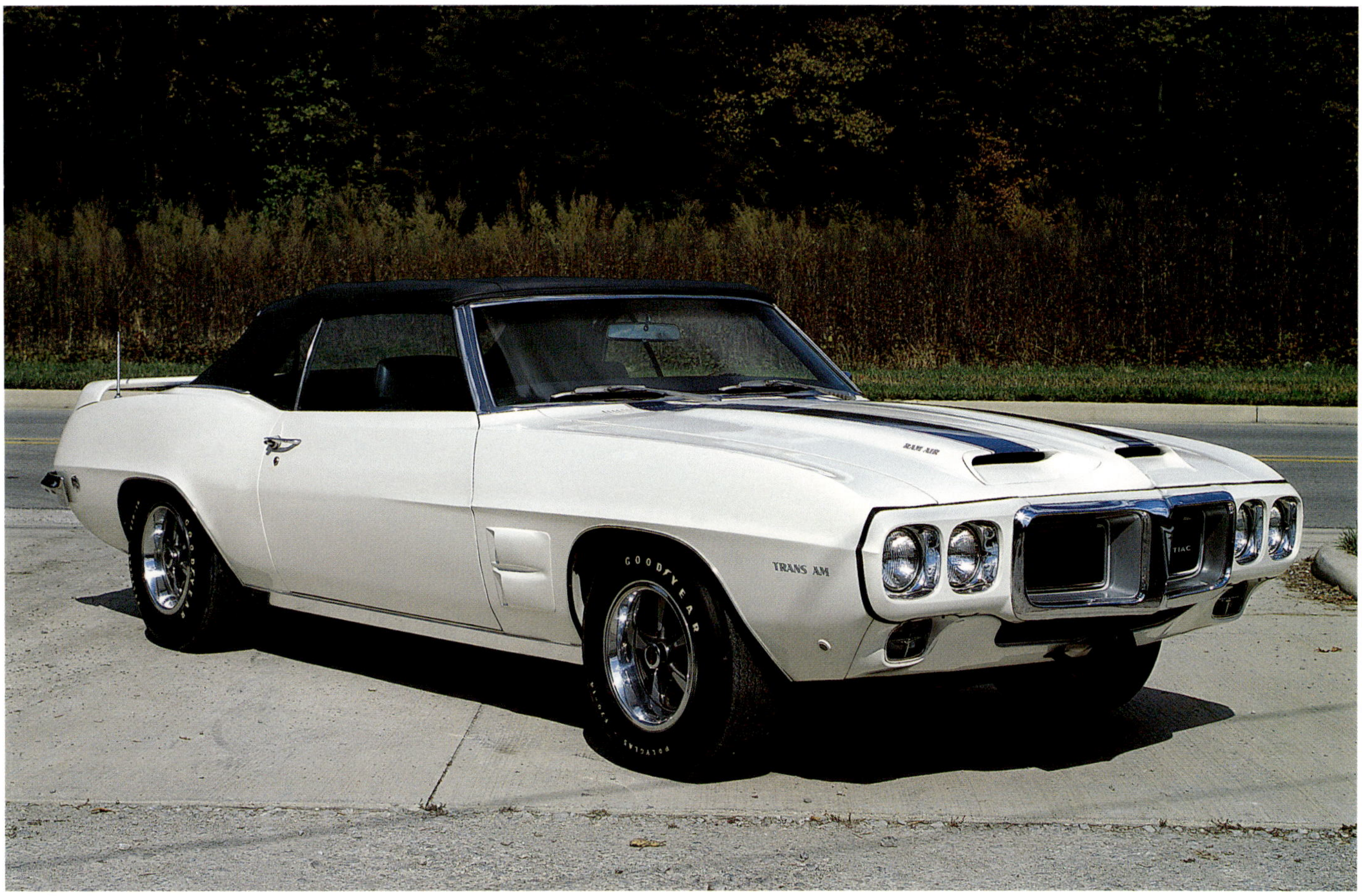

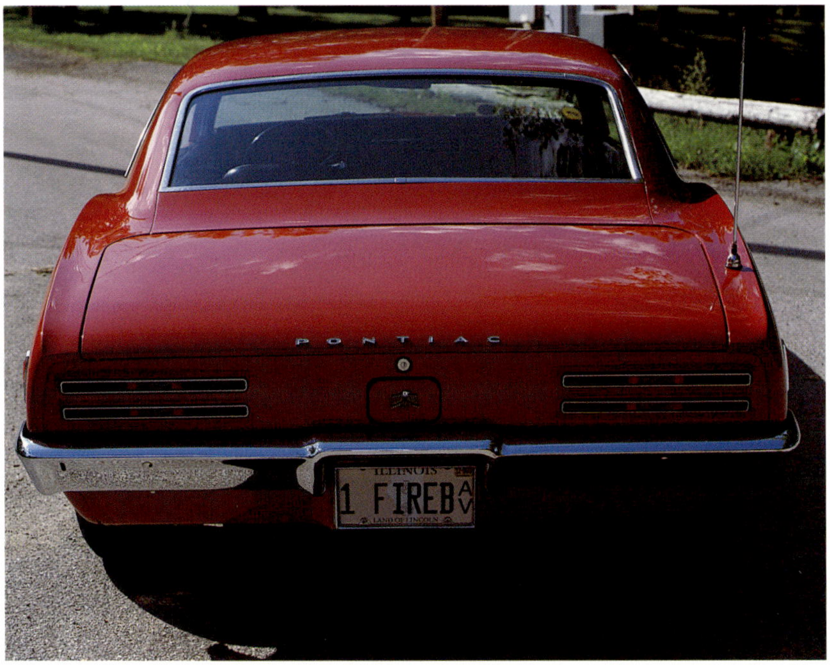

Top: Although only eight 1969 Trans Am convertibles were built, this replica accurately portrays the correct appearance and colors. It is equipped with the optional 14-inch Rally II wheels and white letter F70x14 Goodyear Polyglas tires. The convertible top is dark blue (C), and the body is Cameo Ivory with blue stripes. ***Above:*** This photo shows a rear detail view of a red 1968 Firebird Sprint. Note the distinctive Firebird badge on the fuel filler door and the Firebird nameplate on the deck lid.

easily separate the 1968 from the 1967. The engine option lineup for 1968 was increased to six. The base Firebird 250-ci OHC six, Firebird Sprint OHC six (sales code 342), Firebird 350 (sales code 343), 350 HO (sales code 344) V-8, Firebird 400 (sales code 345), and Firebird Ram Air 400 V-8. The 400 V-8 was again equipped with the twin simulated hood scoops, but the Ram Air option (sales code 347) and 400 HO (sales code 348) made them fully functional. Late in the 1968 model year, a revised engine known as the Ram Air II replaced the Ram Air 400. These are extremely rare and desirable. The same 108.1-inch wheelbase was kept.

Like the 1967, the 1968 Firebird was equipped with five transmission options. The six-cylinder was available with the three-speed manual and two-speed automatic. The Sprint six and V-8 engine options were available with the three-speed manual, four-speed manual, two-speed automatic, and the three-speed automatic with the 400 V-8 only.

The 1968 Firebird was offered with 16 body color choices complemented by four vinyl roof colors, four convertible top colors, and eight vinyl interior trim schemes.

For 1969, the Firebird was treated to minor styling and detail changes that easily identify it from the previous year's models. Most noticeable

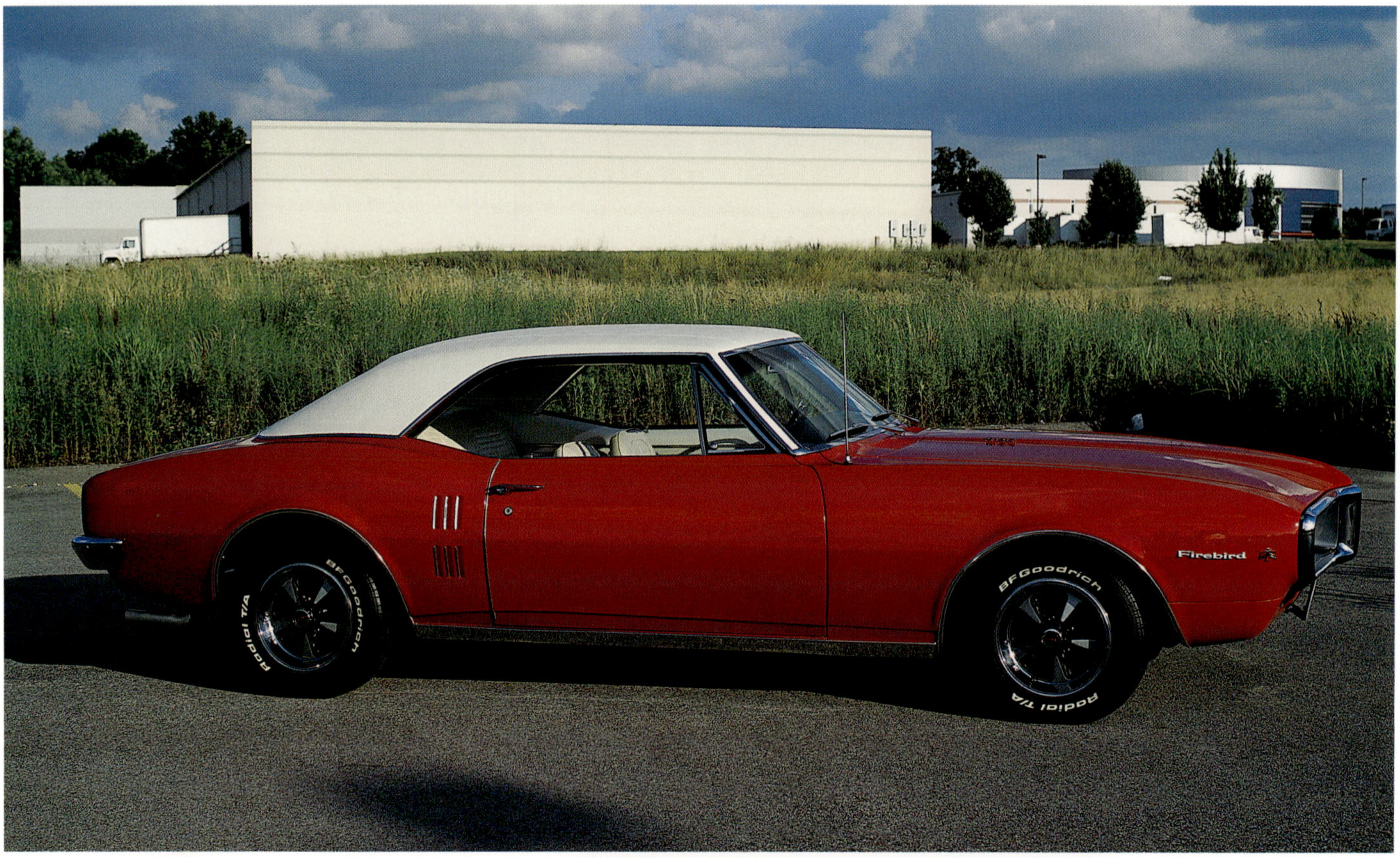

was the grille that divided into a chrome-plated center section and Endura body color bezels for the twin pairs of headlights. The wheel opening shapes were changed, the flares were eliminated, and the fuel filler was moved from the rear deck panel above the bumper to behind the license plate. A distinct horizontal body crease was added just above the wheel openings. There were seven engine options offered for the 1969 introduction, and they included the base Firebird, Firebird Sprint, Firebird 350, 350 HO, base 400, Ram Air III 400, and Ram Air IV.

On March 8, 1969, the new Trans Am option package (UPC WS4) was introduced with great fanfare. The $1,163.74 Trans Am package included the 335-horsepower Ram Air III 400 engine (UPC L74). In addition to the Ram Air III 400 engine, the Trans Am package included a heavy-duty three-speed transmission with floor-shift, 3.55:1 rear axle ratio, heavy-duty shock absorbers, fiberglass belted tires, heavy-duty springs, stabilizer bar, power disc front brakes, variable-ratio power steering, engine compartment heat exhaust extractors on the front fenders, fiberglass rear spoiler, body stripes, and a black textured grille. The 345-horsepower Ram Air IV engine was available as a $558.20 option over the standard Trans Am package. The 1969 Trans Am was only available in Cameo Ivory (50) with twin Nassau Blue full-length wide stripes to correspond with the traditional United States international FIA racing color scheme. The Trans Am took Firebird and Pontiac performance to a higher level, a fact that was not lost to youthful buyers.

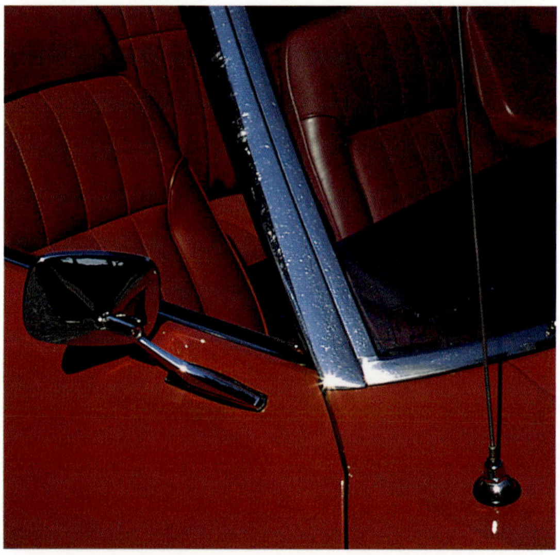

Six hundred ninety-seven Trans Am Firebirds were produced for 1969, consisting of 689 hardtops and eight convertibles. All Trans Am convertibles had the standard UPC L74 Ram Air III engine package; four were four-speed equipped and four were automatics.

The 1969 Firebird was available in 19 body color choices. Five Cordova vinyl roof colors and eight vinyl interior trim schemes complemented the body colors.

Above: This Regimental Red 1967 Firebird sport coupe with optional ivory vinyl Cordova roof and Rally II wheels has six chrome simulated louvers on the rear quarter panel. The tires are aftermarket replacements. ***Left:*** This is a detail view of the right windshield frame and optional outside chrome rearview mirror on a red 1969 Firebird convertible. Note the mounting of the antenna for the optional radio.

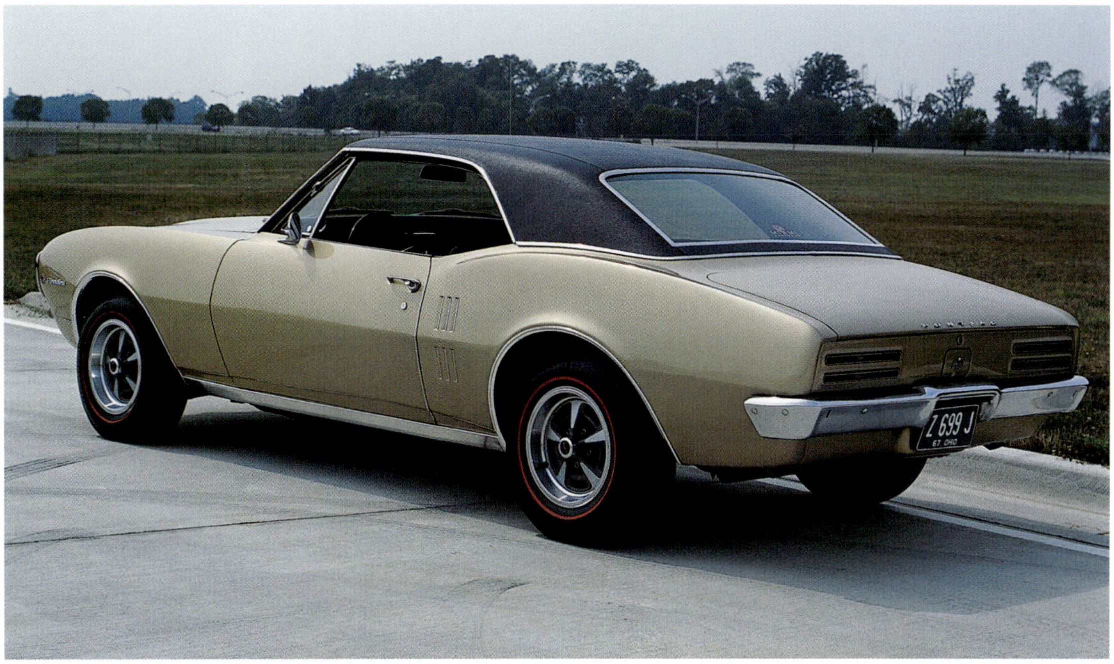

This left rear quarter view shows a Signet Gold 1967 Firebird sport coupe with optional black vinyl roof and 14-inch Rally II wheels with trim rings. Note the distinctive kickup of the rear quarters of the unitized construction body design. The UPC C08 Cordova vinyl roof option includes the bright drip-rail moldings.

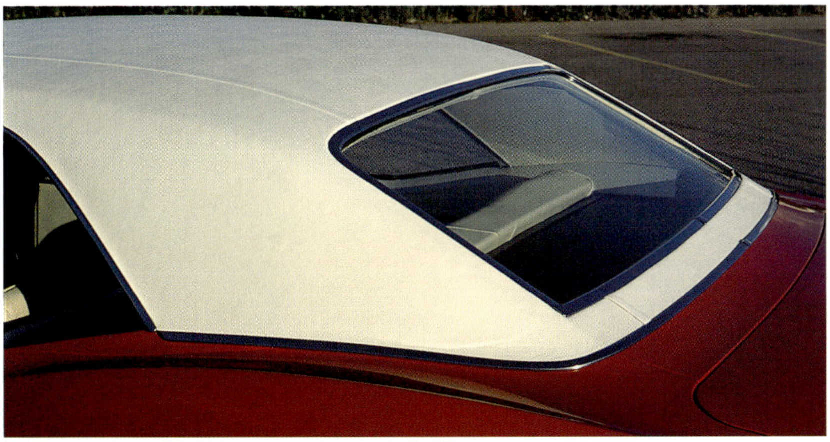

The optional white vinyl roof on this red 1967 Firebird coupe included a two-piece bright body belt molding at the base of the roof. Note the bright molding surrounding the rear window opening.

Body Sheet Metal and Trim

The 1967–1969 Firebird shared its unitized-construction basic body shell with the Chevrolet Camaro, and both used a steel channel front sub-frame to carry the engine and front suspension components. The semigloss-black painted (some may have been bare, unfinished steel) front sub-frame was bolted to the body with four rubber-isolated mounts. The remainder of the welded steel body shell incorporated a steel floorpan with longitudinal parallel rear members to support the suspension and drivetrain. The underside of the body floorpan was coated with a red oxide primer. All 1967–1969 Firebirds had an 18.5-gallon galvanized steel fuel tank mounted at the rear of the body pan. All 1967–1969 Firebirds were based on two basic body configurations—a two-door sport coupe (hardtop) and two-door convertible—all on a 108.1-inch wheelbase.

In addition to the standard steel roof, all 1967–1969 Firebird sport coupes were available with an optional Levant-grain vinyl roof covering (UPC C08). All Firebird sport coupe bodies used a standard bright stainless-steel roof drip rail molding. When the optional vinyl roof was ordered, an additional two-piece bright molding was added at the lower edge of the vinyl roof at the sail panel and wrapped around the lower border of the back glass opening. The 1969 vinyl roof was slightly different in design and fit from the 1967 and 1968 version.

The optional Cordova vinyl roof was available in ivory (1), black (2), and cream (7) in 1967. For 1968, the vinyl roof was available in ivory (1), black (2), teal (5), and gold (8). The 1969 vinyl roof colors were black (B), dark blue (C), parchment (E), dark fawn (H), and dark green (I). The vinyl roof installation was in three sections, with the large center section between two side sections and a longitudinal seam on each side of the roof panel.

The Firebird convertible had a standard manually operated folding top with an electric/hydraulic power top (UPC C06) optional. The rear window was sewn-in clear vinyl, and it folded with the top. A bright trim molding was attached to the outer body opening at the rear of the top. The standard vinyl top boot was generally color-coordinated with the top color, but a gold body color with a white top and gold interior had a gold boot. The top boot was attached by hooking under the edge of the trim molding. The boot was stored in the trunk in a heavy black vinyl boot bag when not used. The convertible body type was available in all models, but only eight 1969 Trans Am convertibles were built. Four were equipped with a four-speed transmission, and the other four had an automatic.

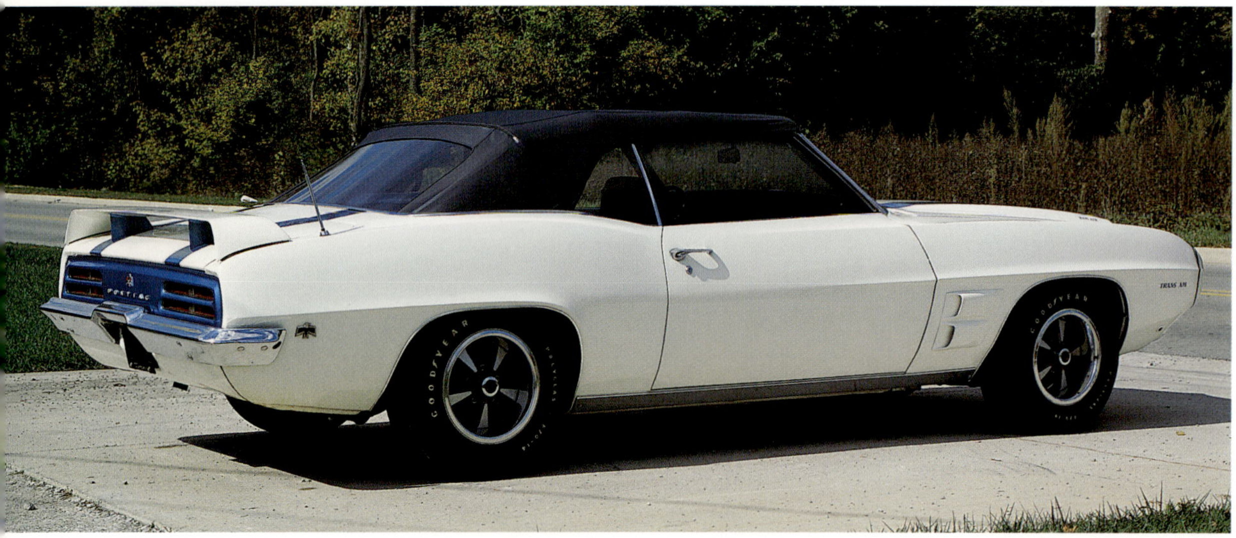

This Cameo Ivory 1969 Trans Am convertible replica has the distinctive horizontal body feature line above the wheel openings unique to the 1969 Firebird and Trans Am body design. Note the wide rear spoiler, Nassau Blue body stripes, and rear deck lower panel.

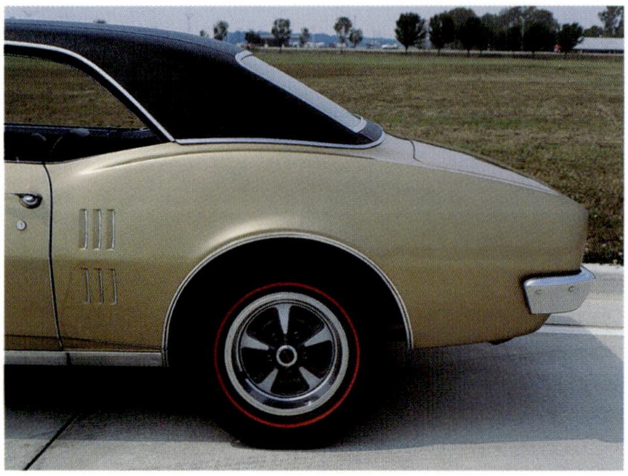

This is a detail view of the left rear quarter panel on a 1967 Firebird coupe finished in Signet Gold with an optional black vinyl Cordova roof. Note the smooth curve of the upper panel over the rear wheel opening and the bright rocker panel molding and the outer end of the rear bumper.

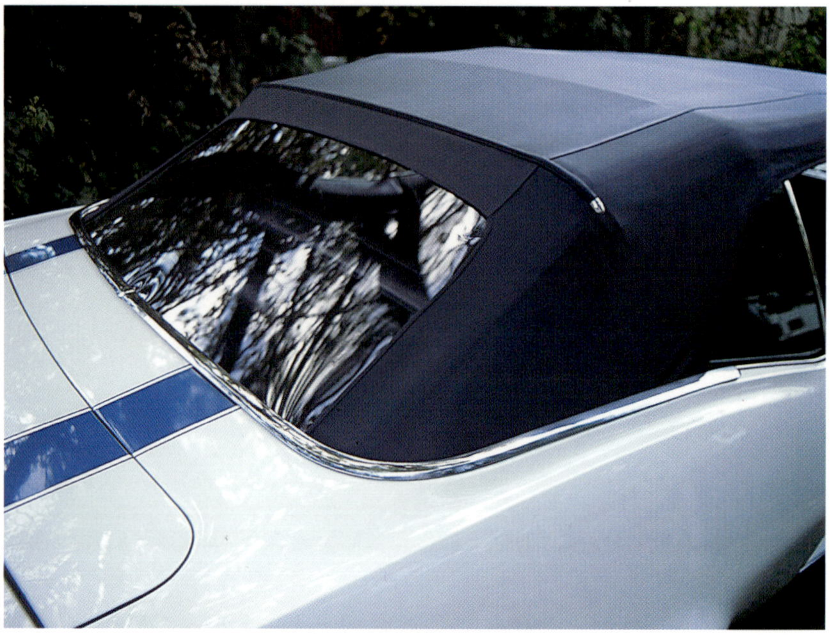

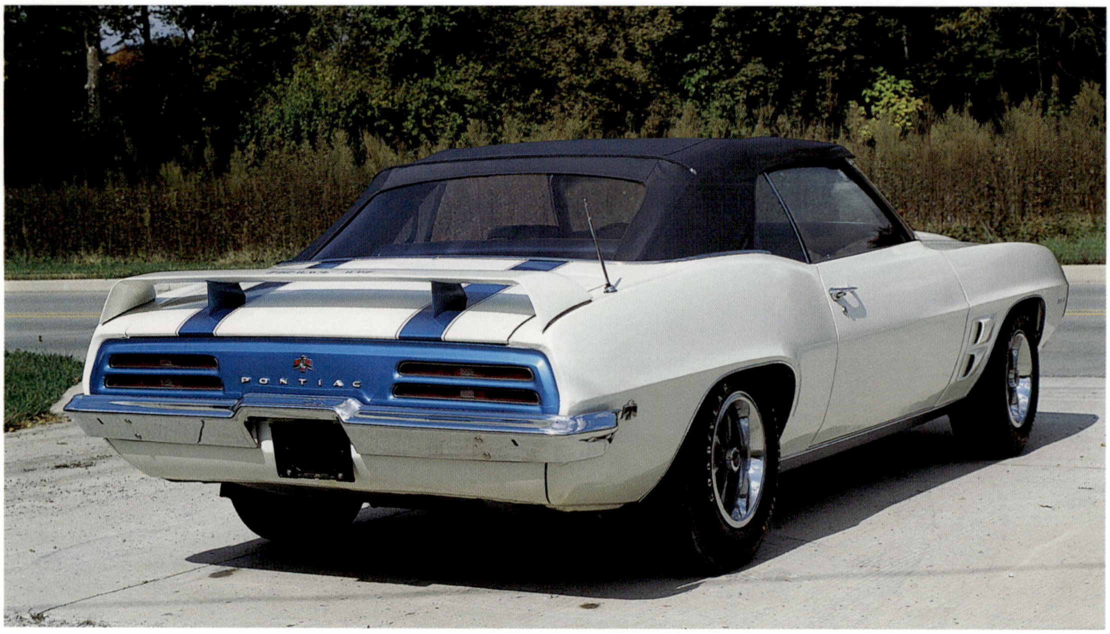

Above: This photo shows a detail view of the right rear of the blue convertible top on a replica 1969 Trans Am convertible. The 1969 Trans was only available in Cameo Ivory with blue stripes. Note the two-piece bright trim surrounding the rear of the top. ***Left:*** Rear view of a replica 1969 Trans Am convertible finished in the standard Cameo Ivory with Nassau Blue stripes. The 1969 Firebird convertible top was available in ivory, black, dark green, or dark blue, as this one is.

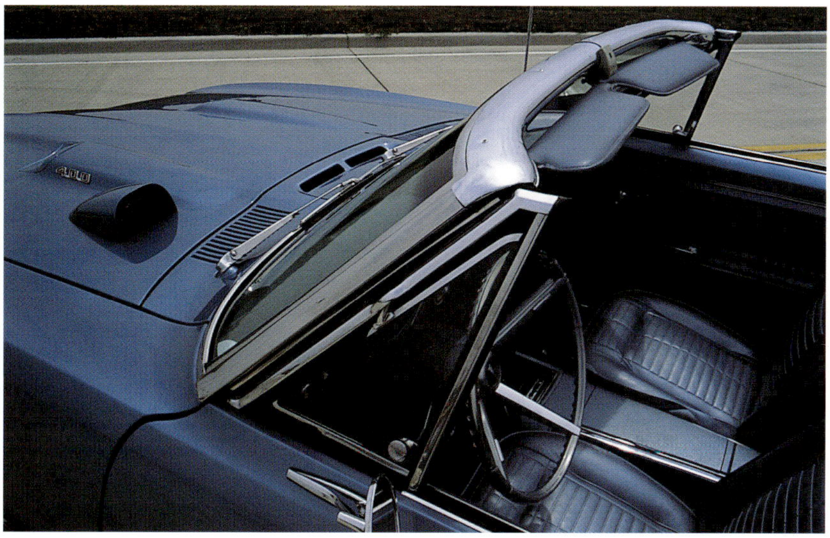

Left: The top of the windshield frame on a convertible is equipped with a special molding to allow the front of the top to seal. This view of a Tyrol Blue 1967 Firebird convertible with optional blue vinyl interior trim shows the optional hood-mounted tachometer.

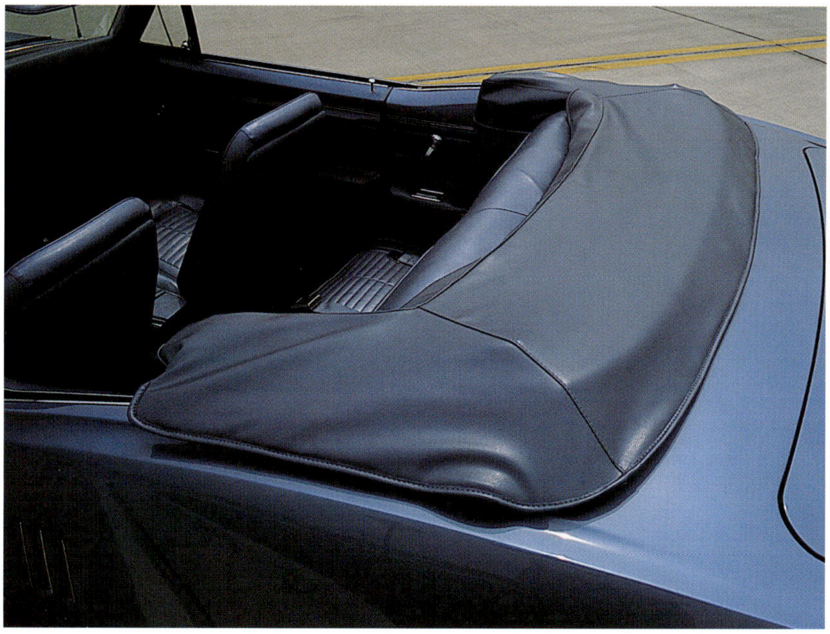

Above: This Tyrol Blue 1967 Firebird convertible had a custom blue vinyl interior and an ivory-white convertible top. The standard vinyl top boot is blue to match the interior trim combination. The outer edges of the top boot clip under the edge of the bright body molding. ***Below:*** The left front quarter view shows the design of the door panel on a red 1968 Firebird Sprint coupe. The 1968 doors differ from the 1967 doors because the earlier vent windows were eliminated as part of the new ventilation system.

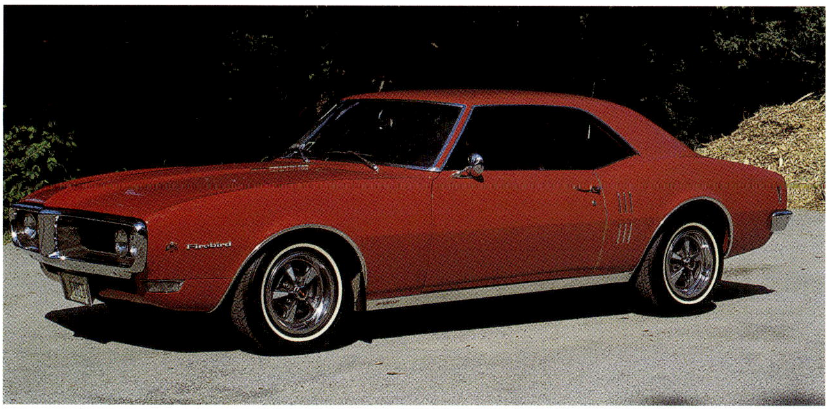

All 1967–1969 Firebirds used the same left and right door shells for each respective year. Changes occurred in the door and door latch design for each year, so components are not interchangeable from year to year. The most obvious changes to the doors were the deletion of the vent windows for 1968 and a redesign of the body side contours for 1969. The doors were operated by chrome-plated push-button-type handles that were identical for all 1967–1969 bodies.

A chrome-plated left outside mirror was standard equipment on all 1967–1969 Firebirds. A chrome-plated remote control left-side mirror (UPC D33) was an option for all models and years. The mirrors were round for 1967 and rectangular for 1968 and 1969.

All 1967–1969 Firebird doors were sealed with black soft sponge rubber weatherstrip that surrounds the outer perimeter of the door shell. The perimeter of the body door opening used a color-coordinated push-on vinyl windlace that also served to secure the inside trim panels. The lower door opening was trimmed with an aluminum sill plate with a Fisher Body badge in the center. The upper end of the body latch pillar has a small rubber cap that seals the front of the quarter window opening. The single-year 1967 triangular vent window has a black rubber seal around its entire perimeter. A body-color Torx-head door latch striker was mounted in the center of the door-opening pillar. A black ABS plastic vent grille was also mounted in both body doorjambs of the 1968 and 1969 models as part of the Astro ventilation system. The vent had a one-way relief valve that allowed air back into the passenger compartment.

All 1967–1969 Firebirds used the same deck lid, hinges, and supports with variations only for trim badges. On all except the 1969 Trans Am, individual block letters spelling Pontiac were mounted in the center rear edge, but the badge was deleted with the dealer-installed rear spoiler option. An appropriate 400 engine option badge was mounted on the right corner. There were no engine badges for any other engine choices. The 1969 Trans Am deck lid deleted the 400 engine badge and Pontiac letters in the center, but a wide functional spoiler was mounted across the full width of the rear deck. The spoiler actually created 100 pounds of down force at high speed. Block decal letters spelling Trans Am were applied to the center top of the spoiler. Part of the 1969 Trans Am package was a unique pair of wide, blue

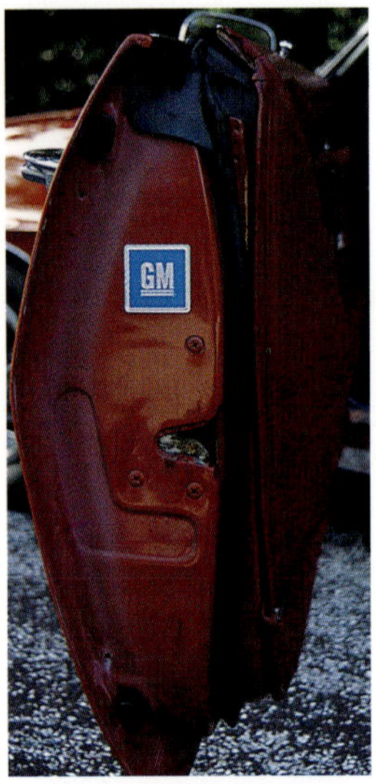

Left: Detail view of the left doorjamb on a Matador Red 1969 Firebird convertible. Note the black rubber door opening weatherstrip attached to the outer perimeter of the door shell. ***Right:*** Detail view of the rear body doorjamb post on the left door of a Matador Red 1969 Firebird convertible. Note the black ABS grille attached to the body as part of the body ventilation system. The molded rubber seal at the top of the door opening is part of the door seal system.
Below left: This is the standard, round, chrome-plated left outside mirror on a Regimental Red 1967 Firebird coupe. A left-hand outside mirror was optional. The door vent window was used only in 1967 on the Firebird.
Below right: The standard chrome-plated left-hand outside mirror was rectangular on the 1968 and 1969 Firebird. Note that this Cameo Ivory 1969 Firebird coupe no longer has the door vent window used in 1967.

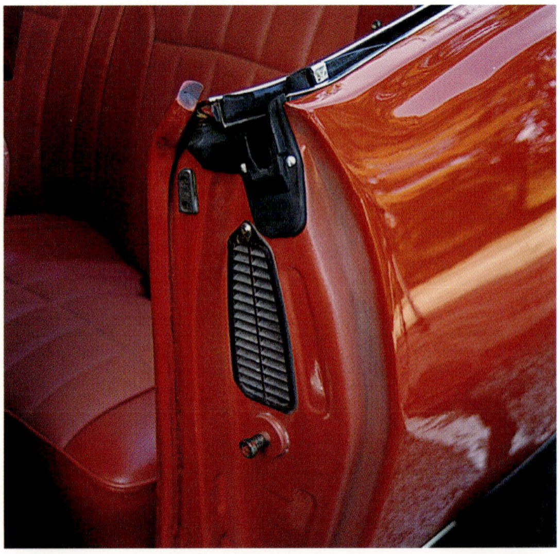

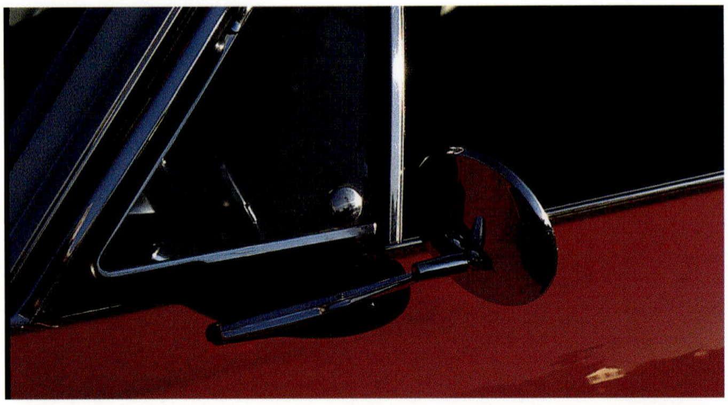

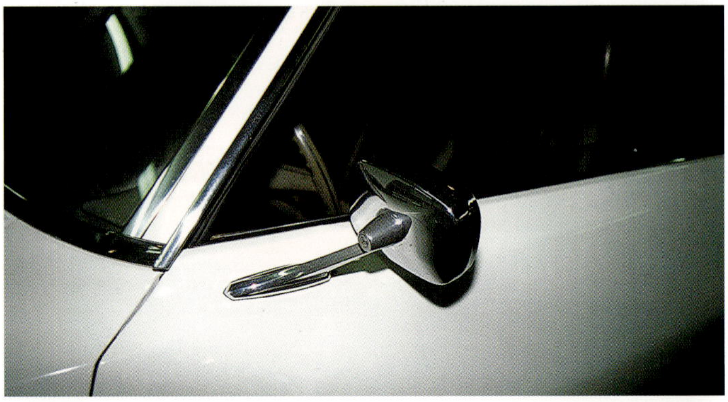

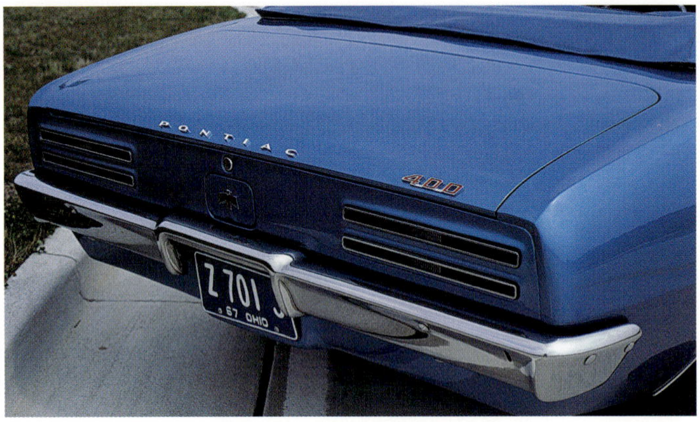

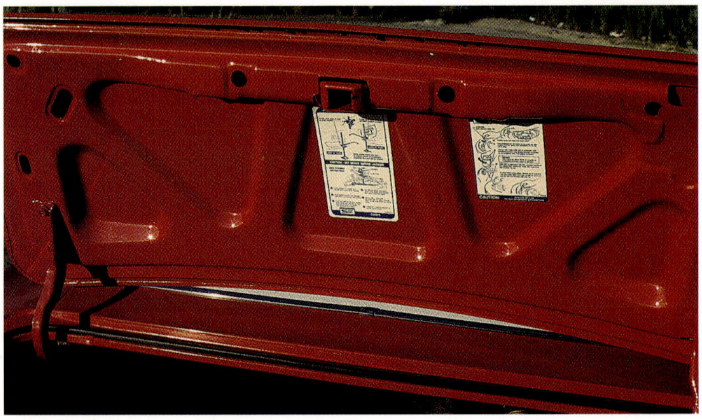

Above left: Detail view of the rear deck lid and rear deck lower panel on a Tyrol Blue 1967 Firebird convertible. Note the 400 engine badge and Pontiac name on the deck lid. The square fuel filler door with Firebird badge was mounted in the rear deck lower panel in 1967 and 1968. ***Above right:*** The inside of the deck lid on a red 1967 Firebird displays the jack instructions decal and operating instructions decal for the standard inflatable compact spare tire.

longitudinal stripes that extended the length of the body from the front of the hood scoops to the rear deck lower panel. The stripes were applied on the deck lid and spoiler pedestals only. Although at least two early-press, or pilot, Trans Ams may have had the blue stripe extend over the top of the spoiler, later, regular production cars did not.

All 1967–1969 Firebirds had a flat trunk floor with a standard space-saver spare tire mounted on the right with its inner side up. The jack base was mounted bottom-side up in the center of the face down spare wheel and secured by a plated wing nut. The jack was held in place by the wheel and tire. The jack in the sport coupe was mounted transversely at the front of the wheel. In the convertible trunk, the jack was mounted at an angle at the lower right of the wheel. A pressure can in a pasteboard canister with a GM instruction label was mounted longitudinally on the right side of the space-saver spare wheel. On some cars,

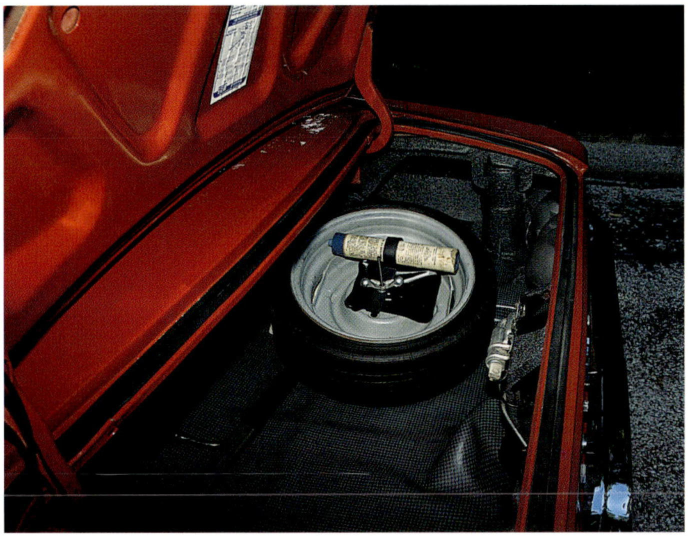

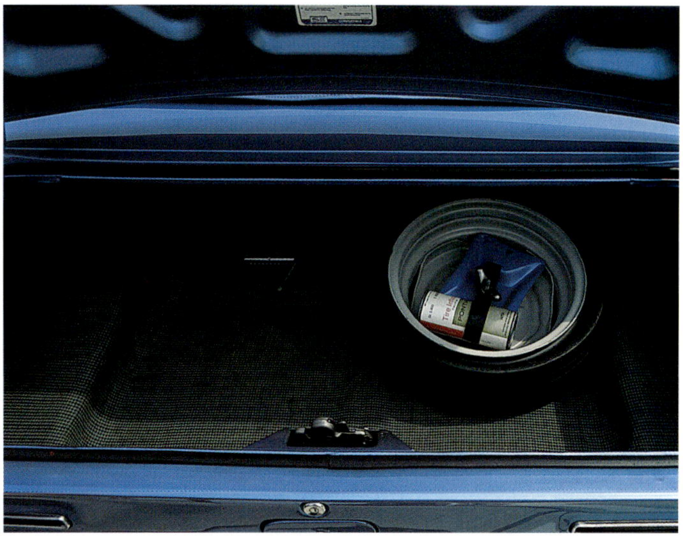

Above left: The 1967–1969 Firebird convertibles had unique oil-filled dampeners installed in the right and left corners of the trunk designed to absorb vibrations from the body structure of the convertible. The inflatable compact spare tire was standard in 1967–1969. ***Above right:*** This is a detail view of the trunk in a Tyrol Blue 1967 Firebird convertible. The standard compact spare tire has the original tire inflator canister mounted at the rear of the wheel. The jack is installed under the spare tire, and the tire and wheel are held in place with the jack base.

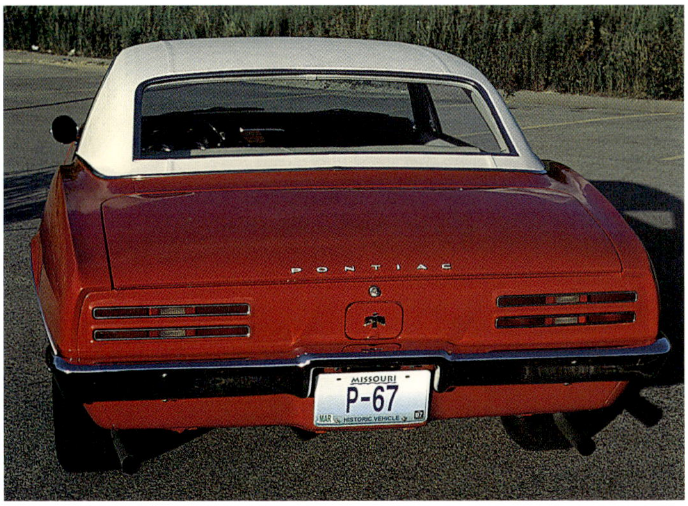

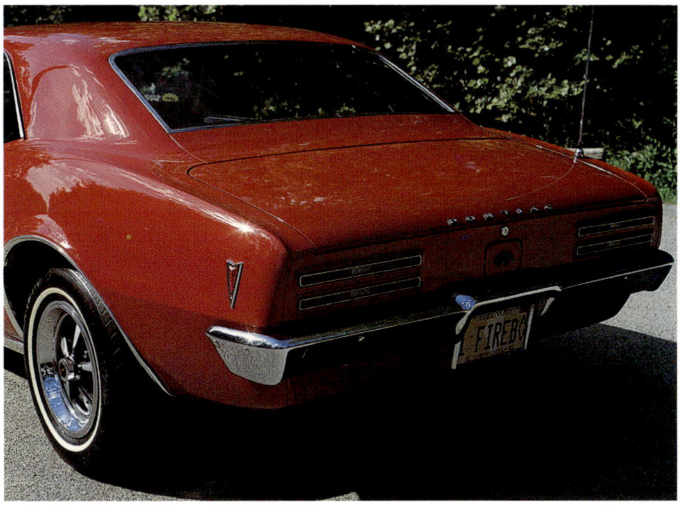

Above left: Rear detail view of the rear deck lower panel, taillights, and deck lid of a Regimental Red 1967 Firebird coupe with a white vinyl Cordova roof. Note the square fuel filler door with Firebird badge. ***Above right:*** Detail view of the deck lid and rear deck lower panel on a Solar Red 1968 Firebird Sprint coupe. Note the arrowhead-design side marker on the rear quarter panel and Pontiac name on the rear of the deck lid. ***Right:*** The rear deck lower panel of this red 1969 Firebird shows the fuel filler door moved from the center of the panel to behind the license plate. Note the Pontiac nameplate moved from the deck lid to rear panel.

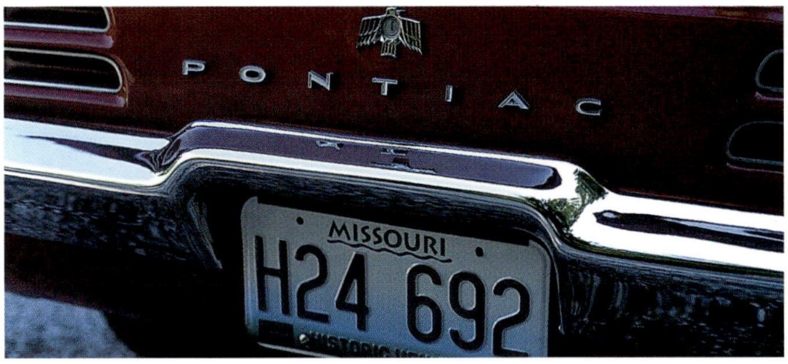

the inflator pressure may have been mounted transversely to the front of the spare wheel. A standard spare wheel was available as a no-cost option with UPC N64.

The flat part of the trunk floor was covered with an aqua-and-black houndstooth pattern vinyl mat, but an optional fitted mat was available with UPC B42. The entire trunk interior was finished with gray speckle paint. The trunk capacity was 9.9 cubic feet for all models. The 1967–1969 Firebird convertibles had an unusual dampener and bracket mounted in each rear corner of the trunk compartment. These dampeners (sometimes called "cocktail shakers" by enthusiasts)

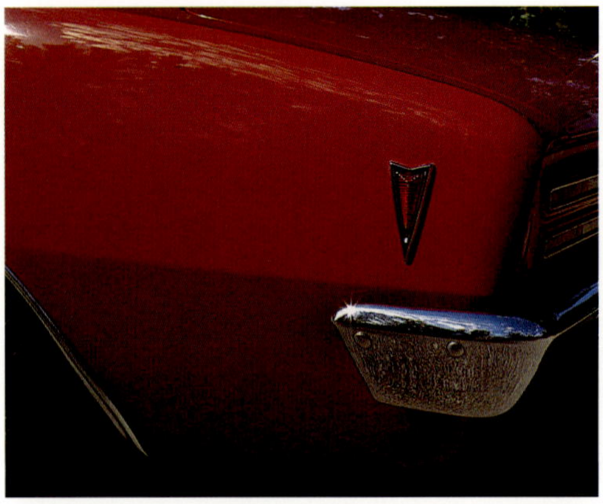

Left: This detail view of the left rear quarter panel of a 1968 Firebird Sprint coupe finished in Solar Red shows the arrowhead side marker light unique to 1968. This Firebird has the optional bright wheel opening moldings. ***Right:*** This is a detail view of the right rear quarter panel on a Matador Red 1969 Firebird convertible. Note the unique 1969 stylized-bird rear side marker light and the different rear bumper design from 1968.

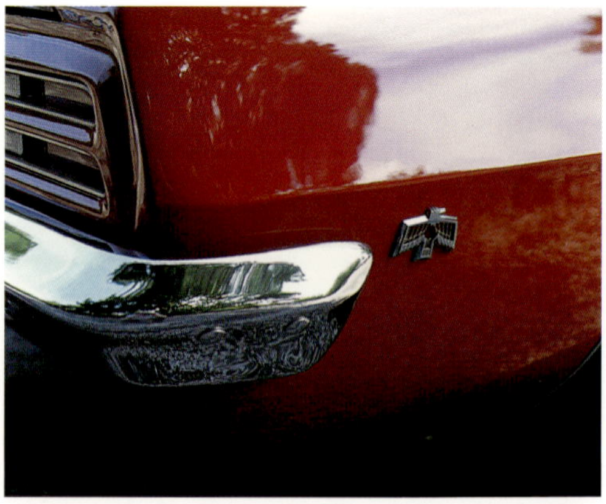

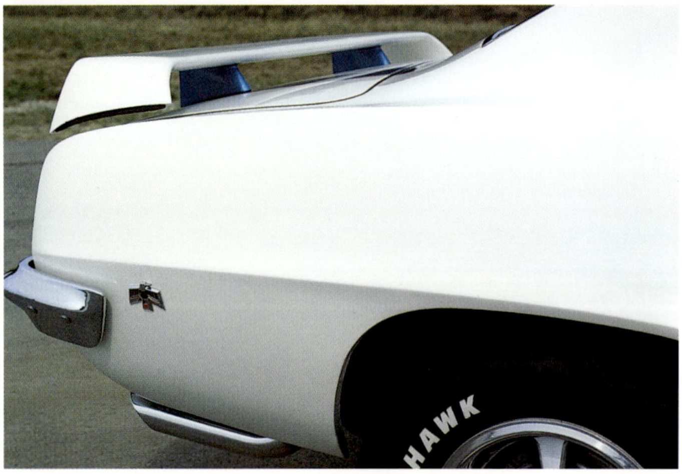

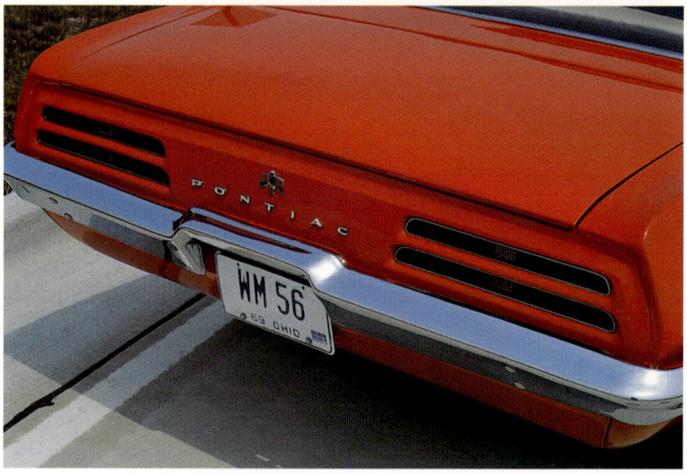

Above left: A detail view of the right rear quarter of a Cameo Ivory 1969 Trans Am coupe shows the design of the wide rear spoiler standard with the Trans Am. The dual Nassau Blue body stripes are not continued over the top of the spoiler. Note the bird design side marker light in front of the bumper end. ***Above right:*** A rear view of a Carousel Red 1969 Firebird convertible shows the rear deck lower panel and deck lid. Note the difference in the design of the taillights from 1968 and the relocation of the fuel filler door.

were painted with gray speckle trunk interior finish and contained 25-pound weights suspended in oil (ATF) that helped to absorb some of the inherent vibrations in the convertible body structure. There were separate dampener part numbers for left and right and different part numbers for each year, and left and right units were not interchangeable. Two additional similar vibration dampeners were installed in each corner of the front subframe.

The rear deck lower panel was flat except for two bright trimmed thin horizontal taillights on each side and the deck lid lock in the upper center. The 1967 and 1968 Firebirds had a square fuel filler door with a Firebird badge mounted in the center on the rear panel. For the 1969 models, the fuel filler door was moved to a location behind the license plate below the rear bumper. The rear deck lower panel had a Firebird badge in its center and the word Pontiac centered in block letters below the badge. The 1969 Trans Am rear deck lower panel (including the taillight surrounds) was finished in Nassau Blue to match the stripe color. A relatively straight chrome-plated bumper with the license plate mounted in its lower center was used for all 1967–1969 Firebirds. The bumper wrapped around the sides of the rear quarter panels.

The rear quarter panels of the Firebird had the distinctive kickup of the Camaro, but the front center of the quarter panel of the 1967 and 1968 Firebird had three unique bright metal vertical hash marks, or chevrons, above and below the horizontal center crease just behind the door opening on each side. For 1968, the quarter panel had a small Pontiac arrowhead badge marker light just in front of the rear bumper ends on each side. The quarter panel was redesigned for 1969. The crease was raised to the top of the wheel opening, and the chevrons were deleted. A small bright-rimmed stylized Firebird-shaped marker light was added to the rear side of the panel just ahead of the rear bumper ends.

All 1967 and 1968 Firebirds had the same front fenders. The right fender had part number 9793816 and the left used part number 9793617. A Firebird script nameplate was mounted in the front center just behind a Firebird badge. Separate lower front extensions were used on all applications.

For 1969, the front fenders were redesigned with a higher horizontal crease and flatter wheel openings. All 1969 models (except the Trans Am) used fenders with part number 9798212 for the right and 9798213 for the left. Two small simulated rectangular extractor louvers were made as part of the fender just behind the wheel opening on the standard and 400 models. The 1969 Trans Am used front fenders with part number 546680 for the right and 546681 for the left. The lower

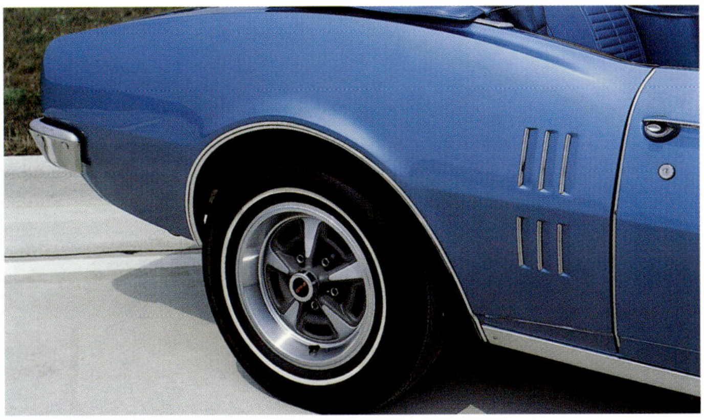

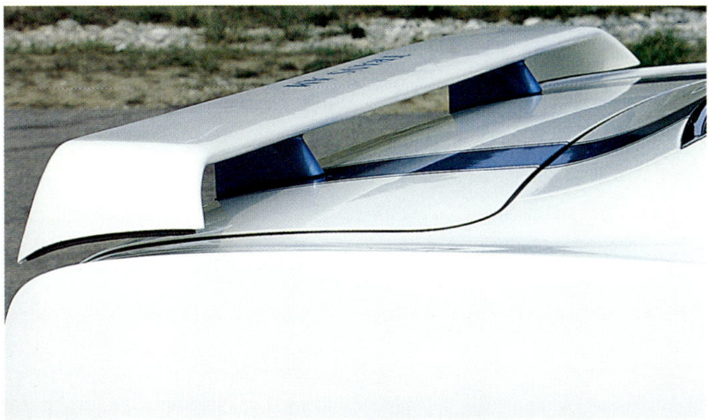

Above left: The right rear view of a Tyrol Blue 1967 Firebird convertible shows the smooth design of the typical 1967 and 1968 rear quarter panel. Note the bright wheel opening molding and rocker panel moldings. This Firebird also has optional UPC B93 door edge moldings. ***Above right:*** Right rear quarter view of a Cameo Ivory 1969 Trans Am sport coupe. The wide deck-lid-mounted spoiler was unique to the 1969 Trans Am.

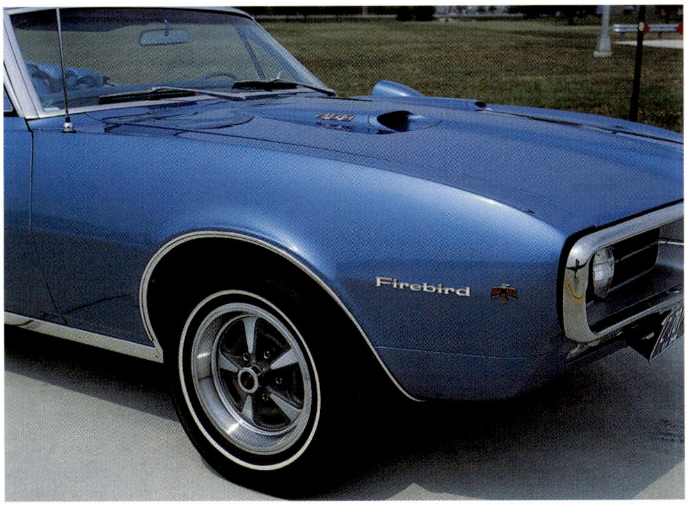

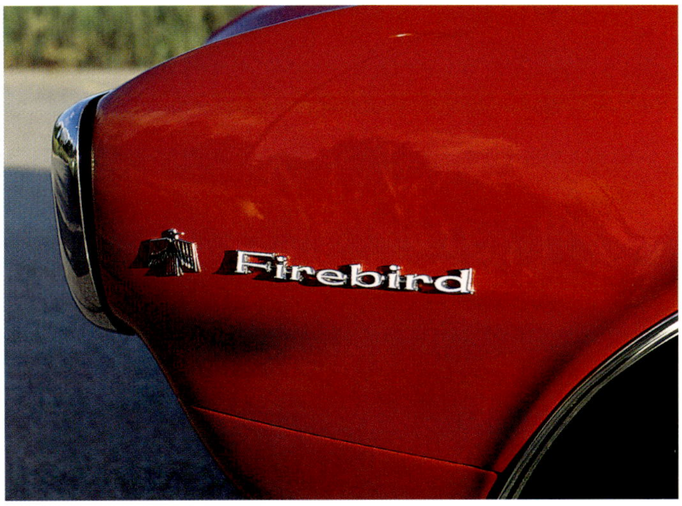

Above left: Right front fender of a Tyrol Blue 1967 Firebird convertible. Note the unique bird design, Firebird nameplate, scoops, and 400 engine badge on the hood. The hood-mounted tachometer was an unusual option (UPC U16) available on the 1967 Firebird. ***Above right:*** This detail view of the left front fender of a red 1967 Firebird coupe shows the bird badge and paint-filled Firebird nameplate. This Firebird is equipped with optional bright wheel opening moldings.

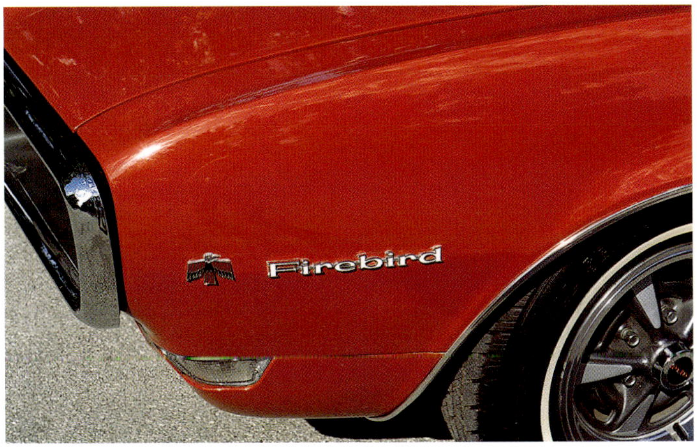

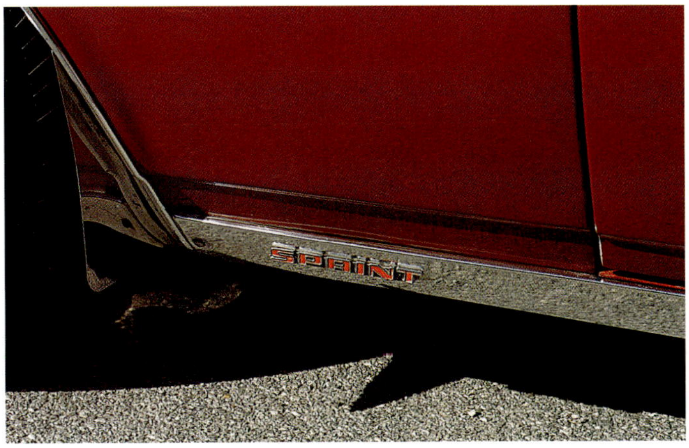

Above left: This Solar Red 1968 Firebird Sprint coupe shows the same paint-filled Firebird nameplate and bird as the 1967 model, but the front parking light wraps around the side of the lower valance panel. ***Above right:*** This red 1968 Firebird Sprint has a unique lower rocker panel molding with a Sprint nameplate. The bright mud flap is an accessory attached over the optional wheel opening molding.

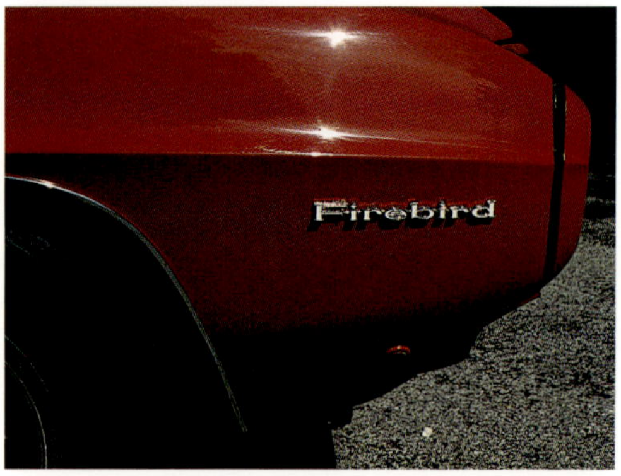

Left: Detail view of the Matador Red 1969 Firebird convertible right front fender showing the paint-filled Firebird nameplate. Note the small round side marker used on the 1969 Firebird. ***Right:*** The rear of the right front fender of a red 1969 Firebird has the chrome-plated simulated extractor vents used on all except the Trans Am. Note the bright lower rocker panel molding.

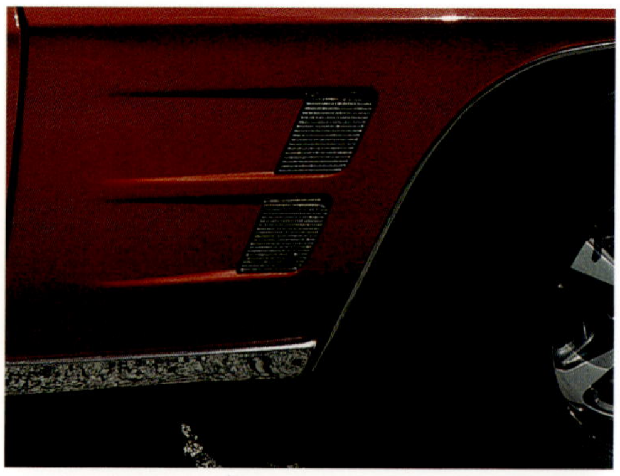

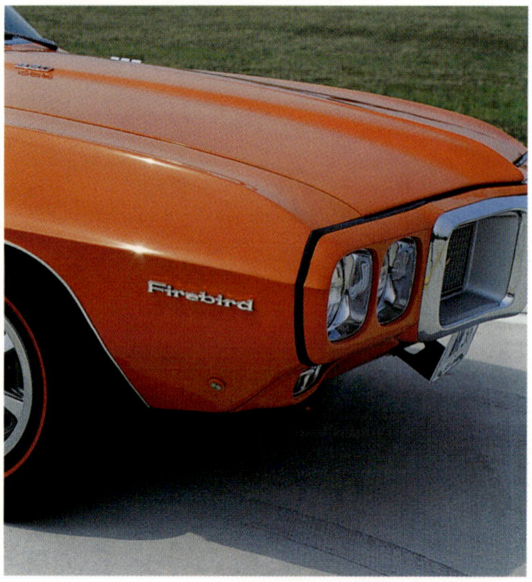

Left: This view of the right front fender of a Carousel Red 1969 Firebird convertible clearly shows the distinctive horizontal character line that identifies the 1969 Firebird body design. Note the black joint seal between the front fascia and fender. Carousel Red was a special-order color for 1969. ***Right:*** The right front fender of a Cameo Ivory 1969 Trans Am has a distinctive Trans Am decal and 1969 round side marker light. Note the 1969 unique horizontal body character crease and black rubber seal between the front fascia and fender edge.

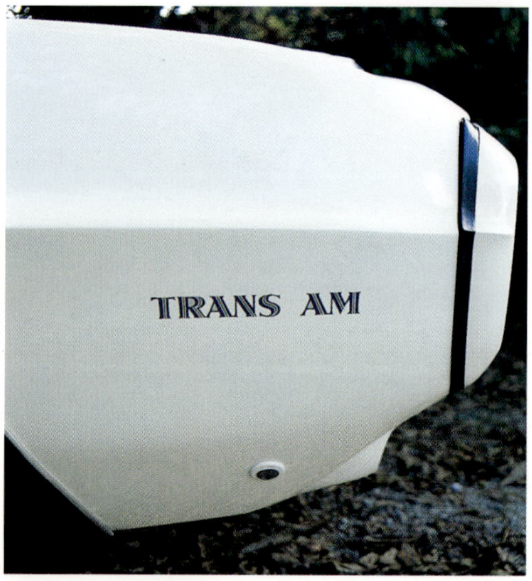

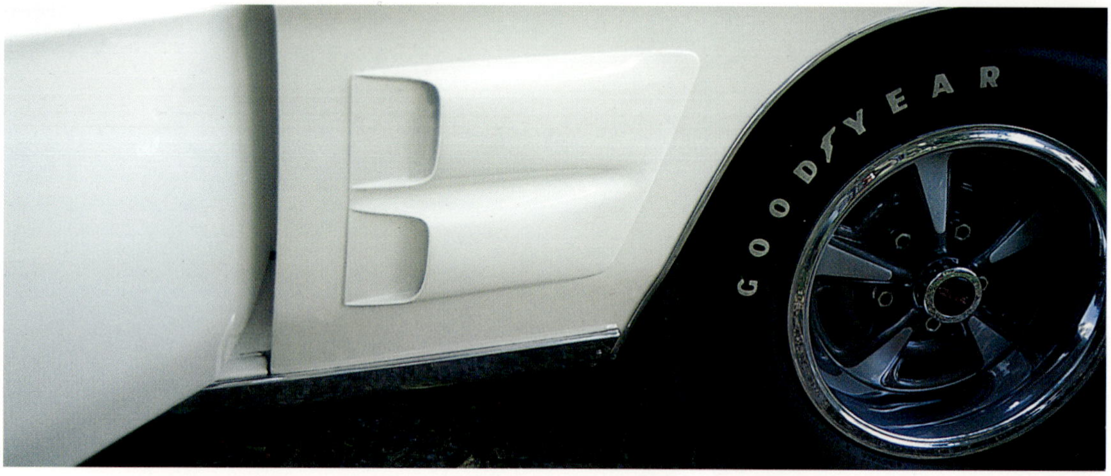

These dual rear-facing simulated extractor scoops were used on the rear of the 1969 Trans Am front fenders. This Trans Am has optional Rally II wheels and trim rings.

extensions used for 1967 and 1968 were eliminated, and the lower front was made part of the fender. When the Trans Am option was ordered in 1969, the extractors were more distinctive bolt-on, rear-opening functional scoops. A script Firebird nameplate was mounted at the front center just below the horizontal crease. Also, on early production cars, a small Trans Am decal was mounted just below the Firebird nameplate as part of the 1969 Trans Am option. The Firebird nameplates may have been deleted some time after initial production began, leaving only the Trans Am decals. A small painted body-color-rimmed round marker light was mounted at the forward lower end of the front fender on all versions.

There were seven different hoods used on the 1967–1969 Firebirds. The standard 1967 Firebird with the 230-ci OHC six used a flat hood with a slightly raised center bulge pointed toward the front (part number 9789969). The 1968 and 1969 Firebird with the 230 six-cylinder or 350 V-8 used a hood with part number 9793429. The 1967 Firebird with a 326 V-8 used a hood with part number 9788846. An appropriate 3.8-liter or

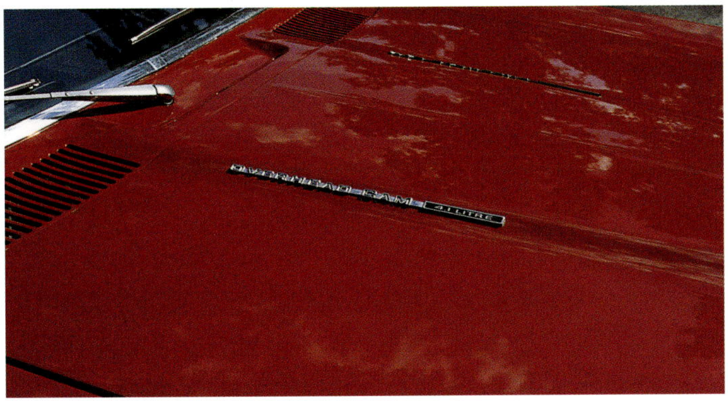

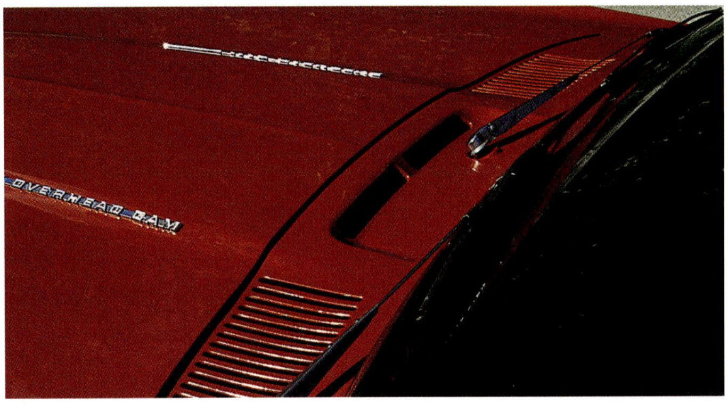

Above left: This is a detail view of the hood and engine badge on a Solar Red 1968 Firebird Sprint. Note the "Overhead Cam 4.1 Litre" identification used on the right side of the hood in 1968. ***Above right:*** This view shows the left side of the hood of a red 1968 Firebird Sprint. The engine badge is the opposite of the one used on the left side and reads: "4.1 Litre Overhead Cam."

4.1-liter engine badge was mounted on each side of the standard six-cylinder hood. A bright-trimmed red "326" or "350" badge was added to each side of the hood when the 326 or 350 V-8 engines were ordered. An optional distinctive body color hood-mounted tachometer was available with UPC U16 in 1967 and 1968 and with UB5 in 1969.

When the 400 engine was ordered, the hood (part number 9789418 in 1967 and 9793430 in 1968 and 1969) had two forward-opening raised simulated scoops stamped into each side with a bright-trimmed red "400" badge on the outside of each scoop. Each scoop had a body color bezel on the front. When the 1969 Ram Air 400 package was ordered (except Trans Am), the scoops were opened and became functional, with foam seals surrounding the carburetor air cleaner backing plate (hood panel part number 9797763). The twin 400 scoops were mounted at the rear half of the hood.

When the UPC WS4 Trans Am package was ordered for 1969, the hood (part number 546014) was redesigned and had two large wide scoops molded toward the front end of the hood. These scoops were open and made functional with soft foam rubber seals on the carburetor air cleaner backing plate. A Ram Air (or Ram Air IV when appropriate) decal was mounted at the rear outside of each scoop. A wide, longitudinal Nassau Blue body stripe was applied down the top center of each of the scoops and extended to the rear of the body to the rear deck lower panel.

All 1967 and 1968 Firebird grilles were in two sections, one on each side of the full-width chrome bumper with quad round headlights. The front bumper had a distinct vertical peak at the center with a silver-and-black-trimmed Pontiac arrowhead badge in the center when the 400 engine was ordered. The 1967 Firebird standard and Sprint six used the standard grille, and the Firebird 400 used its own unique grille design with a bright horizontal bar in the center of each grille section. Both grille designs used bright surrounds. Both used a bright horizontal divider bar in the center. A block Pontiac script name badge was mounted in the upper left grille section. The 1967 lower valance had rectangular parking lights mounted inside of a wide rectangular opening on each side below the grille.

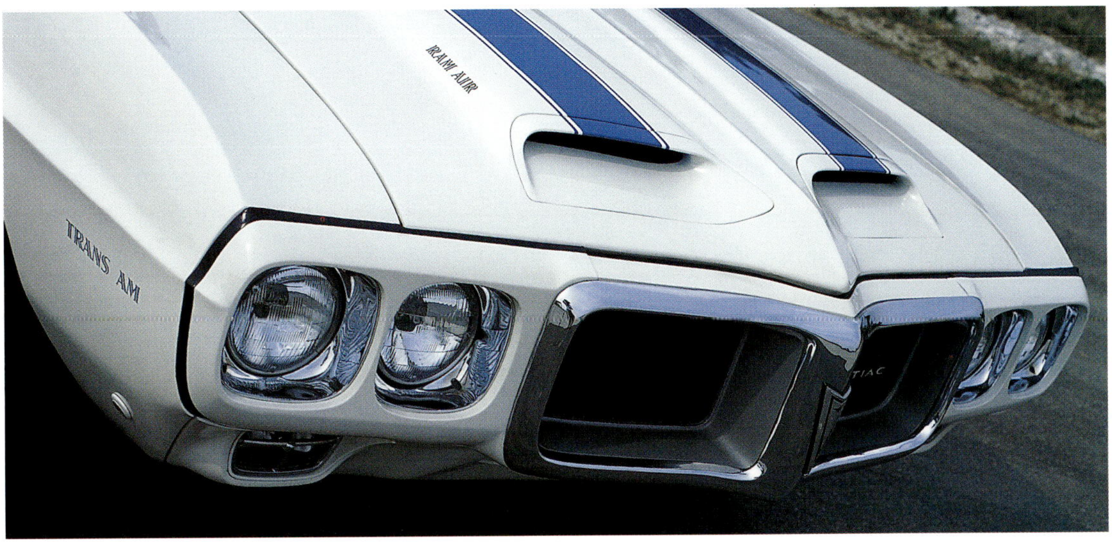

The 1969 Trans Am hood had functional twin scoops when the UPC L74 Ram Air 400 V-8 option was ordered. The Cameo Ivory finish with Nassau Blue stripes was representative of the traditional United States FIA racing colors and standard with the Trans Am.

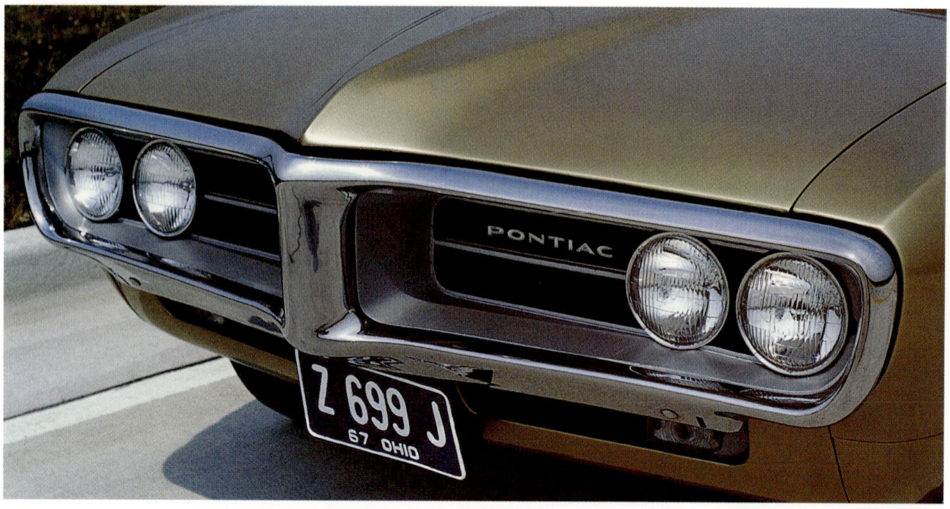

Left: The grille design of the 1967 Firebird included the massive chrome-plated front bumper. This Signet Gold Firebird is equipped with the 326 V-8 engine. Note the side marker and Firebird nameplate on the front fender. ***Below left:*** Detail view of the left side of the grille, front bumper, and original headlights of a red 1967 Firebird with a "T" in a triangle in the center of the lens. ***Below right:*** The 1968 Firebird Sprint grille and front bumper were identical to the 1967 design. This Solar Red 1968 Firebird Sprint is equipped with the unusual overhead-camshaft inline six-cylinder engine.

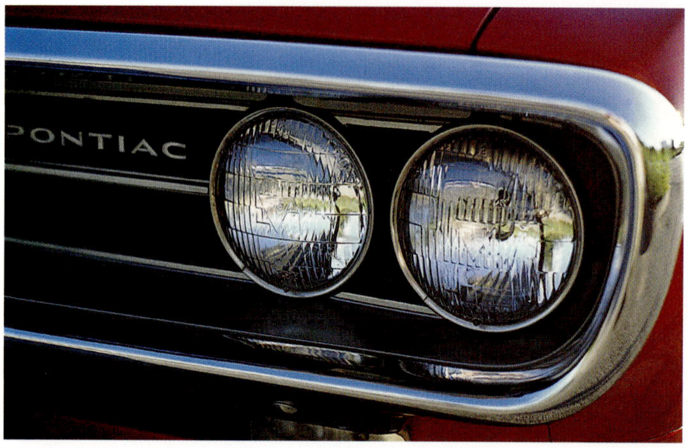

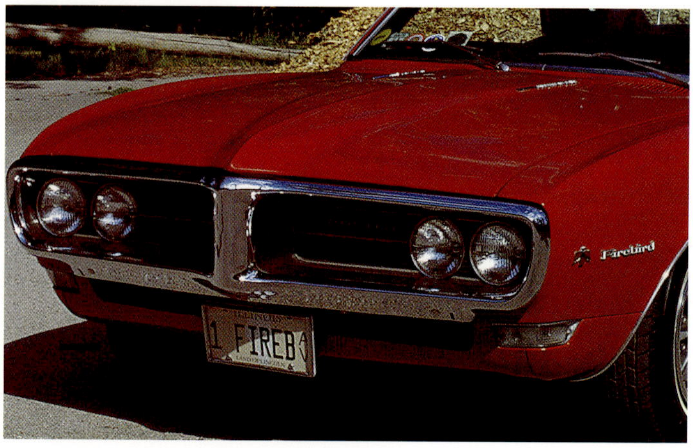

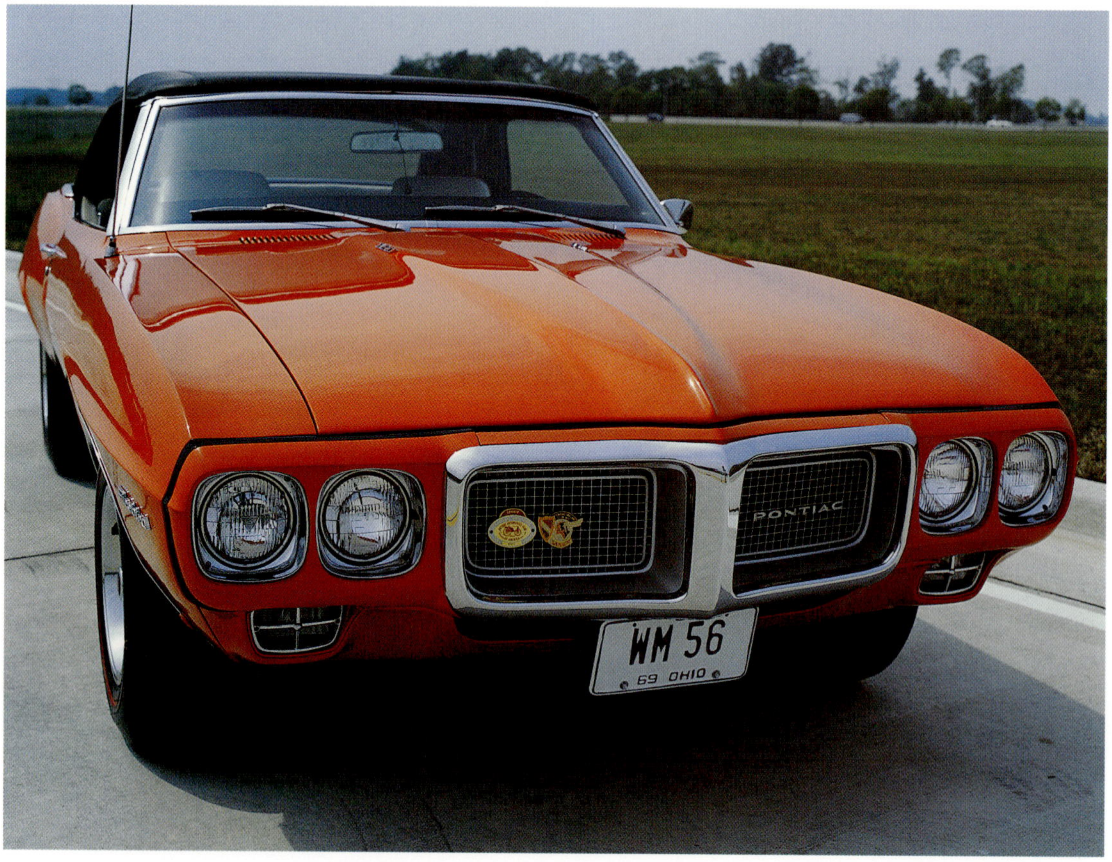

The Firebird grille and front bumper were changed completely for the 1969 model year. This Carousel Red 1969 Firebird convertible shows the silver finish on the standard Firebird grille mesh.

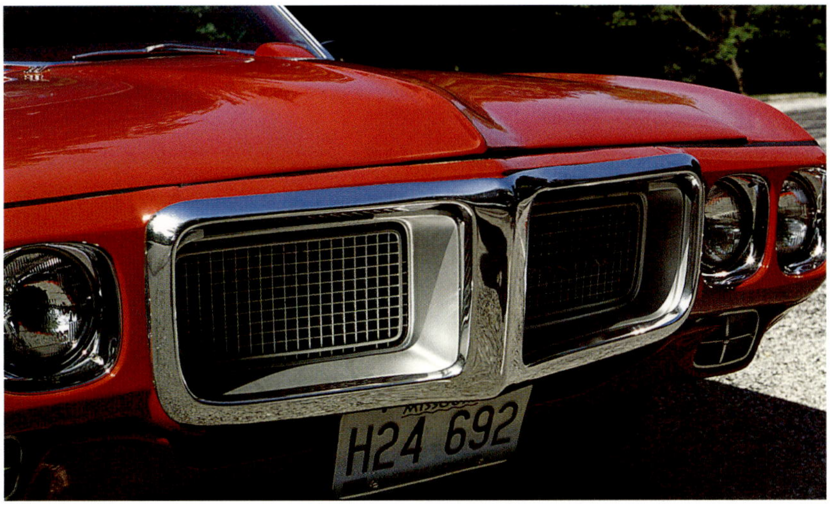

This view of the grille, Endura front fascia, and headlights of a Matador Red 1969 Firebird convertible equipped with the optional 350 HO V-8 engine shows the square mesh of the 1969 Firebird grille and the silver grille surround.

Firebird Production

Model	Production
1967	
Firebird sport coupe	67,032
Firebird convertible	15,528
1968	
Firebird sport coupe	90,152
Firebird convertible	16,960
1969	
Firebird sport coupe	75,362
Firebird convertible	11,649
Trans Am sport coupe	689
Trans Am convertible	8

The 1968 Firebird and Sprint used the standard grille, and the Firebird 400 used its own design with a bright horizontal center bar, both with bright surrounds. Both the Sprint and Firebird also used a script Pontiac name badge on the upper left. The Firebird 400 had an arrowhead badge in the center of the grille. The 1968 lower valance had wide rectangular openings, but they were narrower than the 1967. The rectangular parking lights were now mounted outside of the openings to the outer end of the panel, wrapping slightly around the ends to serve as side markers.

The entire front end of the Firebird was redesigned for 1969. The body color front fascia was formed from energy-absorbing Endura plastic. The twin chrome grilles were mounted in a rectangular peaked chrome bumper with a Pontiac arrowhead badge in its center for the 400 and Trans Am. The arrowhead badge was deleted in the base Firebird grille. The standard Firebirds had a rectangular crate-pattern silver-color grille design with a bright-plated surround and a block-letter Pontiac nameplate in the left section. The 1969 Trans Am grille was a black crate design with Pontiac nameplate and did not have the bright border. The lower valance had air intakes under each of the grille sections and rectangular parking lights in sculptured nacelles at each end.

Interior

The 1967 Firebird was available with a variety of interior trim combinations, all with standard front bucket seats and a bench-type rear seat. A bench front seat with fold-down center armrest (UPC AL4) was available as an extra-cost option in the sport coupe only. All interior trim schemes

Body Colors

1967 Firebird Body Colors
(Two letters indicate lower body and upper body or roof color)

Code	Color
A	Starlight Black
C	Cameo Ivory
D	Montreux Blue
E	Fathom Blue
F	Tyrol Blue
G	Signet Gold
H	Linden Green
K	Gulf Turquoise
L	Mariner Turquoise
M	Plum Mist
N	Burgundy
P	Silver Glaze
R	Regimental Red
S	Champagne
T	Montego Cream

1968 Firebird Body Colors
(Two letters indicate lower body and upper body or roof color)

Code	Color
A	Starlight Black
C	Cameo Ivory
D	Alpine Blue
E	Aegean Blue
F	Nordic Blue
G	April Gold
I	Autumn Bronze
K	Meridian Turquoise
L	Aleutian Blue
N	Flambeau Burgundy
P	Springmist Green
Q	Verdoro Green
R	Solar Red
T	Primavera Beige
V	Nightshade Green
Y	Mayfair Maize

1969 Firebird Body Colors
(Two pairs of numbers indicate lower body and upper body or roof color)

Code	Color
10	Starlight Black
40	Mayfair Maize
50	Cameo Ivory
51	Liberty Blue
52	Matador Red
53	Warwick Blue
55	Crystal Turquoise
57	Midnight Green
59	Limelight Green
61	Expresso Brown
63	Champagne
65	Antique Gold
67	Burgundy
69	Palladium Silver
72	Carousel Red
73	Verdoro Green
76	Goldenrod Yellow
87	Windward Blue

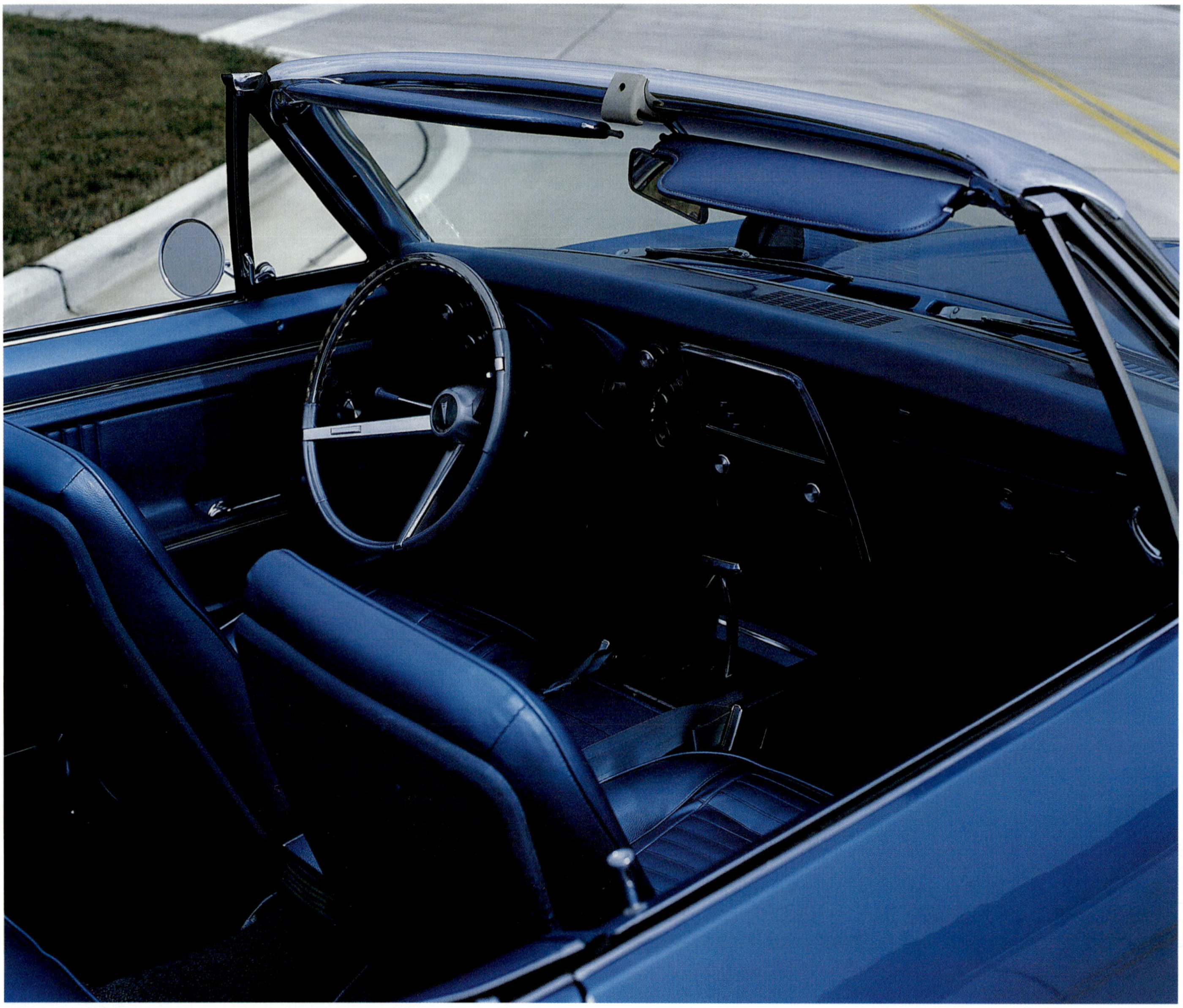

This Tyrol Blue 1967 Firebird convertible has an optional blue custom-vinyl interior (255) with Strato bucket seats, optional color-keyed console with T-handle shifter for the automatic transmission, and a color-keyed deluxe steering wheel with horn buttons on the aluminum spokes.

Interior Trim

1967 Code	Color	1968 Code	Color	1969s Code	Color
255	Medium Bright Blue (custom)	250	Dark Teal	200	Dark Blue
265	Medium Bright Blue (custom, bench seat)	255	Dark Teal (custom)	210	Dark Blue (custom)
256	Dark Turquoise (custom)	251	Medium Gold	202	Medium Gold
251	Medium Gold	257	Medium Gold (custom)	212	Medium Gold (custom)
257	Medium Gold (custom)	252	Medium Red	293	Medium Gold (custom)
271	Medium Gold (bench seat)	258	Medium Red (custom)	214	Medium red (custom)
267	Medium Gold (custom, bench seat)	253	Black	206	Medium Green
253	Black	272	Black (bench seat)	216	Medium Green (custom)
259	Black (custom)	259	Black (custom)	207	Parchment
272	Black (bench seat)	269	Black (custom, bench seat)	217	Parchment (custom)
269	Black (custom, bench seat)	261	Dark Turquoise	227	Parchment (custom, bench seat)
254	Parchment	256	Dark Turquoise (custom)	208	Black
260	Parchment (custom)	262	Parchment	218	Black (custom)
250	Dark Blue	273	Parchment (bench seat)	228	Black (custom, bench seat)
270	Dark Blue (bench seat)	260	Parchment (custom)		
252	Medium Red	275	Parchment (custom, bench seat)		
258	Medium red (custom)				

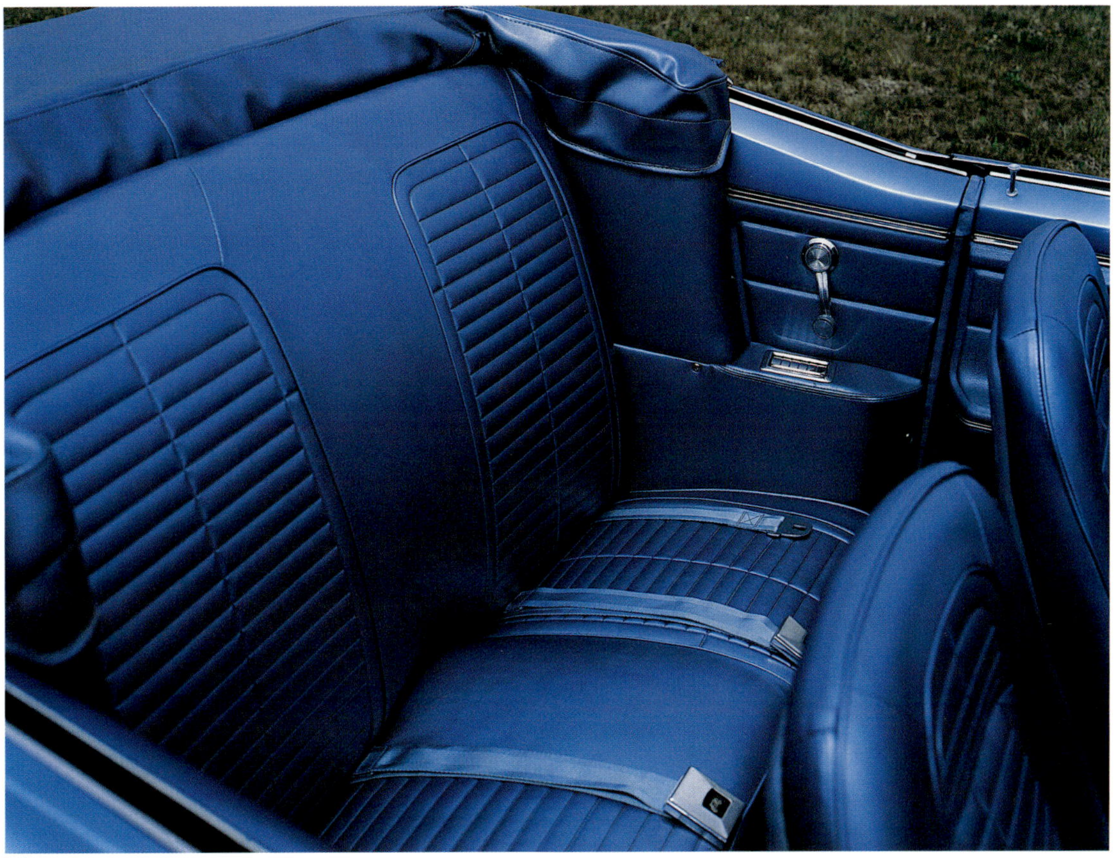

The rear seat trim of this Tyrol Blue 1967 Firebird convertible is the optional blue custom vinyl interior trim. The standard vinyl convertible top boot usually matches the interior trim.

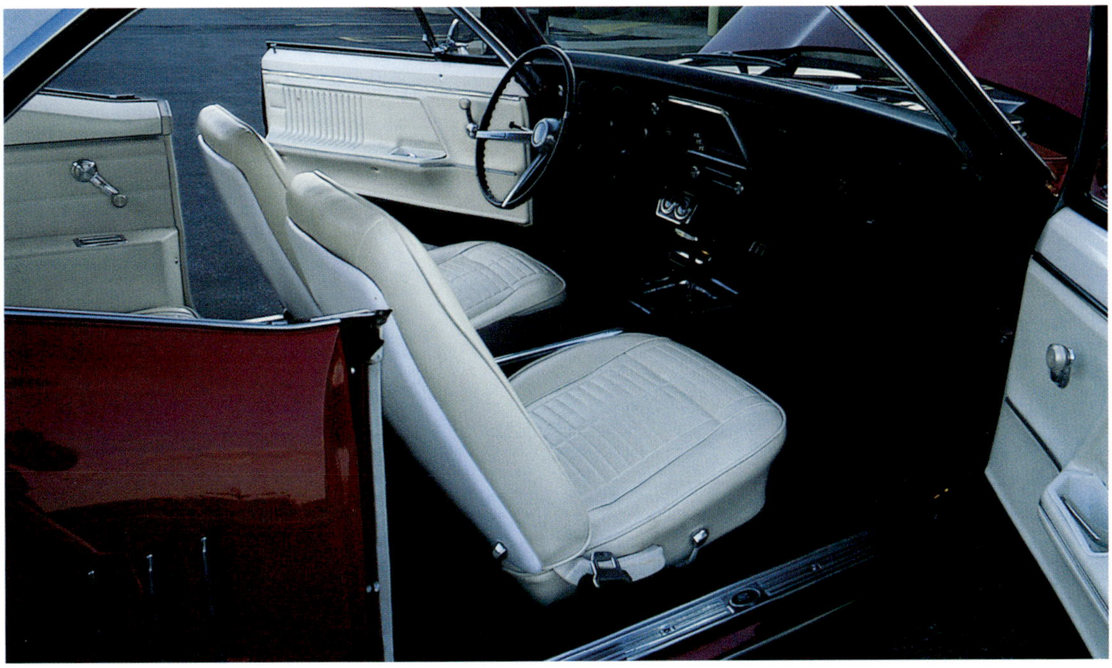

This view shows the custom parchment (260-Z) vinyl interior trim on a red 1967 Firebird coupe with an optional tilt steering wheel (UPC N33) and center floor console with T-handle shifter for the optional automatic transmission. The black carpet is standard with the parchment interior.

were of expanded Morrokide vinyl with narrow transverse Madrid-grain pleats in the seat inserts and smooth bolsters and skirts. The raised center section and folding armrest of the optional bench seat was smooth vinyl. An optional carpeted fold-down rear seat (UPC A67) was available in all models. An optional color-coordinated console with covered compartment was available with the bucket seat interior choices.

The standard bucket seats were available in blue (270), gold (271), and black (272). The optional bench seat interiors were available in blue (250), gold (251), red (252), black (253), and parchment (254). The optional custom bench seat interior schemes were available in blue (265), gold (267), and black (269) in the sport coupe only. The sport coupe and convertible with the custom bucket seat interior were available in blue (255), turquoise (256), gold (257), red (258), black (259), and parchment (260). The door panels for all combinations used a vertically pleated center insert, a smooth upper bolster, and a painted steel horizontal panel at the top. The 1967 deluxe interiors had a molded arm rest extending the length of the door panel.

The 1968 Firebird interior was also available in all-vinyl with transverse Madrid-grain pleats like 1967, but a longitudinal embossed center seam set it apart from the previous design. The custom vinyl interiors had distinctive longitudinal wide pleats with a custom weave design. Front bucket seats were again standard, with an all-vinyl bench seat with fold-down armrest optional. A carpeted folding rear seat was also optional for 1968. A color-coordinated vinyl center console with burled wood-grain top insert was optional with the bucket seat interiors. The vinyl door panel trim extended to the top of the door for 1968.

The standard interior schemes were available in plain vinyl colors of teal (250), gold (251), red (252), black (253), turquoise (261), and parchment (262) with knit-weave vinyl an option available in black (269) and parchment (275) only. The optional custom vinyl interiors were available in dual-pattern designs of knit-weave and

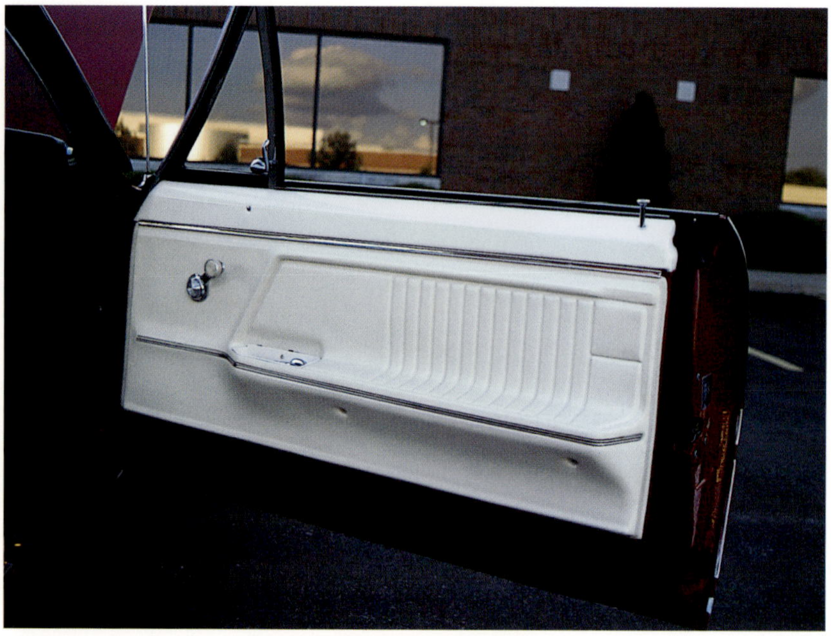

Above: This is the right interior door panel on a Regimental Red 1967 Firebird coupe with optional parchment custom vinyl interior. The painted upper door panel matches the interior trim color. ***Below:*** Detail view of the black vinyl (253) interior with Strato bucket seats in a Solar Red 1968 Firebird Sprint coupe. This Firebird has a deluxe steering wheel with horn buttons on the spokes and a Firebird medallion in its center. The under-dash air-conditioning unit is an aftermarket addition.

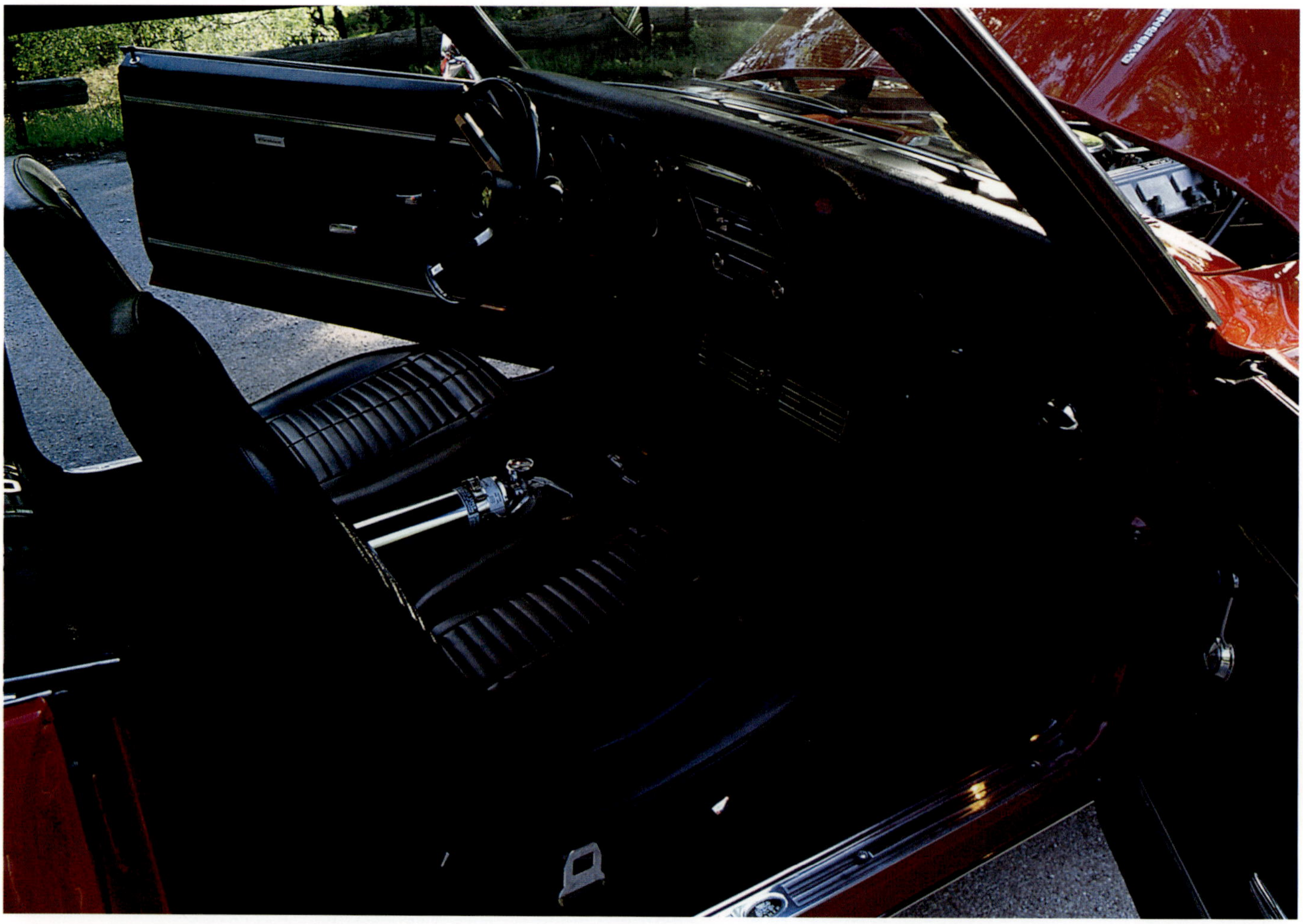

This is a parchment vinyl interior (207) with optional Strato bucket seats in a Carousel Red 1969 Firebird convertible. The black carpet and instrument panel are standard with the parchment interior trim.

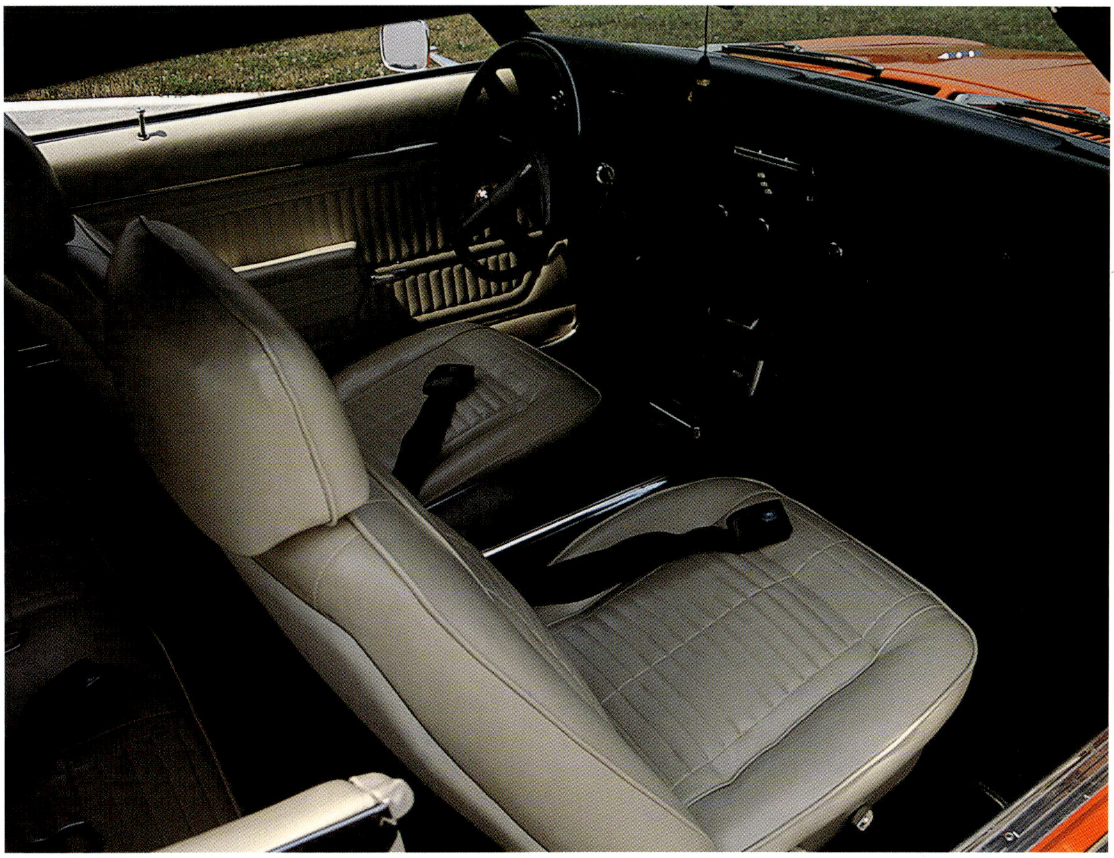

This is a view of a red custom-knit vinyl-weave interior trim (214) in a Matador Red 1969 Firebird convertible. Note the burled wood-grain console insert and instrument panel background. This Firebird is equipped with optional power windows and air conditioning.

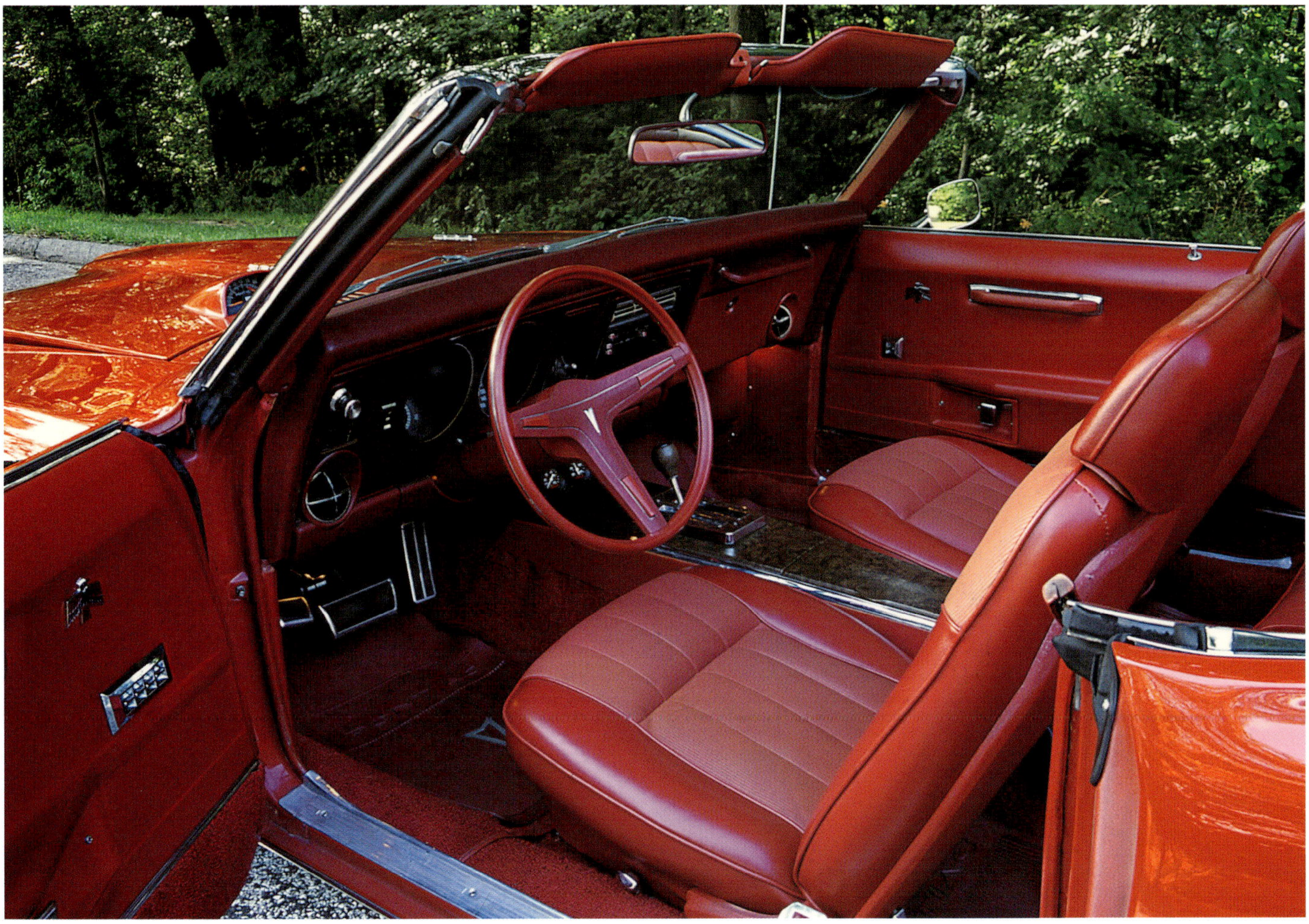

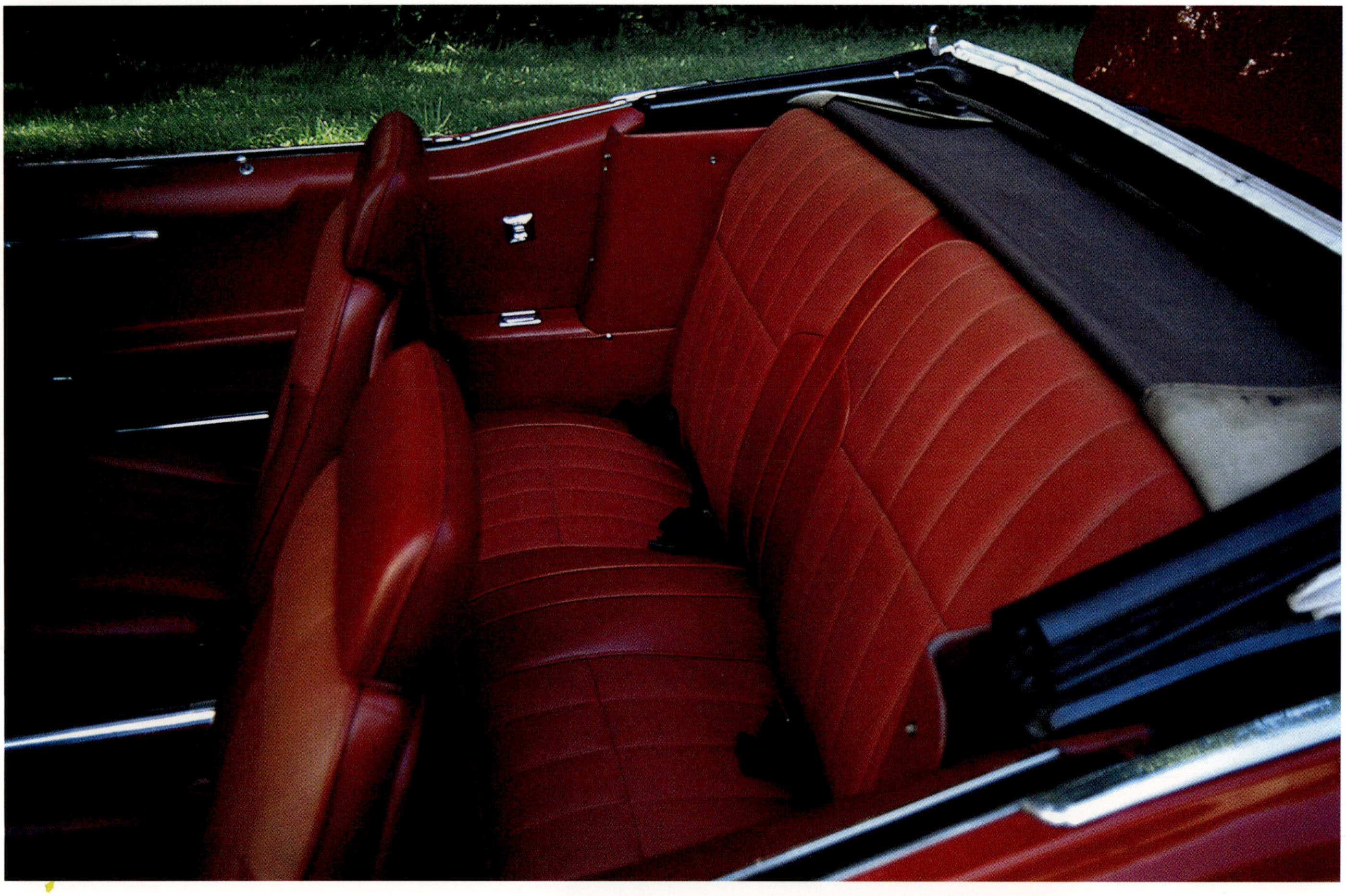

smooth teal (255), turquoise (256), black (259, 272), parchment (260, 273), gold (257), red (258), and saddle (281). The 1968 door panels were smoother than the 1967, as the vertical pleats in the inset were eliminated. The bucket seat backs for the 1967 and 1968 custom interiors were more rounded than those of the standard seats.

The 1969 Firebird interior was available in all-vinyl with transverse Madrid-grain pleats with a longitudinal center seam in the inserts like the 1968 seats. Front bucket seats were standard, with an all-vinyl bench seat with fold-down armrest optional. Like the previous year, a folding, carpeted rear seat was also optional. A color-coordinated center console with burled wood-grain insert and padded door was available with the bucket seat interiors. Front seat headrests were optional at the beginning of the 1969 model year but were made standard by midyear.

The standard interior trim of the 1969 Firebird was available in plain vinyl colors of blue (200), gold (202), green (206), parchment (207), and black (208). The knit-weave and smooth vinyl combination was available in parchment (227) and black (228). The custom vinyl was available in gold (283), and the custom knit-weave vinyl and smooth combination was offered in blue (210), gold (212), red (214), green (216), parchment (217), and black (218).

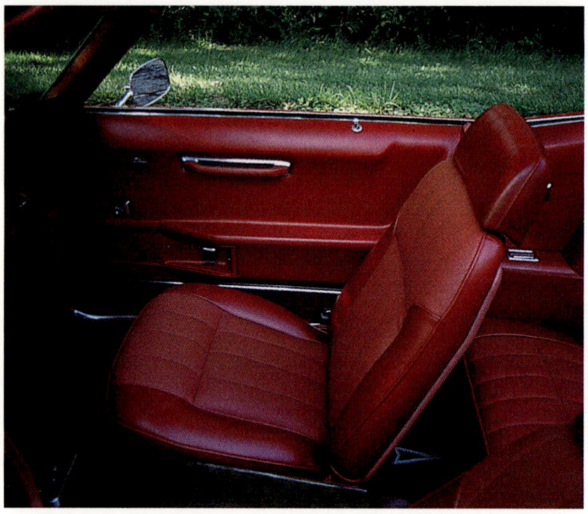

The 1967 and 1968 Firebird instrument panels and clusters were much the same as those used in the Camaros of the same years. There were two large round bezels in the instrument cluster that held the black-faced speedometer, odometer, oil pressure light, and left turn indicator on the left and the fuel gauge, temperature indicator light, and right turn signal indicator on the right.

To the left of the instrument cluster were two round switches: the windshield wiper switch was at the top and the headlight controls at the bottom. To the right of the cluster were two more switches controlling the cigarette lighter at the top

Above: This is a view of the rear seat compartment in a Matador Red 1969 Firebird convertible with the red custom vinyl-weave interior. Note the black carpet and the switches for the optional power windows. The standard top boot is not in place in this photo.
Left: The right front bucket seat of this red 1969 Firebird convertible with optional red vinyl interior trim has woven-pattern vinyl in the center insert of the seat. This Firebird has optional power windows.

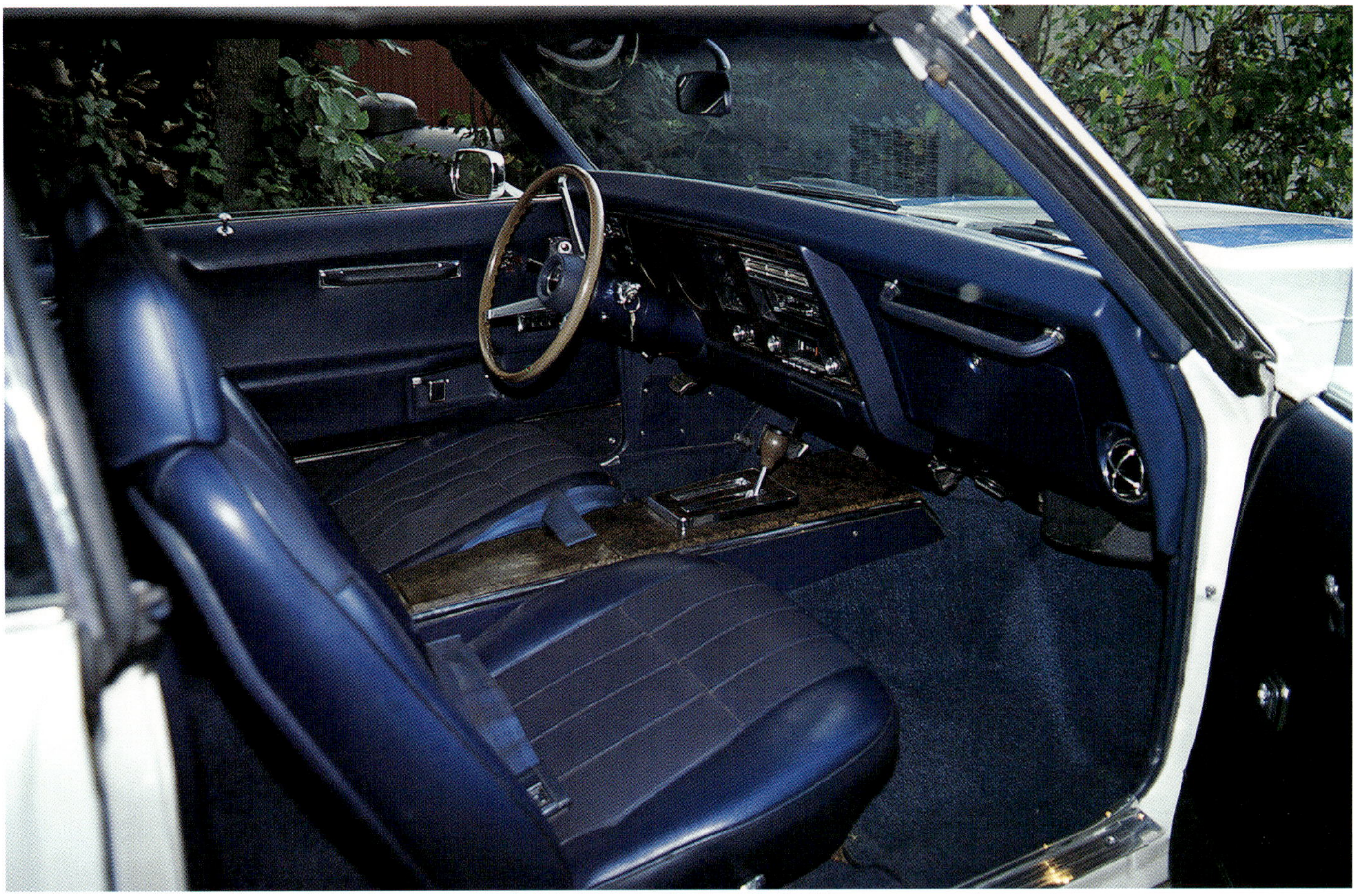

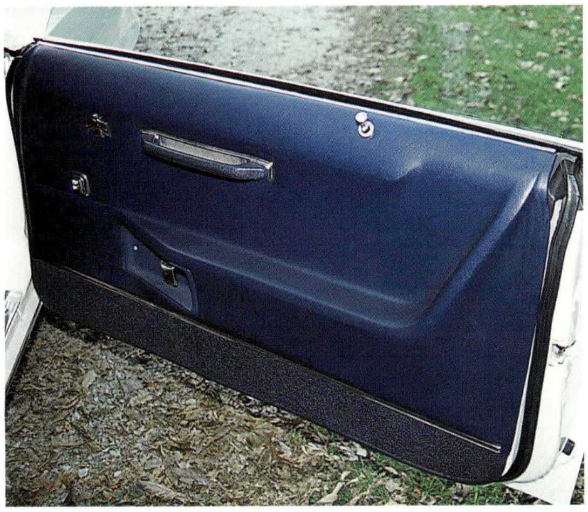

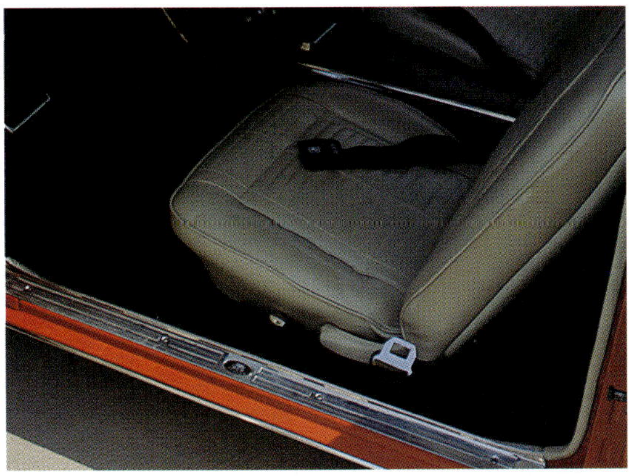

Above: This is the blue custom-knit vinyl-weave interior (210) in a 1969 Trans Am convertible replica with blue carpet, optional floor console, and instrument panel. The steering wheel is a custom sports wheel (UPC N34) with wood-grain rim. ***Right:*** Detail view of the right door panel on a Cameo Ivory 1969 Trans Am convertible replica equipped with the blue custom-knit vinyl-weave interior trim. Note the switches for the optional power windows (UPC A31). ***Right:*** Detail view of the left door opening of a Carousel Red 1969 Firebird convertible with optional parchment vinyl interior and a Fisher Body badge on the door sill molding.

and the ignition switch at the bottom. An optional instrument package (UPC U17) was available at extra cost that included an additional panel with three smaller stacked gauges in the clock panel. An unusual option was the hood-mounted tachometer (UPC U16) that placed the tachometer in a scoop-like bezel on the hood in front of the driver.

The heater and optional air-conditioning controls were mounted in a separate panel at the center of the instrument panel to the right of the cluster. This center panel had a vinyl-simulated straight horizontal-grain wood background and also housed the radio below the heater controls. The radio could have been either the push-button AM radio with front antenna (UPC U63) or a push-button AM-FM with front antenna (UPC U69). An optional stereo tape player (UPC U57) could be mounted in the front of the console under the instrument panel. A manual rear antenna (UPC U73) and rear Sepra-Phonic speaker were also available. A pull-out ashtray was also located in this center panel below the radio.

In addition to the standard three-spoke Firebird steering wheel, a three-spoke deluxe steering wheel (UPC N30) and three-spoke wood-grain-rim custom sport steering wheel (UPC N34) were available in 1967 and 1968. The standard steering wheel in 1967 and 1968 was available in black (w/trim 253, 254, 272), blue (w/trim 250, 270),

Selected 1967–1969 Regular Production Options

UPC	Description
AL4	Strato bench seat with fold-down center armrest (coupe only)
AS1	Front seat shoulder strap (with standard seat belts)
AS2	Head rest
A01	Tinted glass, Soft-Ray (all)
A02	Tinted windshield, Soft-Ray
A31	Power windows
A46	Power bucket seat, LH
A67	Fold-down rear seatback
A90	Remote deck lid release
B32	Front floor mats
B33	Rear floor mats
B42	Fitted trunk mat
B93	Door edge guards
C06	Power convertible top
C08	Cordova roof
C50	Rear window defogger
C57	Power flow ventilation
C60	Air conditioning, custom
D33	Remote-control outside mirror
D34	Visor vanity mirror (RH)
D55	Front console
D98	Rally stripes
D99	Two-tone paint
G80	Safe-T-Track differential
G90	Performance axle
G92	Special rear axle ratio
JL1	Bright pedal trim
J50	Power brakes
J52	Disc front brakes
K08	Heavy-duty engine fan
K30	Cruise control
K45	Heavy-duty air cleaner
K82	55-amp alternator
L30	326 2-bbl V-8 engine
L67	Ram Air IV 400 engine
L72	230 Sprint six engine
L74	Ram Air 400 engine
L76	326 4-bbl V-8 engine (HO)
M12	Three-speed manual transmission with floor shift
M20	Four-speed manual transmission with floor shift
M21	Four-speed manual close-ratio transmission with floor shift
M30	Two-speed automatic transmission, air-cooled
M31	Two-speed automatic transmission, water-cooled
M38	Three-speed automatic transmission
M40	Three-speed automatic transmission
N10	Dual exhaust system
N25	Exhaust pipe extensions
N30	Deluxe steering wheel
N33	Tilt steering wheel
N34	Custom sport steering wheel
N40	Power steering
N41	Variable-ratio power steering
N64	Conventional spare tire and wheel
N95	Wire wheel discs
N98	Rally II wheels
PX2	E70x14 Wide Oval white-line tires
PX3	E70x14 Wide Oval redline tires
P01	Deluxe wheel discs
P02	Custom wheel discs
P17	Spare wheel cover
T60	Heavy-duty battery
U05	Dual horns
U16	Hood-mounted tachometer
U17	Instrument package
U35	Floor-mounted electric clock
U57	Stereo tape player
U63	Push-button radio
U69	AM/FM radio
U73	Rear manual antenna
V01	Heavy-duty radiator
W53	Sprint engine option
W54	Custom trim
W63	Instrument panel gauge cluster
W66	400 sports engine option
Y96	Firm ride and handling package

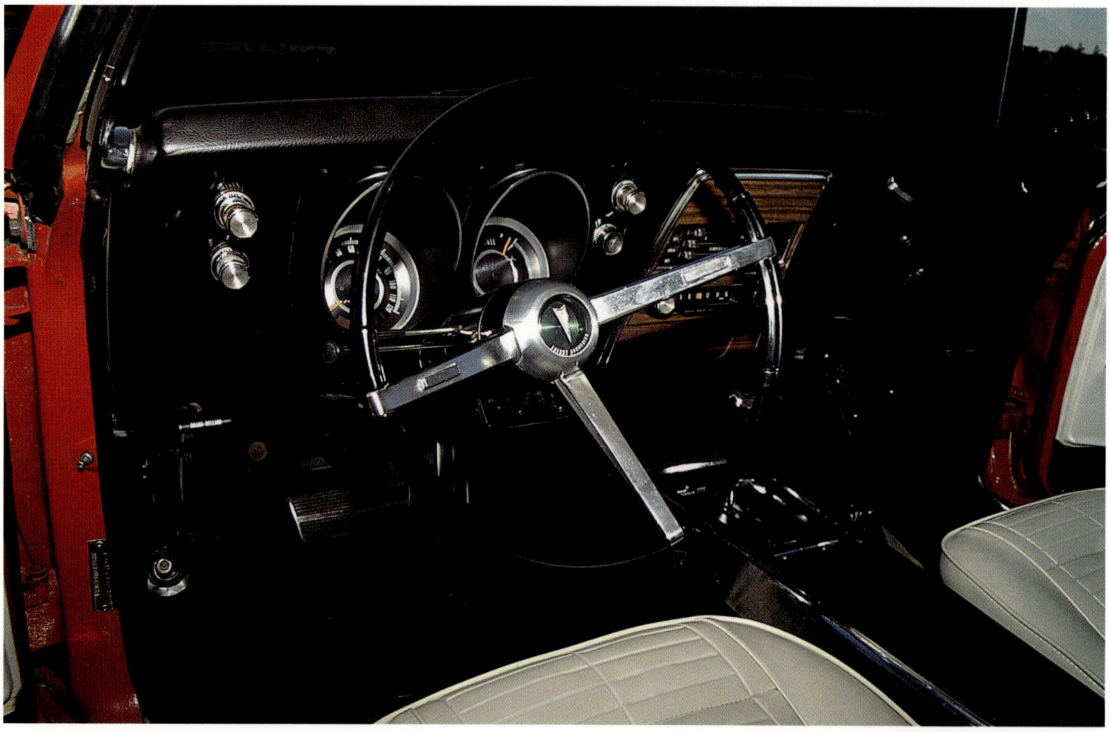

Detail view of the instrument panel and cluster in a Regimental Red 1967 Firebird coupe. Note the optional parchment bucket seat interior and straight horizontal wood-grain finish on the instrument panel center. This Firebird has the optional tilt steering wheel.

gold (w/trim 251, 271), and red (w/trim 252) and had a bright center horn button with an arrowhead badge. The standard and deluxe steering wheels for 1967 were made in two versions. The first type wheel had a diameter of 16½ inches and a 6⅜-inch dish. The second type steering wheel had a diameter of 16 inches and a 5-inch dish.

The 1967 and 1968 deluxe steering wheels had the horn buttons in the spokes and were available in black, blue, gold, and turquoise, depending upon the interior trim scheme. A tilt steering wheel option was also available (except with column-shift manual transmission) with UPC N33. In 1969, the ignition switch was moved to the steering column and locked the wheel when the key was turned off. The steering column also employed a new collapsing mechanism using two sliding tubes rather than the previous cable mesh.

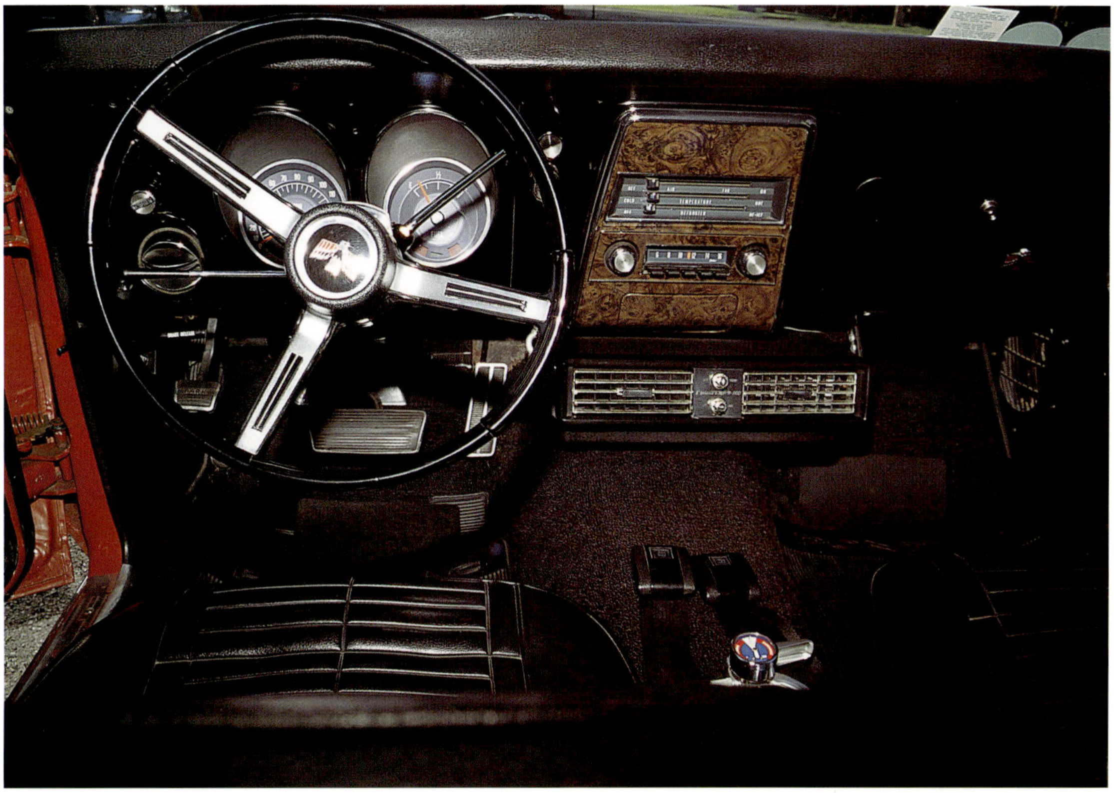

Detail view of the instrument cluster in a Solar Red 1968 Firebird Sprint. The burled woodgrain finish on the center panel was used in 1968 and 1969. This Firebird has a black vinyl interior with Strato bucket seats, but it was ordered without the optional floor console.

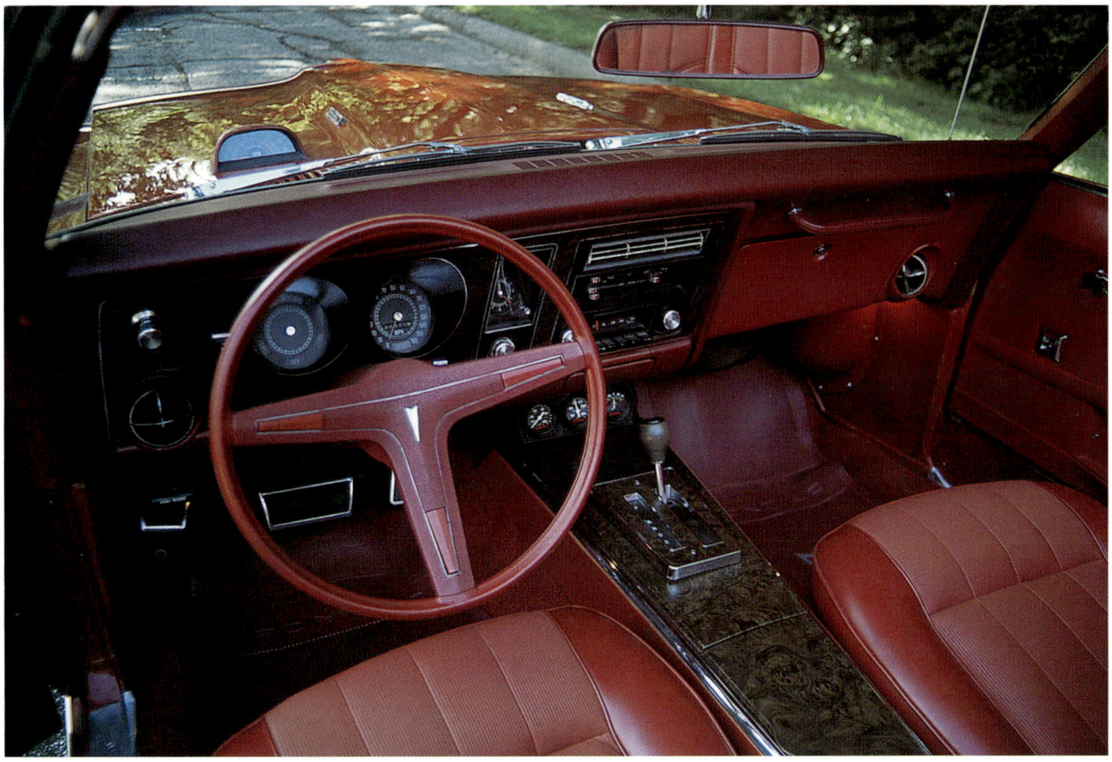

This 1969 Firebird convertible was ordered in red custom vinyl-weave with Strato bucket seats and an optional center console with floor shift. The optional hood-mounted tachometer (UPC UB5) is visible through the windshield.

The instrument panel and cluster were totally redesigned for 1969. The round instrument bezels were further recessed into the tilted flat cluster face. The general layout was very much the same as 1967 and1968, but the gauge layout was swapped side for side. A new burled wood-grain pattern was used for the center panel. In addition to the custom sport steering wheel (part number 9795885), the 1969 Firebird was available with a standard two-spoke wheel in black, blue, gold, and green and a deluxe three-spoke wheel in black, blue, gold, green, and red to match the interior trim. Both the standard and deluxe steering wheels had horn buttons in the spokes. The 1969 Trans Am had a standard 14-inch-diameter thick-rimmed Formula steering wheel (part number

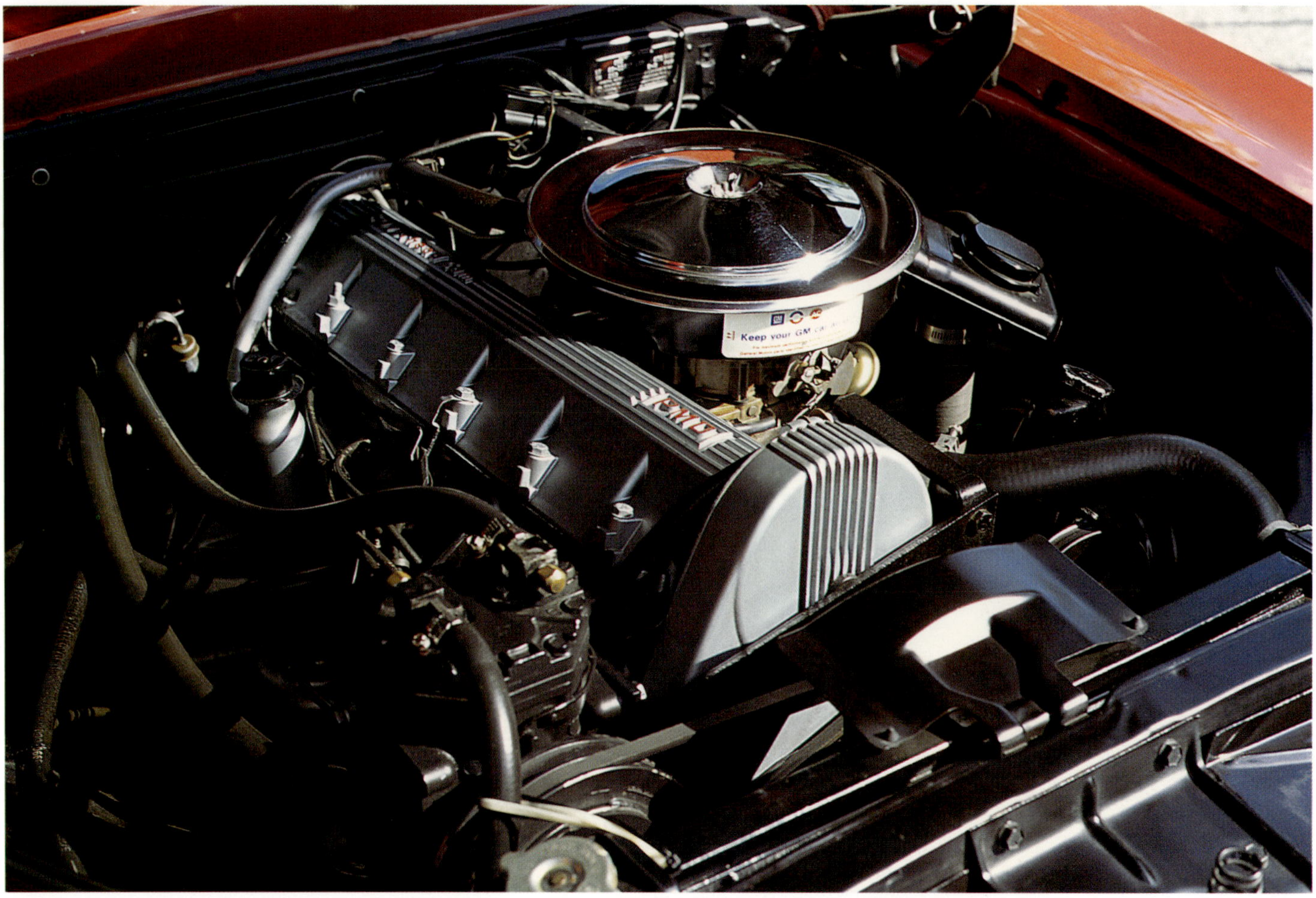

546296) with three flat aluminum spokes, each with two unequal-size holes. The 1969 Formula steering wheel had a unique center horn button.

Engine and Engine Compartment

The 1967 Firebird was available with five engine choices. The standard powerplant was the 230-cubic-inch overhead-cam inline six-cylinder. The optional Sprint version of the 230 six had higher compression with a significant increase in horsepower and torque. The base V-8 was the 326, which was also available in the high output (HO) version. The highest performance engine choice for 1967 was the 400-cubic-inch V-8, which was available in either base or Ram Air versions.

For 1968, engine choices were increased to seven at model year introduction with displacement increases in the six-cylinder and smaller V-8. The Pontiac OHC inline six was increased to 250-ci and was still offered in a standard and Sprint version. The small V-8 was increased from 326- to 350-ci, still in two versions, and the 400 V-8 was now available in three versions: a standard, HO, and Ram Air. Later in the model year, the Ram Air was upgraded to Ram Air II configuration with still higher output.

The 1969 Firebird was also available with seven engine choices. The base OHC inline six was still 250-ci and was still offered in standard and Sprint configurations. The base V-8 was 350-ci and available in standard and HO versions. The 400-ci V-8 was available as a base 330-horsepower version with the 335-horsepower 400 Ram Air III and the 345-horsepower 400 Ram Air IV as options.

OHC Inline Six

The Pontiac overhead-camshaft inline six-cylinder engine was first introduced in the 1966 Tempest. The camshaft was operated by a unique Gilmer-type belt drive mounted under a large front cover. The basic design of the OHC six was developed by Pontiac chief engineer John Z. DeLorean and was based on the 230-cubic-inch overhead-valve Chevrolet six. The engine's intake and exhaust manifolds were both mounted on the left side of the engine like the Chevrolet. The camshaft cover was finned cast-aluminum.

The 1967 Firebird six had 230-cubic-inches displacement in a cast-iron block with a bore and stroke of 3.87 inches x 3.25 inches. The compression ratio was 7.6:1, producing 155 horsepower at 4,700 rpm in the early version (engine codes ZF with manual transmission and ZG with the automatic) and increased to 9:1 and 165

The engine compartment of a 1968 Firebird Sprint with the 4.1-liter (250-cubic-inch) overhead-camshaft six-cylinder engine (UPC L53). The Sprint six was equipped with a four-barrel carburetor and developed 215 horsepower.

horsepower at 4,700 rpm (engine codes ZK/ZS with manual transmission and ZM/ZN with automatic transmission) later in the model year. The standard six developed 216 foot-pounds of torque at 2,600 rpm. The base six had a single-barrel Rochester carburetor and hydraulic valve lifters.

The Sprint version (UPC W53) of the overhead-camshaft six-cylinder was similar to the standard engine, but it had a compression ratio of 10.5:1 and developed 215 horsepower at 5,200 rpm and 240 foot-pounds of torque at 3,800 rpm. The Sprint engine also had a high-performance camshaft, larger valves, and a tuned exhaust system with a split manifold configuration. The engine codes were ZD/ZR with a manual transmission and ZE/ZL with an automatic transmission. The Sprint six had hydraulic valve lifters but used a Rochester Quadrajet four-barrel carburetor. Both six-cylinder engines were painted Pontiac Engine Blue, including the front and camshaft covers.

The 1968 and 1969 overhead-camshaft six-cylinder engine had a longer 3.531-inch stroke and the same 3.87-inch bore of the previous year, increasing the displacement to 250 cubic inches. The compression ratio of the base six was still 9:1, and the engine developed 175 horsepower at 4,800 rpm and 240 foot-pounds of torque at 3,800 rpm with a Rochester model 7028065 single-barrel carburetor. The engine codes were ZK when equipped with a manual transmission and ZN with the automatic.

The 1968 and 1969 250-cubic-inch Sprint six (UPC L53) had a 10.5:1 compression ratio and developed 215 horsepower at 4,800 rpm (5,200 rpm in 1969) and 255 foot-pounds of torque at 3,800 rpm with a Rochester Quadrajet four-barrel carburetor. The 1969 Sprint engine with manual transmission had a redesigned "H" camshaft and developed 230 horsepower at 5,400 rpm and 260 foot-pounds of torque at 3,600 rpm. Sprint engine codes were ZD with the manual transmissions and ZE with the automatic. Both six-cylinder engines continued with hydraulic valve lifters.

Overhead-Valve V-8

The overhead-valve V-8 used in the Firebird was based on the original Pontiac 287-ci Strato-Streak V-8 first used in 1955. The Pontiac offered a number of improvements over the Chevrolet V-8 of the same year. Although the Pontiac was about 75 pounds heavier than the Chevrolet, it had machined combustion chambers for more consistent volume and used a standard oil pan windage tray to prevent crankshaft drag. The Pontiac V-8 engine also used stamped rocker arms similar to the Chevrolet V-8. The Pontiac V-8 differed from the Chevrolet in that it had a dual-pattern camshaft with different duration for the intake and exhaust valves.

The standard V-8 used in the 1967 Firebird was 326 cubic inches (UPC L30). The bore and stroke were 3.72 inches x 3.75 inches with a compression ratio of 9.2:1. The main bearings were 3 inches in diameter. The 326 had a single Rochester two-barrel carburetor and developed 250 horsepower at 4,600 rpm and 333 foot-pounds of torque at 3,300 rpm. The L30 V-8 had engine codes of WC/WH with manual

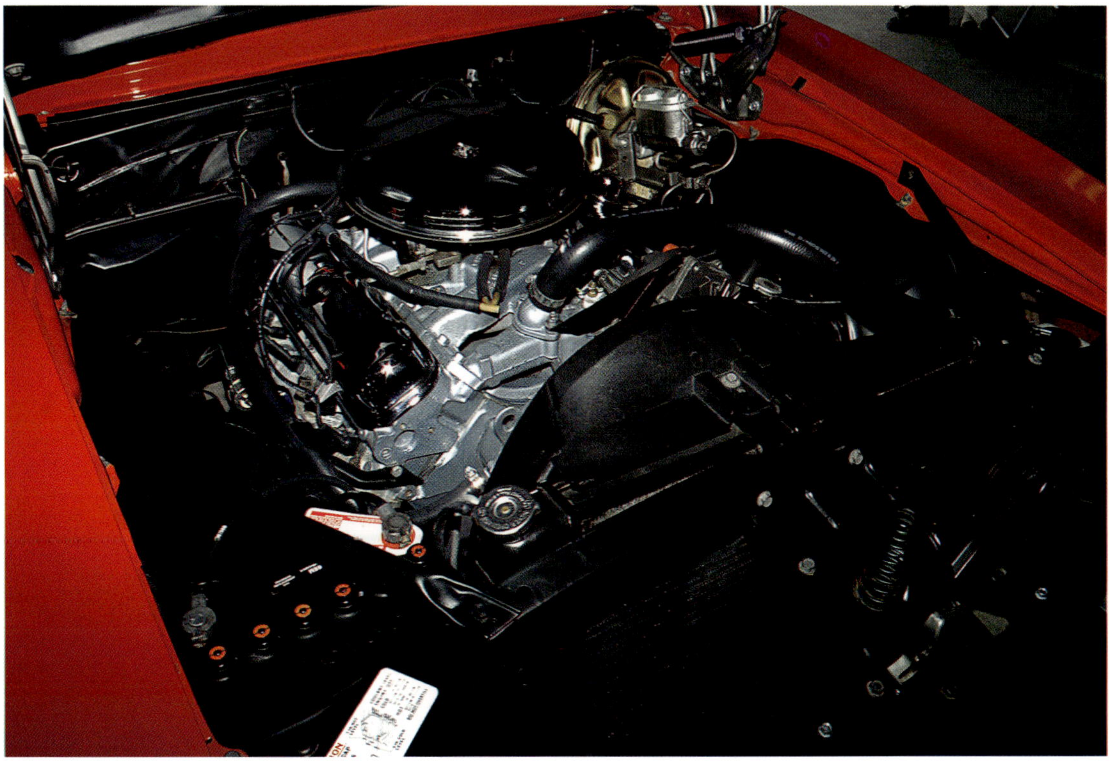

This is the engine compartment of a red 1967 Firebird coupe equipped with the optional 326-cubic-inch HO V-8 engine. This 326 V-8 has a Carter aluminum four-barrel (AFB) carburetor. The Firebird is equipped with optional power brakes (UPC J50).

transmission and XI/XJ with the automatic transmission.

The 326 V-8 was also available as a high-output version (UPC L76). The 326 HO had the same dimensions as the standard engine, but the compression ratio was increased to 10.5:1. The 326 HO used a Rochester four-barrel carburetor and developed 285 horsepower at 5,000 rpm and 359 foot-pounds of torque at 3,200 rpm. The 326 HO had engine codes of WK/WO with a manual transmission and XO/YM with the automatic. Both 326 V-8 engines used hydraulic valve lifters, and both were painted Pontiac Engine Blue.

The base V-8 engine for 1968 and 1969 (UPC L30) was increased in displacement to 350 cubic inches by increasing the bore to 3.875 inches. The compression ratio remained at 9.2:1 with horsepower at 265 at 4,600 rpm and 355 foot-pounds of torque at 2,800 rpm with a Rochester model 7028071 two-barrel carburetor. Engines codes were YJ with the automatic transmission and WC with the manual transmission.

The high-output version of the 350 V-8 (UPC L76) for 1968 and 1969 had a 10.5:1 compression ratio and developed 320 (325 in 1969) horsepower at 5,100 rpm and 380 foot-pounds of torque at 3,200 rpm. The 350 HO had a Rochester four-barrel carburetor. The engine codes were WK with the manual transmission and YM with the automatic.

The larger optional V-8 in the 1967 Firebird was the 400-ci, available in two versions. Both were based on a block with a 4.125-inch bore and a 3.75-inch stroke. The base 400 (UPC W66) had a compression ratio of 10.75:1, hydraulic valve lifters, and a single Rochester Quadrajet four-barrel carburetor. The 400 developed 325 horsepower at 4,800 rpm and 410 foot-pounds of torque at 3,400 rpm for 1967. The engine codes were WI, WQ, WU, or WZ with the manual transmissions and XN or YT with an automatic transmission.

The 400-cubic-inch V-8 was also available in an optional Ram Air version (UPC L67) that developed 335 horsepower at 5,200 rpm and 410 foot-pounds of torque at 3,600 rpm. The 400 Ram Air was essentially identical to the standard 400 engine, but it was equipped with a higher performance hydraulic lifter camshaft, freer flowing exhaust manifolds, and a 750-cfm Rochester model 7037276 Quadrajet four-barrel carburetor fed through functional hood scoops. The actual horsepower output was intentionally limited by a carburetor linkage modification to keep from opening the throttle bores completely and exceeding the power levels of the GTO, according to corporate edicts. The Ram Air 400 was equipped with chrome-plated valve covers. All 1967 Pontiac V-8 engines were painted Pontiac Engine Blue.

For 1968 and 1969, the output of the base 400 V-8 was still 330 horsepower, but the torque was increased to 430 foot-pounds at 3,300 rpm. Engine codes were YW/YN with the automatic transmission and WZ with the manual transmission. The new-for-1968 400 HO (UPC L74) developed 335 horsepower at 5,300 rpm (5,000

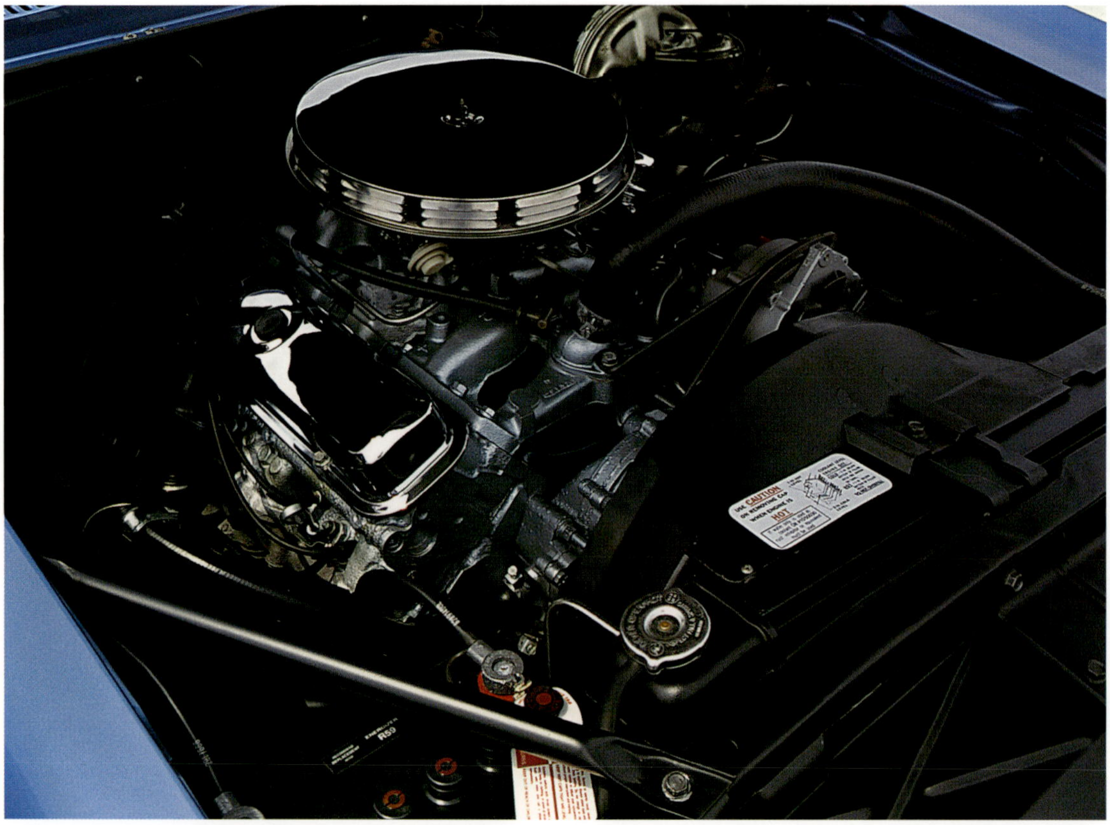

This Tyrol Blue 1967 Firebird convertible is equipped with an optional 400-cubic-inch V-8 engine (UPC W66). Note the correct Delco battery and battery cable clamps and the correct tower clamps on the radiator and heater hoses. The engine is painted Pontiac Engine Blue.

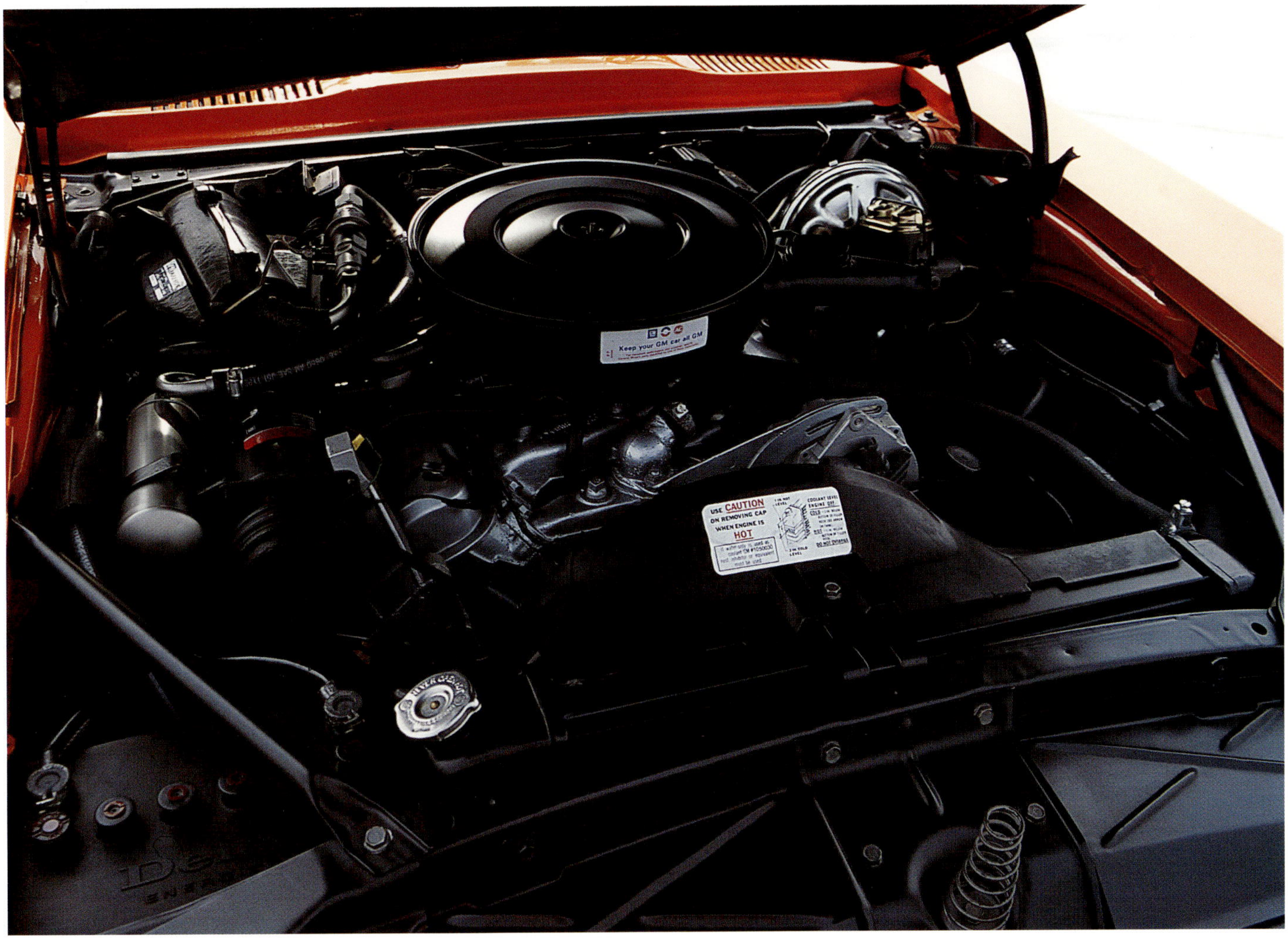

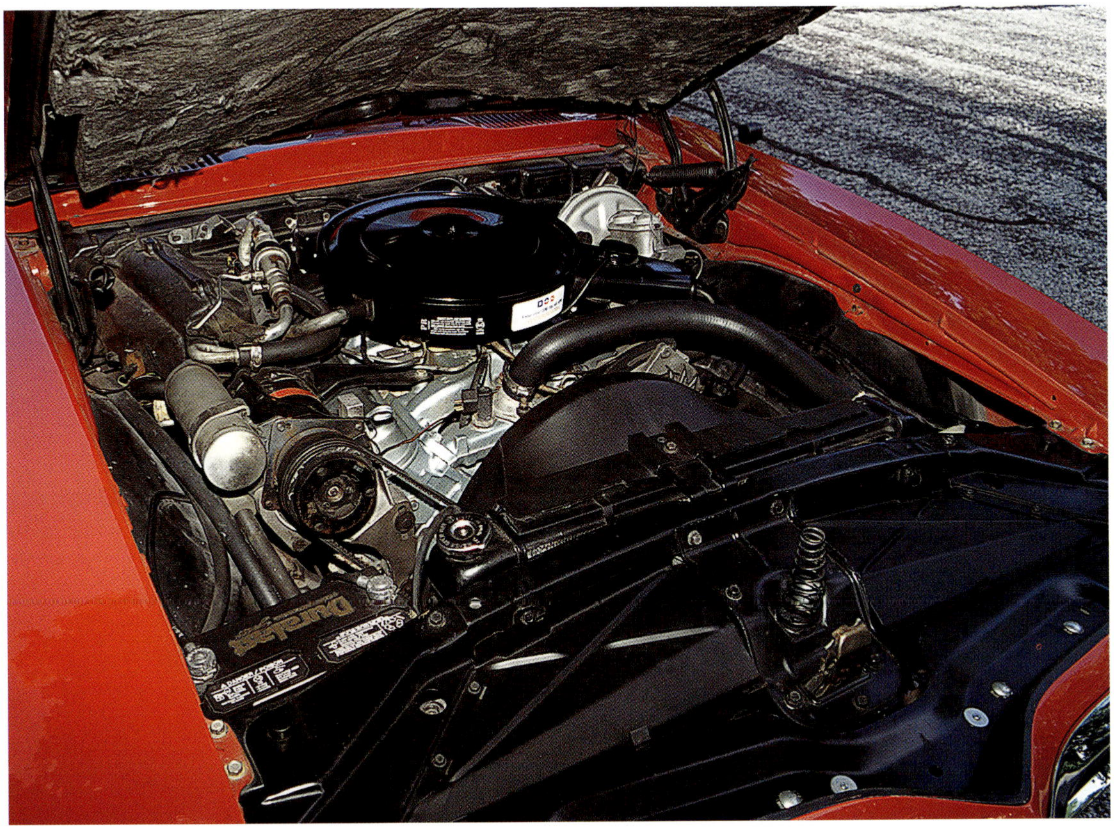

Above: A correctly restored engine compartment in a Carousel Red 1969 Firebird convertible equipped with the optional 350-cubic-inch V-8 engine (UPC L30) finished in Pontiac Engine Blue with a semigloss-black air cleaner assembly. This Firebird has optional power brakes and air conditioning. ***Right:*** The engine compartment of an original Matador Red 1969 Firebird convertible equipped with the optional 350 HO V-8 engine with four-barrel carburetor (UPC L76). This Firebird is equipped with optional power brakes (UPC J50) and air conditioning (UPC C60).

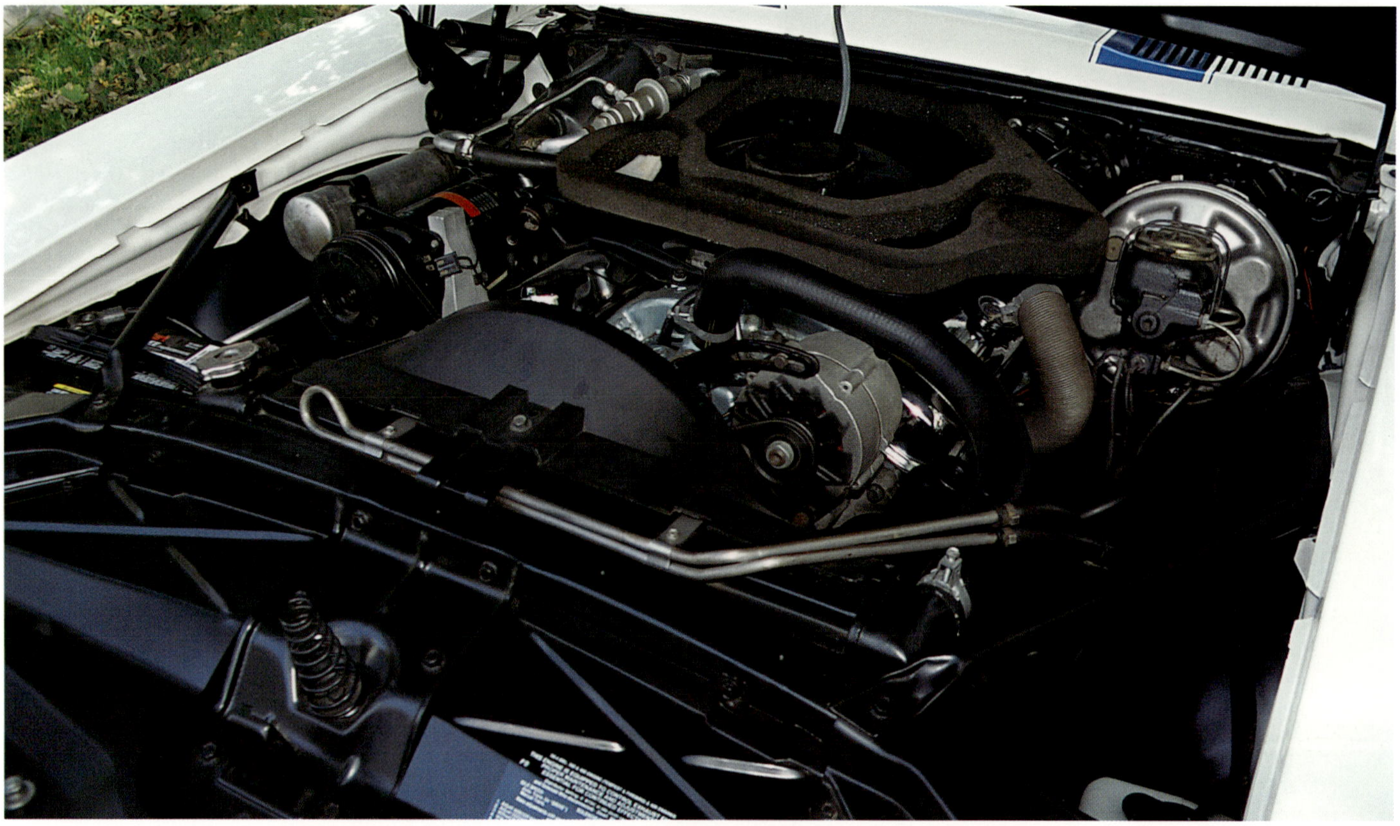

rpm for 1969) and 430 foot-pounds of torque at 3,400 rpm with a single four-barrel carburetor.

The Ram Air 400 (UPC L67) remained essentially unchanged for 1968 but had engine codes of XN for the automatic transmission version and WI for the manual transmission. The Ram Air 400 with the automatic transmission had a dual-pattern camshaft with 0.410/0.413-inch lift and 288/302 degrees duration. Later in the 1968 model year, the Ram Air was replaced by the Ram Air II, and the output was increased to 340 horsepower at 5,300 rpm and engine codes were changed to XT for the automatic and WU with a manual transmission. The 1968 Ram Air 400 used a 750-cfm Rochester 7028276 (automatic transmission) or 7028277 (manual transmission) Quadrajet four-barrel carburetor. There were 413 Ram Air 400 Firebirds ordered in 1968, 321 with a four-speed and 92 with an automatic transmission.

For 1969, the 400 Ram Air II option was available as an upgraded Ram Air IV (UPC L67) that developed 345 horsepower at 5,400 rpm and 430 foot-pounds of torque at 3,700 rpm. The Ram Air IV featured new round-port heads and a redesigned aluminum intake manifold. The Ram Air IV had a 750-cfm Rochester Quadrajet carburetor—a 7029270 was used with an automatic transmission, and a 7029273 was used with the manual transmission. The carburetor was sealed to the hood scoop opening with a hood inlet baffle and a large foam rubber seal. A baffle-to-hood seal with part number 9798061 was used for all but the Trans Am. The Trans Am used a seal with part number 546282. All 1968 and 1969 Firebird V-8 engines were painted Pontiac Engine Blue. All 1967–1969 400 engines had chrome-plated valve covers, air cleaner, and oil filler cap.

Engine Compartment

As with all 1967–1969 General Motors cars, the Firebird firewall, inner fender panels, and radiator support were painted semigloss black. The fenders were attached to the inner fenderwells with black-oxide plated hex-head bolts from the underside, except for the rear upper fender-corner-to-body bolt, which was installed from the top. The driver-side fenderwell was relatively bare as the headlight wiring harness was routed between the inner fenderwell and fender. The square, white plastic windshield-washer reservoir with black plastic cap was attached to the front left side of the fender with a gloss-black steel bracket. The alternator was mounted on the upper left side of the engine. A heavy-duty 55-amp alternator (includes heavy-duty battery) was available as an option with UPC K82.

The passenger-side radiator support front corner held the gloss-black battery support and battery. The standard battery for the six-cylinder and 326 and 350 V-8 was a black 45-amp Delco with top posts. A heavy-duty 61-amp top-post Delco battery was standard with the 400 V-8, standard with air conditioning, and optional (UPC T60) for all others. Side-post batteries may have been used in

This is a view of the engine compartment of a replica 1969 Trans Am convertible equipped with the 400 Ram Air V-8 (UPC L74). Note the foam seal around the air cleaner backing plate for the Ram Air scoops. The tubes at the left front of the radiator support are for the power steering cooler required with the optional 3.55:1 rear axle gears.

some late 1969 models. A six-gauge positive battery cable with red pigtail wire was routed under the battery support. The black negative cable with a long black pigtail wire was grounded to the right fender. The black rubber engine-to-firewall heater hoses were routed across the right side wheelwell and were held together with a dark-gray phosphate clamp. There were a number of radiators used in the 1967–1969 Firebird, depending upon the engine and transmission combinations. The cooling system for the six-cylinder was 12.1 quarts, while the 326 and 326 HO had an 18.6-quart cooling system. The 400 V-8 used a 17.8-quart cooling system. A heavy-duty radiator was available with UPC V01. All radiators had the filler on the right top and the inlet hose on the left side of the top tank. The radiator hoses were secured with plated tower clamps.

The passenger (right) side of the firewall was relatively bare, except for the heater plenum housing and the connections for the heater hoses. If the car was equipped with air conditioning, the hose connections were also located on the right side of the firewall and the heater connections were higher and more toward the center. The heater hoses were secured to the heater and engine fittings with plated tower clamps.

The driver (left) side of the firewall held the brake master cylinder, and the windshield-wiper motor was to the far left. All 1967–1969 Firebird drum brake systems used a dual-reservoir 1-inch-bore Delco Moraine or Bendix master cylinder and power booster (if required). All original Delco master cylinder covers were zinc dichromate finish and stamped "Use Delco Brake Fluid." Master cylinders were finished in semigloss black or natural cast iron, and the vacuum booster was gold cadmium-plated.

The rectangular data code plate was mounted to the firewall with two rivets at the top edge of the firewall between the master cylinder and wiper motor. The data plate was painted black along with the firewall. The gloss-black painted windshield-wiper motor was mounted just to the right of the brake master cylinder. Two-speed wipers were standard for 1967–1969.

The underside of the hood of all 1967–1969 Firebirds was painted semigloss black. The hood hinges and springs were zinc phosphate finish.

Frame, Undercarriage, Transmission, and Driveline

All 1967–1969 Firebirds were welded-steel unitized construction with a separate rubber-cushioned, bolted-on steel front subframe to support the engine and front suspension. The body structure consists of the welded-steel floorpan and side panels integrating the trunk compartment and rear quarter panels. The steel front subframe and related components were finished in either semigloss black or left unfinished bare steel.

A body dampener and bracket was mounted in the left and right front corners of the front subframe behind the headlights on all 1967–1969 Firebird convertibles. The dampeners used different part numbers for the left and right sides and for each year. The dampeners contained weights suspended in oil and were similar to those mounted in the left and right rear corners of the trunk compartment. They were used to absorb body vibrations in the convertible body structure.

Front Suspension

The 1967–1969 Firebird front suspension used unequal-length upper and lower control arms with ball joints, coil springs, and tubular shock absorbers. The stamped-steel upper control arms were used on all Firebirds from 1967 through 1969. The 1967–1969 Firebird upper control arm and ball joint assembly used part numbers 9796890 (right) and 9796891 (left). The upper ball joints were riveted in place, and the pivot joints had steel-encased rubber bushings. The control arms were painted semigloss black except for the outer ends.

All 1967 and 1968 Firebirds used the same lower control arms with part numbers 9794994 (right) and 3938523 (left). In 1969, the part numbers were the same for the right, but the left control arm was changed to part number 9794995. Lower control arm components were painted semigloss black except for the outer ends. The gloss-black-finish front coil springs were mounted between the lower control arm and a pocket in the front subframe. Different coil springs were used depending upon the engine and body type. Front spring rates (at the wheel) were 73 pounds for the six (normal suspension); 85 pounds for the Sprint, 326, and 350; and 92 pounds for the 400 (high-rate suspension) and Trans Am (heavy-duty suspension). Gray Delco spiral-body tubular shock absorbers were mounted in the center of the coil springs.

The standard 0.812-inch front stabilizer bar was mounted between the lower front control arms and rubber-bushed brackets in the front subframe. A 0.937-inch stabilizer bar was standard with the 1969 Trans Am. All front stabilizer bars were finished in black manganese phosphate and attached with natural steel links and rubber bushings. Koni adjustable shock absorbers were available as an option for 1968 and 1969.

The standard front brakes on all 1967–1969 Firebirds were drum-type hydraulic with 9.5-inch cast-iron drums. Standard 2.5-inch-wide brake linings were molded asbestos. Brake drums and backing plates were finished in semigloss black. Power brakes were available as an option with UPC J50.

Front disc brakes were available as an option with UPC J52. Power assist was required with the disc brake option. The 1967 and 1968 brake rotors were vented and 11.1 inches in diameter with natural cast-iron Kelsey-Hayes four-piston calipers and standard metallic pads. For 1969, the optional disc brakes (UPC JL2) were changed to a single-piston floating-caliper design also with a natural cast-iron finish and standard metallic pads.

The standard 1967–1969 Firebird steering gear was a Saginaw unit with three mounting bolts and a ratio of 24:1 with the six-cylinder engines and 28:1 with the V-8. Optional power steering with a 17.5:1 ratio was available for 1967 and 1968. An optional Saginaw gear variable-ratio power steering with a 16:1-12.4:1 ratio was available for 1969, introduced late in the 1968 model year (UPC N41). The steering gear was painted gloss black with a natural-finish side cover and end plug.

Rear Suspension

The 1967–1969 Firebird rear axle was a Salisbury-type (nonremovable center section and removable stamped rear cover) semifloating design available in standard ratios of 2.56:1, 3.08:1, 3.23:1, 3.30:1, and 3.55:1. Special optional ratios (UPC G92-5) were also available in 2.93:1, 2.78:1, 3.36:1, 3.90:1, and 4.33:1. Ratios varied according to the transmission and engine ordered. The 1968 and 1969 Ram Air engines came standard with a 3.90:1 rear axle gear. Rear axles had a 10-bolt cover with an 8.20-inch-diameter ring gear. The ring gear was attached with 3/8-20 bolts until early 1969 when they were changed to 7/16-20. Safe-T-Track limited-slip differential was available as UPC G80 on all models. The Pontiac rear axle housing covers were concave on each side when viewed from the rear. All axles were stamped with a seven-digit, alphanumeric code that identified the axle code, month-and-day build code, and plant letter suffix. The rear axle assembly was finished in semigloss black with paint codes identifying the various configurations.

The 1967 Firebird rear suspension consisted of parallel (angled slightly inward at the front to improve handling) 56-inch-long mono-leaf longitudinal semielliptic springs and dual adjustable rear radius rods (for the Sprint, 326 HO, and 400). Each radius rod (part number 9789801) was attached to the rear axle and enclosed in a U-shaped bracket attached rigidly to the axle housing. The bracket contacts the bar at midpoint only when required to control axle windup. The other end of the radius rod was attached to a bracket on the underside of the body and supported at both ends with large rubber bushings and pivot joints. All other engines (except the base six with 2.56:1 and 3.08:1 axle) had only one radius rod. The radius rods and brackets were finished in semigloss black. The base six-cylinder with 2.56:1 and 3.08:1 axle had no radius rod. Rear spring rates (at the wheel) were 100 pounds for the base Firebird, 115 pounds for the Sprint and 326, and 135 pounds for the 400, 400 HO, and Trans Am. The rear axle was controlled by gray Delco spiral-body tubular shock absorbers.

For 1968 and 1969, the Firebird rear suspension was redesigned and multileaf longitudinal parallel semielliptic leaf springs were used. Spring rates were 100 pounds for the six, 115 pounds for the Sprint and 350, and 135 pounds for the 400 and Trans Am. The springs were natural steel finish. Along with the heavier leaf spring design, the radius rods were eliminated for 1968 and 1969, making the rear suspension more conventional and improving control at the same time. The new design was still supported by gray Delco spiral-body tubular shock absorbers that were now staggered with the right shock absorber in front of the axle and the left one to the rear of the axle. Koni adjustable rear shock absorbers were available as an option for 1968 until mid-1969.

The standard rear brakes on all 1967–1969 Firebirds were drum-type hydraulic with 9.5-inch cast-iron drums. Standard asbestos linings were 2 inches wide. Brake drums (part number 9788681) and backing plates were painted semigloss black.

Tires and Wheels

The standard wheels for the 1967–1969 Firebird were 14x6J steel wheels with five lug nuts. The steel wheels were finished in gloss Starlight Black enamel (A) if full wheel covers were used. If the small standard hubcaps were supplied, the wheels were painted gloss enamel to correspond with the lower body color on the front side only. There were only three body colors available for the body-color steel wheels: Montreux Blue (D), Mariner Turquoise (L), and Seneca Red (T).

Optional wheels for the 1967 Firebird were the slotted 14x6J Argent Silver Rally I wheels with brushed-aluminum trim ring and dark center hub. The steel Rally I wheels were available only in 1967 and only with front disc brakes. Another 1967–1969 option was the 14x6-inch steel mag-styled Rally II wheels (UPC N98), also with brushed-aluminum trim ring. Seven-inch-wide 14-inch Rally II wheels were standard on the 1969 Trans Am. The Rally II wheels were available both with and without front disc brakes.

Standard tires for the 1967 Firebird were announced at introduction as 7.35x14 black sidewall with E70x14 Wide Oval white-line (UPC PX2) and red-line E70x14 optional with UPC

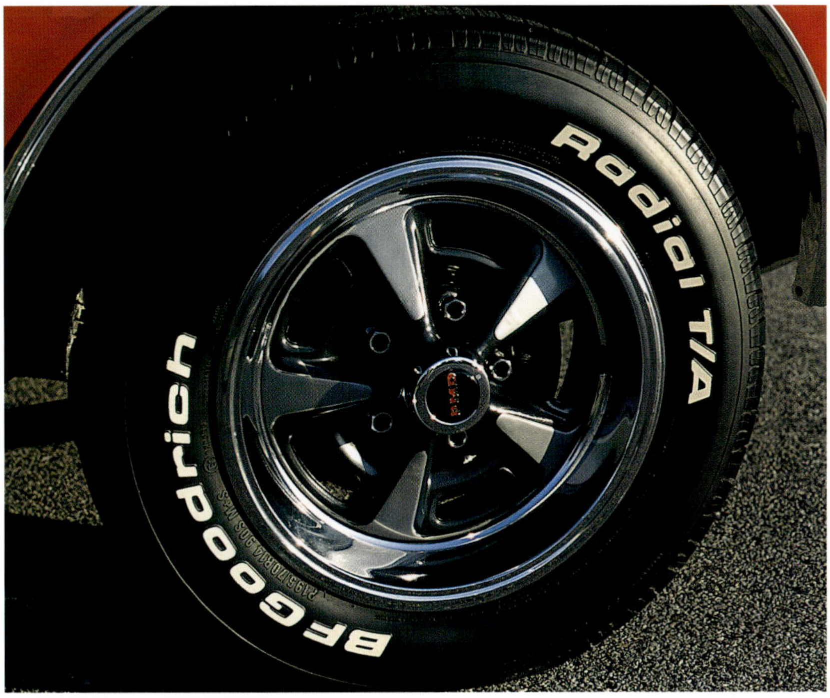

This is a detail view of an optional 1967 Firebird 14-inch Rally II wheel and trim ring (UPC N98). Note the red background on the PMD center cap. The Rally II wheels were available with or without power front disc brakes. The tires are incorrect aftermarket replacements.

PX3. A last-minute change made the E70x14 Wide Oval black sidewall the standard tire for the Firebird coupe and convertible, and the 7.35x14 tire was deleted from the specification list. F70x14 Wide Oval black-sidewall tires were standard with the Sprint, 326 HO, and 400. For 1968 and 1969, the Firebird and Firebird Sprint had standard E70x14 Wide Oval black-sidewall tires. The Firebird 400 and 400 HO had standard F70x14 Wide Oval black-sidewall tires with white-line and red-line Wide Ovals available as an option. For 1968 and 1969, 195Rx14 white-line radial tires were also available.

Small chrome-plated hubcaps with a Pontiac arrowhead badge were standard equipment on all 1967–1969 Firebirds. Deluxe wheel discs (UPC P01) and custom wheel discs (UPC P02) were available as optional choices. The 1967 and 1968 deluxe wheel discs were similar and had 25 small keystone-shaped slots, but a different part number was used for each year. A new design deluxe wheel disc was used for 1969 with six slots and part number 9781045. The 1967 deluxe wheel discs were not available with radial tires.

The custom wheel discs (part number 9787697) had six keystone-shaped slots around the circumference and a raised center hub with PMD in its center. The custom wheel discs (part number 9791006) were redesigned for 1968 and had eight openings rather than six. Simulated wire-wheel covers (UPC N95, part number 9781478) with a recessed center and PMD nameplate were also available on all models until mid-1969, when they were discontinued until 1970. The custom and deluxe wheel discs were not available on the Trans Am.

Transmissions

The 1967–1969 Firebirds were available with a choice of four transmissions. The standard transmission on all models was the cast-iron case, three-speed manual transmission with synchronization in all forward gears. There were three basic versions of the three-speed transmission available, each with optional overdrive (UPC M10). The six-cylinder engines used a transmission with a 2.85:1 low gear. The standard six had a column-mounted shifter, and the Sprint had a floor-mounted shifter. The 326 and 350 V-8 used a transmission with a 2.54:1 low gear and column shifter, and the UPC W66 400 sports option used a heavy-duty three-speed transmission with a 2.42:1 low gear and a floor shifter (UPC M12). All three-speed manual transmissions had a natural cast-iron gray finish. Chrome-plated, floor-mounted shift levers were available with or without an available optional console. A walnut shifter knob was also available as an extra-cost option (UPC M09).

The Muncie all-aluminum case, four-speed manual transmission (UPC M20) was available as an option with the Sprint six and all V-8 engines. The four-speed used with the Sprint six had a 3.11:1 low gear, and the transmission used with the V-8 engines had a 2.52:1 low gear. The 1969 Trans Am used a close-ratio four-speed with a 2.20:1 low gear (UPC M21) and a Hurst floor shifter. The chrome-plated, floor-mounted shifter was available with or without an optional console.

The ST-300 Powerglide two-speed automatic transmission was available with all engines (except the 400 Ram Air), but different versions were used for the six-cylinder (LF), Sprint six (LG), 326 and 350 two-barrel V-8 (MA), 326 and 350 four-barrel V-8 (MB), and 326 and 350 V-8 with air conditioning (MC). The 400 V-8 (except Ram Air) used its own version of the two-speed automatic (NA). The transmission codes appeared on the right side of the transmission case. The water-cooled versions of the two-speed automatic (UPC M31) had natural-steel cooling lines connected from the right side of the transmission case along the frame rail to the radiator fittings. The two-speed automatic transmission was available with either a column shifter or a console-mounted floor shifter with a chrome-plated lever, T-shaped handle, and black push-button release on top.

A three-speed Turbo Hydra-Matic transmission (UPC M40) was available as an option with the 400-cubic-inch V-8. The transmission code was PS with the standard 400 V-8 and PQ with the 400 Ram Air V-8. The case was natural aluminum with a gloss-black oil pan and converter pan.

All transmissions were connected to the rear axle by a natural-finish one-piece welded-steel driveshaft.

Chapter 3

1970–1973

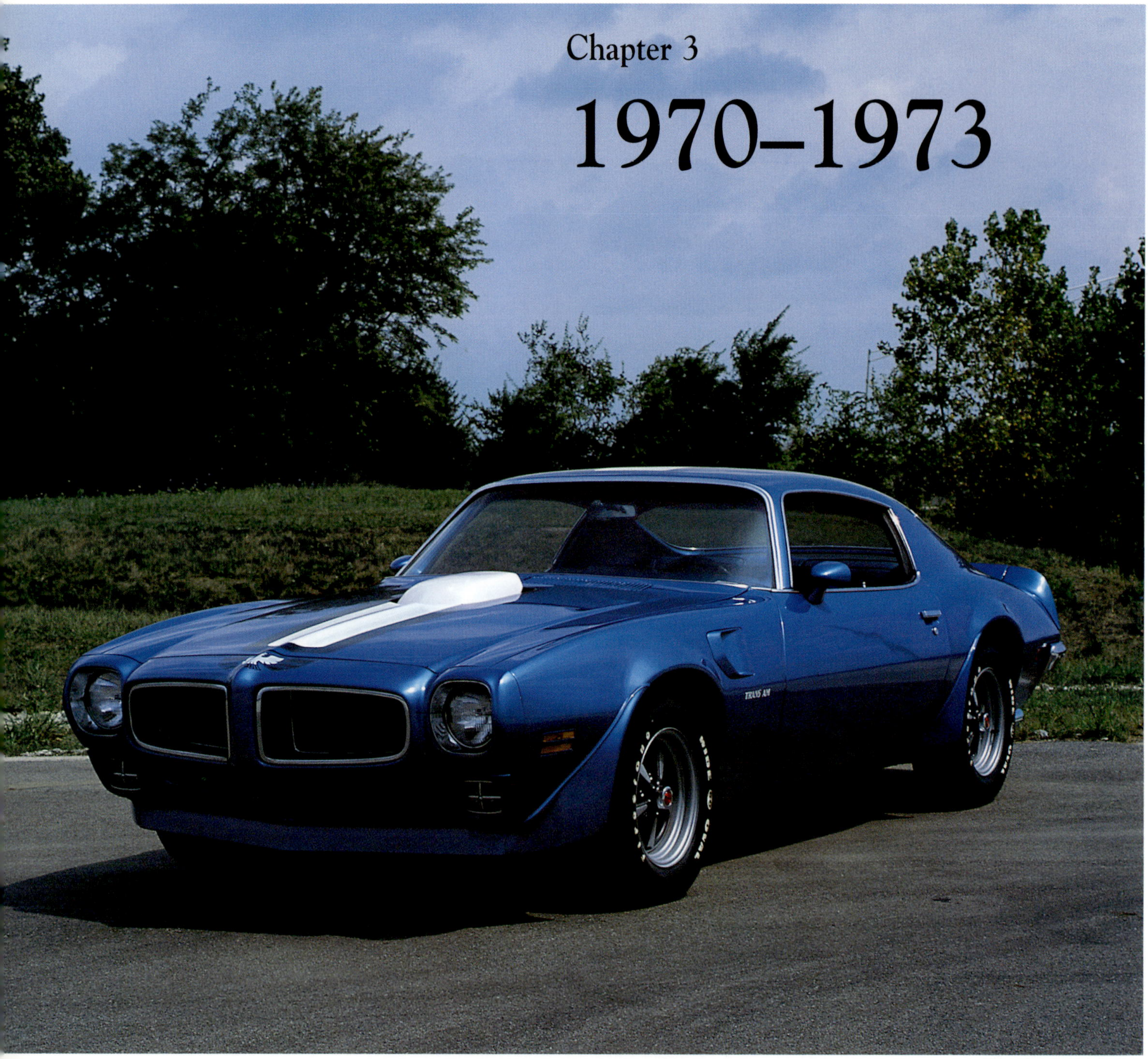

Like its initial 1967 introduction, the February 26, 1970, announcement of the new Firebird for 1970 was late in the model year, making the new evolutionary design a 1970½ model. The reason for the late introduction may be related to the fact that the Chevrolet division called the shots on any new design, and they were surely instrumental in moving the schedule back for the new car.

Regardless of the reasons behind the late introduction, the 1970½ Firebird was clearly an example of Pontiac division's desire to bridge the gap between European styling and American functionality. The new Firebird design was obviously influenced by European sports cars like Ferrari and Maserati and was generally well accepted by the automotive press. Total Firebird production for 1970 was 48,739. For 1971, production totaled 53,125. There were 29,951 Firebirds built for 1972 and 46,313 for 1973.

The new Firebird, now considered "second-generation," appeared smaller due to its single side glass, but it was actually 1.2 inches longer than it predecessor. The 108-inch wheelbase (actually 0.10-inch shorter than 1969) was maintained, but the front and rear wheels were moved 3½ inches forward in relation to the body position. The firewall was also moved back 3½ inches from its 1969 location. The new body was narrower

This 1970 Trans Am sport coupe (2887) is finished in Lucerne Blue (26) with the standard white stripe bordered in black. Note the standard-equipment modified 15-inch Rally II wheels without trim rings. The tires are incorrect aftermarket replacements as the original tires were F60x15 white letter Goodyear Polyglas GT.

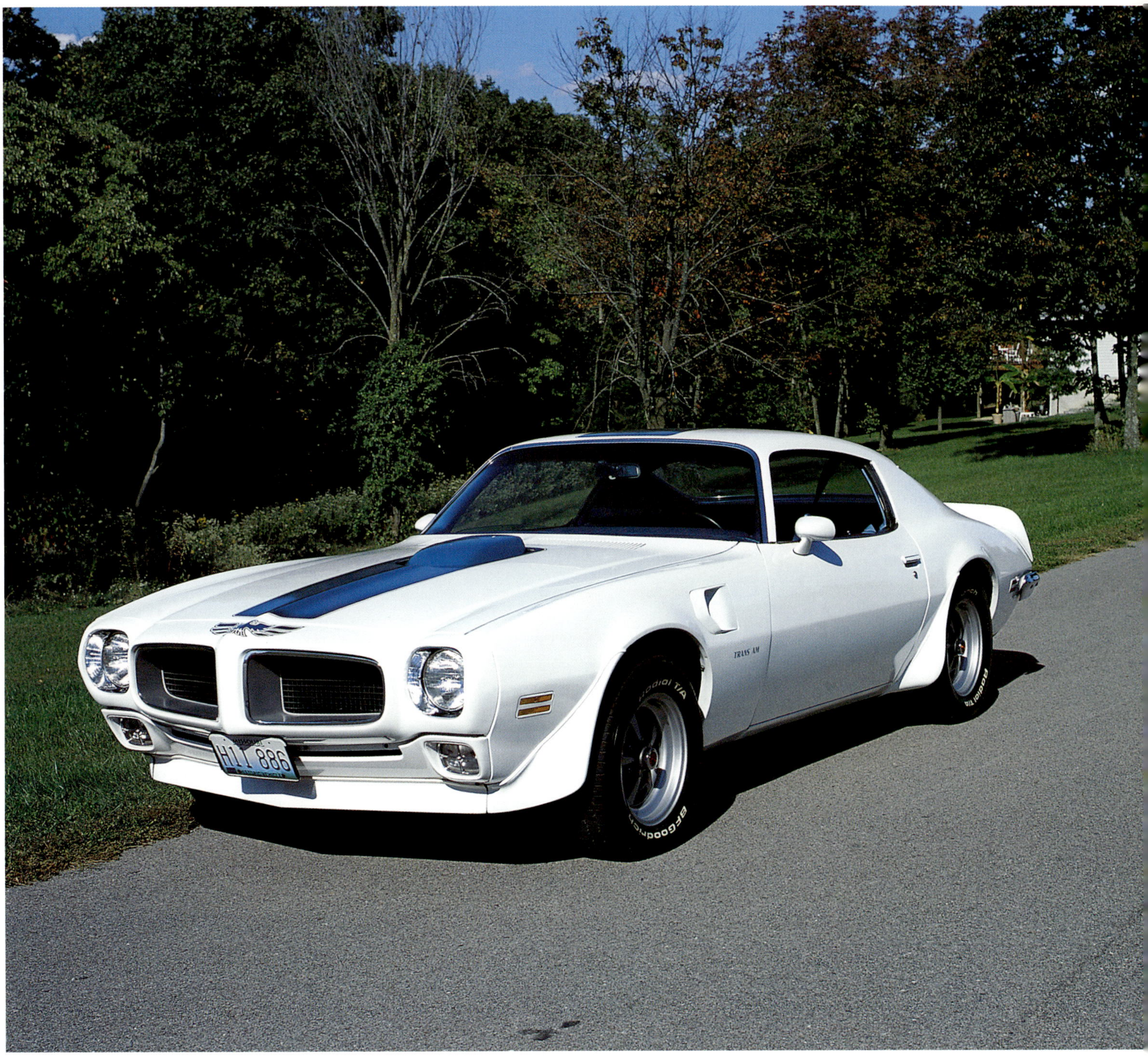

This 1970 Trans Am is finished in Polar White (10) with a blue stripe and blue bird on the front fascia. The car is equipped with the standard-equipment 15-inch Rally II wheels (UPC N98) without trim rings.

than the 1969 model by ½ inch, but the overall height was increased by almost 1 inch, adding to the head and shoulder room in the front seat. Rear seat headroom was reduced by the fastback roof incorporated into the new design, and the driveshaft tunnel was raised ¾ inch.

The fastback roof design of the 1970½ Firebird flowed into a short rear deck and flat deck lid. The body sides were more rounded than those of the earlier models and continued into the long front fenders and full Endura front end fascia. The new nose design consisted of aggressive twin recessed grille openings flanked by single round headlights in squared bezels. Small recessed rectangular parking lights, carried over from the 1969 model, were mounted directly under each headlight.

The model lineup for 1970½ was reduced from the previous year with only four models available, all in two-door hardtop coupe form. The models available included the base Firebird with standard six-cylinder or V-8 engine (2387), the Firebird Esprit with standard V-8 (2487), the Firebird Formula 400 (2687), and the Trans Am (2887). There was no convertible available in the new body style. Available models and engines for 1971 through 1973 were essentially unchanged from 1970, except that the Formula was available with either a 350, 400, or 455 V-8 engine. Styling was

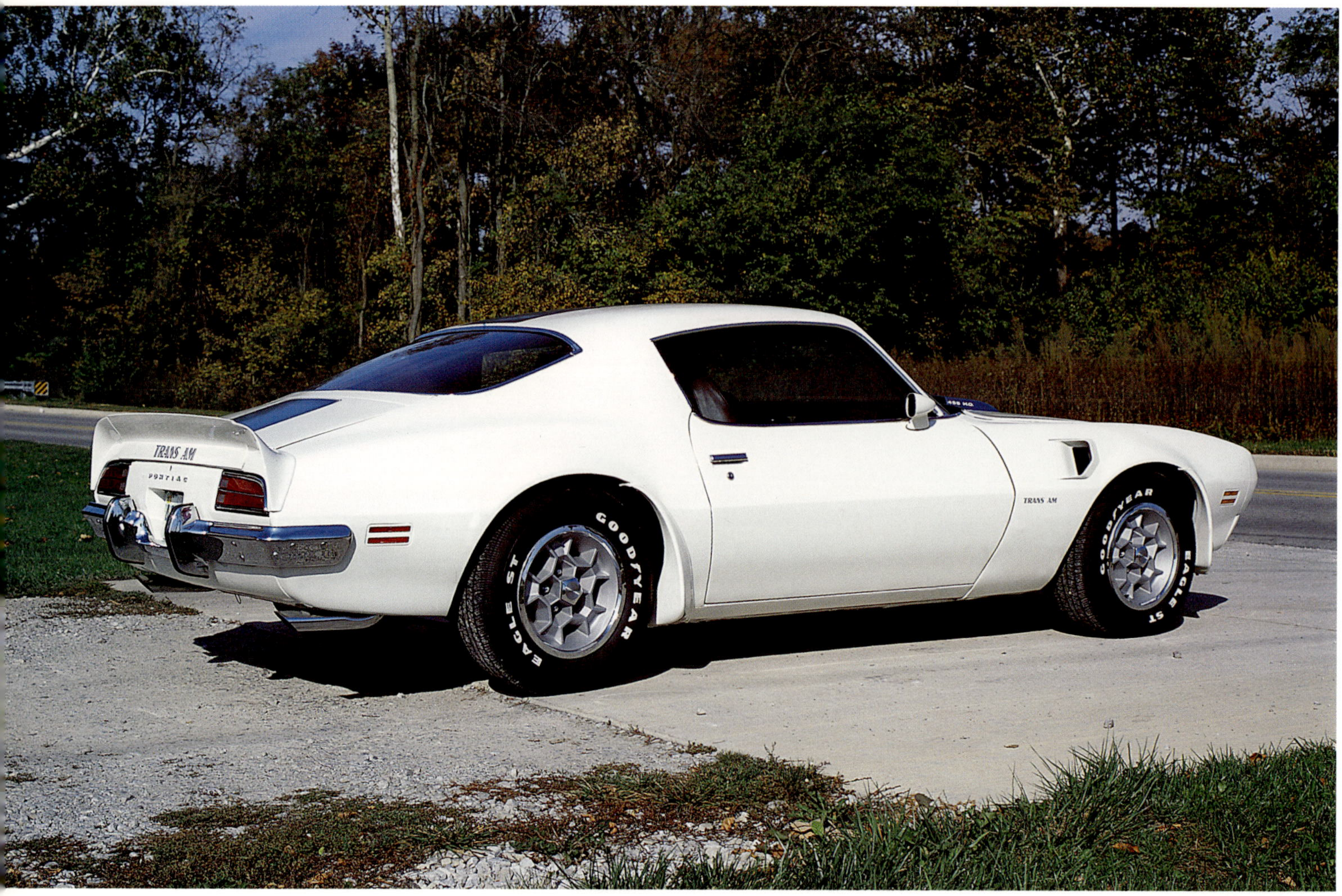

also much the same with only minor updates in the grille mesh.

Firebird engine options for 1970½–1973 still included a standard six-cylinder (Regular Production Option L22) in the base Firebird, but the previous overhead-cam six was replaced by a 250-cubic-inch cast-iron overhead-valve inline Chevrolet engine. The standard V-8 in the 1970–1973 Esprit and in the 1971–1973 Formula was the 350-cubic-inch Pontiac engine with 255 horsepower (UPC L30) in 1970 and 1971, 160 and 175 horsepower in 1972, and 150 and 175 horsepower in 1973 (UPC L30). The reduced power ratings were primarily due to the change to net, rather than gross, horsepower.

The base 400 V-8 was available with 330 horsepower in 1970 (UPC L78), 335 horsepower with the UPC L74 Ram Air III, and 345 horsepower with the Ram Air IV package (UPC LS1). For 1971, the 400 V-8 was available as the UPC L65 with 265 horsepower and the UPC L78 with 300 horsepower. For 1972, the L65 was reduced to 175 horsepower, and the L78 was down to 250 horsepower. In 1973, power was again reduced to 170 for the L65 and 230 for the L78.

A larger, 455-cubic-inch performance V-8 engine was introduced in 1971 and was available in two versions. The UPC L75 had 325 horsepower, and the HO (UPC LS5) had 335 horsepower. For 1972, the 455 was only available as the UPC LS5 at 300 horsepower. In 1973, the 455 was available as the UPC L75 at 250 horsepower, and the UPC LS2 Super Duty 455 was 290 horsepower.

There were four manual and three automatic transmission options available in the 1970–1973 Firebirds. The six-cylinder and V-8 engines were available with a standard and heavy-duty three-speed manual with both column and floor shift. A two-speed automatic was available with the six-cylinder and 350 V-8 until the 1973 model year, when only the three-speed Turbo Hydra-Matic was available as an automatic transmission option. The three-speed Turbo Hydra-Matic was available as an option on the 400 and 455 V-8 engines for 1970–1973.

The 1970½ Firebird was available in 15 body color schemes, complemented with five vinyl roof colors and 14 interior trim combinations. For 1971, the Firebird had 16 body color choices with five vinyl roof colors and 14 interior trim colors. The 1972 Firebird offered 15 body colors with

This Cameo White (11) 1971 Trans Am sport coupe (2887) has optional 15-inch Honeycomb wheels (UPC P05). The new second-generation Firebird unitized body was significantly more aerodynamic than the previous design. The front and rear wheel opening spoilers were standard.

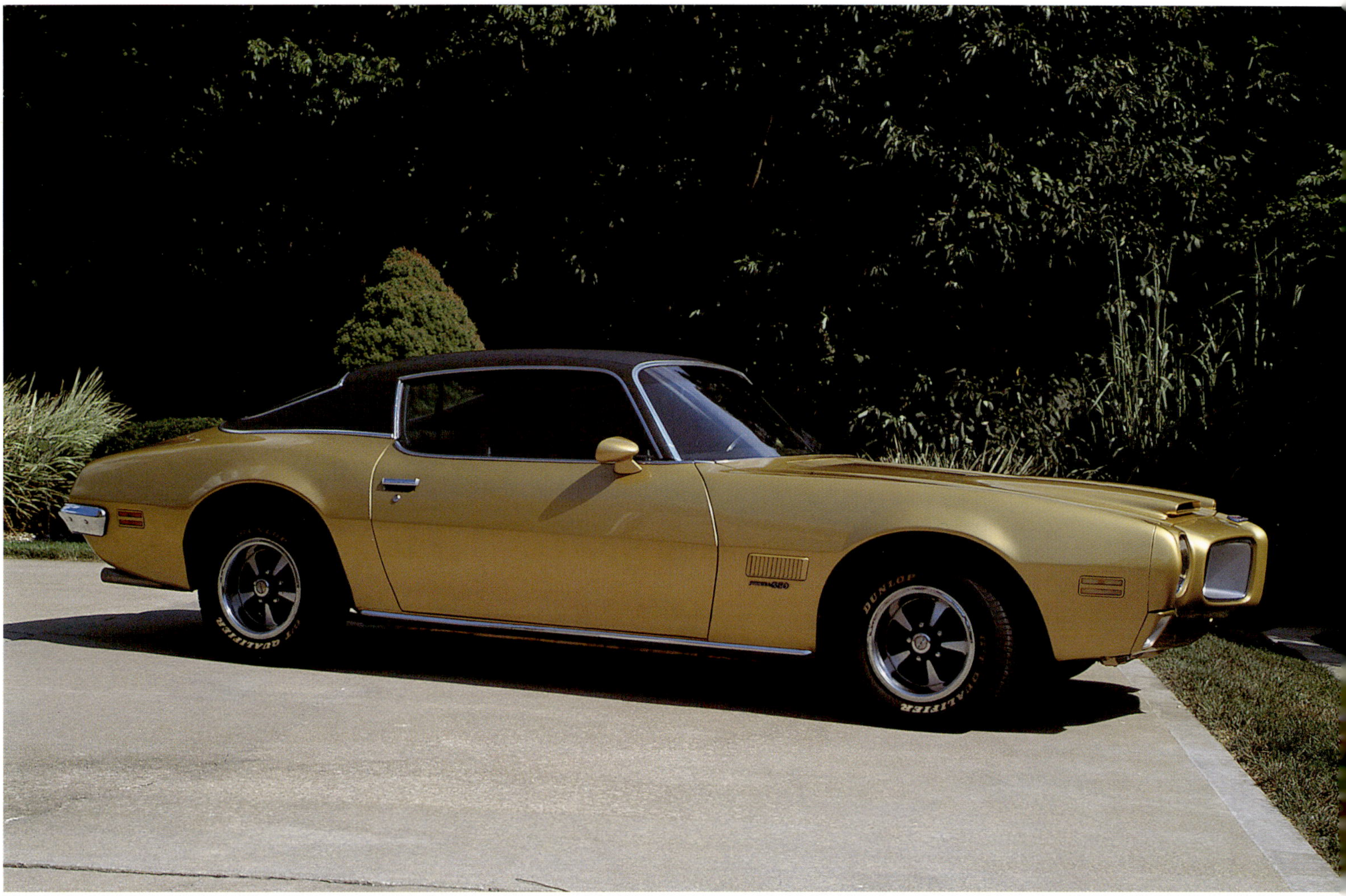

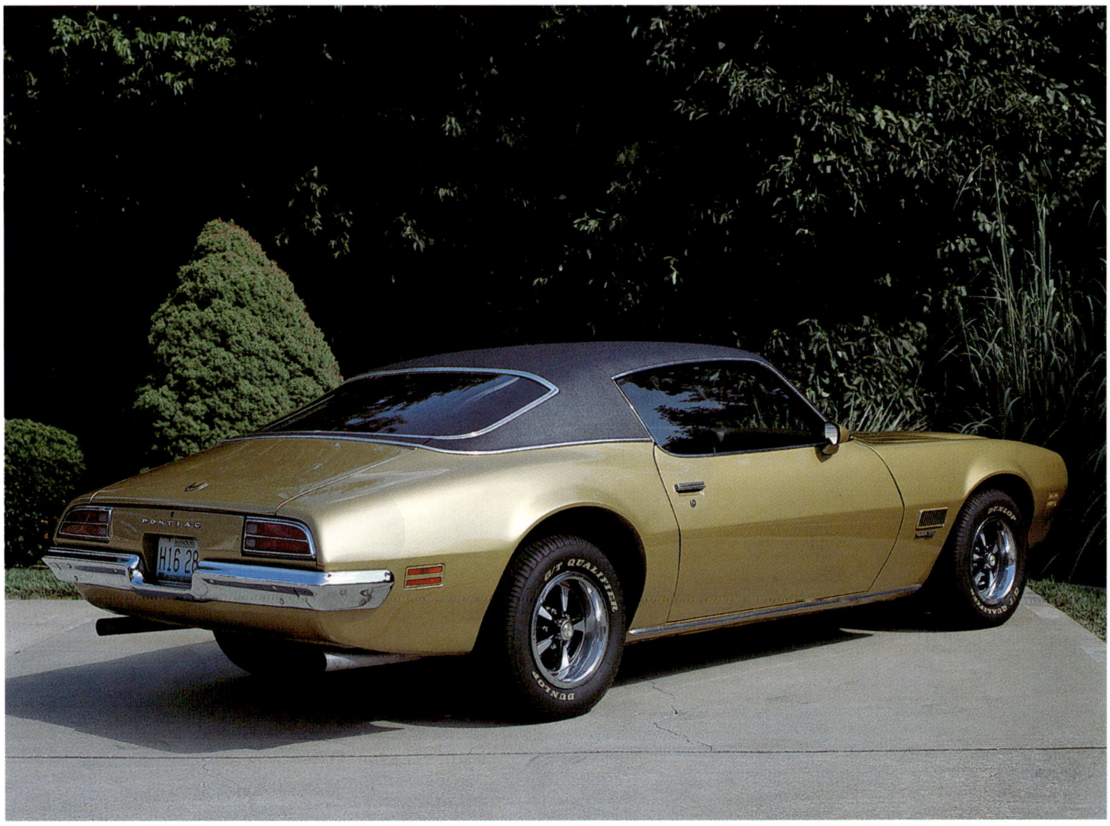

Above: This gold 1971 Firebird Formula 350 sport coupe (2687) with an optional black Cordova vinyl roof (UPC C08) is equipped with optional 14-inch Rally II wheels (UPC N98) with trim rings (UPC P06). Note the 1971-only extractor on the rear of the front fender. ***Right:*** This right rear quarter view shows a Quezal Gold 1971 Firebird Formula 350 with an optional black vinyl roof and optional Rally II wheels. The tires are aftermarket replacements.

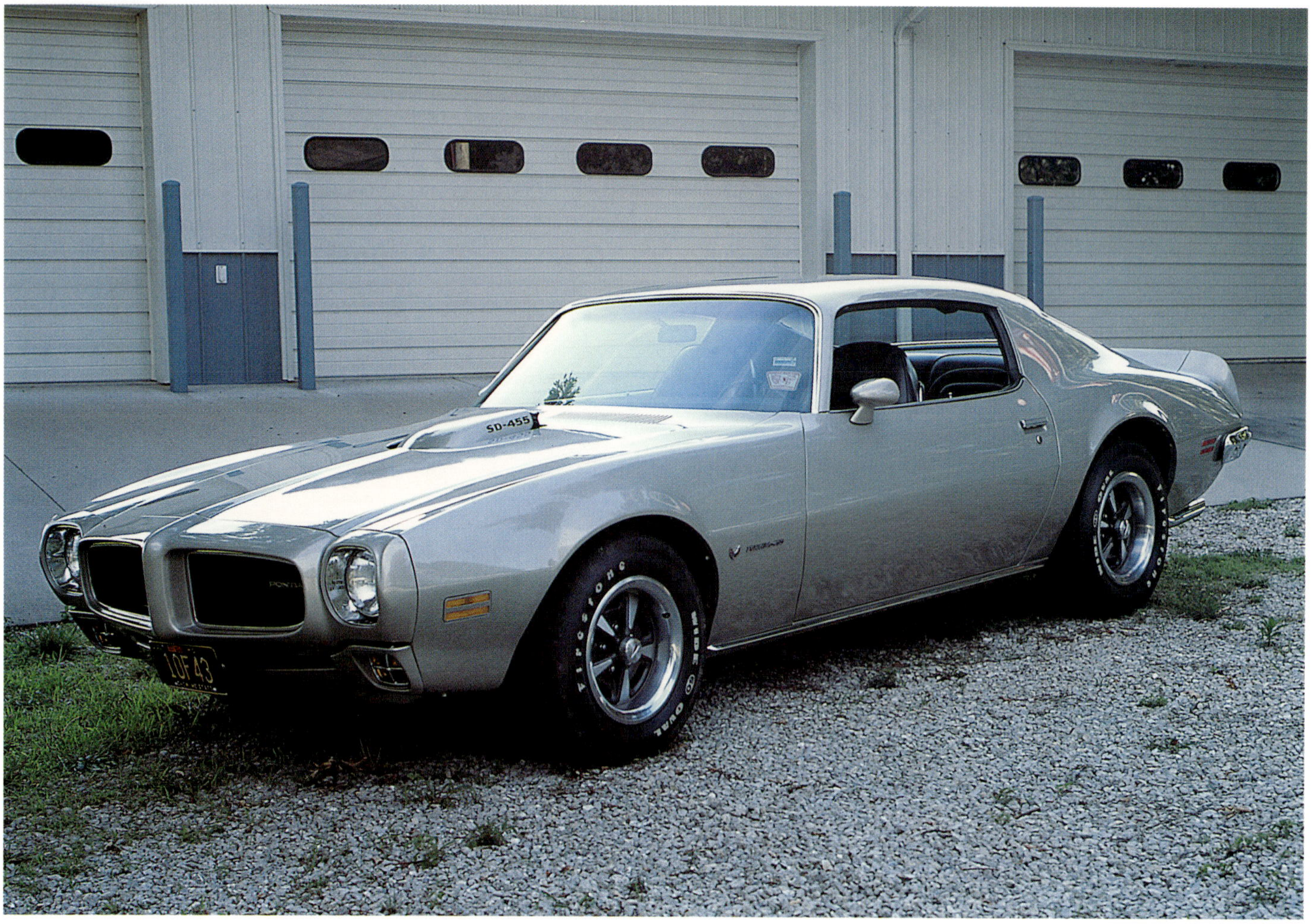

This Ascot Silver (64) 1973 Firebird Formula sport coupe is one of only 43 built with the SD 455 engine (UPC LS2). The shaker scoop and hood was used only with the SD 455 engine in the Formula. This Formula is equipped with optional Rally II wheels and trim rings.

five vinyl roof colors and 12 interior trim schemes. For 1973, there were 16 body color choices with seven vinyl roof colors and eight interior trim choices.

Body Sheet Metal and Trim

As in 1967–1969, the 1970–1973 Firebird shared its unitized body shell and steel channel subframe with the Camaro. The semigloss-black painted (some may have been natural unfinished steel) subframe was bolted to the body with four rubber-isolated mounts and carried the engine and front suspension components. The remainder of the welded-steel body shell used a steel floorpan with parallel longitudinal rear members to support the suspension and drivetrain. The underside of the floorpan was coated with a rust-inhibiting red oxide primer as the entire body was dipped prior to painting. All 1970–1973 Firebirds had an 18.5-gallon galvanized-steel fuel tank mounted at the rear of the body pan. All 1970–1973 Firebirds were two-door hardtop coupes on a 108-inch wheelbase.

The body structure was greatly improved for 1970 with a new roof design that replaced the previous roof rails and longitudinal bows with a one-piece roof inner panel that was pierced with small holes to provide sound absorption. In addition to the standard steel roof, all 1970–1973 Firebird sport coupes were available with an optional Levant-grain Cordova vinyl roof covering (UPC C08). All Firebird Esprit bodies used a standard bright stainless-steel roof drip-rail molding that was available as an option (UPC Y80) on all other models. When the optional vinyl roof was ordered, an additional two-piece bright molding was added at the lower edge of the vinyl roof at the sail panel and wrapped around the lower border of the back glass opening. All 1970–1973 Firebird Esprit models had a small bright Esprit script badge in the sail panel just behind and above the rear of the door opening.

The optional Cordova vinyl roof was available in white (1), black (2), Sandalwood (5), dark gold (7), and dark green (9) in 1970. In 1971, the same codes and colors were used except the dark gold was renamed dark brown. The 1972 vinyl roof colors were black (2), blue (3), parchment (5), fawn (8), and green (9). The available color choices were increased to seven in 1973 and included white (1), black (2), beige (3), chamois (4), green (5), dark burgundy (6), and blue (7). The vinyl roof installation was in three sections

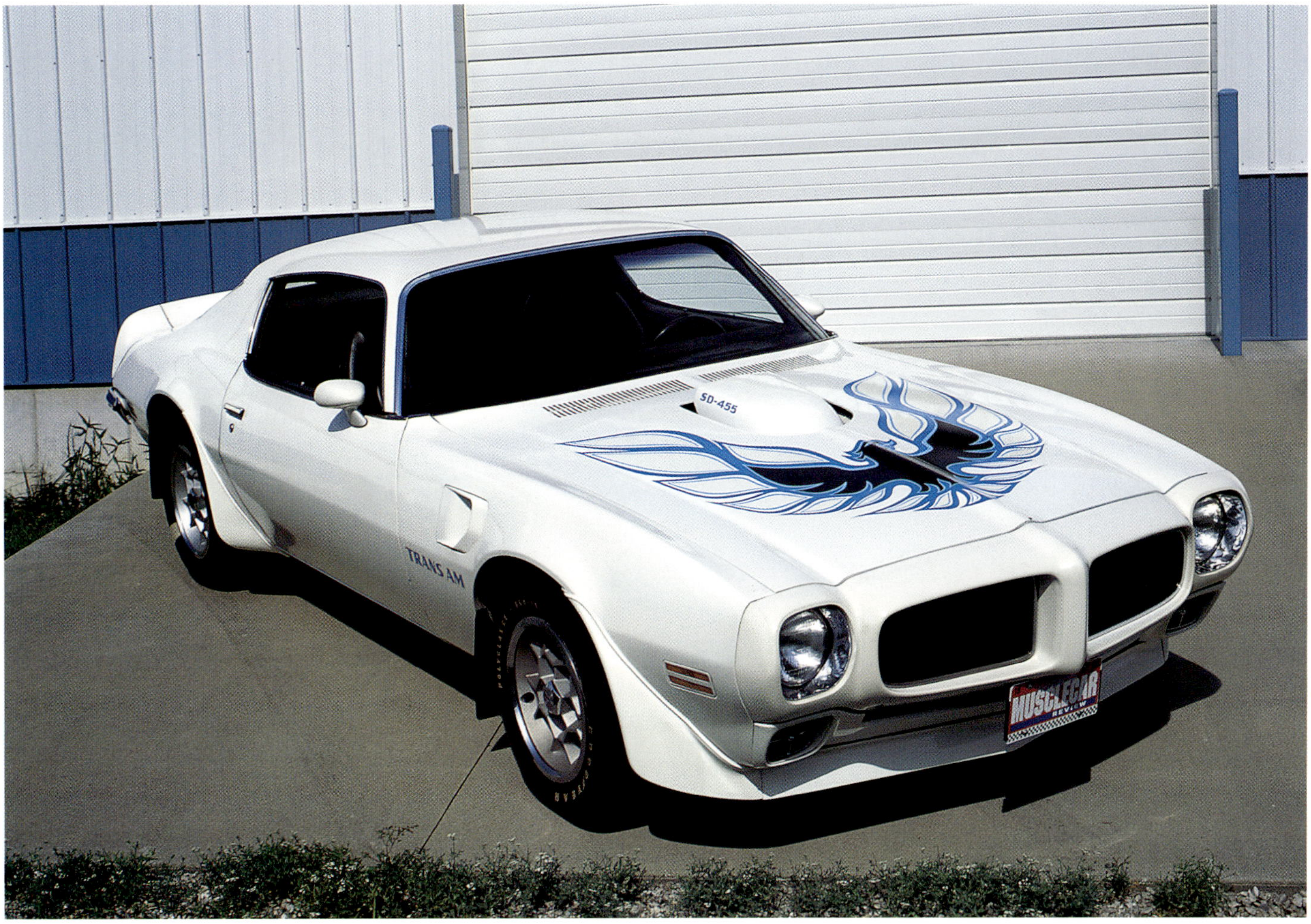

Above: This original Cameo White 1973 Trans Am SD 455 has the distinctive blue Firebird decal on the shaker hood and is equipped with optional 15-inch Honeycomb wheels (UPC P05) and original Goodyear F60x15 Polyglas GT tires. ***Right:*** This Brewster Green (48) 1973 Trans Am sport coupe features the aerodynamic lines of the second-generation body and relatively flat rear glass. This Trans Am is equipped with optional rear bumper guards and standard Rally II wheels and trim rings.

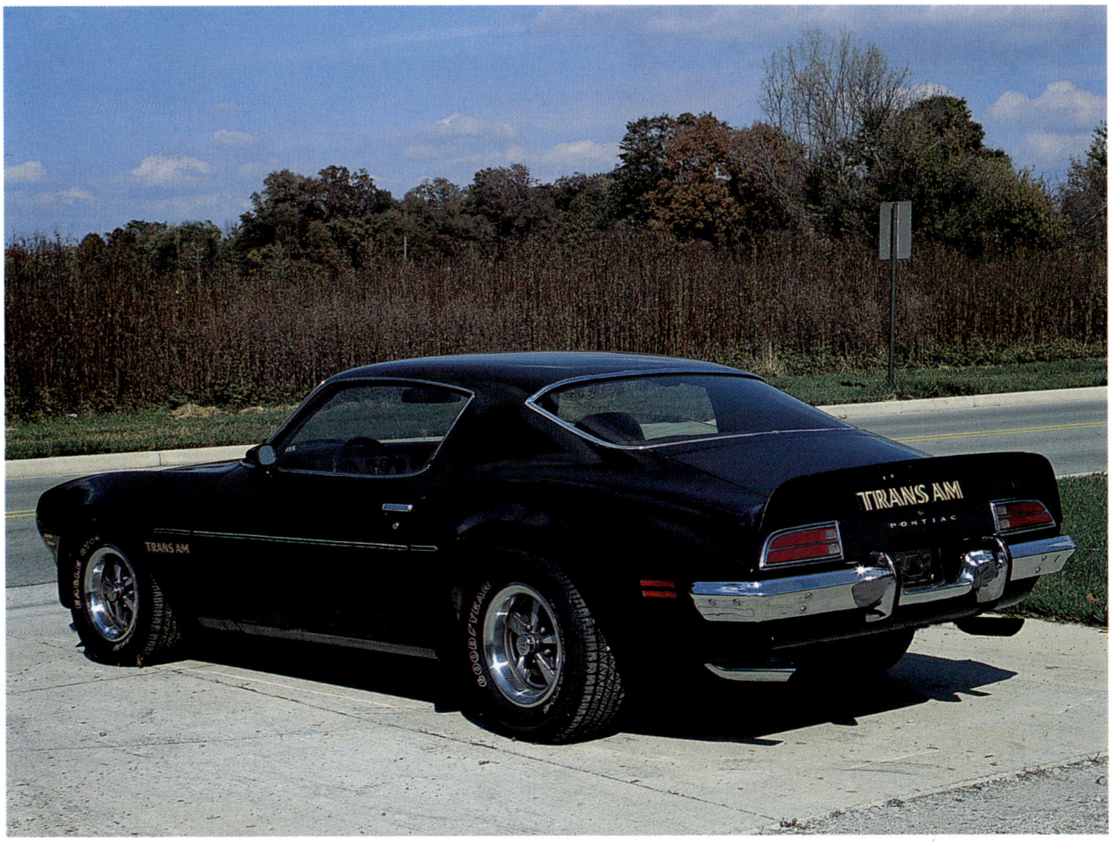

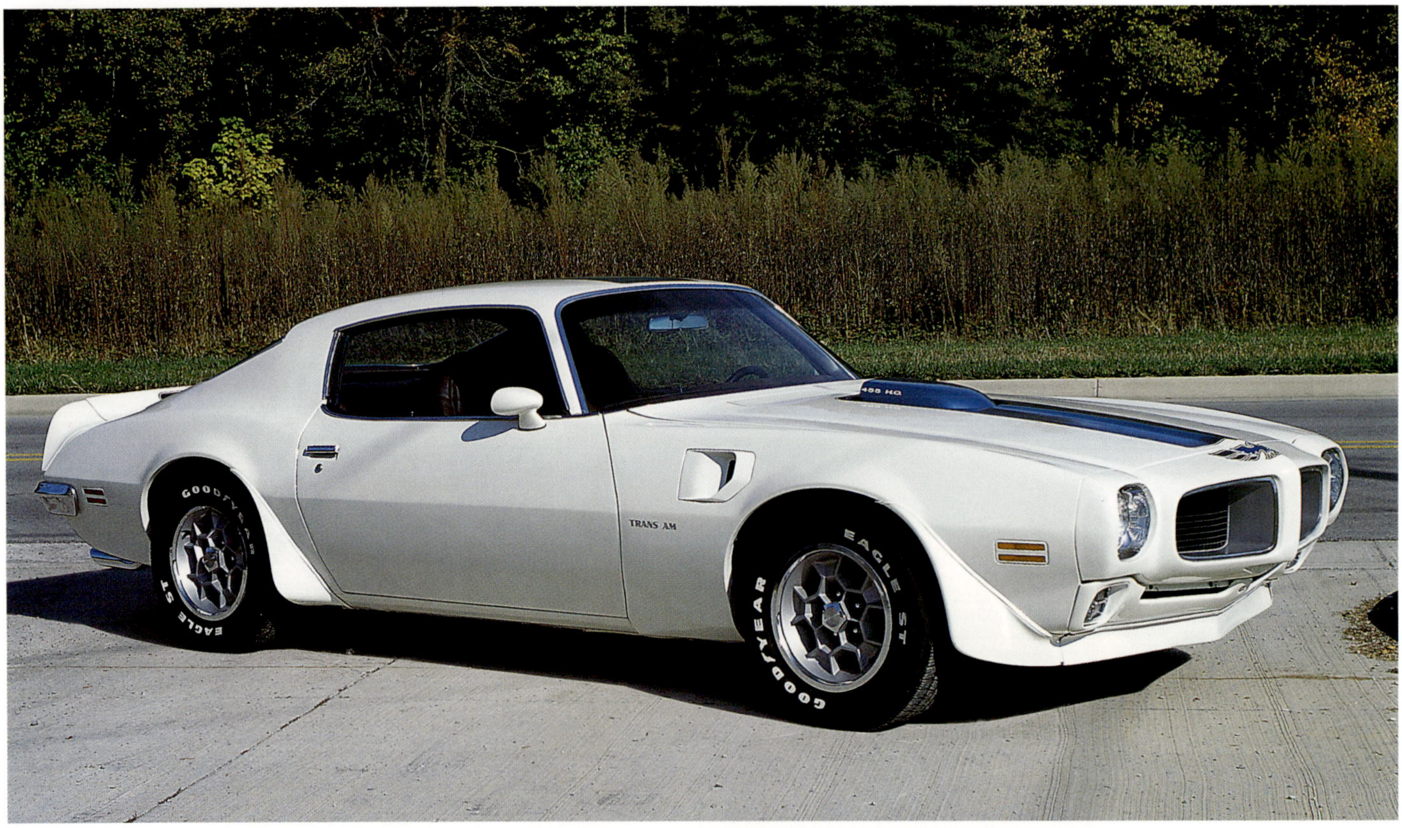

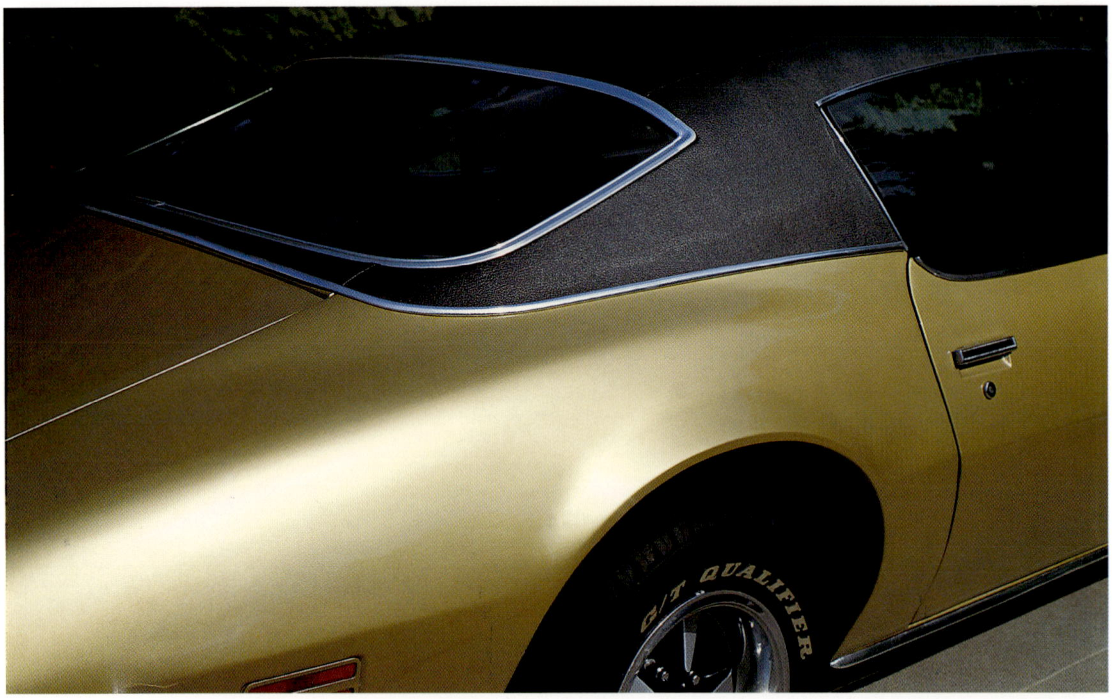

Above: This right front quarter view of a Cameo White 1971 Trans Am 455 HO shows the design of the second-generation sport coupe unitized body. This basic body structure was used with few changes through 1981. ***Left:*** Detail view of the black Cordova roof on a gold 1971 Firebird Formula 350. The Cordova roof option included bright drip-rail moldings and belt-rail moldings. This Formula is equipped with optional Rally II wheels.

with a large center piece between two smaller side sections with a longitudinal seam on each side.

All 1970–1973 Firebirds used the same left and right door shells. There were no vent windows or quarter windows used in any 1970–1973 models, so the side glass was sealed by rubber seals and channels in the front windshield post and the rear roof quarter pillar. The doors were operated by chrome-plated rectangular pull-type lift-bar handles and were identical for all 1970–1973 models.

Left and right outside body-color aerodynamic sport mirrors with a remote-control body-color left side mirror were standard on all 1970–1973 Firebird Esprit, Formula, and Trans Am. Right and left body-color mirrors were available as an option (UPC D35) on the base Firebird.

All 1970–1973 Firebird doors were sealed with black soft sponge rubber weatherstrip that

This original Ascot Silver 1973 Firebird Formula SD 455 displays the design of the door that was used throughout the second-generation Firebird models with little change. This car is equipped with optional rear bumper guards and deck mounted rear spoiler.

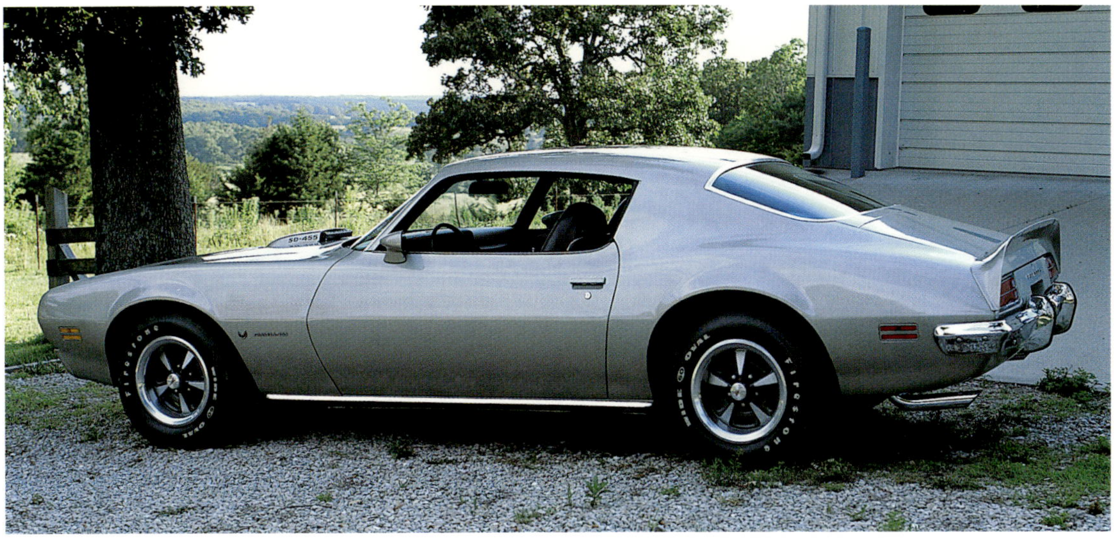

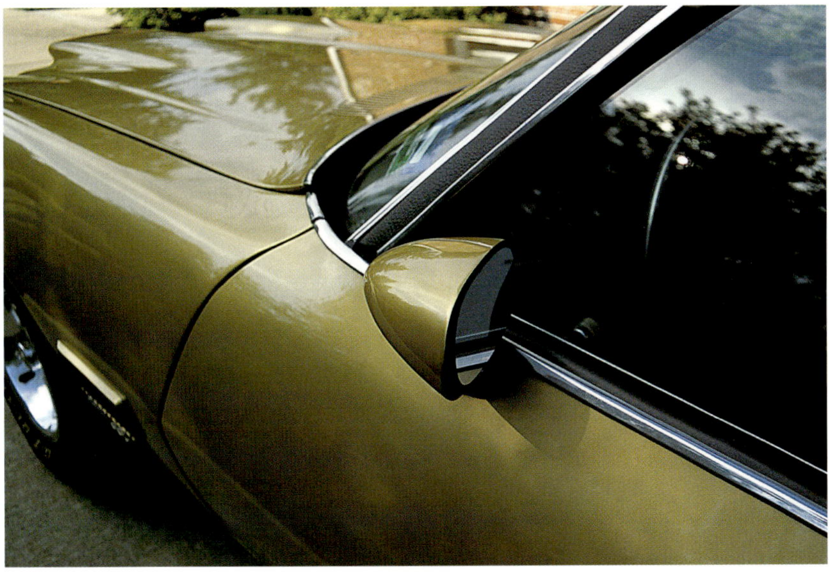

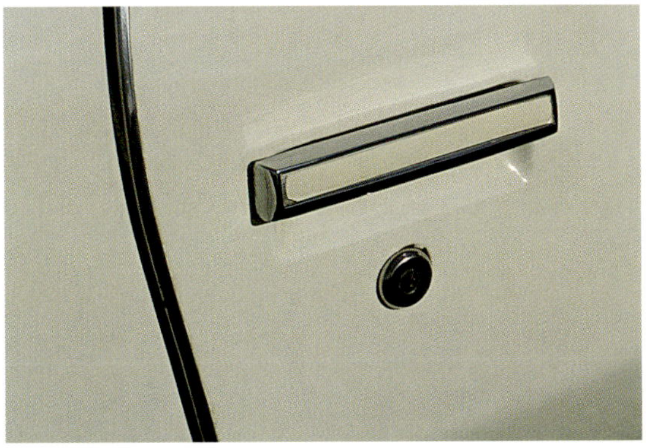

Above: Detail view of the left door and standard outside remote-control sport mirror on a gold 1971 Firebird Formula with optional black vinyl Cordova roof. The bright drip-rail moldings are standard with the Cordova roof. ***Right:*** This original white 1973 Trans Am SD 455 sport coupe door handle has a white insert to match the body color.

surrounded the outer perimeter of the door shell. The lower door opening was trimmed with an aluminum sill plate with a Fisher Body badge glued on at the rear. The badge was riveted in place on some very early models. A black ABS plastic vent grille and a body-color Torx-head latch striker were mounted in the body doorjamb.

All 1970–1973 Firebirds used the same deck lid, hinges, and supports with variations only for trim badges and spoilers. All models, except the Trans Am and those with the optional rear spoiler (UPC D80), had a red-and-black Firebird badge in the rear center of the deck lid. The Trans Am deck lid had no badge but, instead, a three-piece rear deck spoiler was mounted on the deck lid and tops of the rear quarter panels. The outer ends of the wide spoiler wrapped around and down the sides of the rear quarter panels. The spoiler was standard on the Trans Am and optional on the Formula. The rear deck spoiler was also available as a dealer-installed option on the other models. Block decal letters spelling Trans Am were applied to the center of the rear of the spoiler.

All 1970–1973 Firebirds had a flat trunk floor with a standard full-size spare tire and wheel mounted on the right side with its inner side up. The jack base was mounted bottom-side up in the center of the spare wheel and held in place by a plated wing nut, and the jack was held in place by the wheel and tire. A space-saver spare wheel and tire was available as an option with UPC N65. The space-saver spare inflator bottle was mounted in the lower rear of the wheel. The flat part of the trunk floor was covered with a heavy-duty aqua-and-black houndstooth vinyl mat but an optional fitted vinyl mat was available. A spare tire and wheel cover was available with the standard spare with option UPC P17. The entire trunk interior was finished with dark/aqua green paint for Norwood-built cars and most Van Nuys cars, but some Van Nuys–built cars may have had a gray speckle paint.

The rear deck lower panel on all 1970–1973 Firebirds was flat except for two bright-trimmed thin horizontal taillights on each side and the deck lid lock in the upper center. The lower center of the panel had a rectangular opening for the license plate recess. Block chrome-plated letters spelling Pontiac were in the center of the panel. The fuel filler was located under the license plate,

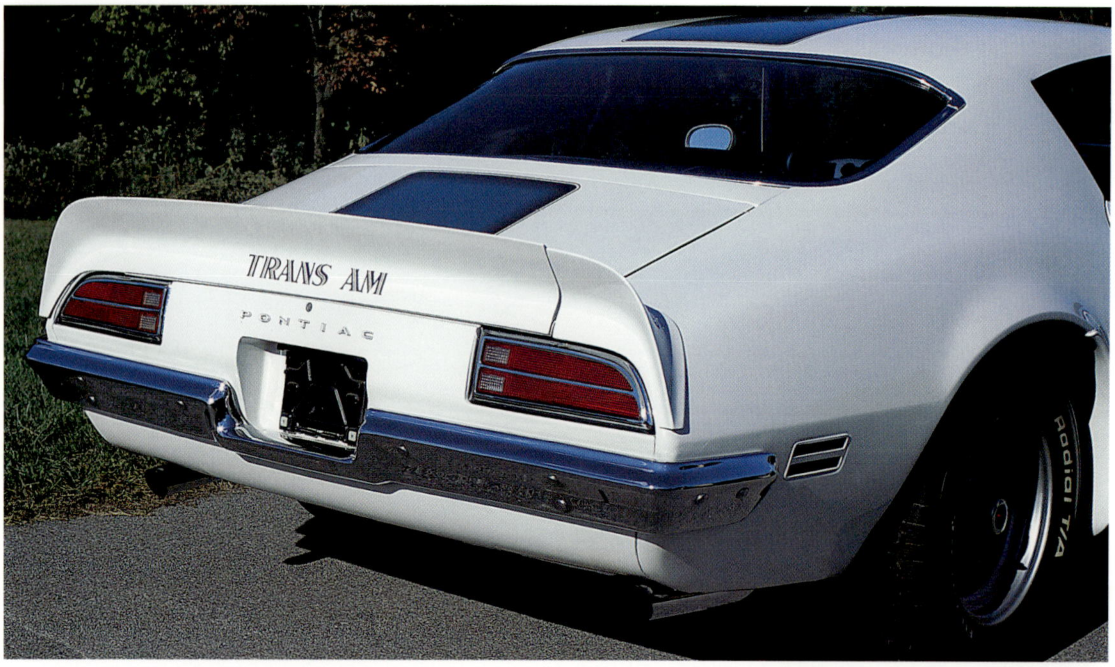

This rear view of a Polar White 1970 Trans Am shows the deck lid and rear spoiler design, the Pontiac nameplate on the lower panel, and the blue Trans Am decal on the rear of the spoiler.

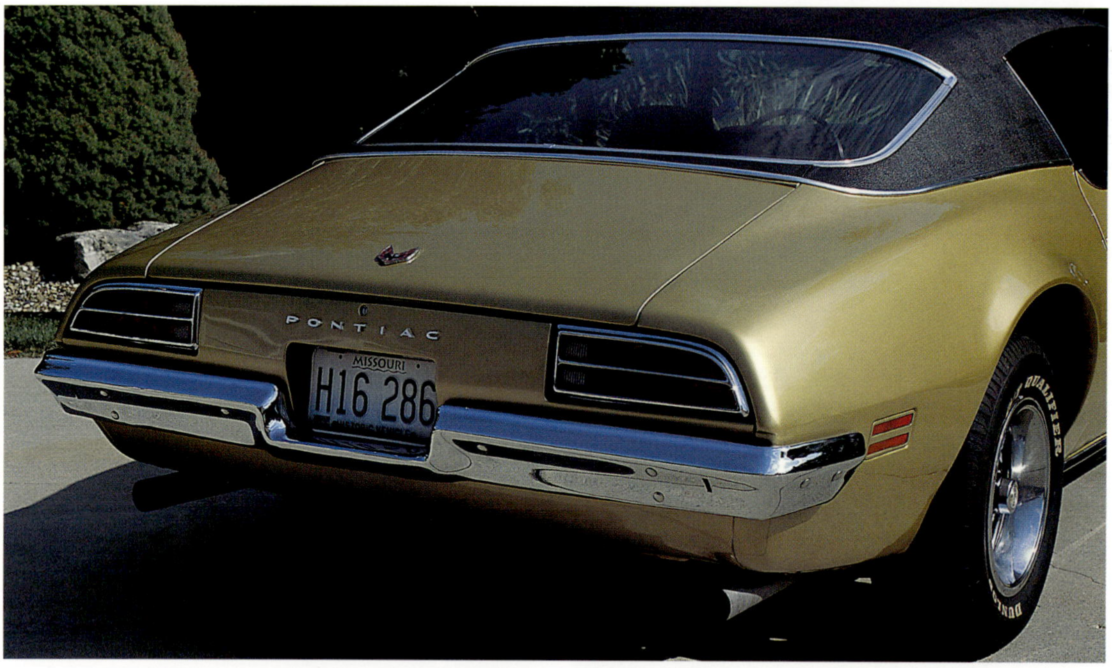

This is a rear view of a gold 1971 Firebird Formula 350 shows the deck lid and rear deck lower panel, the Pontiac nameplate on the lower panel, and Firebird badge on the deck lid. This Formula has an optional black vinyl Cordova roof.

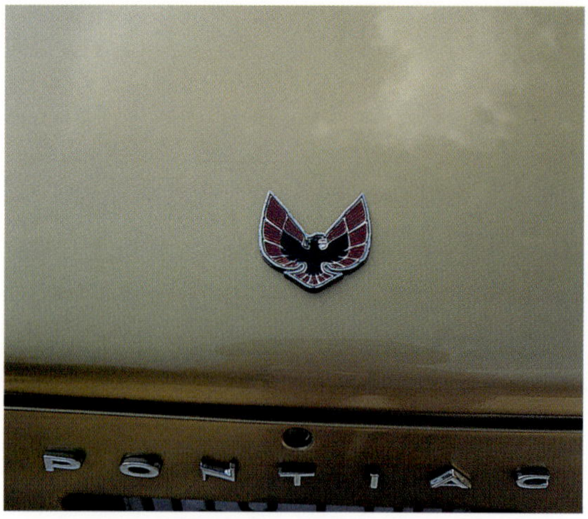

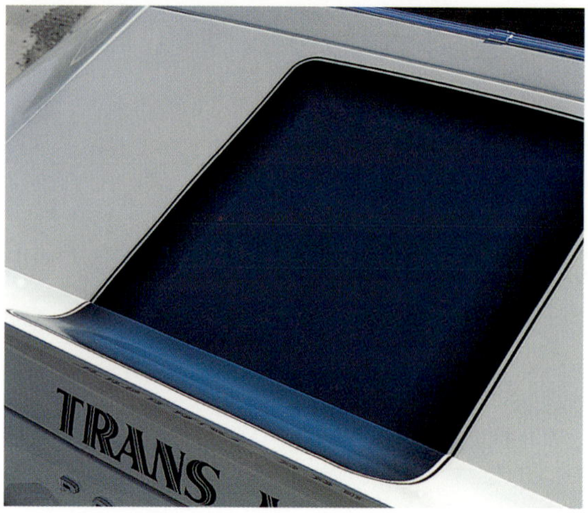

Far left: Detail view of the deck lid of a gold 1971 Firebird Formula 350 showing the Firebird deck lid badge and the Pontiac letters on the rear deck lower panel. ***Left:*** This is a detail view of the blue deck lid stripe on an original white 1971 Trans Am. The stripe continues up the front surface of the rear spoiler.

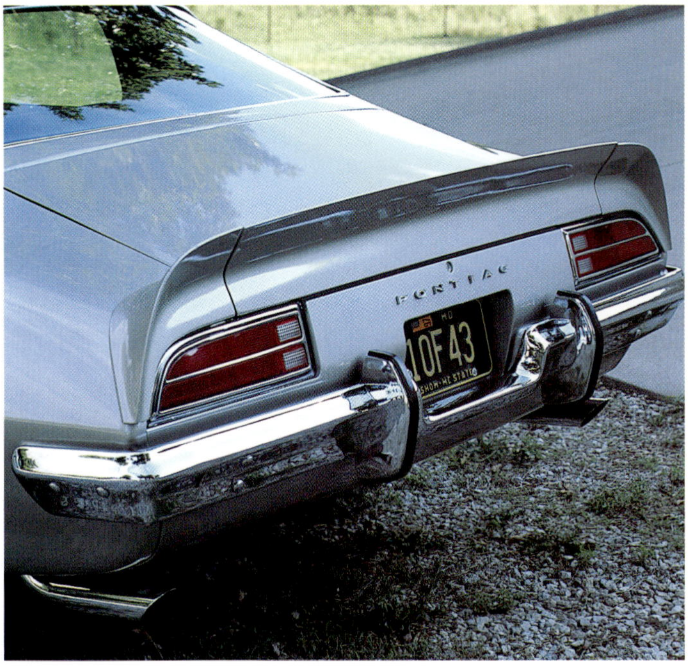

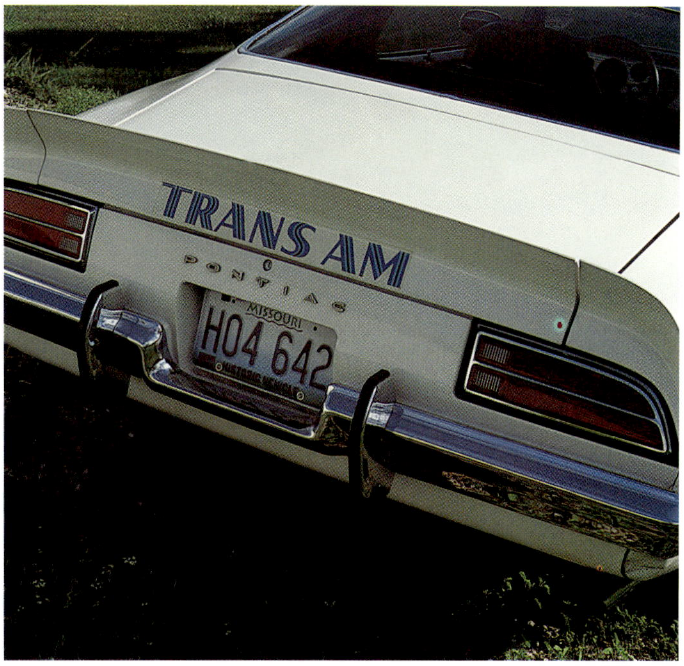

Above left: This rear view shows the deck lid and rear spoiler on an Ascot Silver 1973 Formula SD 455. Note the design and mounting of the three-piece spoiler and optional rear bumper guards. This is one of only 43 1973 Formulas equipped with the UPC LS2 SD 455 engine option.
Above right: Detail view of the deck lid and spoiler on an original white 1973 Trans Am with a blue one-piece Trans Am decal on the rear of the spoiler and the optional rear bumper guards.

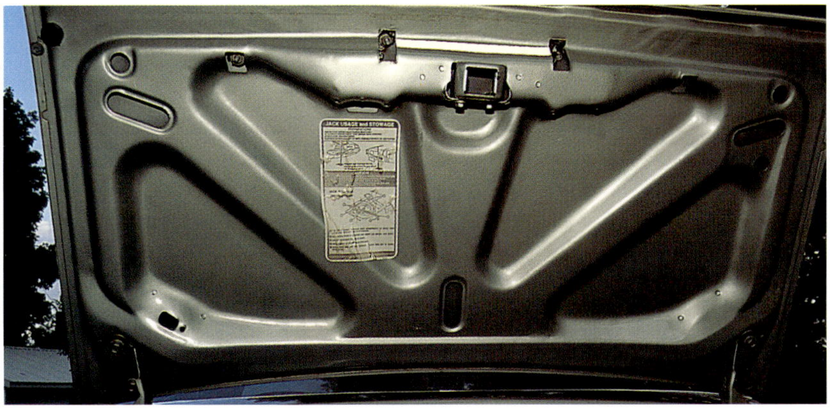

Above: The inside of the deck lid on an original gold 1971 Firebird Formula 350 displays the jack instructions decal. The standard Formula deck lid had different hinge torsion bars than one with a rear spoiler. The standard holes for the optional spoiler fasteners are visible.

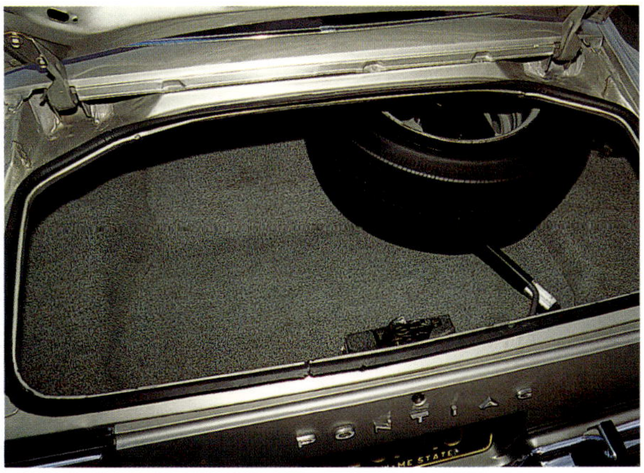

Right: This view of the unrestored original trunk interior of an Ascot Silver 1973 Formula SD 455 sport coupe shows the correct original finish of the trunk mat and interior panels, the spare tire mounting on the floor, and the correct black rubber weatherstrip on the lip.

as it was in 1969. A relatively straight chrome-plated rear bumper had a rectangular notch in its upper center for the license plate mounting. The 1970 Firebird used a bumper impact bar with part number 9799744, and the 1971–1973 models used a similar design with part number 484947. The inner, outer, and intermediate bumper brackets were made slightly longer for 1973 to increase crash resistance. Narrow rubber-faced bumper guards were available as an option. The outer ends of the rear bumper wrapped around the sides of the rear quarter panels.

The relatively short rear quarter panels of the 1970–1973 Firebird had a decided slope to the rear with smoothly rounded sides joining the rear deck area. There were obvious flares around the upper wheel openings. A two-section rectangular side marker light was mounted in the center side of the quarter panel just in front of the rear bumper ends. The Trans Am had separate spoilers in the front of the rear wheel openings. Bright wheel-opening moldings were available as an option (RPO B96) on all models (except the Trans Am) and standard equipment on the Firebird Esprit. A full-length bright rocker panel molding was mounted between the wheel openings and was standard on all but the Trans Am. The bright rocker panel designs were different for the base Firebird (thinner) and the Esprit (wider).

All 1970½ Firebirds except the Trans Am used the same front fenders. The Trans Am used a similar fender with an opening for the rear-facing

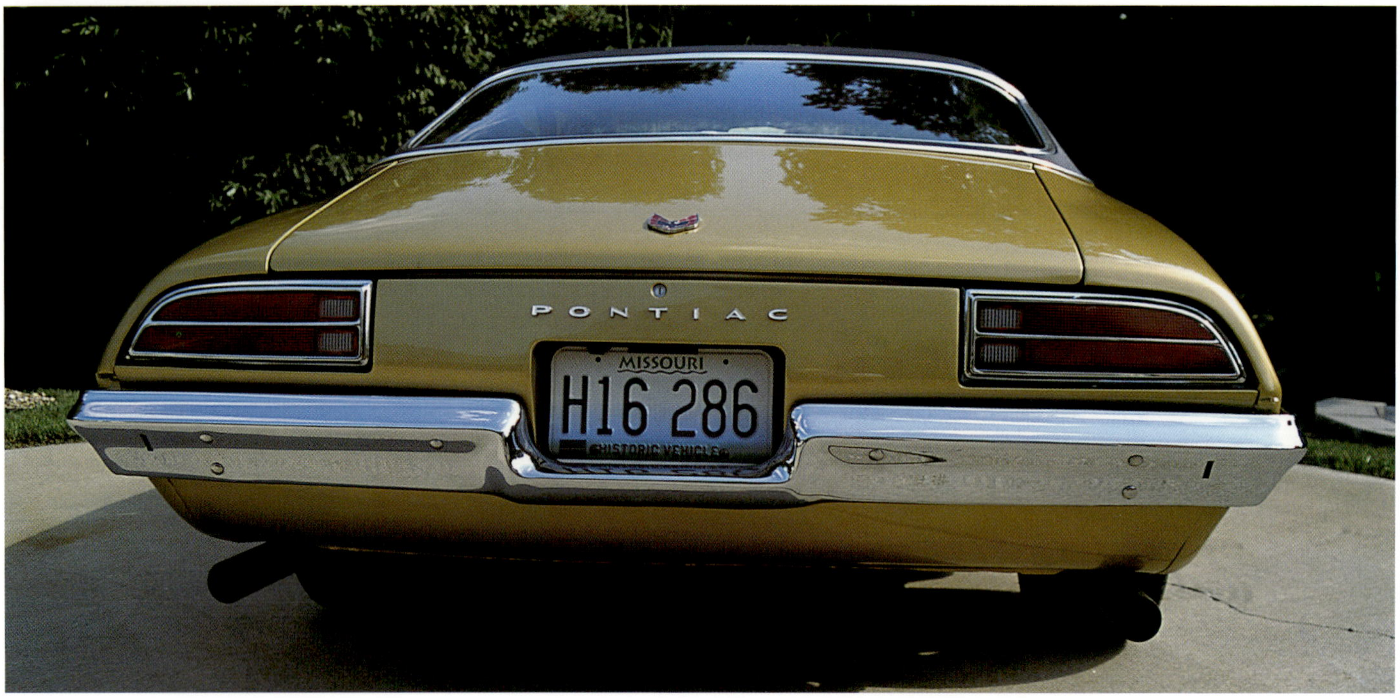

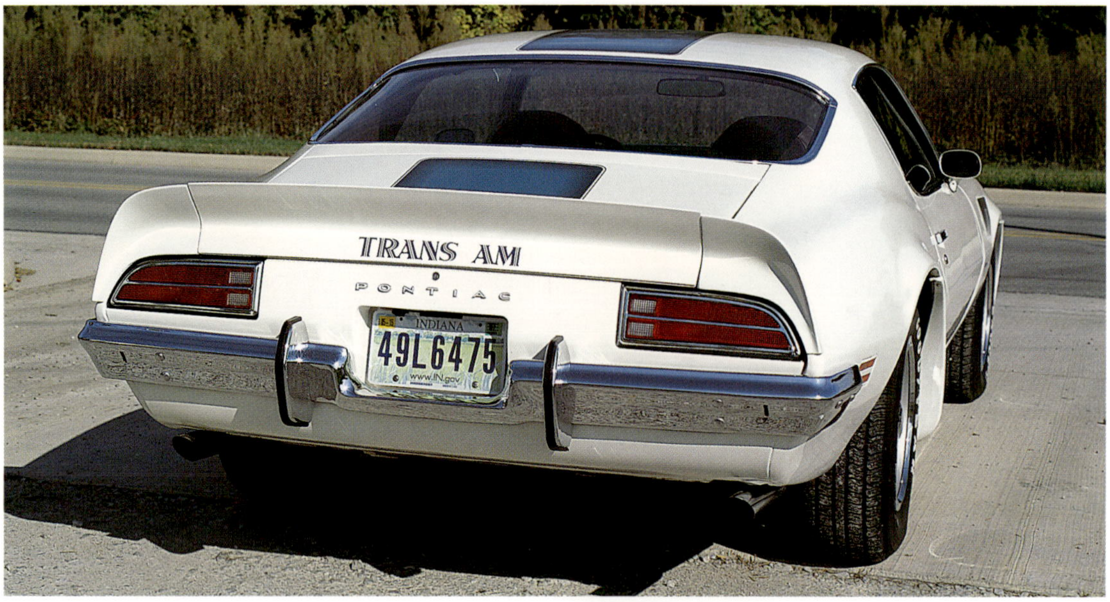

Above: Detail view of the rear deck lower panel and rear bumper of a gold 1971 Firebird Formula 350 sport coupe. Note the straight lines of the rear bumper. ***Left:*** This detail view of a 1971 Trans Am 455 HO shows the rear deck lower panel and standard spoiler, the Pontiac nameplate on the lower panel, and the blue Trans Am decal on the spoiler. This Trans Am is equipped with optional rear bumper guards.

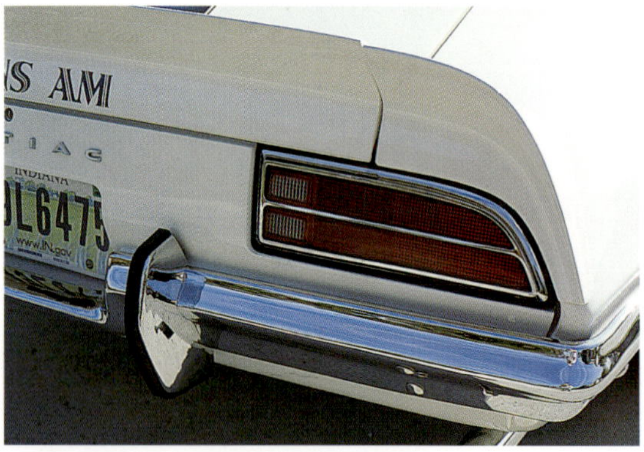

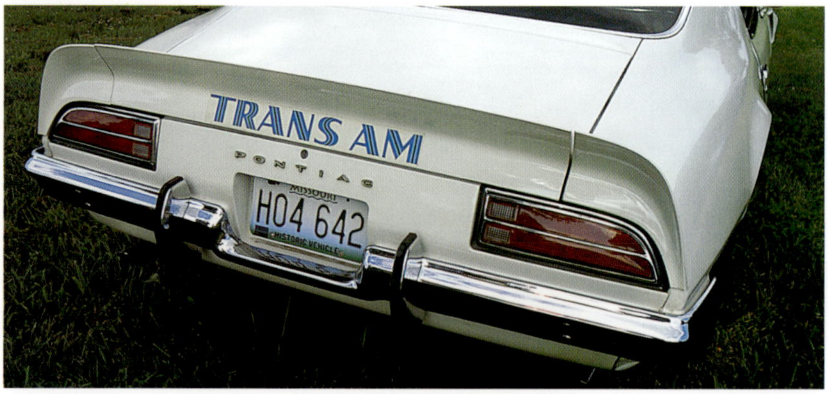

Above left: A detail view of the right taillight and rear deck lower panel on an original white 1971 Trans Am 455 HO with the optional rear bumper guards. ***Above right:*** This view shows the rear deck lower panel and rear bumper on an original white 1973 Trans Am SD 455 sport coupe. Note the design and installation of the three-piece rear spoiler and Trans Am decal.

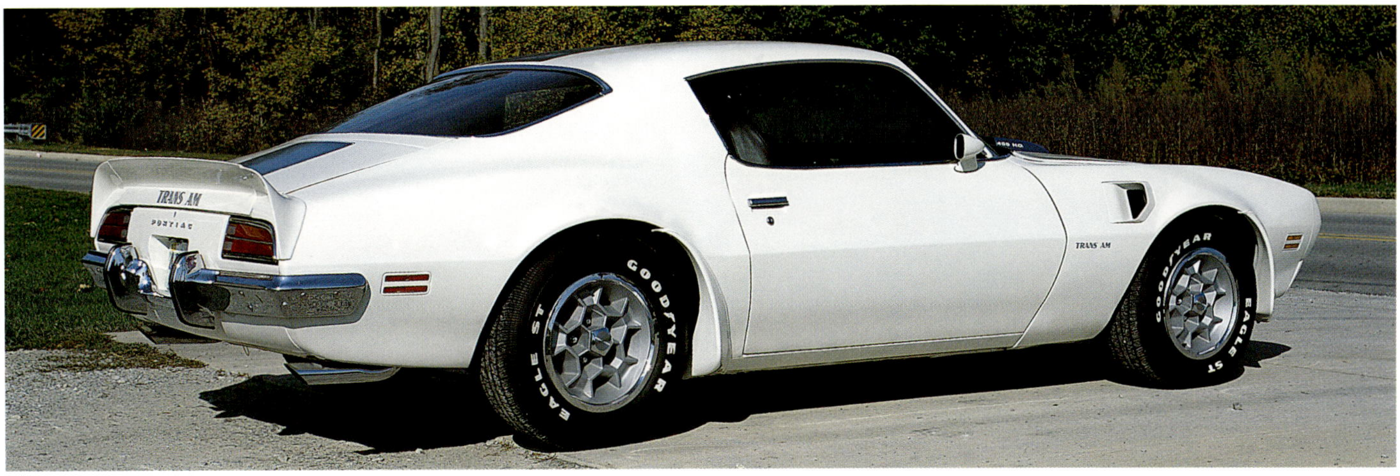

This right rear quarter view shows the rear quarter panel on a white 1971 Trans Am 455 HO. The quarter panel design was used with little change throughout the second-generation Firebird models. Note the distinctive Trans Am fender opening spoilers on the front and rear wheel openings. ***Below left:*** Detail view of the left front fender of a Lucerne Blue 1970 Trans Am sport coupe with distinctive Trans Am extractors and decals on the rear of the fender. This Trans Am is equipped with standard 15-inch modified Rally II wheels without trim rings. ***Below right:*** This view shows the right front fender of a gold 1971 Firebird Formula 350. Note the Formula 350 badge and one-year-only extractor louvers. This Formula has optional 14-inch Rally II wheels and bright trim rings.

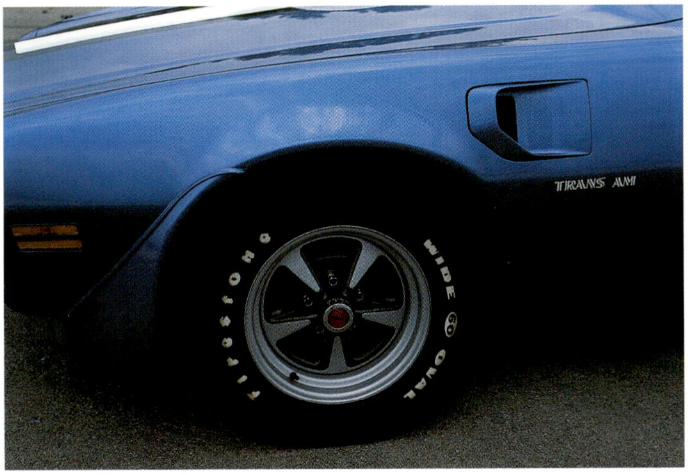

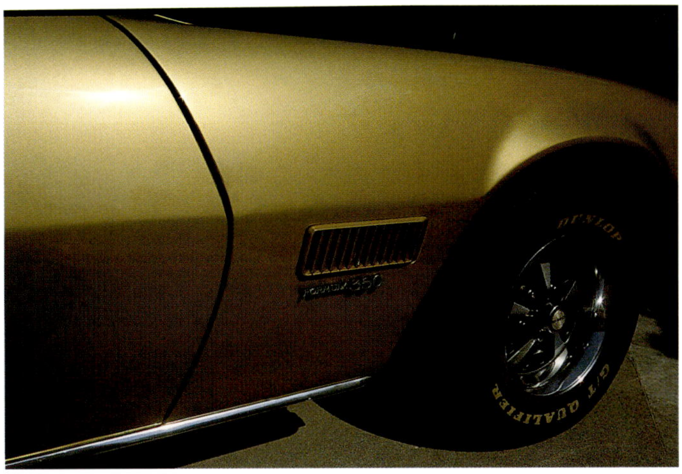

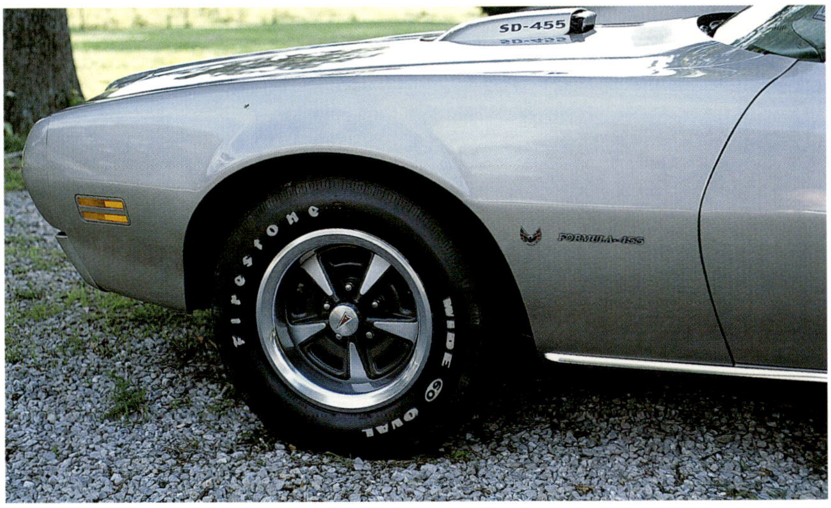

This is the left front fender of an Ascot Silver 1973 Firebird Formula SD 455. The Formula 455 and Firebird badges on the fender side are visible. This shaker hood scoop on the Formula is unique to the SD 455 engine option.

extraction vent at the upper rear. The Trans Am fender had a separate wide spoiler mounted at the front of the wheel opening. The wheel opening spoiler tied to the front lip spoiler at each end and had a body-color seal around its mounting joint with the fender. The Trans Am also had a Trans Am decal just under the body character line and the vent opening. All other models had a bright Firebird badge mounted at the rear center just below the body crease line. The 400 added an identification badge below the Firebird badge. A two-section rectangular marker light was mounted in the front of the fender just below the body crease.

For 1971, the Firebird front fenders were similar to the 1970 fenders but a rectangular simulated extraction vent with vertical louvers was mounted below the body crease line just behind the front wheel opening on all but the Trans Am. Each of the (new for 1971) Formulas carried chrome-plated block letter name plates below these vents

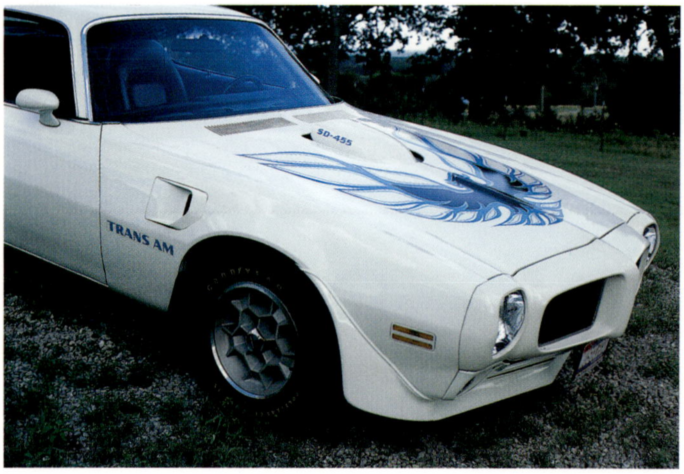

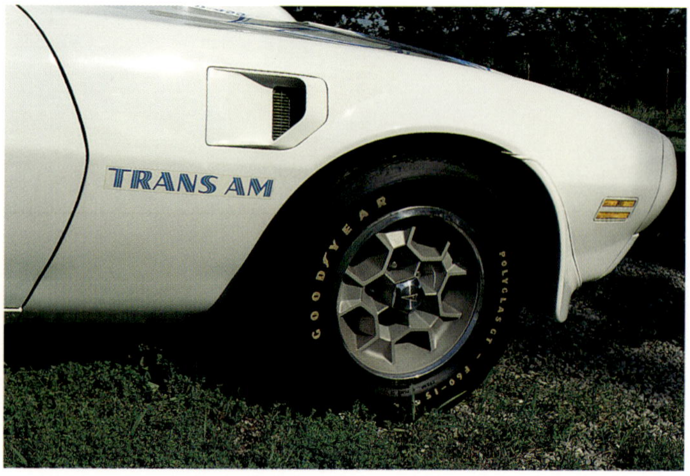

Above left: This Cameo White 1973 Trans Am SD 455 features the distinctive fender air extractor, decal, and wheel opening spoiler used only on the Trans Am. This was the first year for the optional Trans Am bird decal (UPC WW7) on the hood. ***Above right:*** Detail view of the right front fender of a white 1973 Trans Am SD 455 sport coupe with the unique functional Trans Am engine heat extractor and Trans Am decal. This Trans Am has optional 15-inch Honeycomb wheels and standard F60x15 Goodyear Polyglas GT white letter tires.

denoting "Formula 350," Formula 400," or "Formula 455" respectively. In 1972 and 1973, the extraction vent was eliminated and the fenders were plain (except on the Trans Am) as in 1970.

There were four different hoods used on the 1970–1973 Firebirds. The standard Firebird used a flat steel hood with a slightly raised longitudinal center crease (part number 478390). The 1970–1972 Formula used a molded fiberglass hood (part number 480172) with two forward-mounted flat oval scoops with their nonfunctional openings above the hood surface. The standard Formula hood part number was changed to 490660 for 1973. When Ram Air (UPC WU3) was ordered on 1971–1973 Firebird Formula, the Formula hood (part number 490661/superceded 479677) was changed to include functional openings in the scoops. This hood with functional scoops was standard when the 455 engine (except the 1973 SD 455) was ordered in the Formula. The mid-model-year 1973 Formula SD 455 used the same shaker-type hood and rear-facing scoop as the 1970–1973 Trans Am. The shaker hood was used to reduce EPA emissions certifications requirements that would have been necessary on multiple configurations.

The 1970–1973 Trans Am used a hood with part number 485389 or (later) 498391 with an opening in the rear center to allow for the standard rear-facing functional shaker scoop and air cleaner assembly used on the Ram Air engine.

The 1971 and 1972 Trans Am scoop had 455 HO decals. The 1973 Trans Am and 1973 Formula SD used SD 455 decals. The Trans Am 455 used a "455" decal. All of the 1970–1972 Trans Am decals were white-on-blue or blue-on-white depending upon the body color. The Formula used a black or white decal. The center of the

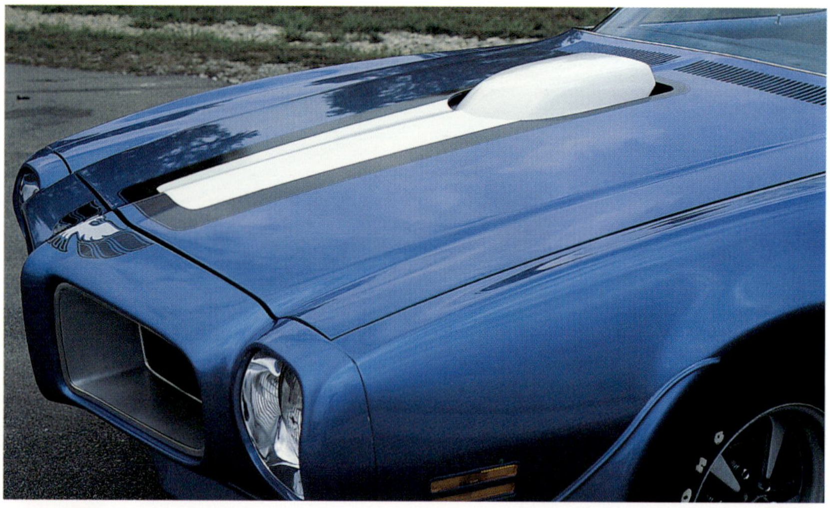

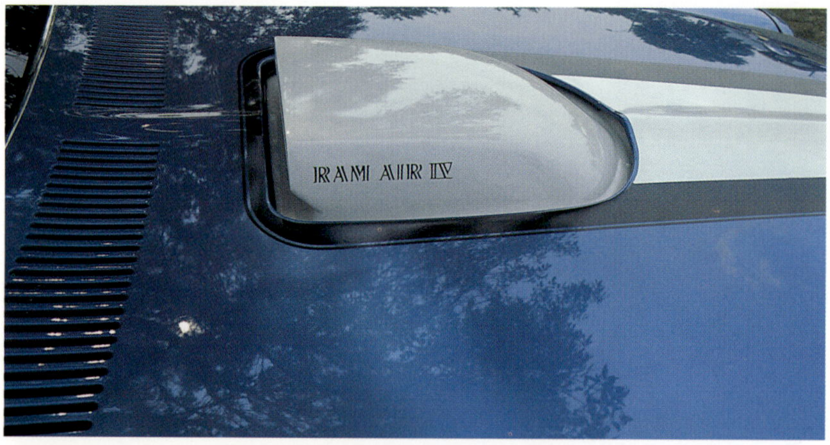

Top: This Lucerne Blue 1970 Trans Am has the standard shaker hood scoop opening. The white stripe with black outline and white bird are used with the blue body color. Note the depth of the 1970 grille surround. ***Above:*** This is a detail view of the hood and shaker scoop on a Lucerne Blue 1970 Trans Am. The black-bordered distinctive wide white stripe used in 1970 is visible. This Trans Am is equipped with the optional Ram Air IV 400 engine.

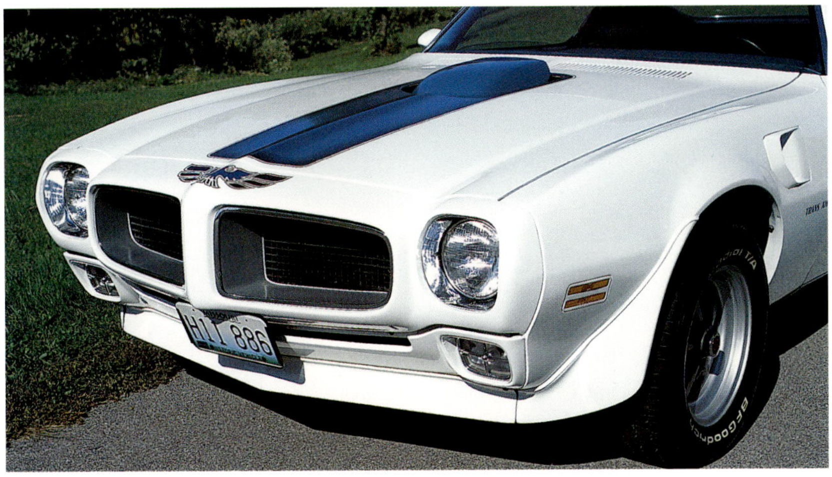

Above: Detail view of the front fascia and hood on a white 1970 Trans Am sport coupe. The hood with shaker scoop opening, blue stripe on the hood and body, and the bird on the nose were standard with the Trans Am. Note the rectangular parking lights and side markers.

1970–1972 Trans Am hood had a wide blue or white (depending upon the corresponding blue or white body color) stripe to match the finish on the scoop. The stripe surrounded the scoop opening, and the blue stripe on the white body color had a thin stripe around its perimeter. The wide white stripe on the Lucerne blue body color was surrounded by a wide black stripe with a thin outer stripe. There were no engine decals or badges on the standard 1971–1973 hoods, but the shaker scoop on the Formula and Trans Am Super Duty carried a SD 455 engine identification decal in the same colors as the stripe. The Formula with the functional Ram Air hood had "Ram Air" decals on the outside of each scoop.

The most noticeable image of the 1973 Trans Am, and all Trans Ams after, was the large bird decal on the hood with its wings surrounding the scoop opening. The bird was an option in 1973 (UPC WW7) and was available in blue (part

Right: The 1971 Formula 350 used a unique fiberglass hood with twin nonfunctional scoops at its front. This Formula is finished in gold. Note the Firebird badge on the top center of the front fascia. ***Below:*** This detail view of the Endura front fascia of a white 1970 Trans Am shows the standard fine-bordered blue stripe on the hood and bird decal on the fascia.

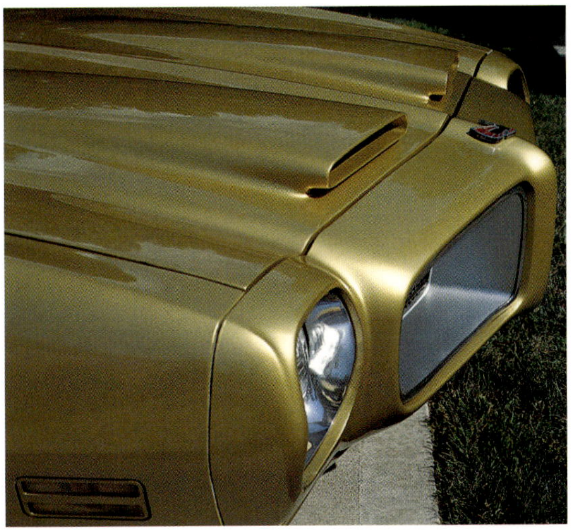

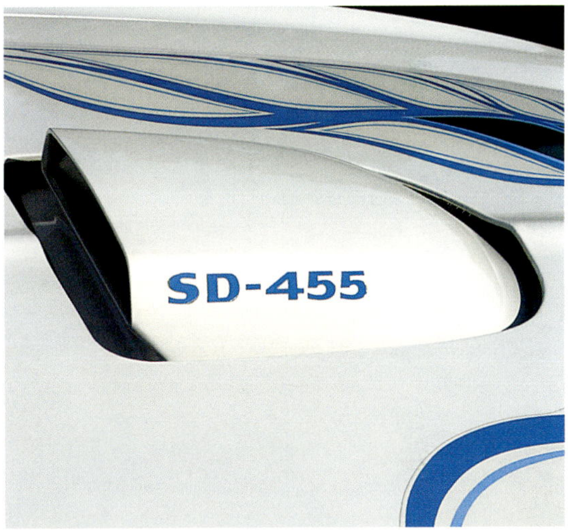

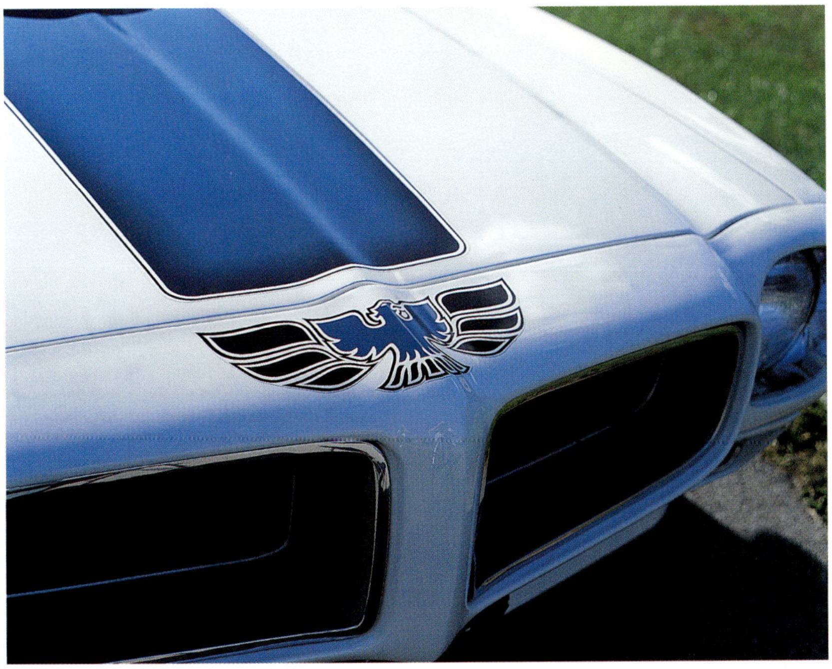

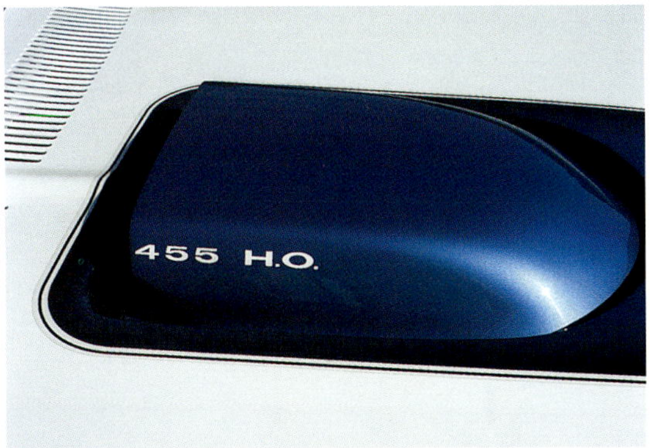

Top: A detail view of the hood and shaker scoop on an original white 1973 Trans Am equipped with the optional SD 455 engine and the optional large bird decal on the hood. ***Above:*** This is a detail view of the hood and rear-facing shaker scoop on a white 1971 Trans Am equipped with the optional 455 HO engine. Note the narrow blue stripe surrounding the wide blue main stripe panel.

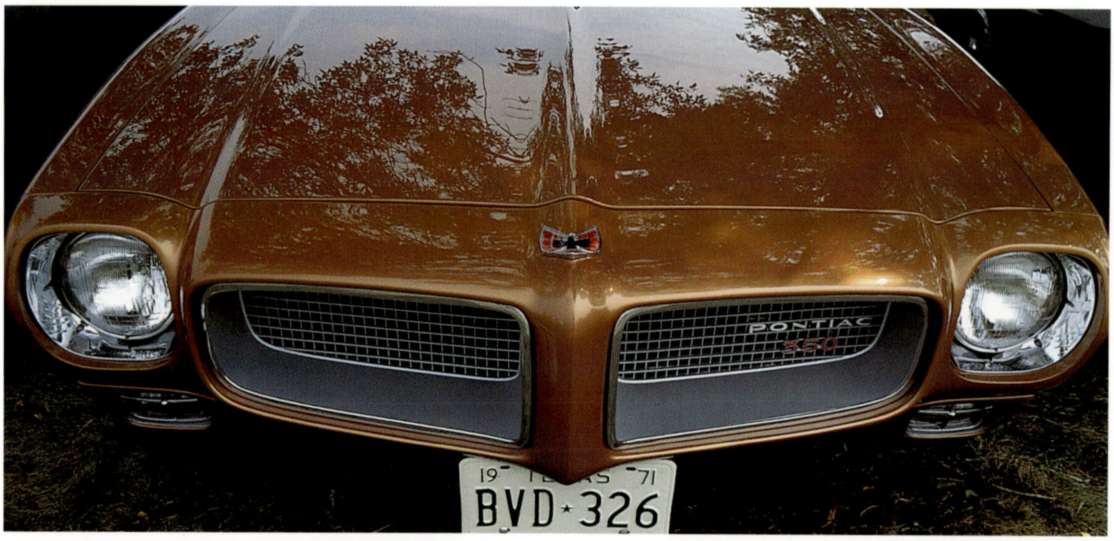

Left: The front fascia of a Canyon Copper (62) 1971 Firebird Esprit sport coupe equipped with an optional 350 V-8 engine. Note the silver finish of the standard Firebird grille mesh and the 350 grille badge.

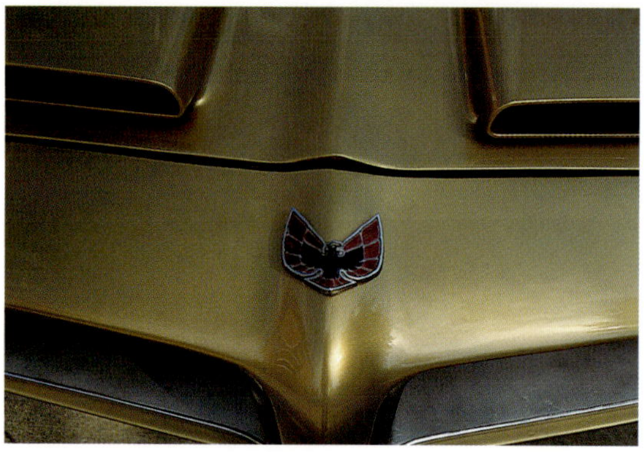

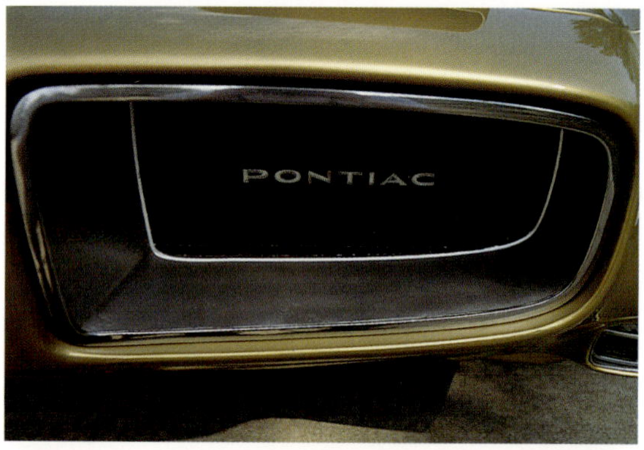

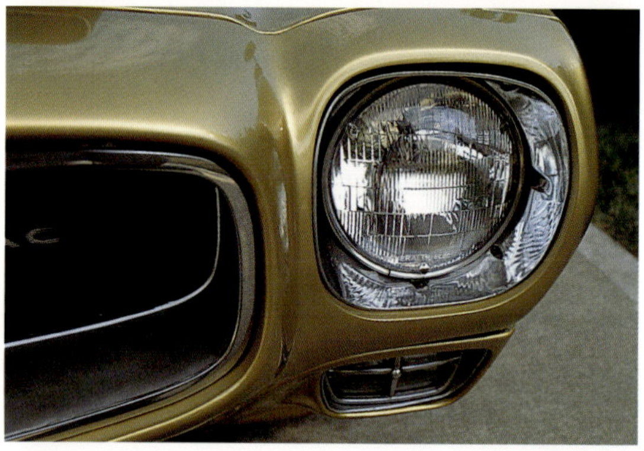

Far left: Detail view of the front fascia of a gold 1971 Firebird Formula 350, including the Firebird badge and distinctive Formula nonfunctional twin scoops on the fiberglass hood. ***Left:*** The grille mesh of a gold 1971 Firebird Formula 350 sport coupe with a bright grille surround and Pontiac nameplate. Note the depth of the grille compared to the redesigned 1973 Firebird grille. ***Lower left:*** A detail view of the left headlight and bezel of a gold 1971 Firebird Formula 350. The 1971 parking light was rectangular.

number 493370) for the white body color; green (part number 493371) with the green body color; and orange (part number 493372) with the red body color.

All 1970–1973 Firebirds had a deep, full body-color flexible Endura rubber front end panel with distinctive dual recessed oval grilles and a divider in the center. There was no separate bumper, but for 1973, the fascia was reinforced with a new inner structure and upper support to better absorb collision forces. The 1973 grille openings were shallower and recessed deeper into the bumper than the earlier design, due to the increased absorption structure required by 1973 government standards.

The 1970 and 1971 grille inserts were rectangular screens and were black on the Formula and Trans Am and Argent Silver on the Firebird and Esprit. The 1972 grille inserts were a horizontally elongated honeycomb design and were black on the Formula and Trans Am. The 1970–1972 grille inserts had a deep silver surround with bright outer rim for all models. For 1973, the grille had a rectangular mesh, was shallower on all models, and did not have the deep silver surround used in the 1970–1972 models. A single round headlamp was mounted at each end of the fascia in a slightly square deep bezel. The

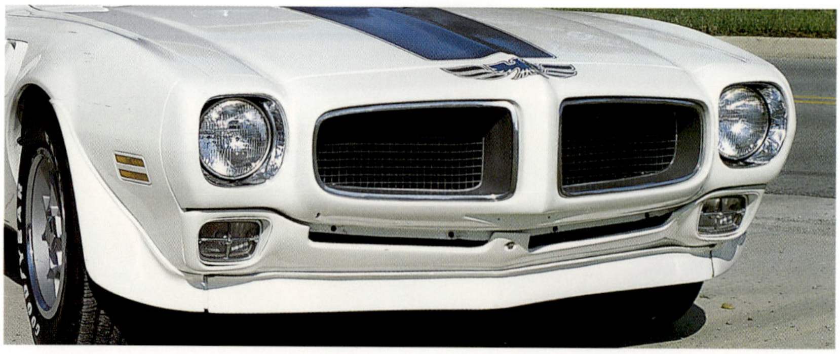

The front fascia on this white 1971 Trans Am has the same stripe and bird decal as those used in 1970. Note the blue shaker scoop with 455 HO decal and standard Trans Am front spoiler.

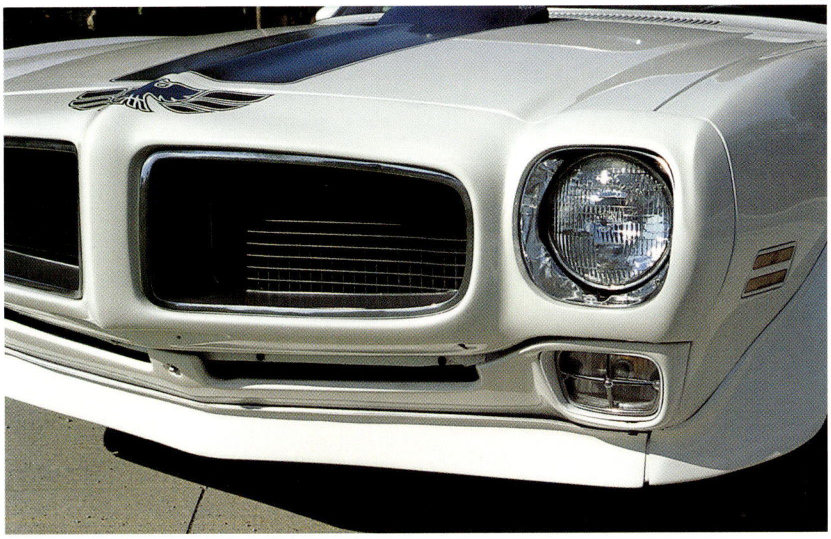

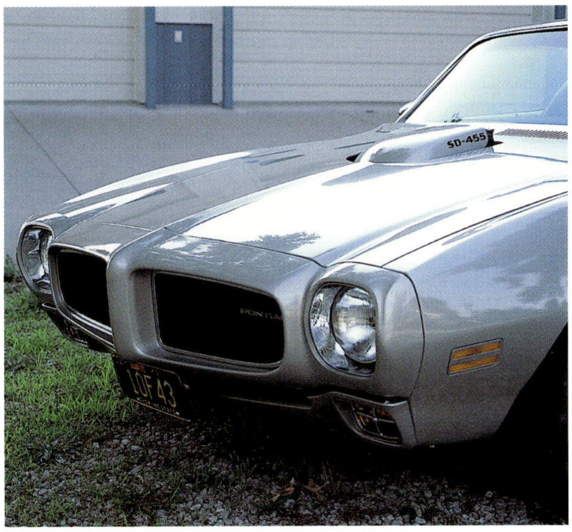

Above: Note the dark grille mesh and rectangular headlight bezel design on this original white 1971 Trans Am sport coupe. The rectangular side marker light is on the outside of the front fender. ***Right:*** The left front quarter of an Ascot Silver 1973 Firebird Formula SD 455; the grille surround is shallower than that of the 1970–1972 Firebirds to allow for the new front fascia design. The 1973 front end was redesigned to satisfy new government crash standards.

license plate was mounted in the lower center of the front fascia. A steel lower valance was mounted beneath the front fascia with a single rectangular parking lamp housing under each headlamp bezel. In early 1972, the valance was changed to plastic. The 1970 and 1971 and some early 1972 parking light lenses were clear, while the 1972 and 1973 lenses were amber. The parking light bezels were the same for 1969–1973.

The Trans Am had an additional lower front spoiler connected to the front fender flares and mounted below the lower valance. The 1970 and 1971 Firebird, Esprit, and Formula had a red-and-black Firebird badge in the top center of the fascia. There was no badge on the 1972 and 1973 models. The Trans Am had a large Trans Am bird decal in the top center the same width as the hood stripe.

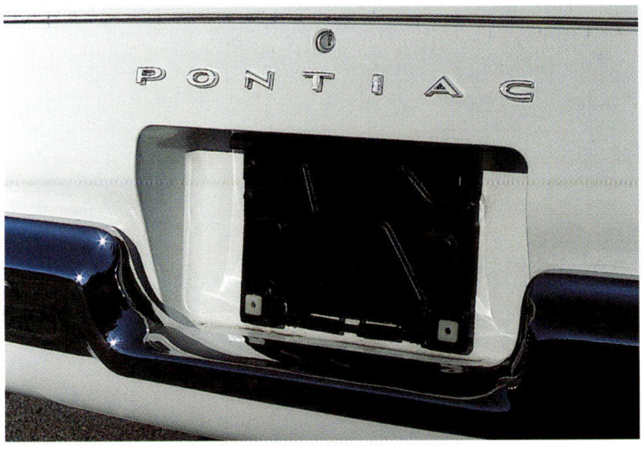

The fuel filler cap is located behind the license plate mounting plate on this white 1970 Trans Am. Note the black finish on the fold-down plate and the Pontiac nameplate on rear deck lower panel.

Firebird Production

1970	
Model	**Production**
Firebird Six	3,134
Firebird V-8	15,740
Esprit	18,961
Formula 400	7,708
Trans Am Ram Air	3,108
Trans Am Ram Air IV	88
1971	
Model	**Production**
Firebird Six	2,975
Firebird V-8	20,047
Esprit	20,185
Formula	7,802
Trans Am 455 HO	2,116
1972	
Model	**Production**
Firebird	12,001
Esprit	11,415
Formula	5,249
Trans Am	1,286
1973	
Model	**Production**
Firebird	14,096
Esprit	17,249
Formula	10,123
Formula SD 455	43
Trans Am 455	4,550
Trans Am SD 455	252

Interior

The 1970–1973 Firebird was available with a variety of interior trim combinations, all with standard front bucket seats and a solid rear seat back with individual seat cushions. The rear seat was divided into two bucket seat sections with a center cover because of the deeper driveshaft tunnel. In 1970, the Firebird, Firebird Formula, and Trans Am had the expanded Morrokide vinyl interior standard. The optional custom (UPC W54) knit-vinyl and vinyl interior combinations were standard on the Esprit and optional on the Formula and Trans Am. The all-vinyl trim was optional with the Esprit.

The 1970 standard interior seat pattern had transverse pleats with smooth bolsters and skirts, all in Madrid-grain vinyl. The bucket seat back was square with relatively straight sides and headrests on the standard seats. Standard vinyl was

Body Colors

1970 Body Colors

Code	Color
10	Polar White
14	Palladium Silver
25	Bermuda Blue
26	Lucerne Blue
28	Atoll Blue
43	Keylime Green
45	Palisade Green
47	Verdoro Green
51	Goldenrod Yellow
53	Coronado Gold
58	Granada Gold
63	Palomino Copper
65	Carousel Red
67	Castillion Bronze
75	Cardinal Red

1971 Body Colors

Code	Color
11	Cameo White
13	Nordic Silver
19	Starlight Black
24	Adriatic Blue
26	Lucerne Blue
42	Limekist Green
43	Tropical Lime
49	Laurentian Green
53	Quezal Gold
59	Aztec Gold
61	Sandalwood
62	Canyon Copper
67	Castillian Bronze
75	Cardinal Red
78	Rosewood

1972 Body Colors

Code	Color
11	Cameo White
14	Revere Silver
24	Adriatic Blue
26	Lucerne Blue
36	Julep Green
43	Springfield Green
48	Wilderness Green
50	Brittany Green
53	Quezal Gold
55	Shadow Gold
56	Monarch Yellow
57	Brasillia Gold
63	Anaconda Gold
65	Sundance Orange
75	Cardinal Red

1973 Body Colors

Code	Color
11	Cameo White
24	Porcelain Blue
26	Regatta Blue
29	Admiralty Blue
42	Verdant Green
44	Slate Green
46	Golden Olive
48	Brewster Green
51	Sunlight Yellow
56	Desert Sand
60	Valencia Gold
64	Ascot Silver
68	Burma Brown
74	Florentine Red
75	Buccaneer Red
97	Navajo Orange

available in blue (201), saddle (205), brown (206), sandalwood (207), and black (208). The custom interior seats had an insert with transverse pleats and a longitudinal seam on each side. The bolsters and skirts were Madrid-grain vinyl, and the insert was Comfortweave knit-vinyl, available in blue (211), brown (213), red (214), saddle (215), green (216), sandalwood (217), and black (218). The custom interior was also available with a cloth insert in sandalwood (227) or black (228). The seat backs for the custom interior were more rounded on the sides and top than the standard seat backs. A color-coordinated front console with padded, covered compartment was available as an option with UPC D55. A color-keyed rear console was available for the 1971–1973 Firebird Esprit, Formula, and Trans Am with UPC D58.

The 1971 standard interior of the Firebird, Firebird Formula, and Trans Am also consisted of Madrid-grain Morrokide vinyl bucket seats in front and separate cushions and a solid back in the rear. The standard high-back bucket seat backs were more rounded at the top than the 1970 models, and the trim pattern was again transverse pleats with smooth bolsters and skirts. The standard vinyl was available in blue (201), saddle (203), jade (206), sandalwood (207), and black (209). The Firebird Esprit had standard custom vinyl with Comfortweave inserts with cloth optional. The cloth-and-vinyl was available in sandalwood (227) or black (229). The custom patterned-vinyl

Interior Trim

1970

Code	Color
201	Medium Bright Blue vinyl
205	Medium Saddle vinyl
206	Midnight Green vinyl
207	Medium Sandalwood vinyl
208	Black vinyl
211	Medium Bright Blue vinyl (custom)
213	Dark Brown vinyl (custom)
214	Medium Red vinyl (custom)
215	Medium Saddle vinyl (custom)
216	Midnight Green vinyl (custom)
217	Medium Sandalwood vinyl (custom)
218	Black vinyl (custom)
227	Medium Sandalwood cloth and vinyl (custom)
228	Black Vinyl cloth and vinyl (custom)

1971

Code	Color
201	Dark Blue vinyl
203	Dark Saddle vinyl
206	Dark Jade vinyl
207	Light Sandalwood vinyl
209	Black vinyl
211	Dark Blue vinyl (custom)
212	Ivory vinyl (custom)
213	Dark Saddle vinyl (custom)
214	Dark Sienna vinyl (custom)
216	Dark Jade vinyl (custom)
217	Light Sandalwood vinyl (custom)
219	Black vinyl (custom)
227	Light Sandalwood cloth and vinyl (custom)
229	Black cloth and vinyl (custom)

1972

Code	Color
121	Ivory vinyl
131	Dark Saddle vinyl
141	Dark Green vinyl
161	Black vinyl
211	Dark Blue vinyl (custom)
221	Ivory vinyl (custom)
231	Dark Saddle vinyl (custom)
241	Dark Green vinyl (custom)
251	Light Beige vinyl (custom)
261	Black vinyl (custom)
351	Light Beige cloth and vinyl (custom)
361	Black cloth and vinyl (custom)

1973

Code	Color
321	White vinyl
331	Saddle vinyl
361	Black vinyl
421	White vinyl (custom)
431	Saddle vinyl (custom)
461	Black vinyl (custom)
471	Burgundy vinyl (custom)
551	Beige cloth and vinyl (custom)

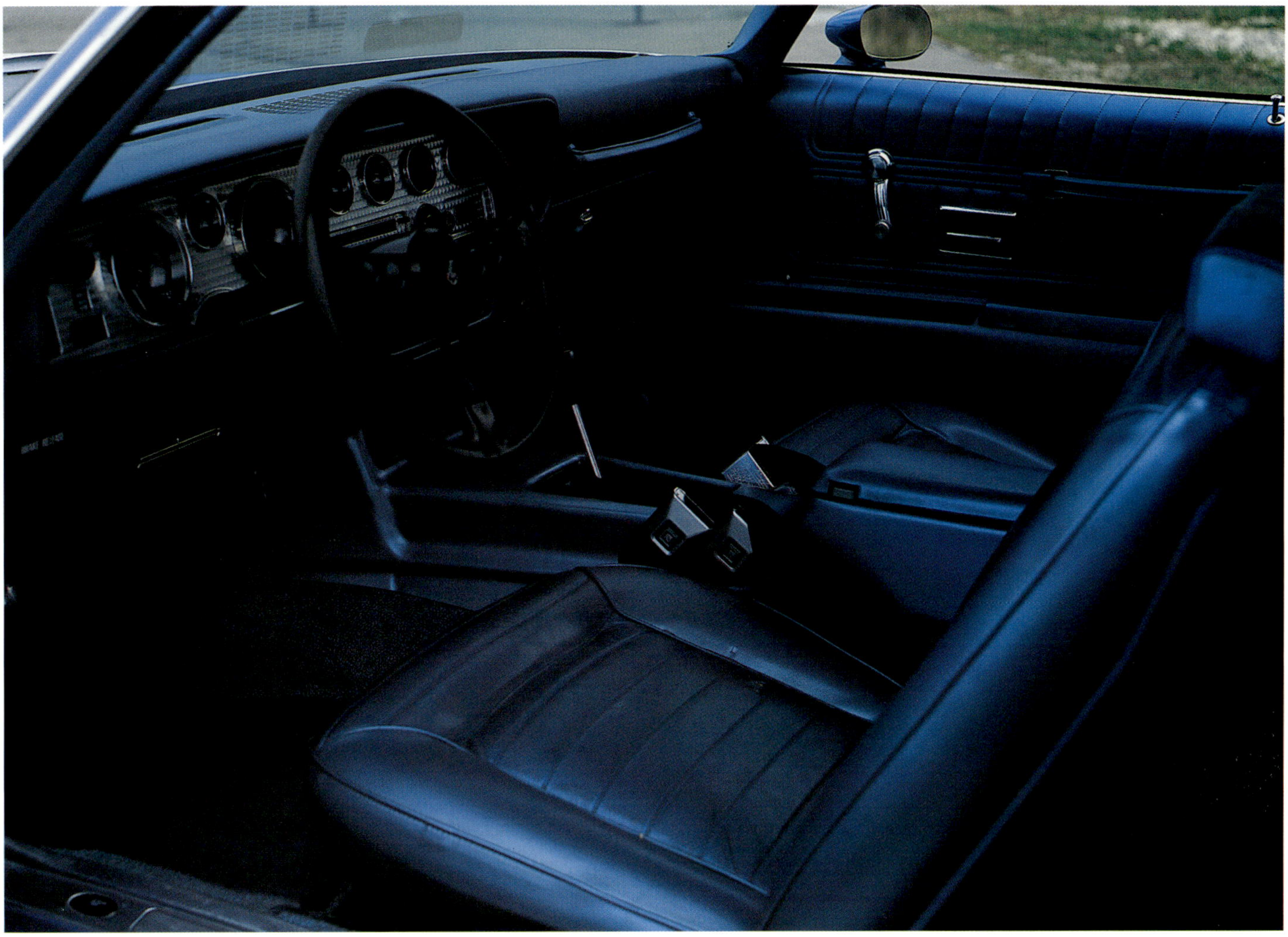

Above: The interior driver's compartment of this Lucerne Blue (26) 1970 Trans Am has blue vinyl interior trim (201) and Strato bucket seats. The Formula steering wheel is standard equipment in the Trans Am. ***Below:*** The left door panel of a Lucerne Blue 1970 Trans Am with blue vinyl interior. This Trans Am has a standard remote-control body-color left side mirror. Left and right side body-color outside sport mirrors were standard with the 1970 Trans Am.

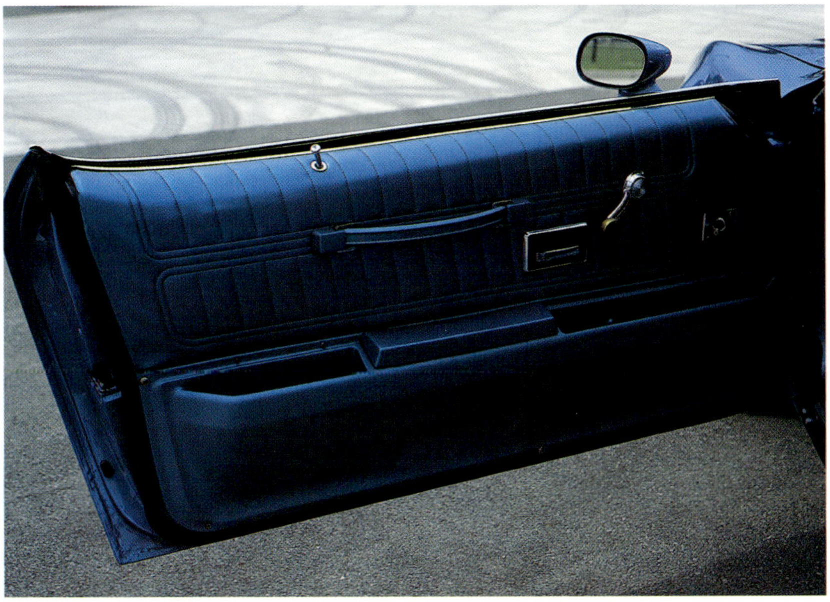

or cloth-and-vinyl interior was optional in the Formula and Trans Am. The custom patterned-vinyl was offered in blue (211), ivory (212), sienna (213), jade (214), sandalwood (217), and black (219).

A color-coordinated console with padded, covered compartment was available with option UPC D55 and only with a floor shifter. A color-keyed rear console was available for the Firebird Esprit, Formula, and Trans Am with UPC D58. Door panels for the 1970 and 1971 standard interiors had Madrid-grain vinyl with inserts of vertical pleats. Door panels for 1970 and 1971 deluxe interiors were Madrid-grain vinyl with a Comfortweave insert.

For 1972, the standard interior for the Firebird, Firebird Formula, and Trans Am was all-vinyl bucket seats in front and separate seat cushions and a solid back in the rear. The bucket seat backs had a rounded top with transverse pleats, twin longitudinal seams and smooth bolsters, and skirts as in the previous year. The standard vinyl interior trim was available in ivory (121, 221), saddle (131, 231), green (141, 241), black (361, 261), and beige (351, 251). The Firebird Esprit had standard vinyl bucket seats with perforated-vinyl

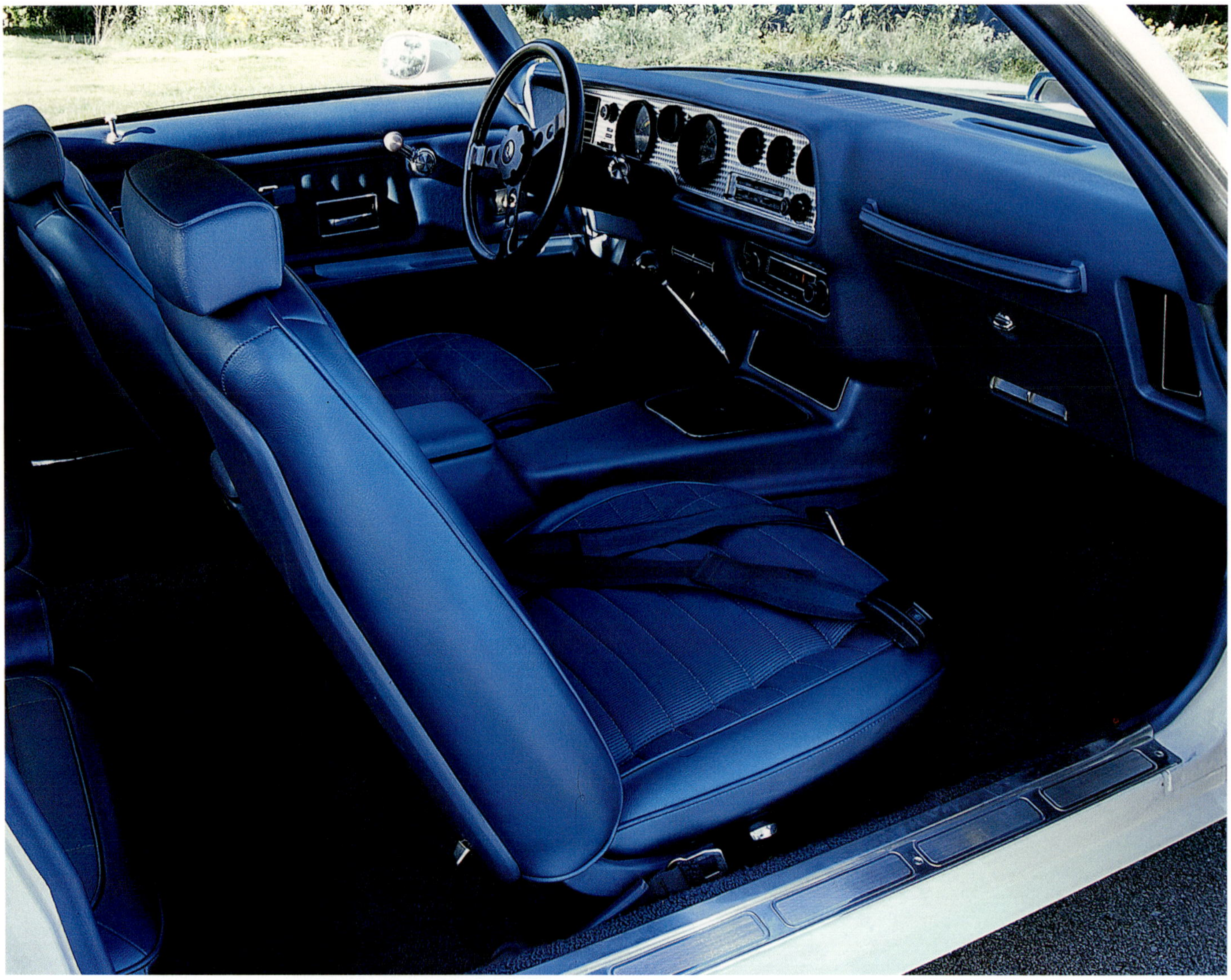

Selected 1970–1973 Regular Production Options

UPC/RPO	Description
AL4	Strato bench seat with fold-down center armrest (coupe only)
AU3	Electric door locks
AU5	Electric door and seatback locks
A01	Soft-Ray glass
A01	Soft-Ray windshield
A31	Power windows
AK1	Custom seatbelts
AK2	Custom front and rear seatbelts
A90	Remote deck lid release
B32	Front floor mats
B33	Rear floor mats
B80	Roof drip moldings
B84	Body side moldings
B93	Door edge guards
C24	Concealed windshield wipers
C08	Cordova top
C60	Air conditioning
C49	Rear window defroster
C88	Convenience lamps
D34	Visor vanity mirror
D35	Body color mirrors, left and right
D55	Floor console
D80	Rear spoiler
D98	Accent stripes
G80	Safe-T-Track rear axle
G90	Performance axle
JL2	Power front disc brakes, 1972 and 1973
J50	Power front disc brakes, 1970 and 1971
K05	Engine block heater
K45	Dual-stage, heavy-duty air cleaner
L30	350 2-bbl 255 horsepower
L65	400 2-bbl 265 horsepower
L74	400 4-bbl Ram Air 345 horsepower
L75	455 4-bbl
L78	400 4-bbl
LS2	455 4-bbl SD
LS5	455 4-bbl HO
M12	Three-speed manual w/floor shift
M20	Four-speed manual
M22	Four-speed manual
M38	Turbo Hydra-Matic, three-speed
M40	Turbo Hydra-Matic, three-speed
M35	Two-speed automatic
N33	Tilt steering wheel
NK3	Formula steering wheel
N30	Deluxe steering wheel
N65	Space-saver spare tire
N95	Wire wheel covers
N98	Rally II wheels
PL3	E78x14 white tires
PX6	F78x14 white tires
PL4	F70x14 white letter tires
PM7	Rally II wheels w/F60x15 white letter tires
PY6	F70x14 black tires
P05	Honeycomb wheels
P06	Trim rings
TP1	Maintenance-free battery
UA1	Heavy-duty battery
U05	Dual horns
U30	Rally gauge cluster
U35	Electric clock
U57	Stereo tape player
U58	Stereo radio, AM/FM
U63	Stereo radio, AM w/windshield antenna
U80	Rear speaker
W54	Custom trim option
W74	Warning lamps and clock
WS6	Power-assist group
WT5	Mountain performance option
WU3	Hood air inlet
WW7	Trans Am hood decal
Y80	Décor moldings group
Y82	Basic group
Y88	Basic group

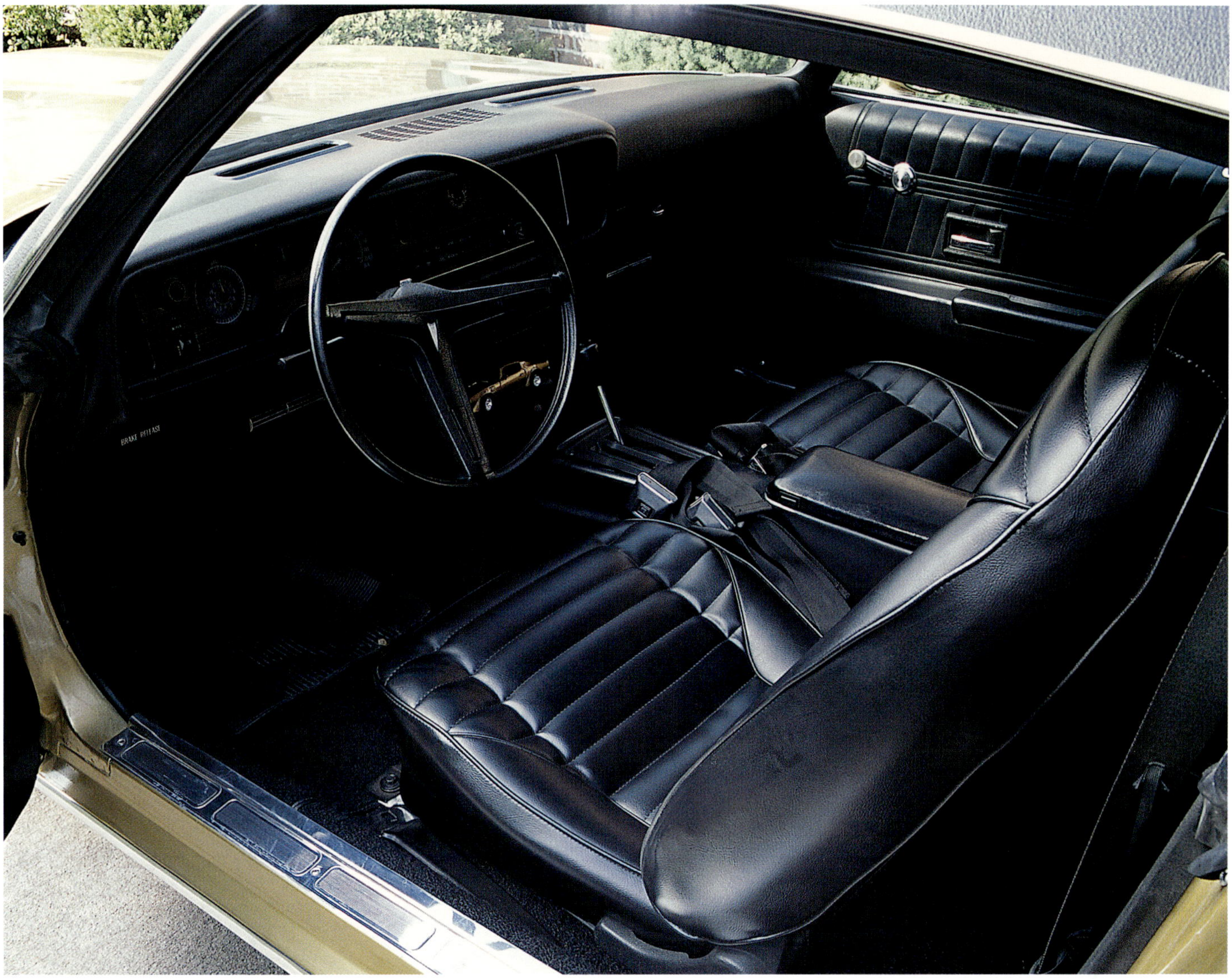

Opposite: The front driver's compartment of this Polar White 1970 Trans Am has the optional blue and knit vinyl (211) interior trim with Strato bucket seats. It is equipped with an optional four-speed manual transmission and optional color-keyed floor console. ***Above:*** The driver's compartment of this gold 1971 Firebird Formula 350 sport coupe has the optional black vinyl interior (209) and Strato bucket seats. This Formula is equipped with a floor console (UPC D55) and optional Turbo Hydra-Matic 350 automatic transmission with console-mounted shifter.

inserts in black (502) and blue (562) and optional cloth. The Firebird Formula and Trans Am were available with optional custom patterned-vinyl or cloth-and-vinyl interior trim. The custom vinyl was available in black (512, 531, 532), green (602), beige (632, 642), and tan (661). A color-keyed console with padded, covered compartment was available as an option with UPC D55 when a floor shift was ordered. A color-keyed rear console was available with UPC D58. The 1972 standard interior door panels were Madrid-grain vinyl with an insert of vertical pleats.

The standard interior for the 1973 Firebird, Firebird Formula, and Trans Am was again all-vinyl front bucket seats and individual seat cushions with a solid back in the rear, but the transverse pleats were wider than the previous years. The Esprit had standard custom vinyl with vinyl-and-cloth as an option. The standard vinyl was available in white (321), saddle (331), and black (361). The optional cloth-and-vinyl and perforated-vinyl was available in white (421), saddle (431), black (461), and burgundy (471). The cloth-and-vinyl was available only in beige (551). A color-keyed front console with padded, covered compartment was available with UPC D55 and a floor shifter. A rear console was also available with UPC D58. Door panels for the 1973 deluxe interior were Madrid-grain vinyl with smooth Tetra-grain inserts.

All models used loop-pile nylon carpet color-coordinated with the interior trim, except the ivory-and-white interiors, which used black carpeting. Power windows were available as an

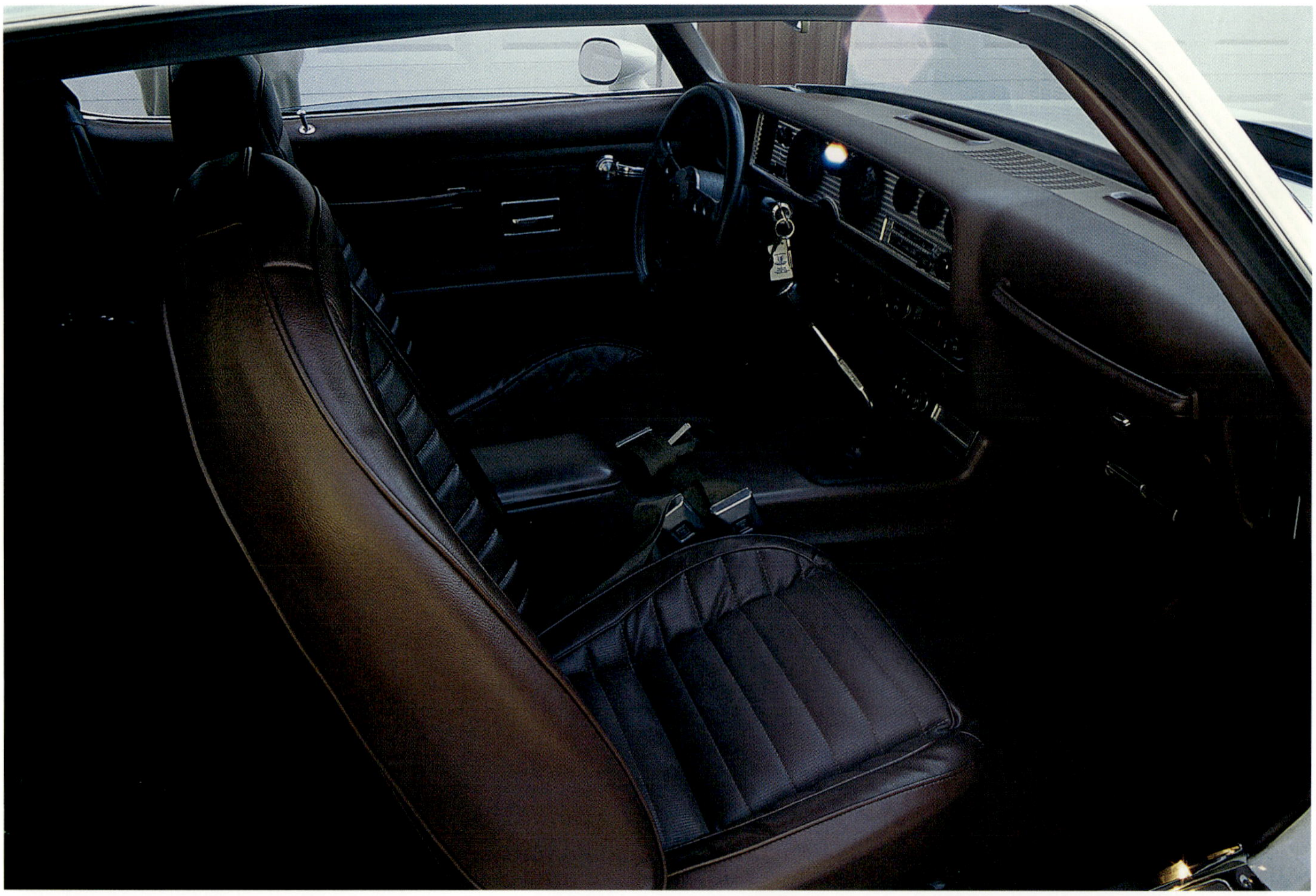

option (UPC A31) in all models equipped with a console because the window control was located in the console. Electric door locks were available as an option (UPC AU5) in all models.

The 1970–1973 Firebird instrument panel was fully padded, color-coordinated vinyl with a rectangular gauge cluster on the left and a large flat glove box door on the right. The instrument cluster panel was flame-chestnut wood-grain vinyl for the Firebird, Formula, and Esprit and damascened (engine-turned) aluminum for the Trans Am. The gauge cluster consisted of one large round gauge on either side of the smaller, and higher, center round gauge. The left large gauge contained the clock on the Firebird and the tachometer and clock on the Firebird Formula and Trans Am with the Rally gauge package. The large round gauge on the right held the speedometer on all models. The smaller center gauge had the coolant temperature and oil pressure.

The Firebird Formula and Trans Am had two more small round gauges to the upper right on the main cluster that held the turn signal indicators on the left and the voltmeter on the right. The Rally gauge cluster and clock were available as an option in the Firebird V-8 and Esprit with UPC W63 and as gauge cluster and tachometer with UPC U30. The heater and air conditioning controls were mounted to the lower right of the main gauge cluster in all models.

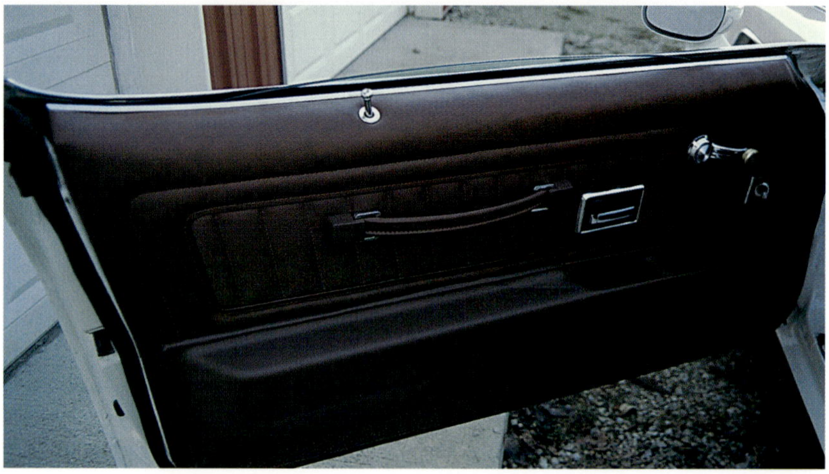

Top: This is the driver's compartment interior of a white 1971 Trans Am equipped with the optional Sienna (213) custom vinyl interior and Strato bucket seats. The car is equipped with an optional four-speed manual transmission (UPC M20) with floor console-mounted shifter. ***Above:*** The right door panel of a 1971 Trans Am with the optional Sienna custom vinyl interior. Note the standard vinyl door-pull handle and remote-control left side mirror.

There was no standard radio on any 1970–1973 Firebird model, but an AM push-button radio (UPC U63), AM/FM radio (UPC U69), or

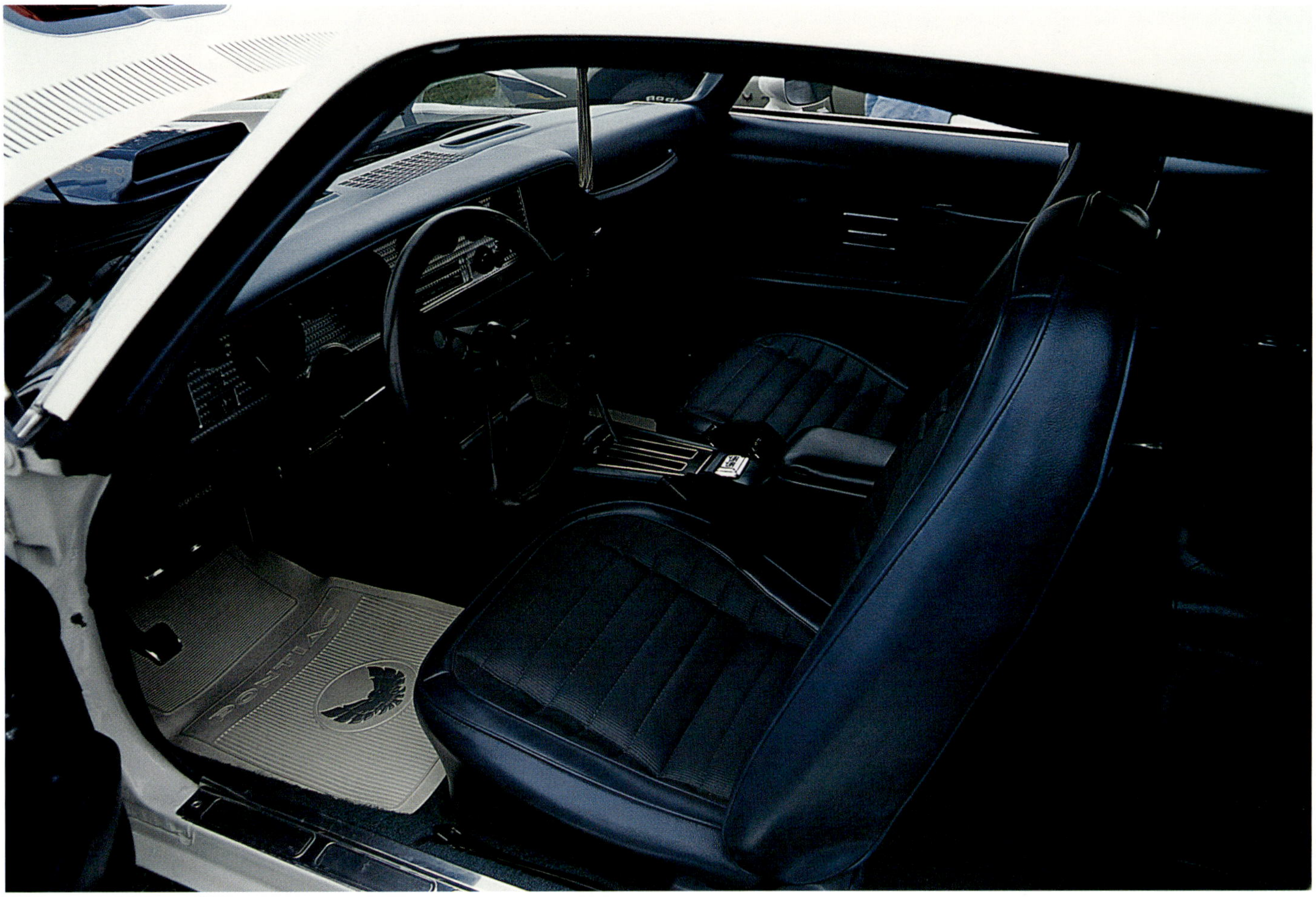

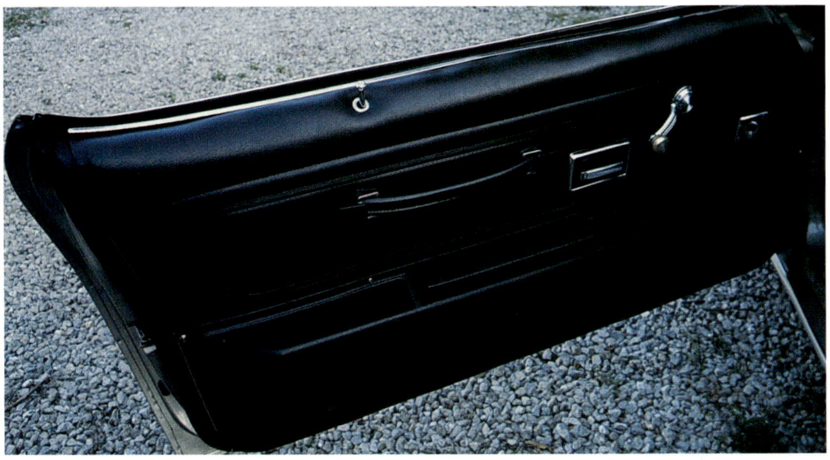

Top: This Cameo White 1971 Trans Am is equipped with an optional blue custom vinyl interior (211) and an optional automatic transmission with console-mounted shifter. The white front floor mat is an accessory. ***Above:*** The left door panel of an Ascot Silver 1973 Formula SD 455 sport coupe with a black vinyl interior. Note the design of the black vinyl door-pull handle and arm rest.

AM/FM stereo radio (UPC U58) were available as options in all models; the radio was mounted in the lower center of the instrument panel. An optional separate cassette tape player (UPC U55) or stereo 8-track tape player (UPC U57) was available in all models and mounted under the center of the instrument panel. A rear speaker was also available with UPC U80 on all except stereo radios or stereo tape players. The basic group option package (UPC Y88) included the push-button AM radio. The radio antenna was integral with the windshield in all 1970–1973 Firebird models equipped with a radio.

The standard steering wheel for the 1970–1973 Firebird was a color-keyed, thin-rimmed plastic, two-spoke shallow-dish design with horn button bars on the end of each spoke and an arrowhead badge in the center. The custom deluxe steering wheel was a color-keyed plastic, three-spoke shallow-dish design with a cushioned vinyl-covered rim and Pontiac arrowhead in the center and a small, narrow triangular horn button on each spoke. In 1970, the wood-rim sport steering wheel was the same as the one used in 1969 and was available as an option with UPC N34. The 14-inch-diameter three-spoke Formula steering wheel (UPC NK3) had a soft-molded urethane foam rim and center horn button and was standard with the Trans Am. The Formula steering wheel was available as an option in the Firebird, Firebird Esprit, and Formula. The Formula steering wheel was only available with power steering.

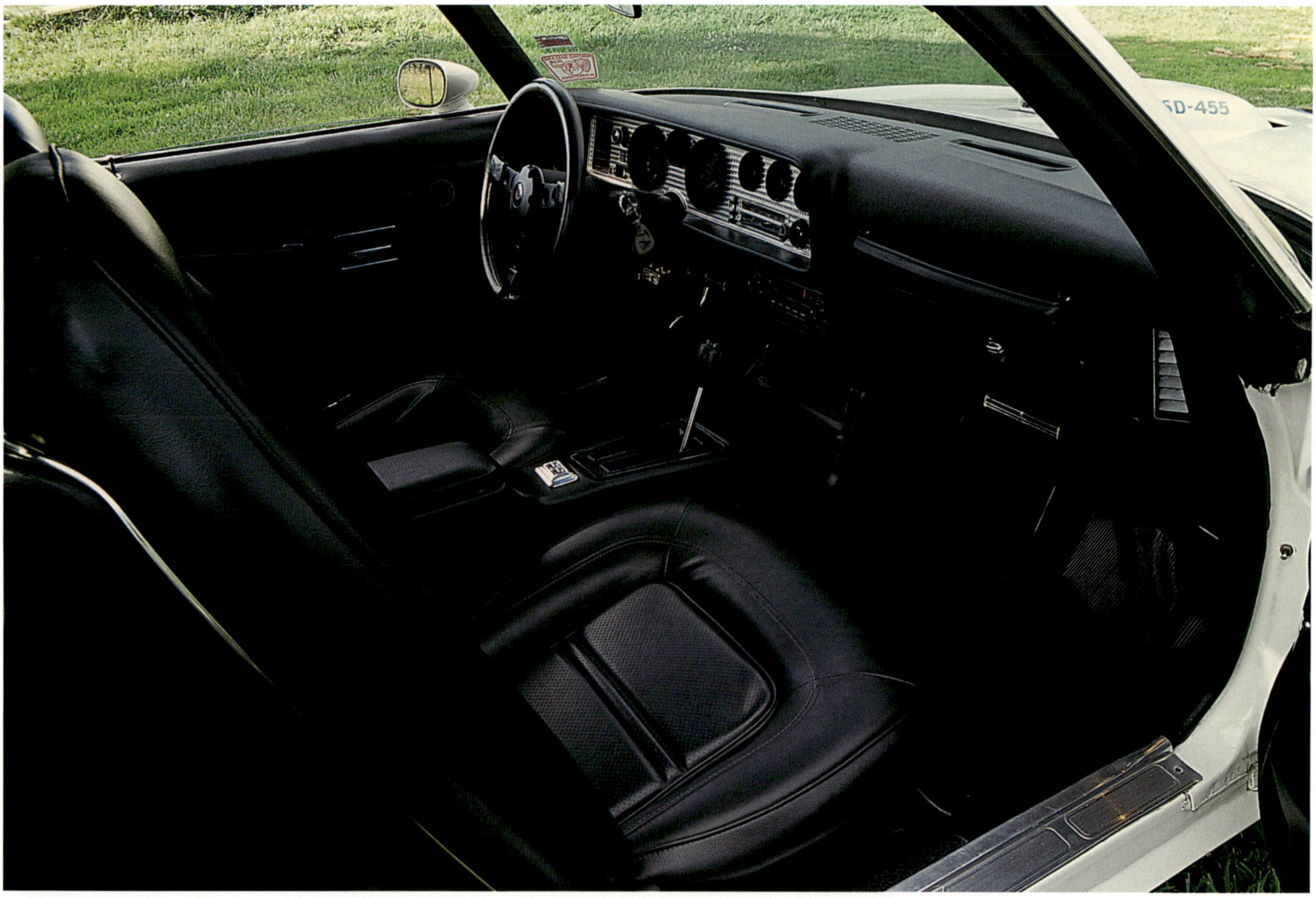

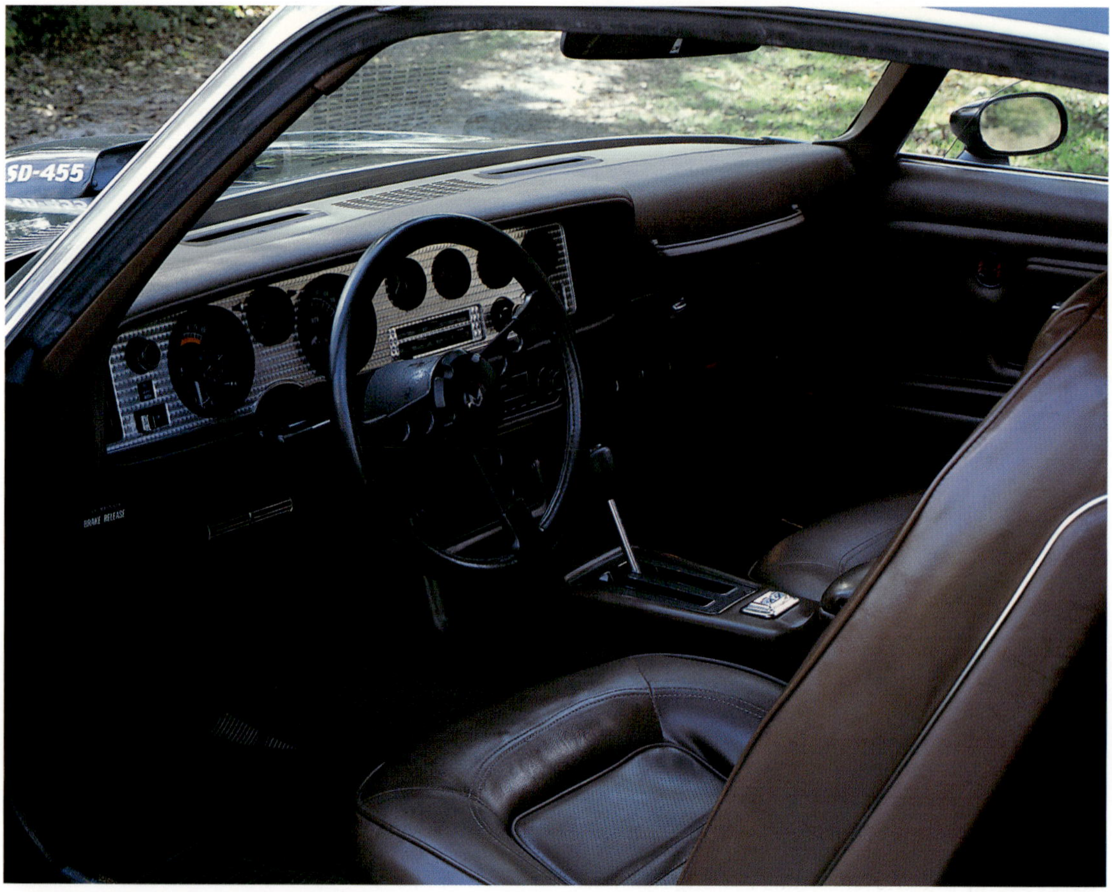

Above: The driver's compartment interior of an original 1973 Trans Am SD 455 with a black vinyl interior and Strato bucket seats. This Trans Am is equipped with the optional three-speed automatic transmission and console-mounted shifter. ***Left:*** This is a detail view of the interior driver's compartment of a Brewster Green 1973 Trans Am with an optional saddle (431) vinyl interior trim. The center seat insert is perforated vinyl in this trim combination.

Right: The instrument panel cluster of the 1973 Firebird Formula has a straight wood-grain finish rather than the engine-turned finish used in the Trans Am. This Formula is equipped with optional Rally gauges with tachometer instrument cluster (UPC WW8) and has a standard deluxe steering wheel (UPC N30). *Below:* This view of the right door panel of an original white 1973 Trans Am SD 455 with black vinyl interior trim (361) includes the Trans Am medallion on the upper door panel.

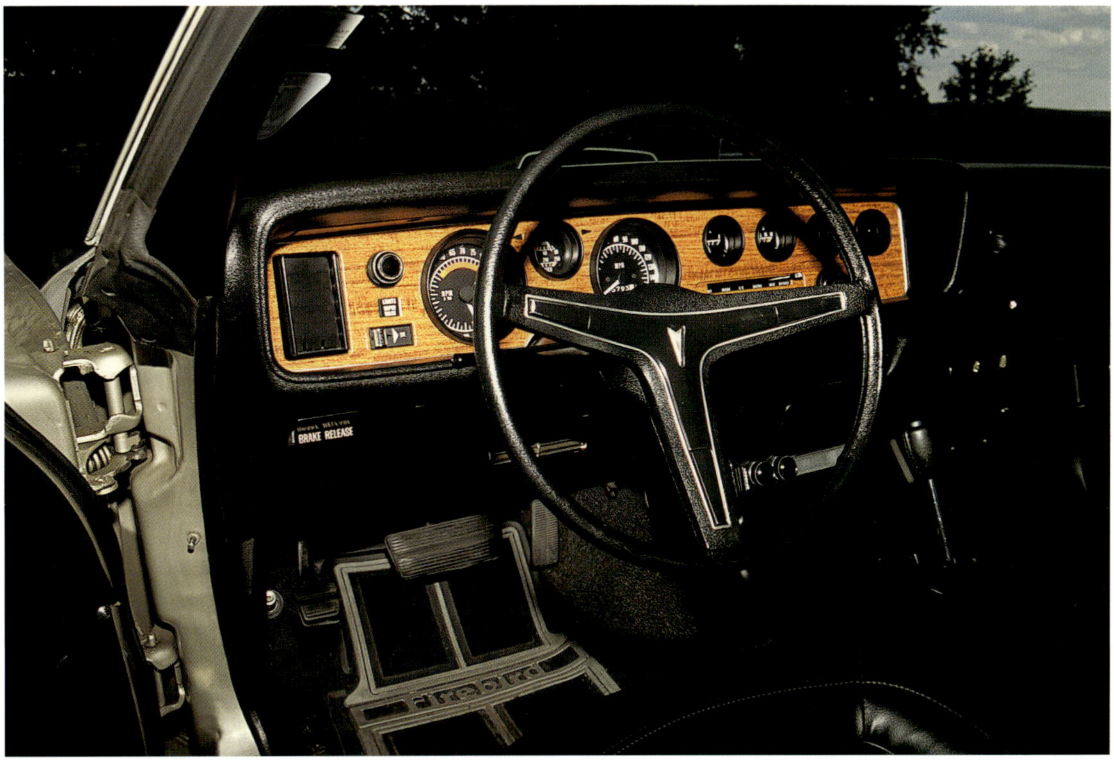

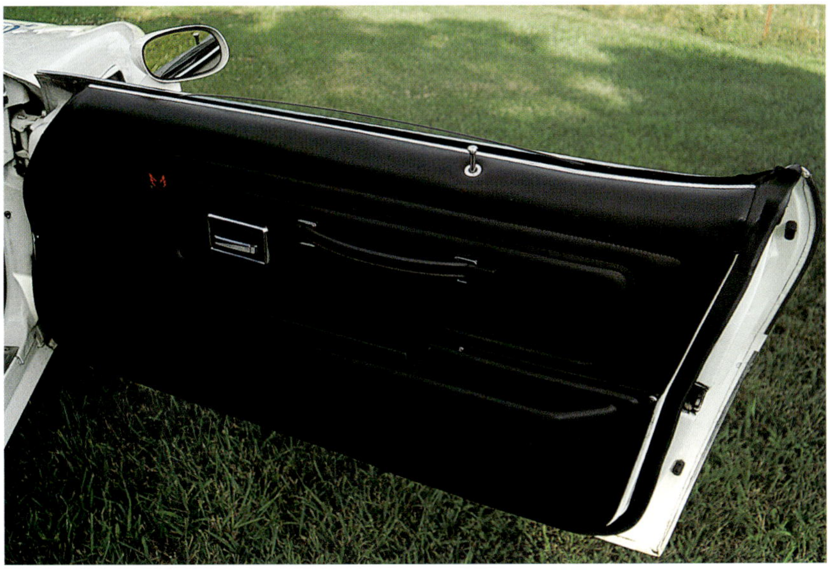

Engine and Engine Compartment

The 1970 Firebird was available with six engine choices. The standard engine in the Firebird was the 250-cubic-inch Chevrolet–built overhead-valve inline six-cylinder. The base V-8 was the 350-cubic-inch overhead-valve with a single two-barrel carburetor. The optional V-8 was 400-cubic-inches and was available in four versions, from the 265 to the 345-horsepower Ram Air IV.

Engine choices were still six in 1971, with the 250-cubic-inch inline six-cylinder standard in the Firebird, but the optional V-8 engines were now available in three displacements from 350 to 455 cubic inches and from 255 to 355 horsepower. Compression ratios had been reduced to 8.4:1 for the 455 HO. For 1972, there were five engines available, from the 250-cubic-inch six to 350-, 400-, and 455-cubic-inch V-8 choices up to 300 horsepower.

Engine choices were increased to eight for 1973, with the 250-cubic-inch inline six still standard in the base Firebird. The 350 V-8 was available in two versions from 150 to 175 horsepower and the 400 V-8 in three versions from 170 to 230 horsepower. The 455 V-8 was still available in a 250-horsepower standard single four-barrel version, but a new single four-barrel Super Duty 455 was available with a special block and heads but rated at only 290 horsepower partly due to a low 8.4:1 compression ratio. All 1971 and 1972 Trans Ams were equipped with 455 HO engines.

Overhead-Valve Six

One of the significant mechanical changes at the introduction of the new Firebird models for 1970 was the replacement of the innovative and unique Pontiac overhead-camshaft inline six-cylinder engine with a more conventional overhead-valve six built by Chevrolet. The new engine maintained the same 250-cubic-inch displacement of the last version of the Pontiac six but was otherwise completely new. The previous engine was actually based on the Chevrolet engine, so the change was not difficult.

The 1970–1973 Pontiac six was only available

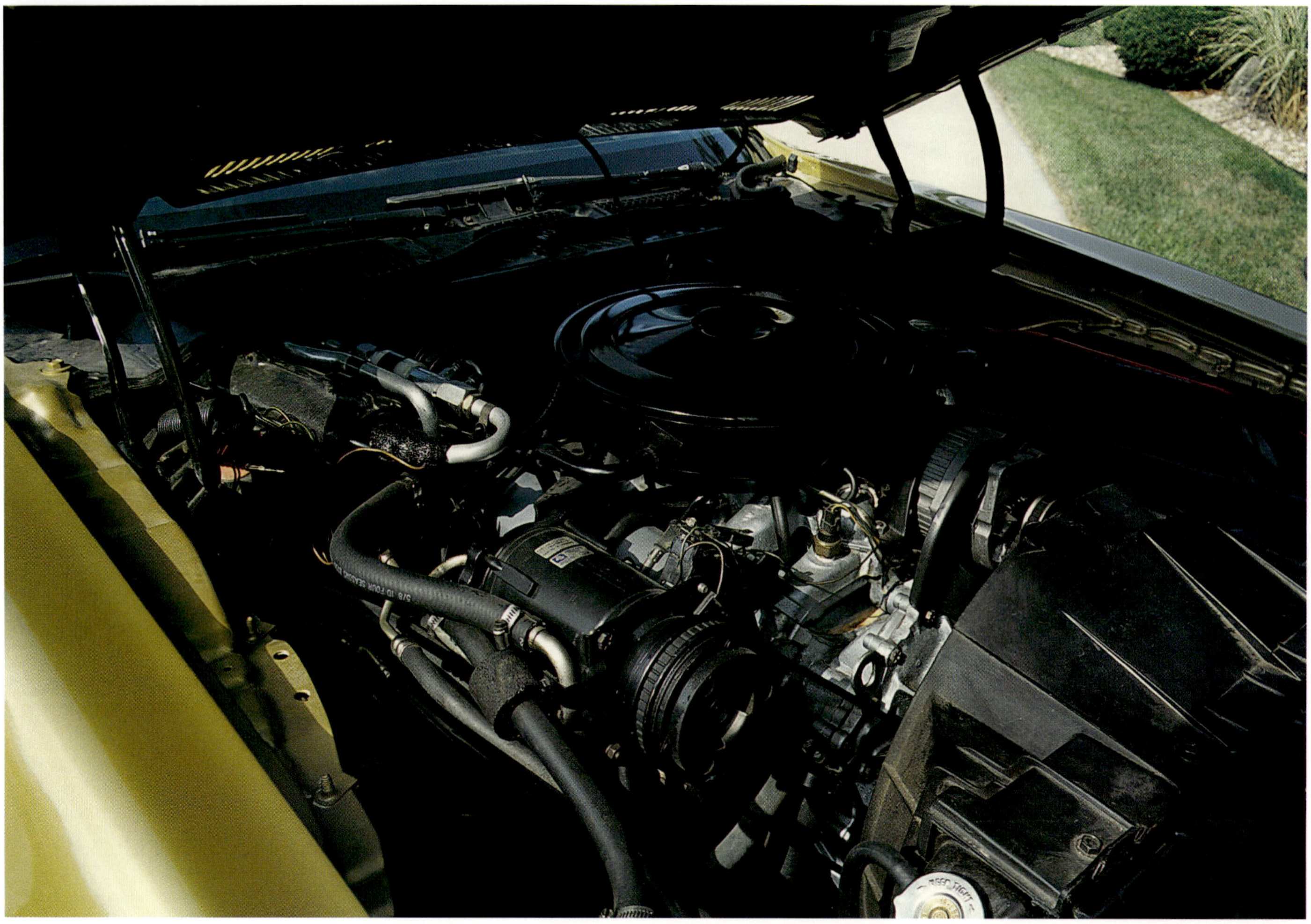

The engine compartment of a gold 1971 Firebird Formula 350 with optional air conditioning. Note the large black plastic fan shroud attached to the top of the radiator support.

in one basic configuration, and it had a cast-iron block with a bore and stroke of 3.875 inches x 3.531 inches, identical to that of the previous six. The compression ratio was 8.5:1 for 1970 and 1971, and the engine developed 155 horsepower at 4,200 rpm and 235 foot-pounds of torque at 1,600 rpm. In 1972, the horsepower rating method was changed, and the six developed 110 horsepower at 4,200 rpm with the same torque as the previous year. In 1973, the horsepower was the same but at 3,800 rpm with torque at 185 foot-pounds at 1,600 rpm. A single-barrel Rochester carburetor and hydraulic valve lifters were used both years. Engine codes were ZB with a manual transmission and ZG with the automatic in 1970, and AA and AB for 1971. The 1972 engine codes were BA, BG, BJ, and BC. For 1973, the engine was identified by a VIN engine code of D. All Pontiac six-cylinder engines were painted Pontiac Engine Blue.

Overhead-Valve V-8

The 1970–1973 Firebird five-main-bearing, overhead-valve V-8 was a continuation of the previous year's design and was available in either 350, 400, or 455 cubic inches. In 1970, the base V-8 (UPC L30) was 350 cubic inches with a bore of 3.875 inches and a stroke of 3.75 inches. The compression ratio was 8.8:1, and it developed 255 horsepower at 4,600 rpm and 355 foot-pounds of torque at 2,800 rpm. The 350 V-8 was only available with a single two-barrel Rochester carburetor and hydraulic valve lifters. All 350 V-8 engines were painted Pontiac Engine Blue. The engine codes for 1970 were WU with the manual transmission and YU with the automatic.

The optional V-8 engines offered in 1970 had 400 cubic inches. The displacement increase was accomplished by increasing the bore to 4.125 inches. The compression ratio of the UPC L65 V-8 was 8.8:1, and using hydraulic valve lifters and a single two-barrel carburetor, it developed 265 horsepower at 4,600 rpm and 397 foot-pounds of torque at 2,400 rpm. The engine code was XX and was available only with an automatic transmission. The UPC L78 version of the 400 V-8 had a 10.25:1 compression ratio and a single Rochester Quadrajet 7040263 (manual) or 7040264 (automatic) four-barrel carburetor to develop 330 horsepower at 4,800 rpm and 430 foot-pounds of torque at 3,000 rpm. The engine code was WT with a manual transmission and YS with an automatic.

There were two high-performance single four-barrel versions of the 400 V-8 available in 1970.

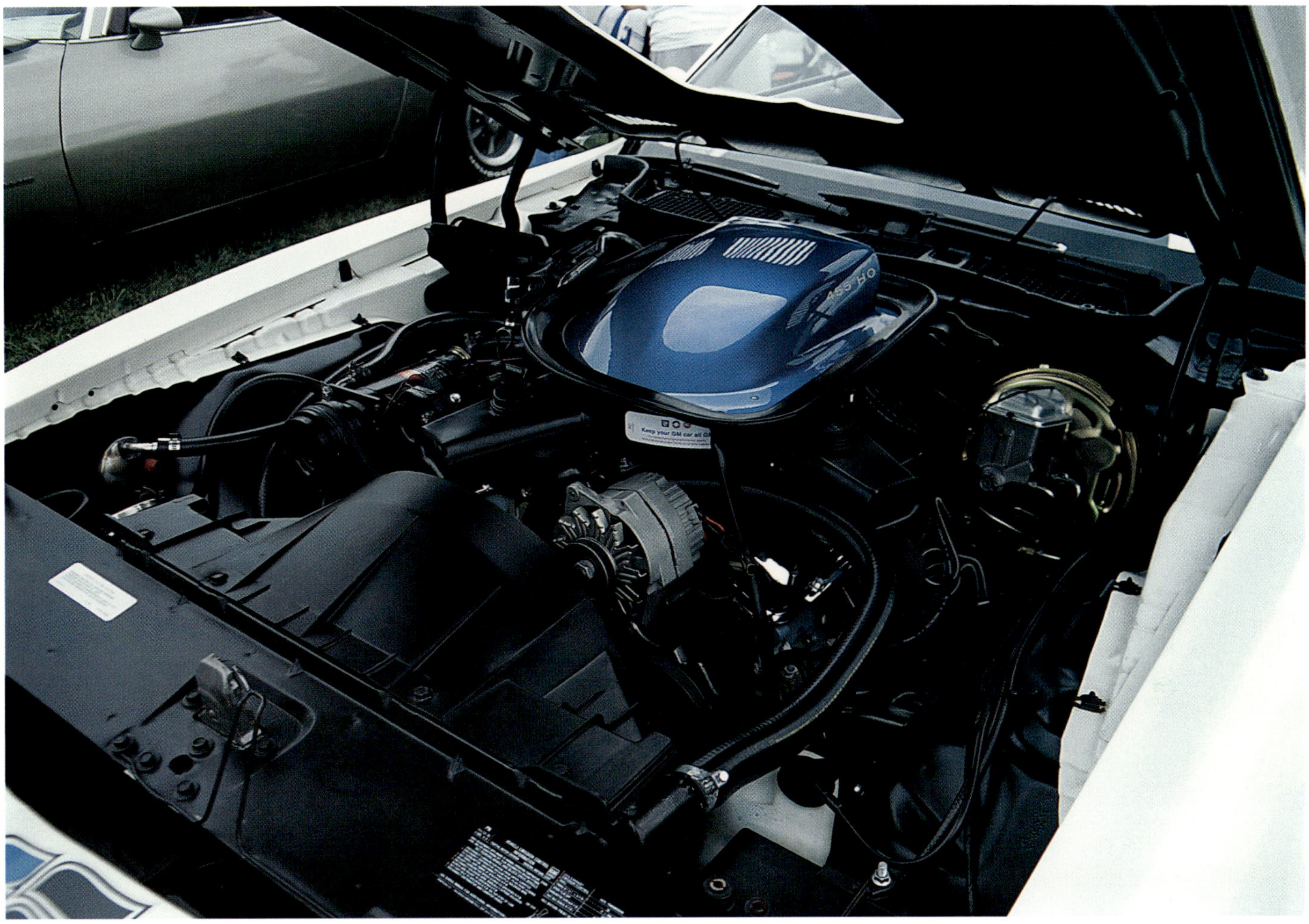

Above: This is the left front view of the engine compartment in a white 1971 Trans Am equipped with the optional 455 HO V-8. Note the decal on the air cleaner and the front of the radiator support valance. The shaker scoop is blue to match the blue stripe on the hood and body. ***Right:*** This view of the left hood hinge and bracket assembly on a white 1970 Trans Am includes the dual-reservoir brake master cylinder and power booster.

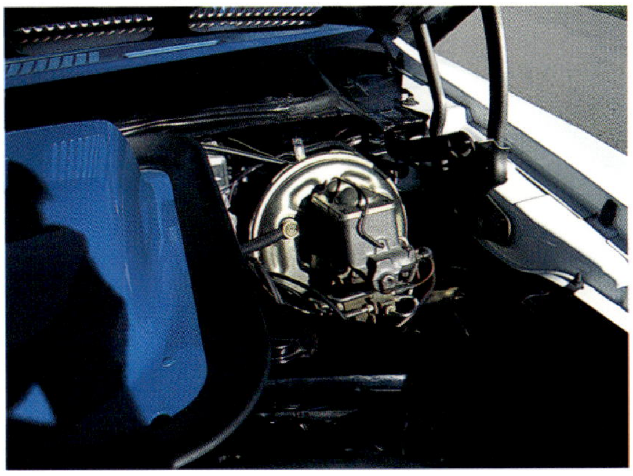

The Ram Air III (UPC L74) had a compression ratio of 10.75:1 and developed 335 horsepower at 5,000 rpm and 430 foot-pounds of torque at 3,400 rpm. Engine codes were WS with a manual transmission and YZ with an automatic. The Ram Air IV (UPC LS1) had a 10.75:1 compression ratio and developed 345 horsepower at 5,400 rpm and 430 foot-pounds of torque at 3,700 rpm. Engine codes for the Ram Air IV were XP with the automatic and WW with a manual transmission. All 1970 Trans Ams with the Ram Air IV V-8 had a 3.73:1 rear axle ratio. Both engines used a single 750-cfm Rochester Quadrajet four-barrel carburetor and hydraulic valve lifters and were painted Pontiac Engine Blue with chrome valve covers and oil filler cap.

For 1971, the 350 (UPC L30) was still the base V-8. The compression ratio was reduced to 8.2:1 for 1971, and the horsepower was 255 at 4,600 rpm with 355 foot-pounds of torque at 2,800 rpm with a single two-barrel carburetor and hydraulic valve lifters. The base 400 V-8 (UPC L65) had an 8.2:1 compression ratio, hydraulic valve lifters with a single four-barrel carburetor, and developed 265 horsepower at 4,400 rpm and 400 foot-pounds of torque at 2,400 rpm. The same XX engine code as 1971 was used, and it was still available with automatic transmission only.

There was a performance version of the 400 V-8 (UPC L78) available in 1971 with an 8.2:1 compression ratio, hydraulic lifters, and a single Rochester Quadrajet four-barrel carburetor (part numbers 7040253/7040264) that developed 300 horsepower at 4,800 rpm and 400 foot-pounds of torque at 3,600 rpm. Engine codes were WK, WT, and YS.

In 1971, two larger-displacement overhead-valve V-8 engines were offered. The 455 engine had a 4.15-inch bore and a stroke of 4.21 inches. The RPO L75 version had an 8.2:1 compression

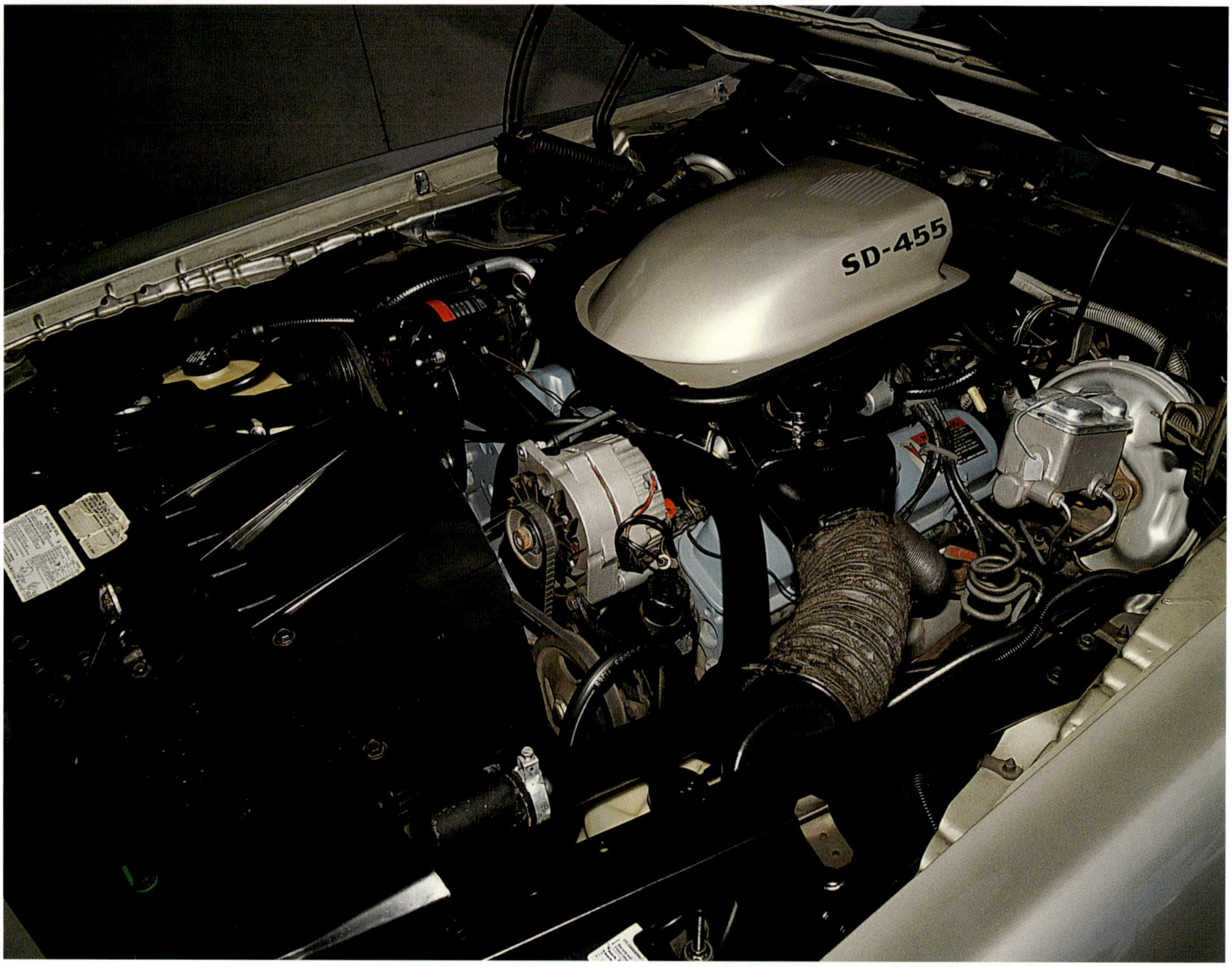

ratio and developed 325 horsepower at 4,400 rpm and 455 foot-pounds of torque at 3,200 rpm. The engine code was YC. The 455 HO engine (UPC LS5) had an 8.4:1 compression ratio and developed 335 horsepower at 4,800 rpm and 480 foot-pounds of torque at 3,600 rpm. Engine codes were WC, WL, and YE. Both engines had hydraulic valve lifters with a single 828-cfm Rochester Quadrajet four-barrel carburetor and were painted Pontiac Engine Blue.

In 1972, the 350 was still the base V-8 in all but the Trans Am. The 1972 (UPC L30) engine had an 8.0:1 compression ratio and developed 160 horsepower (175 in the Formula with dual exhausts) at 4,400 rpm and 270 (275 in the Formula 350) foot-pounds of torque at 2,000 rpm. Both versions had a single two-barrel carburetor and hydraulic valve lifters. Engine codes were WR, YV, and YR.

There were two versions of 400-cubic-inch V-8 for 1972. The base 400 V-8 (UPC L65) in the Firebird and Esprit had an 8.2:1 compression ratio with a two-barrel carburetor and developed 175 horsepower at 4,000 rpm and 310 foot-pounds of torque at 2,400 rpm. Engine codes were YX and ZX. The L65 was only available with a Turbo Hydra-Matic transmission. The UPC L78 version standard in the Formula 400 also had an 8.2:1 compression ratio but used a 750-cfm Rochester Quadrajet four-barrel carburetor and dual exhausts to develop 250 horsepower at 4,400 rpm and 325 foot-pounds of torque at 3,200 rpm. Engine codes were WK, YS, and WS.

The most powerful Firebird engine for 1972 was the 455 HO standard in the Trans Am and the Formula 455. The 455 HO (UPC LS5) had an 8.4:1 compression ratio and developed 300 horsepower at 4,000 rpm and 415 foot-pounds of torque at 3,200 rpm. The 455 HO used hydraulic valve lifters and had a four-barrel carburetor and dual exhausts. The forward air scoops on the Formula 455 were functional. The engine numbers were WD and YE with the older-type breaker-point ignition distributor and WM and YB with the new transistorized breakerless ignition system. All 1972 V-8 engines were painted Pontiac Engine Blue.

This is a view of the left engine compartment of an original Ascot Silver 1973 Formula equipped with the SD 455 engine. Note the unique decal on the left rear valve cover of the 455 engine. This Formula is equipped with optional air conditioning.

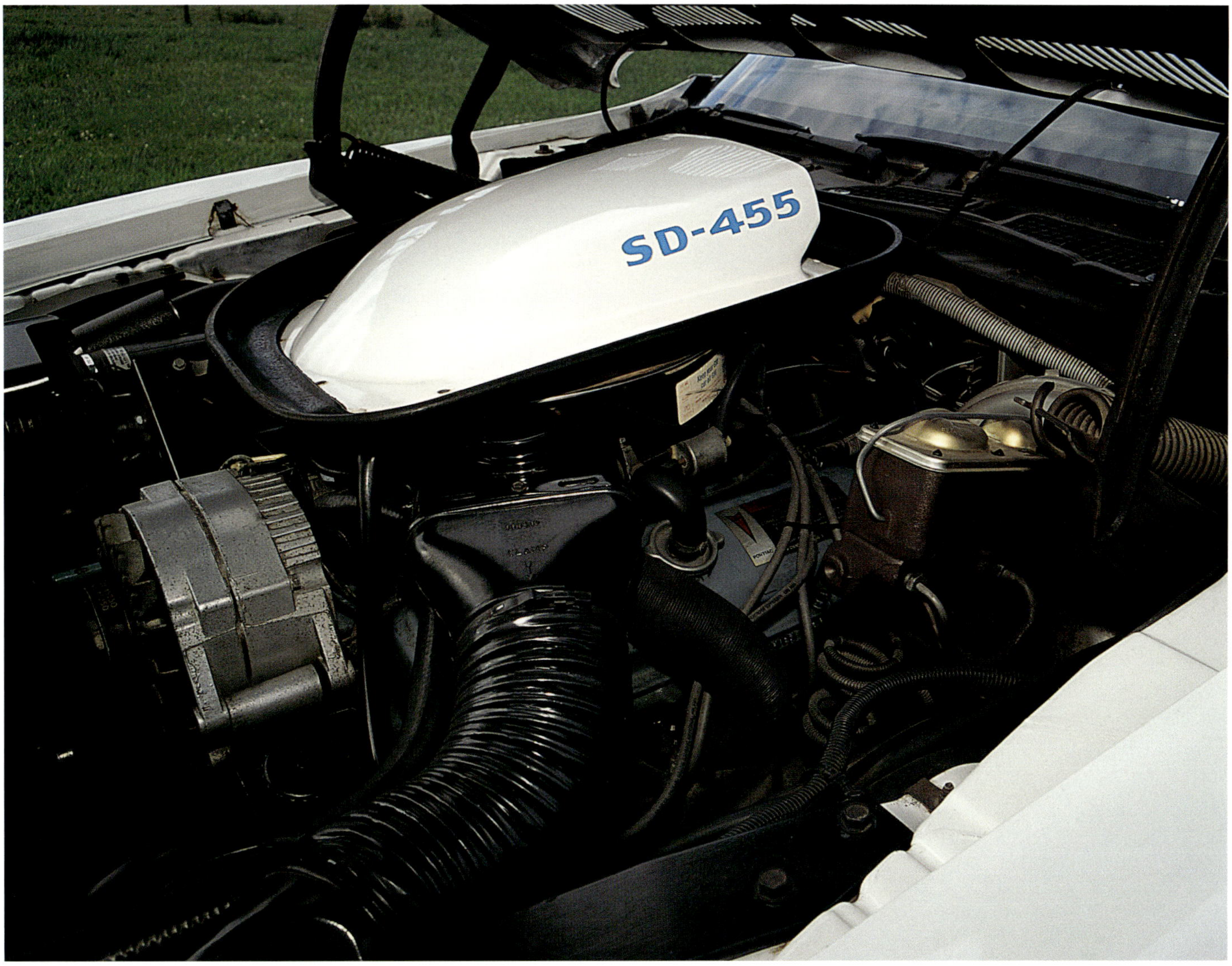

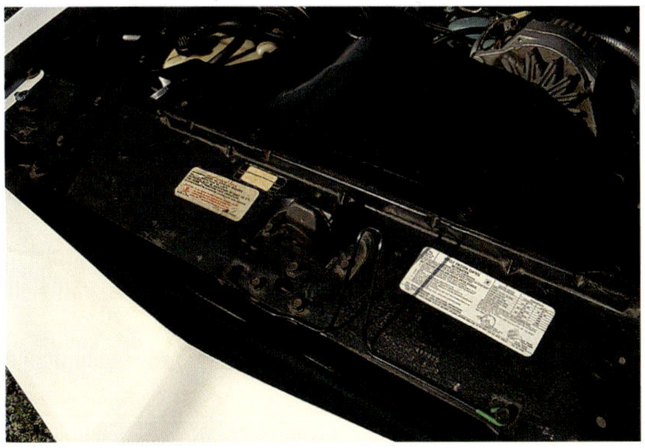

Above: This detail view of the left side of the engine compartment in an original white 1973 Trans Am equipped with an SD 455 engine also shows the black rubber seal and front drain tube on the shaker scoop. ***Right:*** This is a detail view of the radiator valance panel on an original white 1973 Trans Am 455 SD. Note the location and design of the coolant and tune-up information decals.

For 1973, there were again two 350 V-8 engines available. The standard 350 (UPC L30) used in the Firebird and Esprit had a 7.6:1 compression ratio and developed 150 horsepower at 4,000 rpm and 270 foot-pounds of torque at 2,000 rpm with a two-barrel carburetor and single exhaust. The VIN engine code was M. The 350 used in the Formula 350 also had a two-barrel carburetor and 7.6:1 compression, but the dual exhausts raised the output rating to 175 horsepower at 4,400 rpm and 280 foot-pounds of torque at 2,400 rpm. The VIN engine code was N.

There were three versions of the 400 V-8 available in 1973, all with an 8.0:1 compression ratio. The UPC L65 400-cubic-inch V-8 had an 8.0:1 compression ratio and developed 170 horsepower at 3,600 rpm and 320 foot-pounds of torque at 2,000 rpm with a single two-barrel carburetor and single exhaust (VIN engine code R). The same UPC L65 engine was also available as the standard engine in the Formula 400 with a single two-barrel and dual exhaust making 185 horsepower at 4,000 rpm and 320 foot-pounds of torque at 2,400 rpm (VIN engine code P). There was also a four-barrel-carburetor, dual-exhaust version with 230 horsepower at 4,400 rpm and 325 foot-pounds of torque at 3,200 rpm (UPC L78) with VIN engine code T.

The 455 V-8 was available in two forms for 1973. The Formula 455 and Trans Am 455 standard powerplant (UPC L75) had a 750-cfm Rochester Quadrajet four-barrel carburetor with an 8.0:1 compression ratio and developed 250 horsepower at 4,000 rpm and 370 foot-pounds of torque at 2,800 rpm. The VIN engine code was Y.

The 455 Super Duty (SD) V-8 (UPC LS2) had an 8.4:1 compression ratio with an 800-cfm Rochester Quadrajet four-barrel carburetor (part number 7043270) on a low-rise manifold and developed 290 horsepower at 4,000 rpm and 395 foot-pounds of torque at 3,200 rpm. The SD 455 block was based on a standard block, but it had four-bolt main bearing caps, a special casting with a strengthening of the cross valley between the lifter bores, and increased main bearing area webbing. The Super Duty heads had round exhaust ports and required unique exhaust manifolds. The intake ports were modified for constant velocity flow, and the 2.11-inch head diameter intake valves were swirl polished. Both 455 engines had hydraulic valve lifters and a Ram Air III spec camshaft with 0.410-inch lift. The 1973 SD 455 engine used a unique distributor (part number 1112205) with a larger drive gear designed to work with the heavy-duty 80-psi oil pump. All 1973 Firebird V-8s were painted Pontiac Engine Blue, but because the SD 455 was introduced and produced later in the model year (after March 15, 1973), the blue was changed to a darker shade to indicate that it met later emissions requirements. All Pontiac V-8 engines built after that date were painted the darker shade.

All 1973 and 1974 SD 455 engines had the PCV valve outlet in the driver-side oil filler cap rather than the valley cover outlet used on other engines. A rectangular silver, red, and black decal with a red arrowhead logo was mounted at the rear of the left side valve cover of the SD 455. The SD 455 engines have an engine/transmission code stamped on the upper right of the passenger side of the engine block. The codes should be Z1 or XD for 1973. The VIN engine code was X. All 1973 and 1974 455 Super Duty engines were hand-built by two-man teams at the assembly plant.

Engine Compartment

The firewall, inner fender panels, and radiator supports of all 1970–1973 Firebirds were painted semigloss black. The fenders were attached to the inner fenderwells with black-oxide plated hex-head bolts from the underside, except for the rear upper fender-corner-to-body bolts, which were installed from the top. The driver-side fenderwell was relatively bare with only a single black-wrapped headlight wire-loom lying across the front side. The white plastic windshield-washer reservoir with black plastic cap was attached to the front left side of the fender with a black zinc-plated steel bracket. The black rubber washer hose ran along the upper inner fenderwell. The Delco alternator was mounted on the upper left side of the engine for 1970–1973.

The left (driver) side radiator support front corner held the gloss-black battery support and battery. The standard battery for the six and base V-8 was a black 45-amp Delco with side posts (1971–1973). A heavy-duty 61-amp Delco battery was standard with the 400 and 455 V-8, standard with air conditioning, and optional (UPC UA1) for all others. A six-gauge positive battery cable with red pigtail wire was routed under the battery support. The black negative cable with long black pigtail wire was grounded to the right fender. The black rubber engine-to-firewall heater hoses were routed across the right side wheelwell and were held together with a dark-gray phosphate clamp. If air conditioning was ordered, the compressor was mounted at the upper left of the engine.

There were a number of different radiators used in the 1970–1973 Firebird depending upon the engine and transmission combinations. The cooling system capacity for the six-cylinder was 12 quarts, while the 350 V-8 had a 19.4-quart cooling system, and the 400 and 455 V-8 had an 18.6-quart cooling system. A heavy-duty radiator was available. All radiators had the filler on the right top and the inlet hose on the left side of the top tank. The inlet hose exited the engine from the left side and was routed around the rear of the alternator. Both hoses were secured with plated tower clamps. A large black reinforced plastic fan shroud was used on all models. A coolant information label (right) and an emissions control information label (left) were attached to the top of the black painted steel valance in front of the radiator. The wire hood release spring with a green painted hook end was attached to the left side of the steel valance with a hex-head bolt.

The passenger side of the firewall was relatively bare except for the heater plenum housing and the connections for the heater hoses. If air conditioning was ordered, the hose connections were also located on the right side of the firewall, and the heater connections were higher and more toward the center. The heater hoses were secured with plated tower clamps.

The driver (left) side of the firewall held the brake master cylinder, and the windshield-wiper motor was to its left. All 1970–1973 Firebird manual brake systems used a dual reservoir 1-inch-bore Delco Moraine or Bendix master cylinder. When power brakes were ordered, a master cylinder with 1.125-inch bore was used. All original Delco master cylinder covers were gold-zinc-dichromate plated and stamped "Use Delco Brake Fluid." Master cylinders were finished in semigloss black, and the vacuum booster was gold-zinc-dichromate plated. Front disc with rear drum brakes were standard on all 1970–1973 Firebird models, but power brakes were only standard on the Trans Am and optional (UPC J50 in 1970 and 1971 and UPC JL2 in 1972 and 1973) for all others.

The body data plate was attached to the firewall with two rivets or special hex-head screws at the top edge of the left cowl. The data plate was painted black with the firewall. The natural pot-metal-and-steel finish windshield-wiper motor was mounted to the right of the brake master cylinder. All 1970–1973 Firebirds had standard two-speed, electric, parallel-action wipers. Windshield washers were standard on all models.

The underside of the hood of all 1970–1973 Firebirds was painted semigloss black. The hood hinges and springs were black/dark-gray phosphate.

Frame, Undercarriage, Transmission, and Driveline

All 1970–1973 Firebirds used welded-steel unitized construction with a separate rubber-cushioned, bolted-on steel front subframe to support the engine and front suspension. The body structure consists of a welded-steel floorpan and side panels integrating the trunk compartment and rear quarters. The bottom of the floorpan was finished with red oxide primer. The steel front subframe and related components were finished in either semigloss black or natural unfinished bare steel.

Front Suspension

The 1970–1973 Firebird front suspension used unequal-length upper and lower control arms with ball joints, coil springs, and tubular shock absorbers. The stamped-steel upper control arms were used on all Firebirds from 1970 through 1973. The ball joints were riveted in place, and the pivot joints had steel-encased rubber bushings. The control arms were painted semigloss black except for the outer ball-joint ends.

All 1970–1973 Firebirds used the same lower control arms. Lower control arm components were painted semigloss black except for the outer ends. The gloss-black-finish front coil springs were mounted between the lower control arm and a pocket in the front subframe. Different coil springs were used depending upon the engine and model. Gray Delco spiral-body tubular shock absorbers were mounted in the center of the coil springs.

The standard 1970–1973 Firebird Esprit with a 250 or 350 engine had a 1-inch front stabilizer bar (part number 3984557) mounted between the lower front control arms and rubber-bushed brackets in the front subframe. The optional heavy-duty suspension (Formula handling package UPC Y99), standard with the Formula 400 and 455, had a 1.125-inch stabilizer bar (part number 3975523) and firm-control shock absorbers. The Trans Am front suspension was similar except with a 1.250-inch front stabilizer bar (part number 3986480). All front stabilizer bars were finished in black manganese phosphate and attached with natural steel links and rubber bushings.

The standard front brakes for all 1970–1973 Firebirds were 10.9-inch-diameter vented discs with single-piston natural cast-iron-finish calipers and standard metallic pads. Manual disc brakes were standard on all, except the Trans Am, which had standard power brakes. Power brakes were optional on all others with UPC J50.

The standard 1970–1973 Firebird steering gear was a manual Saginaw unit with a ratio of 24:1 with the six-cylinder engine and 28:1 with the V-8. An optional variable-ratio (16:1–12.4:1) power steering Saginaw gear was available with UPC N41. The manual steering gear was painted gloss black with a natural-finish side cover and end plug. The power steering gear was natural cast finish with a dull aluminum cover and end plug. In 1970, the steering linkage was moved to the front of the wheel center rather than behind as in past years.

Rear Suspension

The 1970–1973 Firebird rear axle was a Salisbury-type semifloating design available in standard ratios of 2.73:1 (D), 3.07:1 (M), 3.08:1 (F), 3.31:1 (T), 3.36:1 (H), 3.55:1 (K), and 3.73:1 (R). Rear axles were available in both 10-bolt 8.20-inch ring gear (1970 and 1971) and 8.5-inch (1971–1973) and 12-bolt with 8.875-inch ring gear (1970 only). Ratios and axle size varied according to the transmission and engine ordered. The standard 1970–1973 rear axle had a 10-bolt cover, but in 1970–1972 only when the 3.07:1, 3.31:1, 3.55:1, or 3.73:1 gears were ordered an axle with a 12-bolt cover was used. Safe-T-Track limited-slip differential was available as UPC G80 on all models. The performance axle ratio (UPC G90) option varied according to the engine and transmission. All axles were stamped on the front passenger side of the axle tube with a seven-digit alphanumeric code that identified the axle code, month-and-day build code and plant letter suffix. The rear axle assembly was painted semigloss black with paint codes identifying the various configurations.

The 1970–1973 Firebird rear suspension consisted of parallel multileaf semielliptic leaf springs. The spring rates were reduced by about 10 to 15 percent for 1970 and ride quality was softened accordingly. The springs were semigloss black finish with gloss-black hangers and mounting brackets. The rear suspension was still supported by gray-finished (some may have been semigloss black) Delco spiral-body shock absorbers mounted in a staggered configuration with one behind and the

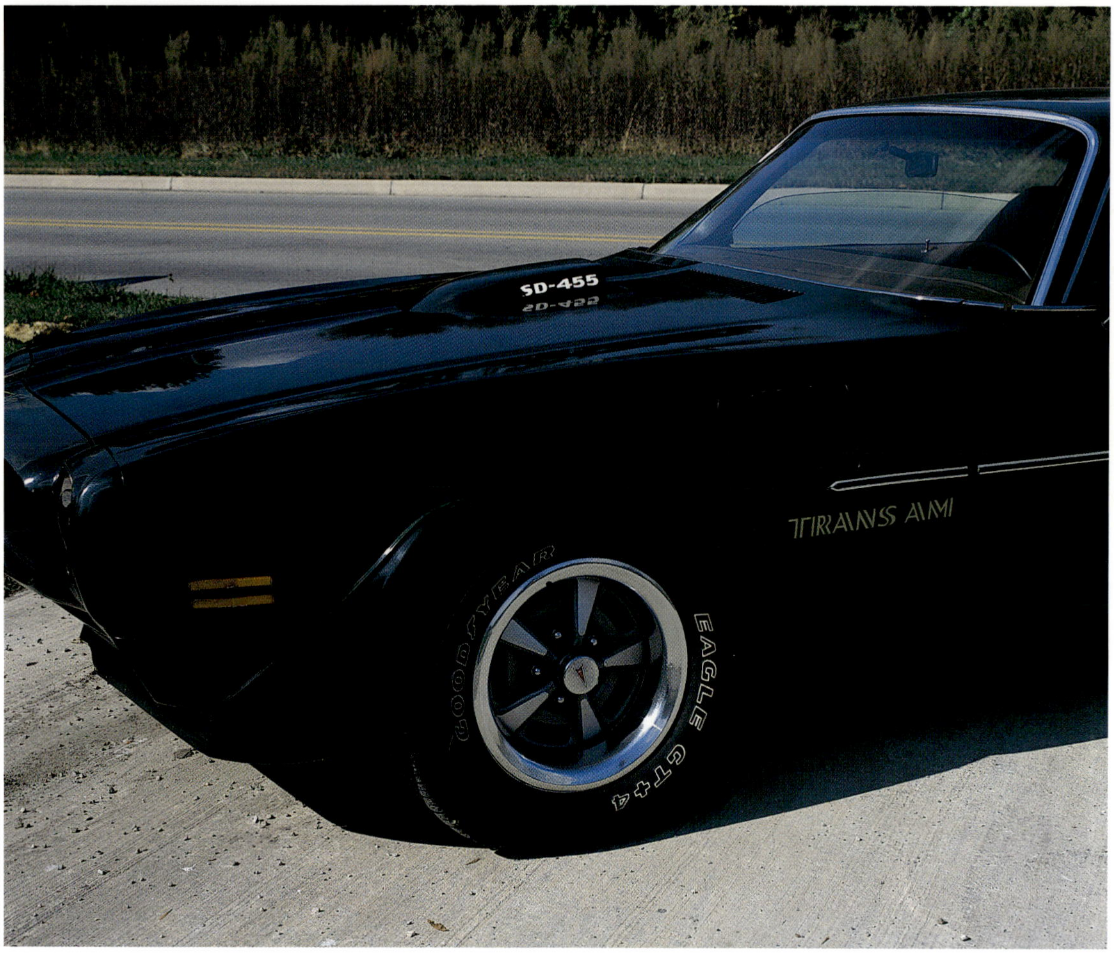

This view of the left front quarter of a Brewster Green 1973 Trans Am shows the Rally II wheels and bright trim rings. This Trans Am is equipped with the optional SD 455 engine and does not have the more-common large bird decal on the hood, but it does have a smaller bird decal on the front fascia.

other in front of the axle. The Formula 400 and 455 had firm-control shock absorbers, and the Trans Am had firm-control shock absorbers and higher-rate springs. There was no standard rear stabilizer bar with the base Firebird or Esprit, but the Formula 400 and 455 had a 0.625-inch bar and the Trans Am had a 0.875-inch rear bar as standard equipment. The stabilizer bar was natural steel or black painted finish.

The standard rear brakes on all 1970–1973 Firebirds were drum-type hydraulic with 9.5-inch cast-iron drums. Standard asbestos linings were 2 inches wide. Brake drums and backing plates were painted semigloss black.

Tires and Wheels

The standard wheels for the 1970–1973 Firebird, Esprit, and Formula were 14x6J steel wheels with five lug nuts. The steel wheels were finished in gloss black enamel if full wheel covers were used, but if the small standard hubcaps were supplied, the wheels were painted gloss enamel on the front side only so as to match the lower body color.

Optional wheels for 1970–1973 included 14x6J Rally II styled wheels (UPC N98), with an optional brushed-aluminum trim ring (UPC P06) available in 1970. In 1971, the Rally II wheels were changed to 14x7JJ. The 14x6 Rally II wheel used a trim ring with part number 9781480, and the 14x7 wheel used part number 9796919. A similar 15x7J Rally II wheel (15x7JW in 1970) with optional brushed-aluminum trim ring was standard on the 1970–1973 Trans Am.

Both wheels had a standard black background center cap with PMD medallion (part number 9787941) through the mid-1970 model year. The mid-1970–1972 wheels used a red background center cap and bright PMD medallion (part number 480302). In 1973, the center cap was bright finish with a Pontiac arrowhead medallion in its center. For 1971–1973, the new unique Bill Porter–designed honeycomb wheel became available with UPC P05. The honeycomb wheel had a polycast-urethane center molded into a steel rim and was available in 15-inch only for the Trans Am and 14-inch for all other models.

Standard tires for the 1970–1973 Firebird and Esprit were E78x14 black sidewall bias-ply with E78x14 and F78x14 white sidewall optional. F70x14 white letter and black sidewall bias-belted tires were also optional on all but the Trans Am, with the F70x14 black bias-belted standard on the Formula. F60x15 white letter bias-belted tires were standard on the Trans Am and optional on the Formula with Rally II wheels only. For

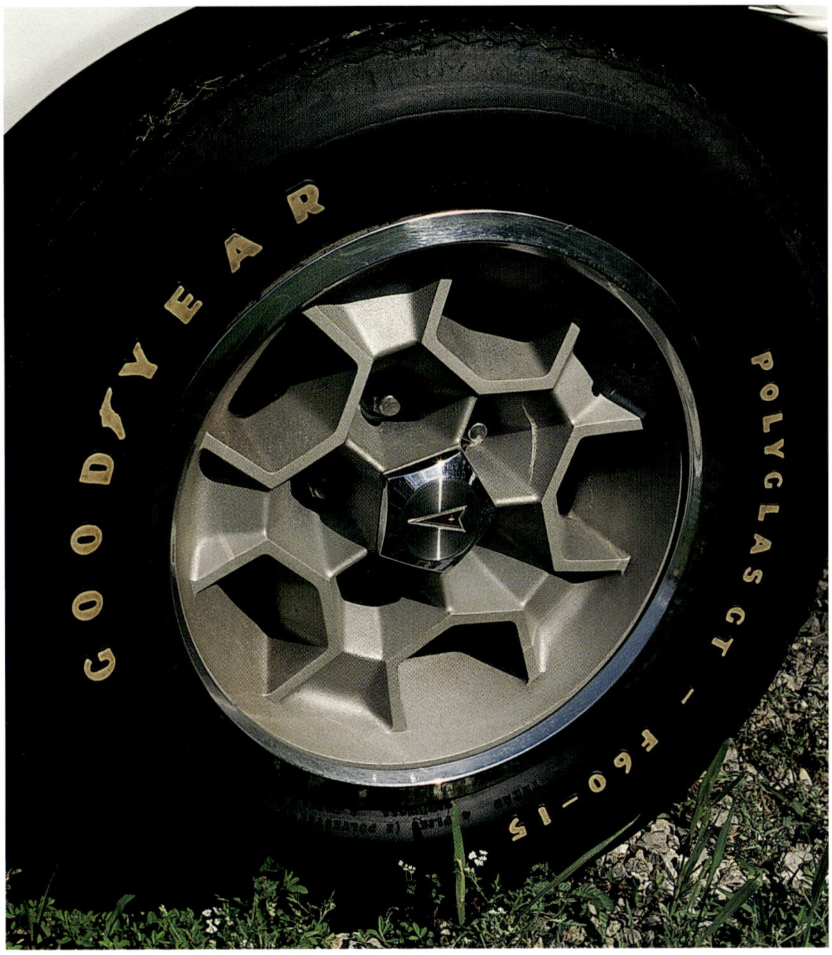

This view shows the right front wheel and tire on an original 1973 Trans Am SD 455 equipped with optional Honeycomb wheels (UPC P05) and standard F60x15 Goodyear Polyglas GT white letter tires.

1973 only, GR70x14 steel-belted radial white-sidewall tires on Rally II wheels were available as an option (UPC P85) on the Trans Am.

Small chrome-plated hubcaps with a Pontiac arrowhead badge were standard equipment for all 1970–1973 Firebirds except the Trans Am. The standard 1970 and 1971 hubcap (part number 5738083) had a dished center in a raised hub with radiating ribs to the outer perimeter. The words Pontiac Motor Division encircled the outer rim of the center hub. The 1972 and 1973 standard hubcaps were redesigned and were a chrome-plated smooth, baby-moon design with a small arrowhead insignia in the center that used part number 485200. The Firebird Esprit had standard bright trim rings that were optional (UPC P06) on all other models.

For 1970–1973, as in previous years, deluxe wheel discs (UPC P01) and custom wheel discs (UPC P02) were available as an option on all but the Trans Am. The 1970–1971 deluxe wheel discs were the same as those used in 1969, but the 1972 deluxe wheel disc had a smooth center with radiating slots and used part number 9890699. The 1970 custom wheel discs were similar to those used in 1969, but for 1971 to early 1972 the custom discs were redesigned and used part number 483526. The late-1972 and 1973 custom wheel discs (UPC N95) had a small center hub with an arrowhead logo and fine radiating lines and used part number 486553. The 1970–1972 wire discs were the same as those used for 1969. The wire-wheel disc option was dropped for 1973. The wire-wheel discs were not available with the Trans Am.

Transmissions

The 1970–1973 Firebirds were available with seven transmission choices. The standard transmission with the six-cylinder and 350 V-8 was the fully synchronized cast-iron-case three-speed manual. Only a column shift was available with the six-cylinder and a floor shift with the 350 V-8. An optional heavy-duty three-speed manual transmission (UPC M13, transmission code DG) with floor shift was standard with the Formula and available with all but the six-cylinder engine. All manual three-speed transmissions had a natural cast-iron finish.

The Muncie aluminum-case four-speed manual transmission (UPC M20) was available as an option with all except the six-cylinder and cars equipped with the UPC WT5 mountain-performance option, which included a Turbo Hydra-Matic transmission. A close-ratio four-speed manual transmission (UPC M21) was available with the 400 and 455 V-8 engines and required the UPC G80 Safe-T-Track rear axle. Both four-speed transmissions had a standard Hurst floor shifter that was available with or without a console.

The two-speed Powerglide automatic (UPC M35) was available as an option on the Firebird and Firebird Esprit with six-cylinder (codes EA 1970, TH 1971, RB 1972) or 350 V-8 (codes EB1970, TS 1971 and 1972) only. The transmission codes appeared on the right side of the transmission case. The two-speed automatic was available with either a column or floor-mounted shifter with console. The two-speed automatic transmission option was dropped in the mid-1972 model year.

A three-speed Turbo Hydra-Matic (Chevrolet–built) transmission was available with the six-cylinder and 350 V-8 (UPC M38). The 400 and 455 V-8 used a Turbo Hydra-Matic 400 transmission (UPC M40). All Turbo Hydra-Matic transmissions used a floor-mounted shifter with a console. Transmission codes were JE for all years with the 250 six-cylinder engine. The Turbo Hydra-Matic 350 and 400 V-8 transmission codes varied according to the engine and axle ratio. The case was natural aluminum with a gloss-black oil pan and converter pan.

All transmissions were connected to the rear axle by a natural-finish one-piece welded-steel driveshaft.

Chapter 4

1974–1981

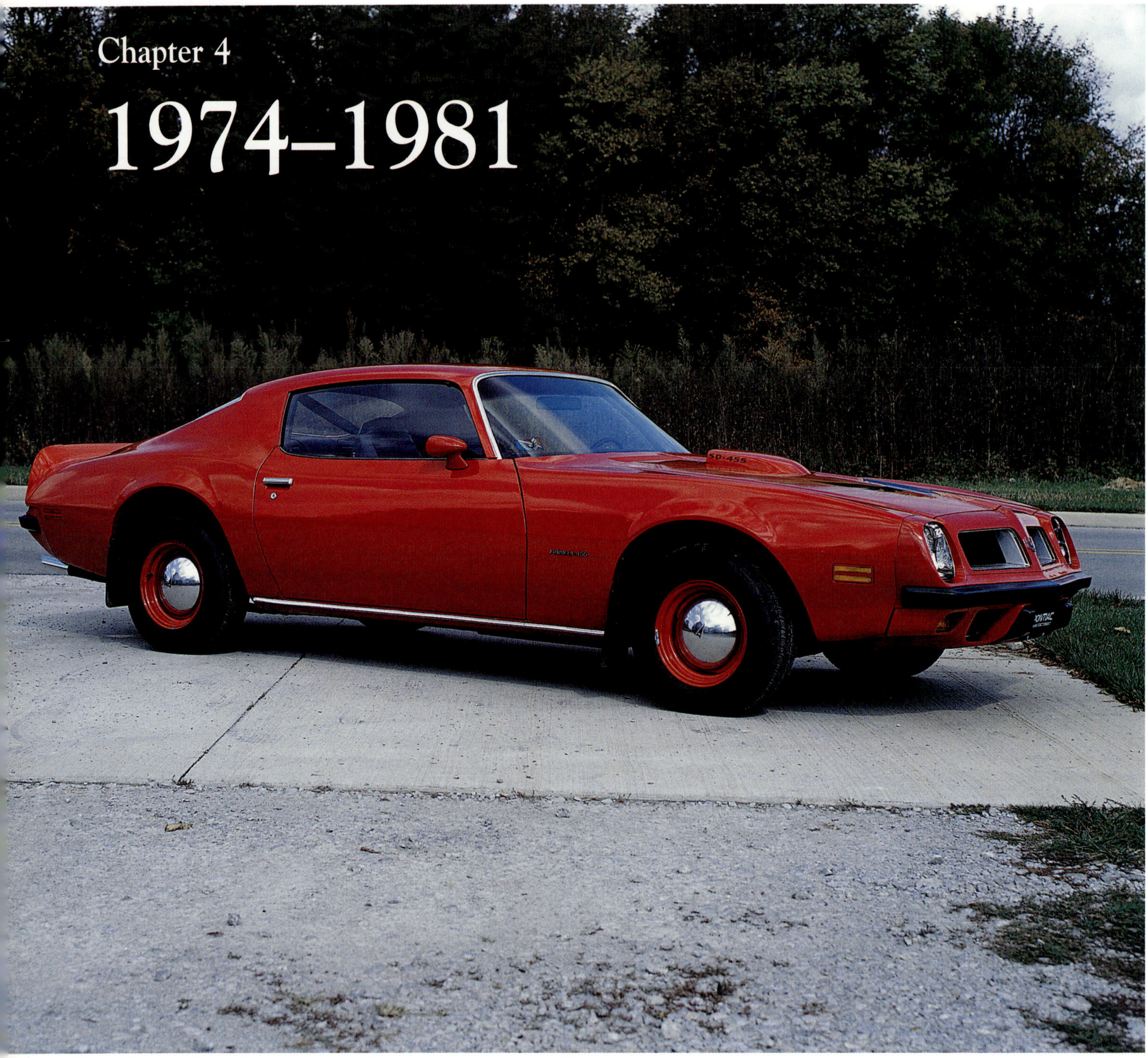

This Buccaneer Red 1974 Firebird Formula SD 455 is equipped with the standard 14-inch painted steel wheels with standard baby-moon-type hubcaps with red Pontiac arrowhead medallion in the center.

Although the new 1974 edition of the Firebird is still considered a second-generation body, and clearly incorporates the basic shell of the 1973, the front and rear fascia were totally redesigned in accordance with the government's mandated 5-mile-per-hour crash impact survival. The new styling theme was created by John Schinella, also known as "Mr. Trans Am." Schinella, along with Pontiac designers Jim Cathcart and Jim Lagergren, developed the newly required and integrated "soft system" into the front and rear of the Firebird. The new design eliminated the chrome bumpers and included a back-tilted, full body-color front end with black rubber bumper and wraparound rear molded bumper with black rubber strip. This new styling was created without changing the basic underlying sheet metal in the front of the Firebird body. The front end design evolved from 1974 to 1981, but the basic concept remained the same.

The new design of the 1974 Firebird continued the fastback roof styling, short rear deck, and relatively flat rear window of the 1970–1973 body, but for 1975 a new wraparound rear window was adopted that increased rear vision. The doors and side windows kept the same appearance as the 1970–1973 Firebirds, and the rear fascia

continued on page 82

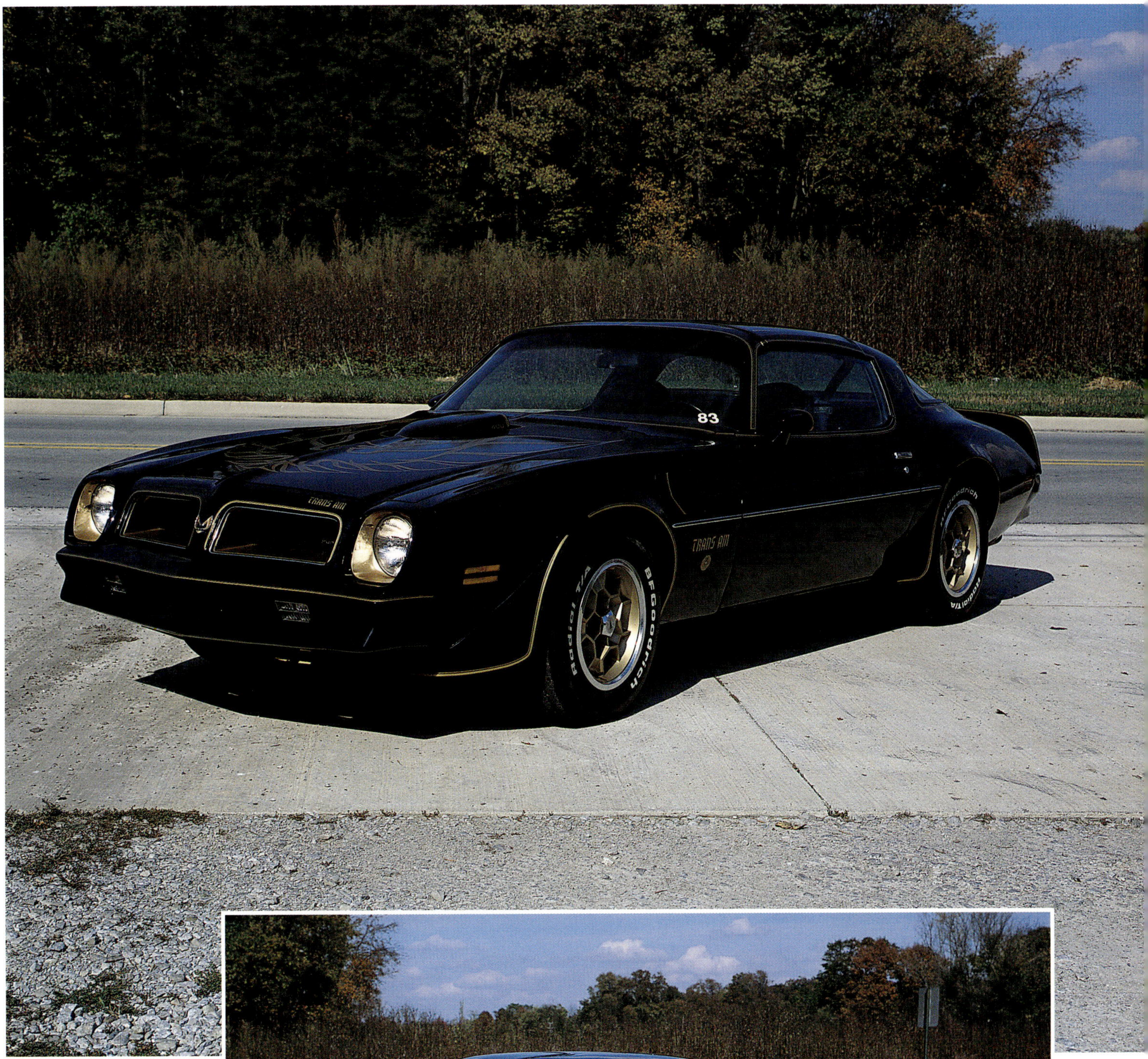

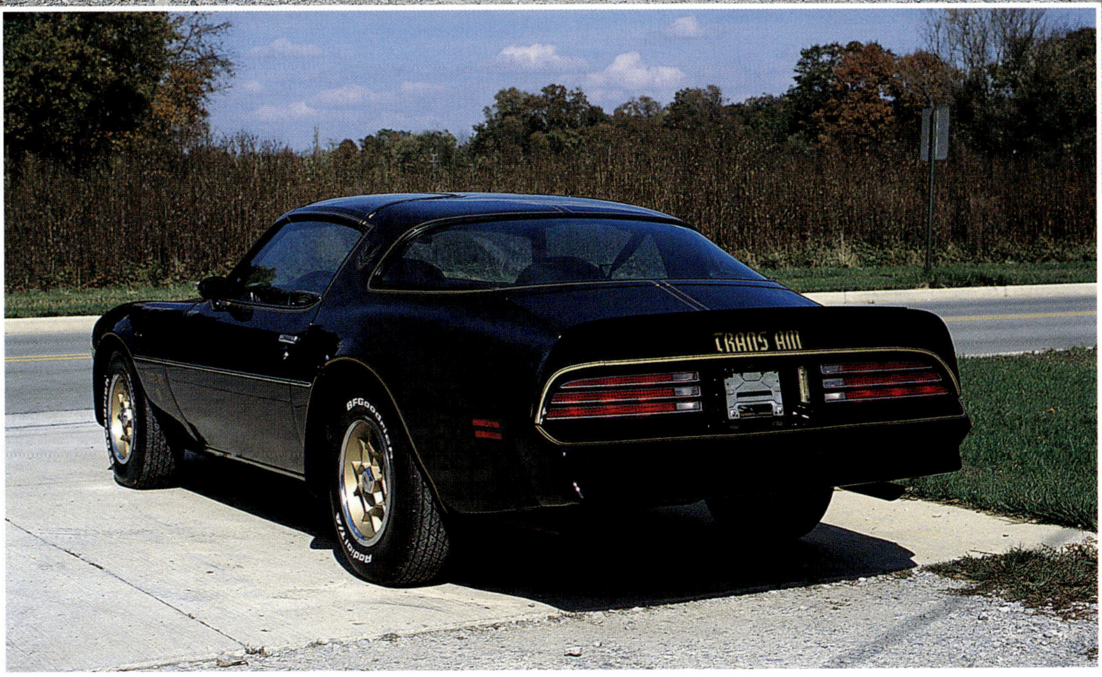

This is a black 50th Anniversary Limited Edition (RPO Y82) 1976 Trans Am. The black body finish with gold trim was part of the Limited Edition package designed by John Schinella. The Hurst-installed T-top was used on only about 25 percent of the 2,590 50th Anniversary Trans Ams produced.

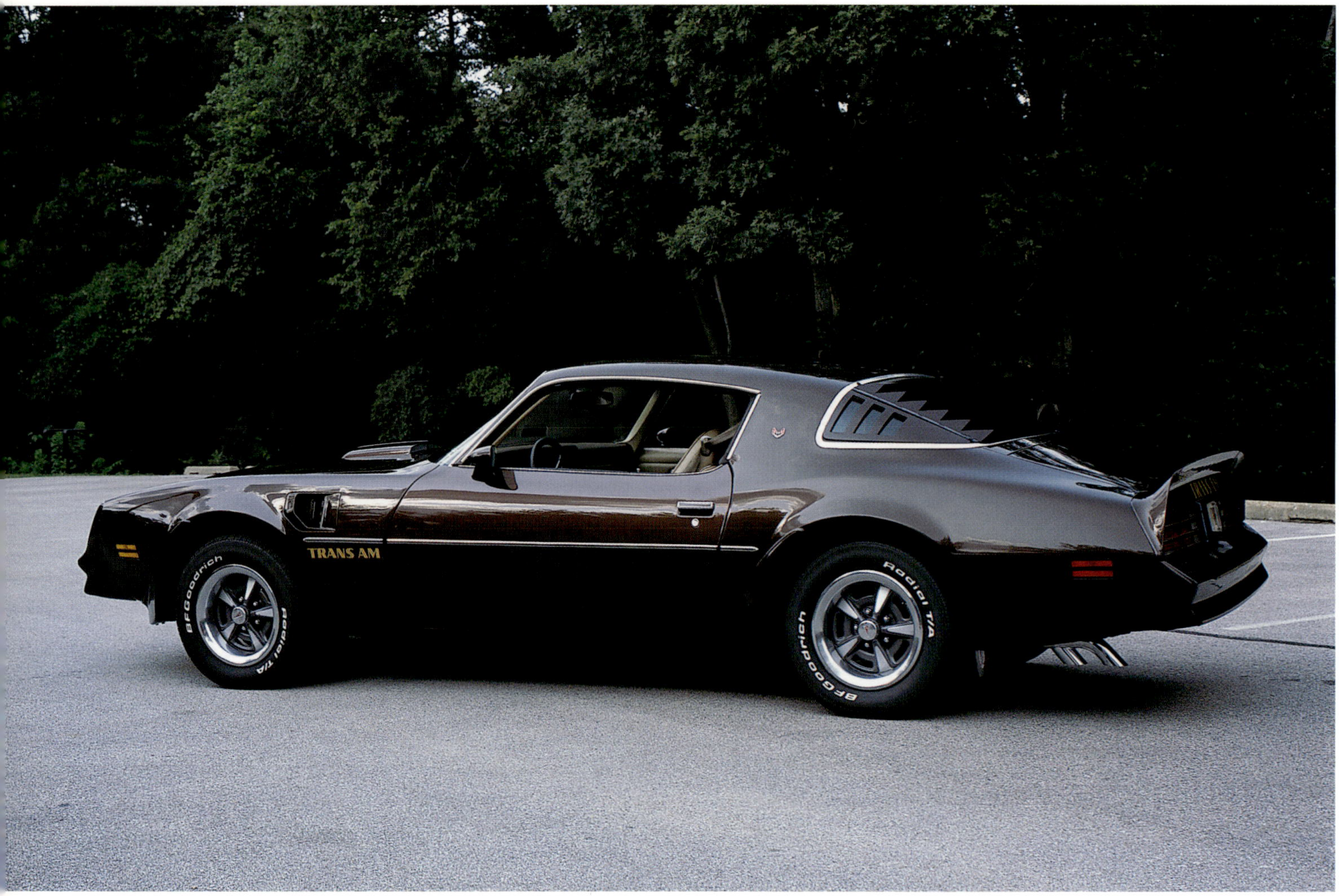

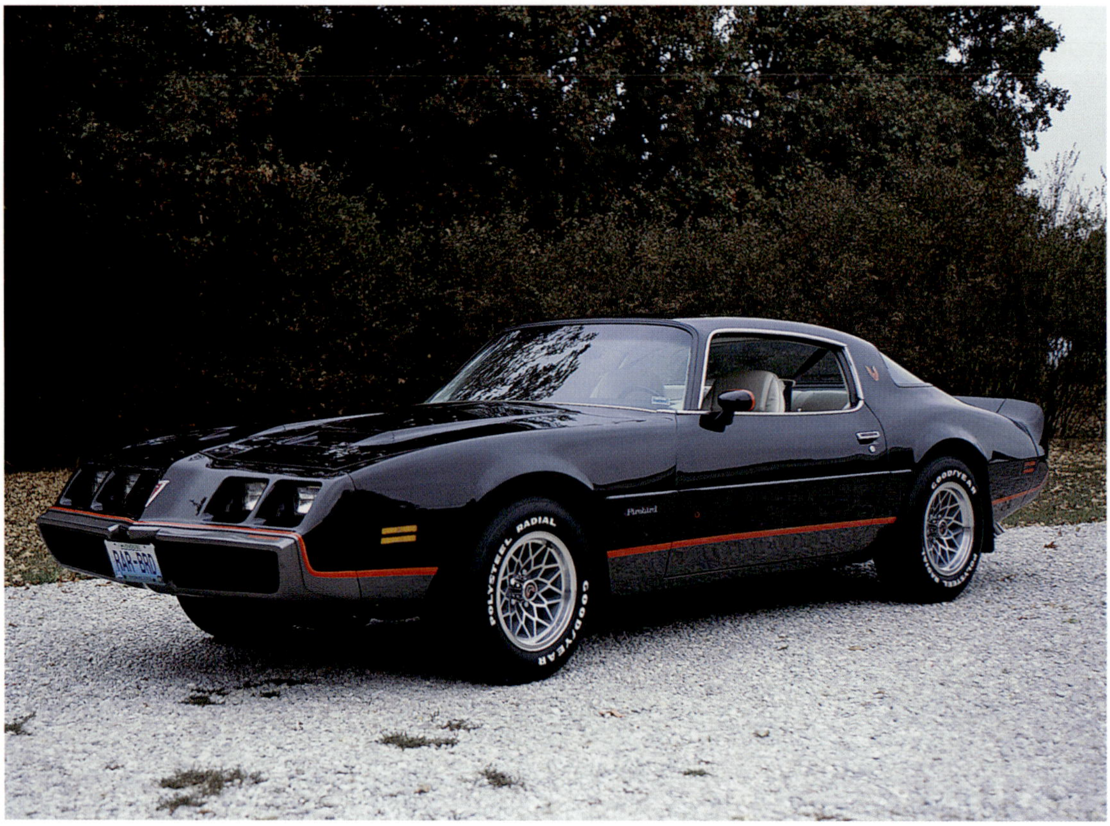

Above: This is a left rear quarter view of a Brentwood Brown (69) 1977 Trans Am. Note the Firebird medallion on the roof B-pillar and Rally II wheels. This view shows the new rear wraparound window design adopted in 1975. ***Left:*** Left front quarter view of an original 1979 Firebird Formula sport coupe (U87) finished in black (19) with optional Honeycomb wheels. The unique red lower body stripe and contrasting silver lower body color were part of the RPO W50 Formula Appearance Package.

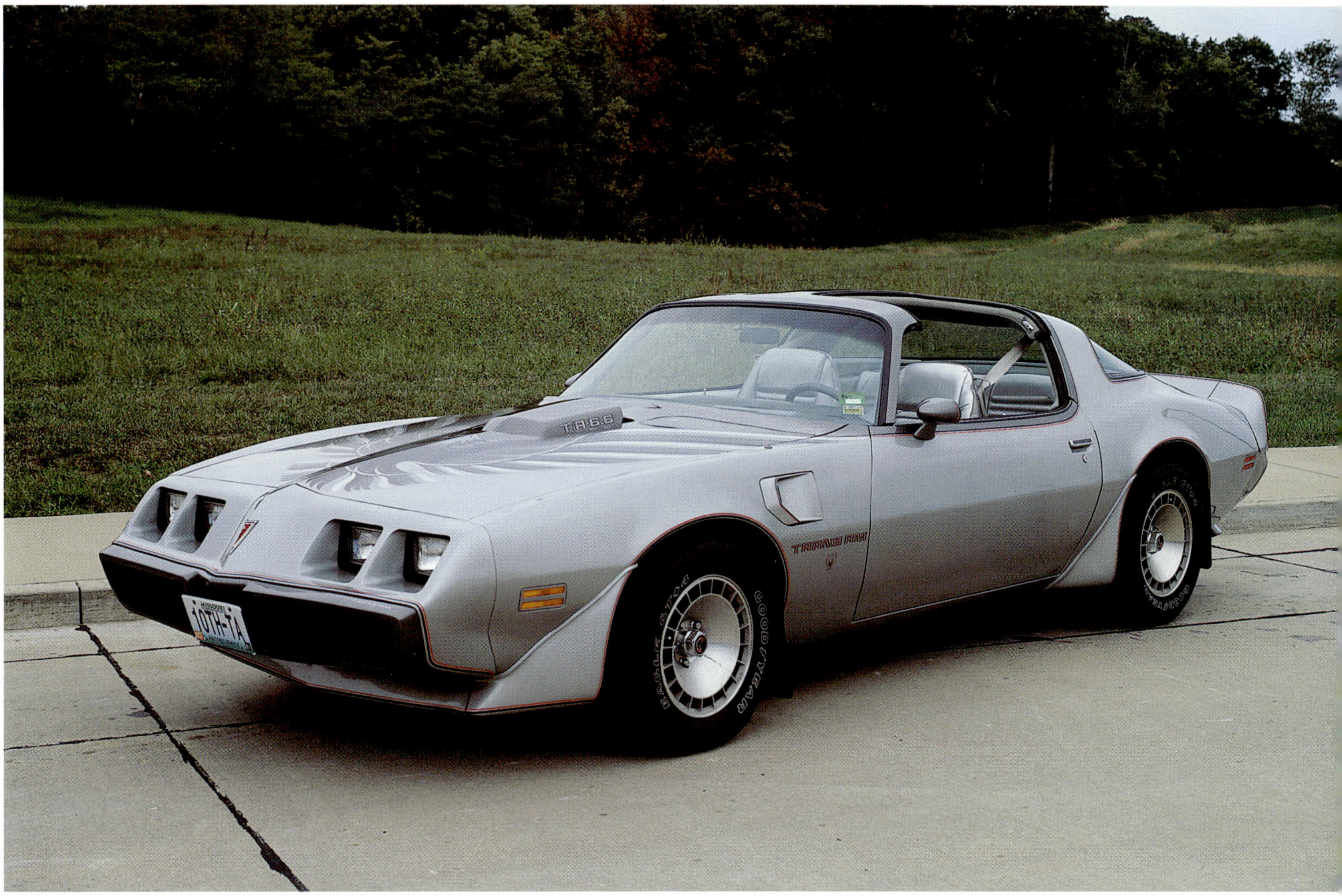

Above: Left front quarter of a 1979 Trans Am 10th Anniversary Edition (X87) finished in Silver Iridescence (15). The 10th Anniversary package was introduced at the Chicago Auto Show on February 24, 1979. *Right:* This 1979 Trans Am sport coupe (W87) finished in Atlantic Blue (24) is equipped with optional snowflake wheels and the 6.6-liter Oldsmobile V-8 engine.

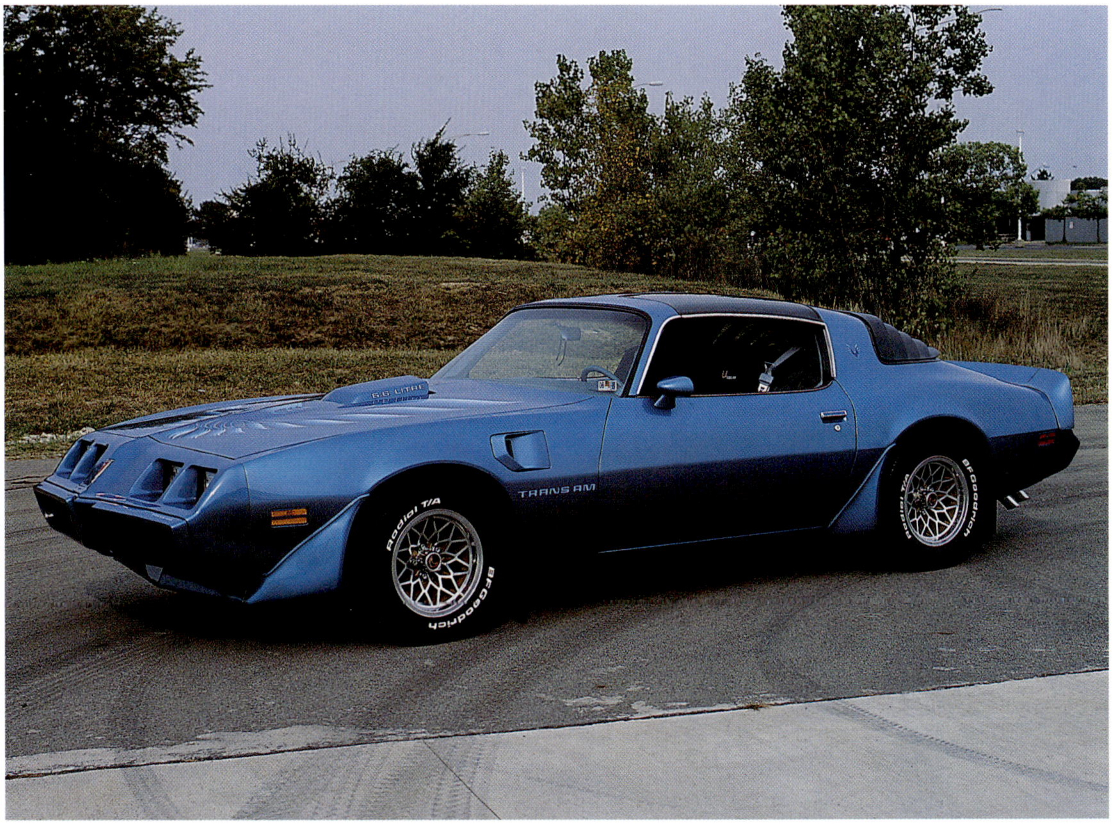

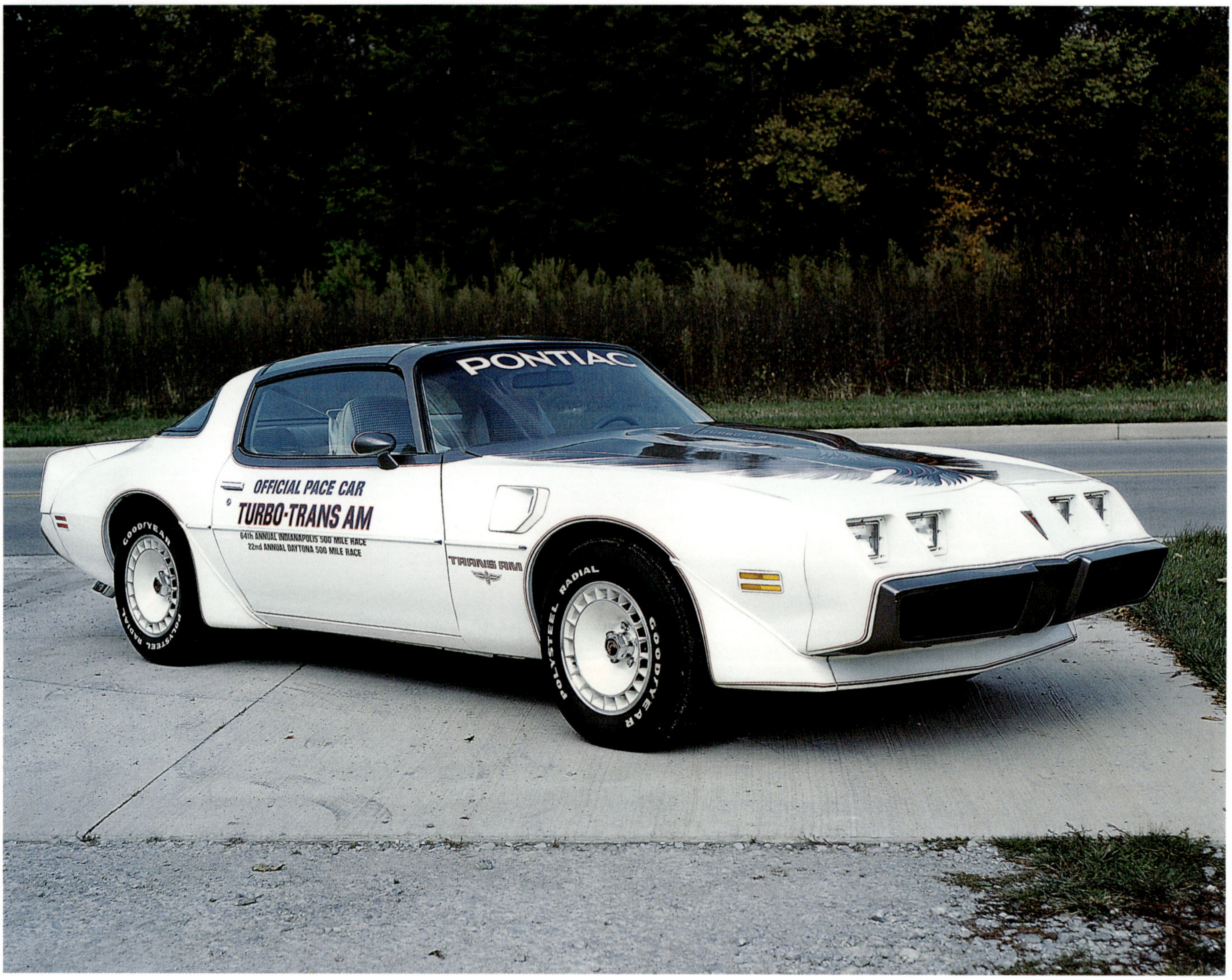

This 1980 Turbo Trans Am Indianapolis 500 Pace Car Edition was finished in white (11) with white painted 15-inch Turbo cast-aluminum wheels. The car is equipped with a 4.9-liter turbocharged Pontiac V-8.

continued from page 78

design was similar through the second-generation years. The basic model lineup continued mostly unchanged with the base Firebird, Firebird Esprit, Firebird Formula, and Trans Am. There were a number of special-edition, limited-edition, and anniversary models during the 1976–1981 model years. Total Firebird production was 73,729 for 1974; 84,063 for 1975; 110,775 for 1976; 155,735 for 1977; 187,294 for 1978; 211,453 for 1979; 107,340 for 1980; and 70,899 in 1981.

Firebird engine options for 1974 and 1975 still included a standard inline OHV 250-cubic-inch Chevrolet six-cylinder available only in the base Firebird. The standard engine for the Esprit and Formula was the 350-cubic-inch Pontiac V-8 (RPO L30). Note that option codes were now identified as RPO (Regular Production Option) rather than UPC, as in the 1967–1973 models. The 1974 and 1975 350 V-8 had a single two-barrel carburetor and 155 horsepower in the Esprit and, in 1975, a four-barrel with 175 horsepower in the Formula.

Optional V-8 engines for 1974 and 1975 included the 400-cubic-inch OHV Pontiac V-8 in three versions of 190 to 225 horsepower (RPO L65 and L78). The 400-cubic-inch V-8 was standard in the Trans Am. In 1975, the 400 V-8 was only available as a 185-horsepower version with a single four-barrel carburetor (RPO L78). In 1974 and 1975, the 455 Pontiac V-8 was still available in two forms. The RPO L75 was available in 1974 (250 horsepower) and 1975 (200 horsepower), but the 290-horsepower Super Duty 455 (RPO LS2) was available only in 1974.

Firebird engines for 1976 again included the 110-horsepower 250-cubic-inch inline Chevrolet six-cylinder as the standard powerplant in the base Firebird. The standard V-8 in the Esprit and Formula was the RPO L30 350-cubic-inch Pontiac V-8 with two-barrel carburetor rated at 160 horsepower. The 350 V-8 was also available with a four-barrel carburetor and 165 horsepower with RPO L76. Optional in the Firebird and standard equipment for the Trans Am was the 185-horsepower 400 Pontiac V-8. The optional

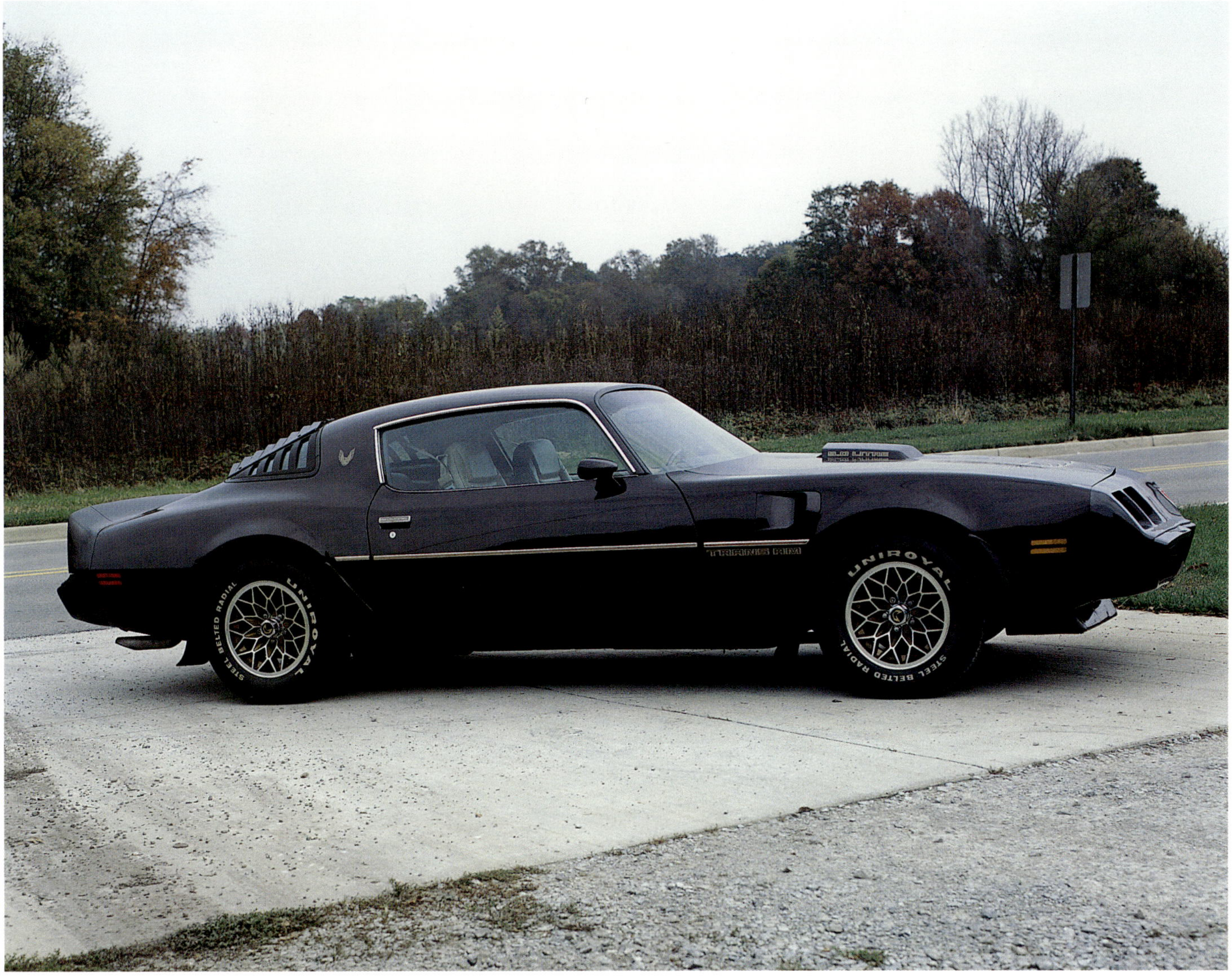

This 1981 Trans Am sport coupe (W87) is finished in Barclay Brown (67) with optional 15-inch cast-aluminum snowflake wheels. Note the gold Trans Am decal on the front fender. The protective body side molding is an option (RPO B84). The rear window louver is an aftermarket accessory.

(RPO L75) 455 Pontiac V-8 was still available in 1976.

Engine choices changed across the Firebird line for 1977. The inline six was gone, and the base Firebird engine was now a 231-cubic-inch Buick V-6 rated at 105 horsepower. The V-6 stayed on as the standard base Firebird engine in various forms through the 1981 model year. The standard engine in the Esprit and Formula (except in California and high-altitude counties) was the 301-cubic-inch Pontiac V-8 with 135 horsepower (RPO L27). The alternate engine for California and special applications was the 350 Pontiac V-8 with a single four-barrel (RPO L76).

The optional V-8 in the 1977 Firebird, Esprit, and Formula and standard in the Trans Am was the 180-horsepower 400-cubic-inch Pontiac V-8 (RPO L78). The standard California Trans Am engine was the 403-cubic-inch Oldsmobile V-8 with 185 horsepower (RPO L80). The Trans Am was also available with an optional 400-cubic-inch (6.6-liter) T/A V-8 with 200 horsepower (RPO L78/W72).

For the 1978 model year, the V-6 was now standard in the base Firebird and Esprit, and V-8 engine options were changed again. The optional V-8 in the base Firebird and Esprit and standard in the Formula was the 305-cubic-inch (5-liter) Chevrolet with a two-barrel carburetor and 145 horsepower. A 350-cubic-inch (5.7-liter) V-8 was optional in the Firebird, Esprit, and Formula. A 350-cubic-inch Oldsmobile V-8 was standard (mandatory) in Trans Ams sold in California or high-altitude areas. The standard V-8 in "Federal" Trans Ams was a 400- or 403-cubic-inch Pontiac V-8 (both called 6.6-liter). Some engines were available exclusively with a Turbo Hydra-Matic transmission.

Engine options for 1979 were similar to 1978, but the Formula now had a standard 301-cubic-inch Pontiac V-8 with mandatory Turbo Hydra-Matic transmission. The standard Trans Am V-8 was the 403-cubic-inch (6.6-liter). For 1980 and 1981, a new turbocharged 4.9-liter (301-cubic-inch) Pontiac V-8 was adopted as optional for the Formula and Trans Am. The standard engine for the

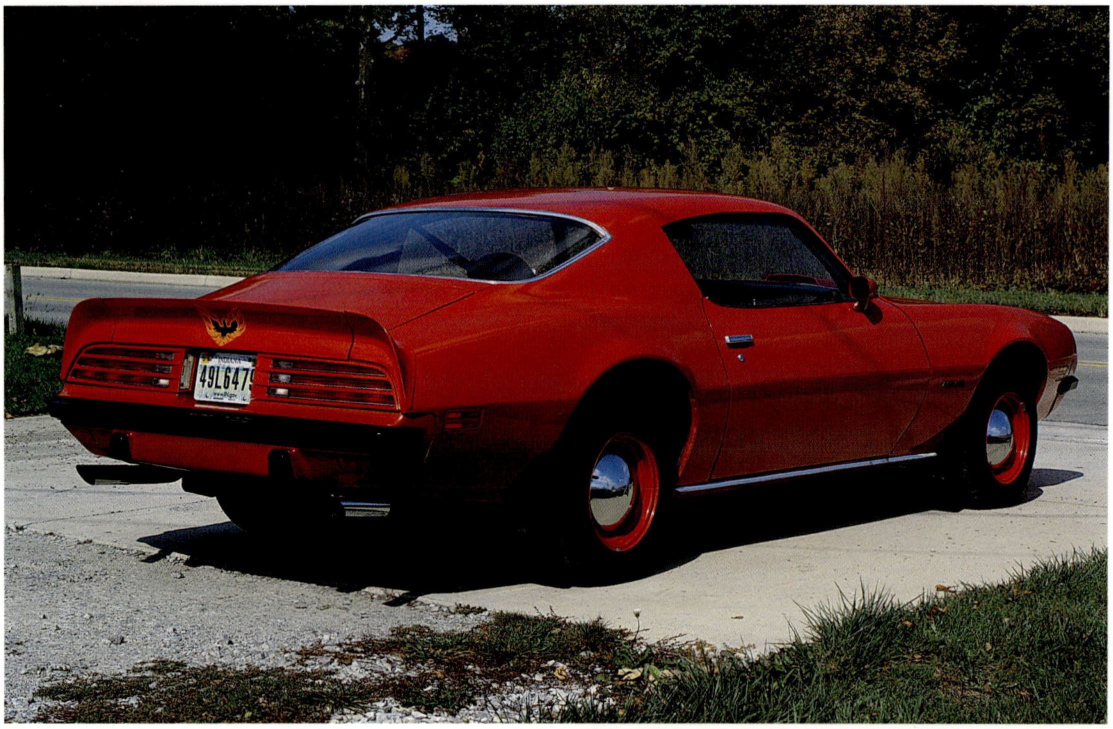

Left: This right rear quarter view of a Buccaneer Red 1974 Firebird Formula shows the body design and flat rear window carried over from 1970–1973. An orange-and-black Formula bird decal appears on the rear spoiler and the black rear bumper. ***Below:*** This is a detail view of the rear window on a Buccaneer Red 1974 Formula SD 455 sport coupe. Nineteen seventy-four was the final year for the flat rear window design used since 1970. Note the bright rear window molding.

1980 and 1981 Trans Am was now the 4.9-liter (301-cubic-inch) Pontiac V-8 with a single four-barrel carburetor and 210 horsepower. The 305-cubic-inch Chevrolet V-8 was available as a delete option in the Trans Am. The 1981 Formula had a 265-cubic-inch Pontiac V-8 as standard equipment with a 4.9-liter (301-cubic-inch) turbocharged V-8 in the Firebird Formula Turbo. The final year for true Pontiac V-8 engines in any Firebird model was 1981.

All 1974 Firebirds were available with four transmission choices that included the three-speed manual, four-speed manual, and Turbo Hydra-Matic 350 and Turbo Hydra-Matic 400 three-speed automatics. The Turbo Hydra-Matic 400 was dropped for 1975, and all 1975–1979 Firebirds had a three-speed manual, four-speed manual, or Turbo Hydra-Matic 350 transmission. The transmission availability was changed for the 1980 and 1981 model years, when a new Turbo Hydra-Matic 200 was adopted for use with the 301- and 265-ci V-8 engines.

The 1974 Firebird was available in 16 body-color schemes, complemented with five vinyl roof colors and 27 interior trim combinations. For 1975, the Firebird had 16 body-color choices with nine vinyl roof colors and eight interior trim combinations. In 1976, there were 14 body colors available with seven vinyl roof colors and 10 interior trim choices. The 1977 Firebird had 17 body colors, seven vinyl roof colors, and 11 interior trim schemes available. For 1978, there were 16 body colors, seven vinyl roof colors, and 10 interior trim combinations offered. In 1979, there were 13 body colors, seven vinyl roof colors, and

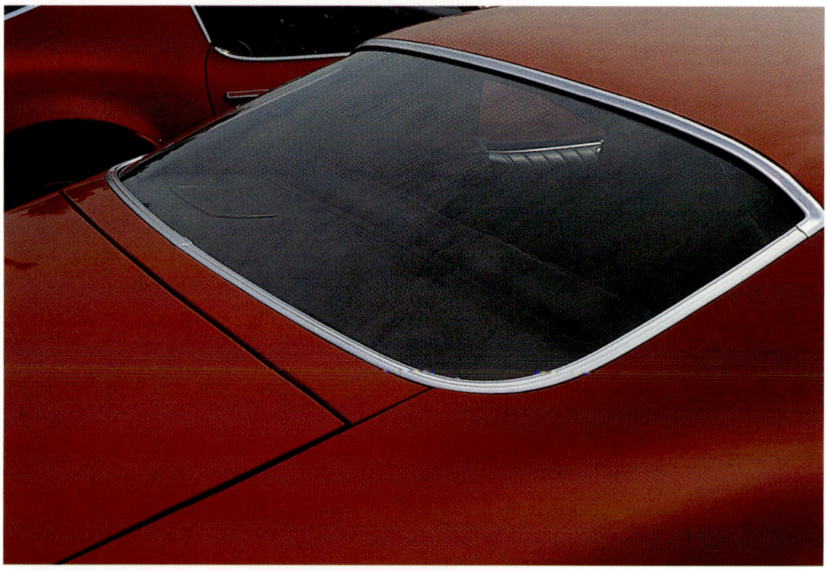

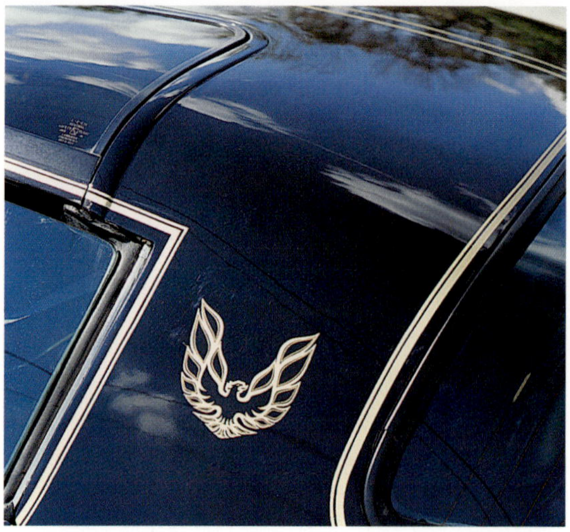

This photo shows the distinctive bird decal and Hurst T-top roof on a black 1976 Trans Am 50th Anniversary Edition. The black finish and gold stripes were part of the 50th Anniversary package. The Hurst T-top is shorter than the later Fisher-designed top.

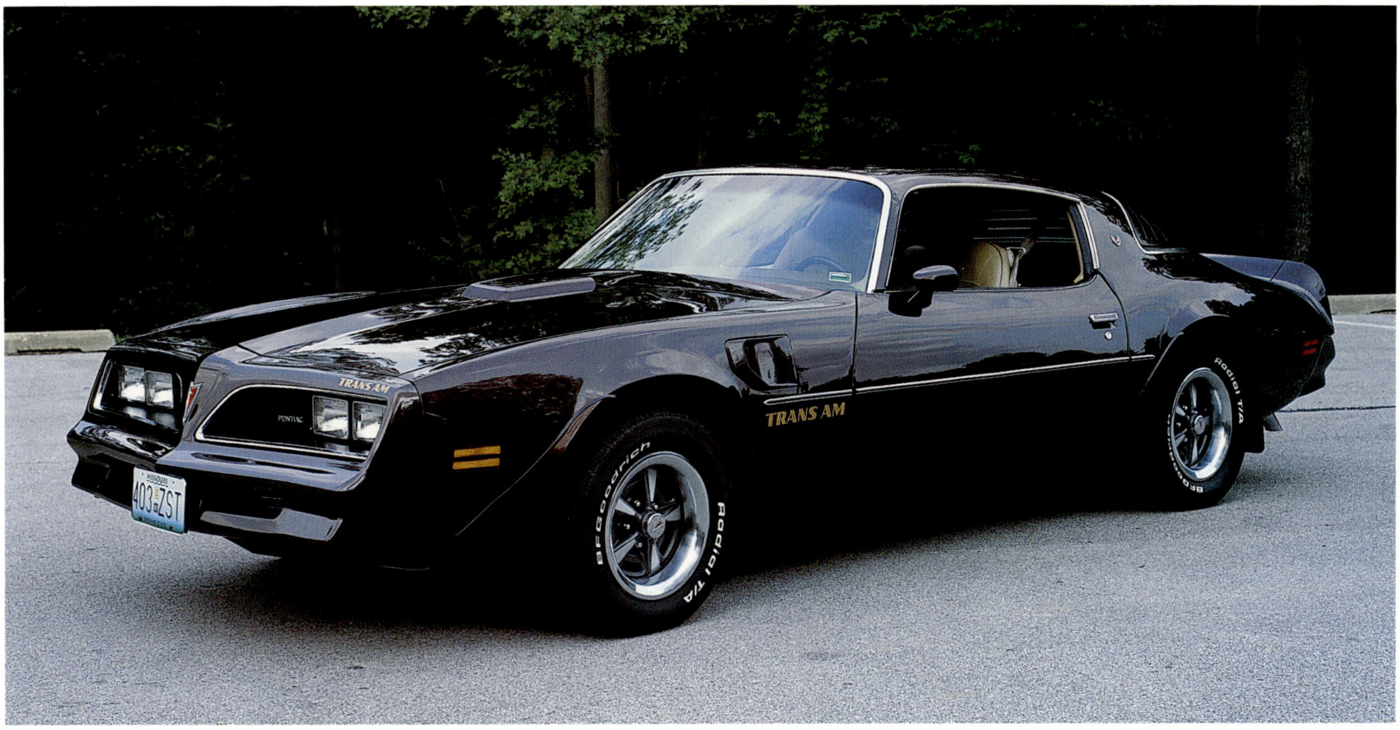

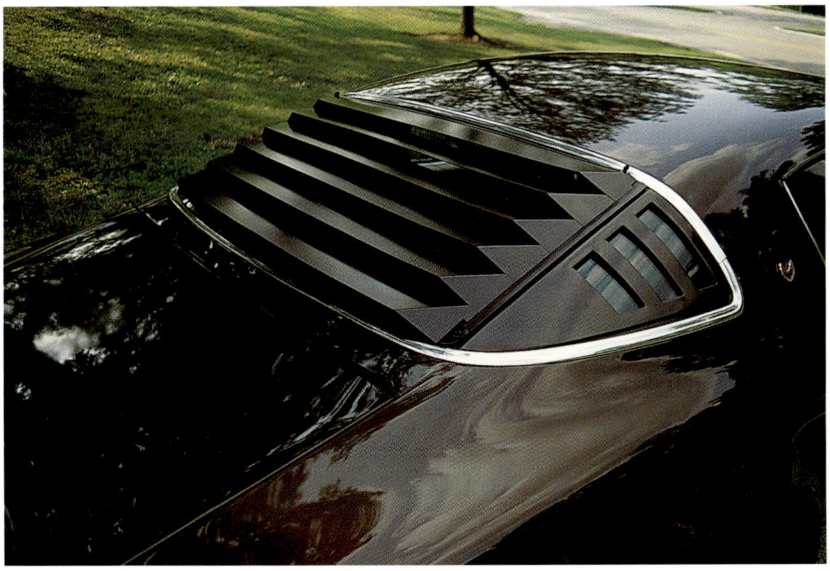

Above: This left front quarter view of a Brentwood Brown 1977 Trans Am shows the second-generation body design. This Trans Am is equipped with standard 15x7 Rally II wheels and bright trim rings. The front and rear wheel opening spoilers are unique to the Trans Am. ***Left:*** The 1975–1981 type rear window used on this Brentwood Brown 1977 Trans Am sport coupe wrapped around the body for better rear visibility than the 1970–1974 design. The rear window louver assembly is an accessory.

10 interior trim combinations. In 1980, 16 body-color choices, eight vinyl roof colors, and 10 interior trim schemes were used. The 1981 Firebird offered 14 body-color schemes, eight vinyl roof colors, and 10 interior trim choices.

Body Sheet Metal and Trim

All 1974–1981 Firebirds used the same unitized-construction body shell and steel-channel front subframe as the previous models. The semigloss-black painted (some may have been bare steel) front subframe carried the engine and front suspension and was bolted to the body shell with four rubber-isolated mounts. The remainder of the steel body shell used a steel floorpan with longitudinal parallel rear members to support the rear suspension and drivetrain. The underside of the body floorpan was finished with red oxide primer. All 1974–1977 Firebirds had a 20.2-gallon galvanized-steel fuel tank mounted at the rear of the body pan. The tank was enlarged to 21 gallons for 1978–1981. All 1974–1981 Firebirds were based on a two-door sport coupe configuration on a 108.1-inch wheelbase.

In addition to the standard steel roof, all 1974 and 1975 Firebird sport coupes were available with an optional Levant-grain vinyl roof covering (RPO C08). All Firebird Esprit bodies had a standard bright stainless-steel roof drip-rail molding that was available as an option (RPO B80) on all other models. When the optional vinyl roof was ordered, an additional two-piece bright molding was added at the lower edge of the vinyl roof at the sail panel and wrapped around the lower border of the back glass opening. Beginning in 1976, the vinyl roof option was replaced with a new canopy top (RPO CB7) that covered only the area of the roof from the rear of the door, opening forward. A narrow bright trim molding was attached at the rear border of the canopy top. An over-the-roof double-stripe option (RPO D98) was available that followed the rear border of the canopy top molding down the rear of the window opening and forward along the door and front fender. The double stripe had a contrasting or complementary color between the stripes. The over-the-roof stripe was also available without the canopy top. All 1976–1978 Firebirds, except the Esprit and Trans Am SE, had a small Firebird medallion on the side of the roof just above and behind the door opening. The 1974 and 1975 Esprit had a bright script Esprit nameplate in the same location.

The optional vinyl roof for 1974 was available in black (2), beige (3), russet (4), green (5), and blue (7). For 1975, the vinyl roof color choices were white (1), black (2), sandstone (3), cordovan (4), green (5), burgundy (6), blue (7), red (8), and silver (9). The 1976 vinyl roofs were available in white (1), black (2), buckskin (3), mahogany (4), firethorn (6), blue (7), and silver (9). For 1977, the canopy top was offered in white (11T), silver (13T), black (19T), blue (22T), firethorn (36T), green (44T), and buckskin (61T). The 1978 colors were white (11T), platinum (15T), black (19T), blue (22T), green (44T), sand (61T), and claret (79T). The 1979 colors were the same except that the green became code 40T. The codes were changed slightly for 1980 and 1981, and the canopy top colors were white (11), silver (13), black (19), blue (21), green (44), camel (63), claret (76), and gray (85). As in the previous years, the vinyl roof installation was in three sections with a large center piece and two smaller side sections with a longitudinal seam on each side.

For the 1976 Limited Edition Trans Am, an optional T-top (Targa) roof was installed by Hurst. The roof was adapted from one used on the 50th Anniversary Grand Prix and was only installed on 643 1976 Trans Am Limited Edition examples. The Limited Edition model was called a Black Special Edition package in 1977 and 1978 and was available either with (RPO Y82) or without (RPO Y81) the T-top option. By 1978, the T-top, or hatch roofs, were made by both Hurst and General Motors and were available in all models with RPO WY9 in 1978 and 1979 and RPO CC1 in 1980 and 1981. The Hurst T-top is shorter than the Fisher Body unit and does not reach to the rear of the door opening. The Hurst top also is narrower, and the body has a wider center section. After the mid-1978 model year, all T-tops were Fisher. The 1979 Trans Am 10th Anniversary model (2FX) used special silver-colored glass T-top hatch roof panels. The hatch roof was standard with the 1980 RPO Y84 special-appearance package.

All 1974–1981 Firebird door panels were interchangeable with those used in the 1970–1973

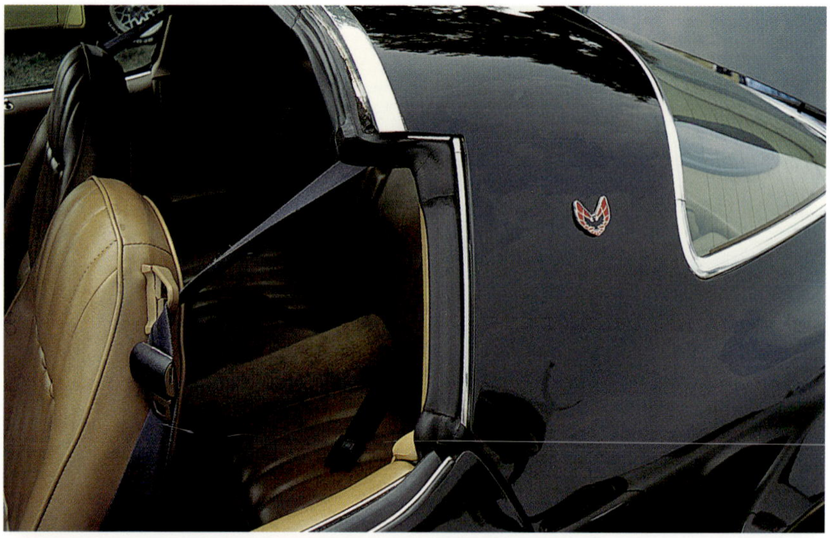

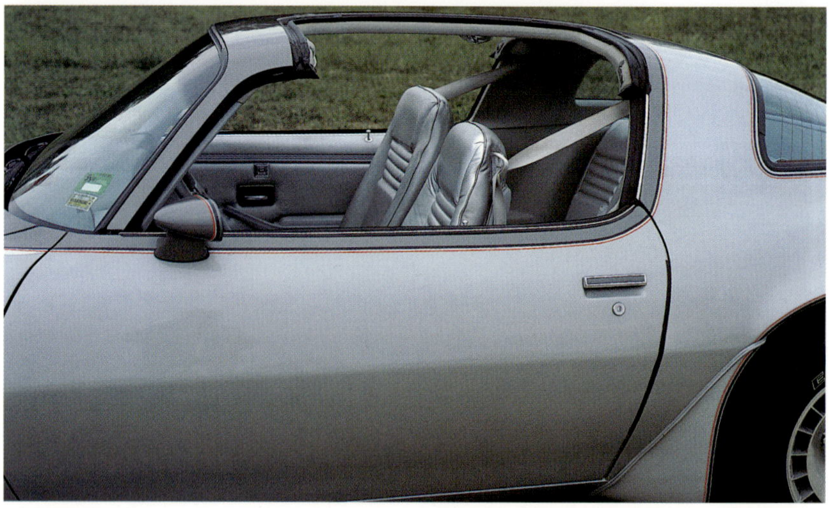

Top: Detail view of the roof and T-top opening on a black 1978 Trans Am. This Trans Am has an optional Camel-Tan vinyl interior trim and the Firebird badge on the roof pillar. ***Above:*** Detail view of the T-top hatch roof on a 1979 Trans Am 10th Anniversary Edition. Note the rubber seal surrounding the top opening. This Trans Am is finished in Silver Iridescence (15) and has the special silver leather interior trim (152) standard with the 10th Anniversary package. ***Below:*** Detail view of the T-top hatch roof on an Atlantic Blue 1979 Trans Am sport coupe. This is the longer Fisher-designed T-top. Note the blue Trans Am decal on the roof pillar.

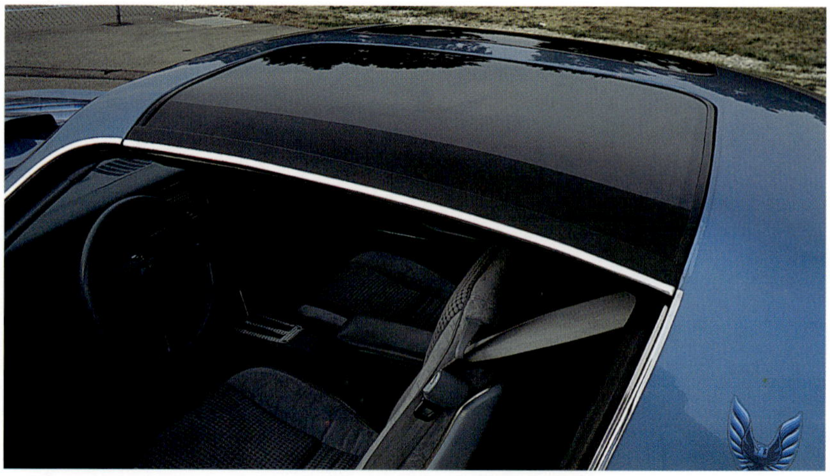

Right: This unique orange-and-red bird decal was used only on the Formula, shown on an original black 1979 Formula sport coupe. The distinctive black rear window molding finish is shown. ***Far right:*** Detail view of the gold roof-pillar bird decal on an original Barclay Brown 1981 Trans Am sport coupe. The gold stripes and decal were used with the brown body finish.

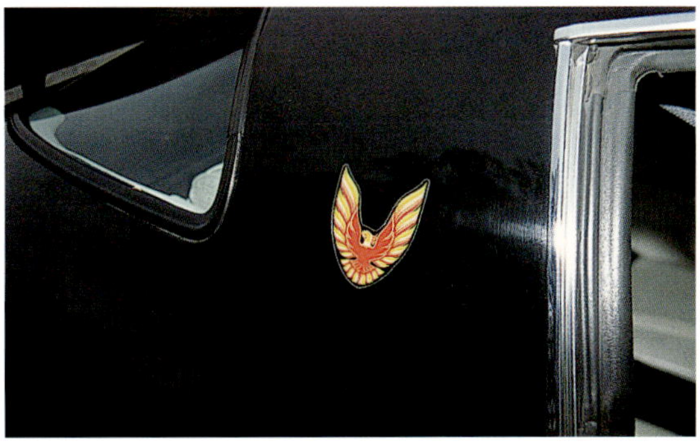

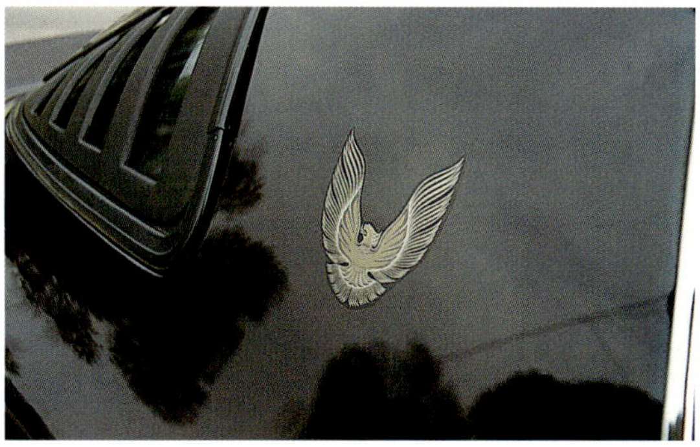

models, but different part numbers were used for 1972–1974 (9681673 L, 9681672 R) and 1975–1981 (20162369 L, 20162368 R). There were no vent windows, so the side glass was sealed by rubber seals and channels in the front windshield post and rear roof quarter pillar. The doors were operated by chrome-plated, rectangular, pull-type, lift-bar handles that were identical for all 1973–1975 models, but a new, slightly shorter design was used for 1976–1981. All outside door handles had a color-coordinated insert appliqué for the custom-trim versions. The 1979–1981 Firebirds equipped with four-wheel disc brakes added an additional decal at each door handle indicating the brake option.

All 1974–1981 Firebird doors were sealed with black soft sponge rubber weatherstrip surrounding the outer perimeter of the door shell. The perimeter of the body door opening used a color-coordinated push-on vinyl windlace that

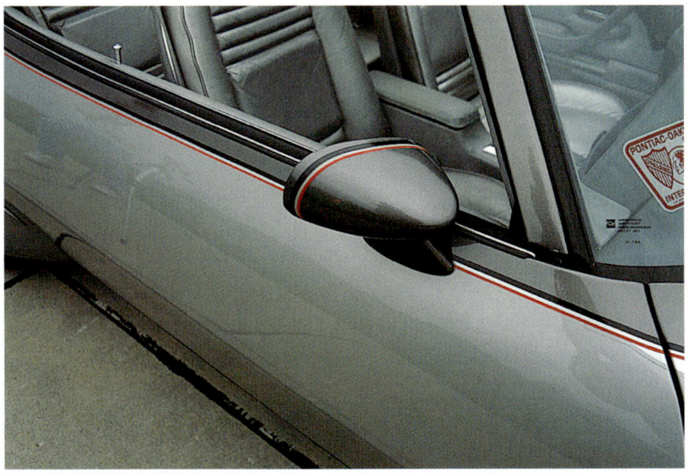

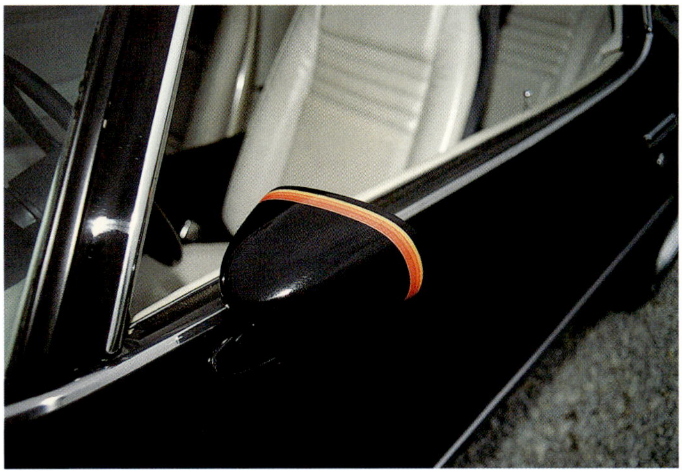

Above left: Detail view of the right side sport mirror on a 1979 Trans Am 10th Anniversary Edition. The body is finished in Silver Iridescence, but the mirrors, roof, and upper body stripes are finished in a darker shade of Gray Iridescence (16). ***Above right:*** This is a detail view of the left outside sport mirror on a black 1979 Firebird Formula with the optional RPO W50 Formula Appearance Package. Note the distinctive stripes on the mirror.

Right: This left outside door handle on a blue 1980 Trans Am equipped with optional four-wheel disc brakes (RPO JL2) has a color-keyed door handle insert. ***Far right:*** This detail view of the left remote-control outside sport mirror on a blue 1980 Trans Am sport coupe shows the distinctive stripes on the mirror body.

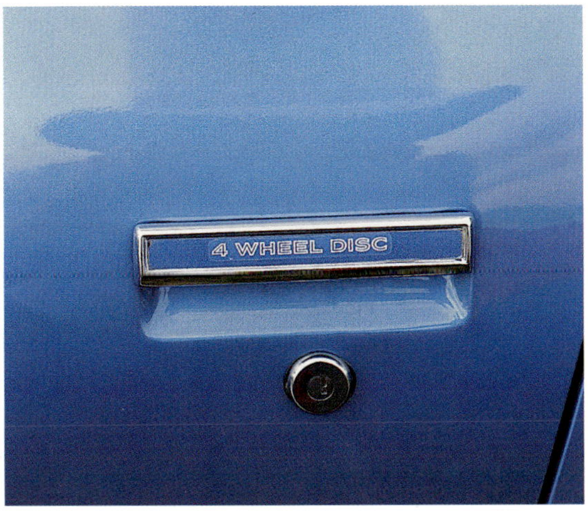

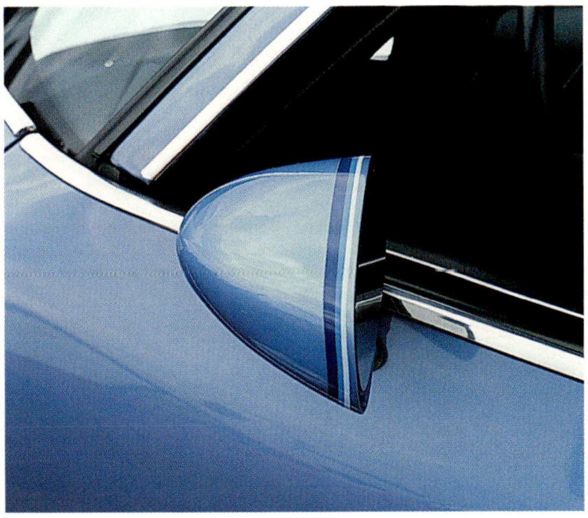

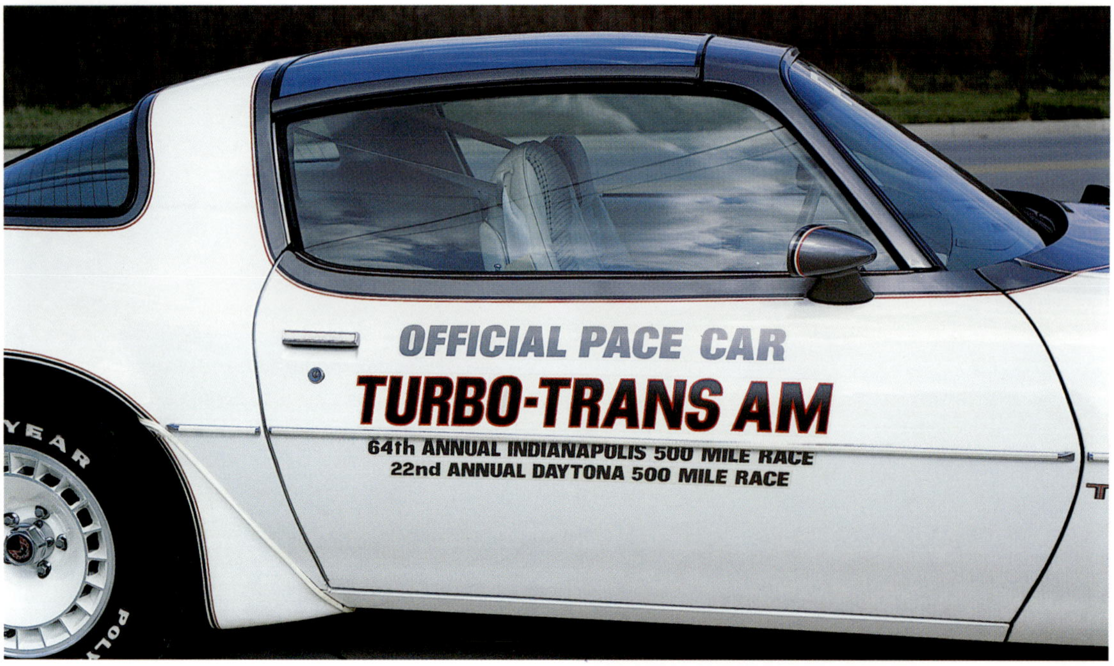

This special door decal package was part of the 1980 Turbo Trans Am Indianapolis 500 Pace Car package. The body and cast-aluminum wheels are finished in white. Note the tinted T-top hatch roof and special body stripe design.

also served to secure the inside quarter trim panels. The lower door opening was trimmed with an aluminum sill plate with a riveted Fisher Body badge at the front end. A black ABS plastic vent grille and a body-color Torx-head latch striker were mounted in the body doorjamb.

All 1974–1981 Firebirds used the same deck lid (part number 9819030), hinges, and supports used for the 1970–1973 models with variations only for trim badges and spoilers. On models without a spoiler, a black-and-red cloisonné Firebird medallion was mounted in the rear center of the deck lid.

All 1974–1980 Firebirds with the optional rear spoiler (other than the Trans Am) had a bird decal mounted in the center of the rear of the spoiler. The decal colors corresponded with the body colors, and for 1974, the decal was available in blue, green, and orange. In 1975, the colors were orange, blue, and charcoal. Red was added for 1976.

All 1974–1981 Trans Ams had a Trans Am decal in the center of the rear spoiler. The Trans Am decal was three colors and in block letters for 1974–1976. Decal colors were determined by the body color and, in 1974, blue-and-black were used for white and blue cars and orange-and-black for red cars. In 1975, charcoal-red-and-black were added for silver cars. For 1976 and 1977, the Trans Am spoiler decals were again three-color with charcoal-red-and-black for white and silver cars; gold-yellow-and-orange for yellow and red cars; and gold-dark-gold-and-black in German-style letters for the black 50th Anniversary Special Edition Trans Am.

In 1978, the Trans Am spoiler decal was available in charcoal-red-and-black for white and platinum cars; gold-yellow-and-black for black, gold, yellow, brown, and red cars; and blue-and-black for bright blue cars. The Special Edition Trans Am had a gold-dark-gold-and-black decal. For 1979, all Trans Am spoiler decals were gold-yellow-and-orange, except for the 10th Anniversary Trans Am, which had a special bird and inscription decal. The 1979 Formula used a unique red-and-orange spoiler bird decal. For 1980, the Trans Am spoiler decals had shades of colors with variations for each body color. The blue decal was used for white, platinum, and blue

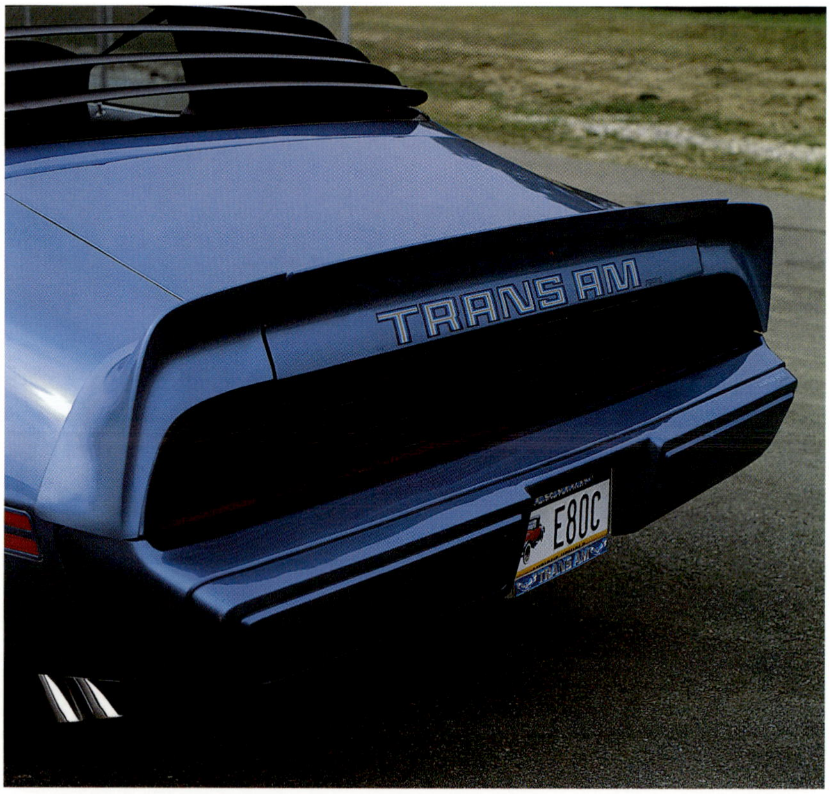

Detail view of the deck lid and rear deck lower panel on an Atlantic Blue 1979 Trans Am sport coupe. The spoiler with color-keyed decal is standard with the Trans Am. The ends of the spoiler are wider and are a different design than earlier Trans Ams.

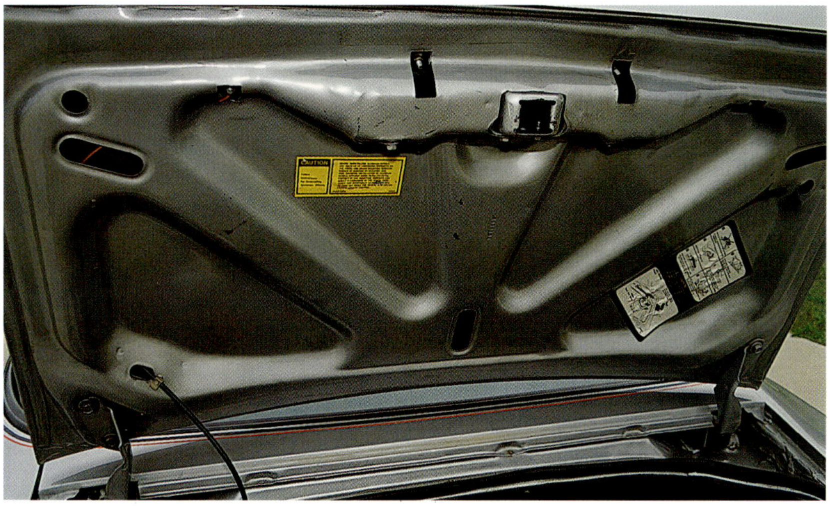

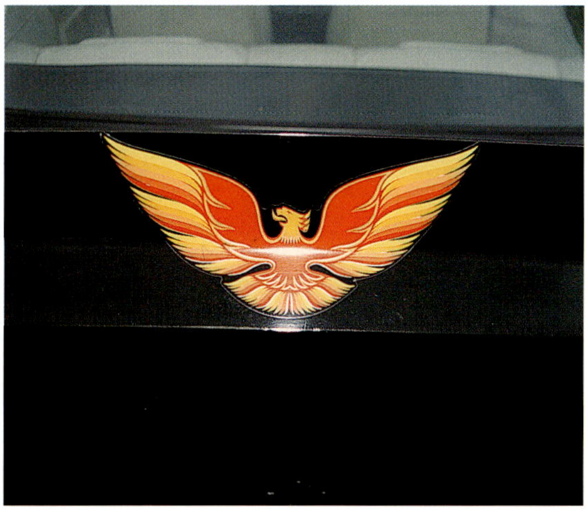

Above: This view of the deck lid on original silver 1979 Trans Am 10th Anniversary Edition includes the placement of the jack instructions decal on the right of the deck lid. ***Right:*** This unique orange-and-red bird decal appears on the rear spoiler of an original black 1979 Firebird Formula with the RPO W50 Formula Appearance Package.

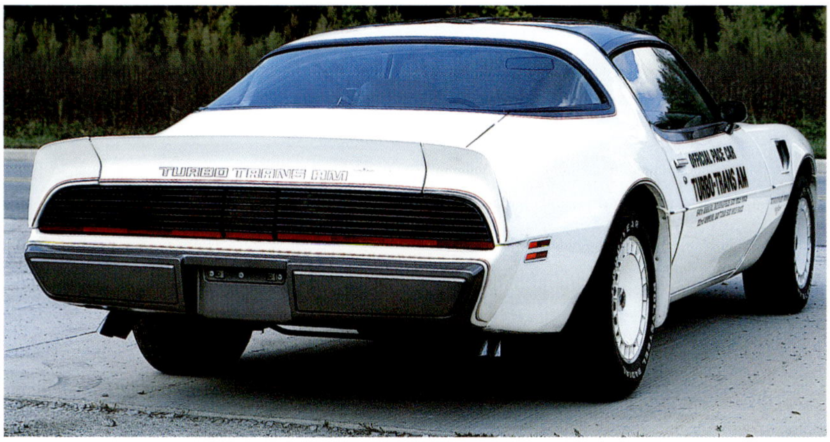

This view shows the rear deck lid and spoiler on a white 1980 Turbo Trans Am Indianapolis 500 Pace Car Edition. Note the silver finish on the bumper, the unique spoiler Trans Am decal, and the unique stripes surrounding the rear window.

cars. Gold was used for gold, yellow, brown, copper, and red cars. Red/orange was used for red cars, and silver/charcoal was used on gray cars.

All 1974–1981 Firebirds had a flat trunk floor (except for a raised area to accommodate the fuel tank) with a standard full-size spare tire and wheel mounted on the right side of the trunk with its inner side up. The jack base was mounted bottom-side up in the center of the wheel and was held in place by a plated wing nut. The jack was held in place by the tire and wheel. The space-saver spare was again available with UPC N65 and had the tire inflator mounted in the lower rear of the wheel. The flat part of the trunk floor was covered with a vinyl mat in either an aqua-and-black or gray-and-white houndstooth pattern. The entire trunk interior was finished with gray speckle paint.

The rear deck lower panel on the 1974–1981 Firebirds was similar in design to the earlier models, but the taillights were wider and the new soft protective bumpers were incorporated into the styling. Each side of the rear deck lower panel had three narrow, horizontal taillamps. The taillamps were the same design from 1974 to 1978, but in 1978, the Trans Am and Formulas with the RPO W50 appearance package had blacked-out taillamp lens dividers with part number 5970348 (right) and 5970347 (left). The taillamp design was restyled with thin horizontal bars for 1979–1981, and a custom extension was used for the Trans Am, the Formula, and the 1980 Esprit. The extension gave the look of a full-width taillamp assembly and added an extra light on each side. The license plate lamp was mounted in the right bezel in 1974 and 1975 but moved to the left side in 1976. The 1974 and 1975 license plate mounting was in the center, partly recessed into the top edge of the bumper. The fuel filler was located under a hinged door behind the license plate.

The rear bumper was redesigned for 1974 and 1975 and was covered with a body-color outer urethane shell and a horizontal black protective strip in its center. For 1976–1978, the bumper was again redesigned and was full body-color urethane with a horizontal crease across its width. The license plate mounting was moved higher into the rear deck lower panel and only projected into the upper bumper edge about 1 inch. The outer ends of the bumper wrapped around the corner of the body and were flush with the body sides for better aerodynamic efficiency. The 1979–1981 rear bumper construction was similar to the 1978 version, but the inner reinforcement was eliminated and replaced with a narrower outer bumper bar. The outer shell was redesigned and featured a raised wide flat horizontal bar across its center. The license plate mounting was moved down into the center of the bumper, and the rear deck lower panel incorporated a separate square fuel filler door. The rear deck lower panel had narrow ribs across its width.

The rear quarter panels of the 1974–1981 Firebird kept the same basic design as the 1973 body and had the same long horizontal body crease. The most significant change was when the wraparound rear window was adopted in 1975. Small rectangular two-section side marker lights were mounted just below the body crease and just ahead of the rear bumper sides. The 1974–1981

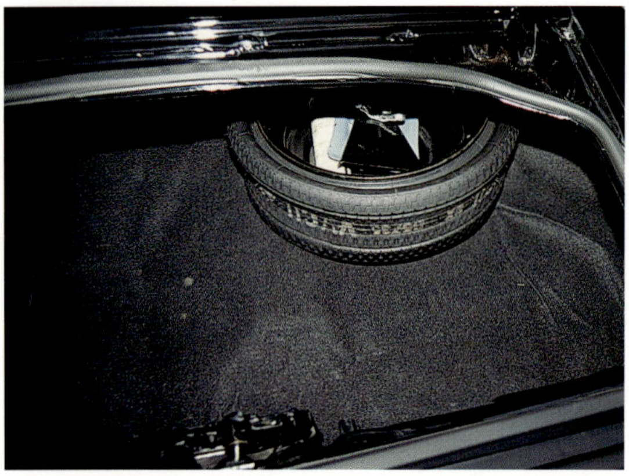

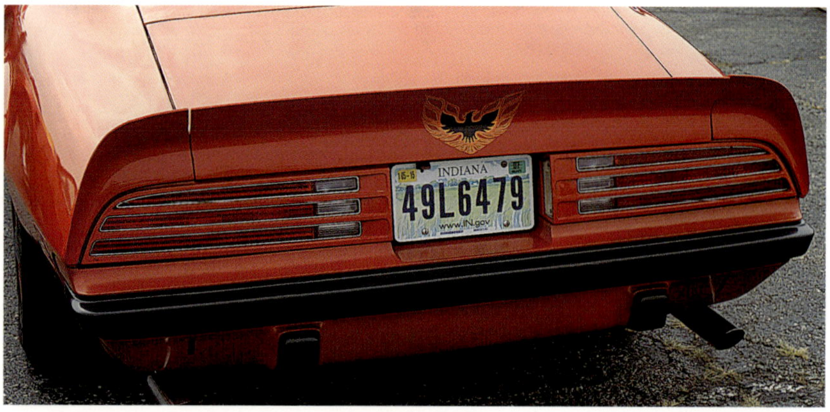

Above left: This detail view of the trunk interior of an original black 1979 Firebird Formula shows the placement of the inflatable compact spare tire held down by the jack base and a wing nut. ***Above right:*** Shown are the rear deck lower panel and taillights of a Buccaneer Red 1974 Firebird Formula with the optional SD 455 engine. Note the design of the rear bumper and lower valance.

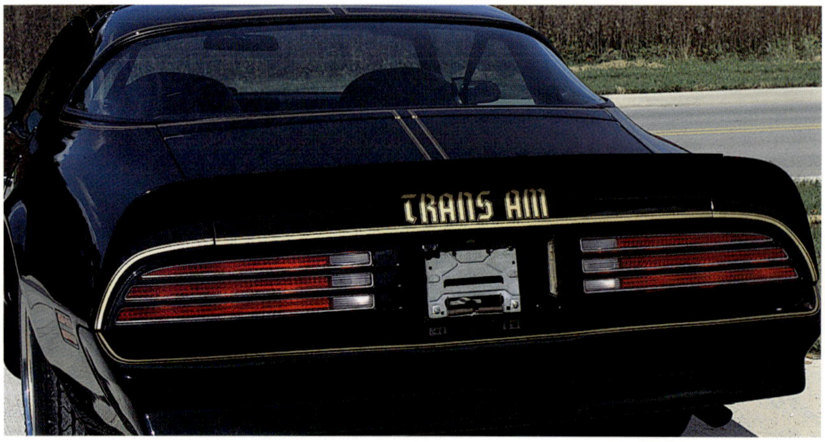

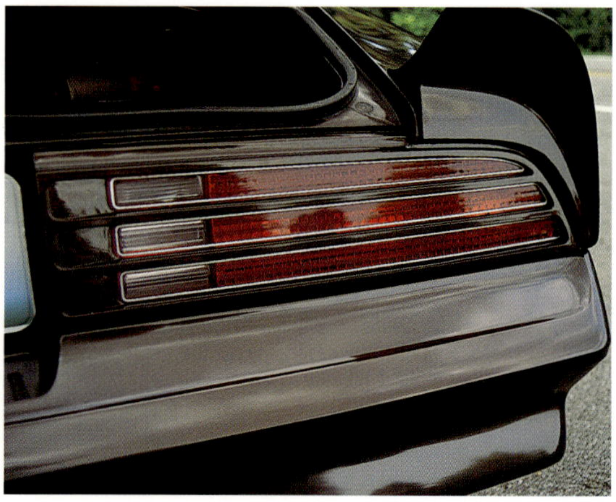

Above left: This view of the rear deck lower panel and deck lid on a black 1976 Trans Am 50th Anniversary Limited Edition highlights the unique gold stripes and German-style lettering on the gold Trans Am decal. This model was the inspiration for the Trans Am used in the 1977 *Smokey and the Bandit* movie with Burt Reynolds and Jerry Reed. ***Above right:*** Detail view of the rear deck lower panel of an original Brentwood Brown 1977 Trans Am sport coupe. The original taillight lenses have a 1974 date identification code.

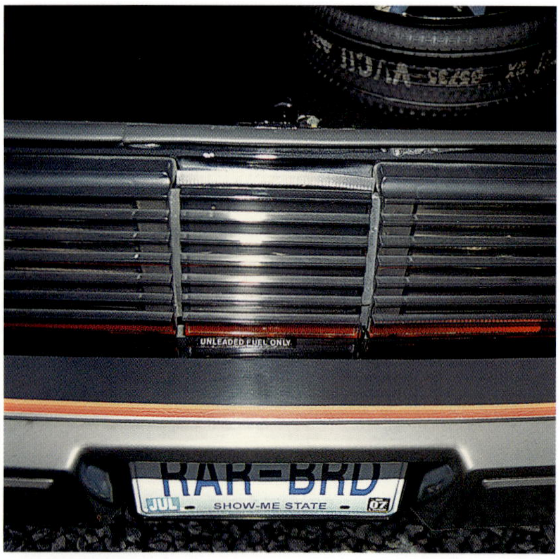

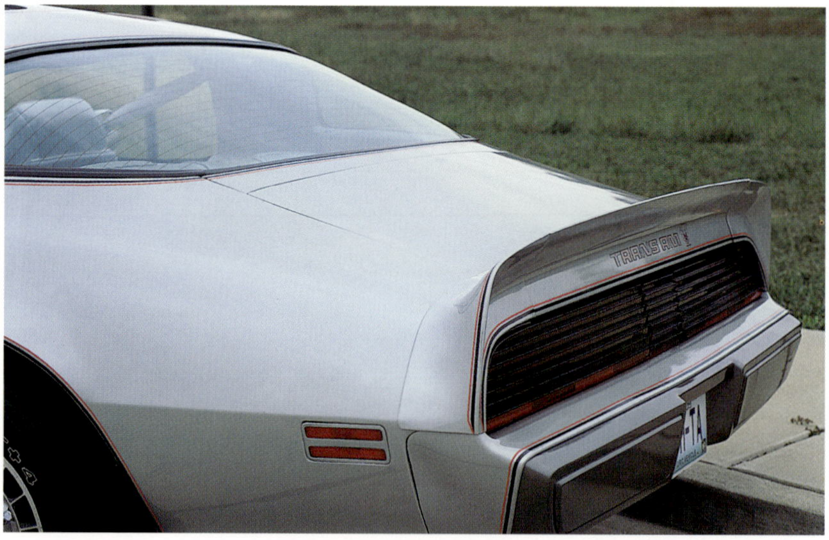

Above left: Detail view of the center of the rear deck lower panel and fuel filler door on a black 1979 Firebird Formula. Note the red stripe at the upper edge of the rear bumper. ***Above right:*** This view shows the details and colors of the rear deck lower panel on a silver 1979 Trans Am 10th Anniversary Edition sport coupe, including the rear bumper design, rectangular side marker lights, and the special stripes on the spoiler.

Right: This right rear quarter view of the rear deck lower panel and deck lid on a Barclay Brown 1981 Trans Am sport coupe shows the Firebird badge on the fuel filler door and "Trans Am Pontiac" decal on the spoiler. The rear window louver is an aftermarket accessory. ***Below:*** A detail view of the front fascia—note the separate square headlight openings and red arrowhead badge.

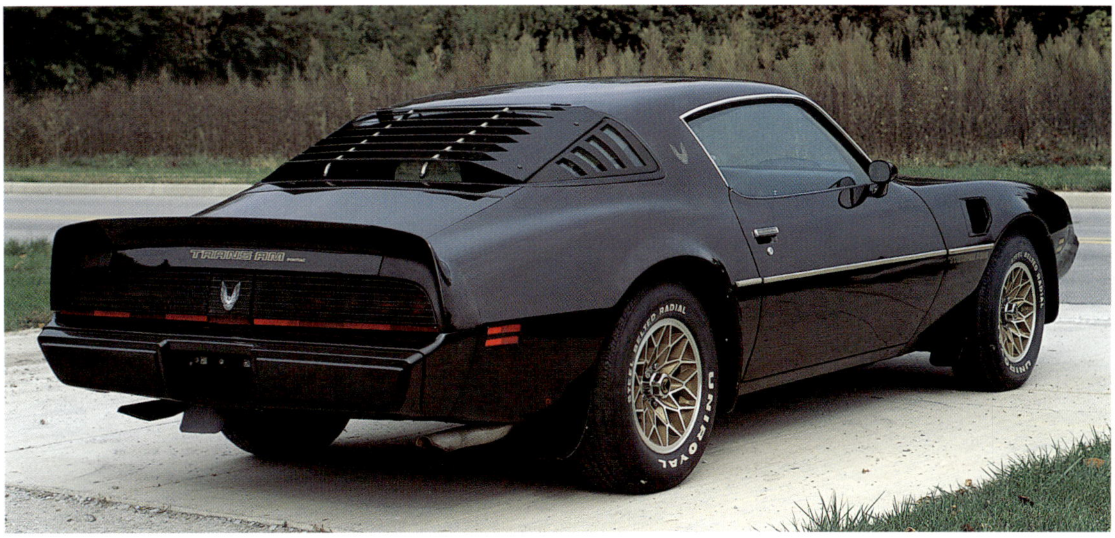

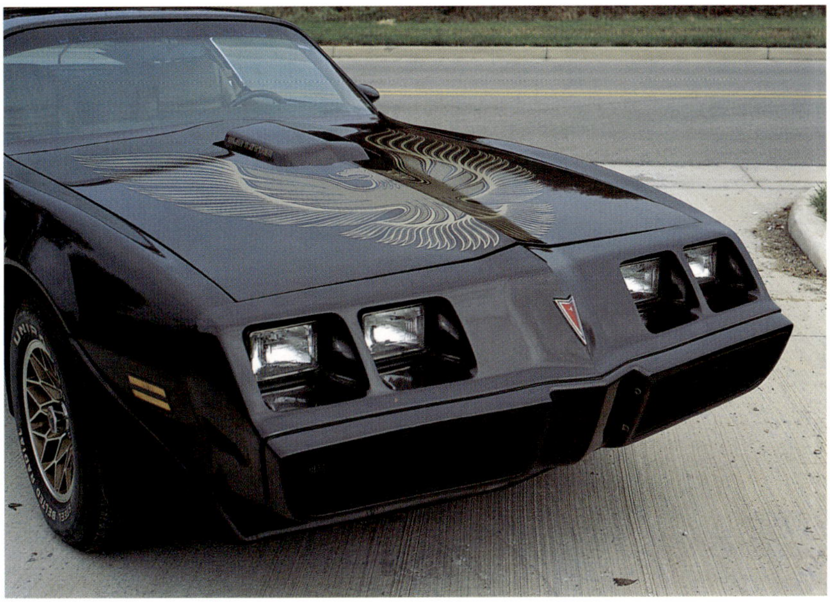

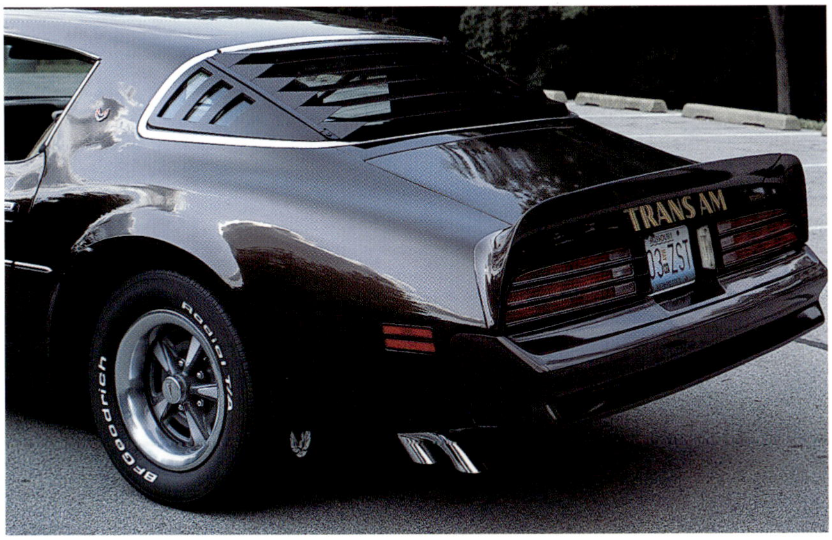

The left rear quarter panel of a 1977 Trans Am sport coupe shows the body design used since 1970 with little change except for the rear window. This Trans Am has an accessory hinged black rear window louver assembly that tilts up to clean.

marker lights were the same design as those used in 1973. As in the 1970–1973 models, the Trans Am had separate spoilers in front of the rear wheel openings. Bright wheel opening moldings were available as an option (RPO B96) on all models, except the Trans Am, and standard equipment on the Esprit. A full-length bright rocker panel molding was mounted between the wheel openings on all but the Trans Am.

All 1974 and 1975 Firebirds, except the Trans Am, used the same front fenders. The fenders were the same as those used in 1973 and had part numbers 492991 (right) and 492922 (left). The standard fenders were redesigned slightly for the 1976 model and used part numbers 546939 (right) and 546937 (left). The 1977–1981 standard front fenders used part numbers 526147 (right) and 526148 (left). The appearance was similar for all versions.

All 1970–1975 Trans Ams used the same front fenders (except for a design change in 1973 for the new fender-to-core support braces) with the opening in the upper rear for the unique rear-facing engine compartment air extractor. The wheelwell openings were also modified for large tire clearance. The 1973–1975 Trans Am front fenders had part numbers 492993 (right) and 492994 (left). The part numbers were changed to 546938 (right) and 546939 (left) for 1976. For 1977–1981, the Trans Am used fenders with part numbers 526149 (right) and 526150 (left). The appearance was similar in all versions. The extractors were redesigned along with the fenders and had different part numbers for 1974 and 1975 and for 1976–1981. The Trans Am front fenders had a separate wide spoiler mounted in the front of the wheel opening. The wheel opening spoiler tied to the front lip spoiler at each end and had a body-color seal around its mounting joint with the fender.

The 1974–1981 Trans Am had a Trans Am

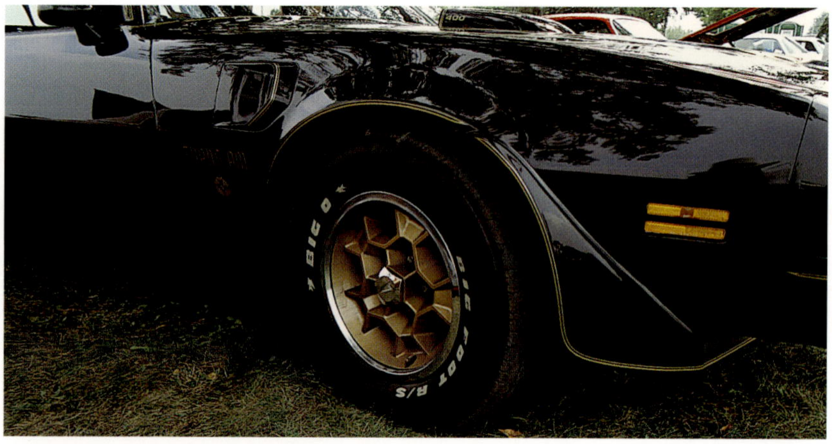

Above left: This detail view of the right front fender of a Buccaneer Red 1974 Formula SD 455 features the one-piece bright Formula 455 badge. ***Above right:*** This view shows the right front fender of a 1976 Trans Am black 50th Anniversary Limited Edition. The gold stripes and accents are part of the 50th Anniversary package. The wheels are gold Honeycomb cast aluminum. ***Below:*** This detail view of the left front fender of a Brentwood Brown 1977 Trans Am sport coupe highlights the distinctive functional extractor vent on the side of the Trans Am fender. The protective body side molding is an option.

decal mounted just beneath the body character line and to the rear of the wheel opening. The 1977 Trans Am Special Edition had a decal in a distinctive Old German-type script. All other 1974 and 1975 Firebird and Esprit models had a bright metal script Firebird badge in the same location. The 1974 and 1975 Formula used unique bright metal Formula nameplates. The 1976–1981 models, other than the Trans Am, had no fender identification. All 1974–1981 Firebird front fenders had a rectangular two-section marker light in the lower front of the fender.

There were three different hoods used on the 1974–1976 Firebirds. The standard Firebird Esprit used a flat steel hood with a slightly raised longitudinal center crease with part number 500085. The 1974 and 1975 Formula 350, 400, and 455 used a fiberglass hood with dual nonfunctional scoops with part number 490660. The 1976 Formula 350 and 400 used a restyled steel hood with twin nonfunctional scoops and part number 499976. The 1974 and 1975 Formula models equipped with Ram Air used a hood with part number 490661. Those with the Super Duty 455 and shaker-type hood used part number 500154, which was standard on all Trans Ams. All hoods used the same hood hinges and springs.

The shaker hoods for 1974–1981 Trans Ams and Formulas continued to use an optional (RPO WW7) large bird decal like the one introduced in 1973. The 1974 and 1975 bird was the same as those used in 1973, except the additional red-and-charcoal color was adopted for the silver body color in 1975 only, and the light-blue-and-dark-blue bird was only used in 1973. Also, the green bird was not used in 1975. For 1976, the bird decal was similar to that used in 1975, but the part numbers were changed to

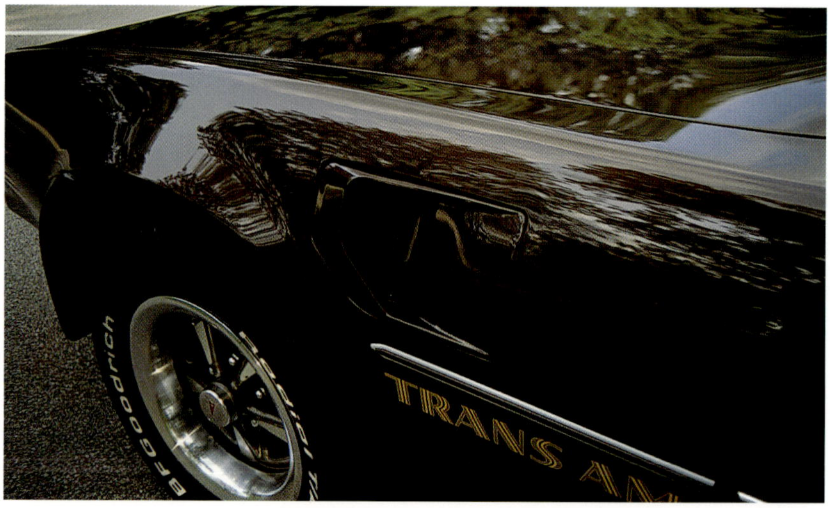

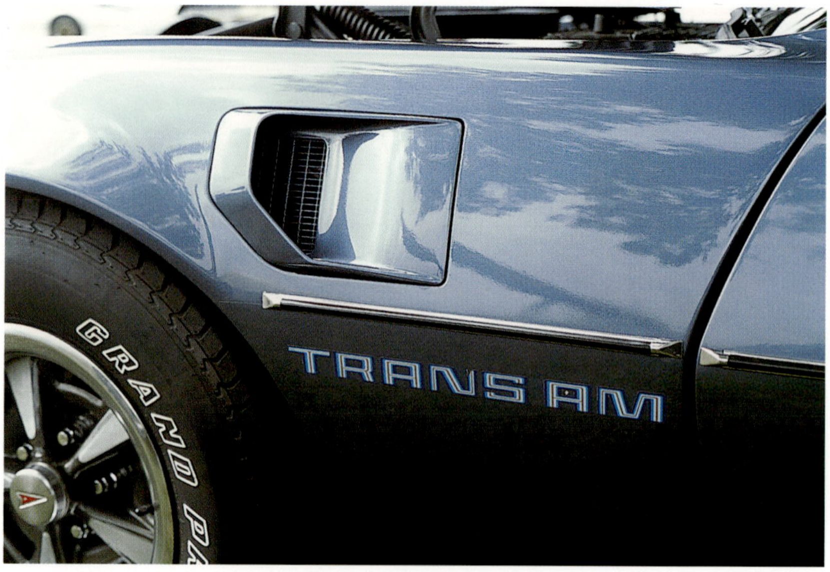

This view shows the details of the left front fender of a blue 1979 Trans Am, the functional heat extractor vent, and the color-keyed blue Trans Am decal.

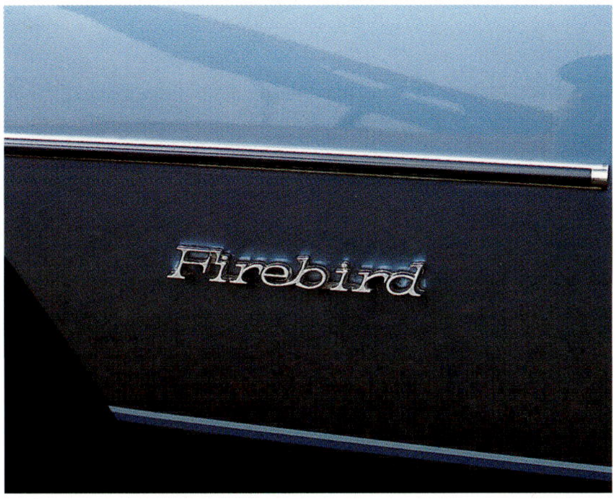

This Bright Blue (24) 1980 Firebird Formula left front fender has the standard bright-filled Formula nameplate and optional color-keyed body side molding (RPO B84).

500666 for the red-and-charcoal, 527047 for the yellow-orange-and-gold on all except silver, 547163 for the yellow-orange-and-gold on black (except the Special Edition), and 547045 for the gold bird used only on the black Special Edition (SE) cars. Due to production quality problems from November 25, 1975, until February 1976, some yellow-orange-and-gold birds on non-SE cars may have been charcoal and red. Color-coordinated engine identification decals for the 400 and 455 were used on the sides of the scoop.

The Firebird front end was restyled for 1977–1979, so new hoods were used across the line. The new standard flat steel hood (part number 10011150) used on all models except the Formula and Trans Am was smoothed, with a less dramatic center crease. There were again three different hoods used across the line. The Formula used a new hood (part number 10012180), with new, flatter, dual simulated scoops. The Trans Am had a standard hood as standard equipment with the shaker hood optional (RPO T48), but few, if any, came without the shaker hood that had part number 10011151. The same hood hinges and latches were continued from the previous year.

The large bird decal was again optional for 1977–1979, except for the Special Edition package with which it was standard. The bird decals were color-coordinated with the body color. Trans Ams with the RPO Y82/RPO Y84 Special Edition package used gold-colored birds. The engine

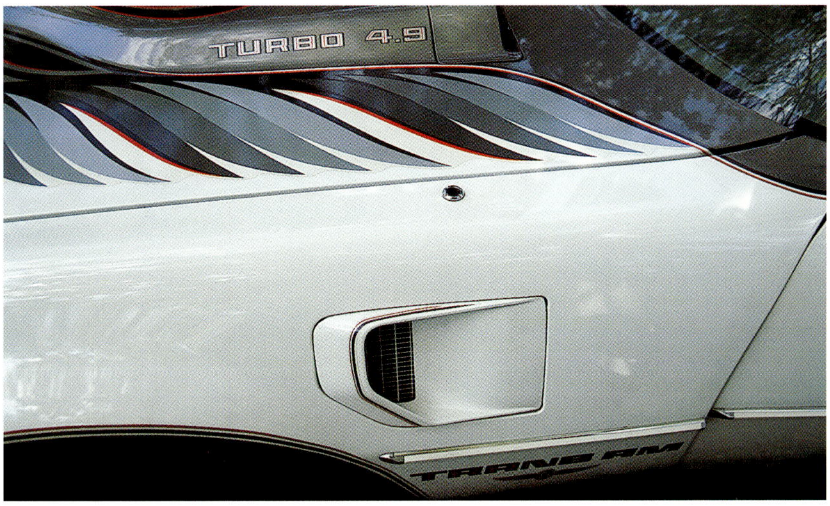

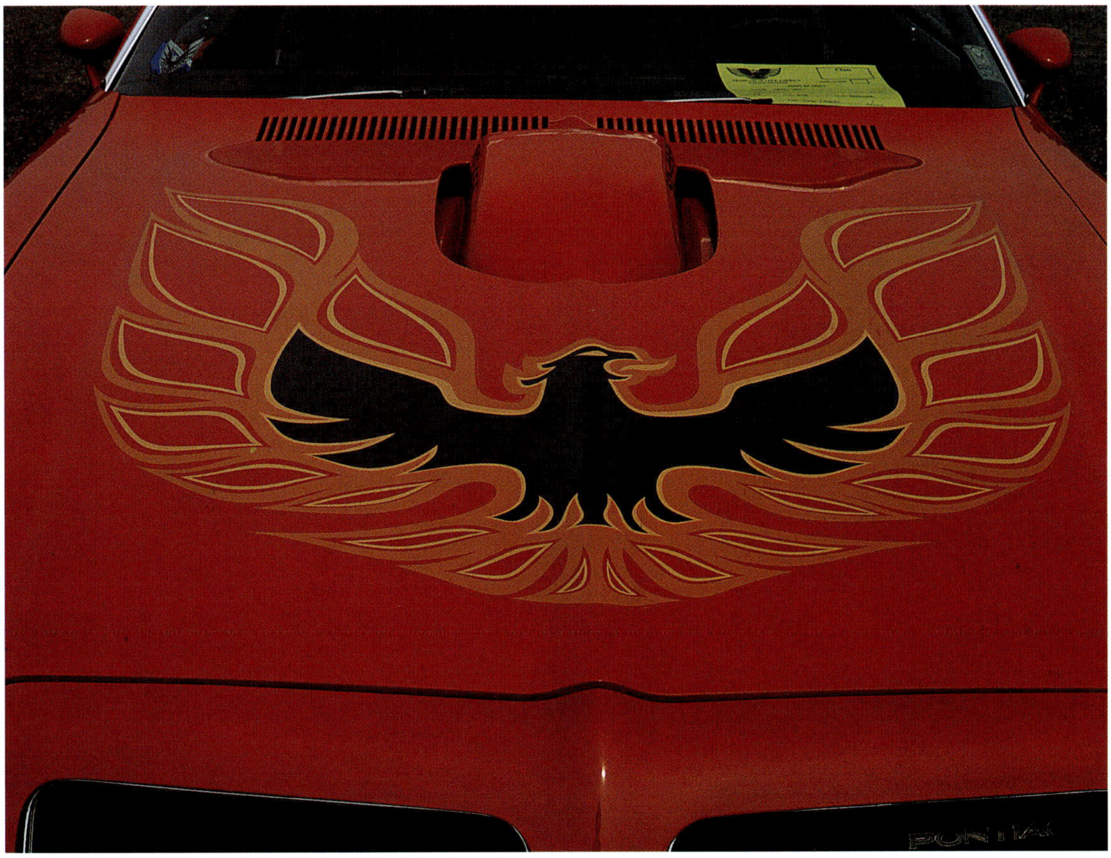

Above: Left front fender of a white 1980 Trans Am Indianapolis 500 Pace Car Edition. Note the special decals on the lower fender panel, the distinctive Trans Am extractor vents, and the opening for the optional power radio antenna (RPO U75). ***Right:*** This yellow-and-black Trans Am bird decal, shown on a Buccaneer Red 1974 Firebird Formula SD 455, was actually only available on the V87 Trans Am, so it is not correct on the Formula.

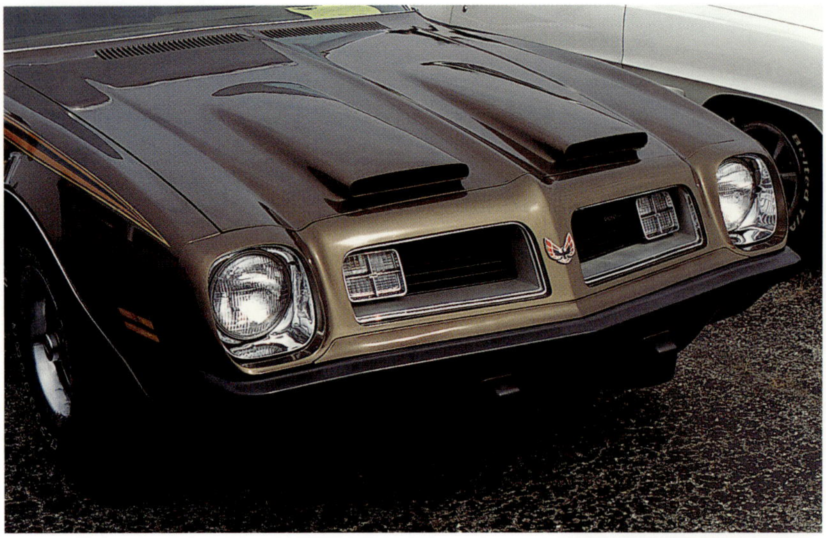

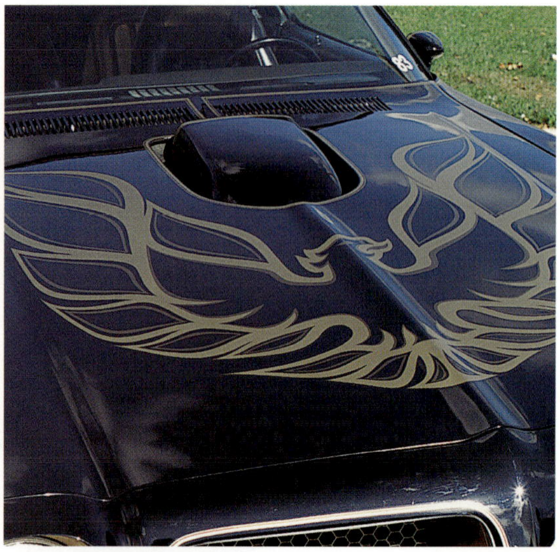

This view shows the front fascia and hood detail of a Ginger Brown (58) 1975 Firebird Formula. The hood and distinctive Formula twin scoops are molded fiberglass.

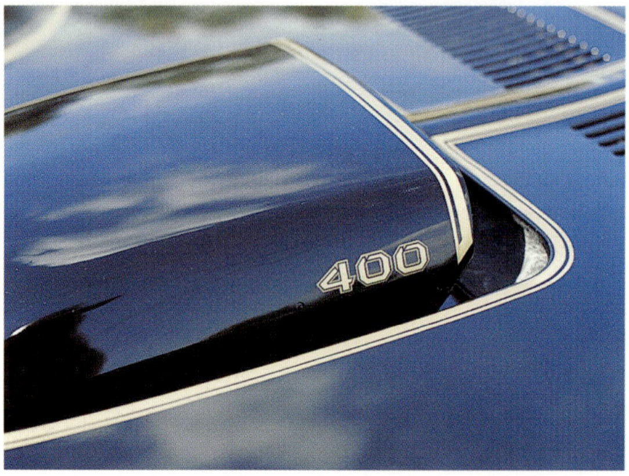

Above: This shows a detail view of the hood and optional gold bird decal on a black 1976 Trans Am 50th Anniversary Limited Edition with gold accents on the grille mesh. ***Left:*** This detail view of the hood and rear-facing shaker scoop on a black 1976 Trans Am 50th Anniversary Limited Edition shows the gold stripes on the hood and the 400 engine decal on the scoop.

identification decals on the optional shaker scoop were also available in colors corresponding with the body color. In 1977–1979, decals that read 6.6 Liter were used on those cars equipped with the Oldsmobile 403-ci engines, while those with the Pontiac 400-ci had decals that read T/A 6.6. The 10th Anniversary Special Edition used charcoal color decals. The charcoal-white-and-silver bird used on the 10th Anniversary Special Edition faced to the right and had wingtips that extended onto the tops of the front fenders.

In 1980 and 1981, the standard hood from 1977–1979 (part number 10011150) was used on the Firebird and Esprit. The standard Trans Am hood was a shaker hood when equipped with the 305-ci or 301-ci V-8. Otherwise, the standard flat hood was used. The shaker hood was not available on any other 1980 or 1981 model. When the turbocharged engine was ordered in the Formula or Trans Am, a new hood (part number 10009232) was used with an off-center (to the left) aerodynamic bulge to clear the turbocharger. The hinges, latches, and springs were the same as those used in 1979.

Hood engine identification and bird decals were changed for 1980 and 1981. The large bird decal was again optional for the Trans Am and

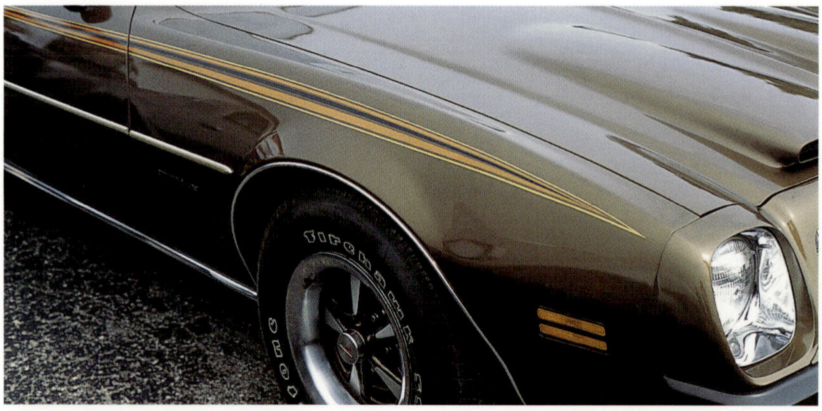

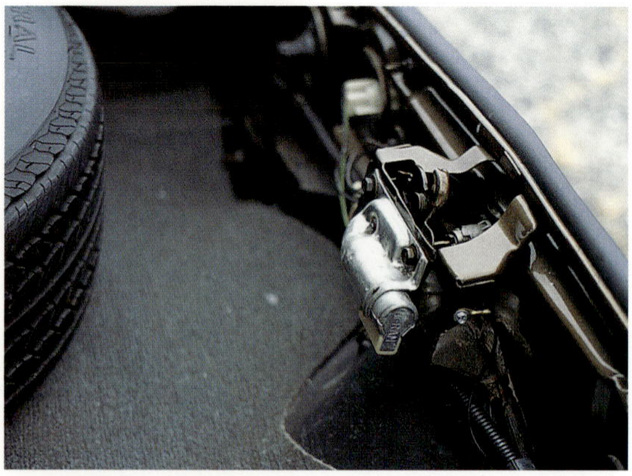

Above left: This is the right front fender of a Ginger Brown 1975 Firebird Formula with optional orange and yellow stripes. The protective body side molding and Rally II wheels and trim rings were optional. ***Above right:*** Detail view of the optional power deck lid release solenoid on a Ginger Brown 1975 Firebird Formula sport coupe. Note the Hi-RAM name and plated finish of the solenoid.

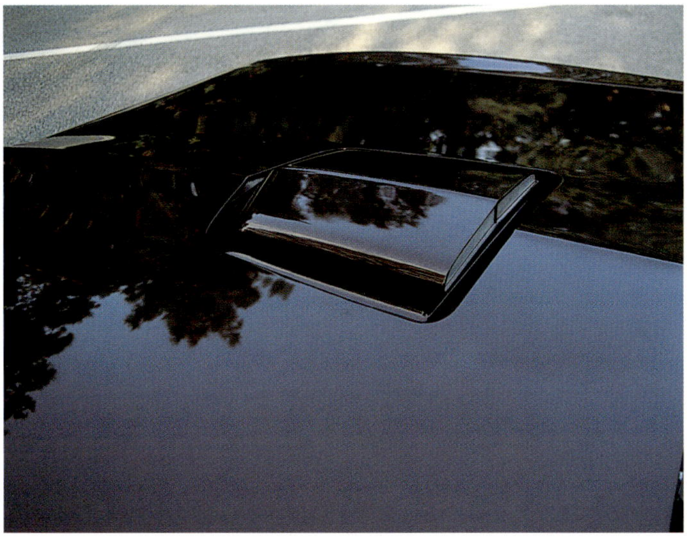

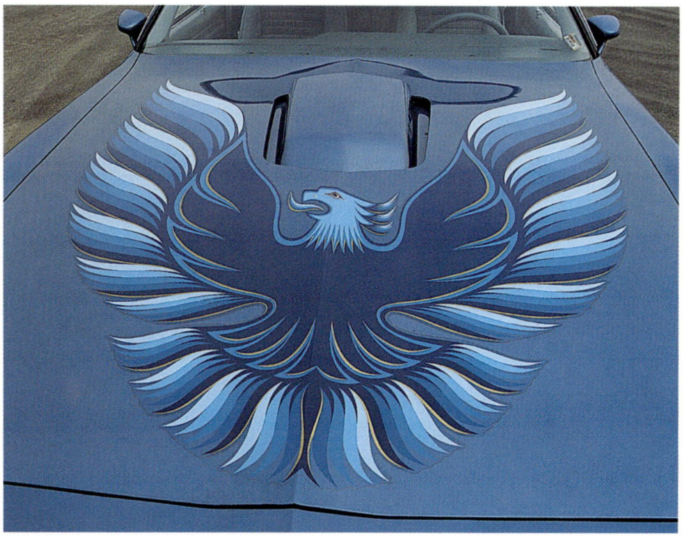

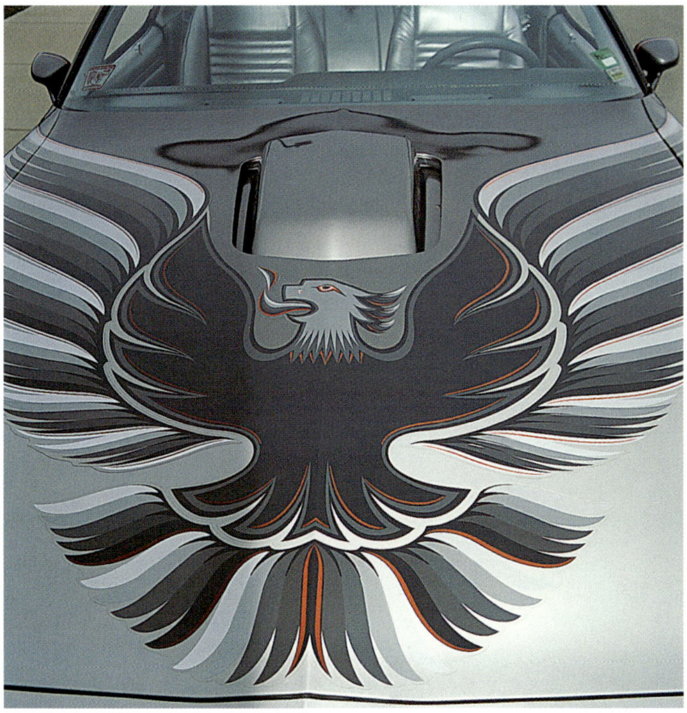

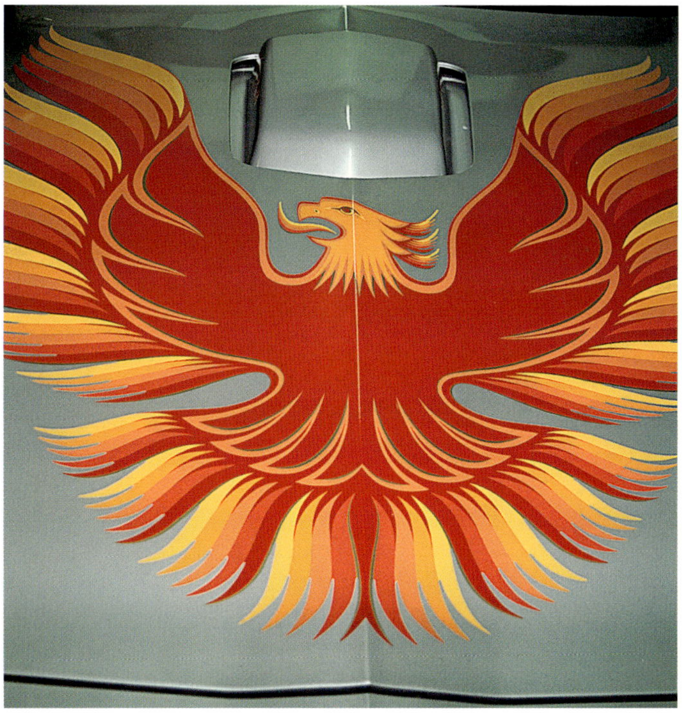

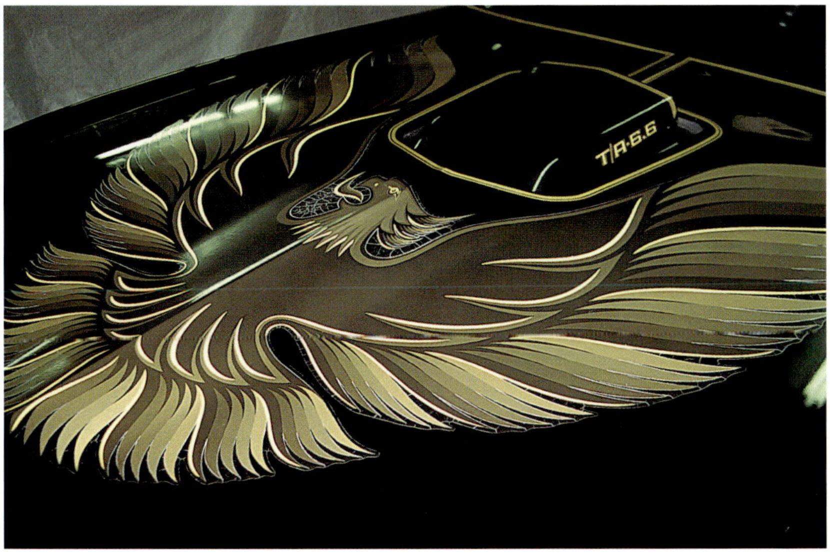

Top left: This is a detail view of the hood and nonfunctional shaker scoop on a Brentwood Brown 1977 Trans Am that does not have the optional decal package. ***Top right:*** This is the optional color-coordinated blue bird decal (RPO D53) on the hood of an Atlantic Blue (29) 1979 Trans Am sport coupe. Note that the bird is facing to the right. ***Above left:*** The standard large gray bird decal used on the 1979 Trans Am 10th Anniversary Edition is in three pieces and extends to the edges of the right and left fenders. ***Above right:*** This silver 1979 Trans Am has an unusual optional red-and-yellow bird decal on the hood. It is slightly smaller and of a different design than the one used on the 10th Anniversary Trans Am. ***Left:*** This 1979 Trans Am had the optional RPO Y84 Black Special Edition package that included the gold bird decal on the hood and gold accents and stripes on the body.

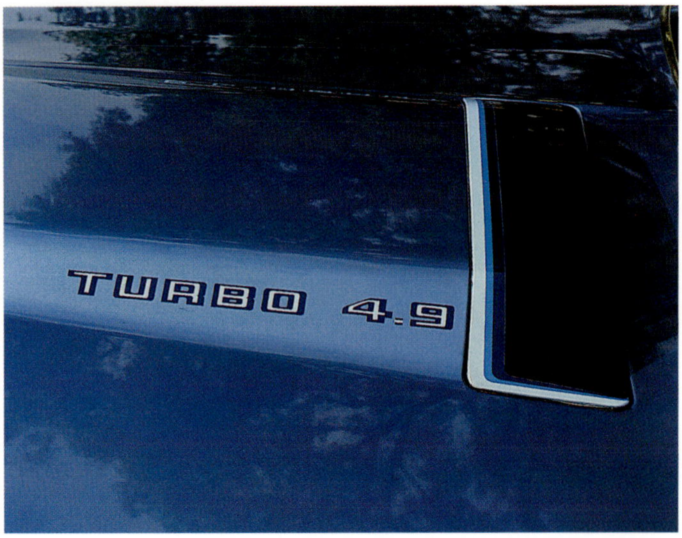

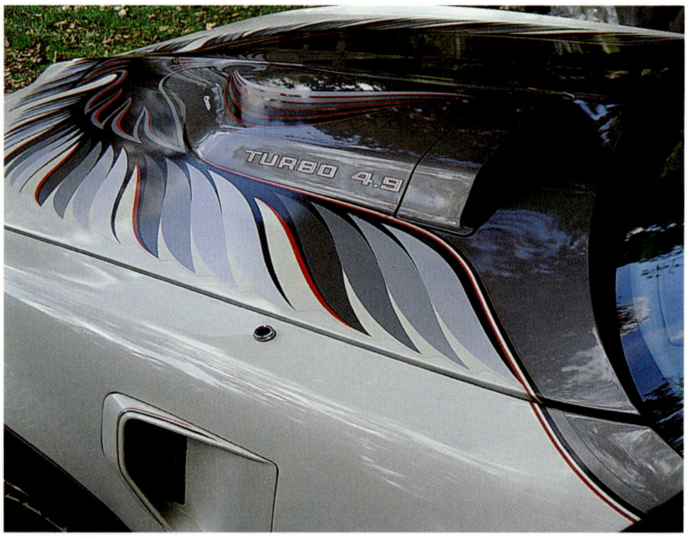

Above left: This blue 1980 Firebird Formula equipped with the 4.9-liter turbo V-8 engine has distinctive stripes and black accents on the hood bubble. ***Above right:*** This is a detail view of the hood scoop and gray bird decal on a 1980 Turbo Trans Am sport coupe. Note the dark gray accent on the body and hood and the red-and-black pinstriping.

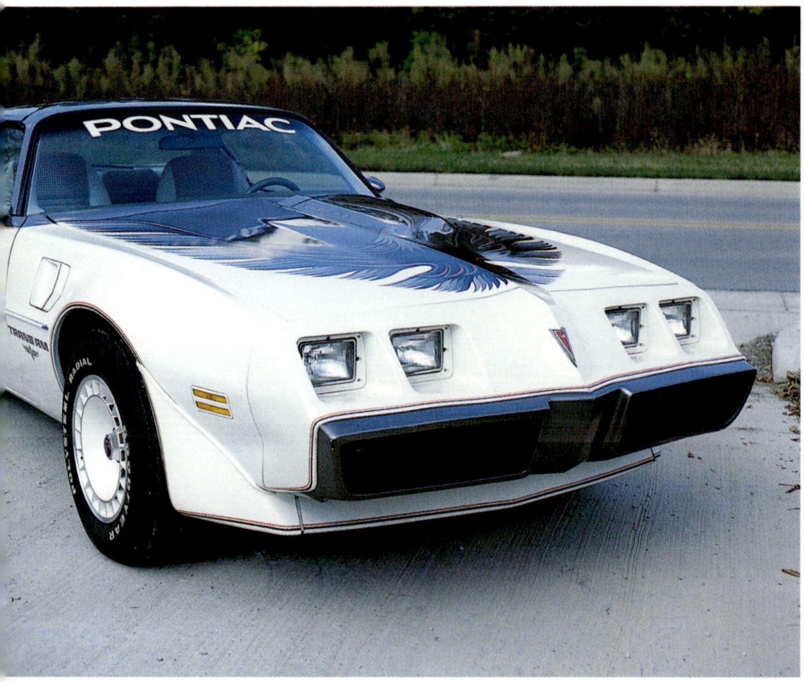

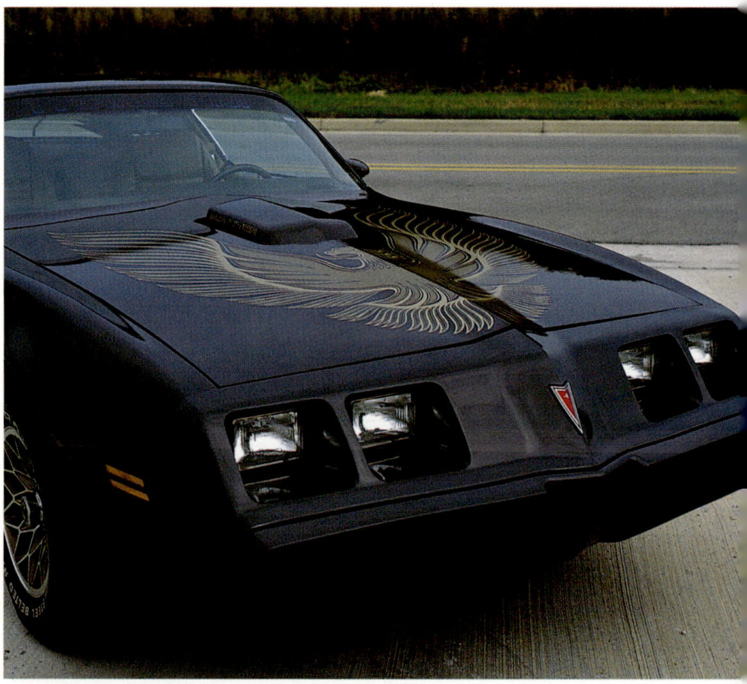

Above left: This view shows the hood and optional gray bird decal on a white 1980 Turbo Trans Am Indianapolis 500 Pace Car Edition. The distinctive windshield Pontiac decal and white-painted cast-aluminum 15-inch wheels are standard with the 1980 Turbo Trans Am Pace Car package. ***Above right:*** This detail view of the hood and optional gold bird decal on a Barclay Brown 1981 Trans Am shows the bird facing left on this design. Note the "5.0 LITRE" engine decal on the shaker hood scoop.

Formula. There were different decals for the turbocharged and nonturbocharged cars. When equipped with the turbocharger, the bird was smaller and faced to the left rather than right as it did with nonturbo engines. The bird used with turbocharged cars had a separate flame decal that emitted from the bird's mouth and across the turbo bulge. The 1981 bird was also a different design than the 1980 version. Again, colors of the decals were coordinated with the body color, and six different colors were used for each year.

The engine identification decals for 1980 and 1981 included a T/A 4.9 for the nonturbocharged engine and TURBO 4.9 for the turbocharged versions. Both decals were on the hood bulge. For 1980, there were no identification decals on the shaker scoop with a 305-ci V-8. In 1981, there was a decal that read 5.0 Liter on the shaker

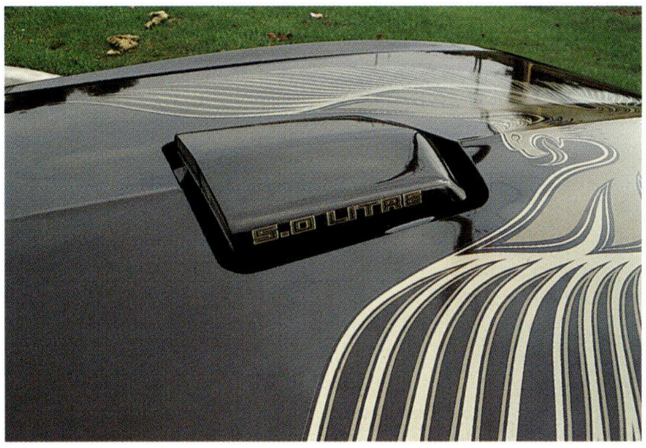

Detail view of the hood scoop of an original Barclay Brown 1981 Trans Am with the optional gold bird decal on the hood (RPO D53) and engine identification decal on the scoop.

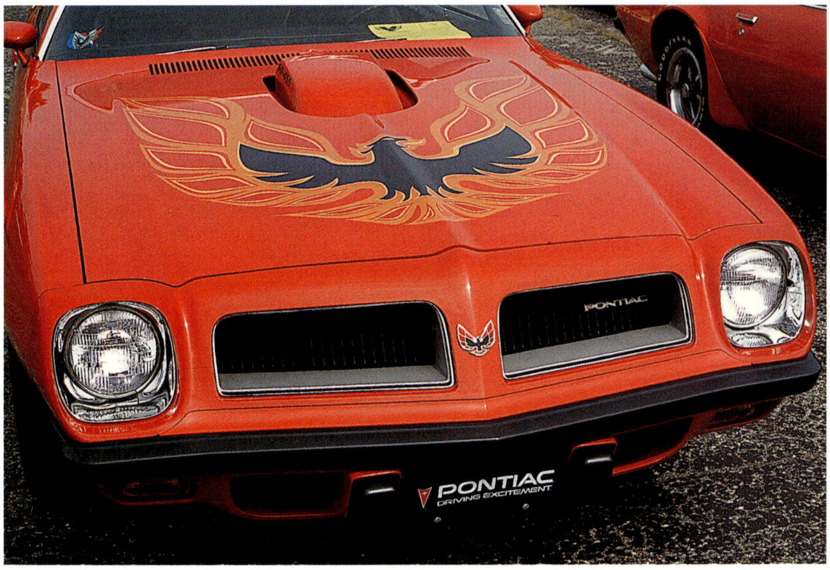

The front fascia of a Buccaneer Red 1974 Firebird Formula SD 455. The front design was entirely new for 1974, but the remainder of the body was similar to the 1973. The bird decal on the hood was intended for the Trans Am and is not correct for the Formula.

scoop. There were also changes in the color shades of the decals between 1980 and 1981.

One of the most significant design changes for the 1974 and 1975 Firebird was the front end panel treatment and grille. The new 1974 and 1975 body-color fiberglass front end panel (part number 4983413) featured a slanted nose with single round headlights on each side encased in rectangular bright bezels. The top center of the fascia had a peak that corresponded with the peak in the center of the hood. The dual rectangular grille openings were divided by a vertical space that included a cloisonné red-and-black Firebird badge. The grille mesh was rectangular and was argent silver for the Firebird and Esprit and flat black for the Formula and Trans Am. A Pontiac nameplate was used in the left hand grille on all models. The front bumper, or impact bar, was a wide black rubber band above a body-color lower panel with dual rectangular openings on either side of the front license plate mounting. A vertical black rubber bumperette was mounted on each side of the license plate. Rectangular parking/turn signal lamps were mounted in the outer ends of the lower panel for 1974, but for 1975, the lights were moved to the outer ends of the grille opening. The Trans Am had an additional lower spoiler under the lower panel that connected to the wheel opening flares.

The 1976 Firebird front end panel and headlamp molding (part number 526351) was redesigned, and a body-color urethane bumper sloped back into the grille openings and wrapped around the sides under the headlight bezels. The peak in the top center of the fascia was like that on the earlier version. The lower panel below the

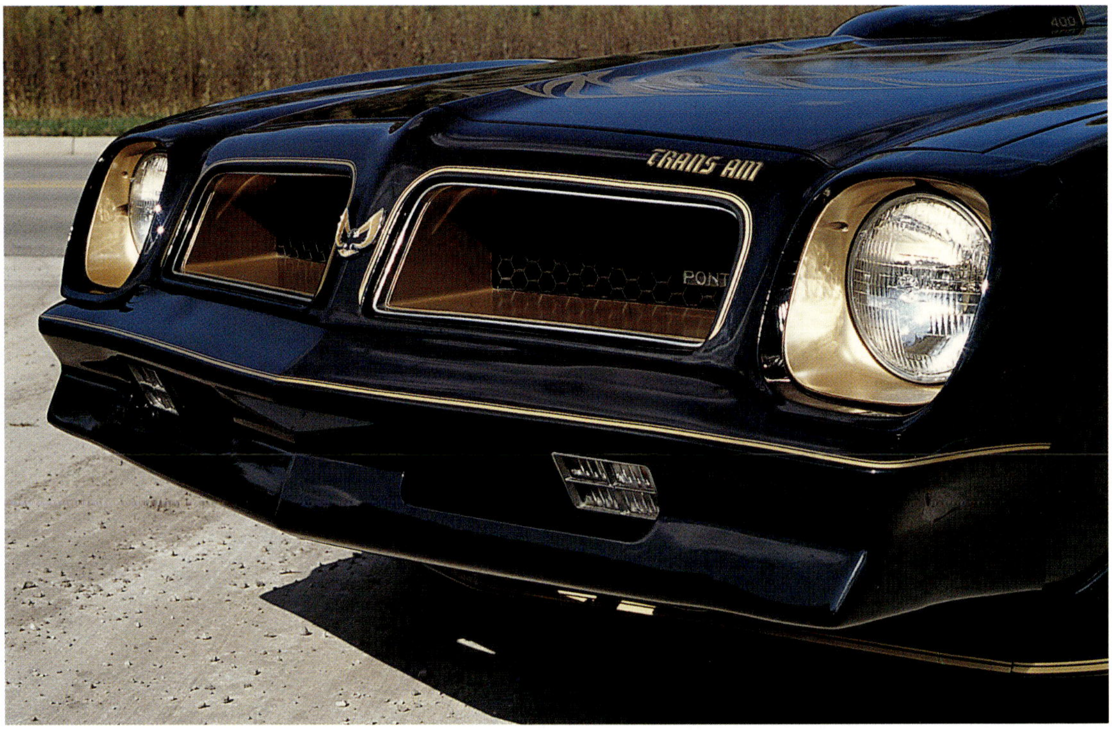

The front fascia on a black 1976 Trans Am 50th Anniversary Limited Edition with the unique gold Limited Edition decals, hood bird, and grille accents.

Firebird Production

1974

Model	Production
Firebird Six	7,603
Firebird V-8	18,769
Esprit	22,583
Formula ex/455 SD	14,461
Formula 455 SD	58
Trans Am 400	4,664
Trans Am 455	4,648
Trans Am 455 SD	943

1975

Model	Production
Firebird	22,293
Esprit	20,826
Formula	13,670
Trans Am 400	26,417
Trans Am 455	857

1976

Model	Production
Firebird	21,206
Esprit	22,252
Formula	20,613
Trans Am 400	37,015
Trans Am 455	7,099
LE coupe 400	1,628
LE coupe 455	319
LE T-top 400	533
LE T-top 455	110

1977

Model	Production
Firebird	30,642
Esprit	34,548
Formula	21,801
Trans Am	68,744

1978

Model	Production
Firebird	32,671
Esprit	36,926
Formula	24,346
Trans Am	93,351

1979

Model	Production
Firebird	38,642
Esprit	30,853
Formula	24,850
Trans Am	109,608
Trans Am 10th Anniv. X87	7,500

1980

Model	Production
Firebird	29,811
Esprit	17,277
Formula	9,356
Trans Am	45,196
Trans Am Turbo Pace Car X87	5,700

1981

Model	Production
Firebird	20,541
Esprit	10,938
Formula	5,927
Trans Am coupe	11,804
Trans Am T-top	14,426
SE coupe X87	121
SE T-top X87	5,142
Trans Am Turbo Pace Car X87	2,000

impact bar now had two long horizontal rectangular openings with the license plate mounting in the center. The parking/turn signal lamps were moved back to the outer ends of the openings in the lower panel. The 1976 rectangular grille openings were similar to 1974 and 1975 and included a honeycomb mesh pattern grille.

For 1977 and 1978, the Firebird front end panel (part number 547092) was redesigned significantly. There were now four rectangular headlights, and the twin grille openings were given a more stylized appearance with a pronounced V-shaped peak and vertical crease in the grille divider. A red cloisonné arrowhead badge (part number 499724) was placed in the center of the V in all 1977 models and in all 1978 models, except the Esprit Redbird package and the Special Edition Trans Am. The outer perimeter of the grille openings in the one-piece unit had a bright trim surround, and each grille insert used a honeycomb design in various colors according to the model. The Firebird and standard Esprit used an Argent silver grille (part numbers 526089 right, 526090 left). The Esprit with the Skybird package (RPO W60) used a blue grille. The Trans Am and Formula used a flat black grille (part numbers 526087 right, 526088 left), and the Trans Am Special Edition used a gold grille. For 1978, the Esprit Skybird package was replaced with the Redbird package (RPO W60) that used a red grille. The black rubber bumper was eliminated for 1977 and 1978 and replaced with a body-color horizontal crease in the fascia with the parking lamps placed into the outer ends of twin

Body Colors

1974 Body Colors

Code	Color
11	Cameo White
26	Regatta Blue
29	Admiralty Blue
36	Gulfmist Aqua
40	Fernmist Green
46	Limefire Green
49	Pinehurst Green
50	Carmel Beige
51	Sunstorm Yellow
53	Denver Gold
55	Colonial Gold
59	Crestwood Brown
64	Ascot Silver
66	Fire Coral Bronze
74	Honduras Maroon
75	Buccaneer Red

1975 Body Colors

Code	Color
11	Cameo White
13	Sterling Silver
15	Graystone
24	Arctic Blue
26	Bimini Blue
29	Stellar Blue
44	Lakemist Green
49	Alpine Green
50	Carmel Beige
51	Sunstorm Yellow
55	Sandstone
58	Ginger Brown
63	Copper Mist
64	Persimmon
74	Honduras Maroon
75	Buccaneer Red

1976 Body Colors

Code	Color
11	Cameo White
13	Sterling Silver
19	Starlight Black
28	Athena Blue
35	Polaris Blue
36	Firethorn Red
37	Cordovan Maroon
40	Metalime Green
49	Alpine Green
50	Bavarian Cream
51	Goldenrod Yellow
65	Buckskin Tan
67	Durango Bronze
78	Carousel Red

1977 Body Colors

Code	Color
11	Cameo White
13	Sterling Silver
19	Starlight Black
21	Lombard Blue
22	Glacier Blue
29	Nautilus Blue
36	Firethorn Red
38	Aquamarine
44	Bahia Green
51	Goldenrod Yellow
55	Gold Metallic
58	Bright Blue
61	Mohave Tan
63	Buckskin
69	Brentwood Brown
75	Buccaneer Red
78	Mandarin Orange

1978 Body Colors

Code	Color
11	Cameo White
15	Platinum Poly
19	Starlight Black
22	Glacier Blue Poly
24	Martinique Blue Poly
42	Redbird Red
48	Berkshire Green Poly
50	Special Edition Gold
51	Sundance Yellow
55	Gold (accent)
58	Blue (accent)
63	Laredo Blue Poly
67	Ember Mist Poly
69	Chesterfield Brown Poly
75	Mayan Red
77	Carmine Poly

1979 Body Colors

Code	Color
11	White
15	Silver Iridescence
16	Gray Iridescence (accent color)
19	Black
24	Bright Blue Iridescence (or Atlantic Blue)
29	Dark Blue Iridescence
50	Gold Iridescence (special order)
51	Bright Yellow
63	Camel Iridescence
69	Dark Brown Iridescence
75	Red
77	Carmine Iridescence
80	Red (special order)

1980 Body Colors

Code	Color
11	White
15	Platinum
19	Black
24	Bright Blue Iridescence
29	Dark Blue Iridescence
37	Accent Yellow (accent color)
51	Bright Yellow
56	Yellow (Yellowbird color)
57	Gold Poly
67	Dark Brown
71	Francisco Red
72	Red
76	Dark Claret
79	Red Orange
80	Rust
84	Charcoal

1981 Body Colors

Code	Color
11	Cameo White
16	Stardust Silver
19	Starlight Black
20	Vibrant Blue
21	Baniff Blue
29	Nightwatch Blue Iridescence
51	Tahitian Yellow
54	Dorado Gold
56	Yellow
57	Navajo Orange
67	Barclay Brown
75	Spectra Red
77	Autumn Maroon
84	Ontario Gray

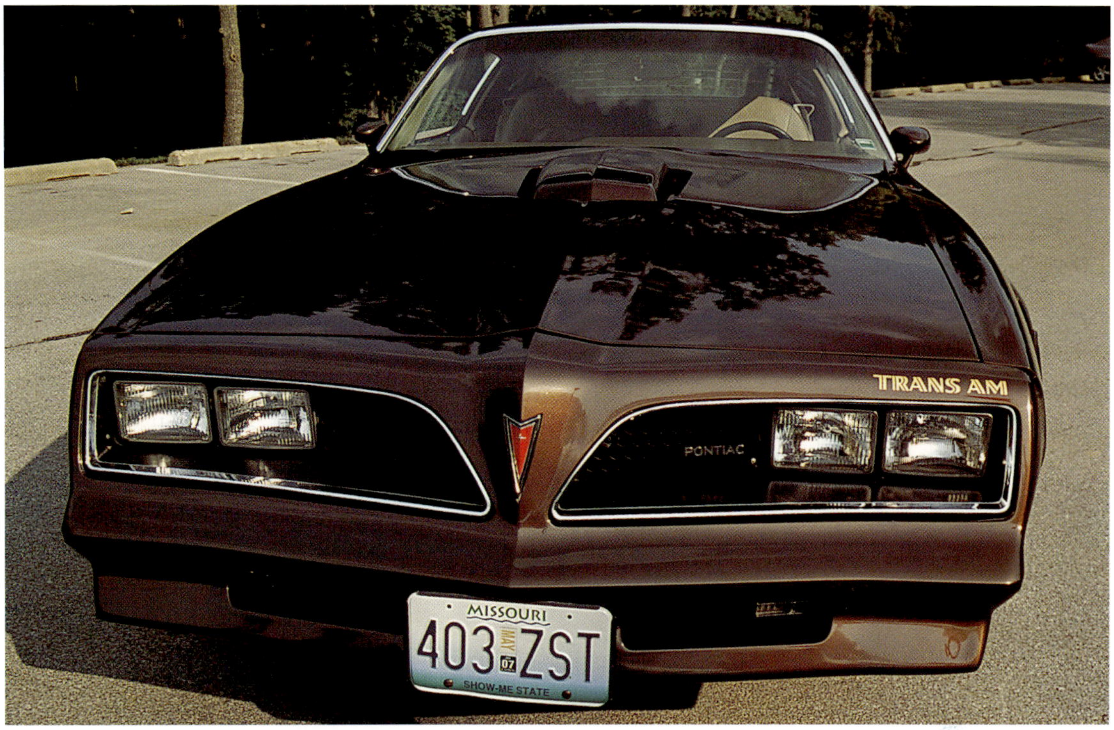

The front fascia of a Brentwood Brown 1977 Trans Am shows the first year for quad headlights on the second-generation Firebirds. Note the black honeycomb grille mesh and distinctive Pontiac peak to the front nose.

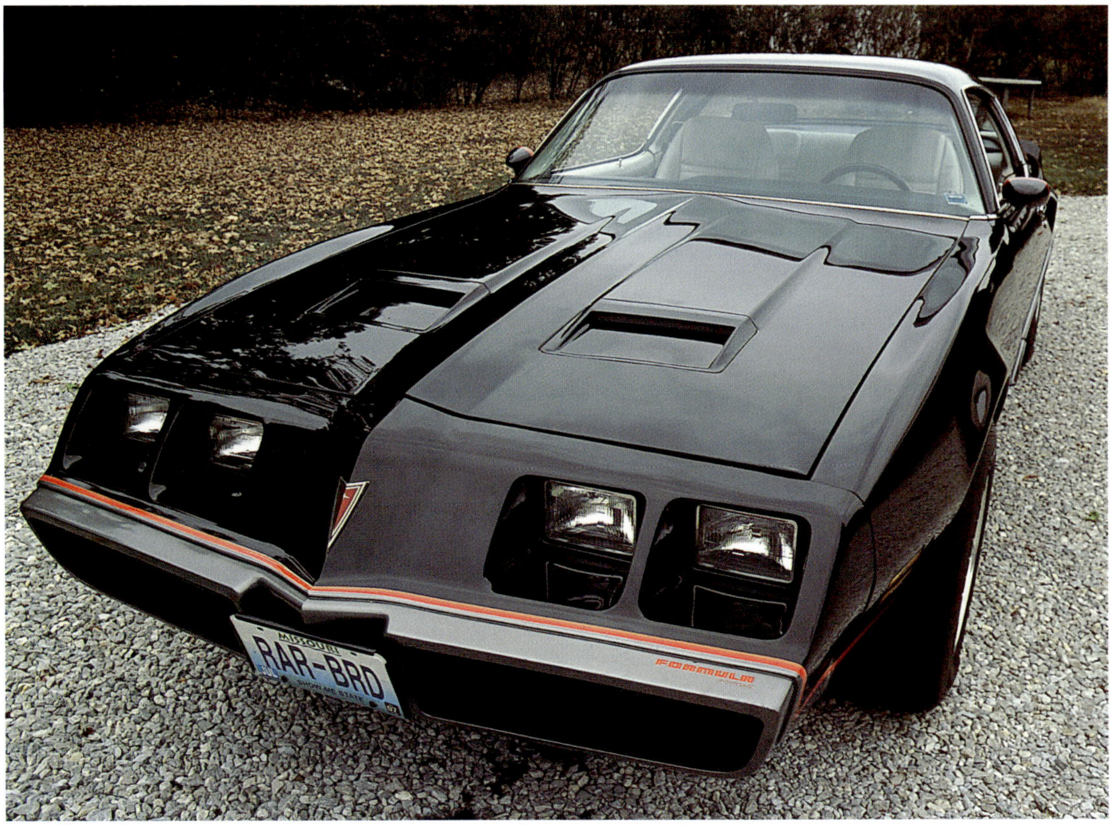

The 1979 Firebird front fascia was a totally new design from the previous year. This view shows an original black 1979 Firebird Formula with optional RPO W50 Formula Appearance Package and a red Formula decal on the left front of the bumper.

openings in the lower panel. The Trans Am again had a lower front spoiler that connected at its outer edges to the wheel opening spoilers.

The Firebird front end panel was again redesigned for 1979–1981 and had part number 10004629. The front end appearance became more massive when the grille openings were eliminated and the quad rectangular headlamps were recessed into individual body-color bezels. The wide flat divider between the headlamps carried a red arrowhead badge on all models, except the Esprit with the Redbird or Yellowbird appearance packages and the Trans Am with the Special Edition package. The special packages used a gold arrowhead badge with part number 1003679. The parking lamps were mounted at the outer ends of

Interior Trim Combinations

1974

Code	Color
721	White vinyl
731	Saddle vinyl
761	Black vinyl
811	Blue/White vinyl
831	Saddle cloth and vinyl (custom)
861	Black cloth and vinyl (custom)
811	Blue vinyl (custom)
901	Red vinyl (custom)
921	White vinyl (custom)
931	Saddle vinyl (custom)
941	Green (custom)
961	Black vinyl (custom)

1975

Code	Color
11V	White vinyl
11W	White vinyl (custom)
19V	Black vinyl
19W	Black vinyl (custom)
26W	Green vinyl (custom)
63V	Saddle vinyl
63W	Saddle vinyl (custom)
73W	Oxblood vinyl (custom)

1976

Code	Color
11N	White vinyl (custom)
11R	White vinyl
19N	Black vinyl (custom)
19R	Black vinyl
64N	Buckskin vinyl (custom)
64R	Buckskin vinyl
71N	Firethorn vinyl (custom)
71R	Firethorn vinyl

1977

Code	Color
11N	White vinyl (custom)
11R	White vinyl
19N	Black vinyl (custom)
19B	Black Cloth
19R	Black vinyl
24B	Blue cloth
24N	Blue vinyl (custom)
64N	Buckskin vinyl (custom)
64R	Buckskin vinyl
71B	Firethorn cloth
71N	Firethorn vinyl (custom)
71R	Firethorn vinyl

1978

Code	Color
11N	White vinyl (custom)
11R	White vinyl
19B	Black cloth
19N	Black vinyl (custom)
19R	Black vinyl
24B	Blue cloth
24N	Blue vinyl (custom)
62B	Camel Tan cloth
62N	Camel Tan vinyl (custom)
62R	Camel Tan vinyl
74B	Carmine cloth
74N	Carmine vinyl (custom)
74R	Carmine vinyl

1979

Code	Color
12N	Oyster cloth
12R	Vinyl
19B	Black vinyl cloth
19N	Black vinyl (custom)
19R	Black vinyl
24B	Blue cloth
24N	Blue vinyl (custom)
62B	Camel Tan cloth
62N	Camel Tan vinyl (custom)
62R	Camel Tan vinyl
74B	Carmine cloth
74N	Carmine vinyl (custom)
74R	Carmine vinyl
152	Silver leather (10th Anniversary)

1980

Code	Color
12N	Oyster vinyl (custom)
12R	Oyster vinyl
19B	Black cloth
19N	Black vinyl (custom)
19R	Black vinyl
26B	Blue cloth
26N	Blur vinyl (custom)
26R	Blue vinyl
62B	Camel Tan cloth
62N	Camel Tan vinyl (custom)
62R	Camel Tan vinyl
74B	Carmine cloth
74N	Carmine vinyl (custom)
74R	Carmine vinyl

1981

Code	Color
15V	Silver vinyl
15W	Oyster vinyl
19B	Black cloth
19N	Black vinyl
19R	Black vinyl
26B	Blue cloth
26D	Blue cloth
26N	Blue vinyl
26R	Blue vinyl
63B	Beige cloth
64B	Camel Tan cloth
64D	Camel Tan cloth
64N	Camel Tan vinyl
64R	Camel Tan vinyl
75B	Red cloth
75N	Red vinyl
75R	Red vinyl

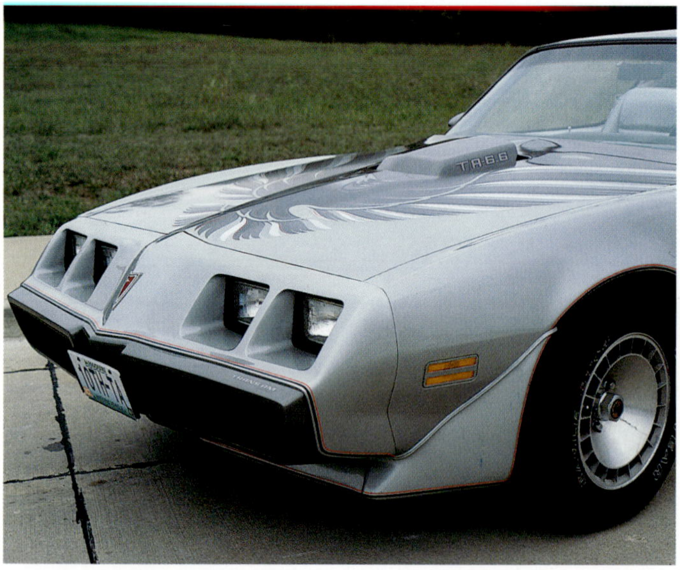

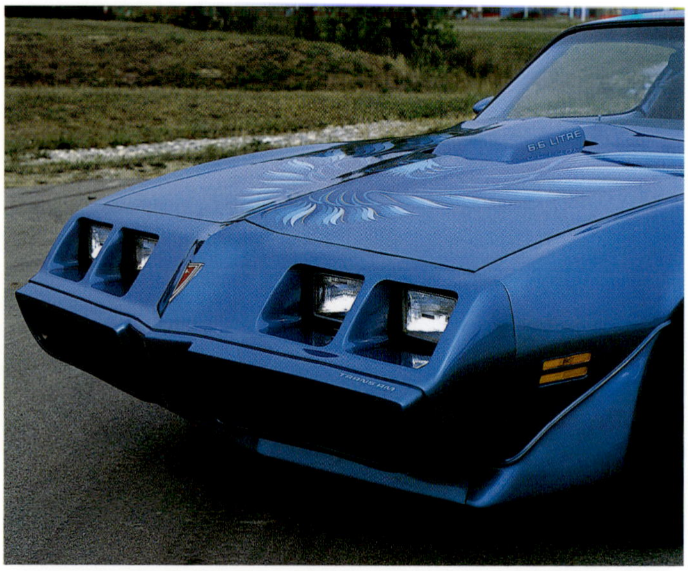

Above left: This view shows the front fascia on a silver 1979 Trans Am 10th Anniversary Edition and the T/A 6.6 engine decal on the shaker hood scoop. The 10th Anniversary Trans Am has the largest bird decal of any model, as it is three pieces and extends onto the tops of the front fenders. ***Above right:*** This Atlantic Blue 1979 Trans Am sport coupe has the 6.6-liter engine and an optional blue bird hood decal that faces to the right.

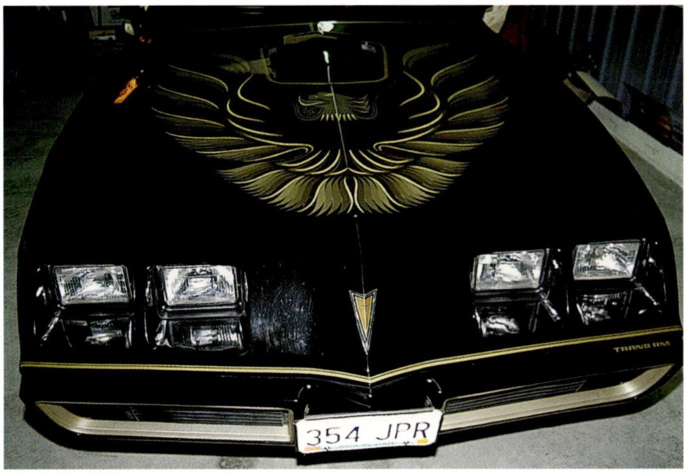

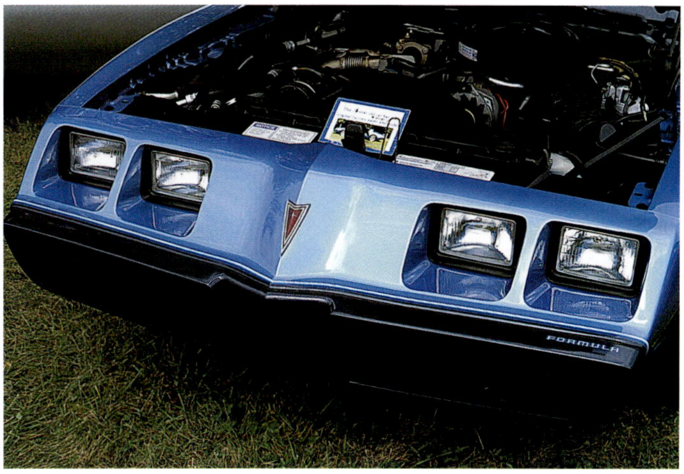

Above left: This is the front fascia of a 1979 Trans Am Black Special Edition. Note the distinctive gold bird decal and accents and the SE unique gold arrowhead badge on the nose. ***Above right:*** Detail view of the front fascia of a Bright Blue (24) 1980 Firebird Formula sport coupe (V87) with black bumper accents and a red arrowhead badge.

the wide rectangular openings below the headlamps. The grille opening surround also served as the primary bumper for the body-color front fascia. The Trans Am had its usual lower spoiler under the front fascia. The Trans Am and Formula used a small nameplate decal on the lower left side of the front fascia below the headlamps.

Interior

The 1974–1981 Firebird was available with a variety of interior trim choices, all with standard front bucket seats and a solid rear seat back with individual seat cushions and a driveshaft tunnel cover. In 1974 and 1975, the Firebird, Formula, and Trans Am had expanded Madrid-grain Morrokide vinyl interior standard. The Firebird Esprit had standard custom trim, also in Madrid-grain Morrokide vinyl. The custom trim with cloth-and-vinyl, or perforated-vinyl was optional in the Firebird, Formula, and Trans Am. The standard interior seat pattern had transverse pleats with smooth bolsters and skirts, and the front seat backs were slightly rounded. The custom interior had wider pleats with three sections in the seat back and two in the cushion. The custom interior had smooth door panels, and the standard interior used vertically pleated door panels.

The 1974 and 1975 standard vinyl interior was available in white (721/11V), black (761/19V), and saddle (731/63V). The custom interior was available in saddle (831/931/63W), black

Selected 1974–1981 Regular Production Options

RPO	Description	RPO	Description	RPO	Description
		JL1	Pedal trim package	N98	Rally II wheels w/trim rings
		JL2	Power front disc brakes	NK3	Formula steering wheel
A31	Power windows	K30	Cruise control	P01	Deluxe wheel covers
AQ1	Soft-Ray glass	LD5	3.8 V-6	P02	Custom, finned wheel covers
AQ2	Soft-Ray glass, windshield only	LG3	5.0-liter V-8	P05	Honeycomb cast wheels
AK1	Seatbelts, tone warning	LM1	5.7-liter V-8	P06	Wheel trim rings
AU3	Electric door locks	L22	250 six	QBU	FR78x15 black, radial tires
BS1	Added acoustical insulation	L27	301 2-bbl V-8	QFL	FR78x14, black, radial tires
B32	Front floor mats	L30	350 2-bbl V-8	TR9	Lamp group
B93	Door edge guards	L34	350 4-bbl V-8	UA1	Heavy-duty battery
B96	Wheel lip moldings	L37	4.9-liter V-8	U35	Clock
B80	Roof drip-rail moldings	L75	455 4-bbl V-8	U57	8-track stereo tape player
B84	Vinyl body side moldings	L76	350 4-bbl V-8	U63	AM radio
B85	Window sill and hood rear edge moldings	L78	400 4-bbl V-8	U69	AM/FM radio
C24	Recessed wipers	L80	403 4-bbl V-8	U75	Power antenna
C49	Rear window defroster	MM3	Three-speed manual	U80	Rear seat speaker
C60	Custom air conditioning	M15	Three-speed manual	VQ2	Radiator super cooling
C09	Cordova top	M20	Four-speed manual	WS6	Trans Am special performance package
D35	Remote-control sort mirror	M21	Four-speed manual, close ratio	WW7	Trans Am hood decal
D55	Front console	M38	Three-speed Turbo Hydra-Matic	WW8	Rally gauges w/clock and tachometer
D58	Rear console	MX1	Three-speed Turbo Hydra-Matic	WY9	Hatch roof
D80	Custom cushion steering wheel	N30	Luxury steering wheel	W63	Rally gauges and clock
D98	Accent stripes	N33	Tilt steering wheel	Y90	Custom trim group
G80	Safe-T-Track axle	N65	Space-saver spare tire		

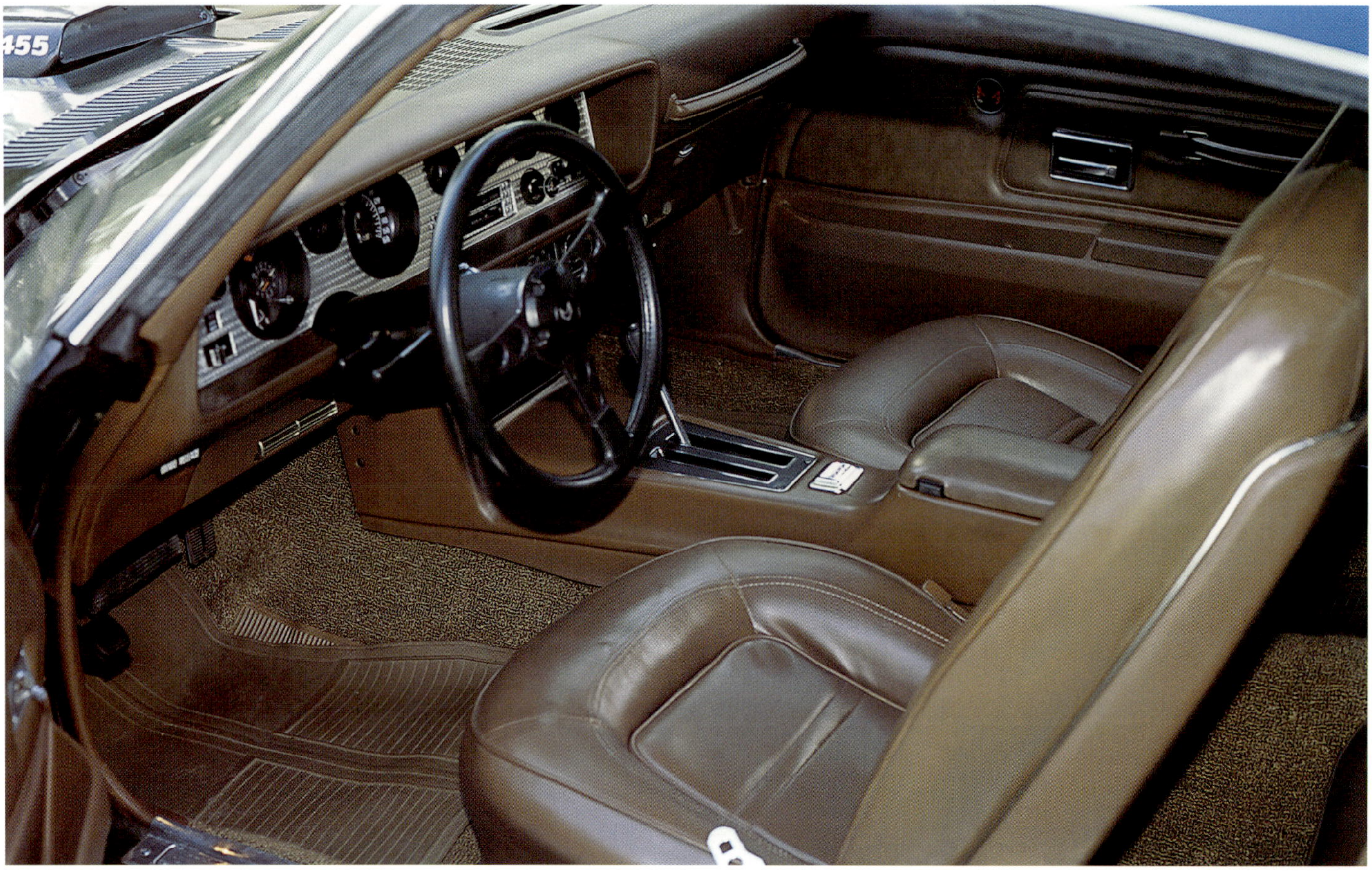

Above: This is the Buckskin vinyl interior with standard bucket seats (64R) in a black 1976 Trans Am Black Special Edition with an optional color-keyed console, automatic transmission with console shifter, and the standard Formula steering wheel. ***Below left:*** This photo shows the left interior door panel on a black 1976 Trans Am with the Special Edition package. The interior trim is Buckskin vinyl. Note the standard remote-control left side mirror and Trans Am medallion on the door panel. This Trans Am has optional power windows so the medallion covers the hole for the unneeded crank. ***Below right:*** The right interior door panel on a Brentwood Brown 1977 Trans Am sport coupe with Buckskin vinyl interior trim (64R) and a vinyl door-pull handle.

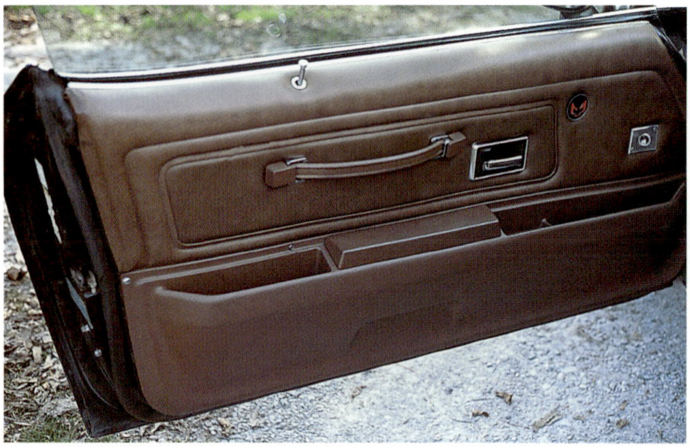

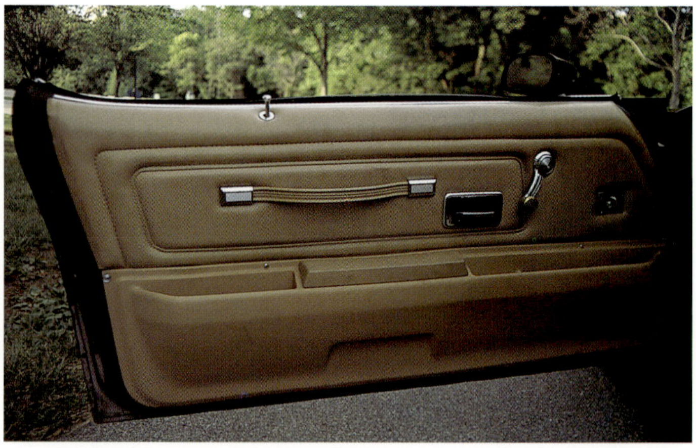

(861/961/19W), blue (1974 only, 811), red (1974 only, 901), white (921/11W), green (1974 only, 941), and oxblood (1975 only, 73W). All trim combinations could have had an optional color-keyed center console (RPO D58). Color-coordinated nylon cut-pile carpet was standard in all trim combinations.

An industry-wide government mandate for 1974 required the addition of a seatbelt interlock system. This system prevented the engine from being started if someone was seated and the seat-belts were not fastened. A button in the engine compartment allowed the system to be bypassed when it malfunctioned. Because of repeated problems and owner complaints, the system was eliminated for the 1975 model year.

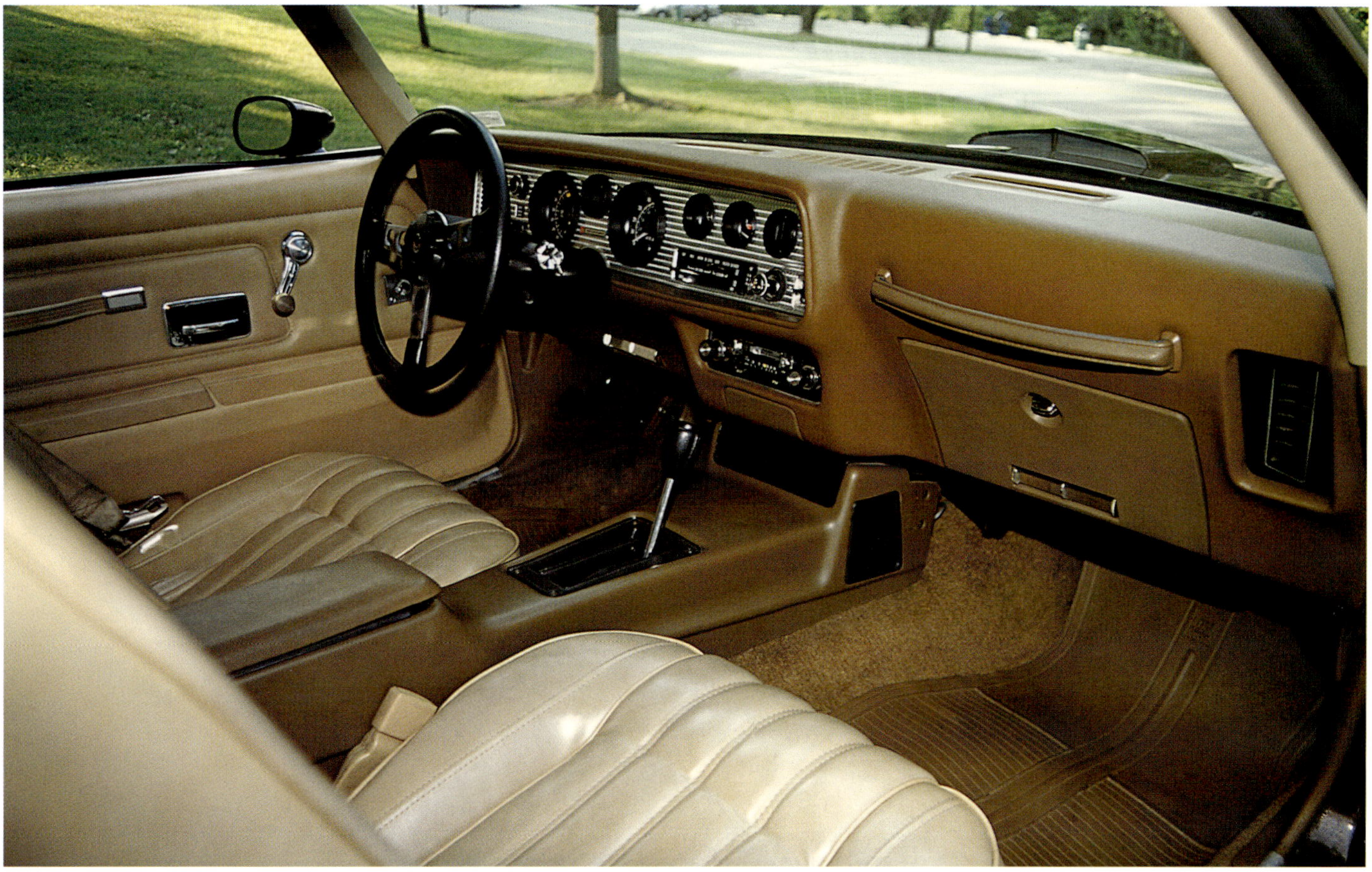

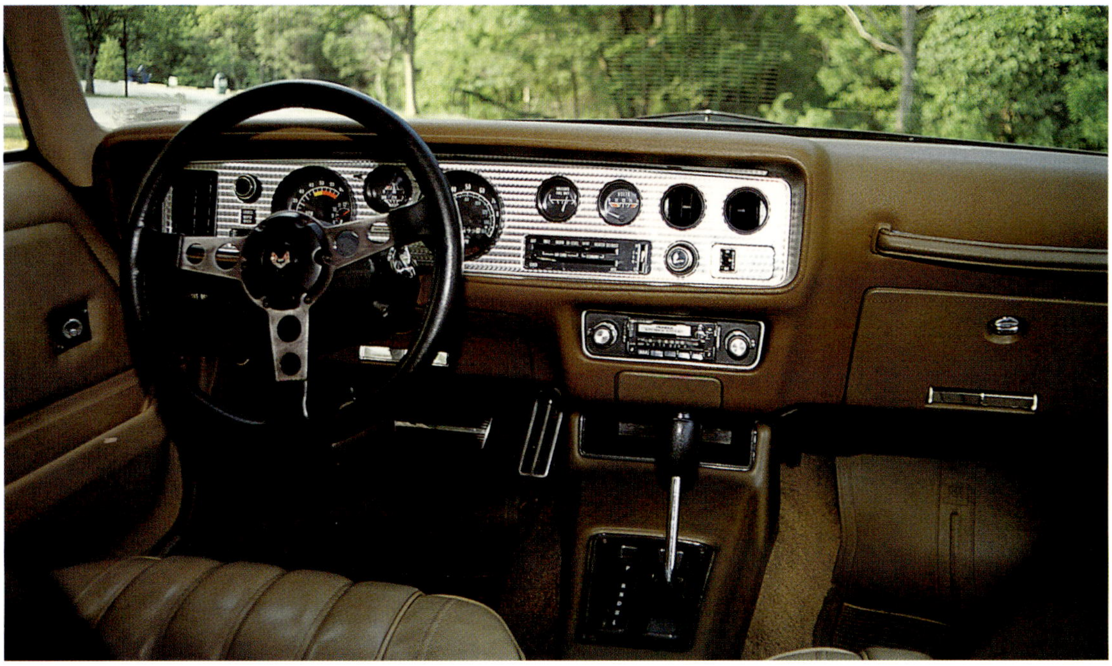

Above: This is the interior of a Brentwood Brown 1977 Trans Am with the optional Buckskin vinyl interior with standard bucket seats, color-keyed center floor console, and automatic transmission shifter. ***Right:*** Detail view of the instrument panel and standard Formula steering wheel on a 1977 Trans Am sport coupe with an optional AM/FM radio with cassette player.

The 1976–1978 Firebirds had all-vinyl standard interior trim with oxen-grain inserts with Madrid-grain skirts and bolsters in 1976 and Sierra-grain inserts and bolsters in 1977–1979. The standard trim had five longitudinal pleats on the cushion and back that extended to the top of the backrest. There were two transverse stamped seams on the backrest and one on the seat cushion.

The custom interior had Tetra-grain inserts with Madrid-grain skirts and bolsters in 1976 and doeskin-grain inserts and Sierra-grain skirts and bolsters in 1977–1979. The custom interior had four wide longitudinal pleats with wraparound backrest bolsters. The 1979 Trans Am 10th Anniversary Edition had a unique cushion design in silver leather trim and silver vinyl seating surfaces with a wide

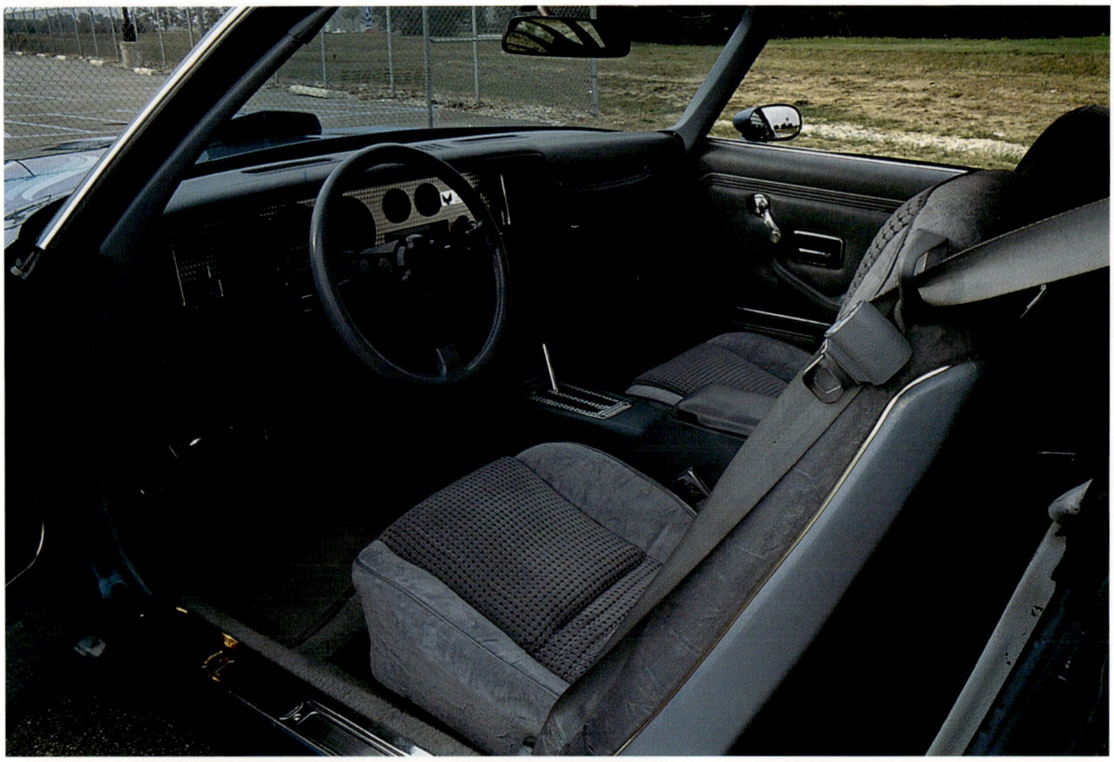

The front driver's compartment of an original Atlantic Blue 1979 Trans Am with optional blue Hobnail-cloth interior trim (24B), the color-keyed steering wheel, and floor console with automatic transmission shifter. ***Below left:*** The left door trim panel of a black 1978 Trans Am with optional camel tan (62R) vinyl interior trim, vertical pleats, and bright trim strip. ***Below:*** The left door panel of a blue 1979 Trans Am with optional blue Hobnail-cloth interior trim. The door panel is blue vinyl with blue carpet at the bottom.

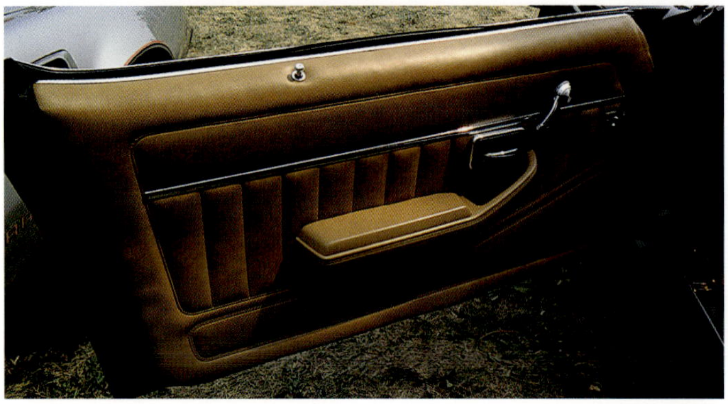

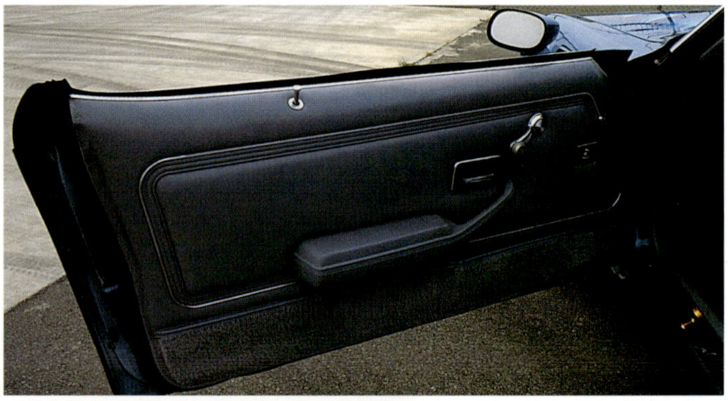

flat panel with narrow transverse pleats on the seat cushion and wide-and-narrow transverse pleated panels on the backrest. The 10th Anniversary Edition door panels had wide flat horizontal panels with an outer bolster and an embroidered red Firebird badge in the center.

The 1976 standard vinyl trim was available in white (11R), black (19R), buckskin (64R), and firethorn (71R). The custom interior was available in white (11N), black (19N), buckskin (64N), and firethorn (71N). For 1977, the standard vinyl trim was available in white (11R), black (19R), buckskin (64R), and firethorn (71R). The 1977 custom interior choices included Lombardy cloth and doeskin vinyl. The cloth was offered in black (19B), blue (24B), and firethorn (71B). The vinyl was available in white (1N), black (19N), blue (24N), buckskin (64N), and firethorn (71N).

Color choices increased slightly for 1978, and the standard oxen-vinyl colors were white (11R), black (19R), camel tan (62R), and carmine (74R). The custom doeskin vinyl was available in white (11N), black (19N), blue (24N), camel tan (62N), and carmine (74N). Lombardy cloth in the custom trim was available in black (19B), blue (24B), camel tan (62B), and carmine (74B). The 1979 colors and codes were the same, except that the white was changed to oyster (12R) and the cloth was now called Hobnail cloth and had

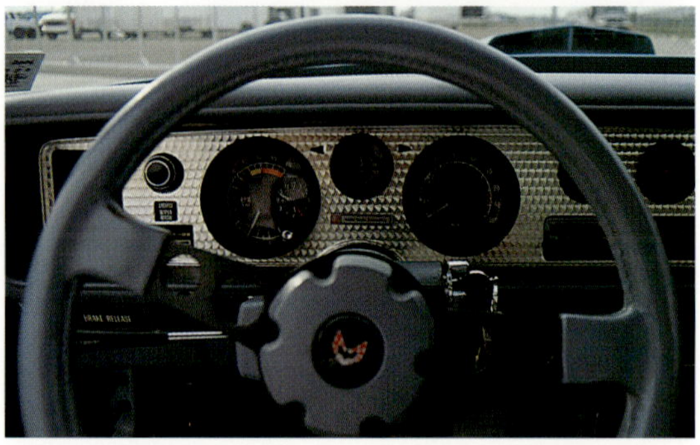

This detail view of the instrument panel and steering wheel of an Atlantic Blue 1979 Trans Am with a blue cloth interior (24B) shows the engine-turned Trans Am instrument panel background and radial-tuned suspension badge.

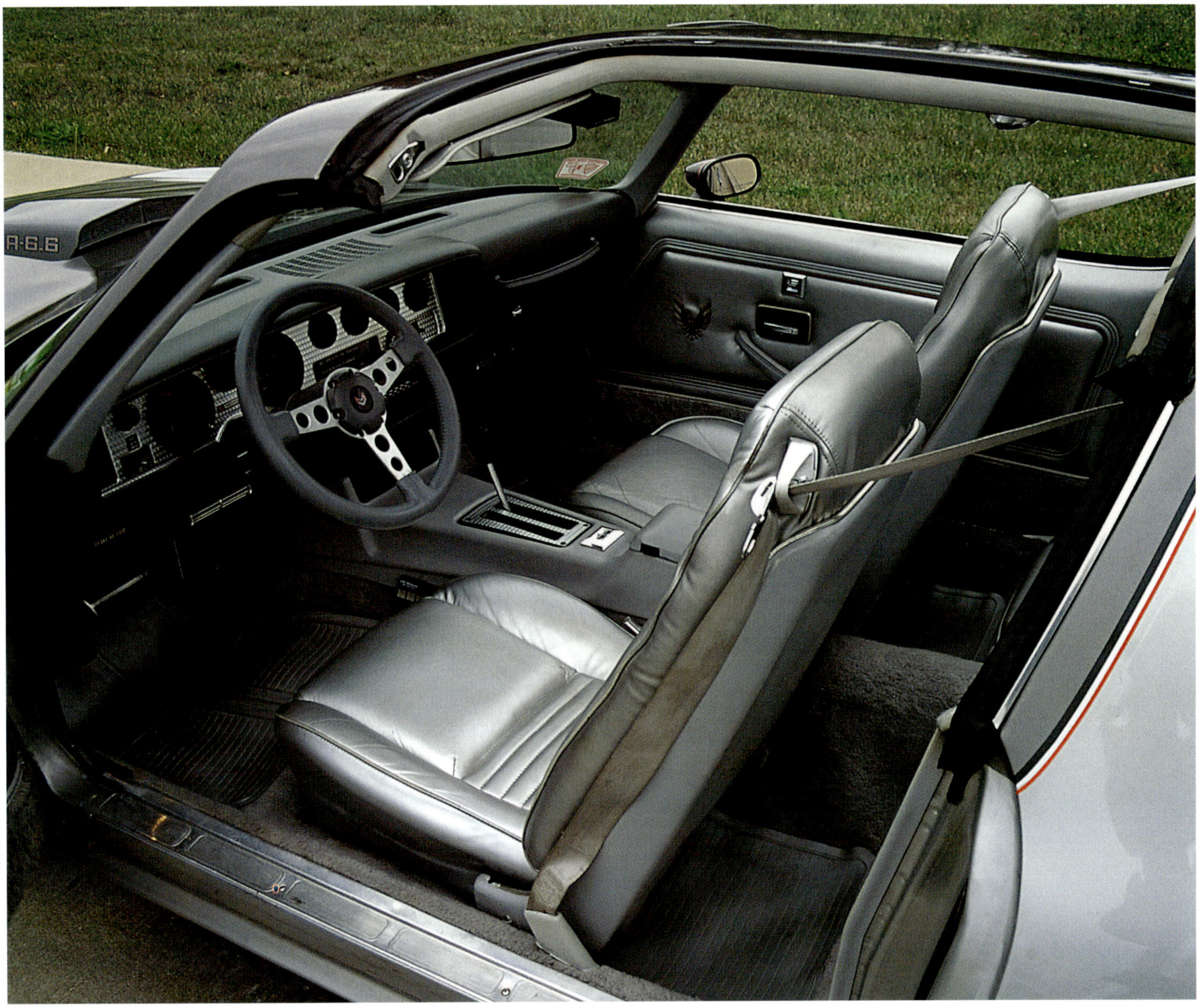

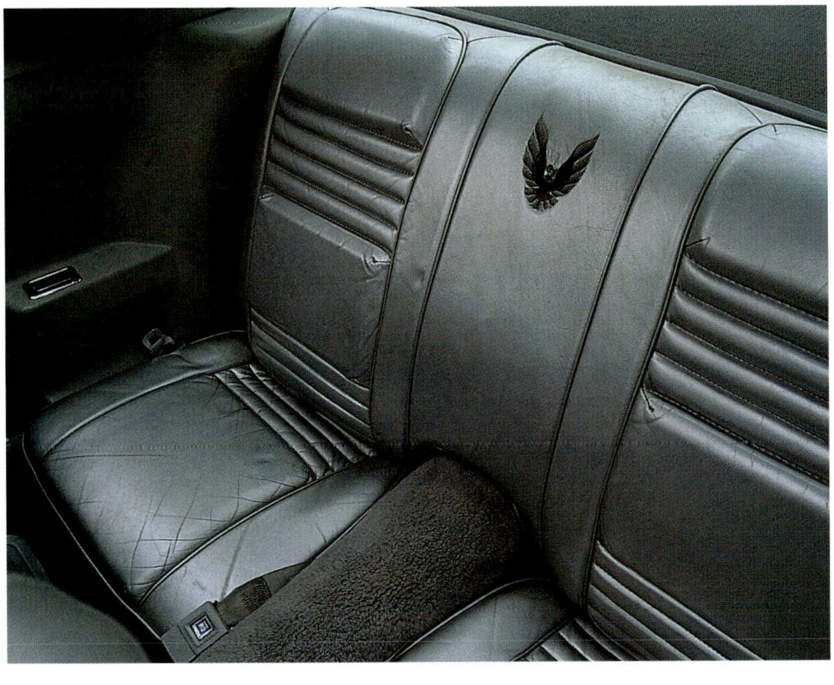

Above: This is the silver vinyl-and-leather-trimmed (152) interior in a 1979 Trams Am 10th Anniversary Special Edition with the color-keyed gray instrument panel and floor console with automatic transmission shifter. ***Left:*** This is the original silver vinyl-and-leather rear seat trim in a 1979 Trans Am 10th Anniversary Edition (X87) equipped with the optional T-top hatch roof (RPO CC1).

a multicolor design pattern in the material.

For 1980, the standard oxen vinyl was available in oyster (12R), black (19R), blue (26R), camel tan (62R), and carmine (74R). The custom interior doeskin vinyl was available in oyster (12N), black (19N), blue (26N), camel tan (62N), and carmine (74N). The custom-patterned Hobnail cloth was offered in black (19B), blue (26B), camel tan (62B), and carmine (74B).

The 1981 interior choices included standard vinyl in silver (15V), black (19R), blue (26R), camel tan (64R), and red (75R). The custom

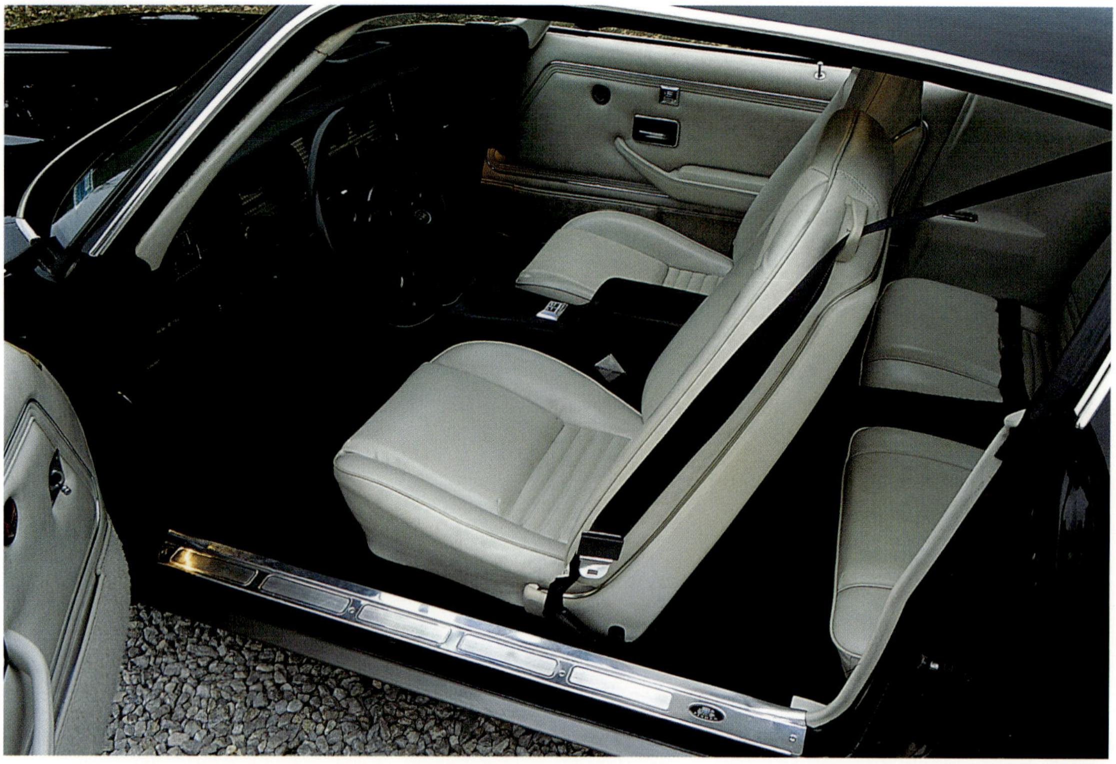

Left: This is the Oyster vinyl interior trim of a black 1979 Formula sport coupe equipped with optional power windows and four-speed manual transmission. ***Below left:*** The right door trim panel of this silver 1979 Trans Am 10th Anniversary Edition has a special bird medallion, power window switch, and smooth bordered insert panel. ***Below:*** The right door panel of a black 1979 Firebird Formula with Oyster vinyl interior trim. This Formula has optional power windows and light gray carpet trim at the bottom of the door panel.

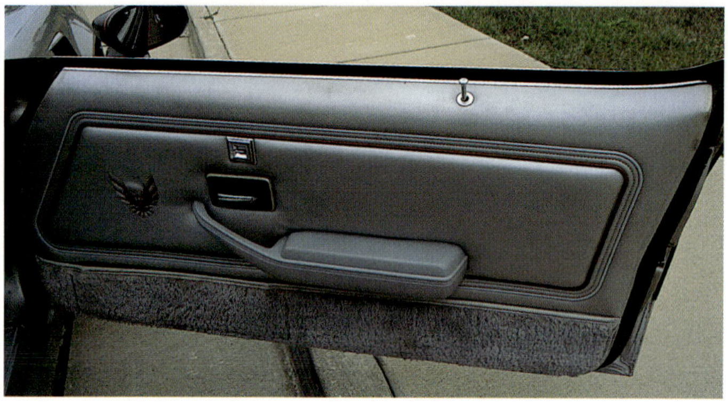

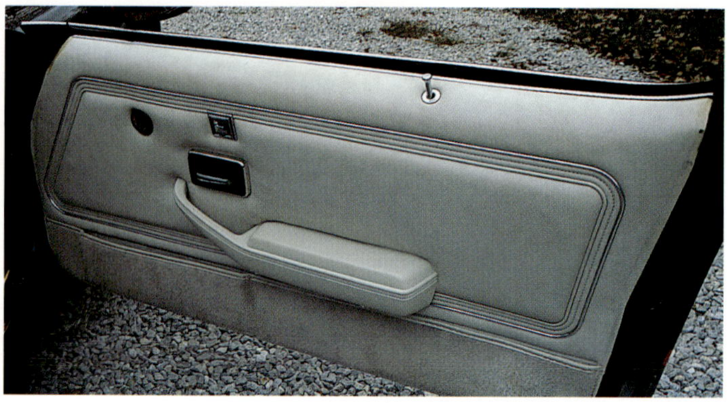

interiors included Millport cloth in blue (26D) and camel tan (64D). Pimlico cloth was available in black (19B), blue (26B), beige (63B), camel tan (64B), and red (75B). The custom doeskin vinyl was offered in oyster (15W), black (19N), blue (26N), camel tan (64N), and red (75N).

The 1974–1981 Firebird instrument panel and cluster was much like the 1970–1973 and similar throughout the years except for a minor restyling of the outer panel in 1978. The generic black replacement pad part numbers are 496352 for 1970–1977 and 10018005 for 1978–1981. The same glove box door (part number 483468 without a/c and 483462 with a/c) was used for all 1974–1981 models but was molded in colors matching the interior trim scheme. Cars with the custom trim group had a color-keyed vinyl assist strap attached to the panel above the glove box door.

The 1974–1981 instrument panel cluster was the same for all years with three basic types used. The instrument cluster panel for the Firebird, Esprit, and Formula was wood grain, and the Trans Am with Rally cluster had a panel of damascened aluminum. There were three different types of clusters available. All had a layout consisting of two large round bezels, one on either side of a smaller and higher center round gauge. The large left gauge housed the warning lamps on the Firebird and a tachometer on the Formula and Trans Am with the Rally gauge package. The right large bezel held the speedometer with a fuel gauge in the center on all standard models. The smaller center gauge had the coolant temperature and oil pressure on those clusters with the RPO W30 clock and Rally cluster. The clock and Rally cluster option moved the fuel gauge to the far right of the speedometer.

The Formula and Trans Am had two more small round gauges to the upper right on the main cluster that held the turn signal indicators on the left and ammeter on the right. The Rally gauge cluster and clock were available as an option on

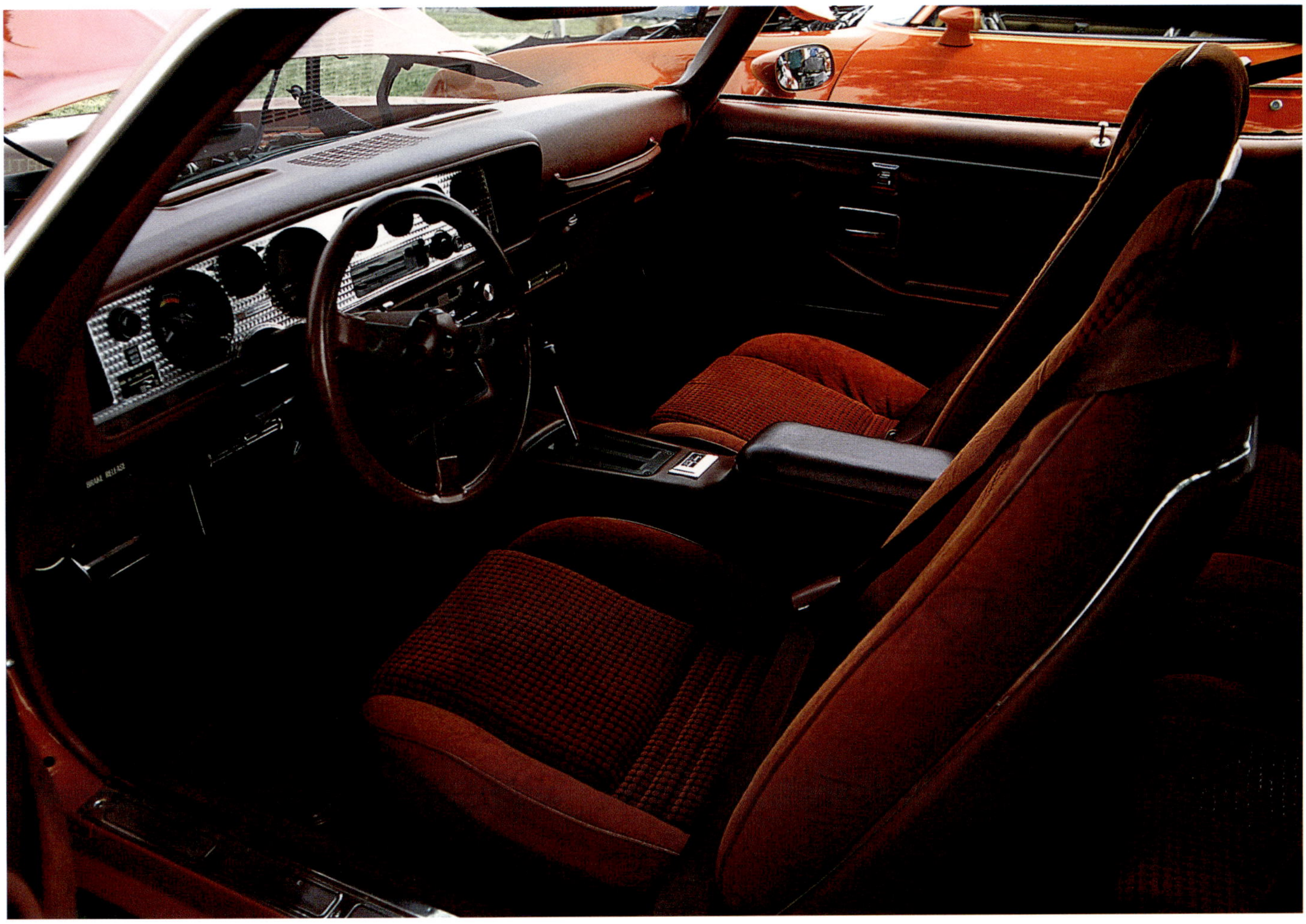

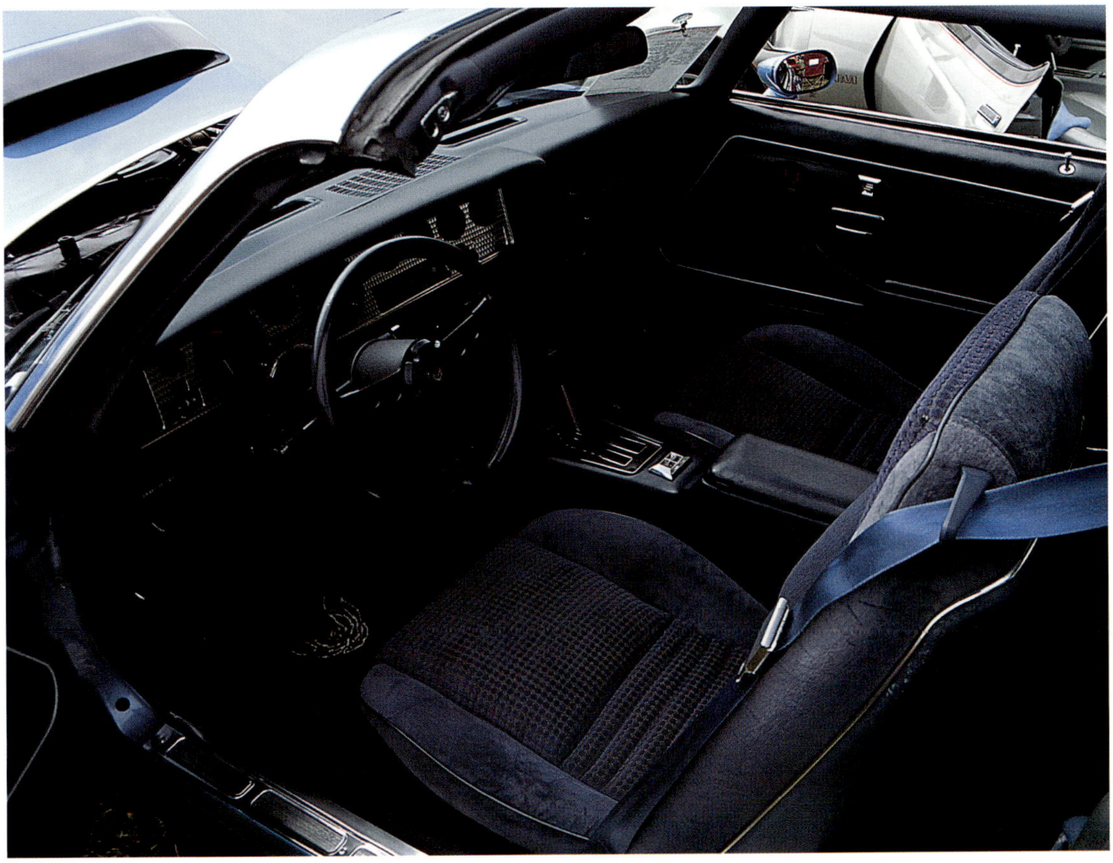

Above: The interior of a red (75) 1979 Trans Am equipped with optional Carmine (74B) Hobnail cloth trim, color-keyed steering wheel, instrument panel, center console, and optional power windows. ***Right:*** The interior of a 1980 Firebird Formula with optional blue Hobnail-cloth custom interior (26B), color-keyed steering wheel, instrument panel, floor console, and optional power windows.

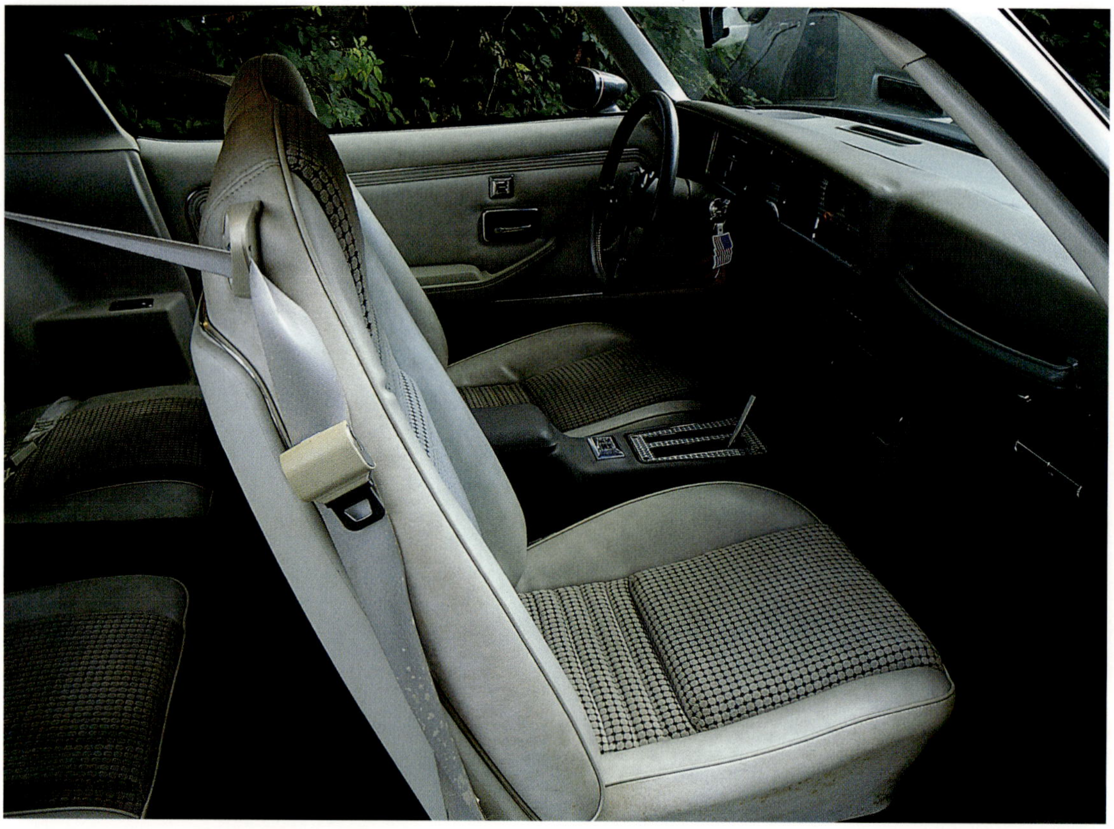

Left: The interior of a white 1980 Turbo Trans Am Indianapolis 500 Pace Car Edition with special Oyster Hobnail-cloth-and-vinyl custom interior trim, light gray Formula steering wheel, instrument panel, and floor console.

the Firebird V-8 and Esprit with RPO W63 and as a gauge cluster and tachometer with RPO U30. The heater and air conditioning controls were mounted to the lower right of the main cluster on all models.

On all models, the optional radio was mounted in the lower center of the instrument panel. There was no standard radio on any 1974–1981 Firebird models, but an AM push-button radio (RPO U63), AM/FM radio (RPO U69), or AM/FM stereo radio (RPO U58) was available as an option in all 1974–1981 models. An optional separate cassette tape player (RPO U55) or stereo 8-track tape player (RPO U57), mounted under the center of the instrument panel, was available in all 1974–1977 models. For 1978–1981, new optional AM/FM stereo radios with 8-track tape player (RPO UM1), stereo cassette player (RPO UN3), or 40-channel CB (RPO UP6) integral with the radio were available. There was also an optional AM/FM stereo radio with digital clock (RPO UY8). If no radio was ordered, a radio accommodation package could be ordered with RPO UN9 that featured the wiring and antenna required for an aftermarket radio installation. The radio antenna was integral with the windshield in all 1974–1981 Firebird models equipped with a radio. A power antenna was also available with RPO U75.

The standard steering wheel for all 1974–1976 Firebirds, referred to as a deluxe wheel, was a color-keyed thin-rimmed plastic two-spoke shallow-dish design with horn button bars on each spoke and an arrowhead badge in the center. In 1977, the standard steering wheel for the base Firebird, Esprit, and Formula became a three-spoke color-keyed plastic design.

The standard steering wheel for the 1974–1976 Firebird Esprit and Formula (and optional on the base Firebird) was the three-spoke custom cushion steering wheel, a shallow-dish design with a cushioned vinyl-covered rim and Pontiac arrowhead badge in the center. For 1975, the custom cushion steering wheel was redesigned and had wider spokes and a vertical wood-grain strip in the center lower spoke.

The standard steering wheel for the 1974 and 1975 Trans Am was the same simulated leather-covered 14-inch-diameter Formula steering wheel (RPO NK3) with three flat black aluminum spokes and center horn button used since 1970 (although the rim thickness was changed in 1977). The 1977–1981 Black Special Edition models (except the 1979 Y89 package) had a steering wheel with a black simulated-leather-covered rim and gold spokes (part number 100013871). The RPO Y89 package and the 1980 and 1981 pace car editions had a steering wheel with a gray simulated-leather rim and silver spokes (part number 1009536). The Formula steering wheel was optional in the other Firebirds, but the Esprit used a special center hub. The Formula steering wheel was only available with power steering.

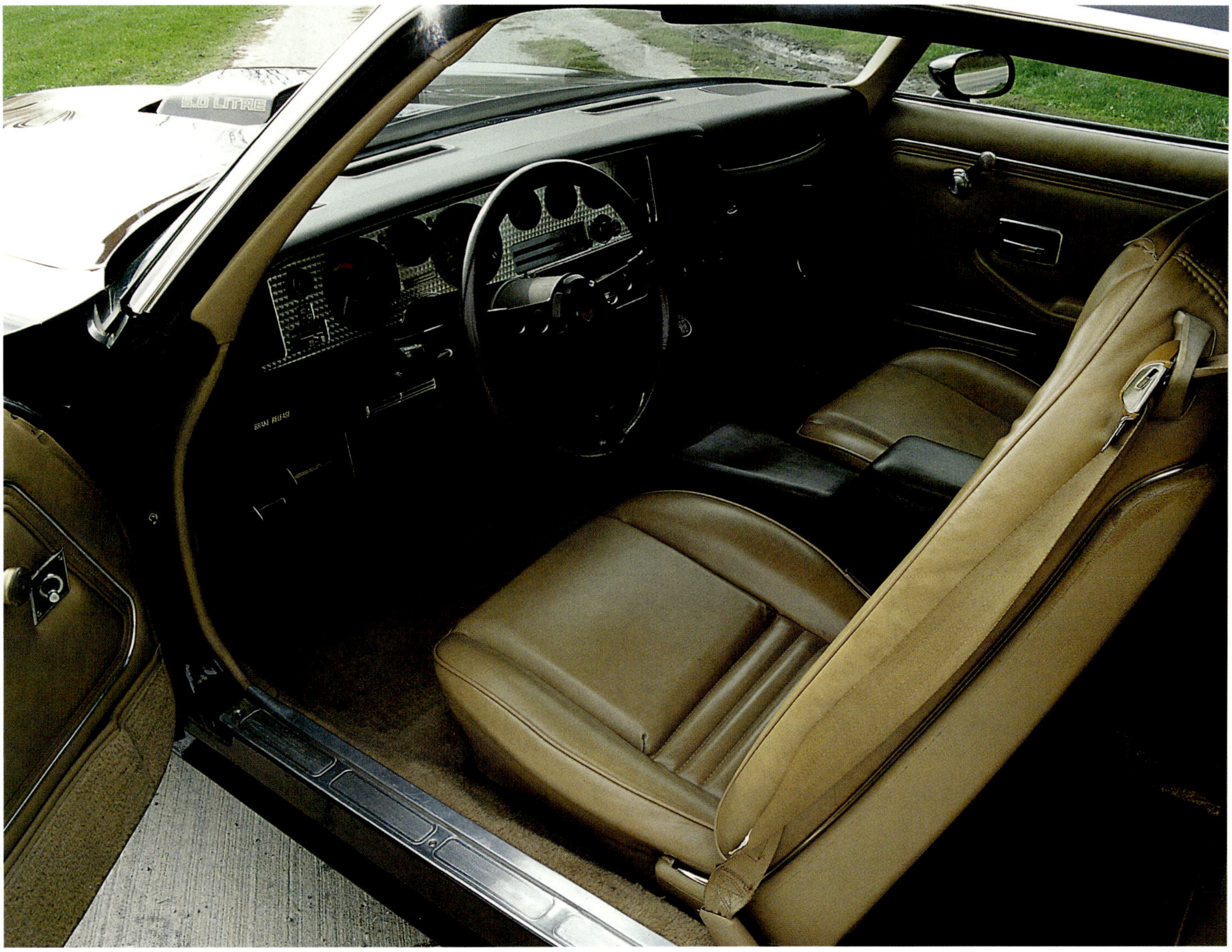

Above: This interior view of a Barclay Brown 1981 Trans Am with the optional Camel Tan (64N) doeskin-vinyl trim combination shows the design of the bucket seats and contrasting colors of the instrument panel and steering wheel. This Trans Am also has a floor console and four-speed manual shifter. ***Below left:*** The right door panel of a white 1980 Turbo Trans Am Pace Car Edition with Oyster vinyl trim equipped with power windows. Note the distinctive badge on the door panel. ***Below right:*** The left door-panel trim of a brown 1981 Trans Am sport coupe with a Camel Tan doeskin-vinyl interior. This Trans Am has standard manual window control and remote-control left outside mirror.

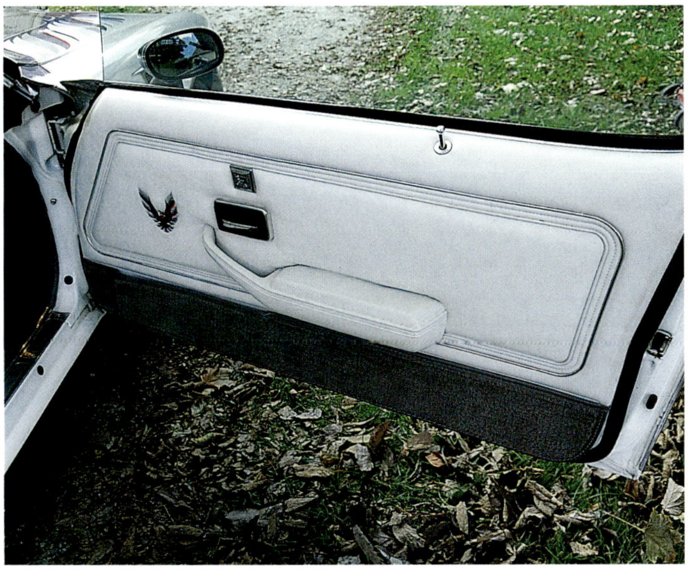

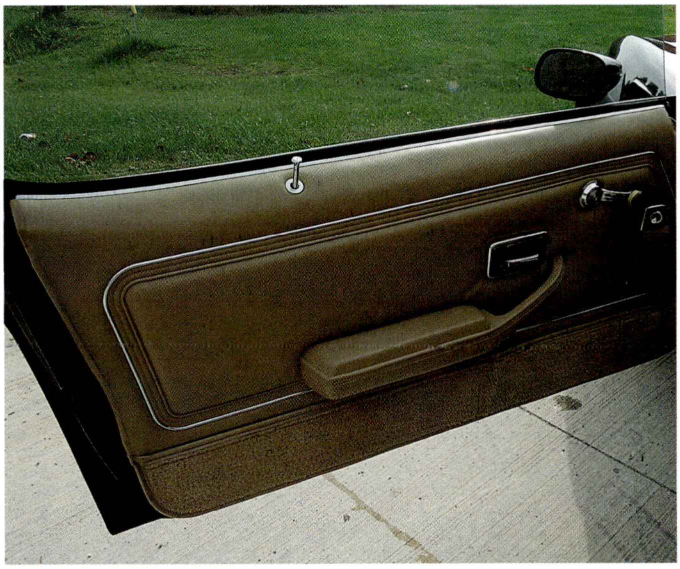

Engine and Engine Compartment

The 1974 Firebird was available with eight engine choices. The standard engine in the base Firebird was the Chevrolet–built 250-cubic-inch overhead-valve inline six-cylinder. The base V-8 was a 350-cubic-inch overhead-valve Pontiac with a single two-barrel carburetor. Optional V-8s included three versions of the 400-cubic-inch V-8 and two versions of the 455 V-8.

For 1975 and 1976, engine choices were reduced to four, with the 250-cubic-inch inline six still standard in the Firebird. The standard V-8 was the 175-horsepower 350-cubic-inch Pontiac. Optional V-8s were the 185-horsepower 400-ci and 200-horsepower 455-ci engines. Compression ratios were decreased to 8.25:1 in the six and 7.6:1 in some V-8s because of emissions and fuel mileage requirements.

Engine choices were increased and changed significantly for 1977, with seven variations offered. The inline six-cylinder was dropped as the standard Firebird powerplant and replaced with a 231-cubic-inch Buick V-6 with 105 horsepower. Base V-8 power consisted of a 301 Pontiac V-8 and a 305 Chevrolet V-8. Optional engines included a 350 Oldsmobile V-8 (available only in California as a mandatory option), two 400-cubic-inch Pontiac V-8s and a 403 Oldsmobile V-8. Power ranges for V-8 engines were from 135 to 185 horsepower. Engine choices for 1978 were still eight and similar to 1977, except the 301 was dropped and there were now four variations of 305-cubic-inch Chevrolet V-8. There were still two 400-cubic-inch Pontiac V-8s and the California 350 Oldsmobile V-8 available.

For 1979, there were seven engines available starting with the 231 Buick V-6. V-8 engines included two variations of the 301 Pontiac V-8, one 305 Chevrolet, a 350 Chevrolet V-8, a 400 Pontiac, and a 403-cubic-inch Oldsmobile V-8. Horsepower ranged from 105 for the V-6 to 185 horsepower for the 403 V-8. Power choices for 1980 were reduced to six, with the Buick 231-cubic-inch V-6 still standard in the base Firebird. V-8 engine choices ranged from the 265 and three variations of a 301-cubic-inch Pontiac V-8 to a 305-cubic-inch Chevrolet. The highest output came from the 301-cubic-inch (4.9-liter) turbocharged Pontiac with 200 horsepower. The engine was assisted by a TBO 305 AiResearch Corporation turbocharger. For 1981, engine choices were reduced to five. The 110-horsepower V-6 was again standard, with a 265, two 301 Pontiac V-8s, and a 305-cubic-inch Chevrolet V-8 available.

Overhead-Valve Inline Six

The 250-cubic-inch Chevrolet inline six-cylinder (RPO L22) was carried over virtually unchanged from 1973. The 1974 version still had a cast-iron block with 3.875-inch bore and 3.531-inch stroke with a compression ratio of 8.2:1 (reduced from 8.5:1 in 1973). The six was rated at 100 horsepower at 3,600 rpm and 175 foot-pounds of torque at 1,600 rpm. For 1975, the compression ratio was 8.25:1, and the horsepower was increased to 105 at 3,800 rpm with 185 foot-pounds of torque at 1,200 rpm. In 1976, the horsepower was increased again to 110 at 3,600 rpm, but the torque remained the same as the previous year. The six had a single-barrel Rochester carburetor and hydraulic valve lifters. Nineteen seventy-six was the final year for the inline six-cylinder. The VIN engine code is D for all years. The six-cylinder was painted Pontiac Engine Blue.

Overhead-Valve Buick V-6

The 231-cubic-inch Buick V-6 (RPO LD7) had a cast-iron block with a bore and stroke of 3.80x3.40 inches and a compression ratio of 8.0:1. The 1977 V-6 developed 105 horsepower at 3,200 rpm and 185 foot-pounds of torque at 2,000 rpm. The VIN engine code was C for 1977. The 1978 and 1979 version of the V-6 (RPO LD5) also developed 105 horsepower but at 3,400 rpm. For 1980, everything was the same except the horsepower rating was increased to 115 at 3,800 rpm and the torque to 188 foot-pounds at 2,000 rpm. In 1981, the horsepower was 110 at 3,800 rpm and the torque was 190 foot-pounds at 1,600 rpm. All versions had a single two-barrel carburetor. The VIN engine code was A for 1978–1981.

Overhead-Valve V-8

There were a variety of different V-8 engines available in the 1974–1981 Firebirds that may have been built by Pontiac, Chevrolet, or Oldsmobile. The Pontiac V-8 was based on the previous years' designs and was available in 265-, 301-, 350-, 400-, and 455-cubic-inch displacements. The smallest version of the Pontiac V-8 was the 265-cubic-inch example first used in 1980. The 301 V-8 (RPO L27, L37, and W72) had a bore and stroke of 4.00x3.00 inches and a compression ratio of 8.2:1 in 1977 and 8.1:1 in 1979–1981.

The 265-cubic-inch Pontiac V-8 had a bore and stroke of 3.75x3.00 inches and a compression ratio of 8.3:1. The 265 (RPO LS4) was only available in 1980 and 1981 and developed 120 horsepower and 205/210 foot-pounds of torque with a two-barrel carburetor and hydraulic valve lifters. The VIN engine code was S.

In 1980 and 1981, the turbocharged version

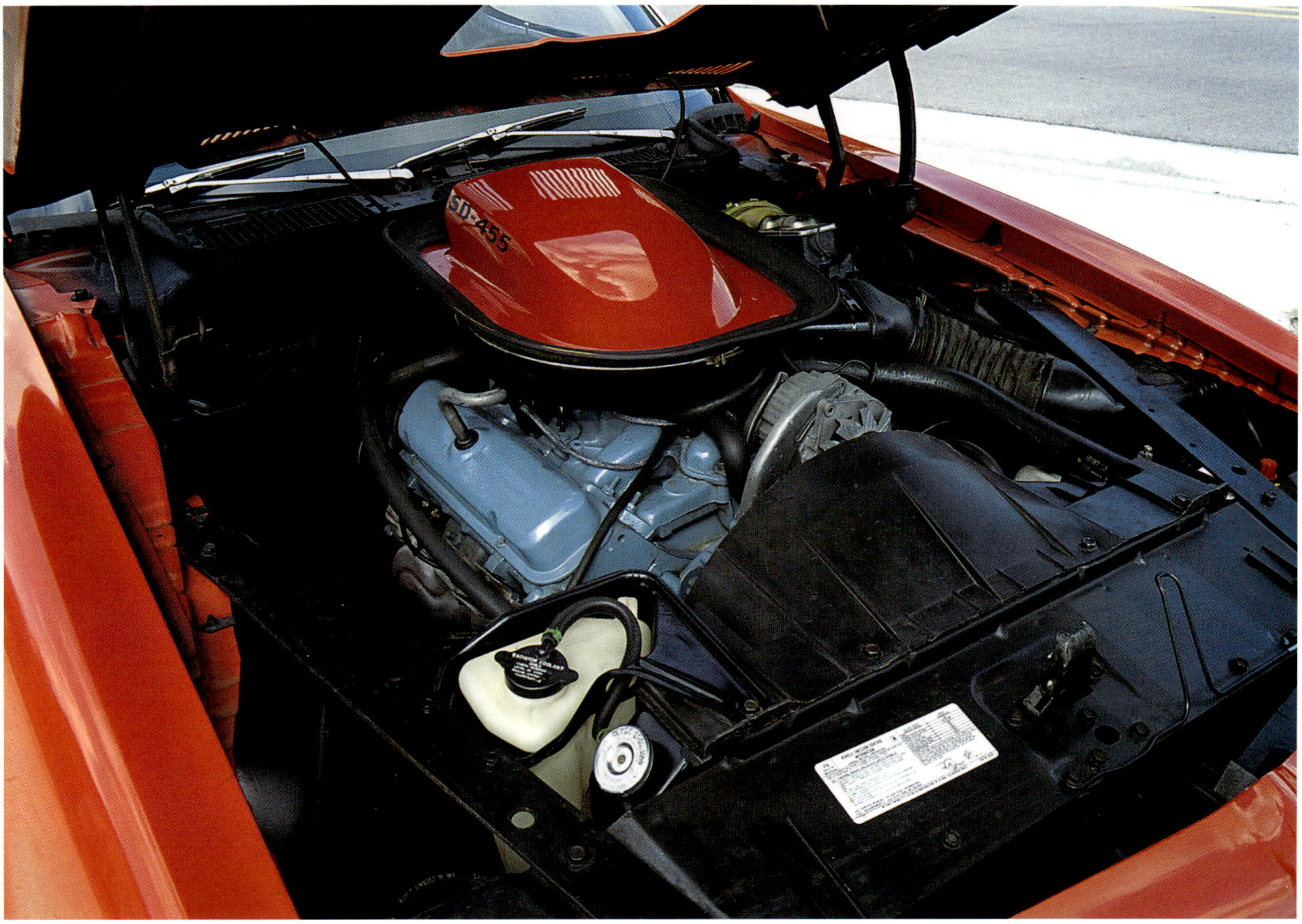

The right view of the engine compartment of a Buccaneer Red 1974 Firebird Formula equipped with the optional SD 455 engine. Note the body-color shaker-scoop air cleaner assembly and the correct clamps on the heater and radiator hoses.

of the 301 was called the 4.9-liter Turbo V-8 and used RPO LU8. The LU8 had a 7.6:1 compression ratio and developed 210 horsepower at 4,000 rpm and 345 foot-pounds of torque at 2,000 rpm. The 4.9 Turbo V-8 was equipped with a Garrett AiResearch TBO 305 turbocharger feeding a Rochester Quadrajet four-barrel carburetor through an aluminum plenum. The system was similar to that used on the contemporary Buick Turbo Regal, but the Trans Am unit had a larger compressor and had 9 psi boost pressure. Air intake was through a 4-inch duct above the front air dam. The Turbo V-8 had reinforced main bearing webs and larger ½-inch main bearing cap bolts for added strength. A 60-psi oil pump and baffled oil pan were also added for increased reliability. The 4.6 Turbo V-8 was only available with an automatic transmission and air conditioning.

The 301-ci L27 V-8 had 135 horsepower at 4,000 rpm and 235 foot-pounds of torque at 2,000 rpm for 1977. The 1979 examples had 140 horsepower at 3,600 rpm and 235 foot-pounds of torque at 2,000 rpm with a two-barrel carburetor (L27), and 150 horsepower and 240 foot-pounds of torque with a four-barrel (L37). In 1980, the L37 had 140 horsepower and 240 foot-pounds of torque, and the W72 with a four-barrel had 155 horsepower and 240 foot-pounds of torque. The 1981 L37 V-8 had 150 horsepower and 245 foot-pounds of torque. The RPO LU8 4.9 Turbo V-8 had a 7.6:1 compression ratio, 210 horsepower at 4,000 rpm, and 345 foot-pounds of torque at 2,000 rpm in 1980. In 1981, the 4.9 Turbo V-8 had a 7.5:1 compression ratio and developed 200 horsepower and 340 foot-pounds of torque.

The next-largest-displacement Pontiac V-8 was the 350-cubic-inch with a bore and stroke of 3.875x3.75 inches. The RPO L30 350 V-8 had a compression ratio of 7.6:1 in 1974 and 1975, and developed 155 horsepower at 3,600 rpm and 275/280 foot-pounds of torque at 2,400/2,000 rpm or 170 horsepower at 4,000 rpm and 290 foot-pounds of torque at 2,400 rpm, both with a two-barrel carburetor. In 1976, the L30 produced 160 horsepower and 280 foot-pounds of torque. In 1975, the 350-cubic-inch V-8 was available with a four-barrel carburetor (RPO L76) and had 175 horsepower and 280 foot-pounds of torque. For 1976, the horsepower was reduced to 165 and the torque to 260 foot-pounds. In 1977, the final year for the Pontiac 350, the horsepower was increased to 170. All versions had hydraulic valve lifters.

The Pontiac V-8 was also available as a 400-cubic-inch version from 1974 to 1979. The 400

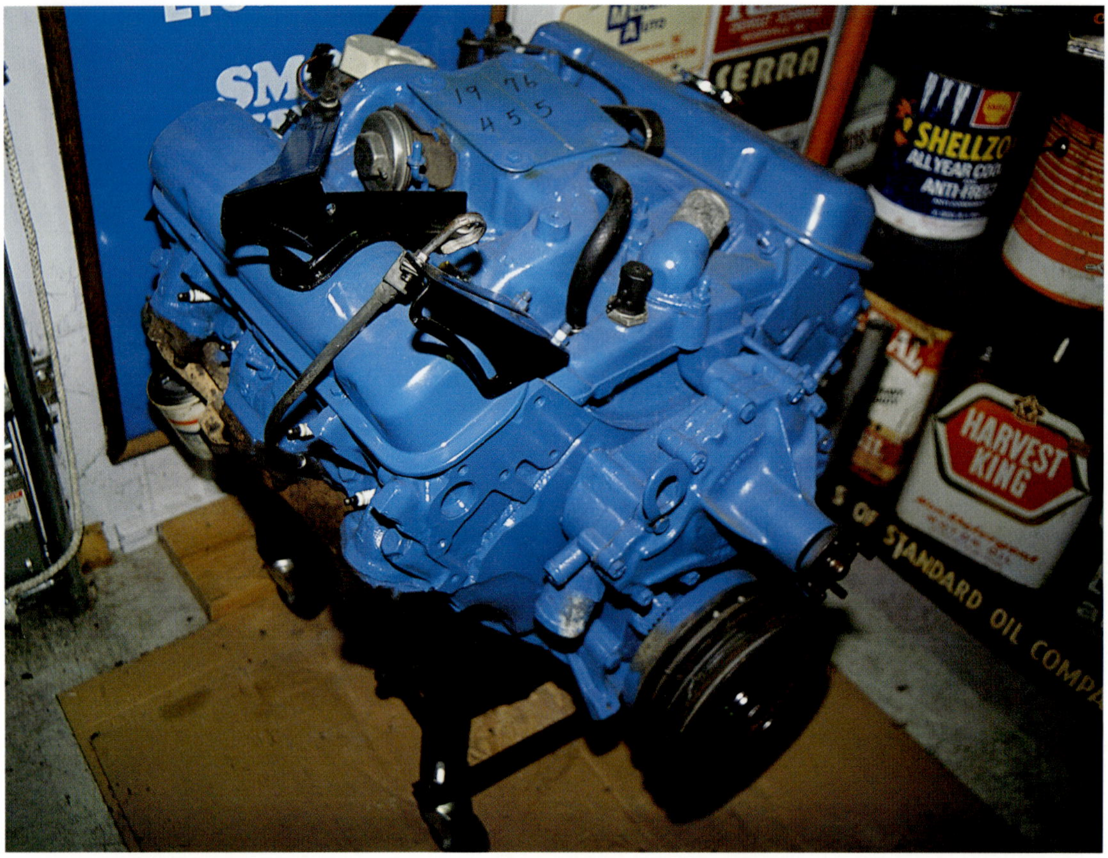

This restored 1976 Firebird 455 V-8 engine is painted standard Pontiac Engine Blue and has the brackets attached for the air-conditioning compressor on the right side of the engine block.

Pontiac V-8 had a bore and stroke of 4.125x3.75 inches. In 1974, the 400-cubic-inch V-8 was available as the RPO L65 with a compression ratio of 8.0:1, developing 190 horsepower at 4,000 rpm and 330 foot-pounds of torque at 2,400 rpm with a single two-barrel carburetor (VIN code P). There were two RPO L78 four-barrel versions of the 400 available with the same compression ratio, developing 200 (single exhaust) and 225 horsepower (dual exhaust).

By 1975–1977, only the L78 version was available: with 185 horsepower and 310 foot-pounds of torque in 1975 (VIN Code R and S) and 1976 (VIN code Z) and 180 horsepower and 325 foot-pounds of torque for 1977 and 1978. The 1975 L78 was the first Trans Am engine to be fitted with a catalytic converter. The change required a switch to the TH350 transmission from the TH400. In 1977–1979, the RPO L78/W72 engine was called a 6.6-liter and had an 8.1:1 compression ratio and 200/220 horsepower and 325/320 foot-pounds of torque. The VIN code was Z for all 6.6-liter engines. The 400 V-8 was not available for 1980 or 1981. All 400 Pontiac engines were painted Pontiac Engine Blue.

The Pontiac V-8 was still available with 455 cubic inches for 1974–1976. The 455 was similar in design and construction to the 400, but it had a bore of 4.15 inches and a stroke of 4.21 inches. The 455 was available in two 8.0:1 compression ratio versions for 1975, both with dual exhaust and a single four-barrel carburetor. The RPO L75 had 250 horsepower and 380 foot-pounds of torque (VIN code Y), and the RPO L82 (called Super Duty in 1974) had 290 horsepower and 395 foot-pounds of torque (VIN code X). The SD 455 engines had the PCV valve outlet in the driver-side oil filler cap rather than the valley cover, as in the other engines. In 1975, the L82 was dropped, and the L75 with a 7.6:1 compression ratio was now called an HO (1975 only) with 200 horsepower and 330 foot-pounds of torque. The L75 was available in 1975 and 1976, and had tuned exhaust with splitters and a single four-barrel carburetor. All 455 Pontiac engines were painted Pontiac Engine Metallic Blue.

Beginning in 1977, the Firebird was available with optional or standard engines made by General Motors divisions other than Chevrolet. In addition to the Buick V-6 already discussed, there were V-8 powerplants made by Chevrolet and Oldsmobile. The smallest corporate V-8 in 1977–1979 was the Chevrolet 305-cubic-inch (RPO LG3) first used February 1, 1977, in the base Firebird and Esprit V-8. The Chevrolet 305 had a bore and stroke of 3.74x3.48 inches and a compression ratio of 8.4:1. The LG3 had a two-barrel carburetor and single exhaust and developed 145 horsepower at 3,800 rpm and 245 foot-pounds of torque at 2,400 rpm. In 1978, there were four versions of the 305 Chevrolet V-8 with 135 (RPO LG3) to 170 horsepower (RPO LM1),

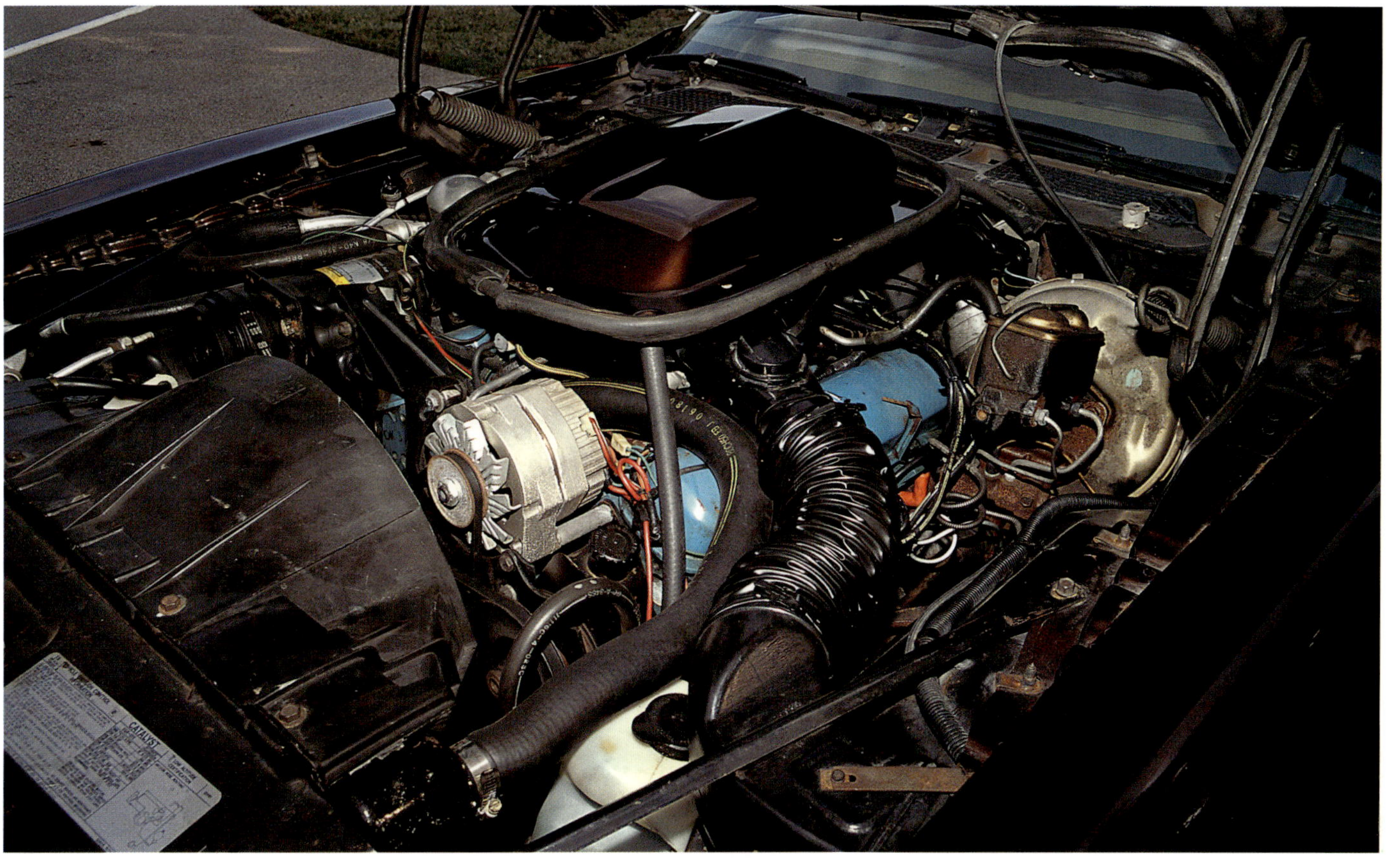

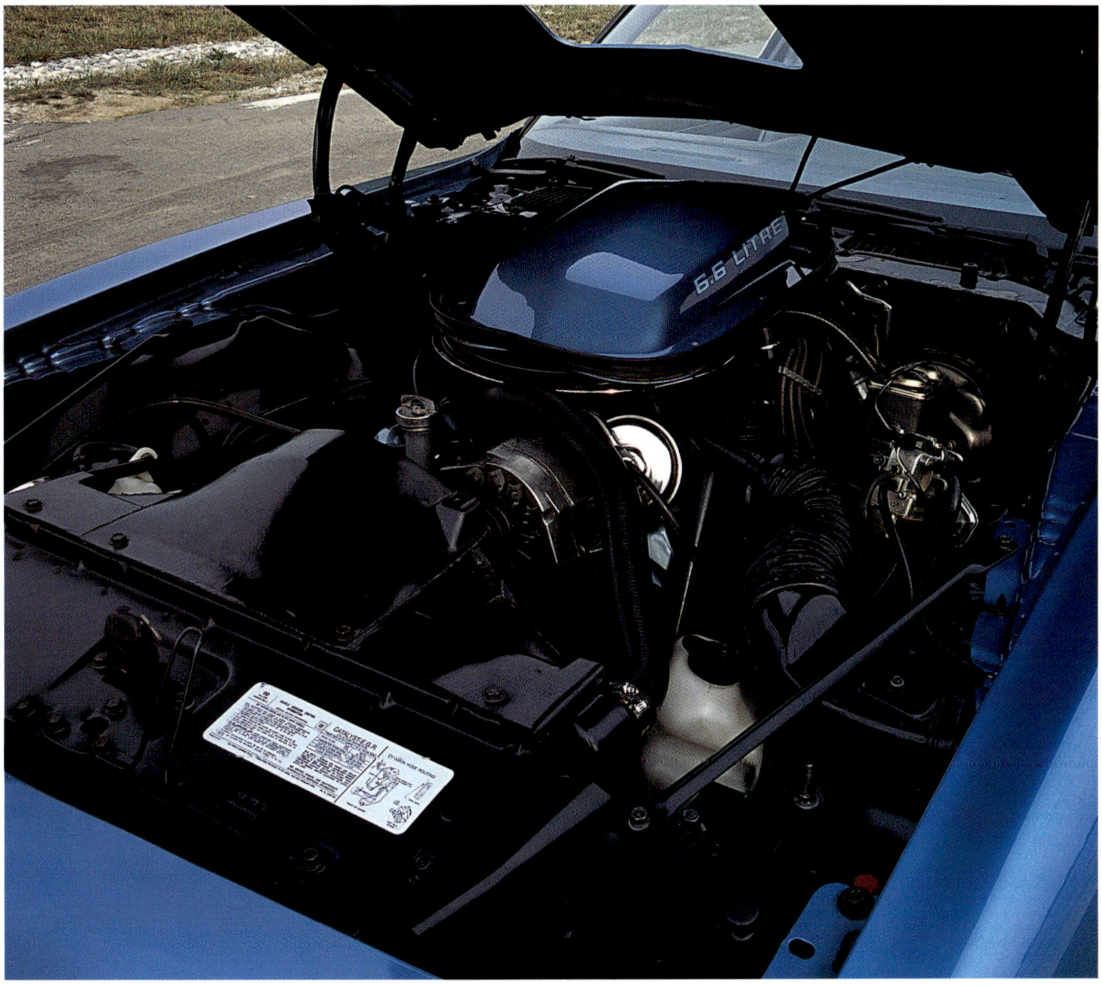

Above: The left view of the engine compartment of an original Brentwood Brown 1977 Trans Am equipped with a 400 Pontiac V-8 engine. Note the flexible hose for the air intake and the mounting of the alternator and air-conditioning compressor. ***Right:*** This is a view of the engine compartment of an Atlantic Blue 1979 Trans Am sport coupe equipped with the 6.6-liter (403-cubic-inch) Oldsmobile-built V-8 engine. The radiator hose is routed correctly. The hose clamps are incorrect replacements.

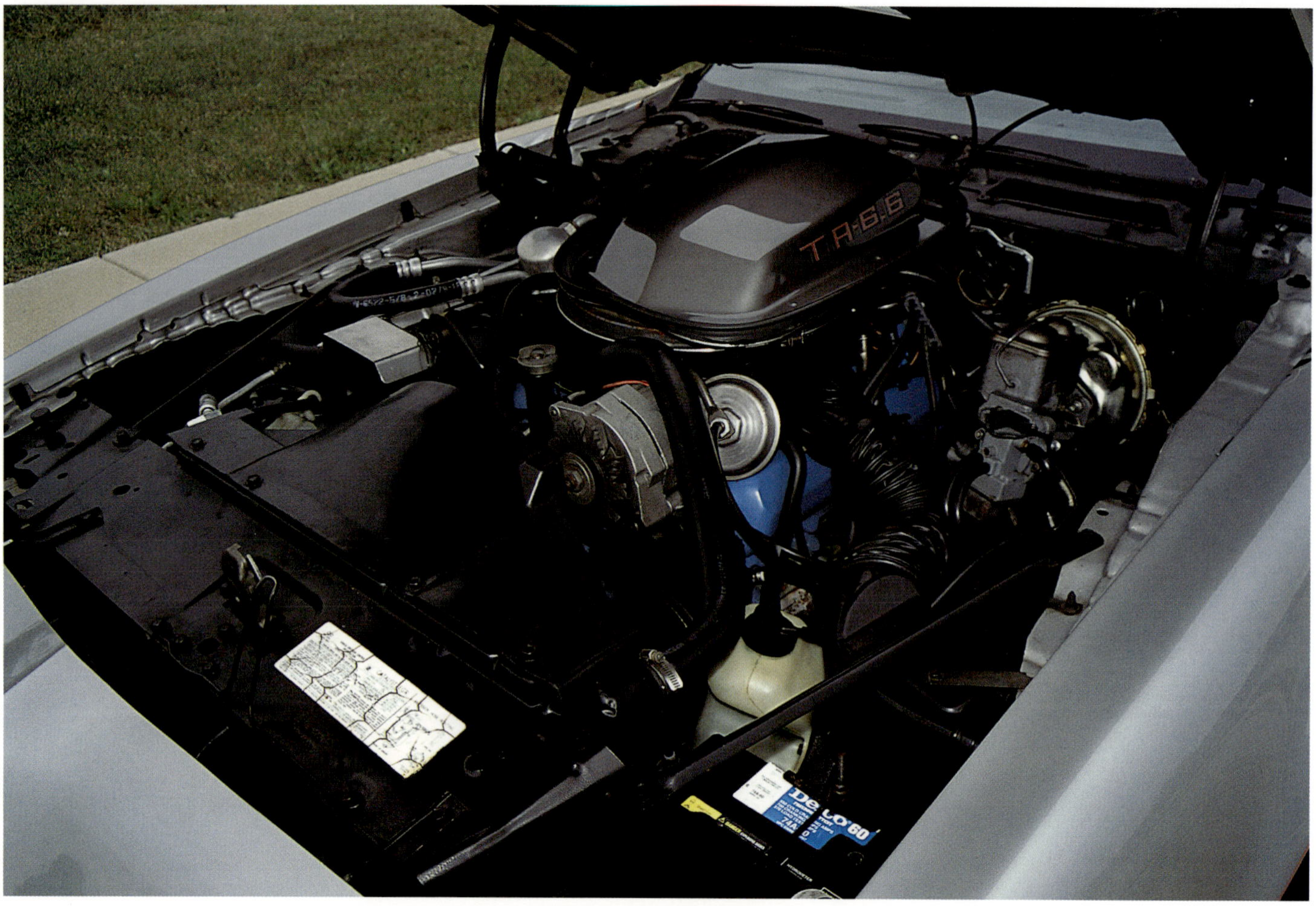

The engine compartment of a 1979 Trans Am 10th Anniversary Edition houses the Oldsmobile-built RPO L80 403-cubic-inch V-8. The shaker scoop is incorrectly marked as a 6.6-T/A engine. The engine is painted Pontiac Engine Blue.

depending upon the application and carburetion. The VIN engine code was U for LG3 and L for the LM1. The 305 Chevrolet V-8 was identified by RPO LG4 in 1980 and 1981 and had 150 horsepower and 230 foot-pounds of torque.

Firebirds sold in California in 1977–1979 had an optional 350-cubic-inch Oldsmobile V-8 (RPO L34) available with a bore and stroke of 4.06x3.39 inches and a compression ratio of 8.0:1. The L34 V-8 had a single four-barrel carburetor and hydraulic valve lifters and developed 170 horsepower and 275 foot-pounds of torque. The VIN engine code for the L34 was R.

Trans Ams sold in California and high-altitude counties in 1977–1979 used a 403-cubic-inch Oldsmobile V-8 (RPO L80) in place of the Pontiac 6.6-liter V-8. The 403 had a bore and stroke of 4.35x3.385 inches and a compression ratio of 8.0:1. The L80 engine developed 185 horsepower at 3,600 rpm and 320 foot-pounds at 2,200 rpm with a four-barrel carburetor. The L80 V-8 was also the optional V-8 in the Formula when sold in California. The VIN engine code was K.

Engine Compartment

The firewall, inner fender panels, and radiator support of all 1974–1981 Firebirds were painted semigloss black. The fenders were attached to the inner fenderwells with black phosphate-coated hex-head bolts from the underside, except for the rear upper fender-corner-to-body bolts, which were installed from the top. The driver-side fenderwell was bare except for a single black-wrapped headlight wire-loom lying across the front side. The white plastic windshield-washer reservoir with black plastic cap was attached to the front left side of the fender with a gloss-black steel bracket. The black rubber washer hose ran along the upper fenderwell. The Delco alternator was mounted on the upper left side of the engine for 1974–1981.

The passenger-side radiator support front corner held the gloss-black battery support and battery. The standard battery for the six and base V-8 was a black 45-amp Delco with side posts. A heavy-duty 61-amp Delco was standard with the 400 and 455 V-8, with air conditioning, and optional (RPO UA1) for all others. A six-gauge positive battery cable with red pigtail wire was routed under the battery support. The black negative cable with long black pigtail wire was grounded to the right fender. The black rubber engine-to-firewall heater hoses were routed across the right side wheelwell and were held together with a dark-gray phosphate clamp. If air conditioning was ordered, the compressor was mounted at the upper left of the engine.

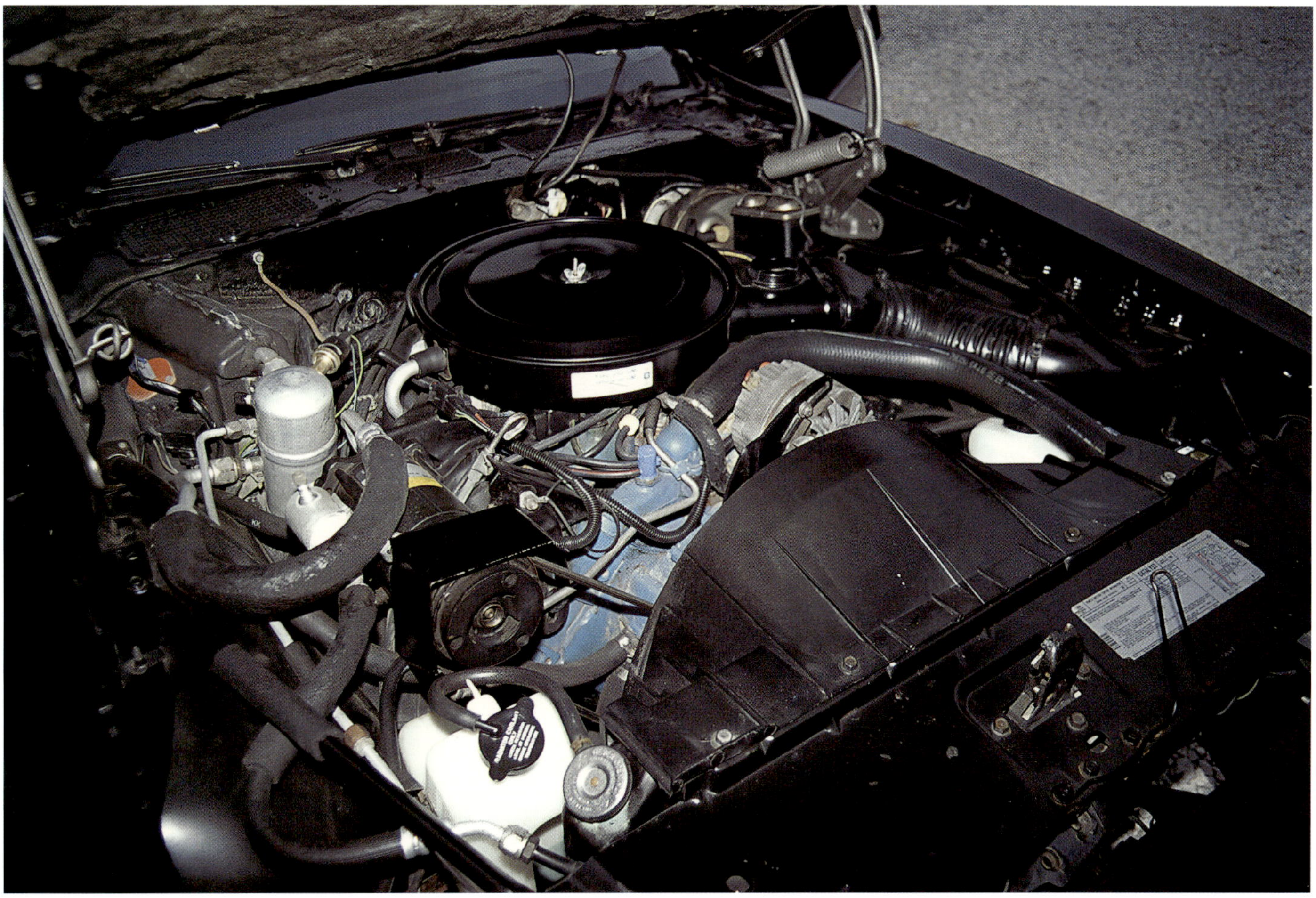

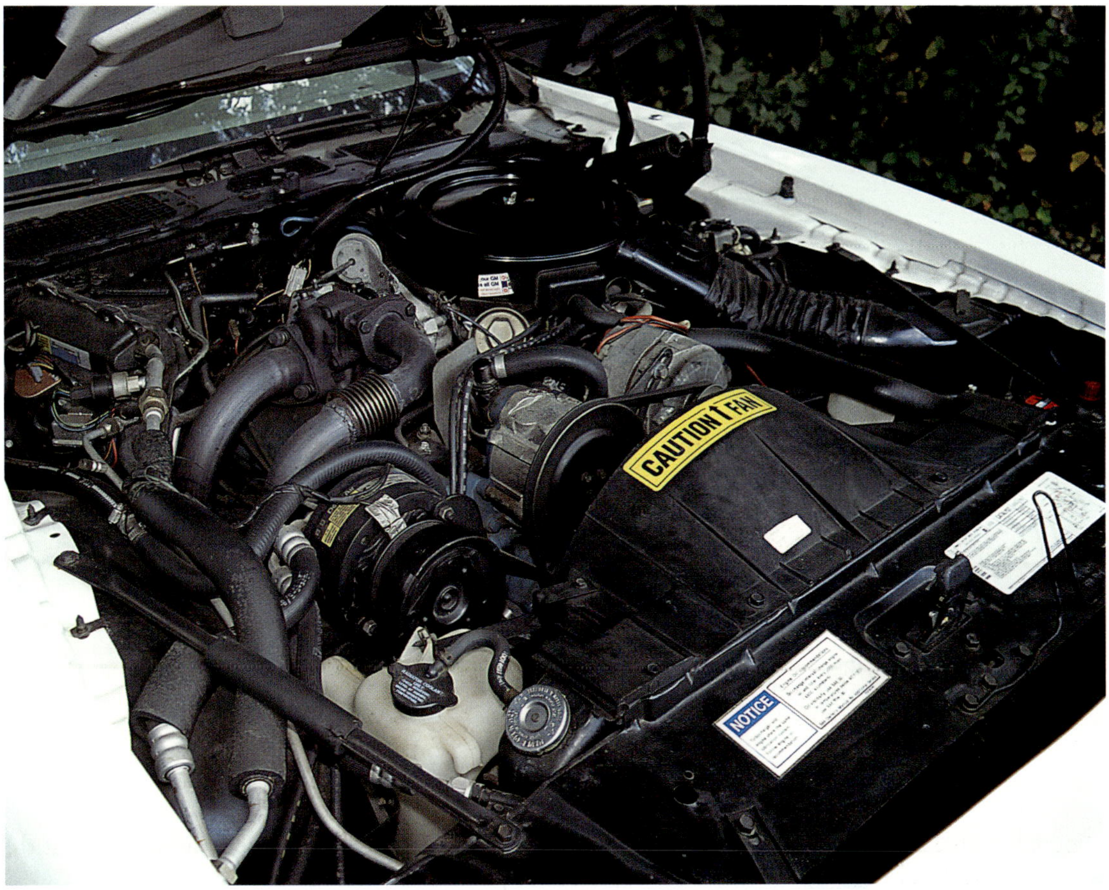

Above: The engine compartment of an original black 1979 Firebird Formula with the 4.9-liter (301-cubic-inch) RPO L27 V-8 with two-barrel carburetor. The cover over the air-conditioning compressor is an aftermarket accessory to prevent the loss of the belt if it should break. ***Right:*** The engine compartment of a 1980 Trans Am Indianapolis 500 Pace Car Edition equipped with the 4.9-liter (301-cubic-inch) turbocharged Pontiac V-8 (RPO LU8). The metal heat shield mounted on the underside of the hood protects from the heat of the turbocharger on the right side of the engine.

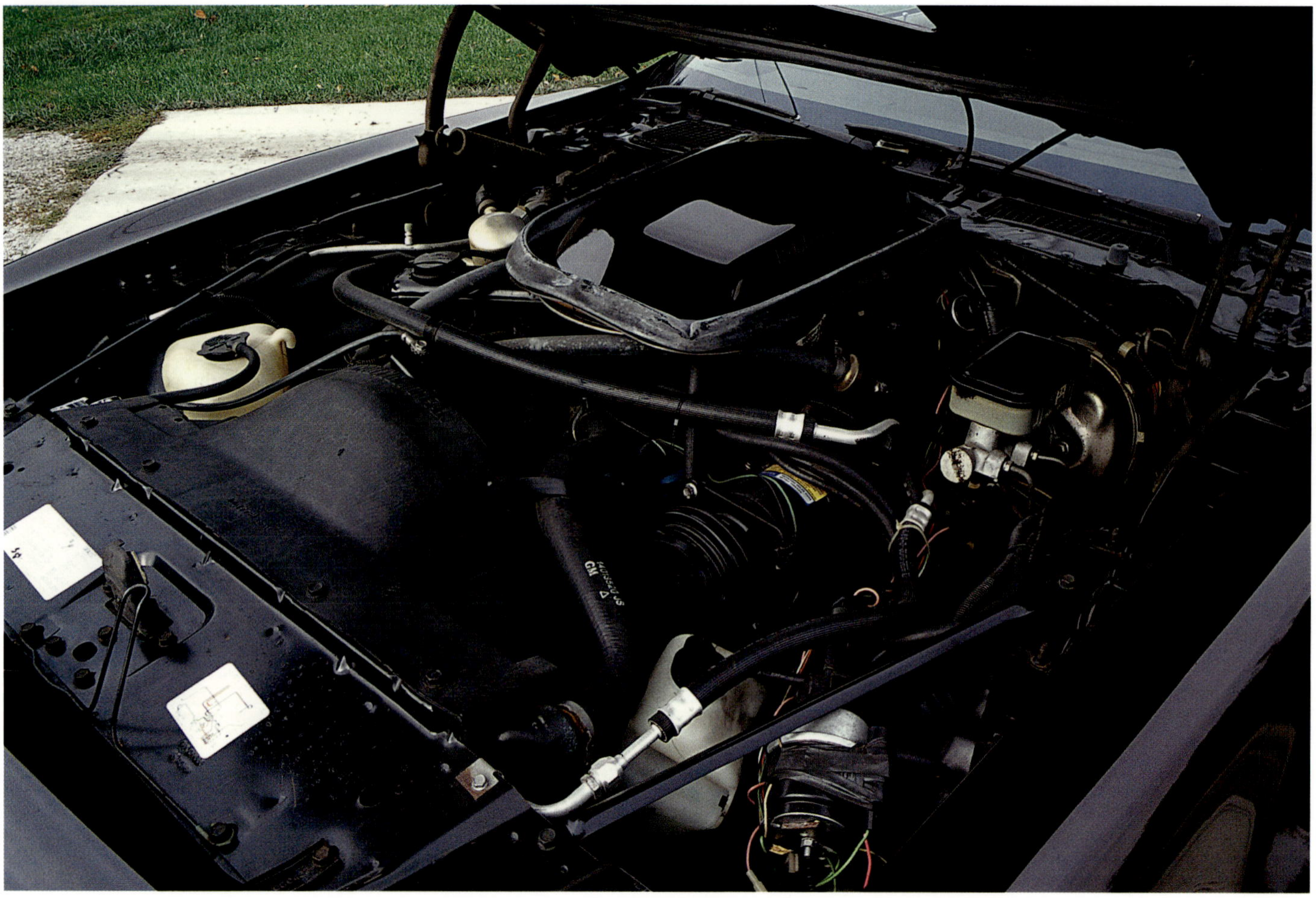

There were a number of different radiators used in the 1974–1981 Firebird, depending upon the engine and transmission combinations. The cooling system capacity for the six-cylinder was 12 quarts. The 350 V-8 had a 19.4-quart cooling system, and the 400 and 455 V-8 had an 18.6-quart system. A heavy-duty radiator was available. All radiators had the filler on the right top and the inlet hose on the left side of the top tank. The inlet hose exited the engine from the left side and was routed around the rear of the alternator. A large black reinforced-plastic fan shroud was used on all models.

The passenger side of the firewall was bare except for the heater plenum housing and the connections for the heater hoses. If air conditioning was ordered, the hose connections were also located on the right side of the firewall, and the heater connections were higher and more toward the center.

The driver (left) side of the firewall held the brake master cylinder, and the driver-side windshield wiper was to its left. All 1974–1980 Firebird manual brake systems used a dual reservoir 1-inch-bore Delco Moraine or Bendix master cylinder. Power brakes used a master cylinder with a 1.125-inch bore. All original 1974–1980 Delco master cylinder covers were gold-cadmium plated and stamped "Use Delco Brake Fluid." The 1974–1980 master cylinders were finished in semigloss black or natural cast iron, and the vacuum booster was gold-cadmium plated. A new power brake booster was adopted for 1978 with part number 18003895. In 1979 and 1980, two different boosters were used depending upon whether rear disc brakes were ordered.

For 1981, a new master cylinder was adopted with an aluminum cylinder assembly and translucent plastic reservoir with a black plastic cover. Four different master cylinders were used with or without the 1981 turbocharged option and with or without rear disc brakes. Front disc with rear drum brakes were standard on all 1974–1978 Firebird models, but power brakes were only standard on the Trans Am and optional (RPO JL2) for all others. Rear disc brakes became available as an option in 1979.

The body data plate was attached to the firewall with two special hex-head screws at the top edge of the firewall between the master cylinder and wiper motor. The data plate was painted semigloss black with the firewall. The gloss-black-painted windshield-wiper motor was mounted to the right of the brake master cylinder. All 1974–1981 Firebirds had standard two-speed electric parallel-action wipers. Windshield washers were standard on all models.

The engine compartment of a Barclay Brown 1981 Trans Am equipped with the 5-liter (305-cubic-inch) Chevrolet V-8 (RPO LG4). The cruise-control unit on the left side of the engine compartment is an aftermarket accessory.

The underside of the hood of all 1974–1981 Firebirds was painted semigloss black. The hood hinges were black/dark-gray phosphate, and the hood springs were natural unfinished steel.

Frame, Undercarriage, Transmission, and Driveline

All 1974–1981 Firebirds used welded-steel unitized construction with a separate rubber-cushioned, bolted-on steel front subframe to support the engine and front suspension. The body structure consists of the welded-steel floorpan and side panels integrating the trunk compartment and rear quarters. The steel front subframe and related components were finished in either semigloss black or natural unfinished bare steel.

Front Suspension

The 1974–1981 Firebird front suspension used unequal-length upper and lower control arms with ball joints, coil springs, and tubular shock absorbers. The stamped-steel upper control arms were used on all Firebirds from 1974 through 1981. The ball joints were riveted in place, and the pivot joints had steel-encased rubber bushings. The control arms were painted semigloss black except for the outer ball-joint ends.

All 1974–1981 Firebirds used the same lower control arms. Lower control arm components were painted semigloss black except for the outer ends. The gloss-black-finish front coil springs were mounted between the lower control arm and a pocket in the front subframe. Different coil springs were used depending upon the engine and model application. Gray painted Delco spiral-body tubular shock absorbers were mounted in the center of the coil springs.

The standard 1974 Firebird and Esprit 0.938-inch-diameter front stabilizer bar was mounted between the lower front control arms and rubber-bushed brackets in the front subframe. The optional (1974 only) radial-tuned suspension (RPO TGJ/TGK) had firm-control shock absorbers and a 1.00-inch-diameter bar that was standard with the Formula in 1974. Rally-tuned suspension was standard in the 1974–1981 Trans Am and radial-tuned suspension became standard in all models in 1975. The 1.00-inch front stabilizer bar was standard with the base Firebird and Esprit for 1975 and 1976, and the Formula had a 1.125-inch bar. For 1977–1981, the base Firebird, Esprit, and Formula all had a 1.125-inch front stabilizer bar. The 1974–1981 Trans Am front suspension was similar, except it used a 1.250-inch-diameter front stabilizer bar. All front stabilizer bars were finished in black phosphate and attached with natural steel links and rubber bushings.

The standard front brakes for all 1974–1981 Firebirds were 10.9-inch-diameter vented discs with single-piston cast-iron-finish calipers and standard metallic pads. A different caliper housing and part number was used respectively for model years 1975–1976, 1977, 1978, 1979–1980, and 1981. Manual front disc brakes were standard on all 1974–1976 models, except the Trans Am, which had standard power brakes. Power brakes were optional on all other models with RPO JL2 and standard on all 1977–1981 models with V-8 engines.

The variable-ratio Saginaw power steering with 16.5:1: to 14.3:1 ratios was standard equipment for all 1974–1981 Firebirds. For 1975, special valves were added to increase road feel. The manual steering gear was painted gloss black with a natural-finish side cover and end plug. The power steering gear was natural cast finish with a dull aluminum cover and end plug.

Rear Suspension

The 1974–1981 Firebird rear axle was a Salisbury-type semifloating design with an 8.5-inch ring gear and 10-bolt cover. The axle was available in 1974 in standard ratios of 2.73:1 (CA), 3.42:1 (CM), and 3.08:1 (GY) in Safe-T-Track (RPO G80), and 2.73:1 (GZ), 3.42:1 (CL), and 3.08:1 (GX) in open differential. For 1975, the axle codes were changed to 2.73:1 (PA/PU), 3.08:1 (PC/PW), and 2.56:1 (PG/PT). Axle codes for 1976–1981 were similar except new 2.41:1 (PJ/PS) and 3.23:1 (PX/PD) ratios were added, and some additional codes were used. The axle code plus a code identifying the month-and-day built and plant letter suffix are stamped on the front passenger side of the axle tube. The rear axle assembly was painted gloss black with paint codes identifying the various configurations. The 1974–1981 Trans Am had standard Safe-T-Track

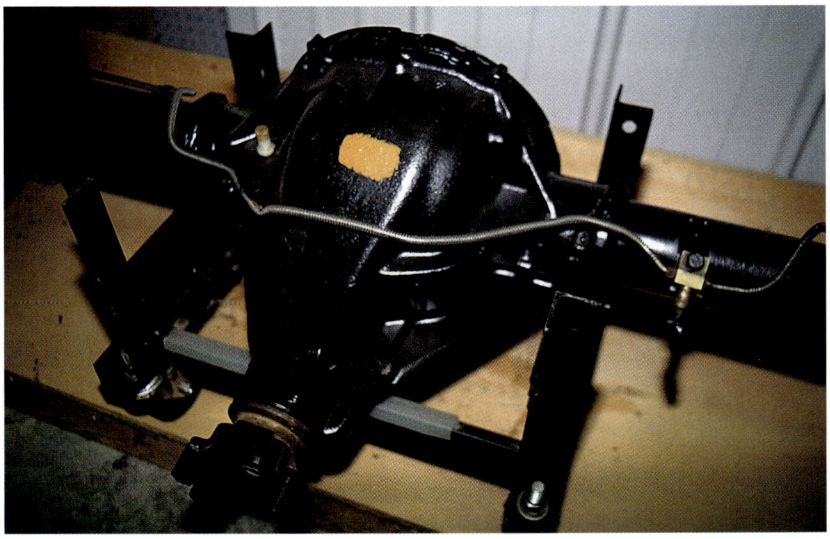

This original, unrestored, 10-bolt General Motors rear axle assembly from a 1976 Firebird is finished in semigloss black, and the original green-and-orange paint markings indicate the axle ratio and Safe-T-Track differential.

limited-slip differential.

The 1974–1981 Firebird rear suspension consisted of parallel multileaf semielliptic leaf springs. Springs were natural-steel finish with gloss black mounting brackets and hangers. The spring rates varied according to engine and option combinations. The rear suspension was supported by gray painted Delco spiral-body shock absorbers (some may have had a semigloss black finish) mounted in a staggered configuration with one behind the axle and the other in front. All 1975–1981 Firebirds had radial-tuned suspension, and 1974–1981 Trans Ams had Rally-tuned suspension with firm-control shock absorbers.

The rear stabilizer bar was optional for the base Firebird and Esprit in 1974 but standard in the Formula and Trans Am. For 1975–1981, the rear stabilizer bar was standard in all models and included in the radial-tuned suspension (RTS). The standard rear stabilizer bar for the RTS in the 1974–1981 Firebird, Esprit, and Formula was 0.625 inch in diameter. The Trans Am rear bar was 0.812 inch in diameter. In 1975, the Trans Am rear bar was increased to 1.250 inches in diameter. The stabilizer bar was natural steel finish.

The standard rear brakes on all 1974–1981 Firebirds were drum-type hydraulic with 9.5-inch cast-iron drums. Standard asbestos linings were 2 inches wide. Brake drums and backing plates were painted semigloss black. Beginning in 1979 and through the 1981 model, rear disc brakes were available as an option, with RPO J65 on the Formula and Trans Am, and standard with the 1979 10th Anniversary Trans Am model. The rotor used part number 10005272, and the rear calipers were part number 18006748 (left) and 18006749 (right). Front and rear power disc brakes were also included in the RPO WS6 Special Performance Package in the 1979–1981 Trans Am.

Tires and Wheels

The standard wheels for the 1974 Firebird, Esprit, and Formula were 14x6J steel wheels with five lug nuts. In 1974, there were also 14x5 and 14x7 painted steel wheels with either 0.20 inch or 0.34 inch offset used depending upon the tire equipment. The standard wheel for 1975–1981 Firebird and Esprit and 1975–1977 Formula was a 15x6 painted steel wheel. The steel wheels were finished in gloss black enamel if full wheel covers were used, but if the small standard hubcaps were supplied, the wheels were painted gloss enamel on the front side only to match the lower body color.

Optional wheels for 1974 included the silver 14x7JJ Rally II wheels with argent silver background (RPO N98) with standard aluminum trim ring. The 15x7JJ Rally II wheels with trim ring were available as an option on all 1975–1981

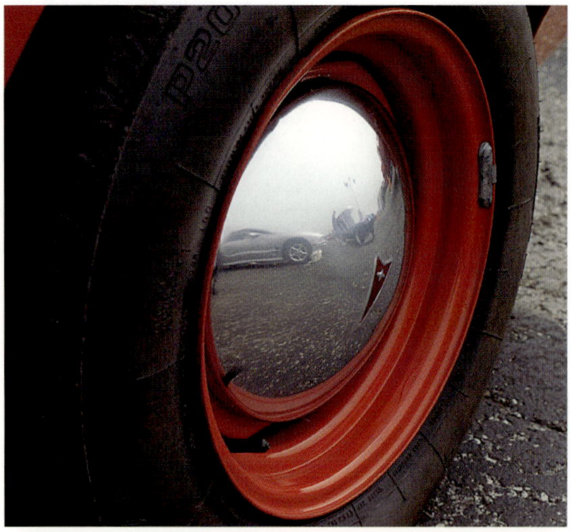

This is an original, standard, 14-inch-steel, painted right front wheel on a Buccaneer Red 1974 Firebird Formula equipped with an SD 455 V-8 engine. The hubcap is the standard baby-moon style with a red Pontiac arrowhead medallion.

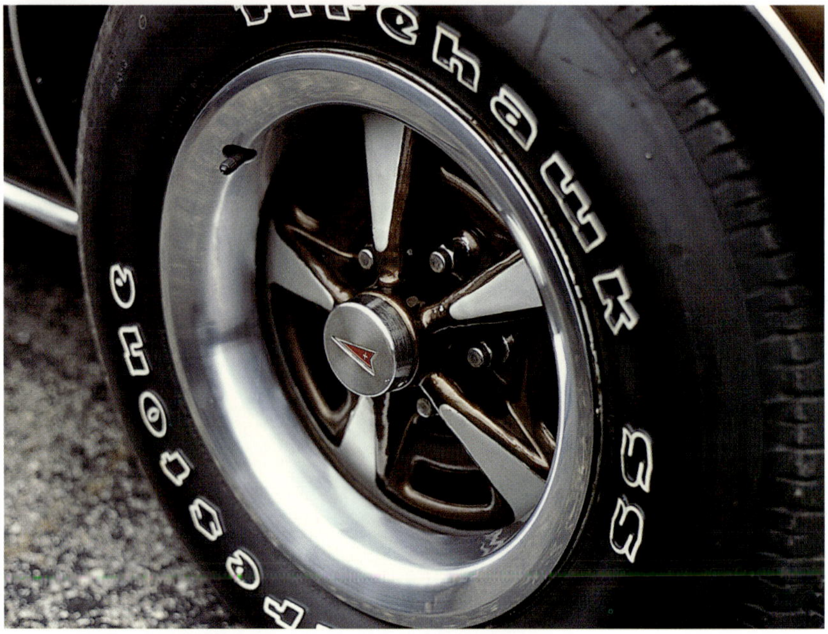

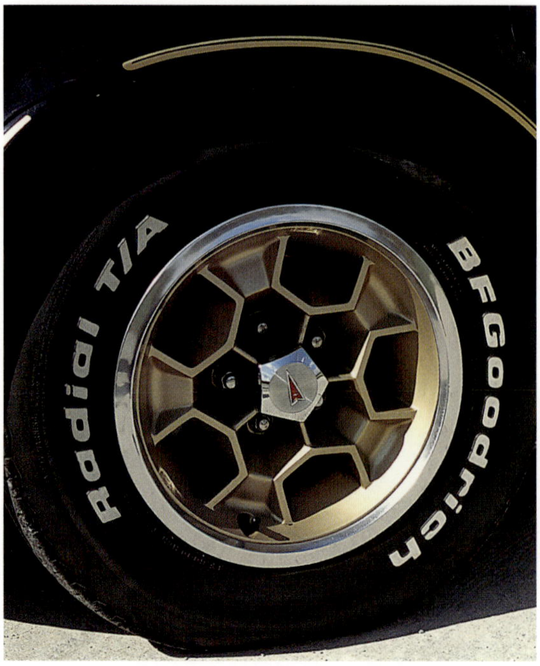

Above: This is a detail view of a body-color-coordinated 15-inch Rally II wheel and bright trim ring (RPO N67) on a Ginger Brown 1975 Firebird Formula. The tire is an incorrect aftermarket replacement. ***Left:*** Detail view of the standard 15-inch gold finish Honeycomb wheels (RPO P05) on a 1976 Trans Am black Limited Edition. The 1976 Limited Edition Trans Am package included a number of gold-accented components.

Right: This is a gold-accented cast-aluminum 15-inch snowflake wheel on a black 1978 Trans Am with the distinctive red-and-black Firebird medallion in the center. *Far right:* This is the 15-inch Turbo cast-aluminum wheel standard on the silver 1979 Trans Am 10th Anniversary Edition. The wheels were made by Appliance Wheel Company. Note the red-and-black Firebird medallion in the center.

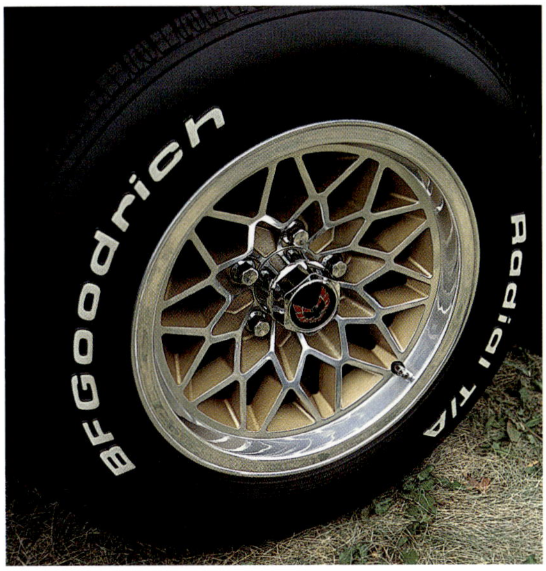

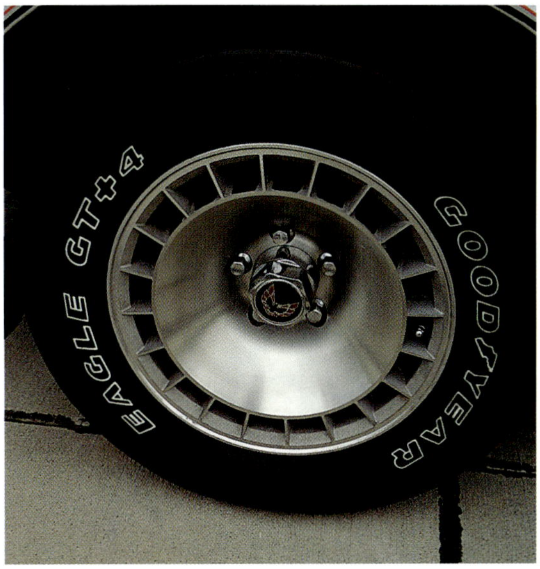

models and standard on the 1974–1981 Trans Am and 1978–1981 Formula. In 1976, 15x7 Rally II wheels with body-colored backgrounds (RPO N67) became available on all models. All 1974–1981 Rally II wheels had a standard dark-rimmed bright center hub with red Pontiac arrowhead badge.

An additional optional wheel for 1974–1976 was the cast-aluminum honeycomb wheel (RPO P05) in both 14x7 and 15x7 sizes first introduced in 1971. In 1977, new 15x7 (15x8 with the 1978–1981 WS6 handling package) cast-aluminum wheels, commonly referred to as "snowflake wheels" (RPO YJ8), replaced the honeycomb wheels as an option for all models. There was a change in design of the 15x7 snowflake wheel in 1979, which reduced the thickness of the spokes and eliminated the step from the bolt circle to the snowflake pattern. The 15x8 wheel had a noticeable recess to the pattern, separating it from the outer rim. The background finish of the snowflake wheel was gold (Trans Am SE), silver, or red (1978 and 1979 Esprit W68 Redbird package), depending upon the specific model, but the outer spoke surface (except for the 1978 SE 15x8 wheels) and outer rim was always machined aluminum.

For 1980 and 1981, the Formula and Trans Am were available with optional 15x8 Turbo cast-aluminum wheels (RPO N90). The Turbo cast-aluminum wheels had a smooth dished center with turbine-like fins around the circumference and were introduced as an exclusive part of the 1979 10th Anniversary Trans Am Special Edition (2FX).

The standard tires for the 1974 Firebird and

Right: This is a detail view of a 15-inch cast-aluminum snowflake wheel (RPO N90) with gray painted accents on an original black 1979 Firebird Formula with the RPO W50 Formula Appearance Package. *Far right:* This is a detail view of a left front wheel on an Atlantic Blue 1979 Trans Am. This is the optional cast-aluminum snowflake wheel. The tires are aftermarket replacements.

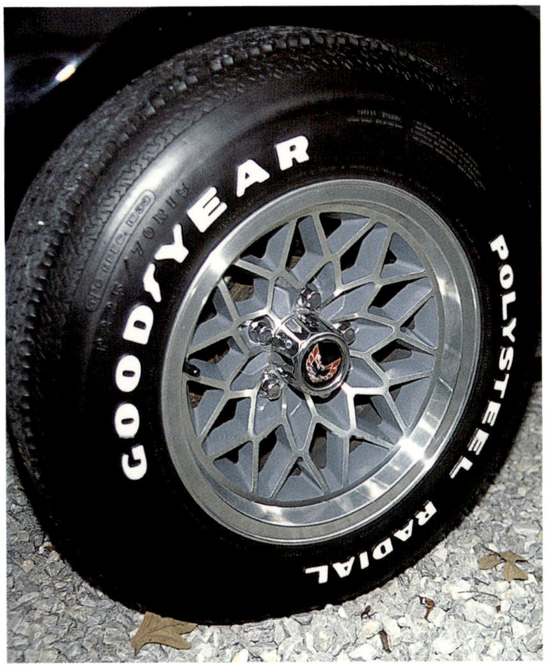

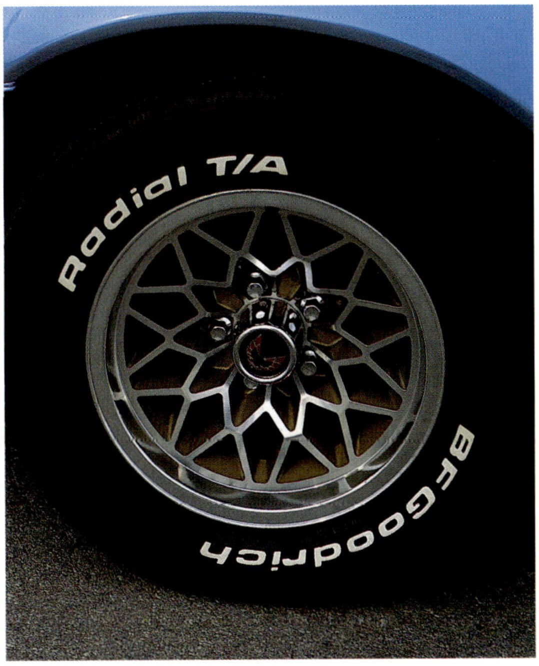

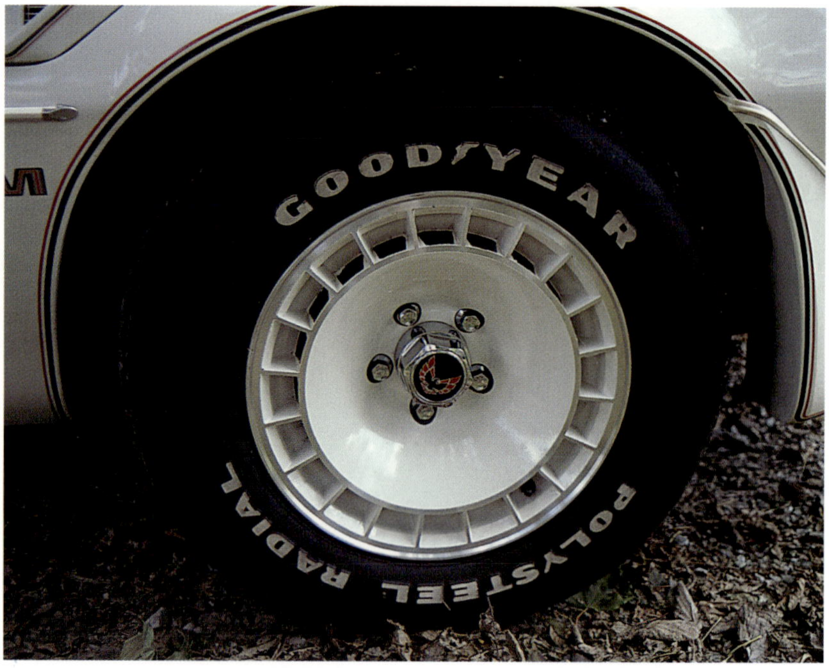

Above: This is the standard 15x8 white-accented Turbo cast-aluminum wheel on a 1980 Trans Am Turbo 4.9 Indianapolis 500 pace car. The center and inside of the spokes of the wheel are painted white to match the body finish, and distinctive stripes carry over to the wheel opening spoiler. ***Below:*** This is a detail view of the 15x7 gold-accented cast-aluminum snowflake wheel on a Barclay Brown 1981 Trans Am with the unique gold-and-black Firebird center hub. The rear mud flap is an accessory.

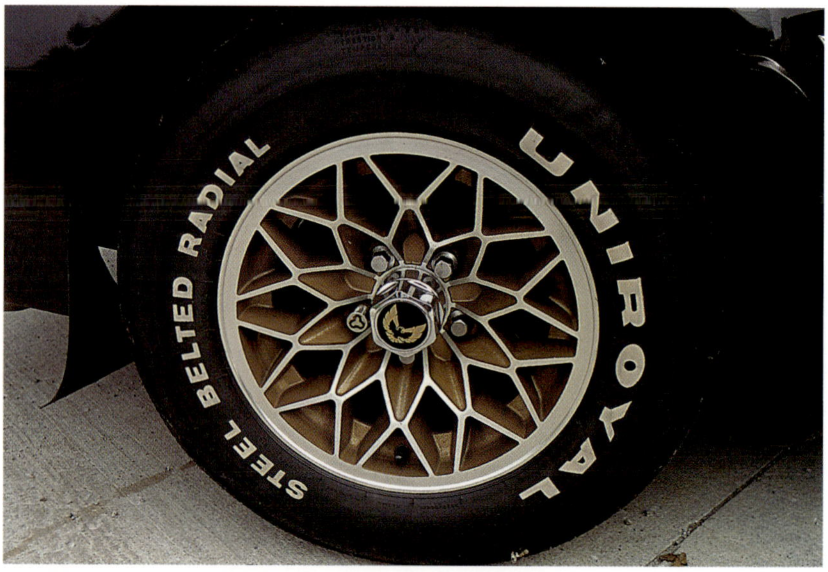

Esprit were E78x14 black sidewall bias-ply with E78x14 white letter (RPO THB), white sidewall (RPO TGR), F78x14 black sidewall (RPO TGF), and F70x14 white letter (RPO TML) available as options. Standard tires for the 1974 Formula were F70x14 bias-ply black sidewall with optional F70x14 white letter and GR70x15 steel-belted radial (TGH) available. The optional radial-tuned suspension package (RPO TGJ) included FR78x14 steel-belted radial white-sidewall tires, and the RPO TGK version replaced them with FR78x14 white letter tires. The RPO TVH radial-tuned suspension package included GR70x15 tires. The 1974 Trans Am had F60x15 white letter bias-ply tires standard, with GR70x15 white letter tires available.

Standard tires for the 1975–1979 Firebird and Esprit and 1975–1977 Formula were black-sidewall FR78x15 steel-belted radials. Optional tires for the 1975–1979 Firebird, Esprit, and Formula were FR78x15 white letter steel-belted radial, FR78x15 white-sidewall steel-belted radial, and GR70x15 steel-belted radials in either black sidewall (RPO QBX) or white letter (RPO QCY). F78x14 white-sidewall or black-sidewall fiberglass bias-belted tires were also an option in the base Firebird and Esprit for 1975 and 1976. Standard tires for the 1975–1979 Trans Am were GR70x15 black-sidewall steel-belted radials with white letter GR70x15 radials optional.

Tire equipment changed significantly for 1980, when metric-sized radial tires were adopted for most models. The standard tires for the base 1980 and 1981 Firebird and Esprit were 205/75R-15 black-sidewall steel-belted radials. Standard tires for the 1980 and 1981 Formula and base Trans Am were 225/70R-15. Special Edition, Turbo, and Pace Car 1980 and 1981 Trans Ams (Y84, LU8) had standard GR70x15 steel-belted radial black-sidewall tires. Optional tires for the 1980 and 1981 base Firebird and Esprit were 205/75R-15 white letter steel radials (RPO QGR/QMC) and 205/75R-15 white-sidewall steel radials (RPO QJW). The Trans Am and Formula were available with optional 225/70R-15 steel-belted white letter radials (RPO QQR).

Small chrome-plated hubcaps with a Pontiac arrowhead badge were standard equipment for all 1974–1981 base Firebirds. The baby-moon design used since 1972 (part number 485200) was standard in 1974, but in 1975–1981, the hubcap was changed to a flatter design (part number 498800) with a small center rim around a small arrowhead medallion.

The 1974–1981 Firebird Esprit had standard deluxe wheel discs that were optional (RPO P01) on the base Firebird and 1974–1977 Formula. The 1974 14-inch deluxe wheel disc (part number 496031) had a small flat center section surrounded by a smooth disc with small radiating fins around its circumference. For 1975 and 1976, the deluxe wheel disc was a 15-inch design (part number 496972) with a smooth outer circumference and a wide flat center section with an arrowhead medallion, surrounded by letters spelling "Pontiac Motor Division" inside a darker rim.

The deluxe wheel cover (RPO P01) for 1977 and 1978 (part number 527060) was completely redesigned and had a relatively flat surface with numerous small holes and a smaller center and

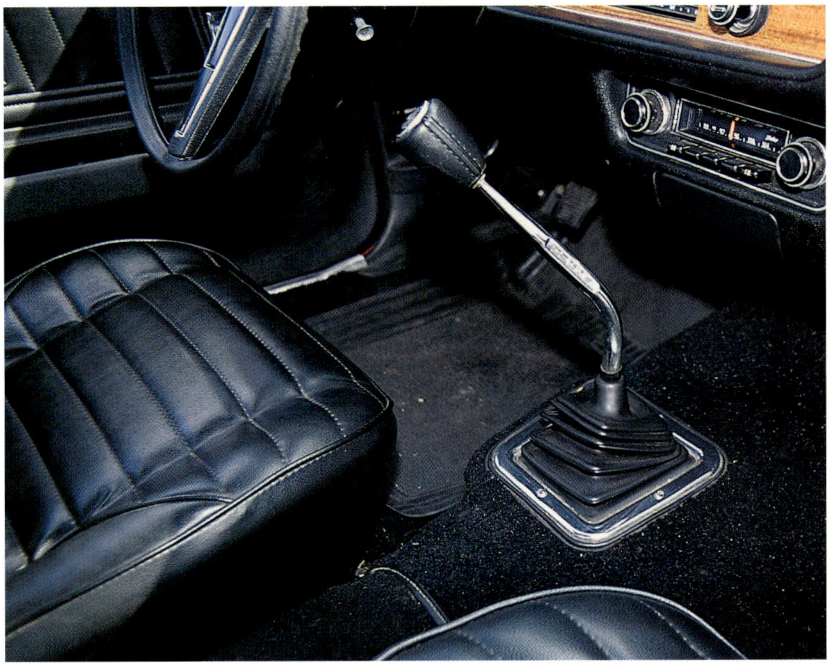

This 1974 Firebird Formula SD 455 is equipped with an optional four-speed manual transmission (RPO 36E). This view shows the Hurst floor shift and rubber boot, the straight horizontal wood-grain finish on the instrument panel, and the optional radio mounted beneath the center.

arrowhead medallion. For 1979–1981, the deluxe wheel cover (part number 20005598) was again redesigned and had a dished center with a small hub and arrowhead logo.

The 1974–1981 custom wheel covers were available as an option with RPO P02 on all models except the Trans Am and the 1978–1981 Formula. The 1974–1976 custom wheel cover (part number 486554) had a small center with an arrowhead medallion and fine fins radiating to the outer rim. In 1977–1981, the custom wheel covers were dropped and replaced with optional chrome-plated wire-wheel covers (RPO N95). The wire-wheel covers (part number 549372) were not available on the Formula or Trans Am. The wire-wheel covers had a hexagon-shaped center hub with an arrowhead medallion.

Transmissions

The 1974–1981 Firebirds were available with a variety of transmission choices depending upon the year, model, and engine. In 1974, the standard transmission in the Firebird and Esprit equipped with the six-cylinder and 350 V-8 was the three-speed manual with floor shift (RPO M12). The four-speed manual transmission with floor shift (RPO M20) was optional with the 350 V-8. The 400 four-barrel V-8 and 455 SD V-8 were also available with the four-speed. For 1975, the three-speed manual (RPO M15) was also standard with the six, but it was not available with any other engine. The four-speed was available with the 250 six, 350 two-barrel, 400 and 455 V-8s. For 1976, the four-speed was no longer available with the 350 V-8 and was not available in California.

In 1977, the three-speed manual transmission (RPO M15) was standard on the Firebird and Esprit with the 231 V-6. The three-speed manual was also available with the 350 V-8 (RPO M38) and the 305 V-8 (RPO M15). The four-speed manual transmission (RPO M20) was standard on the Formula and available with the 231 V-6 and 301 V-8. The 400 V-8 was available with the Muncie close-ratio four-speed transmission (RPO M21). Manual transmissions were not available in California. In 1978, choices were changed again, and the M15 three-speed was only available with the 231 V-6. The M21 close-ratio four-speed was only available with the 400 V-8, but the M20 four-speed was available with the 231 six, 305 V-8, and 350 V-8.

For 1979, the three-speed manual transmission was again available only with the 231 V-6. The M20 wide-ratio four-speed was available with the 231 V-6, 301 V-8, and 305 LG3 V-8. The M21 close-ratio four-speed was available with the 301 L37 V-8 and 400 L78 V-8. In 1980 and 1981, the three-speed manual (RPO MM3) was only available with the LD5 231 V-6. The wide-ratio four-speed manual (RPO MM4) was only available with the 5.0-liter V-8 in the Formula and Trans Am.

There were three basic types of three-speed Turbo Hydra-Matic transmissions offered in the 1974–1981 Firebirds. In 1974, the Turbo Hydra-Matic TH350 was optional (RPO M38) in the Firebird and Esprit with the 250 six and standard with the 350 V-8. The TH400 transmissions were optional (RPO M40) with the 400 four-barrel V-8 and 455 SD V-8 and standard with the 400 two-barrel engines. For 1975, the TH400 was no longer available, and the TH350 was optional for all applications except the 455 V-8. The TH400 was dropped in 1975 because the 400 engine was fitted with a catalytic converter, and the converter's size and mounting location did not allow space for the larger transmission case.

In 1976, the TH350 was optional with the 250 six and standard with the 350 V-8. The 400 V-8 with 3.08:1 and 3.23:1 rear axle and 400 four-barrel V-8 also used the TH350 transmission. For 1977–1979, the TH350 (RPO M40) was available or standard with all applications. For 1980, a new TH200 version of the Turbo Hydra-Matic (RPO MV9) was introduced and used with the 301 and 265 V-8 engines only. The 231 V-6 and all other V-8 engines used the TH350 (RPO M38). In 1981, only the 265 V-8 used the TH200. All Turbo Hydra-Matic transmission cases were natural aluminum with a gloss-black oil pan and converter pan.

All transmissions were connected to the rear axle by a natural-finish one-piece welded-steel driveshaft.

Chapter 5

1982–1992

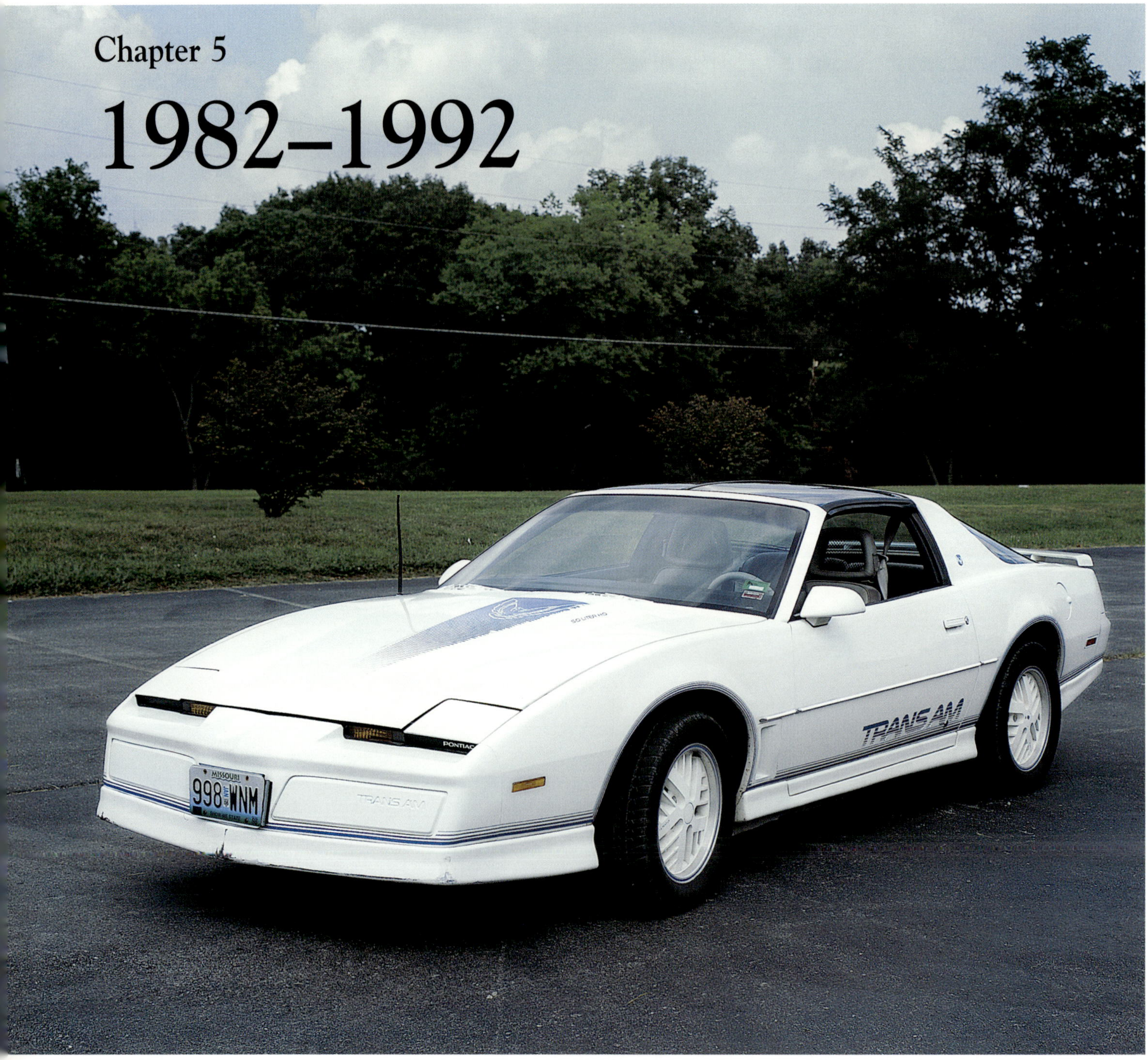

This original white 1984 Trans Am 15th Anniversary Edition has blue accent stripes and decals. Special panels were used to fill in the grille openings in the standard Firebird front fascia.

Nineteen eighty-two was a significant year for major changes in the F-body Firebird line. Not only were the bodies restyled, the chassis and body construction was also changed dramatically. The new Firebird shared 65 percent of its parts (compared to about 25 percent in the second generation) with the third-generation Chevrolet Camaro. Along with the styling and mechanical changes, the wheelbase of what is now considered the third-generation Firebird was reduced by 7 inches, to 101 inches, thus reducing the weight to improve fuel efficiency and handling qualities. Pontiac advertising began to emphasize fuel economy alongside performance and style. The slogan for 1982 was "Now the excitement really begins," but the message was the necessary compromise between performance and efficiency. Pontiac Chief Engineer Robert L. Dorn proudly announced this "balance of acceleration, handling and efficiency" in the 1982 brochures.

The new styling of the Firebird included retractable headlights and was described as pure aerodynamics with a "saber-like nose and rakish tail." The new 1982 Firebird windshield had a 62-degree slant that helped produce the lowest drag coefficient (0.323 Cd) of any production car in General Motors test history. The new design, directed by the Pontiac II Studio headed by John

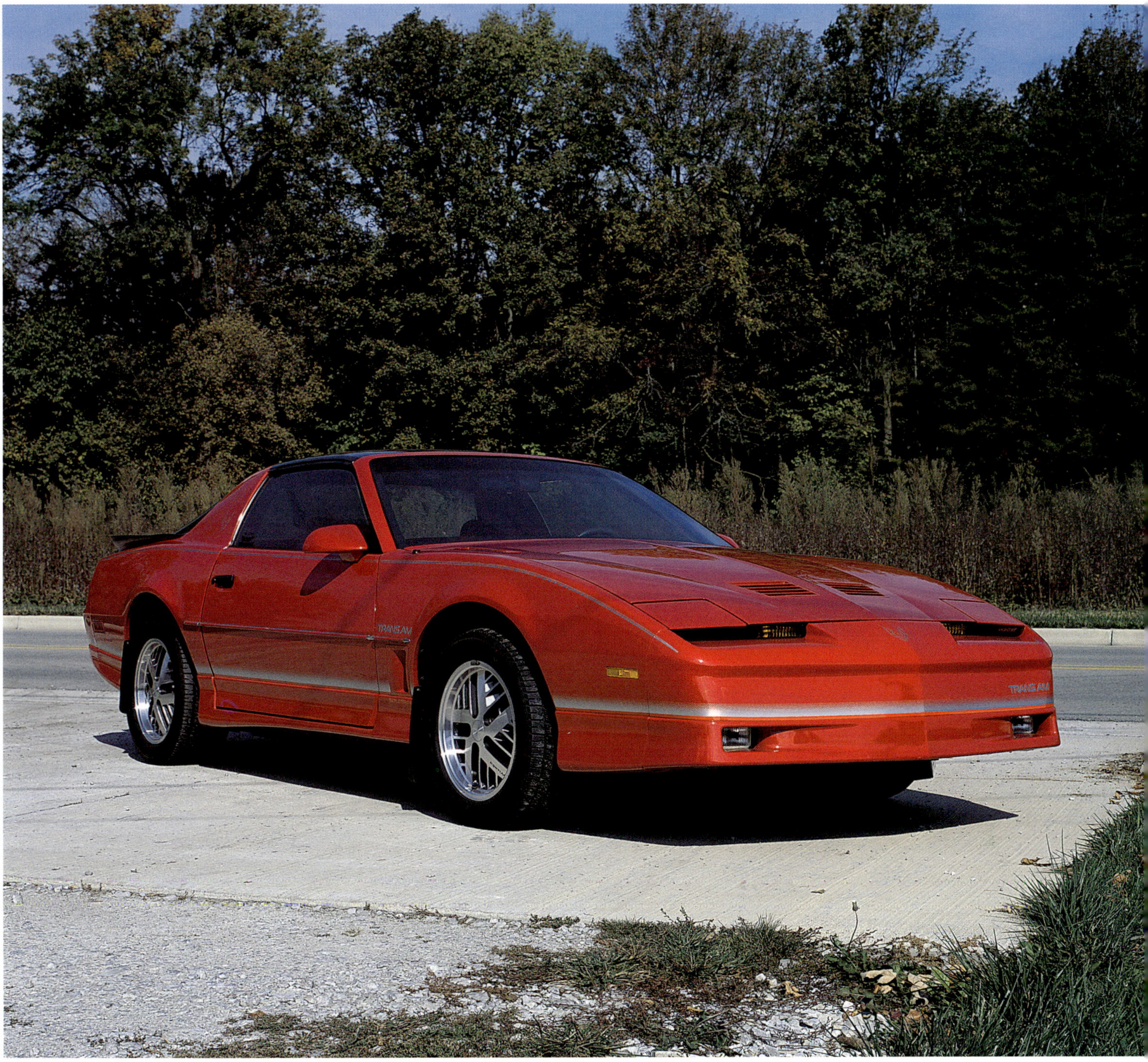

This is the right front quarter of a Bright Red (81) 1986 Trans Am sport coupe with 15x7 High-Tech Turbo cast-aluminum wheels and special silver body accent stripe.

Schinella, managed to reduce the overall length by 10 inches and the width by 2 inches, creating a new, sleeker look while maintaining the same passenger compartment space. Of course, overall weight was also reduced by almost 500 pounds. The new design featured a standard rear hatch and deck lid that allowed easier access to the cargo compartment. The hatch was equipped with a frameless window that was said to be the most complex piece of automotive glass ever made with compound and convex curves.

The model lineup for 1982–1986 was reduced along with everything else, and the Esprit and Formula were dropped. The new models consisted of the base Firebird, Firebird Trans Am, and Firebird S/E. The base Firebird continued as the economy choice, while the Trans Am led the performance choices. The S/E was the luxury model with more comfortable ride and trim. The model lineup was changed further for 1987–1992, when the S/E model was eliminated and the Formula name was resurrected in the form of two Formula option packages (RPO W61/W63/W66) on the base 1987 Firebird with either a 5.0-liter or 5.7-liter V-8. In 1988–1992, the Formula became a separate model line available only as a two-door hatchback. Another addition for 1987 was the GTA, introduced as an option package (RPO

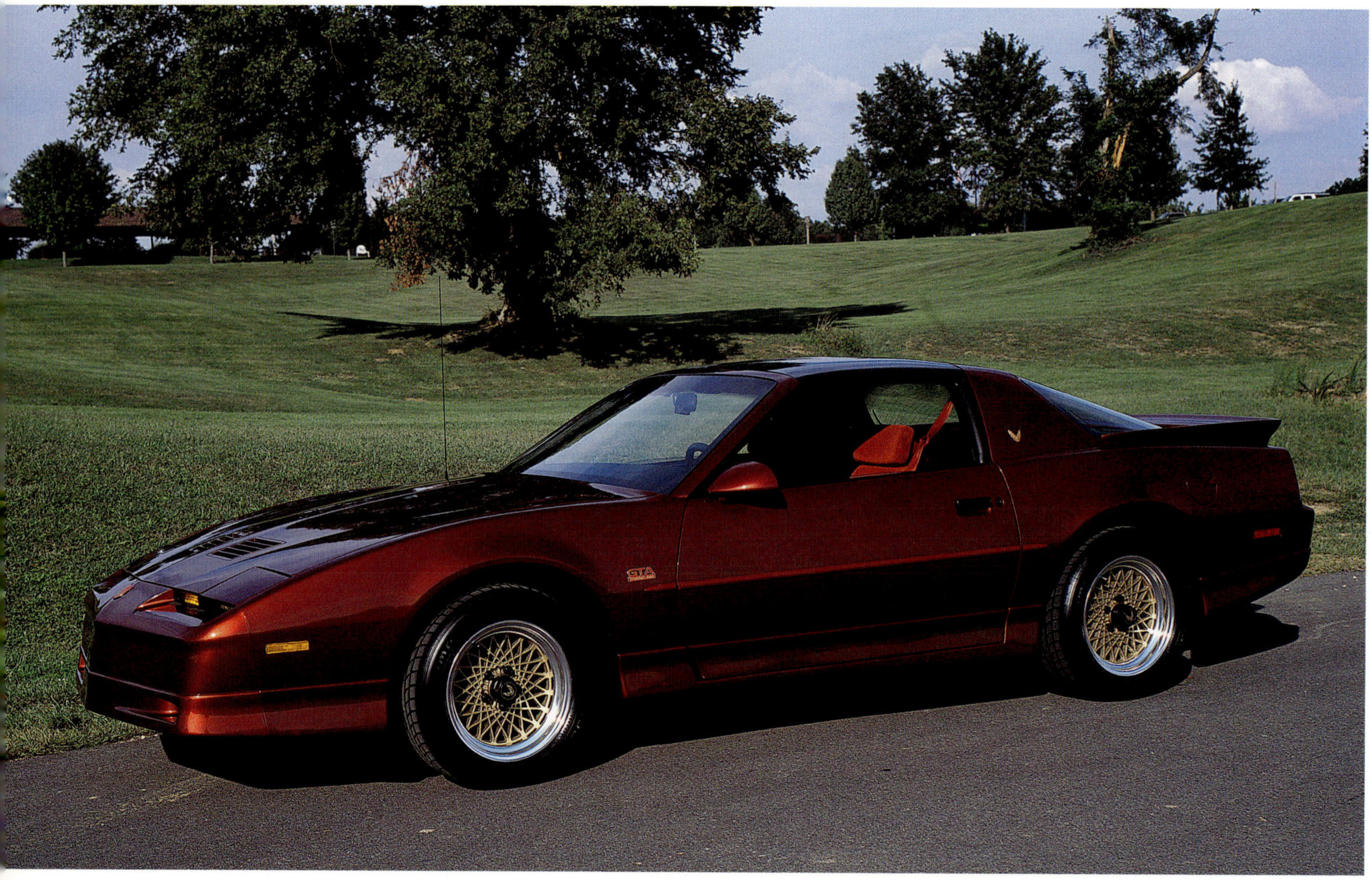

Y84) on the Trans Am. Within the basic Trans Am models were additional special packages that included the 1983 Daytona 500 Pace Car replicas, 1984 15th Anniversary Trans Am, and the 1989 20th Anniversary Turbo Trans Am GTA Indy Pace Car.

An exciting addition was made in 1991 by reintroducing convertibles to the model lineup. Two thousand base Firebird and Trans Am convertibles were made in 1991, with 1,948 built in 1992. The 1991 and 1992 convertibles were actually American Sunroof Corporation (ASC) conversions. Another 1992 addition to Firebird choices were the Street Legal Performance (SLP) Formula Firehawks (RPO B4U) with high-performance engine and drivetrain modifications. Only 25 Firehawks were built, including one Trans Am–based convertible, and all but four were red.

Firebird engine choices were also reduced and changed for the third-generation 1982 Firebird with all engines (except the Pontiac four-cylinder) now considered "GM Corporate," although they were essentially Chevrolet engines. The base Firebird for 1982–1986 was equipped with an economical 151-cubic-inch (2.5-liter) throttle-body electronic-fuel-injected four-cylinder. The standard engine for the Special Edition (S/E) and the 1987–1989 base Firebird was a 173-cubic-inch (2.8-liter) OHV V-6 with a two-barrel carburetor. The four-cylinder was a delete option in the S/E through 1986. The base V-6 was increased in displacement to 191 cubic inches in 1990. A 305-cubic-inch (5.0-liter) OHV V-8 with a four-barrel carburetor was standard in the Trans Am, with an electronic Crossfire fuel-injected version available as an option.

Engine choices stayed much the same from 1982 to 1992, except that a special 125-horsepower HO version of the 173-cubic-inch V-6 became available in 1983 and 1984. The HO V-6 was replaced by a third, 190-horsepower HO version of the 5.0-liter V-8 for 1985. This engine was kept but downgraded in 1987, when a new 210-horsepower 350-cubic-inch (5.7-liter) V-8 was adopted. In 1988 only, the two versions of the 305 V-8 were both called "HO," and the 5.7-liter V-8 was considered the GTA engine. The 5.0 HO designations were dropped for 1989, only to return for 1990 and be dropped again for 1991 and 1992. Engine sizes and availability remained much the same.

Transmission choices were also changed for 1982. A wide-ratio four-speed manual transmission (RPO MM4) was standard with the base Firebird, Trans Am, and S/E. In 1983, a new

This original 1987 Trans Am GTA sport coupe finished in Flame Red Metallic (74) has gold 16x8 diamond-spoke aluminum wheels (RPO PW7). The Trans Am GTA has a special aero body package.

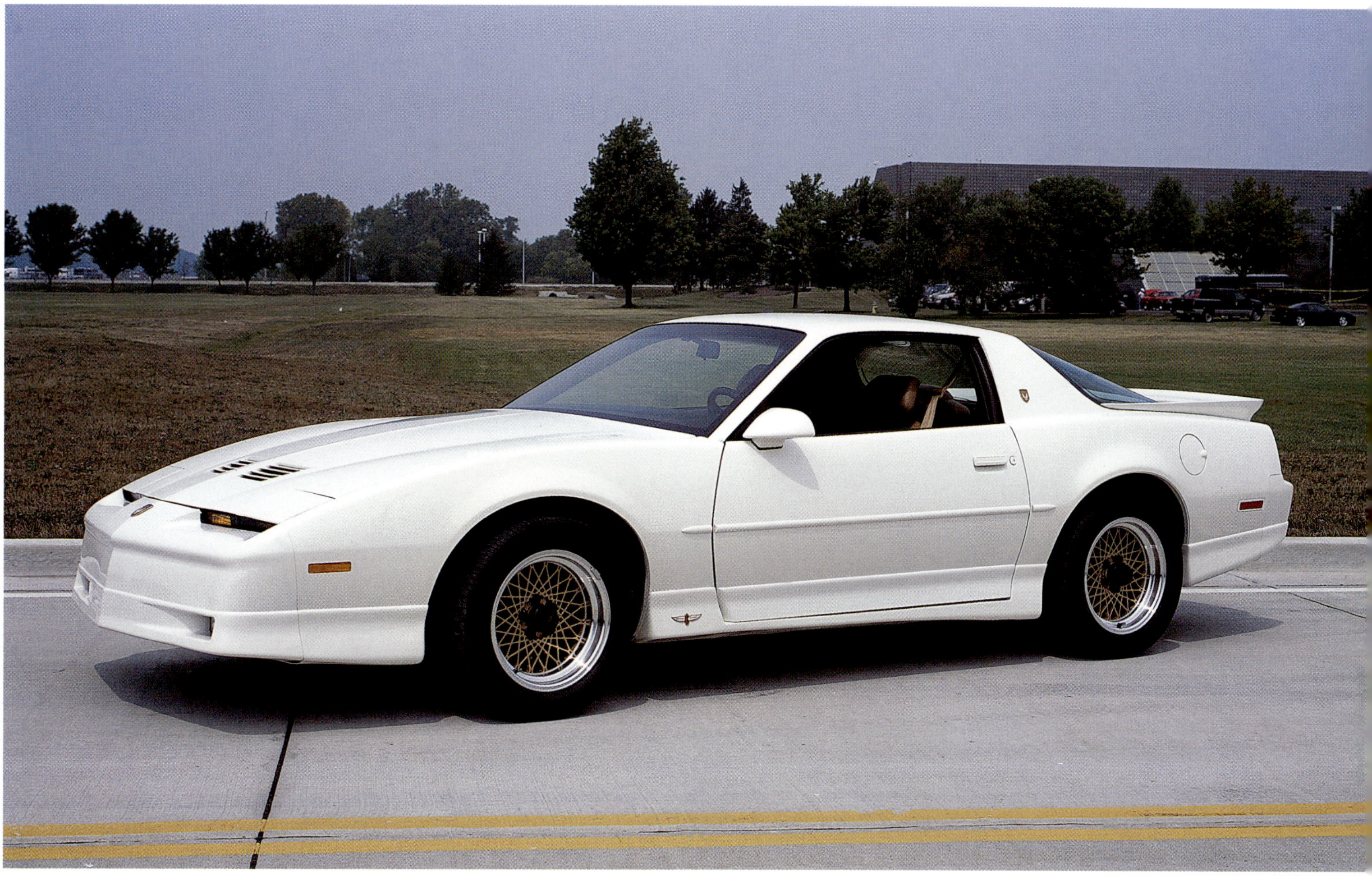

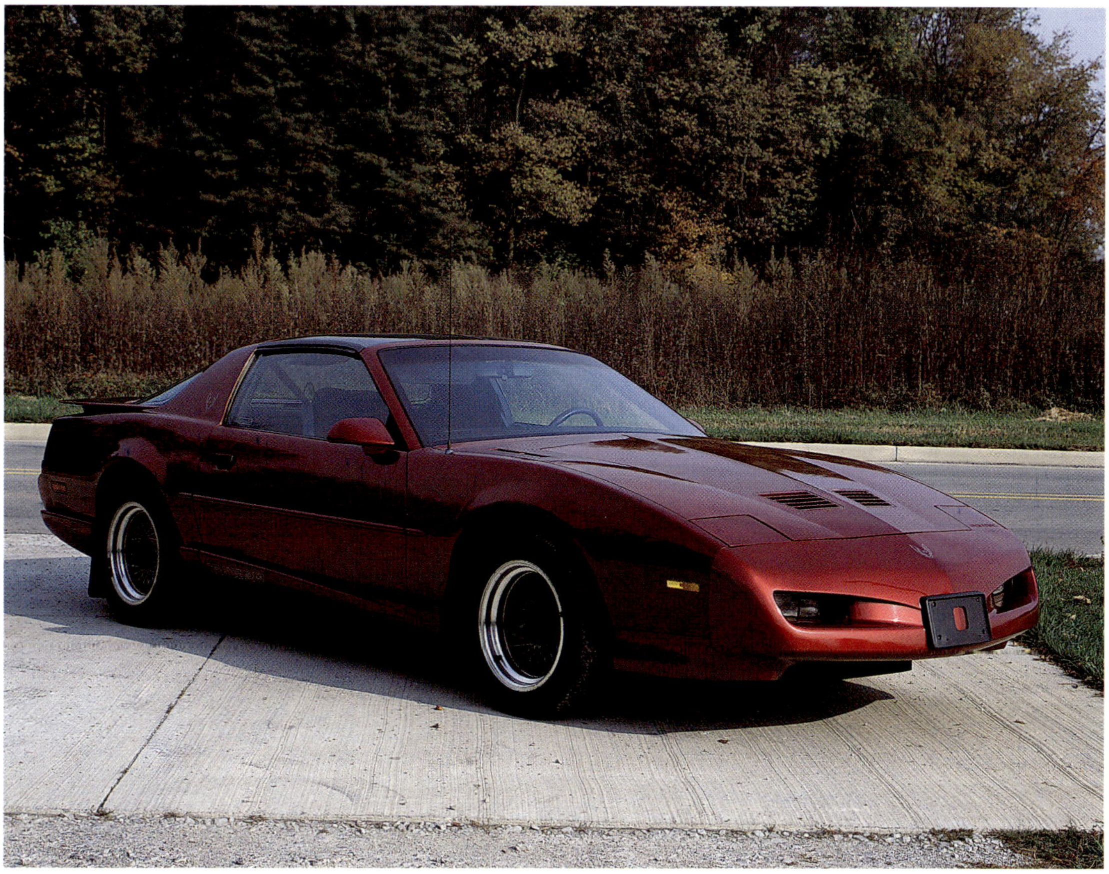

Above: This is a left front quarter view of an original white 1989 20th Anniversary Trans Am GTA Indianapolis Pace Car Special Edition equipped with a special turbocharged V-6 engine. The 20th Anniversary Trans Am GTA has a camel vinyl interior trim (662). ***Right:*** The front fascia of the 1991 Trans Am immediately identifies it from the earlier third-generation styling. This design was only used in 1991 and 1992. This Trans Am sport coupe is finished in Brilliant Red Metallic (75).

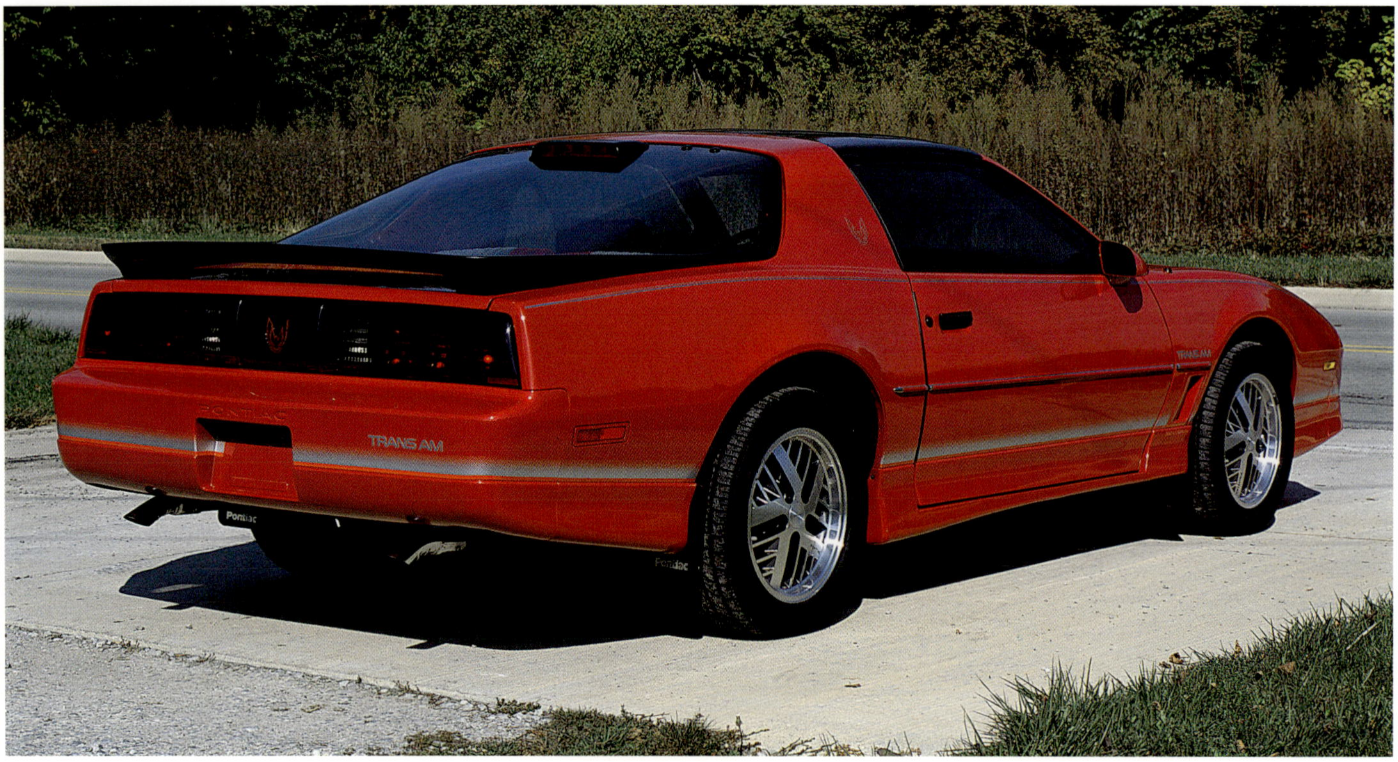

This rear view of a Bright Red 1986 Trans Am shows the new third-generation Firebird body design. The hinged liftgate rear hatch with curved window in dark tinted glass was part of the new body styling. Note the black deck-mounted spoiler and high stop lamp used in 1986. This Trans Am is equipped with an optional T-top roof (RPO CC1).

five-speed manual transmission with overdrive became standard in the S/E and Trans Am. For 1985, the five-speed manual transmission (RPO MM5) became standard equipment in all models. Automatic transmission choices were also changed significantly. In 1982, the only automatic available was the TH200 in all engines, but in 1983, the new TH700-R4 four-speed automatic (RPO MX1) became available with all but the 173-cubic-inch four-cylinder. By 1984, the TH700-R4 was the only automatic transmission available with all engines until 1989. For 1989, only a new TH200-R4 became available with the 231-cubic-inch turbocharged V-6. In 1990–1992, the TH700-R4 was the only automatic available.

The 1982 Firebird was available in 12 color combinations with 12 interior trim choices. For 1983, there were 10 body-color schemes and 13 interior trim combinations. For 1984, body-color choices were increased to 22 and interior trim combinations were 12. There were 15 body colors and 12 interior trim colors available in 1985. In 1986, body-color schemes were reduced to 12 and interior trim choices to 10. Body colors were reduced to 11 and interior trim combinations to seven for 1987. There were 13 body colors and seven interior schemes for 1988. There were 10 body-color choices and 10 interior colors for 1989. Body colors were reduced to seven and interior trim to six for 1990. There were eight body colors and six interior trim choices in 1991 and 1992.

Firebird production increased significantly from 1981 numbers to a total of 116,364 in 1982, but for 1983, production dropped back to 74,884. Production for 1984 climbed back to a high of 128,304 and then dropped to only 95,880 for 1985. Production for 1986 jumped back up to 110,463 and slipped back to 88,587 in 1987. Sales were down for 1988, when only 62,455 were built. Nineteen eighty-nine totals were similar, with 64,404 Firebirds produced. Nineteen ninety production dropped even further, and total U.S. production was 20,532. Firebird production for 1991 was 50,454, and 27,567 were built for 1992.

Body Sheet Metal and Trim

All 1982–1992 Firebirds used a new-for-1982 full unitized body construction that eliminated the separate front subframe previously used. The front suspension, rear suspension, and drivetrain support were now built into the body structure, and the entire body shell assembly was painted the body color. All 1982–1984 Firebirds had a 16-gallon galvanized-steel fuel tank mounted at the rear of the body pan. Fuel tank capacity was reduced to 15.5 gallons for 1985 and 1986. In 1987, the fuel tank held 15.5 gallons when equipped with the Tuned Port Injection V-6 and 16.2 gallons with the V-8. In 1988–1992, fuel tank capacity was 15.5 gallons for all applications. All 1982–1992 Firebirds were based on a two-door sport coupe configuration (except for the 1989 PAS convertible conversion and the 1991 and 1992 ASC convertible conversions) on a 100-inch wheelbase.

In addition to the standard steel roof, all 1982–1992 Firebird sport coupes were available

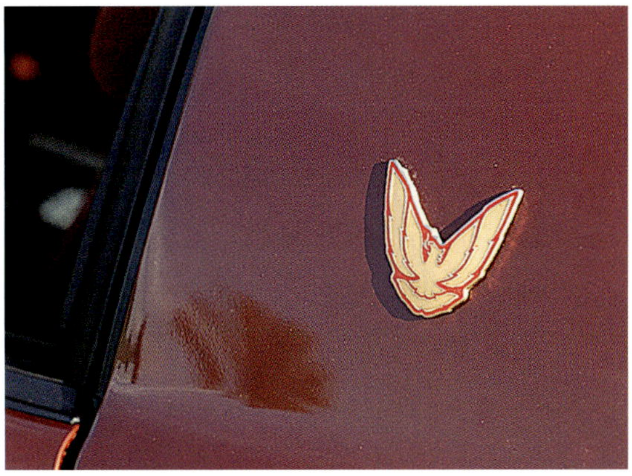

The gold-roof B-pillar decal on an original Flame Red Metallic 1987 Trans Am GTA equipped with an optional T-top hatch roof with tinted glass panels.

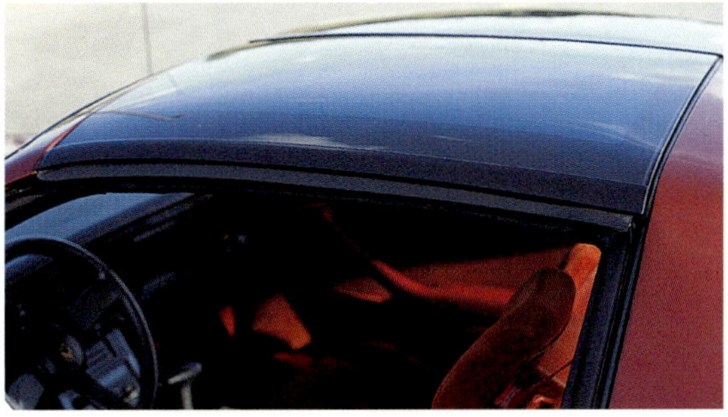

This is a detail view of the dark tinted glass panels in an original Flame Red Metallic 1987 Trans Am GTA sport coupe and the black rubber seal at the top of the opening.

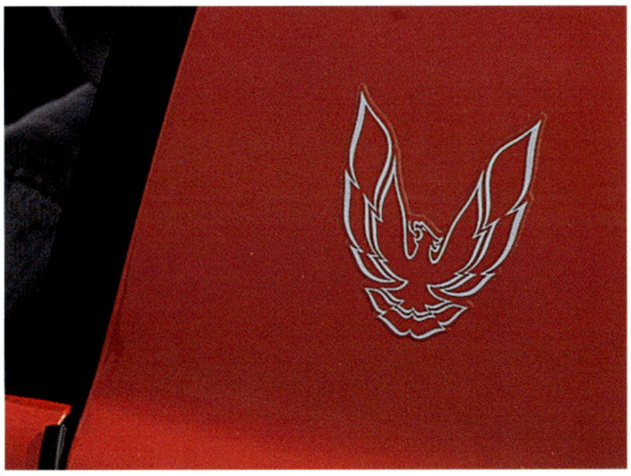

This is the bird decal on the roof B-pillar of a red 1987 Formula 350. Note the optional black door edge molding (RPO B91) and black rubber door window seal.

with an optional T-top (hatch) roof with two removable dark-tinted glass panels and no roof drip moldings (RPO CC1). The hatch roof was also part of the RPO Y84 Recaro Trans Am Package and RPO B57 custom exterior group option package that included a remote-control left-hand mirror. When removed, the glass roof panels were stored in slots for that purpose in the rear cargo compartment. Although technically available, orders for T-top hatch roofs were discouraged on Firebirds with the 5.7-liter V-8 due to problems with body flexing. No vinyl roof options were available with the 1982–1992 Firebirds. The sail panel roof behind the side window had either an S/E badge on the S/E or a bird decal on the Trans Am. A unique red or black shield medallion was used for the 1987–1992 Trans Am GTA, and a special blue shield medallion was used for the 1984 15th Anniversary Edition Trans Am.

All 1982–1992 Firebird door panels were similar in design, but the 1982–1984 used part numbers 20493186 (right) and 20493187 (left). The 1984–1990 used part numbers 10114498 (right) and 10114497 (left). For 1991 and 1992, the door part numbers were 10160406 (right) and 10160407 (left). There were no vent windows, and the side glass was sealed with black sponge rubber and channels in the front windshield post and rear roof quarter pillar. The doors were operated by chrome rectangular pull-type handles with body-color tape inserts. In 1985, an optional Special Black Appearance Package (RPO W51) became available that included black door handles and lock cylinders. The 1987–1992 Formula had standard black door handles and locks. An optional horizontal soft protective molding was available on all 1982–1992 Firebird bodies.

continued on page 130

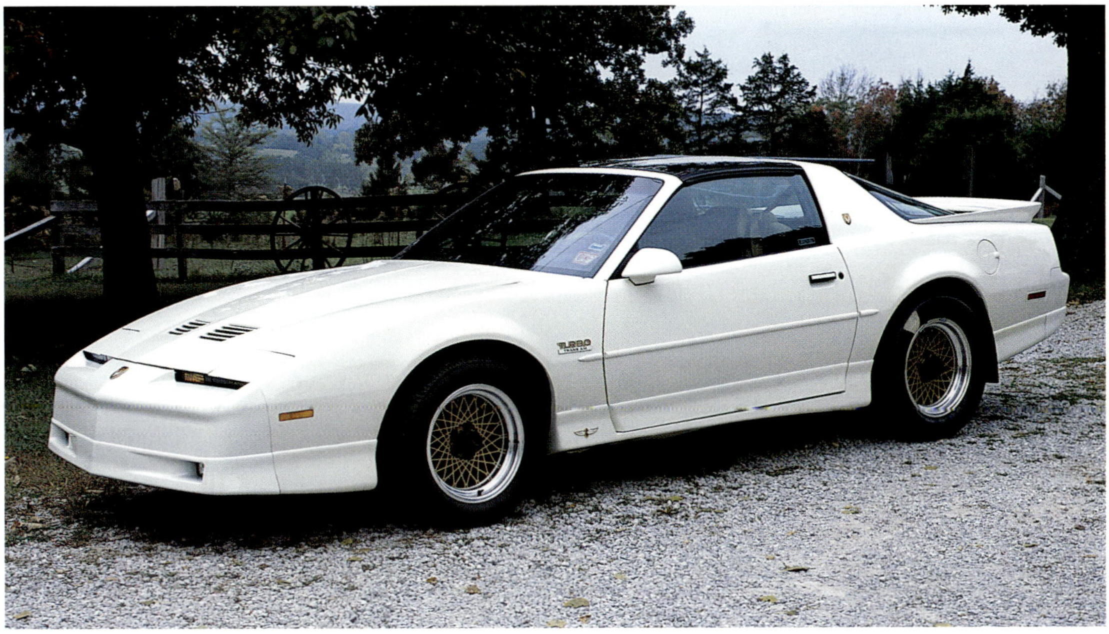

The left front quarter of a white 1989 Turbo Trans Am GTA 20th Anniversary Edition showing the design of the third-generation Firebird body. The new wheelbase was 101 inches, and the aerodynamic styling created the lowest drag coefficient of any GM car.

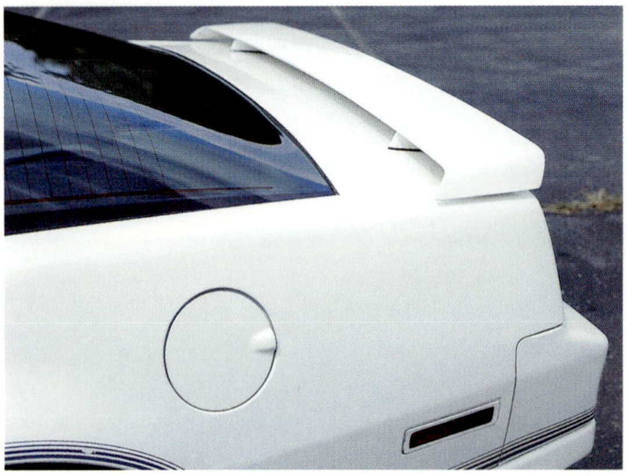

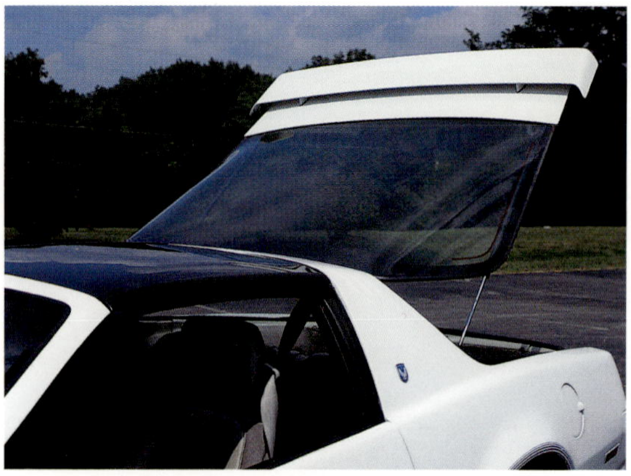

Far left: Detail view of the rear liftgate and spoiler on a white 1984 Trans Am 15th Anniversary Edition with the new round fuel filler door on the left rear quarter. ***Left:*** This view shows the raised rear liftgate with dark tinted glass and integral spoiler on a white 1984 Trans Am 15th Anniversary Edition sport coupe. The rear hatch covers a deep, carpeted, cargo compartment.

Right: The rear spoiler was redesigned for 1987 and had a center stop lamp in the spoiler mounting pedestal shown on a Flame Red Metallic (74) 1987 Trans Am GTA sport coupe.

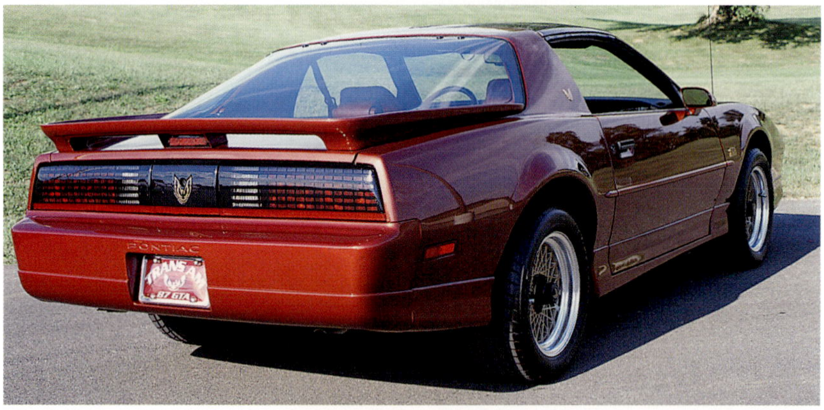

Below: This left front quarter view of an original Flame Red Metallic 1987 Trans Am GTA sport coupe shows the raised rear liftgate with integral spoiler. This GTA has a red cloth interior trim.

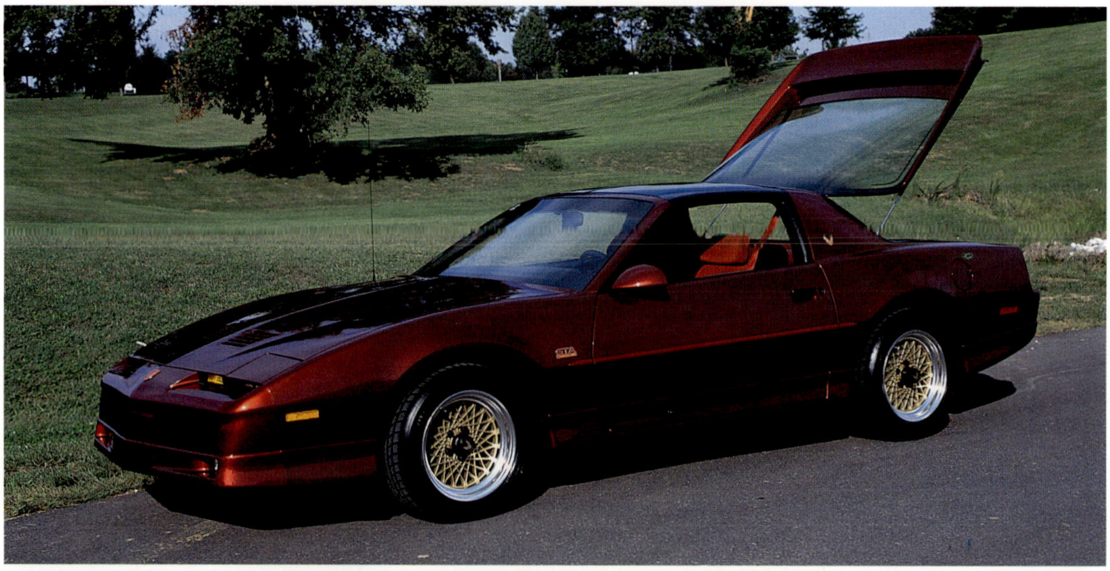

Below left: Rear view of the tan convertible top on a Medium Green Metallic (45) 1992 Trans Am GTA convertible (FV3). Note the flexible rear window sewn into the folding top. ***Below right:*** Right side view of a tan convertible top on a Medium Green Metallic 1992 Trans Am GTA convertible. Nineteen ninety-one and 1992 were the only years a standard convertible model was available in the third-generation Firebird and Trans Am.

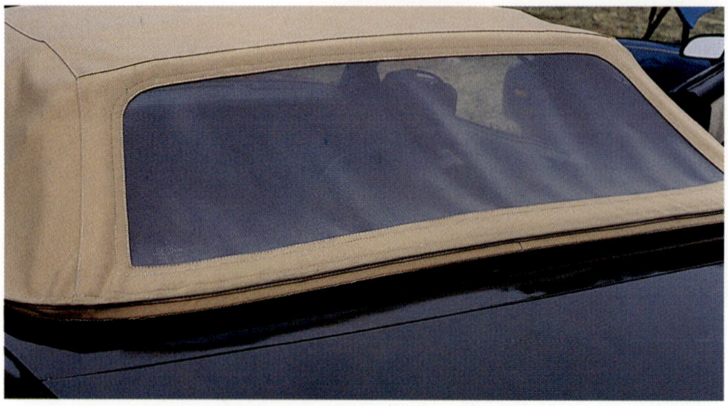

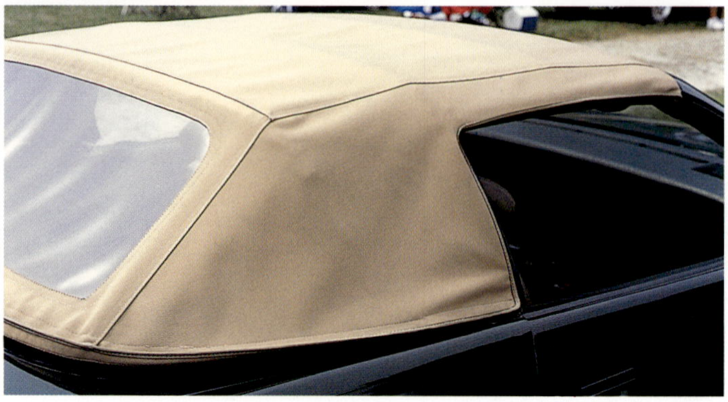

Right: Detail view of the right door on a 1984 Trans Am 15th Anniversary Edition with the unique blue body decal, stripes, and lower air dam. ***Far right:*** This is a detail view of the black finish door handle and fine silver accent stripes on a Bright Red 1986 Trans Am sport coupe. Note the optional vinyl body side molding (RPO B84). ***Right:*** The right side door of a Flame Red Metallic 1987 Trans Am GTA has the black door handle and optional vinyl side molding (RPO B84). ***Far right:*** Detail view of the left door on a Bright Red (81) 1989 Firebird Formula 350 (RPO W66) showing the unique door decal and optional vinyl body side molding.

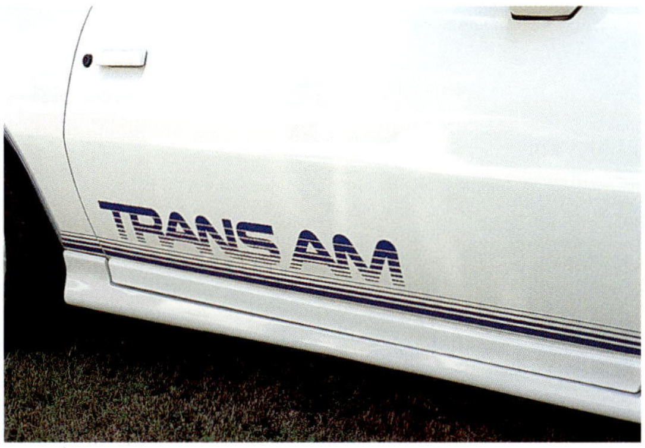

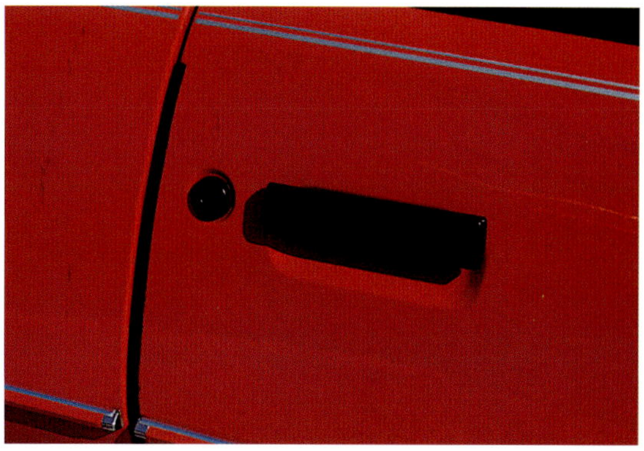

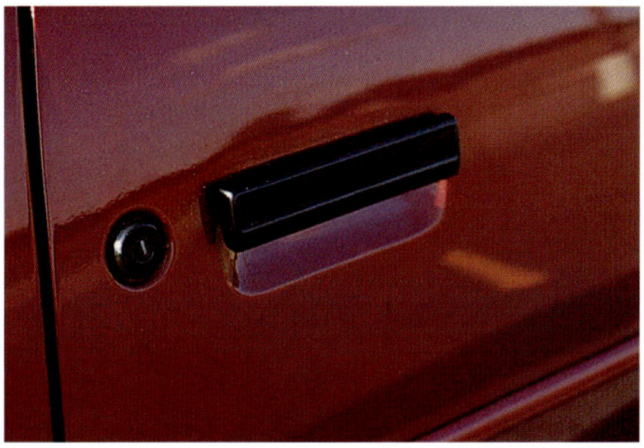

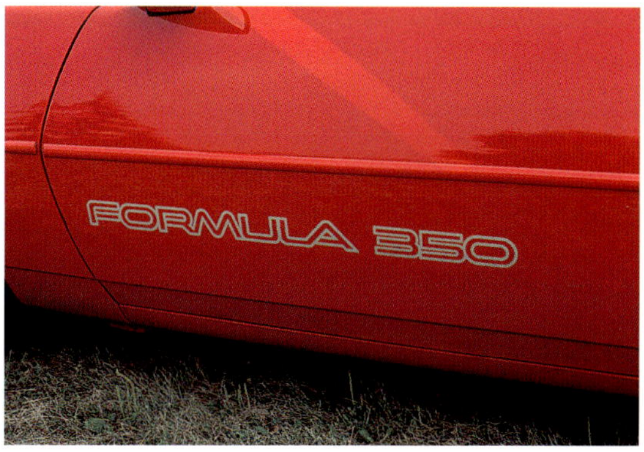

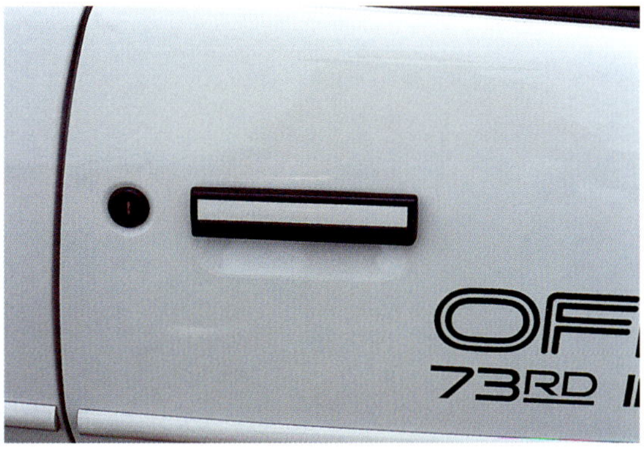

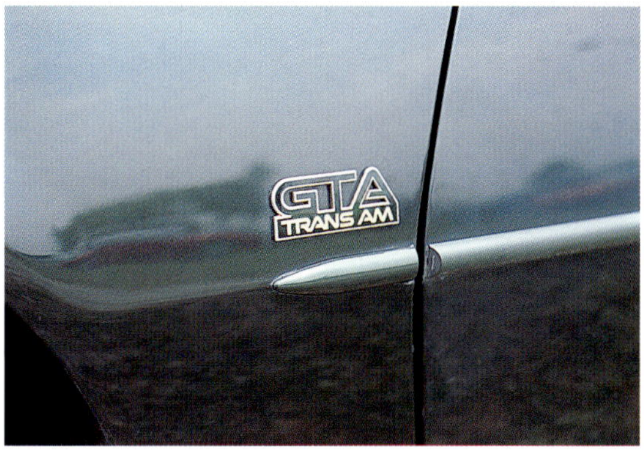

Above left: This detail view of the right door on a white 1989 Turbo Trans Am GTA Indianapolis 500 Pace Car Edition shows the white door handle insert. ***Above right:*** Detail view of the unique green-and-gold left side fender badge on a Medium Green Metallic (45) 1992 Trans Am GTA convertible.

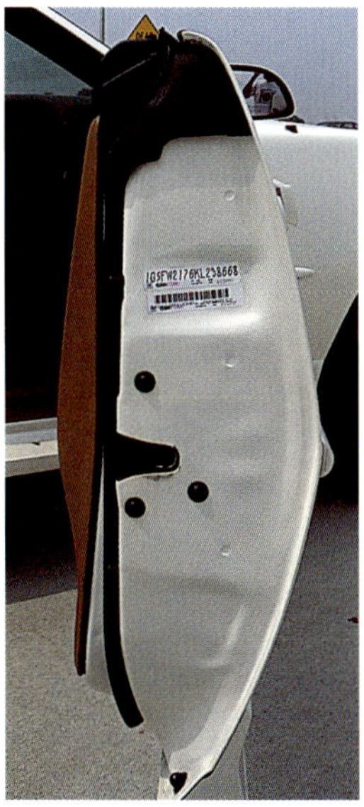

The outer jamb of the right side door on an original white 1989 Turbo Trans Am GTA Indianapolis 500 Pace Car Edition. The white VIN decal is visible on the upper door panel.

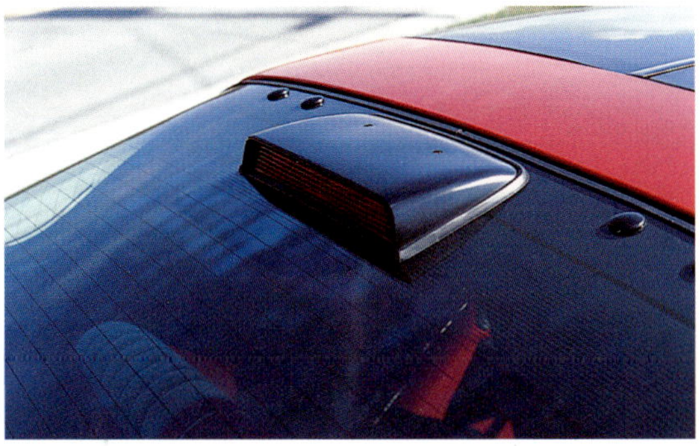

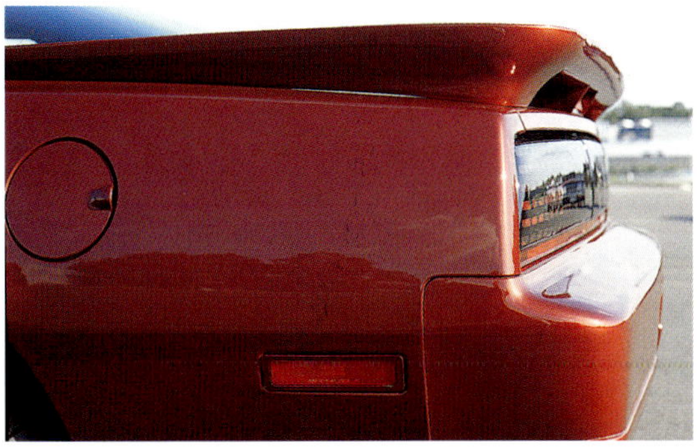

Above left: This is the upper liftgate-mounted rear stop light on a red 1986 Trans Am sport coupe. Nineteen eighty-six was the only year that the light was mounted at the top of the hinged rear window. ***Above right:*** Detail view of the unique rear spoiler and liftgate hatch design used on a 1987 Trans Am GTA. The 1987 spoiler included a center-mounted stop light in the spoiler pedestal.

continued from page 127

All-white 1989 20th Anniversary Turbo Trans Am Indianapolis 500 Pace Cars (RPO Y82) had a special "Official Pace Car" decal on each door, but the owner could have deleted the entire dealer-installed decal package (part number 12397715). The 1991 and 1992 Firebirds with the optional aero package had distinct raised side skirting that flowed from the front to the rear, including the lower door panels.

All 1982–1992 Firebird doors were sealed with black soft sponge rubber weatherstrip surrounding the outer perimeter of the door shell. The weatherstrip was made in left and right parts because of the molded upper rear door seal construction. The perimeter of the body door opening used a color-keyed push-on vinyl windlace that also served to secure the inside quarter trim panels. A Torx-head latch striker was mounted in the center of the rear doorjamb.

All 1982–1992 Firebirds had a standard front-hinged rear liftgate that included the large curved-glass backlight and a short body-color panel. Long, thin, black-finish gas struts supported the hatch. A luggage compartment trim package was available with RPO B48 that included a storage well cover, deluxe carpeting, rear panels, and a spare tire cover. In 1986 only, a high-mounted brake lamp was attached to the top center of the rear hatch glass. In 1988, a notchback option (RPO AA8) was available on the Trans Am GTA. This option replaced the standard glass liftgate with a fiberglass rear hatchback deck lid (part number 10070763) that included a special integral deck lid spoiler (part number 10065170). Only 624 were built in 1988 and one in 1989. The option was cancelled on August 30, 1988, partly due to paint quality problems.

There was no separate deck lid on the 1982–1992 Firebird, as the rear compartment was covered with a forward-hinged liftgate with curved Soft-Ray tinted glass. The rear hatch design was similar for all models (except the AA8 notchback option), but the 1982–1984 Trans Am had a bolt-on body-color aero-wing rear spoiler with two mounting stands and turned-down ends. The spoiler was also optional on the base Firebird and S/E (RPO D80). A rear window defogger (RPO C49) and wiper-washer system (RPO C25) were optional on all models. A remote-control deck lid release was also available with RPO A90. The rear hatch was sealed with a black sponge rubber seal around the perimeter of the body opening.

The rear deck spoiler was redesigned for the 1985 Formula and Trans Am and was now semi-gloss black and wrapped the sides of the rear liftgate to the lower corners of the rear glass. The optional rear spoiler for the base Firebird continued to be the earlier version. Both types of spoiler were made body color for 1986. In 1987, a new center rear brake lamp was incorporated into the center mounting post of the spoiler. The body-color rear spoiler for the Trans Am was redesigned again for 1991 and was wider and flatter while still wrapping around to the front of the rear hatch. The base Firebird continued to use

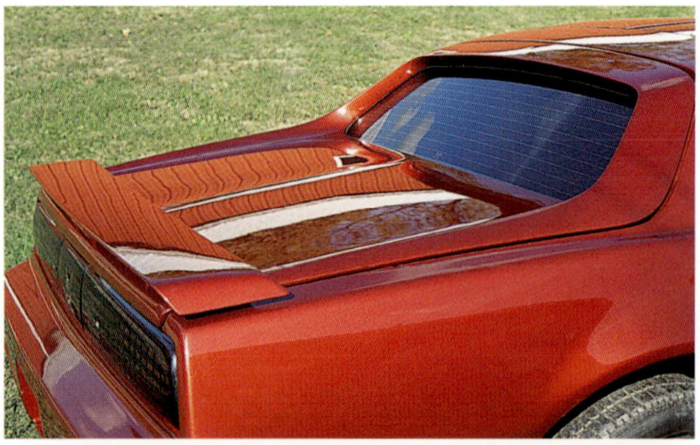

In 1988, an optional notchback liftgate was available on the Trans Am GTA (RPO GQ9). The spoiler is unique to the notchback design. This is a Flame Red Metallic 1988 GTA.

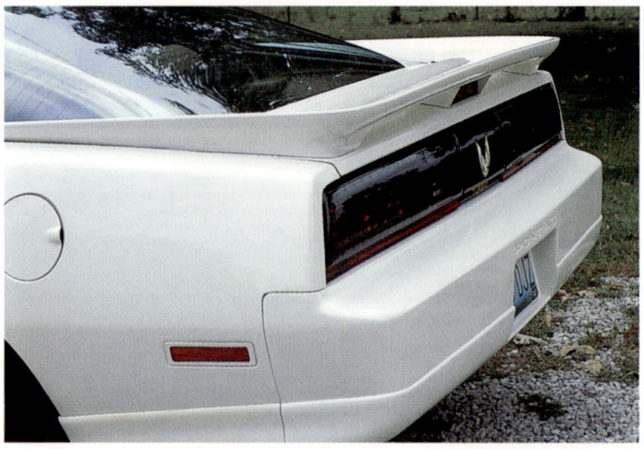

Detail view of the left side of the rear deck and spoiler on a white 1989 Turbo Trans Am GTA 20th Anniversary Edition. The spoiler wraps around the width of the rear liftgate hatch and has a stop lamp mounted in its center.

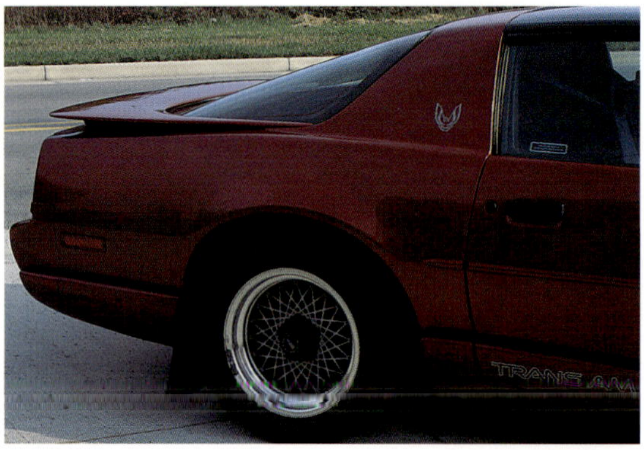

Right rear quarter of a Brilliant Red Metallic 1991 Trans Am sport coupe showing the design of the rear liftgate, spoiler, and tinted rear window. The bird decal on the roof pillar is visible.

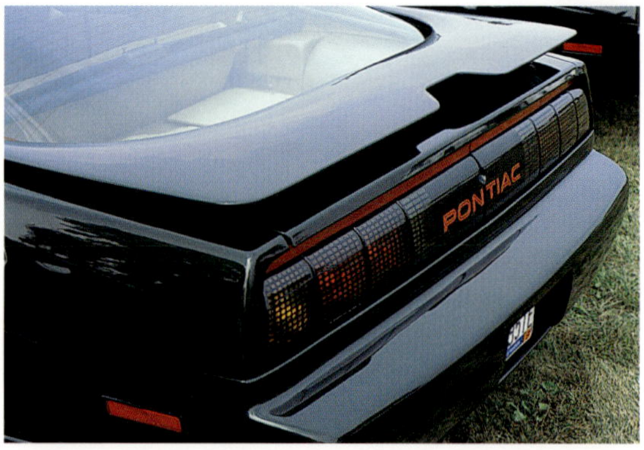

This is a detail view of the liftgate and rear spoiler on a Medium Green Metallic 1991 Trans Am GTA sport coupe. Note the Pontiac nameplate on the taillight panel and the notch in the center of the rear spoiler.

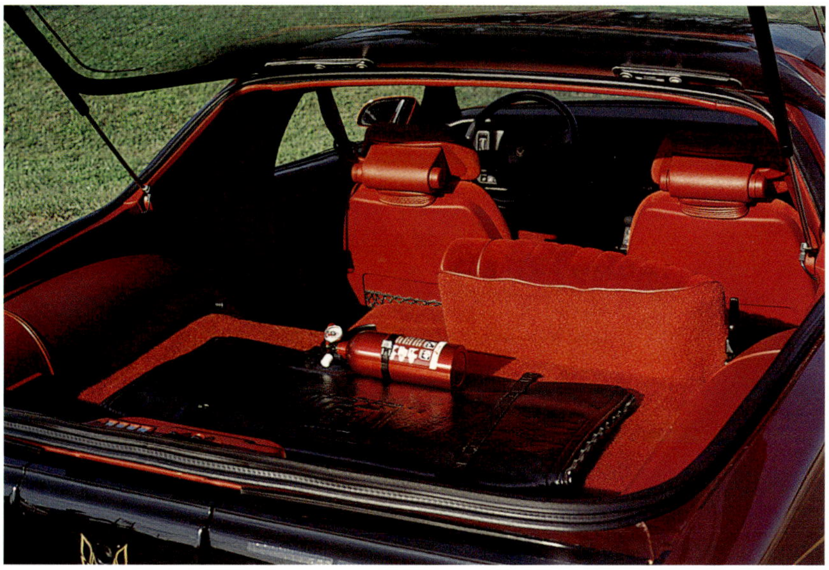

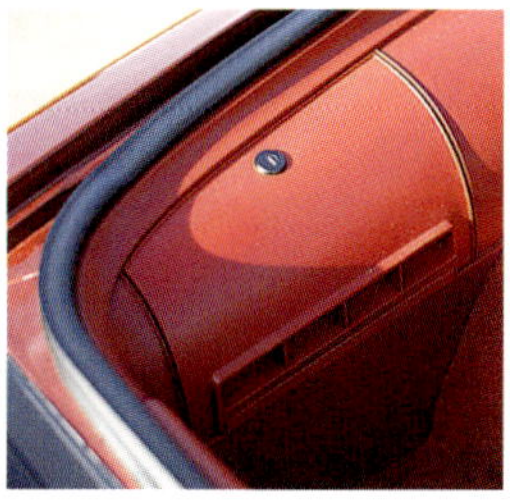

Above: This interior view of the rear cargo compartment of a Flame Red Metallic 1987 Trans Am GTA sport coupe with optional red cloth interior trim shows the black vinyl bag used to hold the T-top roof panels when not in place. ***Left:*** The left side of the rear cargo compartment of a red 1987 Trans Am GTA has a lockable molded red plastic small storage compartment. The black rubber seal for the rear liftgate is visible.

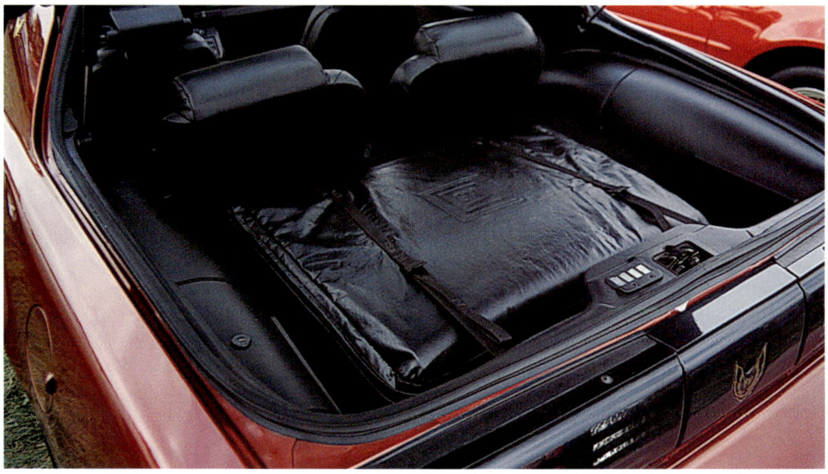

Above: This is the rear cargo compartment of a red 1988 Trans Am GTA with optional black vinyl interior trim. The black vinyl bag is for the T-top roof panels. The removable right molded-plastic side cover is for spare tire storage. ***Right:*** This view shows the proper folded arrangement for the black vinyl roof panel storage bag when not in use. Note the GM logo on the bag. This is the tan vinyl interior of a 1989 Turbo Trans Am GTA 20th Anniversary Edition.

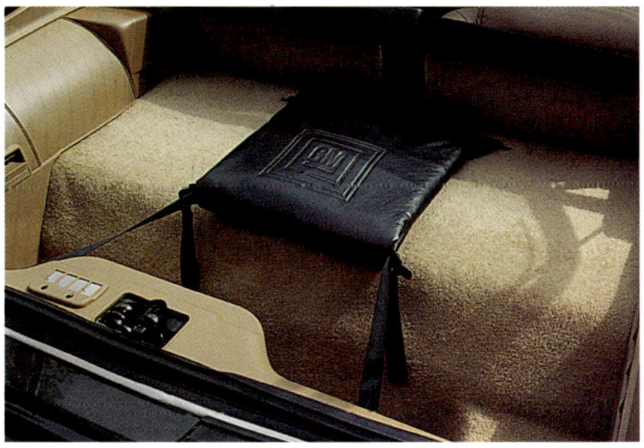

the earlier-design optional pedestal-mounted spoiler.

The 1982–1992 Firebird did not have a conventional trunk like the earlier models. The entire carpeted rear compartment was exposed when the rear liftgate was opened. There was a deeper well to the rear of the axle hump and a hinged smaller storage compartment on the left side. The deeper well also held the T-top roof panels when they were removed. The T-top storage bag was suspended with elastic straps across the length of the compartment. The rear seatbacks folded separately, creating even more storage space.

The rear deck lower panel on the 1982–1984 Firebird was relatively flat and vertical with six fine horizontal ribs running across the full width, with the horizontal taillights on either side of a separate matching rectangular center panel with the rear hatch lock in its center. Although the center panel looks like a fuel filler door, the filler was no longer located at the rear. The 1982 and 1983 Firebird center panel had a bird medallion and a Pontiac logo at its bottom edge. The Trans Am center panel had a bird medallion and Trans Am logo at its lower edge. The rear panel design was changed for 1984, and the center panel had a red plastic lens panel at the bottom with "Pontiac" in block letters on all models. In 1984, the optional W62 Aero Package on the Trans Am added rear fascia side extensions. The remainder of the rear panel was similar to the 1982 and 1983. In 1985, the entire rear deck panel was redesigned, and the taillights consisted of a smooth lens across each side, giving the rear fascia an integrated appearance. The Aero Package became standard on the Trans Am. The Trans Am and S/E taillamp lenses were dark smoked gray. There were three or four dividers behind the smooth lenses on each side depending on the year.

The 1982–1984 Firebird rear bumper was urethane-covered and finished in body color. The bumper was relatively flat, with the license plate mounted in the lower center. For 1985–1988, the Trans Am used a body-color rear bumper, but the Firebird, Formula, and S/E had a black protective flat strip on either side. For 1985–1989, block letters spelling "Pontiac" were embossed into the bumper just above the license opening, and the Pontiac logo in the rear deck center panel red lens was eliminated. For 1989–1992, the rear bumper was body-color urethane on all models.

The rear quarter panels of the 1982–1992 Firebird were redesigned from the previous years, and the roofline no longer blended smoothly into the quarters. The rear wheel opening was still rounded and slightly flared, but there was a clear separation between the roof and curved upper-body line. The outer ends of the rear bumper were flush with

continued on page 134

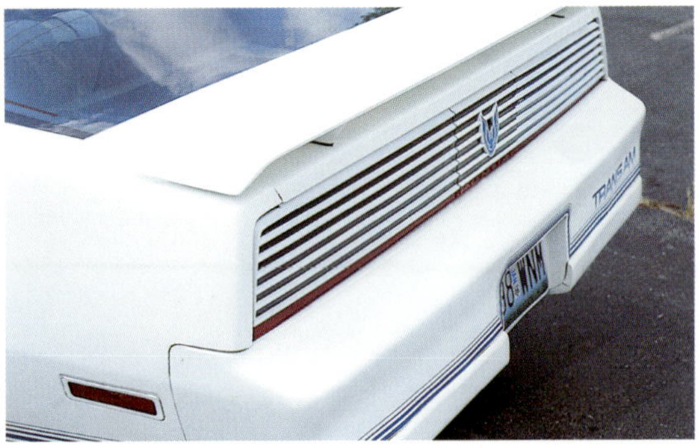

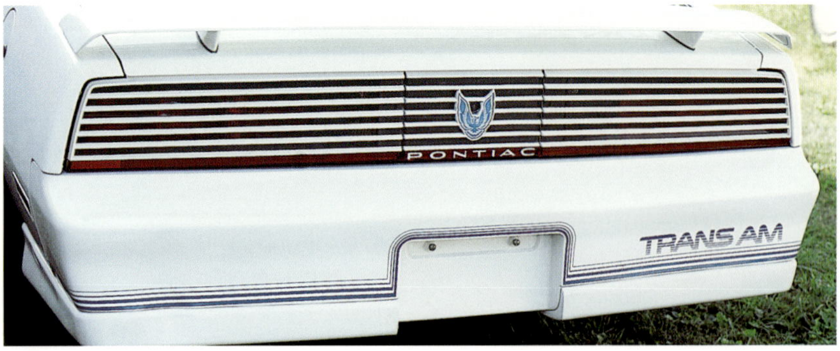

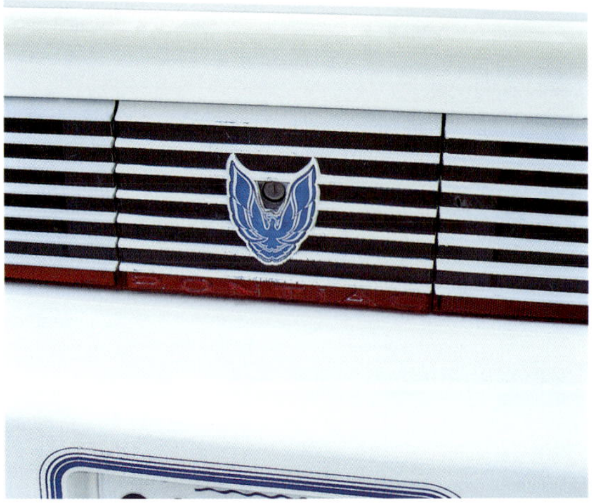

Above left: This view shows the rear deck lower panel and bumper on an original white 1984 Trans Am 15th Anniversary Edition, including the design of the spoiler and the Trans Am decal on the right side of the bumper. ***Above:*** This shows the rear deck lower panel on an original 1984 Trans Am 15th Anniversary Edition. The red Pontiac nameplate and unique blue 15th Anniversary badge in the center of the panel are visible. ***Left:*** Detail view of the center of the rear deck lower panel on an original white 1984 Trans Am 15th Anniversary Edition. The blue bird medallion is unique to this special-edition package.

Below left: Detail view of the rear deck lower panel of a red 1986 Trans Am sport coupe. Note the design and finish of the black spoiler and the full-width taillight lens with red bird medallion. ***Below right:*** Detail view of the rear deck lower panel and bumper on a Flame Red Metallic 1988 Trans Am GTA sport coupe. The center-mounted stoplight on the spoiler pedestal and gold GTA bird medallion on the center of the panel are visible.

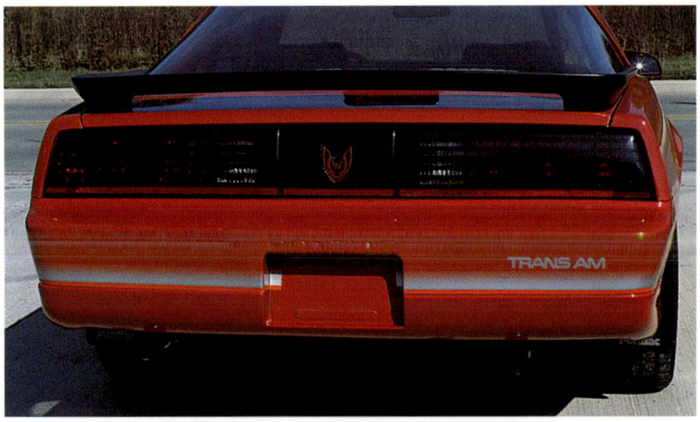

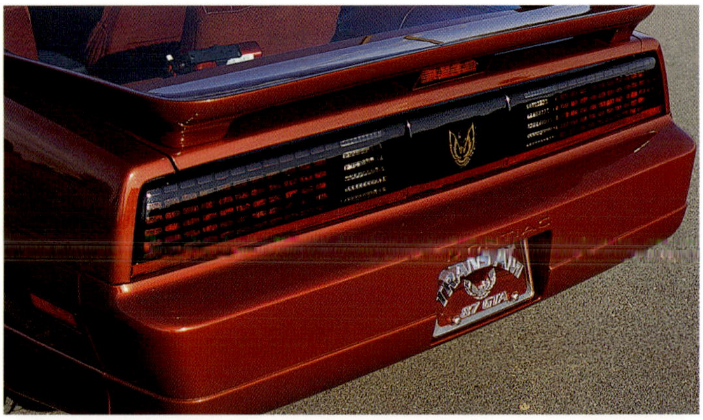

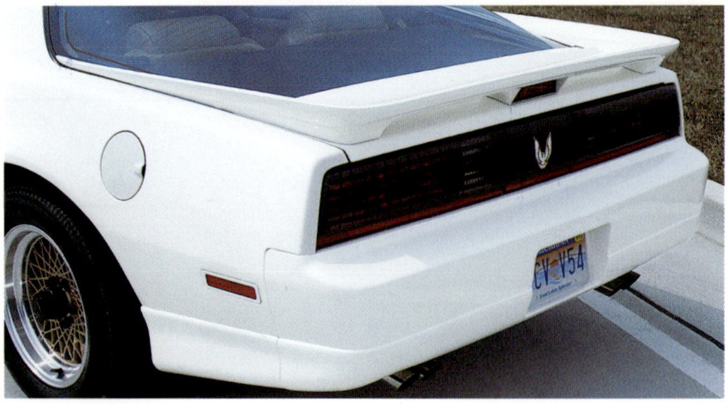

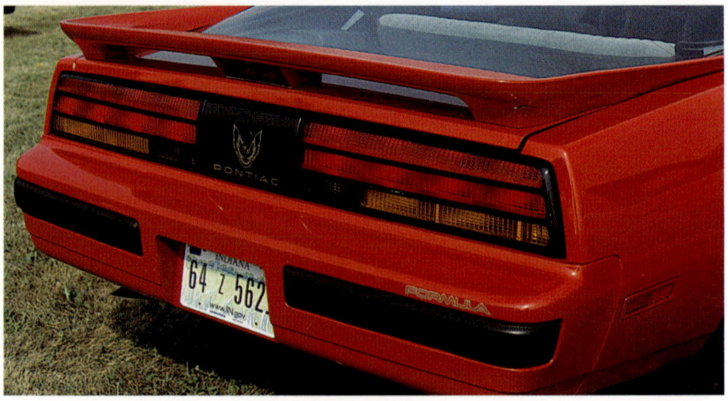

Above left: This is a detail view of the rear deck lower panel and bumper of an original white 1989 Trans Am GTA 20th Anniversary Edition. The lower air dam wraps around the sides of the body. Note the unique white bird medallion in the center of the rear panel. ***Above right:*** This view of the rear deck lower panel and rear bumper design on a Bright Red (81) 1989 Firebird Formula 350 sport coupe (RPO W66) shows the design of the spoiler and the black center panel with bird badge.

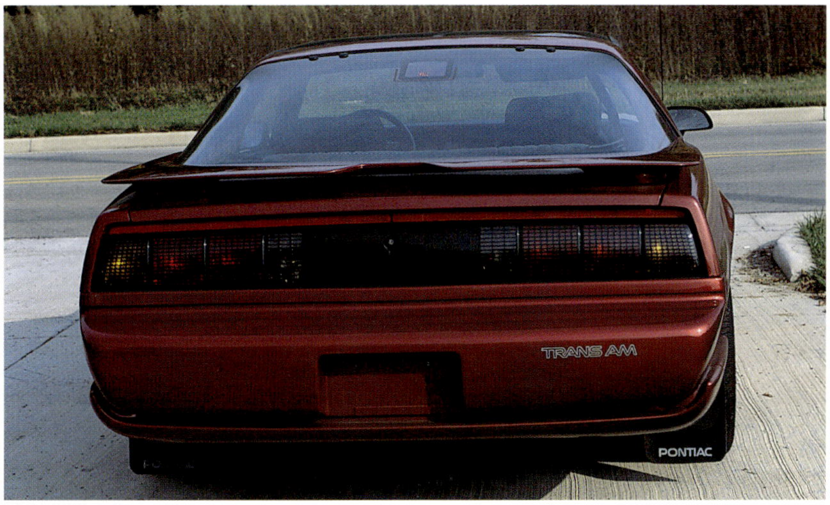

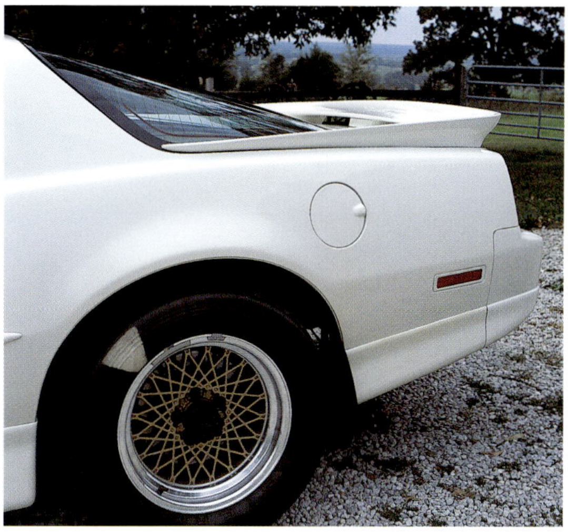

Above left: This is the rear deck lower panel and bumper on a Brilliant Red Metallic 1991 Trans Am sport coupe. Note the smooth center panel and the small Trans Am decal on the lower right side of the bumper. ***Above right:*** This photo shows a detail view of the left rear quarter panel on a white 1989 Trans Am GTA 20th Anniversary Edition, the round fuel filler door, and the unique spoiler design.

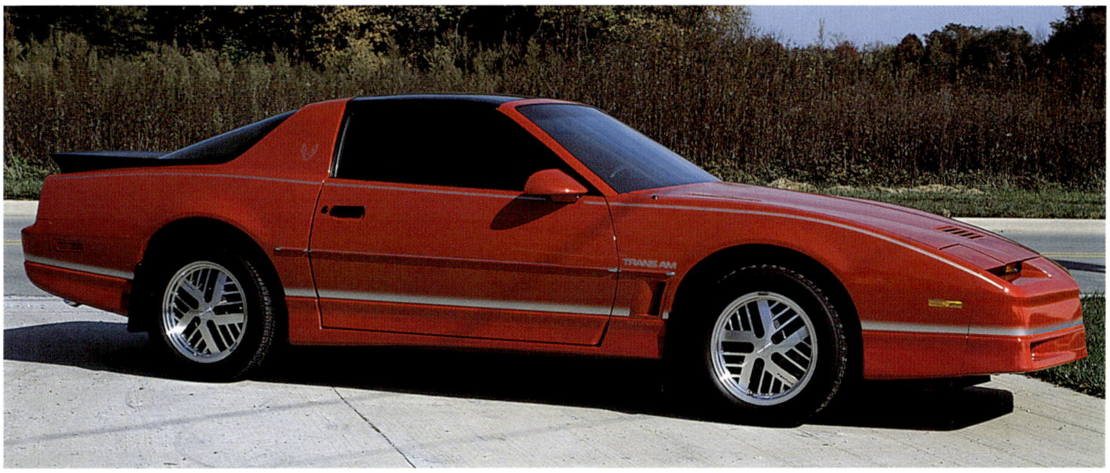

This right side view of a red 1986 Trans Am sport coupe shows the design of the front fender. Note the distinctive extractor vent on the rear of the fender, the full-length silver accent stripe, the black outside door handle, and the optional T-top hatch roof.

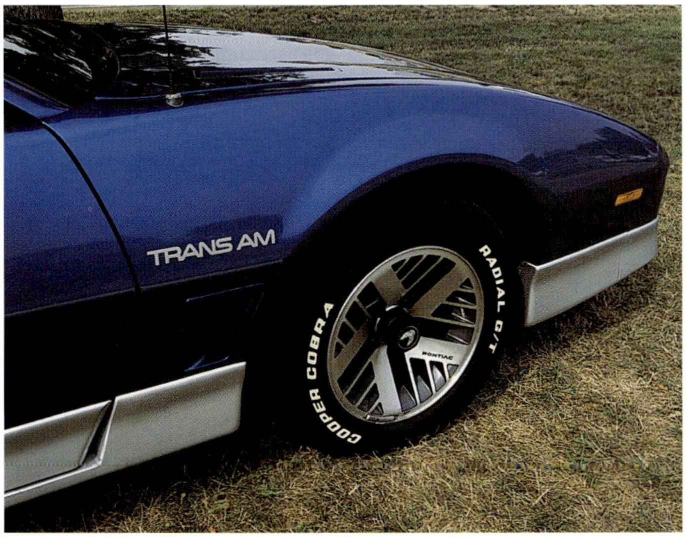

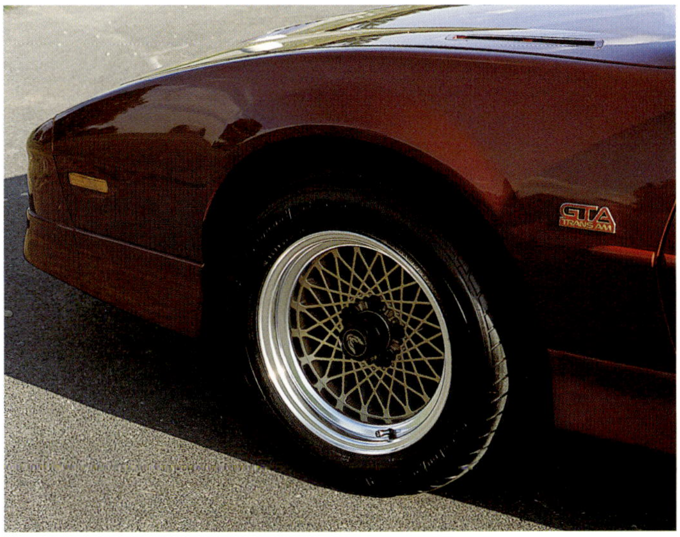

Above left: This view of the right front fender of a Bright Blue Metallic (23) 1986 Trans Am sport coupe shows the distinctive extractor vent and Trans Am decal on the rear of the fender. The lower air dam is finished in silver metallic (13S). ***Above right:*** Detail view of the left front fender and wheel opening on an original Flame Red Metallic 1987 Trans Am GTA sport coupe. Note the distinctive gold GTA Trans Am badge.

continued from page 131

the body sides. The round body-color fuel filler door was located at the upper left rear quarter panel just above and behind the wheel opening. A rectangular side marker lamp was mounted on each side just below the centerline of the quarter panel ahead of the rear bumper ends. The marker lamps were different left and right. On some models, a different color paint finish was used on the lower rocker panel and wrapped around the lower portion of the rear bumper.

All 1982–1984 Firebirds (except Trans Am, RPO WS4) used the same front fenders with a design that featured a long, sloping front. The Firebird used front fenders with part numbers 10020750 (left) and 10020749 (right). The 1982–1984 Trans Am front fenders used part numbers 10020752 (left) and 10020751 (right). For 1985–1992, the Firebird and Formula front fenders were part numbers 10081964 (left) and 10081963 (right). The 1985–1992 Trans Am used front fenders with part numbers 10081966 (left) and 10081965 (right). The 1988 and 1989 Trans Am with the RPO Y84 package used front fenders with part numbers 10081961 (left) and 10081962 (right). All 1982–1992 Firebird and Trans Am front fenders had a rectangular marker lamp at the front side just below the horizontal character line.

There were a number of different hood designs used on the 1982–1992 Firebirds. The standard hood for the 1982–1992 Firebird and S/E was relatively flat and smooth with no vents or scoops and used part number 10030760. The 1982–1984 Trans Am had a similar hood with a raised, aerodynamically styled, rear-facing scoop on its left side (part number 14103677). The 1985 and 1986 Trans Am, GTA, and S/E had a similar design (part number 10030794) but with two columns of five wide transverse louvers on either side of the center of the hood and a single small longitudinal vent at the rear of each side. For 1987–1992, the Trans Am used a redesigned hood with part number 10030761. The 1987–1992 Formula hood was the same as that used on the 1982–1984 Trans

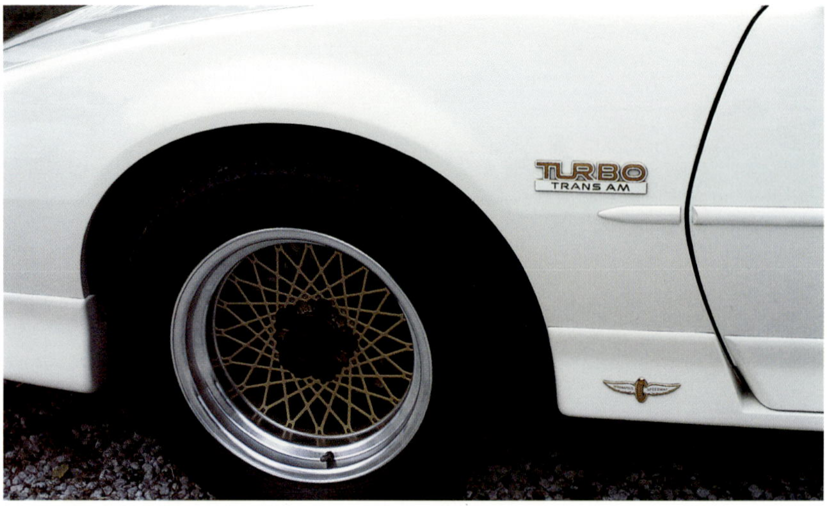

This view of the left front fender on a white 1989 Turbo Trans Am 20th Anniversary Edition shows the unique gold badge and white body side molding.

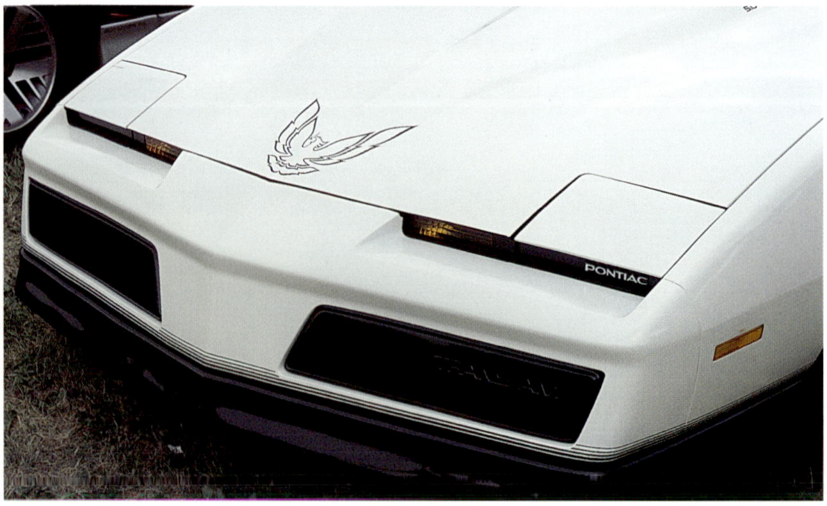

This view shows the hood on a white 1984 Trans Am equipped with the 5.0-liter V-8 engine and the standard Firebird grilles used only in the 1982–1984 models. The 1982–1984 Trans Am used the same front fascia as the Firebird except for some special editions. ***Below left:*** Detail view of the hood on an original white 1984 Trans Am 15th Anniversary Edition with the unique 15th Anniversary Edition blue hood scoop decal and 5.0-liter engine identification decal. ***Below right:*** This is a detail view of the two rows of louvers on a red 1986 Trans Am hood. Note the crease in the center of the hood and the silver bird badge on the top of the front fascia.

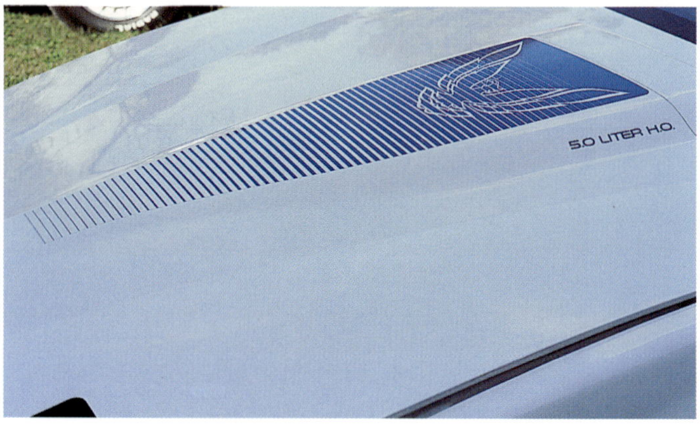

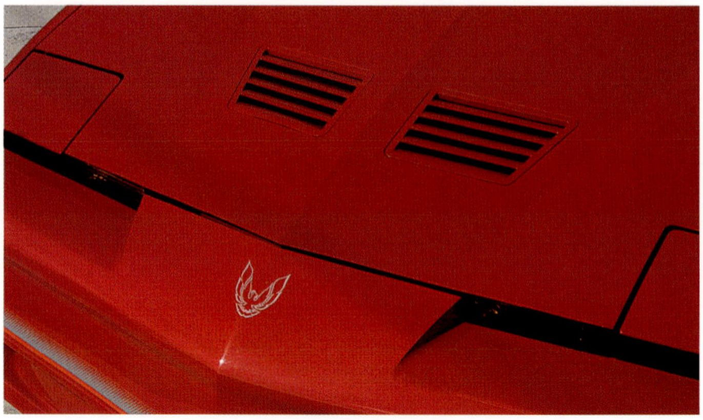

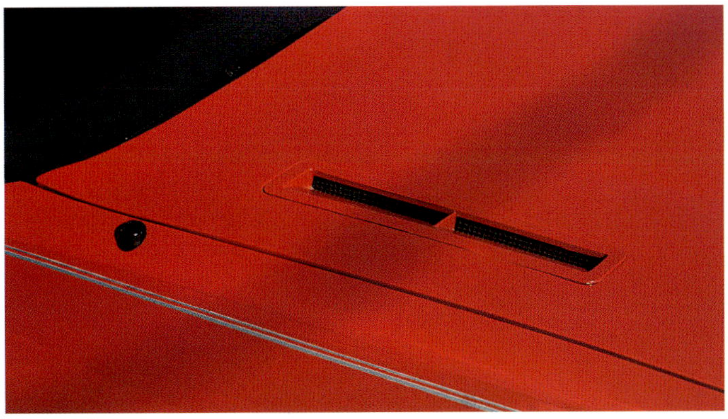

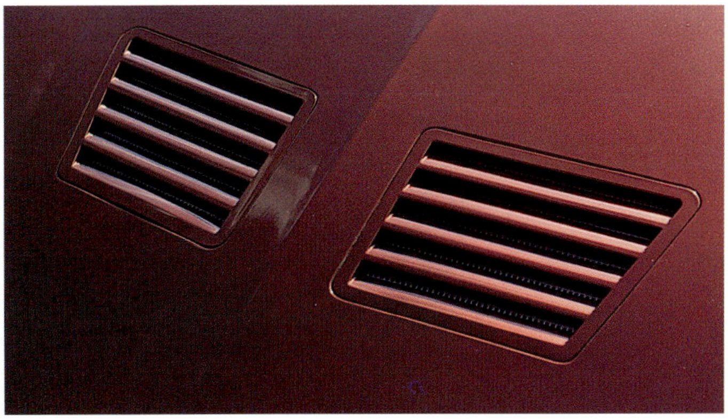

Above left: This is a detail view of the longitudinal vents on the right rear of the hood on a red 1986 Trans Am sport coupe. Note the black radio power antenna opening and silver accent stripes. ***Above right:*** Detail view of the two rows of hood louvers on an original one-owner Flame Red Metallic 1987 Trans Am GTA sport coupe.

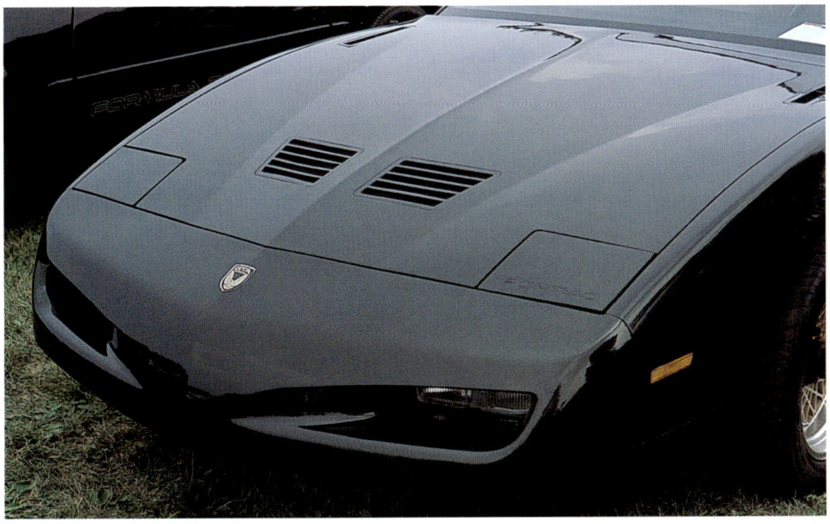

This shows the hood and front fascia of a Medium Green Metallic (45) 1991 Trans Am GTA sport coupe with the Pontiac name molded in the left headlight cover.

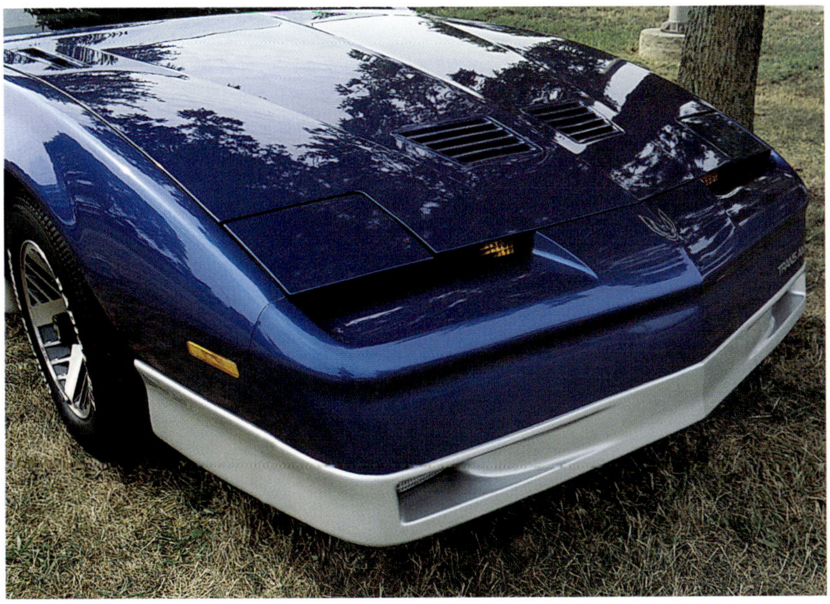

This is a detail view of the fascia of a Bright Blue Metallic 1986 Trans Am with silver metallic accent on the lower air dam and a silver bird badge on the top of the nose.

Am (part number 14103677) with a raised aerodynamic rear-facing scoop on its left side. The 1982–1992 hoods with the rear-facing nonfunctional scoop had a separate body-color ornament and seal attached to the rear of the raised scoop bubble. The outer front corners of all 1982–1992 hoods had an opening for the concealed rectangular headlamp doors. All 1982–1992 Firebirds (except the GTA) had a block letter Pontiac emblem on the left headlamp door.

The 1983 and 1984 Trans Am had a unique bird decal with a louvered appearance on the top of the hood blister. The decal was available in gold, silver, or black, in addition to charcoal on the 1983 Daytona Pace Car Special Edition. For 1984, the bird was available in gold, silver, and black, plus a special blue decal that was used on the white 15th Anniversary Special Edition Trans Am (part number 10031483). For 1985–1987, a large optional bird decal was used on the hood. This decal was available in gold, silver, black, charcoal, and brown with varied bordered accents depending upon the body color.

The body-color urethane front fascia of the 1982–1984 Firebird and Trans Am (part number 10020286) was changed significantly from the previous model and featured a sloped top surface with a full-width horizontal crease and sharply angled nose. Both sides of the upper surface had a recessed opening for the concealed rectangular quartz-halogen headlamps. The lower section of the front fascia had twin rectangular black grilles (part numbers 10017729 right and 10017730 left) with horizontal louvers. The Trans Am had a front air dam beneath the standard front fascia with the optional RPO W62 Aero Package available in 1984. The Aero Package had blanked front air intakes and a different lower air dam to lower the drag coefficient. The 1983 Daytona 500 Special Edition and the 1984 15th Anniversary Trans Am included special white covers over the grille openings and a lower air dam extension as

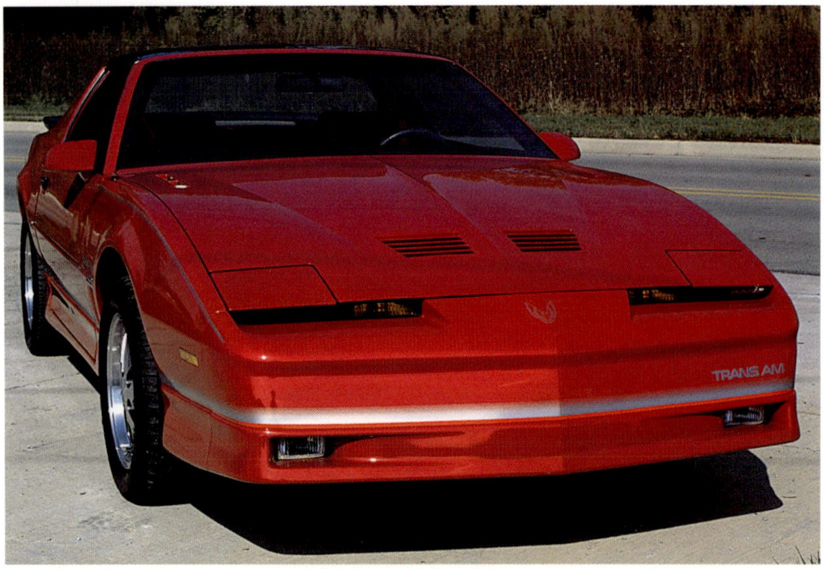

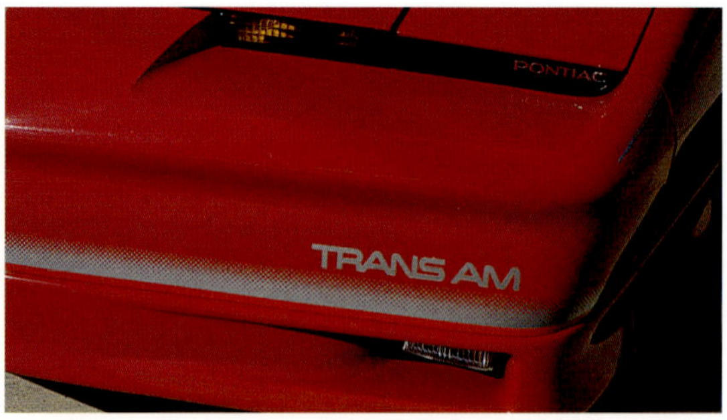

Left: This front fascia on a red 1986 Trans Am sport coupe was a different design from that used on the base Firebird. ***Above:*** Detail view of a red 1986 Trans Am sport coupe showing the silver Trans Am decal on the left front and full-body silver accent stripe.

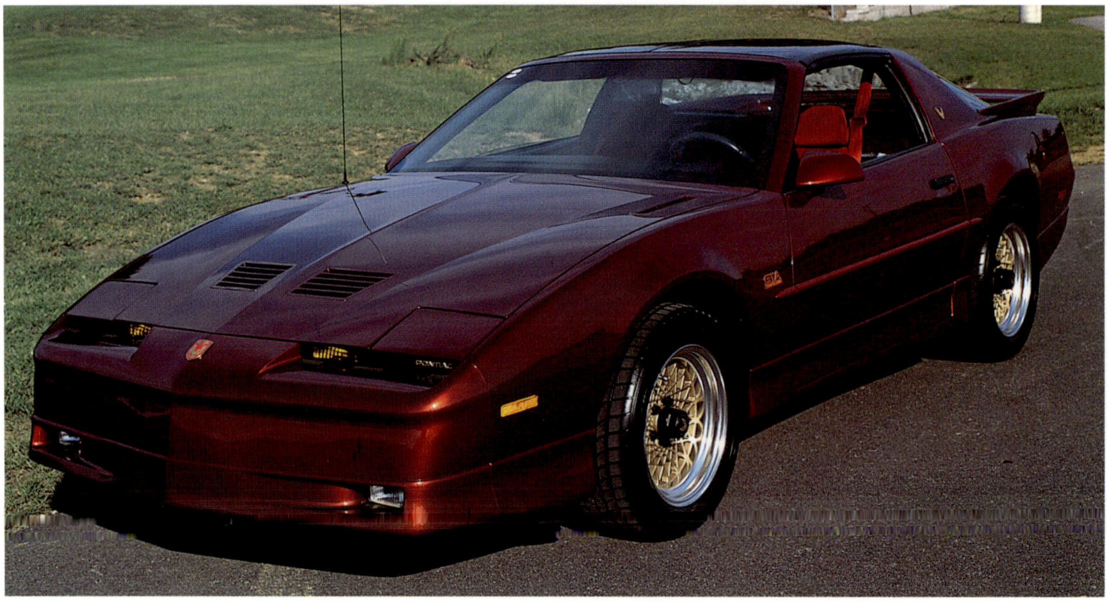

This is an original Flame Red Metallic 1987 Trans Am GTA showing the front fascia with the retractable headlights, rectangular side marker light, and distinctive red GTA badge on the center of the nose.

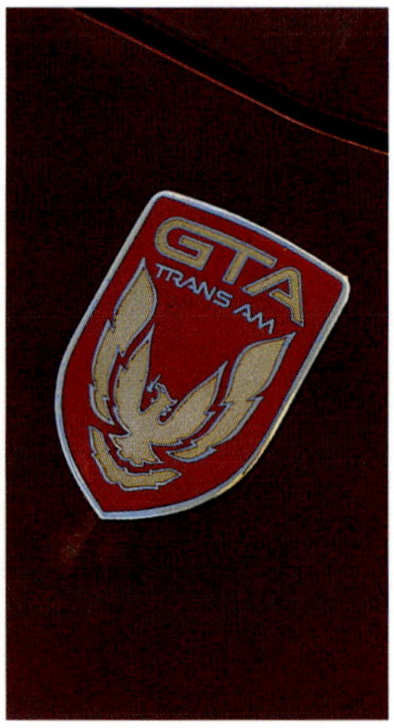

Detail view of the distinctive gold-and-red GTA badge on top of the front fascia of a Flame Red Metallic 1987 Trans Am GTA sport coupe.

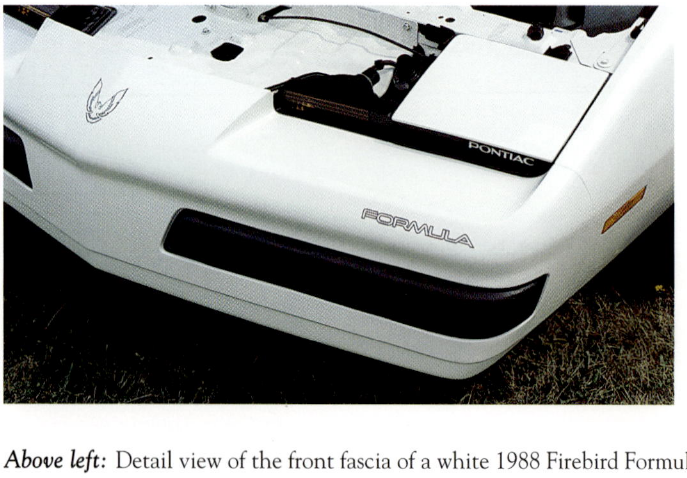

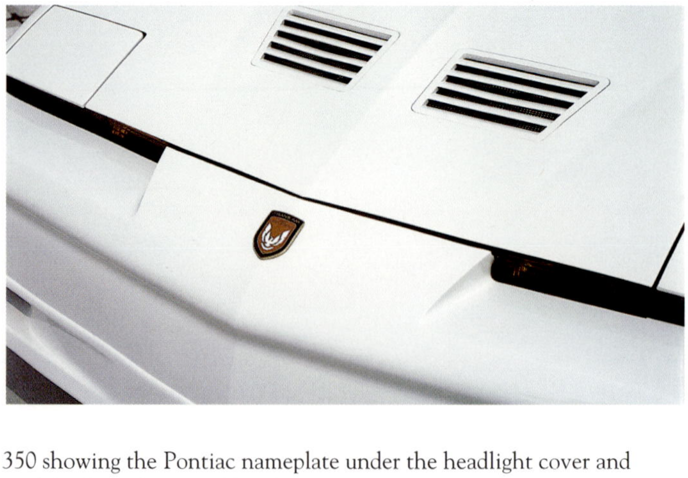

Above left: Detail view of the front fascia of a white 1988 Firebird Formula 350 showing the Pontiac nameplate under the headlight cover and Formula decal on the left front of the nose. ***Above right:*** This is a detail view of the front fascia and hood on an original white 1989 Turbo Trans Am GTA 20th Anniversary Edition. Note the unique gold 20th Anniversary GTA badge.

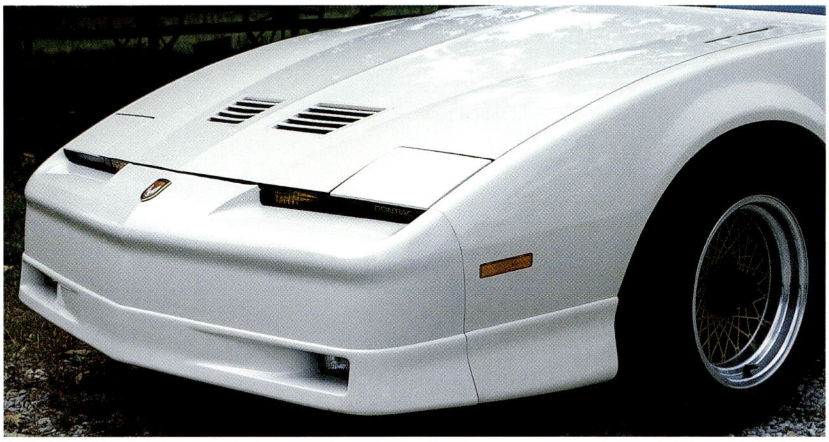

The front fascia and hood of an original white 1989 Turbo Trans Am GTA 20th Anniversary Edition sport coupe. Note the flat front design and lower air dam without any grille openings and the small, smooth, amber side marker light.

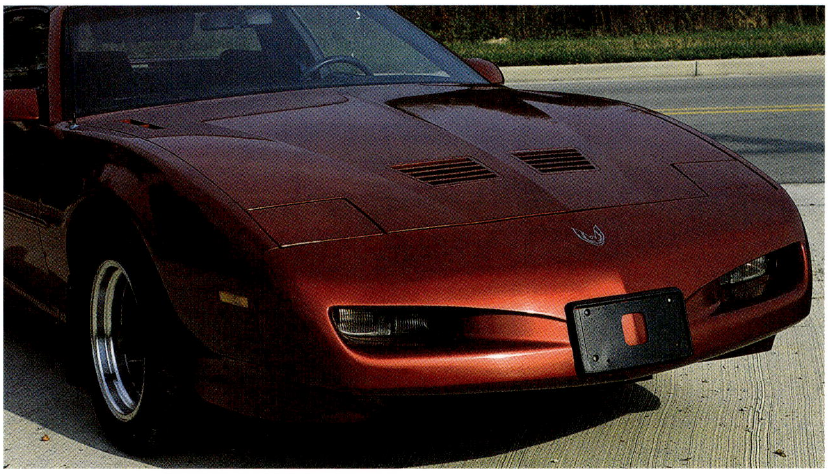

The 1991 Firebird and Trans Am front fascia was totally redesigned and featured a stylized cat's-eye look to the outer openings. This Brilliant Red Metallic 1991 Trans Am has driving lights and parking lights in the outer ends of the panel.

part of the Aero Package. Redesigned panels behind the front fascia created a bottom-breather air intake system.

The Firebird front fascia (part number 16509377) was redesigned for 1985–1990, and the twin grille openings were eliminated, creating a smoother appearance. The Aero Package became standard on the 1985–1990 Trans Am front fascia (part number 16509378). Rectangular parking lights were mounted in the outer ends of the lower front panel. The base Firebird and S/E had black fascia pads, but the Trans Am had body-color Endura for the entire front end treatment. The base Firebird, 1985 and 1986 S/E, and 1987–1990 Formula still had black-painted fascia pads, and the Trans Am and GTA continued with body-color finish.

For 1991 and 1992, the Firebird received a dramatic redesign that included a smoother and more aerodynamic peaked, body-color Endura front end treatment with cat's-eye-shaped openings on either side and integral parking lights in their outer corners. All 1991 and 1992 Firebird and Formula front fascias (part number 10118416) had an integral air dam and right (part number 10118514) and left (part number 100118515) black grille inserts. The 1991 and 1992 Trans Am used a slightly different front fascia design (part number 10118417) without grille inserts. Trans Am parking lights were larger than those used on the Firebird and Formula. Rectangular concealed headlamps were still part of the front design, but they were blended into the upper hood line and top of the front fascia to become almost invisible when closed.

Interior

The 1982–1992 Firebird was available with a variety of interior trim choices, all with standard reclining front bucket seats (RPO AR9) and a solid rear seatback with deep individual seat cushions on either side of the driveshaft tunnel. A front center floor console was standard equipment on all 1982–1992 Firebird models. A pull-up hand-brake lever with vinyl boot was mounted on the right side of the console on all models.

The standard 1982–1984 seat designs featured well-formed back and cushion bolsters with inserts of longitudinal sewn pleats forward to about ⅔ of the lower cushion. As in the past, the interior trim was available in standard, custom, and deluxe versions. The Firebird S/E had standard luxury Viscount-cloth trim, which was optional (RPO B20) with the Firebird and Trans Am and included a leather map pocket on the instrument panel. The Encore or Regal cloth was a velour-like material, and the vinyl trim was Madrid-grain. Leather-faced seats were available as an option in all models. The 1982–1984 Trans Am trim was available in two-tone color combinations. In 1983 and 1984, Lear Siegler adjustable custom bucket seats were also available (RPO AQ9) with the luxury interior group (RPO B20).

The 1982 standard interior trim was available in Pompey cloth and Derma vinyl in light slate gray (13B), charcoal (18R), dark blue (26B, 26R), medium jadestone (47B), camel tan (64B, 64R), and maroon (79B, 79R). The custom and deluxe interiors were available in Parella cloth and doeskin vinyl in light slate gray (13C, 13D), charcoal (18C, 18D), dark blue (26C, 26D), medium jadestone (47C, 47D), camel tan (64C, 64V, 64N), and maroon (79N, 79C, 79D). The deluxe interior was also available in leather and vinyl in camel tan (642) and maroon (792).

For 1983, the interior trim choices included standard Pompey-cloth and Sierra-vinyl interiors in dark charcoal (17R, 17B), dark royal blue (22B,

Firebird Production

1982

Model	Production
Firebird	41,683
Firebird S/E	21,719
Trans Am	52,962

1983

Model	Production
Firebird	32,020
Firebird S/E	10,934
Trans Am	31,930

1984

Model	Production
Firebird	62,621
Firebird S/E	10,309
Trans Am	55,374

1985

Model	Production
Firebird	46,644
Firebird S/E	5,208
Trans Am	44,028

1986

Model	Production
Firebird	59,334
Firebird S/E	2,259
Trans Am	48,870

1987

Model	Production
Firebird	42,552
Formula	13,160
Trans Am	21,779
Trans Am GTA	11,096

1988

Model	Production
Firebird	28,973
Formula	13,475
Trans Am	8,793
Trans Am GTA	11,214

1989

Model	Production
Firebird	32,376
Formula	16,670
Trans Am	5,727
Trans Am GTA	9,631

1990

Model	Production
Firebird	13,204
Formula	4,832
Trans Am	1,054
Trans Am GTA	1,442

1991

Model	Production
Firebird	39,906
Formula	5,549
Trans Am coupe	2,409
Trans Am conv.	555
Trans Am GTA	2,035

1992

Model	Production
Firebird coupe	23,099
Firebird conv.	1,265
Formula	1,052
Trans Am coupe	980
Trans Am conv.	663
Trans Am GTA	508

Body Colors

1982 Body Colors

Code	Color
11	White
16	Silver Metallic
19	Black
21	Light Blue Metallic
29	Dark Blue Metallic
45	Light Jadestone Metallic
49	Dark Jadestone Metallic
55	Goldwing Metallic
74	Autumn Maple
75	Spectra Red
78	Dark Claret Metallic
84	Charcoal Metallic

1983 Body Colors

Code	Color
11	White
15	Silver Sand Iridescence
19	Black
22	Light Royal Blue Iridescence
27	Medium Dark Royal Blue
55	Gold Metallic
62	Light Briar Brown Iridescence
67	Dark Briar Brown Iridescence
75	Spectra Red
82	Dark Sand Gray Metallic

1984 Body Colors

Code	Color
11	White
15	Silver Sand Gray Metallic
19	Black
22	Light Royal Blue
27	Medium Dark Royal Blue
59	Cream Beige
62	Light Briar Brown Metallic
67	Dark Briar Brown Metallic
75	Spectra Red
65	Dark Goldwing Metallic
82	Midnight Sand Gray Metallic

1985 Body Colors

Code	Color
11	White
12	Silver Metallic
15	Medium Gray Metallic
19	Black
26	Dark Blue
30	Bright Blue Metallic
50	Yellow Gold
54	Yellow Beige
60	Light Chestnut Metallic
69	Russet Metallic
75	Blaze Red
78	Dark Red

1986 Body Colors

Code	Color
13S	Silver Metallic
23	Bright Blue Metallic
28	Black Sapphire Metallic
40	White
41	Black
51	Yellow Gold
60	Champagne Gold Metallic
66	Russet Metallic
68	Medium Russet Metallic
74	Flame Red Metallic
81	Bright Red
84	Gunmetal Metallic

1987 Body Colors

Code	Color
13	Silver Metallic
23	Bright Blue Metallic
28	Black Sapphire Metallic
40	White
41	Black
51	Yellow Gold
60	Champagne Gold Metallic
68	Midnight Russet Metallic
74	Flame Red Metallic
81	Bright Red
84	Gunmetal Metallic

1988 Body Colors

Code	Color
11	White
12	Silver Metallic
13S	Silver Metallic
15	Medium Gray Metallic
19	Black
23	Medium Maui Blue Metallic
40	White
41	Black
51	Yellow Gold
63	Medium Orange Metallic
74	Flame Red Metallic
81	Bright Red
87	Gunmetal Metallic

1989 Body Colors

Code	Color
19	Black
23	Medium Maui Blue Metallic
40	White
41	Black
74	Flame Red Metallic
81	Bright Red
82	Medium Rosewood Metallic
87	Gunmetal Metallic
98	Bright Blue Metallic

1990 Body Colors

Code	Color
23	Medium Maui Blue Metallic
40	White
41	Black
75	Brilliant Red Metallic
81	Bright Red Metallic
87	Medium Gray Metallic
98	Bright Blue Metallic

1991 Body Colors

Code	Color
10	White
23	Medium Maui Blue Metallic
41	Black
45	Medium Green Metallic
75	Brilliant Red Metallic
81	Bright Red Metallic
87	Medium Gray Metallic
98	Ultra Blue Metallic

1992 Body Colors

Code	Color
10	Arctic White
37	Dark Bright Teal Metallic
41	Black
45	Medium Green Metallic
52	Jamaica Yellow
75	Brilliant Red Metallic
80	Medium Quasar Blue Metallic
81	Bright Red Metallic

22R), light sand gray (60B, 60R), camel tan (64R, 64B), and dark briar brown (67R, 67B). The Pallex-cloth and vinyl custom interiors were available in dark charcoal (17C), dark royal blue (22C), light sand gray (60C), camel tan (64C), and dark briar brown (57C). The custom interior was also available in leather and vinyl in camel tan (642) and dark briar brown (672). The custom-leather Recaro seat interior (also part of the RPO Y84 Trans Am S/E package) was available only in camel tan (643).

The 1984 standard Pompey-cloth and Sierra-vinyl interior trim was available in the same colors as 1983: dark charcoal (17R, 17B), dark royal blue (22R, 22B), light sand gray (60R, 60B), camel tan (64R, 64B), and dark briar brown (67R, 67B). The deluxe Pallex-cloth and vinyl trim was available in dark charcoal (17C), dark royal blue (22C), light sand gray (60C), light sand gray leather (604), camel tan (64C), and dark briar brown (67C). The deluxe leather and vinyl was available in camel tan (643). There was also a special 1984 interior trim available only with the 15th Anniversary Trans Am. It had two-tone gray seats with a white leather-wrapped steering wheel. The seat inserts had multiple embossed Trans Am logos on the cushion and backrest.

The 1985–1992 Firebird interiors featured sculptured front bucket seats and individual bucket seat cushions with a solid backrest. The designs had longitudinal pleats and were similar to those used in 1982–1984, with relatively square backs on the standard seats and a rounder shape for the deluxe interiors. The bucket seat backrests had solid plastic backs finished in

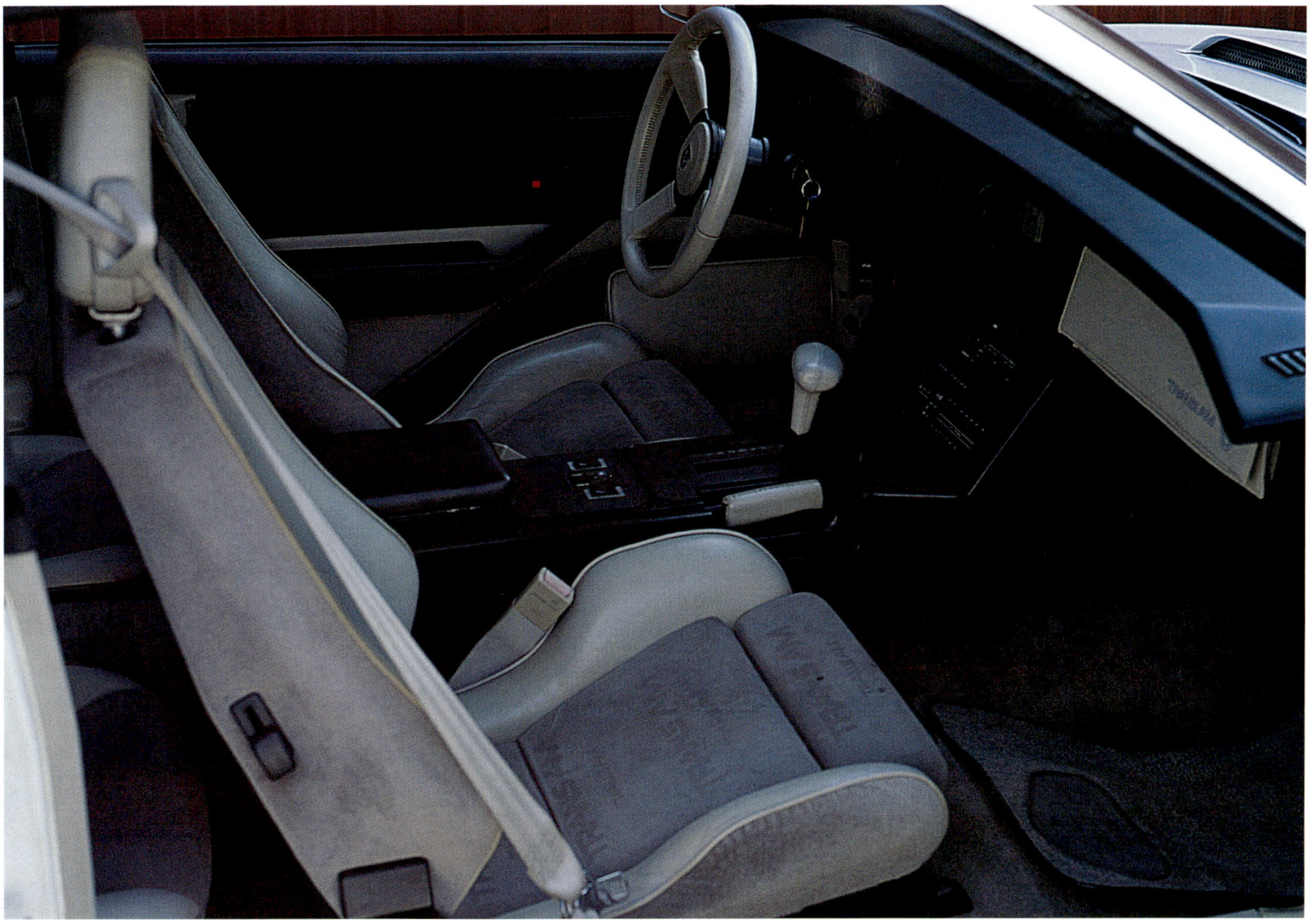

Above: This is a view of the special white-and-gray cloth-and-vinyl interior in an original 1984 Trans Am 15th Anniversary Edition. The center inserts of the seats have transverse Trans Am logos embossed into the material. The white vinyl storage envelope on the right side of the instrument panel is visible. ***Right:*** This is the carmine-and-gray deluxe Genor-cloth interior trim (72B) in a red 1986 Trans Am sport coupe. Note the gold Trans Am and performance suspension badges on the right side of the instrument panel.

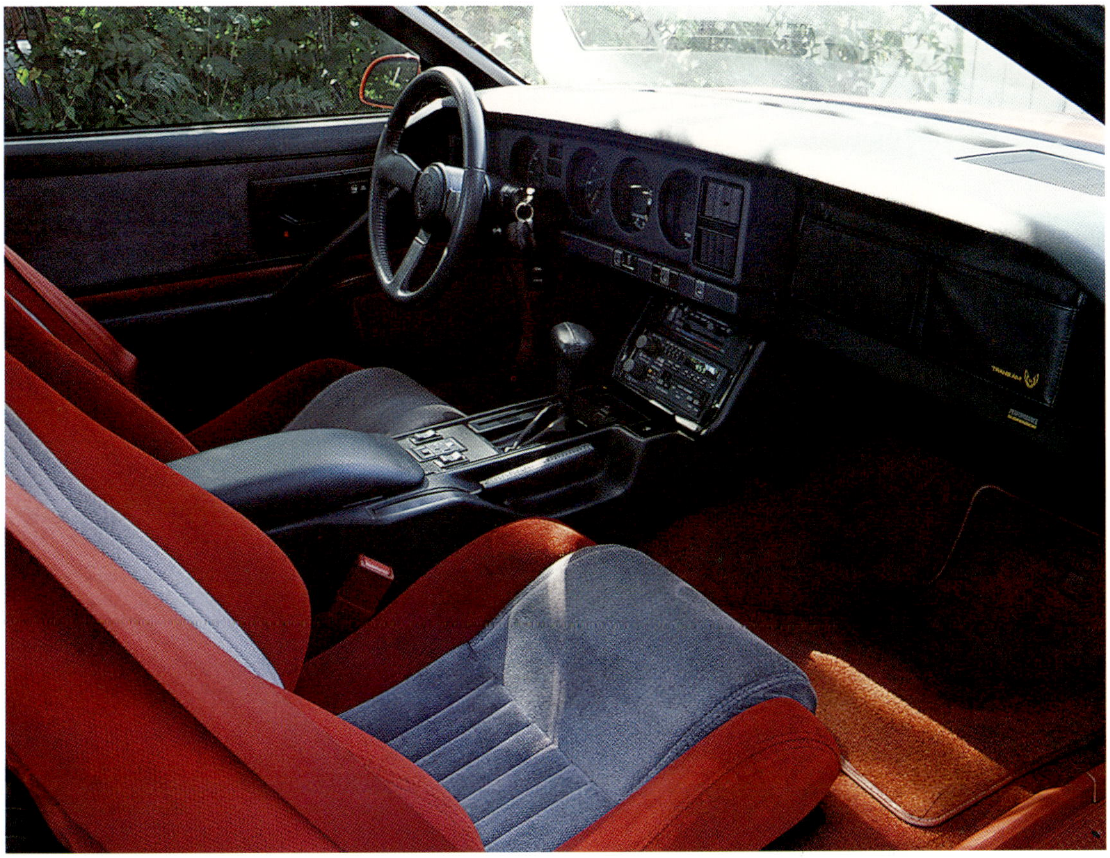

interior trim color. The Lear Siegler adjustable custom bucket seats were again available as an option (RPO AQ9) in 1985 and 1986 with the luxury interior group (RPO B20). The luxury trim group included a split folding rear seat and door map pockets. The Recaro bucket seats with split folding rear seat were also still an option (RPO AS5) in 1985 and 1986.

The 1985 and 1986 standard Genor-cloth and Sierra-vinyl interiors were available in black (19R, 19B), camel (62R, 62B), russet (68R, 68B), medium dark carmine (72B), and medium dark gray (82R, 82B). The custom and deluxe interiors in Pallex cloth and vinyl were available in black (19C), camel (62C, 62D), russet (68C), medium dark carmine (72C), and medium dark gray 82C). The custom interior trim was also available in leather and vinyl in camel (622) and medium dark gray (822).

For 1987, the standard interior Ripple-cloth interior trim was available in black (19B), light saddle (62B), dark carmine (72B), and dark gray (82B). The custom and deluxe Pallex-cloth interiors were available in black (19E, 19C, 19D), light saddle (62E, 62C, 62D), dark carmine (72C, 72D), and dark gray (82C, 82D 82E). For 1988 and 1989, the standard cloth interior trim was available in black (19B), camel (66B), dark carmine (72B), and medium dark gray (82B). The custom and deluxe Metrix-cloth interiors were available in the Trans Am and GTA in black (19C, 19D), camel (66C, 66D), dark carmine (72C), and medium dark gray (82C, 82D). The deluxe trim was also available in leather and cloth

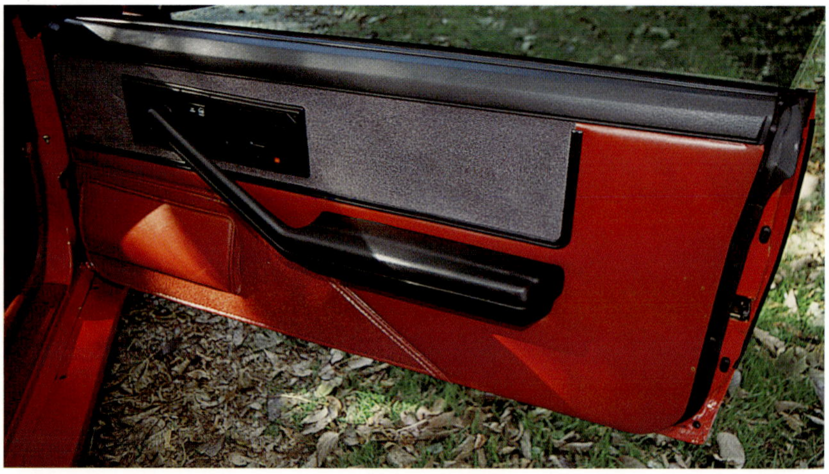

This is a detail view of the door panel on a carmine-and-gray deluxe Genor-cloth interior in a red 1986 Trans Am sport coupe. This Trans Am has power windows and power door locks.

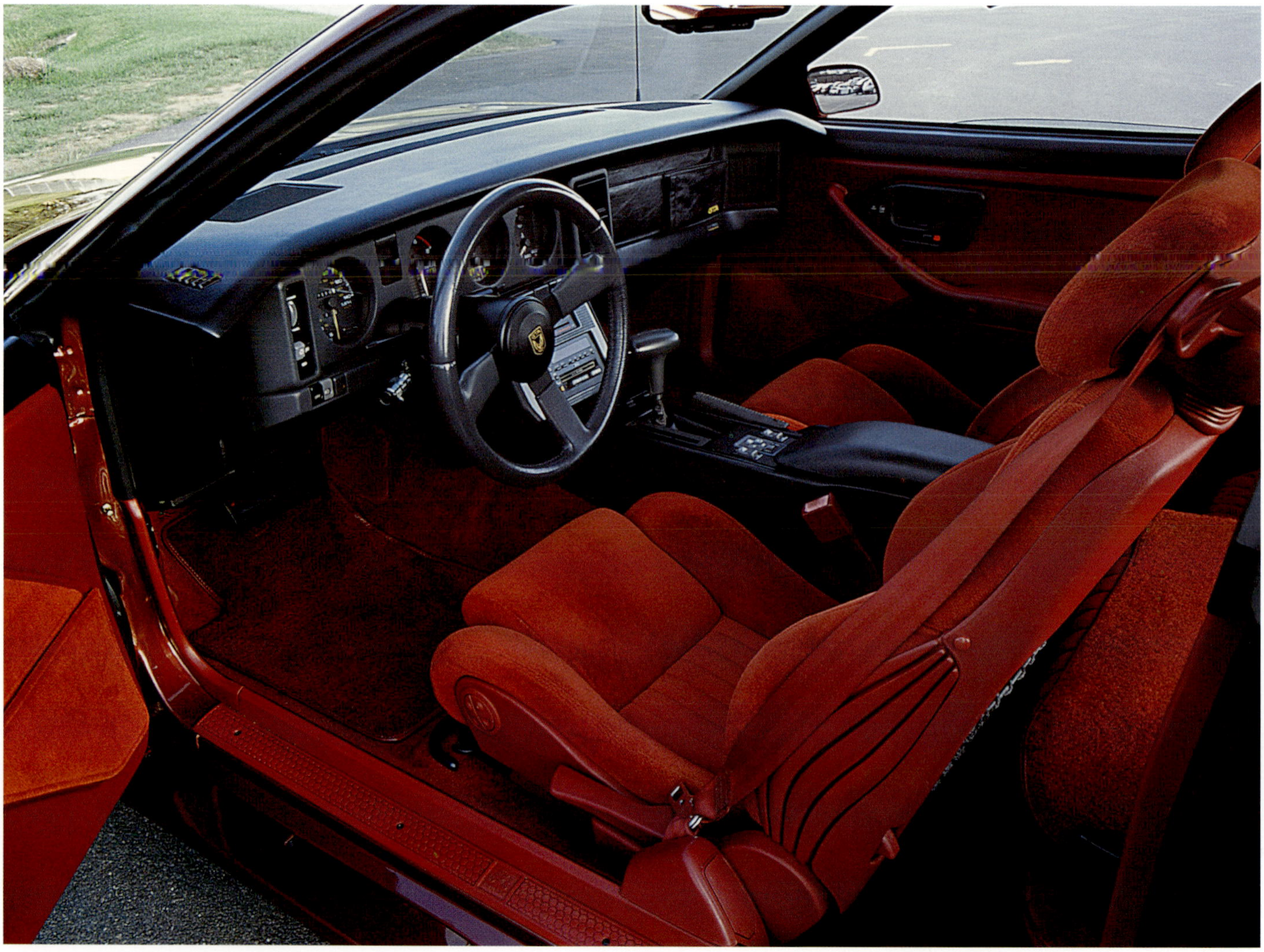

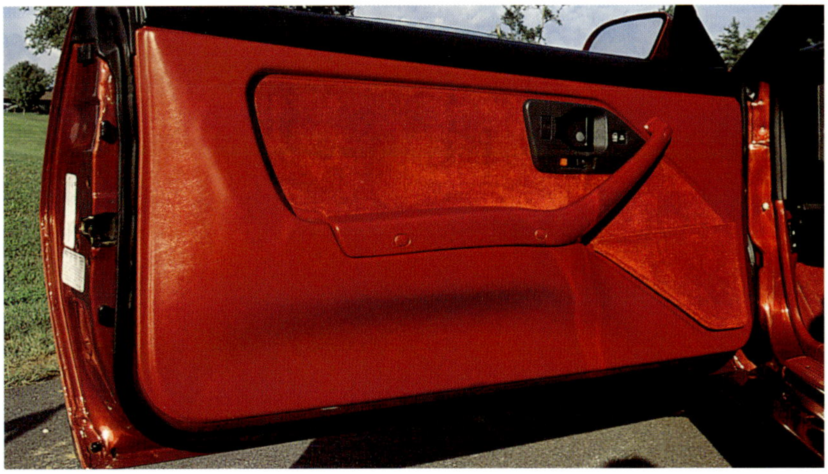

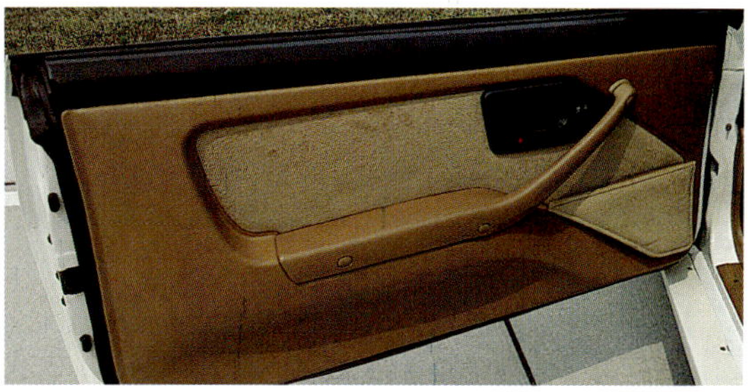

Detail view of the left door panel in an original 1989 Turbo Trans Am GTA 20th Anniversary sport coupe. The interior trim is tan leather (662), and the door panel is finished in tan vinyl with cloth trim and a black upper panel.

This is a detail view of the left door panel on an original 1987 Trans Am GTA with Pallex cloth and red vinyl. Note the black finish on the upper door panel. This GTA has power windows and door locks.

in black (192), camel (662), and medium dark gray (822). New articulated bucket seats became available for GTA in 1988.

The 1990 standard Pallex-cloth interior trim was available in all models in black (19C), camel (66C), and medium gray (82C). The Trans Am and GTA were available with leather in black (192), camel (662), and medium gray (822). For 1991 and 1992, all models were available with standard Pallex cloth in black (19B), camel (66B), and medium gray (82B). The Firebird, Trans Am, and GTA were available with custom and deluxe Metrix cloth in black (19C, 19D), camel (66C, 66D), and medium gray (82C, 82D). The GTA was available with leather in black (192), camel (862), and medium gray (822).

The 1982–1992 Firebird instrument panel was completely redesigned and had a wide rectangular

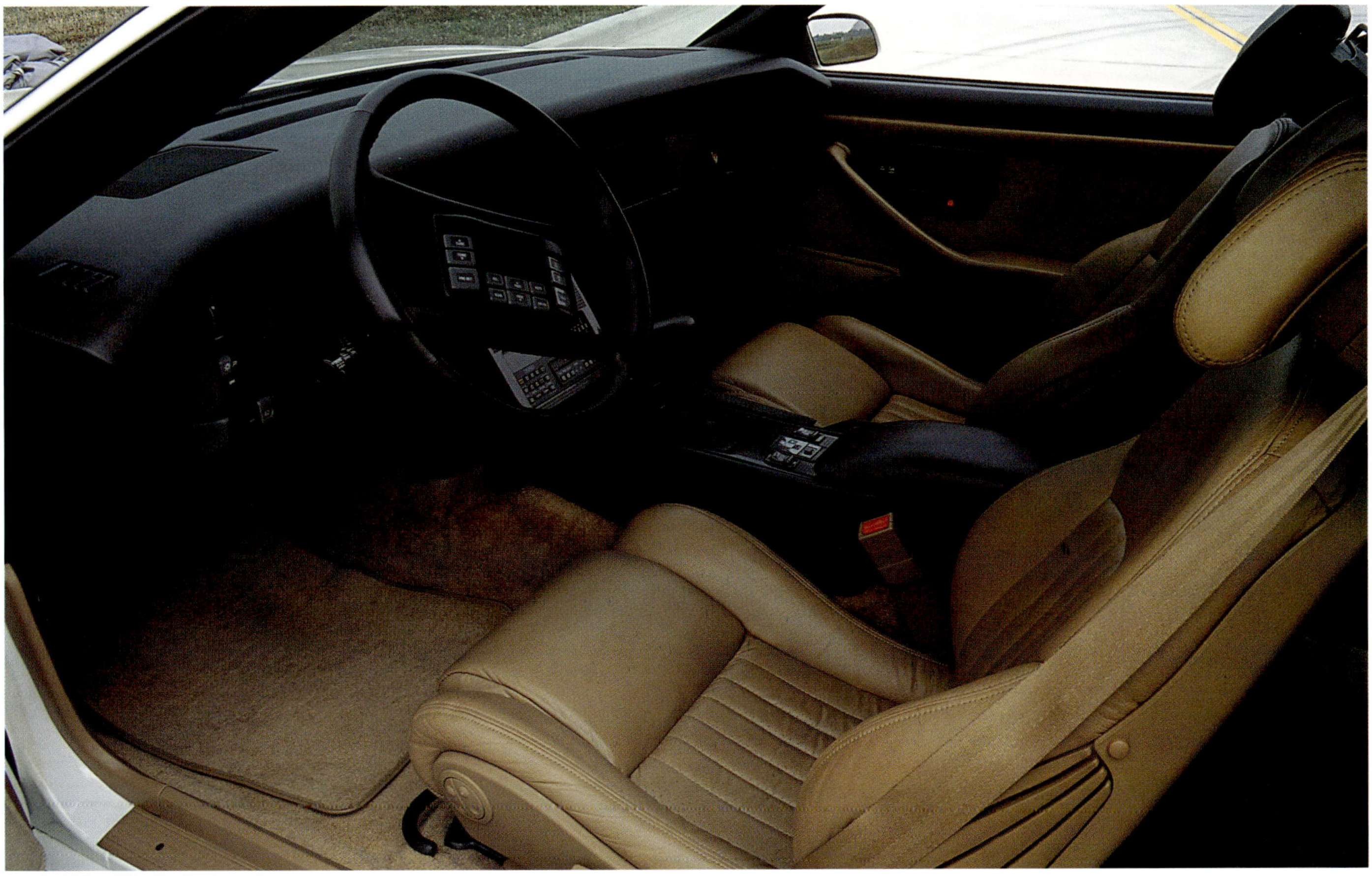

Opposite: This view of the carmine Pallex-cloth (72D) interior of a Flame Red Metallic 1987 Trans Am GTA shows the matching red carpet and dark gray finish on the instrument panel and floor console. Note the gold GTA medallion on the steering wheel center. ***Above:*** The tan leather (662) interior trim in an original white 1989 Turbo Trans Am GTA 20th Anniversary sport coupe is paired with matching tan carpet and radio controls in the dark gray steering wheel.

flat black cluster with four separate, square gauge panels housing large round gauges. Each of the four square panels had simulated Allen-head screws at each corner for a distinctive aircraft-panel appearance. The gauges had black backgrounds with white numerals and bright red/orange indicators. Beginning in 1984, the gauges were lighted in orange with red/orange indicators.

The left round gauge housed the dial speedometer with odometer that had a 120-mile-per-hour limit for the base Firebird and standard Rally panel (RPO U21 in 1982–1988 or UB3 in 1989–1992) and 140-mile-per-hour limit for the 1991 and 1992 Special Performance Rally panel. The second round gauge had a clock in the standard panel and a 6,000-rpm tachometer in the Rally panel, standard in the S/E, Formula, and Trans Am. The third round gauge held the voltmeter at the top and oil pressure gauge at the bottom for 1982–1990 and the voltmeter and fuel gauge for 1991 and 1992. The far-right round gauge held the fuel gauge and coolant temperature gauge for 1982–1990 and the oil pressure and coolant temperature gauge for 1991 and 1992. The Rally and Performance Rally cluster was available as an option in the base Firebird.

The windshield wiper/washer and lighting switches were in a separate black panel to the left of the speedometer, and a square air outlet was to the right of the right round gauge. The heater, air conditioning, and radio or other sound equipment controls were mounted in a flat black center panel below the instrument panel and just above the integral center floor console.

A radio was not standard in any 1982–1984 Firebird. For 1985, a Delco GM AM monaural push-button radio (RPO U63) with dual front speakers became standard equipment in all models. For 1988–1990, the standard radio was a Delco ETR AM/FM stereo (RPO UM7). For 1991 and 1992, the standard Firebird radio was upgraded to an AM/FM cassette stereo. The Formula added a clock, and the GTA added a graphic equalizer to the package.

There were a variety of optional radios and sound systems available with the 1982–1992

Opposite: This detail view shows the optional cloth interior trim in a Brilliant Red Metallic 1991 Trans Am sport coupe and the steering wheel with standard air bag SRS.

Interior Trim Combinations

1982

Code	Color
13B	Gray cloth and vinyl
13D	Gray cloth
18D	Charcoal cloth
18R	Charcoal vinyl
26B	Blue cloth and vinyl
26D	Blue cloth
26R	Blue vinyl
47B	Jadestone cloth and vinyl
47D	Jadestone cloth
64B	Camel Tan cloth and vinyl
64D	Camel Tan cloth
64R	Camel Tan vinyl
64V	Camel Tan vinyl
642	Camel Tan leather
79B	Maroon cloth and vinyl
79D	Maroon cloth
79R	Maroon vinyl
79V	Maroon vinyl
792	Maroon leather

1983 and 1984

Code	Color
17B	Charcoal cloth and vinyl
17C	Charcoal cloth
17R	Charcoal vinyl
22B	Dark Royal Blue cloth and vinyl
22C	Royal Blue cloth
22R	Royal Blue vinyl
60B	Light Sand Gray cloth and vinyl
60C	Light Sand Gray cloth
60R	Light Sand Gray vinyl
64B	Camel Tan cloth and vinyl
64C	Camel Tan cloth
64R	Camel Tan vinyl
642	Camel Tan leather and cloth
643	Camel Tan leather and cloth
672	Dark Brown leather
67B	Dark Brown cloth and vinyl
67C	Dark Brown cloth
67R	Dark Brown vinyl

1985

Code	Color
19B	Black cloth
19C	Black cloth
19R	Black vinyl
62B	Camel cloth
62C	Camel cloth
62D	Camel cloth (Racaro)
62R	Camel vinyl
622	Camel leather and cloth
68B	Russet cloth
68C	Russet cloth
68R	Russet vinyl
72B	Carmine cloth
72C	Carmine cloth
72R	Carmine vinyl
82B	Medium Gray cloth
82C	Medium Gray cloth
82R	Medium Gray vinyl
822	Medium Gray leather and cloth

1986

Code	Color
19B	Black cloth
19C	Black custom vinyl
19R	Black cloth
62B	Camel cloth
62C	Camel custom vinyl
62R	Camel cloth
68B	Russet cloth
68C	Russet custom vinyl
72B	Carmine cloth
72C	Carmine custom vinyl
82B	Medium Gray cloth
82C	Medium Gray custom vinyl
82R	Medium Gray vinyl

1987

Code	Color
19B	Black ripple cloth
19C	Black Pallex cloth
19D	Black Pallex cloth
19E	Black leather and cloth
62B	Camel ripple cloth
62C	Camel Pallex cloth
62D	Camel Pallex cloth
62E	Camel leather and cloth
72B	Carmine ripple cloth
72C	Carmine Pallex cloth
72D	Carmine Pallex cloth
82B	Medium Gray ripple gray
82C	Medium Gray Pallex cloth
82D	Medium Gray Pallex cloth
82E	Medium Gray leather and cloth

19788 and 1989

Code	Color
19B	Black cloth
19C, D	Black cloth
192	Black leather
66B	Camel cloth
66C, D	Camel cloth
662	Camel leather
82B	Medium Gray cloth
82C, D	Medium Gray cloth
822	Medium Gray leather

1990

Code	Color
19C	Black cloth
66C	Camel cloth
82C	Medium Gray cloth
192	Black leather
662	Camel leather
822	Medium Gray leather

1991 and 1992

Code	Color
19C	Black cloth
192	Black leather
66C	Camel cloth
662	Camel Leather
82C	Medium Gray cloth
822	Medium Gray leather

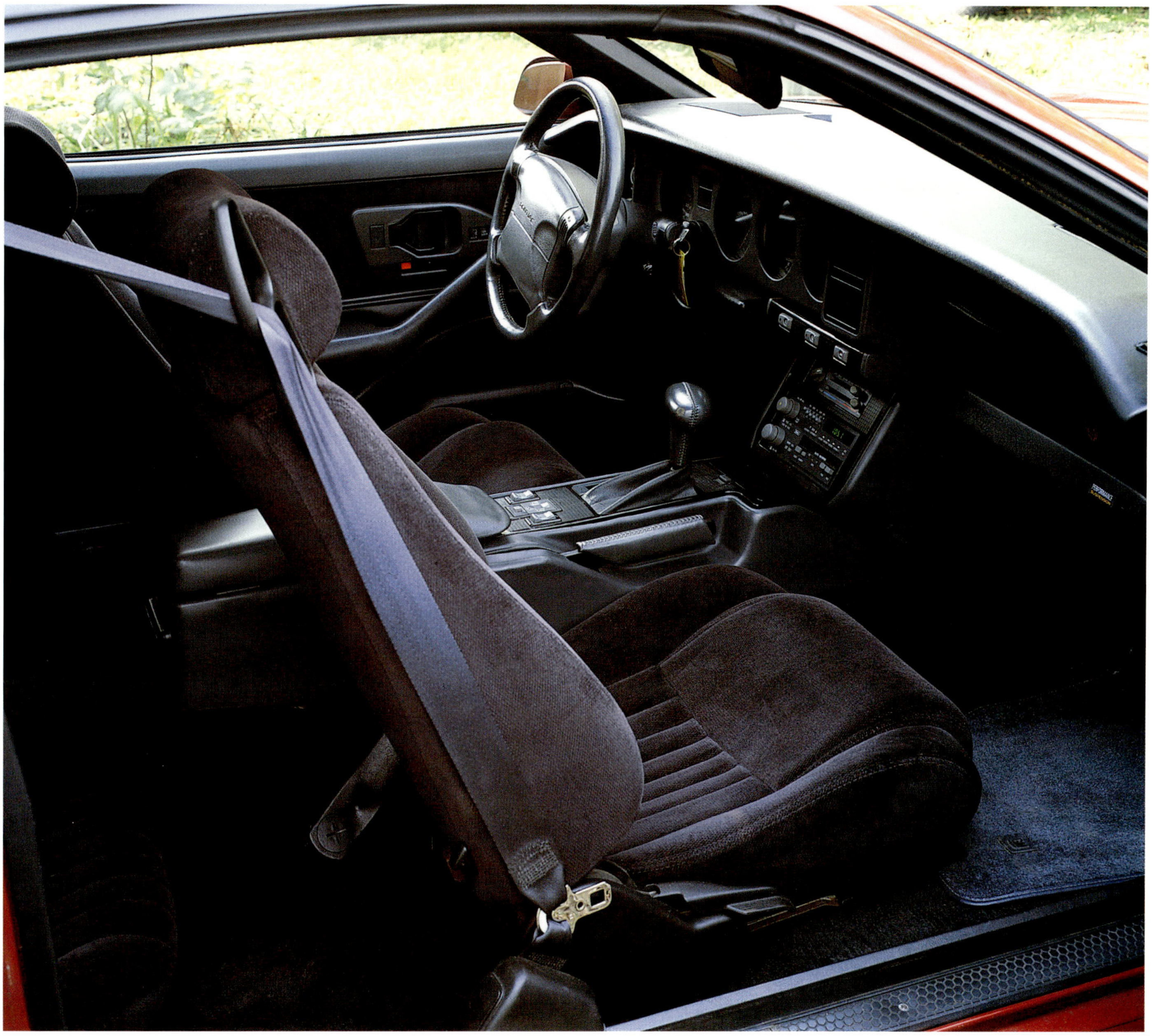

Selected 1982–1992 Regular Production Options

RPO	Description				
		C60	Air conditioning	N91	Wire wheel covers
		D35	Dual sport mirrors	PE5	Rally V wheel covers
AC3	Six-way power driver's seat	D42	Cargo security screen	P06	Wheel trim rings
AK1	Custom front and rear seatbelts	D80	Rear spoiler	P20	Bright aluminum hubcaps
AR9	Reclining bucket seats	G80	Safe-T-Track axle	TR9	Lamp group
AU3	Power door locks	J65	Front and rear power disc brakes	UA1	Heavy-duty battery
A01	Soft-Ray glass	K30	Cruise control	UM6	AM/FM ETR cassette system
A31	Power windows	K73	Heavy-duty generator	UN3	AM/FM stereo cassette system
A90	Remote deck lid release	K81	Heavy-duty generator	UP8	Dual front and rear speakers
B20	Luxury trim group	K99	Heavy-duty generator	U21	Rally gauges and tachometer
B34	Carpeted front mats	LC1	173-ci V-6	U63	Am radio system
B48	Luggage compartment trim	LG4	305 4-bbl V-8	U75	Power antenna
B57	Custom exterior group	LQ9	151-ci L-4	V08	Heavy-duty radiator
B80	Drip-rail moldings	LU5	305-ci V-8	WS6	Special performance package
B84	Vinyl body side moldings	MM4	Four-speed manual	WS7	Special performance package
B91	Door edge moldings	MX1	Automatic transmission	Y84	Recaro Trans Am package
CC1	Hatch roof (T-top)	N24	15x7 cast-aluminum wheels	Y99	Rally-tuned suspension
CD4	Controlled cycle wipers	N33	Tilt steering wheel		
C49	Rear window defroster	N90	Cast-aluminum wheels		

Firebird. In 1982, the Delco AM radio was optional in addition to a Delco AM/FM radio system (RPO U69). RPO U58 brought a Delco AM/FM stereo radio system. A radio accommodation package was also available with RPO UN9. An optional power antenna was available with RPO U75. For 1983–1985, the optional radio was the Delco GM ETR AM/FM stereo radio with cassette-tape player, digital clock, seek and scan, and five-band graphic equalizer available with RPO UU6. The same package without the graphic equalizer was available with RPO UU7. A Delco GM ETR stereo with digital clock was available with RPO UL1. The same radio without the clock was UU9. Dual front and rear speakers were available with RPO UP8.

Additional radio options for 1985 included a new Delco GM ETR AM/FM radio with seek and scan and auto-reverse cassette player with digital clock (RPO UM6). There was also a new Delco GM ETR AM/FM stereo with all of the above plus cassette search, replay, graphic equalizer, and clock (RPO UT4). For 1986–1992, a new optional package included everything in the AM/FM stereo with seek and scan and clock, adding a subwoofer and six-speaker system with extended frequency response. The equipment was similar, but some RPO codes changed slightly from 1988 to 1992.

The standard steering wheel for the 1982–1986 Firebird was the graphite-color Formula steering wheel (RPO NK3), which had three flat spokes with a large round, flat center horn button with Firebird badge. For 1983–1986, a graphite-color leather-wrapped three-spoke Formula steering wheel (RPO NP5) was optional in all models. The 1984 15th Anniversary Trans Am had a white leather-wrapped Formula steering wheel with a blue shield badge in its center. The spokes were redesigned and made wider for 1985–1987, and an interior-color-coordinated leather-wrapped Formula wheel was standard for the S/E. The GTA steering wheels had a special GTA badge in the center. In 1988 and 1989, a new optional four-spoke graphite-color wheel, standard in the GTA, was available with radio controls for the RPO UT4 system in the center of the wheel.

In 1990–1992, a new four-spoke graphite-color leather-wrapped sport steering wheel with tilt (RPO N36) was optional on the Firebird and standard on the Trans Am and GTA. The standard Firebird steering wheel was a graphite-color four-spoke with tilt. The 1990–1992 steering wheels were redesigned to incorporate the new driver-side air bag supplemental restraint system. The sport four-spoke wheel was standard in the Firebird and Formula, and the sport leather-wrapped wheel was standard in the Trans Am and GTA. Both were graphite color.

Engine and Engine Compartment

The 1982 Firebird was available with four engine choices. The standard engine in the base Firebird was the Pontiac 151-cubic-inch (2.5-liter) four-cylinder with throttle-body fuel injection. Optional engines included a 173-cubic-inch Chevrolet V-6 and two versions of 305-cubic-inch Chevrolet V-8s. For 1984, engine options were increased to five as a new 125-horsepower HO version of the V-6 was added to the line. All engines except the four-cylinder were carbureted.

In 1985 and 1986, engine choices were five, but the HO V-6 was dropped and replaced by another version of the 305 V-8. The RPO LB8 V-6 and LB9 305-ci V-8s had electronic fuel injection. The other two V-8 engines still had carburetors.

For 1987 and 1988, engine options changed again, and the four-cylinder was dropped. The base engine was now the 173-cubic-inch V-6 with electronic multiport fuel injection. There were two versions of 305 V-8s, one with fuel injection and the other with a four-barrel carburetor. The standard engine in the Trans Am GTA, and optional in the Trans Am, Firebird, and Formula, was a 350-cubic-inch V-8 (RPO L98 and B2L) with tuned-port fuel injection. A visual change for 1988 was the exchanging of the alternator and air-conditioning compressor locations left and right and the adoption of a serpentine belt system.

There were five engines available in 1989, but the choices changed in a number of areas. The base engine in the Firebird was still the 173-cubic-inch V-6, and there were still two variations of 305 V-8s, all with throttle-body electronic fuel injection. The 5.7-liter (350-ci) V-8 with 225 horsepower was standard in the GTA. A special 231-cubic-inch 250-horsepower V-6 with turbocharger (RPO LG3) was standard in the Indy Pace Car Turbo V-8.

There were still five engine choices for 1990 and 1991, including the base V-6 (now 191 cubic inches), three 5-liter V-8s, and the 240-horsepower 5.7-liter V-8 standard in the GTA. For 1992, one version of 305-ci (5-liter) V-8 was dropped, leaving only four engine options.

Overhead-Valve Inline Four

The 151-cubic-inch (2.5-liter) Pontiac cast-iron inline four-cylinder (RPO LQ9) had a bore and stroke of 4.00x3.00 inches and a compression ratio of 8.2:1. The four-cylinder developed 90 horsepower at 4,000 rpm and 134 foot-pounds of torque at 2,400 rpm with hydraulic valve lifters. The compression ratio was increased to 9:1 in 1984, and the horsepower increased to 92. Rated

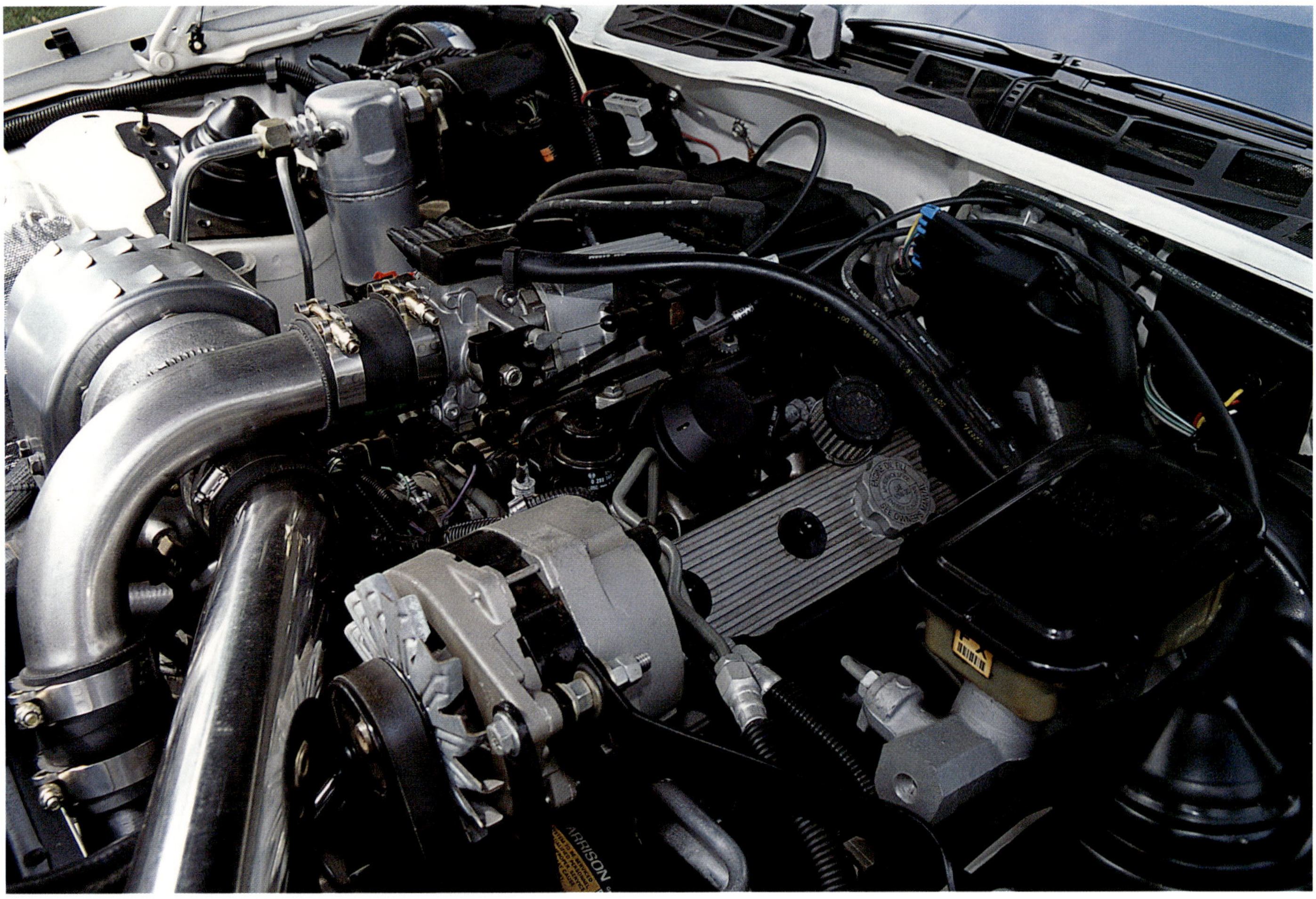

This is a view of the engine compartment of an original 1989 Turbo Trans Am GTA 20th Anniversary Pace Car Edition. The engine is a specially prepared 3.8-liter V-6 with a Garrett T3 turbocharger developing 250 horsepower. The turbocharger and heat shield are visible on the right side of the engine compartment.

power was reduced to 88 at 4,400 rpm for 1985 and 1986. The induction system was throttle-body fuel injection. The VIN engine code was 2.

Overhead-Valve Chevrolet V-6

The 173-cubic-inch overhead-valve Chevrolet V-6 (RPO LC1) was introduced in the Firebird in 1982. This engine was originally used in the 1980 Chevrolet Citation front-wheel-drive X-body, but the F-body application reduced horsepower by 10 due to the use of an engine-driven cooling fan. The V-6 had a bore and stroke of 3.50x3.00 inches and a compression ratio of 8.5:1, developing 105 horsepower at 4,800 rpm and 142 foot-pounds of torque at 2,400 rpm. Horsepower was increased slightly to 107 in 1983 and 1984. The V-6 had hydraulic valve lifters and a Rochester two-barrel carburetor. In 1985, the RPO was changed to LG4, electronic throttle-body fuel injection was added, and horsepower was increased to 135 at 5,100 rpm. The RPO was again changed to LB8 for 1986–1988. The VIN engine code was S in 1982 and X or 1 in 1983. The VIN engine code was S in 1985–1987 and E in 1988. The VIN engine code was W or S in 1989 and T in 1990.

In 1983 and 1984, another V-6 was introduced with RPO LL1. The LL1 HO V-6 had an 8.9:1 compression ratio and developed 125 horsepower at 5,400 rpm and 145 foot-pounds of torque at 2,400 rpm using a two-barrel Rochester E28E. The VIN engine code was L.

In 1990, the displacement of the V-6 (RPO LB8) was increased to 191 cubic inches by enlarging the stroke to 3.31 inches. The compression ratio was also increased to 8.75:1. Horsepower was 140 at 4,400 rpm, and torque was 180 foot-pounds at 3,600 rpm with electronic fuel injection (EFI/MFI). The VIN engine code was T. For 1991 and 1992, the 191-cubic-inch (3.1-liter) V-6 was given a new RPO of LHO. The horsepower was still 140, and the VIN engine code was still T.

In 1989, a special 231-cubic-inch V-6 (RPO LG3) was standard and exclusive in the 20th Anniversary Indy Pace Car Turbo V-6 Trans Am. The LG3 engine was specially built by PAS in Industry, California, for the 20th Anniversary Trans Am. The engines were sent to the final assembly plant in Van Nuys, California, to be installed in Trans Ams originally intended to have a V-8. This engine had a cast-iron block, aluminum intake manifold, and a bore and stroke of 3.80x3.40 inches. The compression ratio was 8.0:1, and it developed 250 horsepower at 4,000 rpm and 340 foot-pounds of torque at 2,800 rpm. Induction was electronic sequential fuel injection

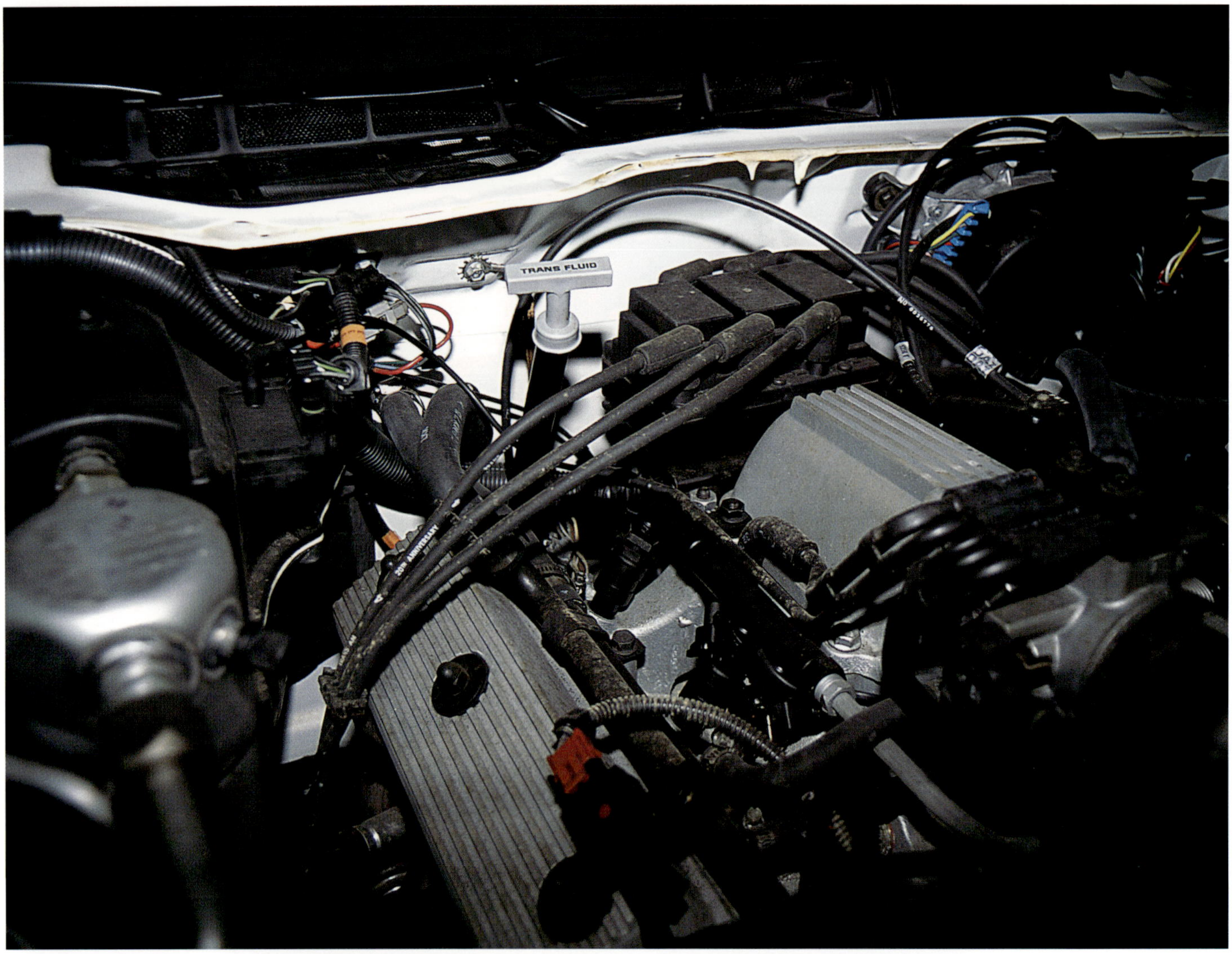

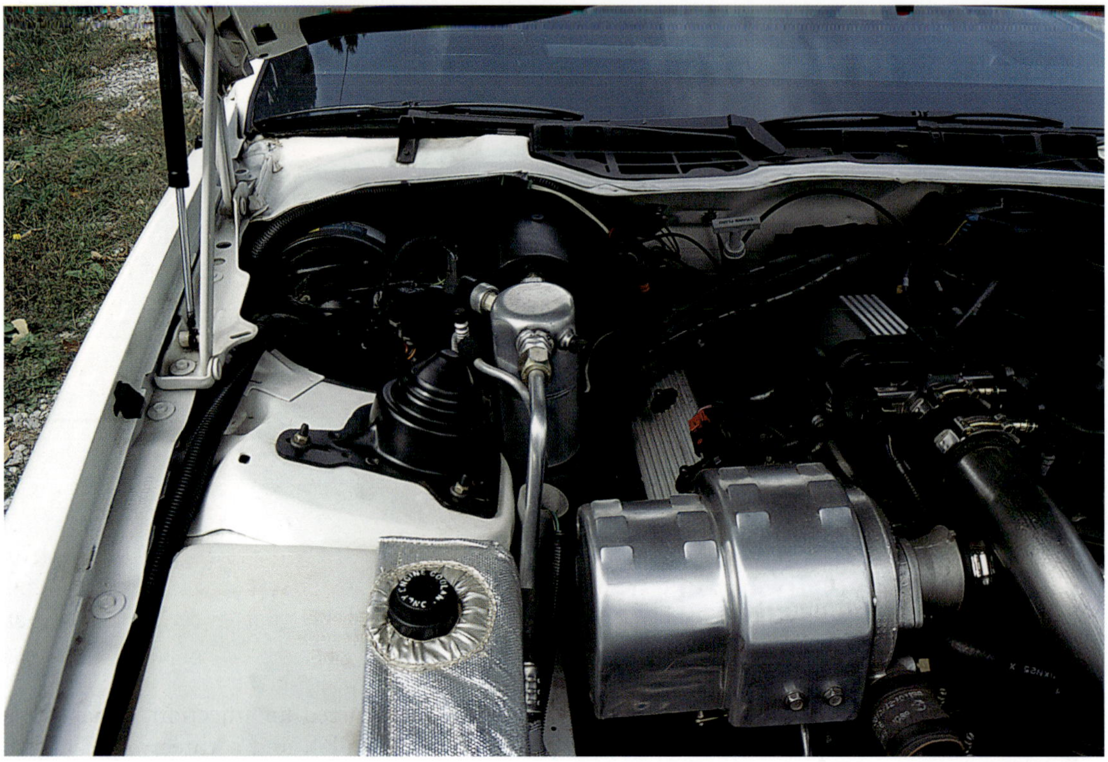

Above: This is a detail view of the rear of the engine compartment of the 3.8-liter V-6 in a 20th Anniversary Turbo Trans Am GTA. The black original spark plug wires are printed in white with "20th Anniversary," and each is numbered on this original engine. ***Left:*** Detail view of the Garrett T3 turbocharger on the 3.8-liter V-6 in a 1989 Turbo Trans Am GTA 20th Anniversary Edition. Note the heat shield cover over the engine coolant reservoir on the right side of the engine compartment. This is an original, unrestored Trans Am.

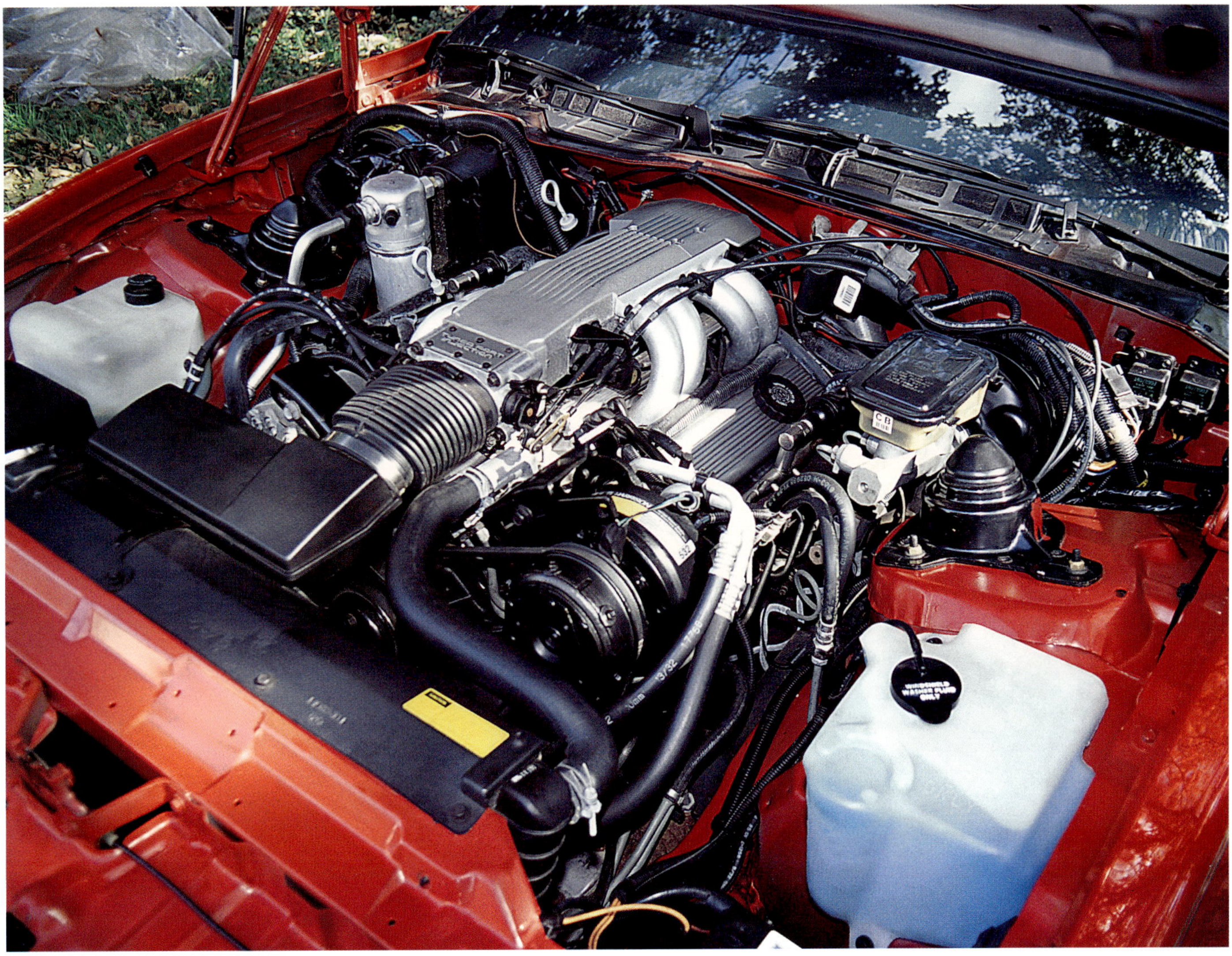

This detail view of the engine compartment of a red 1986 Trans Am with a 305-cubic-inch Chevrolet V-8 equipped with electronic fuel injection (RPO LB9) shows the air-conditioning compressor on the left front of the engine.

(EFI/SFI) enhanced by an intercooled Garrett T3 turbocharger. The VIN engine code was W, S, or 9. The 20th Anniversary Trans Am with the Turbo V-6 was considered the fastest currently available automobile in the United States in 1989 with 0–60-mile-per-hour times of 4.6 seconds and quarter-mile elapsed times of around 13 seconds. This model was the first Indianapolis 500 pace car that did not require modifications for pace car duty.

Overhead-Valve Chevrolet V-8

There were two basic sizes of overhead-valve V-8s used in the 1982–1992 Firebirds, with a number of variations depending upon the model application and year. The smallest V-8 was the 305-cubic-inch Chevrolet V-8 with a bore of 3.74 inches and a stroke of 3.48 inches. The base V-8 for 1982 was the RPO LG4 with 8.6:1 compression ratio and hydraulic lifters. The LG4 developed 145 horsepower at 4,000 rpm and 240 foot-pounds of torque at 2,000 rpm with a single Rochester E4ME four-barrel carburetor. The VIN engine was H. The horsepower was increased to 150 for 1983 and 1984. In 1985, the compression ratio was increased to 9.5:1, making the horsepower 160 at 4,200 rpm. In 1986 and 1987, the power dropped to 155, but specifications stayed essentially the same.

For 1988–1992, the base V-8 in the Formula and Trans Am was the 305-cubic-inch RPO LO3 with a 9.3:1 compression ratio developing 170 horsepower and 225 foot-pounds of torque with electronic fuel injection on an aluminum intake manifold. The VIN engine code was E or F.

The next-most-powerful V-8 for 1982 and 1983 was the 305-cubic-inch RPO LU5 with a 9.5:1 compression ratio developing 165/175 horsepower at 4,200 rpm and 240/250 foot-pounds of torque at 2,400 rpm. The LU5 was equipped with Rochester Crossfire fuel injection controlled by an electronic engine management center. The Crossfire system used two 255-cfm TB401 throttle-body fuel injection units that supplied air/fuel mixture through tuned runners to opposite cylinder banks. The new Crossfire system also included air injection, exhaust gas recirculation (EGR), and a three-way catalytic

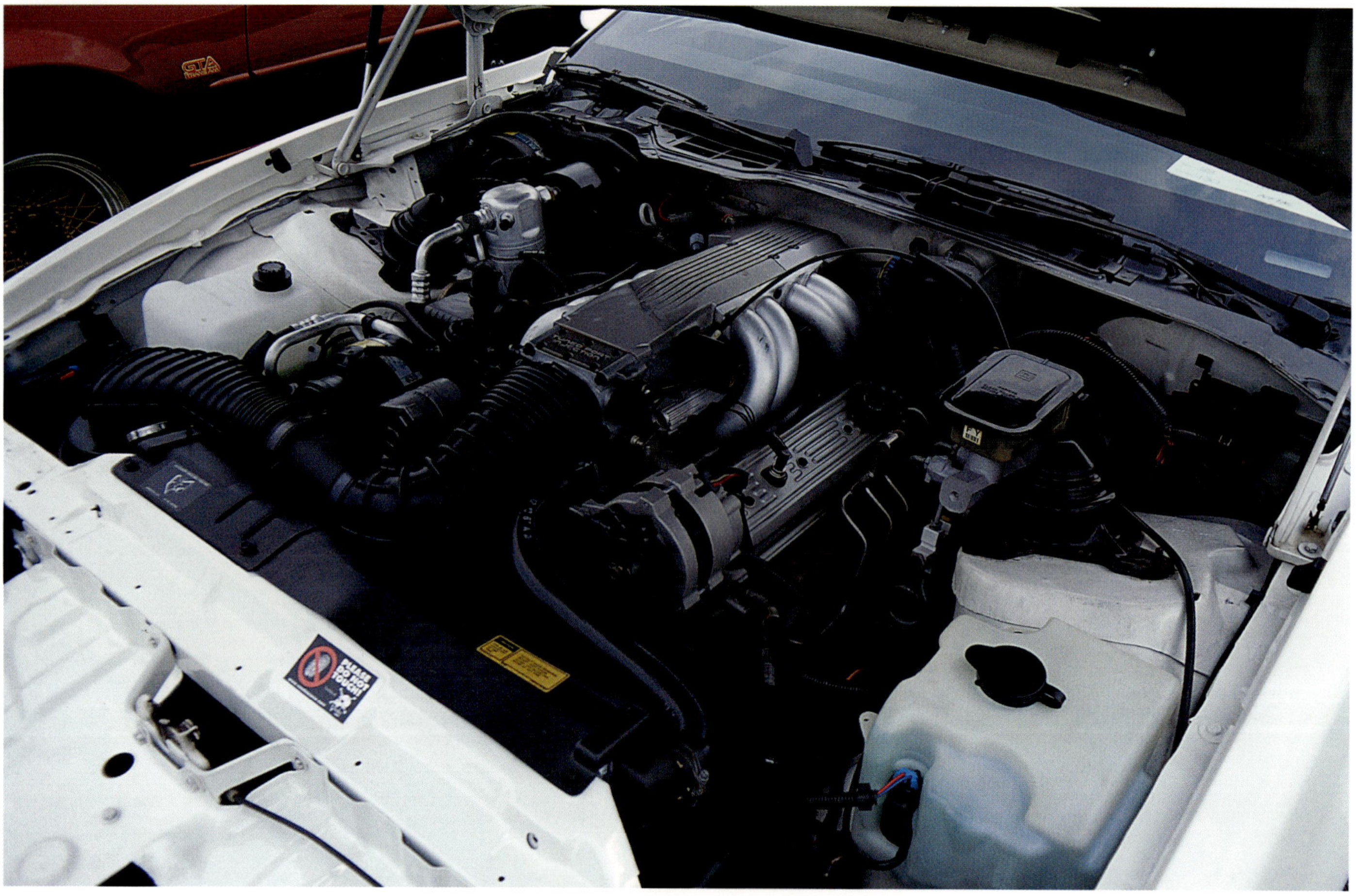

converter. The VIN engine code was 7. For 1984, the LU5 was dropped, and the RPO L69 (HO) was introduced with a four-barrel carburetor and 190 horsepower at 4,800 rpm and 240 foot-pounds of torque at 3,200 rpm. The horsepower was increased to 205 in 1985 and dropped back to 190 for 1986. The L69 was optional in the Trans Am and had a VIN engine code of G.

Another version of the 305 V-8 was introduced in 1985 as the RPO LB9 with a 9.5:1 compression ratio, 205 horsepower, and 275 foot-pounds of torque. The LB9 had electronic tuned-port fuel injection. The VIN engine code was F. The LB9 was used through 1992, and the horsepower increased to as much as 230 when it was optional in the 1986–1992 Trans Am, GTA, and Formula. The horsepower varied on some models depending on the transmission and model application.

The largest overhead-valve V-8 offered in the 1987–1992 Firebird was the 350-cubic-inch (5.7-liter) Chevrolet with a bore and stroke of 4.00x3.48 inches. In 1987, the UPC L98 version was the base engine in the Trans Am GTA and optional in the Trans Am and Formula. The L98 had a 9.5:1 compression ratio and developed 210 horsepower at 4,000 rpm and 315 foot-pounds of torque at 3,200 rpm with electronic tuned-port fuel injection. The L98 also had hydraulic-roller valve lifters, a special hardened-steel camshaft, and a low-restriction exhaust system.

For 1988–1990, the 350 was called a 5.7-liter GTA V-8 (RPO B2L) and was standard in the GTA with automatic transmission and optional in the Trans Am and Formula. The B2L had a 9.3:1 compression ratio and developed 225/235 horsepower and 330 foot-pounds of torque with a low-profile aluminum intake manifold and tuned-port electronic fuel injection. The B2L had a low-restriction exhaust system and a VIN engine code of 8. Horsepower was increased to 240 for 1990–1992 with the addition of the Performance Enhancement Group (RPO WS6), which included dual catalytic converters, engine oil cooler, and performance axle ratio.

Engine Compartment

The firewall, inner fender panels, and radiator support of all 1982–1992 models were finished in body color, as the new unitized body and chassis design was painted as a unit. The fenders were attached with body-color hex-head bolts and washers from the top. The most significant component in the driver-side fenderwell was the large tower mounting the upper attachment of the suspension strut. The conical strut housing was painted semigloss black and attached to the tower with three large studs and cadmium-plated nuts

This is the engine compartment of a white 1988 Firebird Formula 350 equipped with a 350-cubic-inch Chevrolet V-8 with tuned-port electronic fuel injection (RPO B2L) and optional air conditioning.

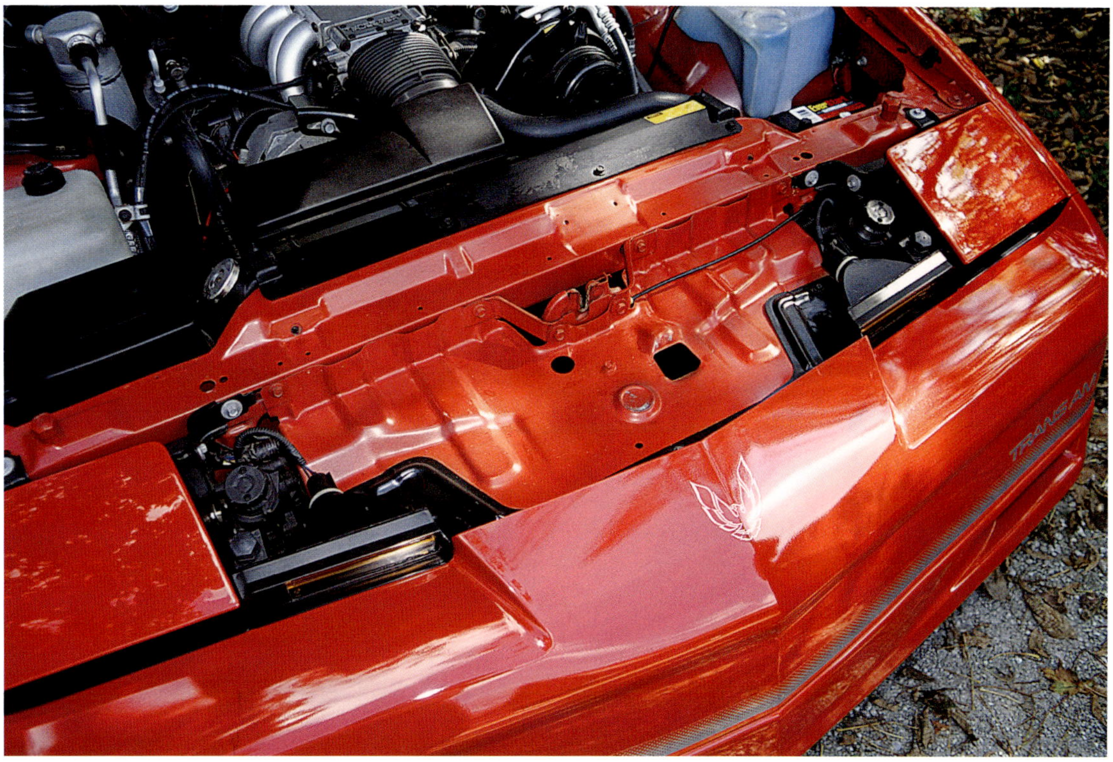

This view of the front valance of the engine compartment of a Bright Red 1986 Trans Am equipped with the 305-cubic-inch Chevrolet V-8 also shows the finish on hood latch and the mounting of the retractable headlight motors.

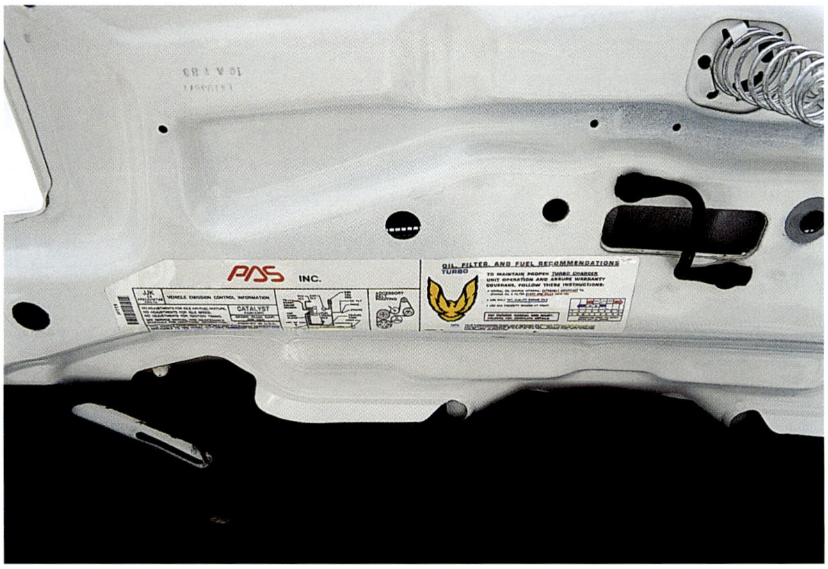

This detail view of the front underside of the hood on a white PAS–built 1989 Turbo Trans AM GTA 20th Anniversary Edition shows the emissions and belt information label with gold bird logo.

through slotted holes used for suspension alignment adjustment. To the front of the strut tower was the molded white plastic windshield-washer reservoir with black plastic cap. The black Delco Freedom battery was mounted at the forward left corner of the engine compartment behind the radiator support.

The horizontal flow radiator had its plated filler cap on the right side and the inlet hose exiting the left side, curving sharply around the front of the alternator mounted on the upper left side of the engine. When air conditioning was present, the compressor was mounted on either the upper left or upper right of the engine, and the alternator was relocated depending on the engine application. On a 1987 GTA with a 305 V-8 engine, the semigloss black compressor was mounted on the upper left and the A/C lines routed toward the front of the engine compartment. The 1989 Formula 350 V-8 had the A/C compressor on the upper right of the engine and lines mounted toward the front right. The standard power steering pump was mounted on the lower left side of the engine. A black plastic shroud was attached to the top of the radiator support, and the flexible black plastic air intake hose was routed across the top of the shroud to the right side of the engine compartment.

The turbocharged V-6 used in the 1989 Special Edition had the turbocharger mounted transversely on the upper right of the engine compartment and the flexible air intake hose routed across the front of the engine to the left side fenderwell. The aluminum induction tubing was routed across the front center of the engine to the intake manifold.

The right front corner of the Firebird engine compartment held the white plastic radiator-overflow reservoir with black plastic cap. The reservoir used on the 1989 turbocharged V-6 had an aluminum insulation shield on the inside to protect it from the heat of the turbocharger. The aluminum shield was mounted just to the outside of the black filler cap, and a hole was provided in the shield for the filler spout. The black plastic emissions system vacuum canister with its hoses and wiring was mounted forward of the coolant reservoir partially under the right front corner of the radiator support. The right fenderwell with black upper strut support was just to the rear of the reservoir.

The passenger-side firewall contained the heater hose connections and hose connections for the air conditioning, if present. The aluminum vertical air-conditioning receiver/dryer was mounted just ahead of the semigloss-black plenum on the right side of the firewall. A large black flexible wiring conduit was routed across the top of the plenum.

The driver (left) side of the firewall held the brake master cylinder and power brake booster, and the windshield-wiper motor was to its right. The master cylinder was a Delco Moraine unit that used part numbers 18009127 w/J50 or 18001926 w/J65 in 1982 and 1983, and part numbers 18014286 w/J50 and 18014287 w/J65 in 1984–1992. The power brake vacuum booster for 1983–1986 used part number 1801911, but the 1987–1992 booster varied according to the engine application and model year. The standard windshield wipers were controlled-cycle variable speed. A semigloss-black wiring junction box and bracket were mounted to the far left side of the firewall. The dual-reservoir master cylinder was bare cast finish, and the reservoir was tan plastic. The master cylinder cap was gloss-black flexible plastic. The body-data code plate was mounted on the upper left side of the firewall with special hex-head screws until 1985, when the information was moved to a printed white decal in the glove compartment. Hood hinges and springs were painted body color along with the hood and body.

Frame, Transmission, and Driveline

All 1982–1992 Firebirds used welded-steel unitized construction with an integral front subframe to support the engine and suspension. The body structure consisted of a welded-steel floorpan and side panels integrating the trunk compartment and rear quarters. All components but the underside of the lower body pan were finished in body color. The lower body floorpan underside was finished in light gray primer with body-color overspray.

Front Suspension

The 1982–1992 Firebird independent front suspension used modified MacPherson struts with lower control arms and nonconcentric coil springs. The upper ends of the MacPherson struts were attached to adjustable semigloss-black towers inside the engine compartment. The Firebird (and concurrent Camaro) system differs from a conventional MacPherson strut design in that the coil springs are not mounted around the struts but between the lower lateral links and the engine/transmission crossmember. This unique design allowed the engineers to lower the front end of the car.

The control arms and coil springs were painted semigloss black, and the same control arms were used on all models. The Firebird front spring rates were 365 pounds (standard) or 548 pounds (optional with Firebird and standard with Trans Am, S/E, and Formula). The standard 1982–1992 Firebird front suspension included a 1.106-inch-diameter (28-millimeter) steel anti-roll bar. A 1.185-inch-diameter (30-millimeter) front stabilizer bar was standard with the 1982–1992 Trans Am, S/E, and Formula (level II suspension). The optional level III suspension with the 1982–1984 UPC WS6 Special Performance Package replaced the standard front bar with a 1.26-inch-diameter (32-millimeter) bar. In 1985, the WS6 package enlarged the front stabilizer bar to 1.34 inches (34 millimeters). In 1991, a larger 1.42-inch (36-millimeter) front bar was available with the WS6 package. All front stabilizer bars were finished in black phosphate and attached with natural steel links and rubber bushings.

The standard front brakes for all 1982–1992 Firebirds were 10.5-inch-diameter vented power discs with single-piston cast-iron-finish calipers and standard metallic pads.

The variable-ratio Saginaw power-assisted steering gear with a recirculating ball design was standard with all models. The standard steering gear ratio was 15/13:1 with the Firebird and 14:1 with the Trans Am and S/E, but with the optional WS6 package, the ratio was quickened to 12.7:1. The power steering gear was natural cast finish with a dull aluminum cover and end plug.

Rear Suspension

The 1982–1984 Firebird rear axle was a Salisbury-type semifloating design with a 7.5-inch ring gear and 10-bolt cover. The axle was available in 1982 with standard ratios and open differential of 2.41:1, 2.73:1, 3.08:1, 3.23:1, and 3.42:1. The ratios available in Safe-T-Track (UPC G80) were 2.73:1, 2.93:1, 3.08:1, and 3.23:1. For 1983, the open 2.73:1 ratio was dropped, and the open differential was available in 2.93:1, 3.08:1, 3.23:1, 3.42:1, and 3.73:1. Safe-T-Track was available with 2.73:1, 2.93:1, 3.08:1, 3.23:1, 3.42:1, and 3.73:1. For 1984, axle codes were changed and standard open differential axle ratios were 3.08:1, 3.23:1, 3.42:1, and 3.73:1. Safe-T-Track ratios were available in 3.08:1, 3.23:1, 3.42:1, and 3.73:1.

The 1985–1990 Firebird had a Salisbury-type semifloating axle with a 7.75-inch ring gear and 10-bolt cover. In 1985, the 7.75-inch axle had ratios of 3.27:1, 3.45:1, and 3.70:1 in open and Safe-T-Track with new codes. An axle with a

7.625-inch ring gear and 10-bolt cover was also available in open and Safe-T-Track ratios of 3.08:1, 3.23:1, 3.42:1, and 3.73:1. Codes and ratios were changed again for 1986, with 7.625-inch axles available in 2.73:1, 3.23:1, 3.42:1, and 3.73:1. The 7.75-inch axle was available with ratios of 2.77:1, 3.08:1, 3.27:1, 3.45:1, and 3.70:1. In 1987–1990, available axle ratios were 2.73:1, 3.08:1, 3.23:1, 3.42:1, and 3.73:1 with the 7.625-inch rear axle. The 7.75-inch axle had ratios of 2.77:1, 3.27:1, and 3.45:1. For 1991 and 1992, the ratios were similar, but the 3.45:1 was dropped.

Axle sizes, ratios, and codes varied each year according to model and engine/transmission configuration. The axle code was stamped on the front passenger side of the axle tube or on an identification tag attached to the carrier cover. The rear axle assembly was painted semigloss black and had paint codes identifying the various configurations.

The 1982–1992 Firebird rear suspension was completely redesigned from the previous year and consisted of outboard semitrailing lower control arms with coil springs, tubular shock absorbers, and an aft-mounted track (Panhard) bar to stabilize the axle location. The rear suspension also included a semigloss-black-painted torque arm, linking the transmission and rear axle, to control windup. The standard Firebird rear suspension (level I) did not include a stabilizer bar. In 1982 and 1983, the Firebird S/E and Trans Am standard Rally-tuned rear suspension (level II, RPO Y99) had a 12-millimeter-diameter (0.47-inch) rear stabilizer bar. The optional level III suspension (RPO WS6) upgraded the bar to a 21-millimeter (0.829-inch) rear bar. For 1984, the WS6 package included a 23-millimeter (0.908-inch) rear bar. For 1985–1992, the rear stabilizer bar was increased in size to 23 millimeters for the Y99 package and 24 millimeters (0.948 inch) for the WS6. The 1987–1992 Trans Am GTA had the WS6 suspension as standard equipment. The rear stabilizer bar was natural steel finish.

The standard rear brakes on all 1982–1992 Firebirds were drum-type hydraulic with 9.5-inch cast-iron drums. Standard asbestos linings were 2 inches wide. Brake drums and backing plates were painted semigloss black. The 1982–1992 optional WS6 Special Performance Package included rear disc brakes (four-wheel power-assisted) as standard equipment. The vented rear rotors were 10.5 inches in diameter and worked in conjunction with single-piston calipers. Four-wheel power disc brakes were also standard with the 1983 Trans Am Recaro Special Edition. The four-wheel power disc brakes were optional on other models with RPO J65.

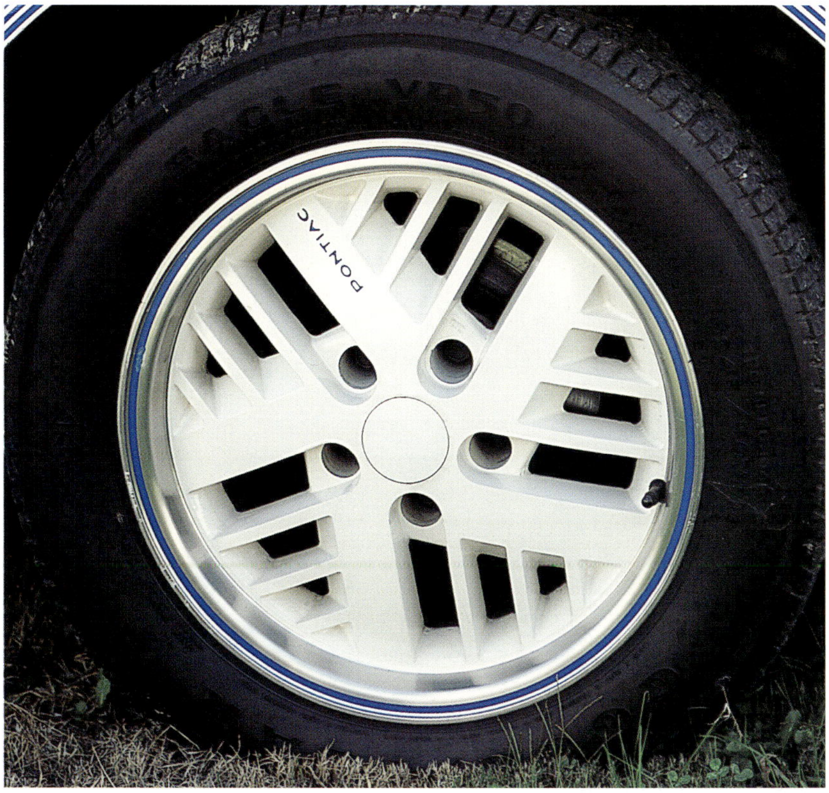

This right front wheel on a 1984 Trans Am 15th Anniversary Edition is a white 16-inch High-Tech cast aluminum (RPO N78).

Tires and Wheels

The standard wheels for the 1982 base Firebird were 14x6J steel wheels with five lug nuts. The standard steel wheels were finished in gloss black enamel if full Rally V wheel covers (RPO PE5) were used, and lower body-color gloss enamel on the front side, only if the standard small hubcaps (RPO P20) were supplied. Bright wheel trim rings were optional with the small hubcaps (RPO P06). Wire-wheel covers were also available on the base Firebird with RPO N91.

Standard wheels for the 1982 Firebird Special Edition were 14-inch Turbo cast-aluminum with body-color flush covers (RPO N90). The 1982 Trans Am used the same 14-inch Turbo cast-aluminum wheels but with black covers. Both wheel covers had a red Pontiac arrowhead in the center. The 1982 Trans Am Recaro edition used gold-color 15x7 Turbo cast-aluminum wheels (RPO N24). The Turbo cast-aluminum wheels were not available with the base Firebird.

Firebird standard wheels for 1983 were 14-inch Rally wheels with black caps and lug nuts. Standard painted steel wheels were also available with small hubcaps and optional trim rings, PE5 Rally V wheel covers, or N91 wire-wheel covers. Standard wheels for the 1983 Firebird S/E were 14-inch Turbo cast-aluminum with body-color caps (RPO N90). The Trans Am used similar Turbo cast-aluminum wheels with a black cover. The Trans Am Recaro edition had 15-inch gold-finish Turbo finned-aluminum wheels (RPO N24). The 1983 25th Anniversary Daytona 500

Limited Edition Trans Am had 15x7 Turbo Aero-aluminum wheels. The cast-aluminum wheels were not available on the base Firebird.

For 1984, the standard Firebird wheels were 14x6 Rally with black center caps and black lug nuts. Painted steel wheels were also available with hubcaps and trim rings, UPC P02 five-port wheel covers, or N91 wire-wheel covers. Standard wheels on the Firebird S/E were 14-inch Turbo cast-aluminum with body-color caps (RPO N89). The Trans Am had standard 14-inch Turbo cast-aluminum wheels with black covers. The Trans Am Recaro Edition had 15x7 Turbo finned-aluminum wheels (N24). The 1984 15th Anniversary Trans Am had standard 16x7 High Tech cast-aluminum wheels finished in white (RPO N78).

The 1985 standard Firebird wheels were 14x6 Rally wheels with black caps and black lug nuts. Painted steel wheels were still available with hubcaps and trim rings or five-port wheel covers. The S/E standard wheels were 14x7 deep-dish High Tech aluminum with light chestnut or charcoal finish (RPO N24). Trans Am standard wheels were 15x7 diamond-spoke (RPO N90, PE1). For 1986, the standard Firebird wheels were 15-inch Rally II, but painted steel wheels were still available with hubcaps and trim rings or five-port wheel covers. S/E standard wheels were 15-inch diamond-spoke aluminum (RPO N90). The Trans Am had deep-dish 15x7 High Tech Turbo wheels in gold or silver finish (RPO N24).

The 1987 standard Formula wheels were 16x8 High Tech aluminum (RPO N96). Trans Am wheels were 15x7 gold-and-silver-finish High Tech Turbo cast-aluminum (RPO N24). GTA standard wheels were 15x8 diamond-spoke in gold or silver (RPO N90). For 1988, standard Firebird wheels were 15x7 deep-dish High Tech Turbo cast-aluminum (RPO N24). The 1988 Formula standard wheels were 16x8 High Tech Turbo cast-aluminum (RPO N96) that were also standard with the WS6 package. Standard Trans Am wheels were 15x7 deep-dish High Tech Turbo cast-aluminum or diamond-spoke. GTA wheels were gold-finish lightweight diamond-spoke cast-aluminum (RPO PW7).

The 1989 Firebird wheels were 15-inch High Tech Turbo cast-aluminum. The Formula had standard 16-inch deep-dish Turbo cast-aluminum wheels. The Trans Am had 15x7 High Tech Turbo cast-aluminum, and the Trans Am 20th Anniversary Edition had 16-inch gold lightweight diamond-spoke wheels. The GTA had standard 16-inch lightweight cross-laced aluminum wheels.

For 1990, the standard Firebird had 15-inch High Tech Turbo cast-aluminum wheels with locks. The Formula had 16-inch deep-dish High Tech Turbo cast-aluminum wheels with locks. The Trans Am had standard 15-inch deep-dish High Tech Turbo wheels with machined faces and charcoal ports. The GTA standard wheels were diamond-spoke aluminum. The 1991 standard Firebird wheels were 15x7 High Tech cast-aluminum. The Formula had 16x8 deep-dish High Tech Turbo cast-aluminum. The Trans Am and GTA came with 16x8 diamond-spoke wheels.

For 1992, standard Firebird wheels were 15-inch High Tech Turbo cast-aluminum. The Formula had 16x7 deep-dish High Tech aluminum, and the Trans Am had 16x8-inch diamond-spoke cast-aluminum.

Optional wheels for the 1982 Firebird included gold and silver cast-aluminum (RPO N90), available on all but the base Firebird. The 15x7 finned Turbo cast-aluminum wheels (RPO N24) were available with the WS6 package. Bright aluminum hubcaps (RPO P20) were available with the Firebird S/E and Trans Am only with the WS6 or WS7 package.

For 1983, optional wheels included silver cast-aluminum wheels (RPO N90) or finned Turbo cast-aluminum wheels (RPO N24) available with the base Firebird with the Y99 package and available with the Trans Am and S/E replacing the standard Turbo cast-aluminum wheels. For 1984, Turbo Aero cast-aluminum wheels (RPO N89) were available with the Firebird S/E and Trans Am. Finned Turbo cast-aluminum wheels (RPO N24)

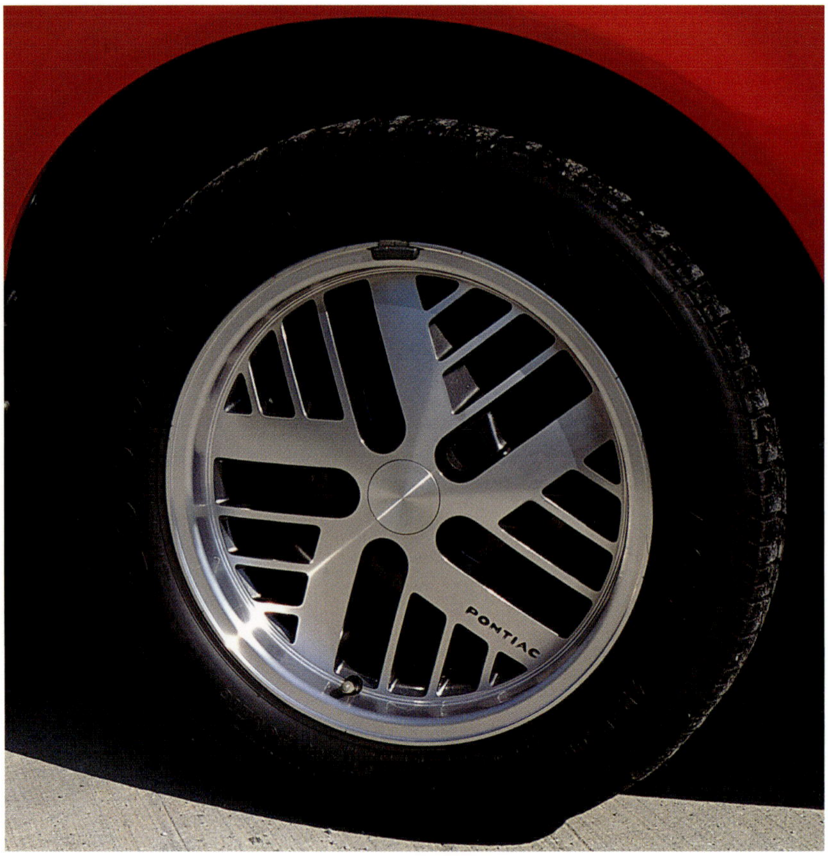

This is a detail view of a silver 15x7 High-Tech Turbo cast-aluminum wheel on a Bright Red 1986 Trans Am (RPO N24).

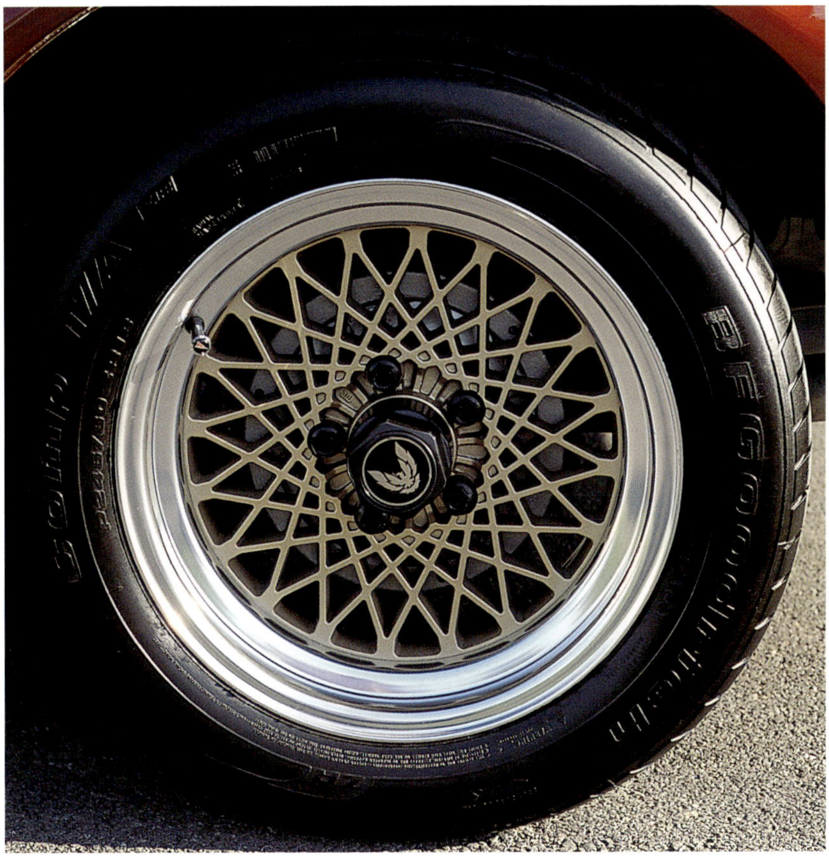

This is a detail view of a gold-finish deep-dish 16x8 diamond-spoke cast-aluminum wheel (RPO PW7) that is standard on this Flame Red Metallic 1987 Trans Am GTA sport coupe. Note the gold-and-black bird medallion in the center.

were available with the S/E, Trans Am, and base Firebird without the WS6 and WS7 packages.

Optional wheels for 1985 were 14-inch cast-aluminum diamond-spoke (RPO PE1) available on the Firebird and S/E. The S/E, Trans Am, and base Firebird with Y99 packages had the 15-inch cast-aluminum diamond-spoke wheels (RPO N90) that were required with the Y99 package. Cast-aluminum 15-inch deep-dish High Tech Turbo wheels (RPO N24) were required with the Y99 package. Cast-aluminum 16-inch High Tech wheels (RPO N96) required the WS6 package on the Trans Am.

In 1986 and 1987, 14-inch cast-aluminum diamond-spoke wheels (RPO PE1) were available on the base Firebird and S/E. The diamond-spoke wheels are sometimes referred to as "cross-laced" wheels. Cast-aluminum 15-inch diamond-spoke wheels were required with the Y99 package and available with RPO N90. RPO N24, along with the required Y99 package, brought 15-inch cast-aluminum deep-dish High Tech Turbo wheels. Cast-aluminum 16-inch High Tech Turbo wheels were available with RPO N96. The same choices were available in 1987 with the N24 and N90 wheels color-coordinated and with anti-theft lock packages.

For 1988 and 1989, deep-dish 15-inch charcoal High Tech cast-aluminum wheels with locks were available with RPO N24 on all but the Formula and GTA. Cast-aluminum diamond-spoke wheels were also available in 15- and 16-inch sizes. RPO PW7 16-inch diamond-spoke cast-aluminum wheels with anti-theft lock package in black, silver, or gold were available with the GTA and Trans Am.

In 1990 and 1991, 15-inch deep-dish charcoal High Tech cast-aluminum wheels (RPO N24) were available on all but the Formula and GTA. Deep-dish 16-inch High Tech Turbo cast-aluminum wheels with locks were available with RPO PE0. RPO PW7 brought 16-inch color-coordinated diamond-spoke cast-aluminum wheels with locks. For 1992, these were charcoal on the Trans Am and Formula and gold on the GTA. The 1992 Trans Am convertible had RPO 52P gold diamond-spoke wheels with gold decals, with the beige convertible roof only.

The standard tires for the 1982 base Firebird were 195/75R14 glass-belted black sidewall. The 1982 Special Edition and Trans Am had 205/70R14 steel-belted black-sidewall tires. Standard tires for the 1982 Trans Am Recaro edition were 215/65R15 steel-belted black sidewall. The 1983 base Firebird still had 195/75R14 glass-belted black-sidewall tires. The 1983 Special Edition had standard 215/65R15 steel-belted black-sidewall tires. The 1983 Trans Am had standard 205/70R14 black-sidewall steel-belted tires, but the Recaro Special Edition Trans Am and 25th Anniversary Daytona 500 Special Edition had 215/65R15 black sidewall. The 1984 base Firebird standard tires were 195/75R14 steel-belted black sidewall, and the Special Edition and Trans Am had 205/70R14. The WS6 Special Performance Package included Goodyear Eagle GT

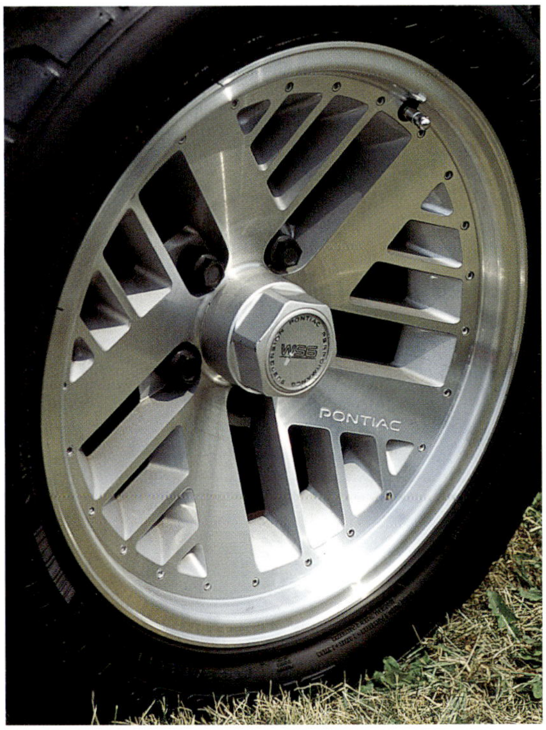

This is a detail view of the standard 16x8 High-Tech Turbo cast-aluminum wheel on a white 1988 Firebird Formula. The center cap has a logo for the WS6 Performance Suspension Package.

215/65R15 black-sidewall steel-belted tires in all three years. The Firebird with the Y99 package included 205/70R14 black-sidewall tires. White-letter performance tires were also available in various sizes. A space-saver spare was standard with all models.

Standard base Firebird tires for 1985 were 195/75R14 steel-belted black sidewall. The S/E had 205/70R14 steel-belted black-sidewall tires, and the Trans Am had 215/65R15 steel-belted black sidewall. Trans Ams with the optional L69 or LB9 engine had 235/60VR15 black sidewall, and the Trans Am with the WS6 package included 245/50VR16 Goodyear Eagle GT black-sidewall tires. White-letter performance tires were also available in various sizes. A space-saver spare was standard with all models.

For 1986, standard Firebird, S/E, and Trans Am tires were 215/65R15 black-sidewall steel-belted radials. The previous 195/75R14 tires in black sidewall, white sidewall, or white letter were also available with the standard steel wheels. The 205/70R14 black-sidewall, white-sidewall, or white-letter tires were also available as an option. The Trans Am with the L69 or LB9 engine had standard 235/65R15 black sidewall, and the WS6 package on the Trans Am included 245/50VR15 black-sidewall tires. A space-saver spare was standard with all models.

The 1987–1992 Firebird had standard 215/65R15 black-sidewall steel-belted radials, and the Formula had 245/50VR16 Goodyear Eagle GT black-sidewall tires. Standard tires on the 1987–1992 Trans Am were 215/65R15 steel-belted black sidewall. The 1987 GTA had standard 245/50VR15 Goodyear black-sidewall radials. The 1988–1992 GTA tires were upgraded to 245/50ZR16 steel-belted black-sidewall radials. The WS6 package included 245/50VR16 black-sidewall steel-belted radials. A space-saver spare was standard with all models.

Transmissions

The 1982–1992 Firebirds were equipped with a variety of transmission choices depending upon the year, model, and engine. In 1982, the standard transmission in the Firebird was a four-speed manual with Pontiac floor-shift linkage. The Muncie four-speed was standard in the Firebird and optional (RPO MM4) in the S/E with the 2.5-liter four-cylinder. The four-speed was standard in the S/E with the 2.8-liter V-6 (not available in California) and standard in the Trans Am with the 305 V-8 and four-barrel carburetor. The LG4 V-8 came with a four-speed that was not available with the Crossfire fuel-injected LU5 305 V-8.

For 1983 and 1984, the four-speed manual transmission was still standard with the 2.5-liter four-cylinder. However, the V-6 and V-8 engines had a five-speed manual transmission that was standard with the S/E and LL1 V-6 and with the Trans Am with the LG4 305 V-8 and optional (RPO MM5) on the S/E with the 305 V-8. The five-speed was also optional with the four-cylinder engine in the base Firebird.

In 1985 and 1986, the four-speed manual transmission was no longer available, and the five-speed manual became the standard transmission for the four-cylinder Firebird, S/E with the LB8 V-6, and Trans Am with the LG4 and L69 305 V-8s. The five-speed manual was optional with the V-6 in the base Firebird.

For 1987–1991, the four-cylinder engine was no longer available. The standard transmission for the Firebird, Formula, and Trans Am with 2.8-liter V-6 and 5.0-liter V-8 was the five-speed manual with Pontiac floor shifter. The 5.7-liter V-8 standard in the GTA was not available with a manual transmission.

The only automatic transmission available with the 1982 Firebird line was the General Motors three-speed Turbo Hydra-Matic 200. The three-speed automatic was optional on the 2.5-liter four-cylinder Firebird, V-6 S/E, and Trans Am with the LG4 V-8, and optional with the V-6 and LG4 V-8 in the Firebird. The LU5 V-8 was available only with the three-speed automatic transmission. The Turbo 200 transmission had an eight-digit code located below the build date on an identification plate on the right side of the transmission case. The code identified the year, vehicle application, and month built.

In 1983, the three-speed Turbo Hydra-Matic 200 was optional (RPO MX1) with the 2.5-liter four-cylinder and 2.8-liter V-6. A new four-speed 700-R4 four-speed automatic was optional (RPO MD8) with the V-6 and 305 V-8. For 1984–1992, the 700-R4 four-speed automatic became optional with all engines (except the 1989 231-ci Turbo Trans Am V-6), and the three-speed automatic was dropped. The four-speed automatic transmission had a transmission code on the right rear of the oil pan that included the year, model, Julian build date, and shift. The 1989 20th Anniversary Turbo Trans Am used a 200-R4 automatic transmission built at the GM Three Rivers assembly plant. The 200-R4 had an application code of TAF and a transmission code on the right side of the case. All Turbo Hydra-Matic transmission cases were natural aluminum with a gloss-black oil pan and converter pan. All Trans Am GTA models had a standard-equipment transmission oil cooler.

All transmissions were connected to the rear axle by a natural-finish one-piece welded-steel driveshaft.

Chapter 6

1993–2002

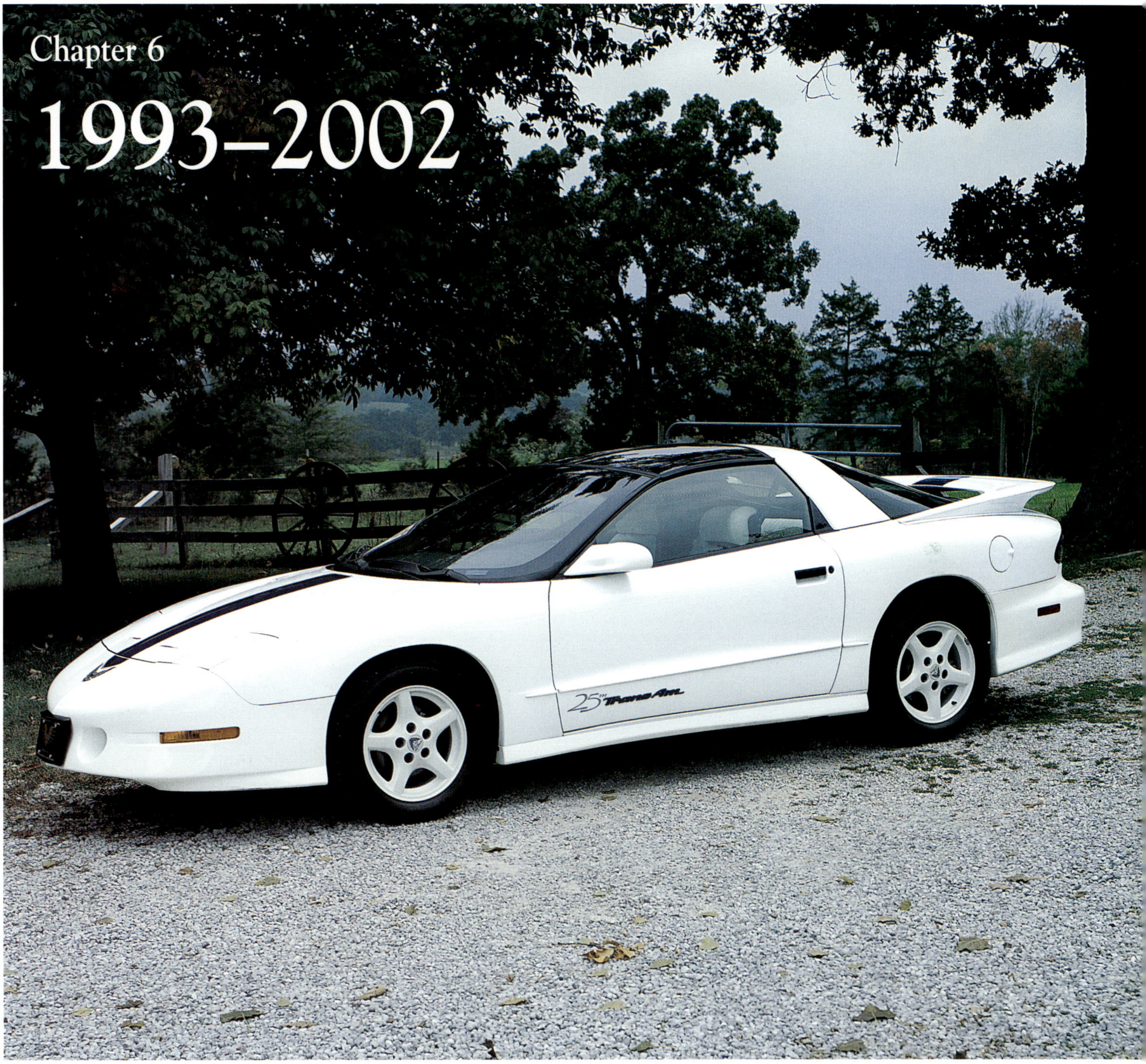

This white 1994 Trans Am GT 25th Anniversary Edition hatchback coupe (FV2) is an example of the fourth-generation Firebird and Trans Am styling introduced in the 1993 model year. The new design used the same wheelbase as the previous model, but the body and chassis structure were totally new.

The new Firebird, introduced for the 1993 model year, represented a significant restyling effort and was 90 percent a totally new car from top to bottom compared to the 1992 model. Development of the new fourth-generation Firebird was late compared to previous years, with production beginning at the St. Therese, Quebec, Canada, plant in November 1992. Delivery to Pontiac dealer showrooms did not take place until early in calendar-year 1993.

Although changes for the fourth-generation Firebird were carried across all aspects of the new car, the radical styling under the direction of Chief Designer John R. (Jack) Folden was the most obvious. It was clear that the styling of the new Firebird was based on two distinctive GM concept cars: the 1988 Banshee IV concept car, described as a "futuristic performance coupe," and the 1989 ACC "California" Camaro designed by GM's Advanced Concept Center in Thousand Oaks, California. The front fascia was uniquely rounded, with a deeply sloping hood and an integrated, deeply sculpted front air dam. The new design had concealed headlamps with no visible grille opening (Trans Am only) and featured low recessed round running lights on either side of the sharply pointed nose. The sculpted body sides flowed smoothly into the aero

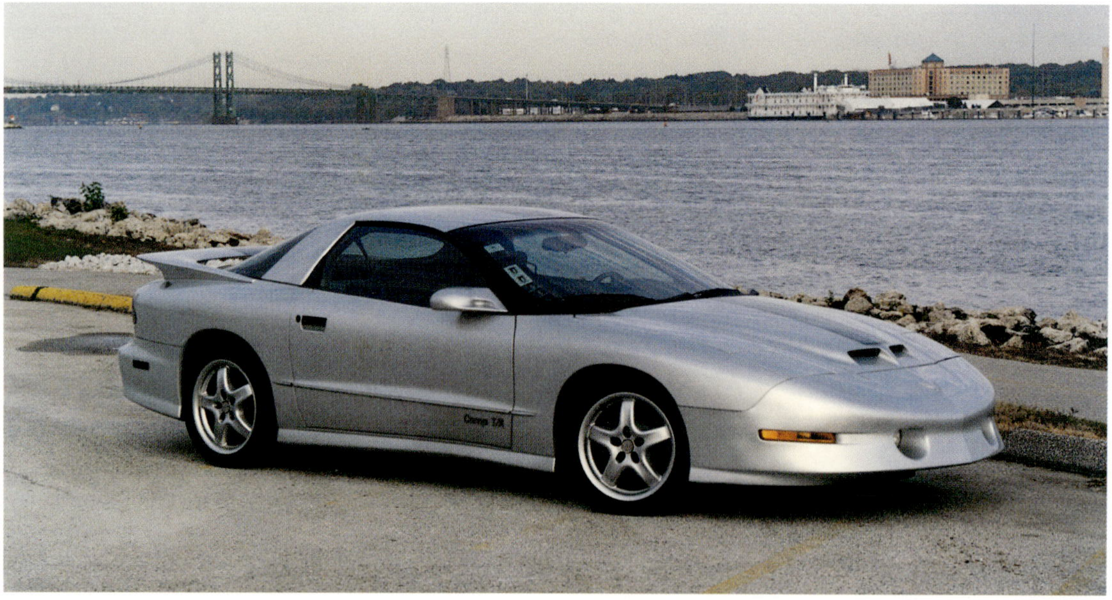

This is a right front quarter view of a Bright Silver Metallic 1995 Trans Am Comp T/A hatchback coupe. The Comp T/A had a list of special equipment including B.F. Goodrich Comp T/A tires, 17x9 Speedline wheels, and unique graphics. Only 72 Comp T/As were built in 1995. The hood inlet design differed from the SLP Firehawk and Pontiac's Ram Air version. This is the first mule car used for development. *Dean Fait*

rear spoiler. The new body used a combination of steel and composite (sheet-molded compound and reaction-injection-molded polyurea) panels for lighter overall weight. The Firebird bodies were finished in a modern durable basecoat/ clearcoat acrylic urethane paint system. The new interior design offered increased head, leg, and hip room, and the rear compartment provided increased cargo capacity.

Mechanically, the new Firebird was based on the previous front-engine rear-drive design, but improvements were made in every area of the chassis and drivetrain. The wheelbase maintained the same 101 inches as the 1992 model, while the overall length was increased. The width was slightly more than the 1992 model, and the height was increased about 2.3 inches. The front suspension was redesigned to use a high-arm

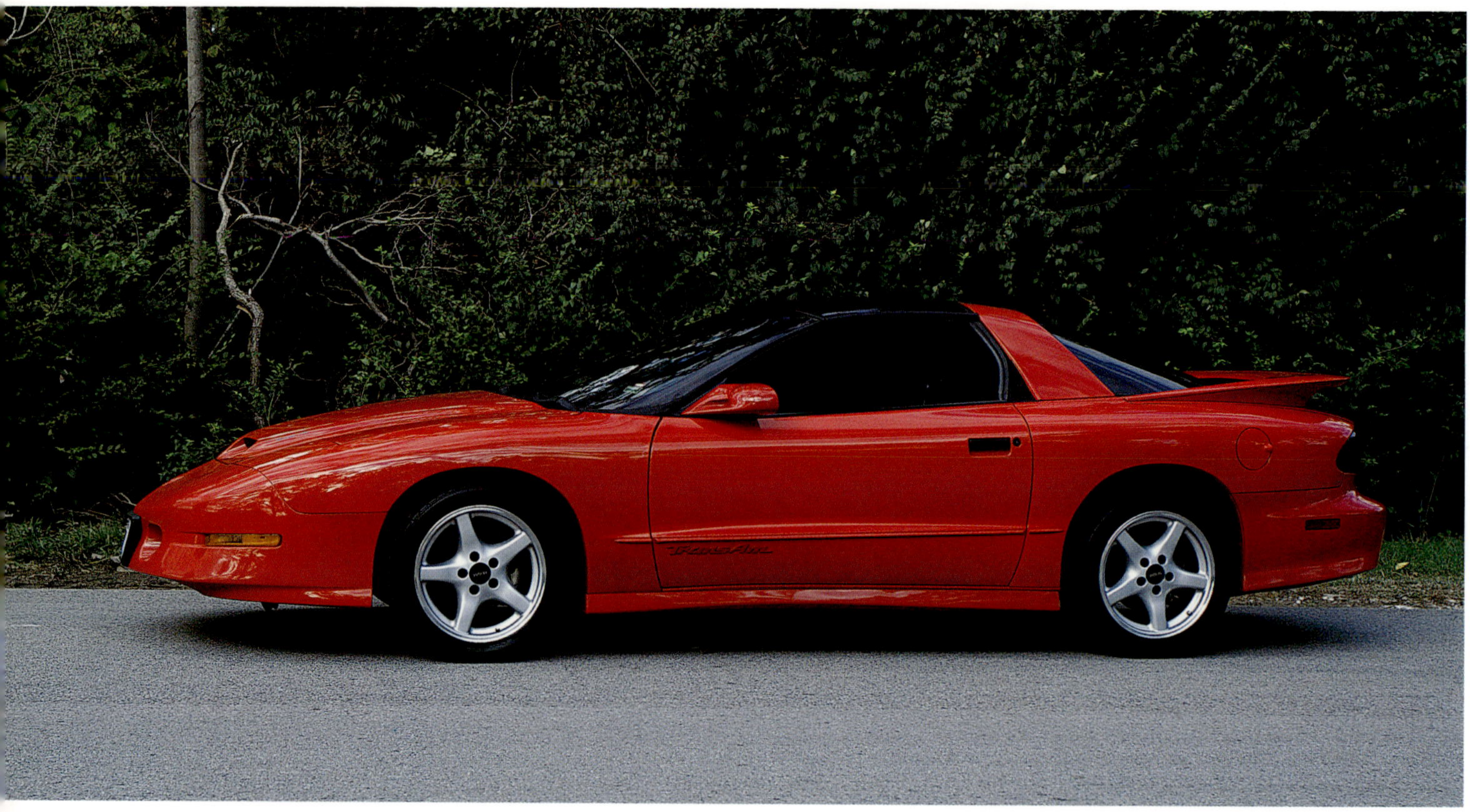

This left side view of a Bright Red (81) 1996 Trans Am equipped with a 5.7-liter Ram Air V-8 shows the lines of the body that includes molded composite components for all but the left and right rear quarters. This Trans Am has an optional T-top hatch roof.

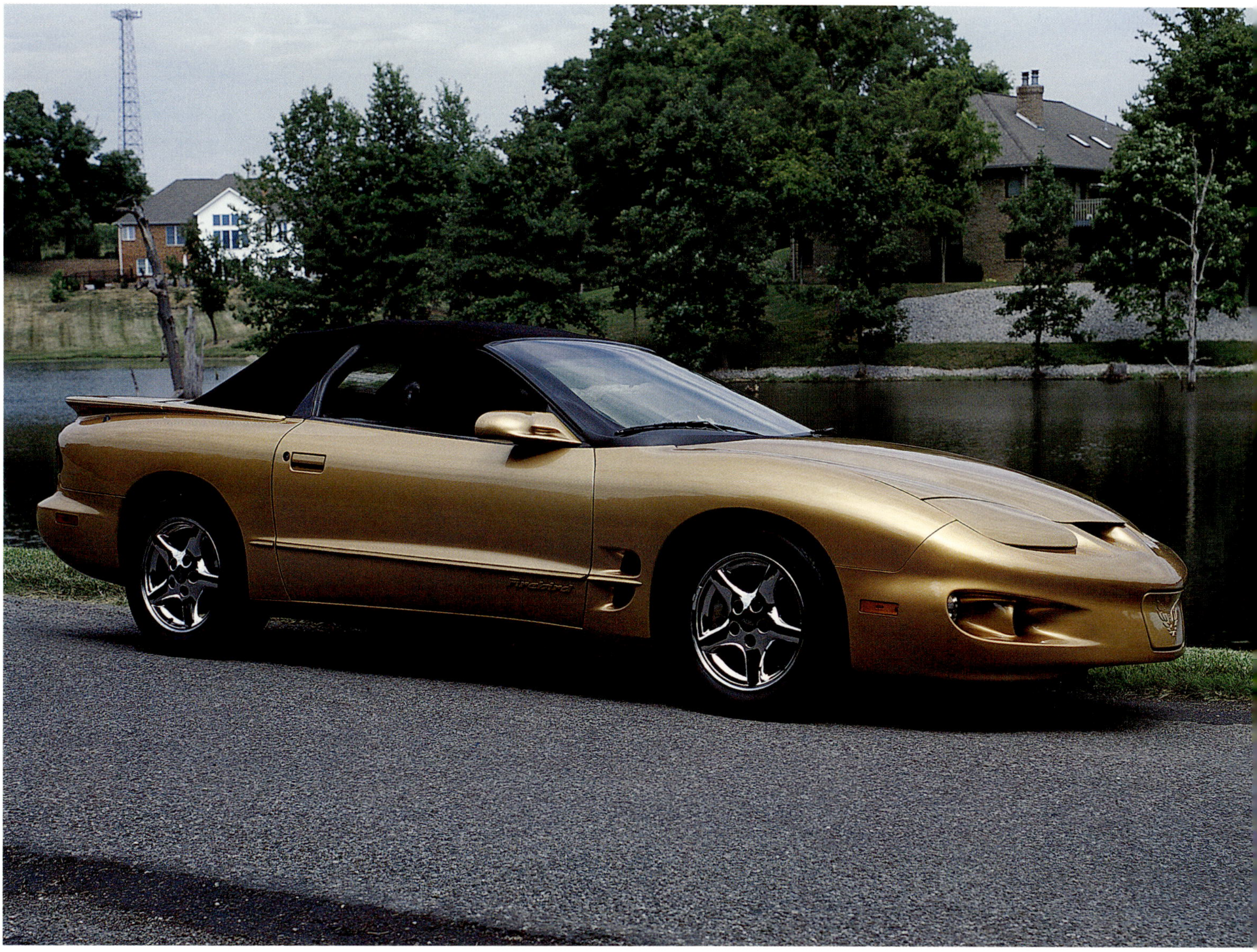

This Sport Gold Metallic (63) 1998 Firebird convertible (S67V) is one of only 704 Firebird convertibles built for the 1998 model year. It has a standard 231-cubic-inch V-6 engine and the body-color Firebird nameplate on the door.

short/long arm (SLA) upper and lower control arm design with power-assisted rack-and-pinion steering. Rear suspension included dual lower trailing links and a torque arm with coil springs. All models ran on standard 16-inch wheels with anti-lock braking (ABS), and the entire package was decidedly stiffer with less torsional stress.

As an illustration of the performance potential of the fourth-generation Firebirds, they were selected for use in the 1996 International Race of Champions (IROC) Series. These twenty-four specially built race cars were constructed around full-tube chassis designs and had 500-horsepower LT1 V-8 engines.

The model lineup for 1993–2002 consisted of the base Firebird (S/F), Formula (2/F), Trans Am (F/V), and 1994 Trans Am GT, with later variations of collector and anniversary editions, NHRA package, Harley Davidson Edition, pace car editions, and additional special Street Legal Performance (SLP) Firehawk and GT models, all with distinctive individual styling and/or trim details. There were also the special silver-finish 1995–1997 Comp T/A models. The new Firebird was available in sport coupe with and without T-top roof in all years, and in convertible models from 1994 to 2002. Engine choices consisted of the base 160-horsepower 231-cubic-inch (3.8-liter) V-6 and the 350-cubic-inch (5.7-liter) V-8, which delivered 270 horsepower for the standard 1993 V-8 and 325 horsepower for the 2001 and 2002 Ram Air version.

There were two manual transmissions and two automatic transmissions available with the 1993–2002 Firebirds. The Firebird with V-6 had a standard aluminum-case Borg-Warner T5 five-speed. The Formula and Trans Am V-8 had two variations of a new Borg-Warner T56 six-speed manual transmission. Both transmissions were equipped with a floor shift synchronized in all speeds. A 4L60 or 4L60-E four-speed Turbo Hydra-Matic was optional with all engines and models and was standard with the 1995–2002 Formula and Trans Am.

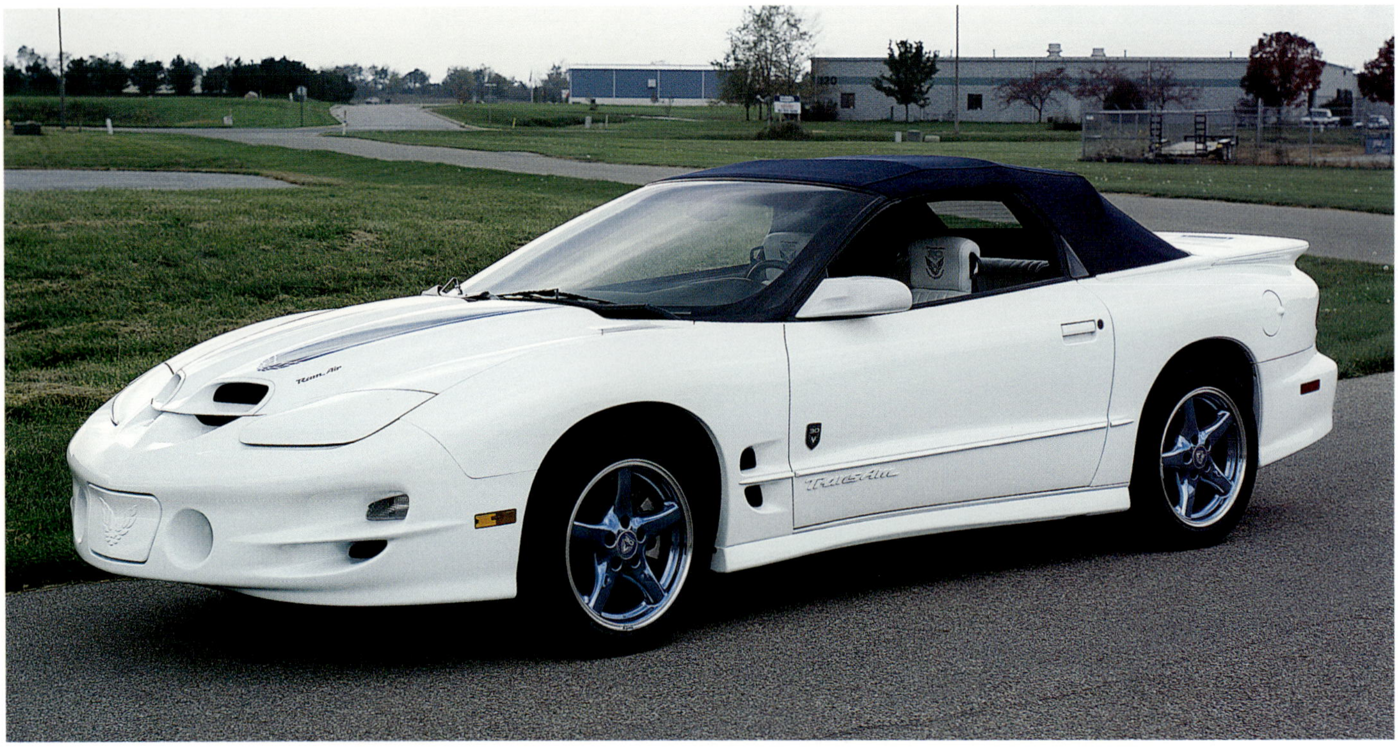

Above: This 1999 Trans Am convertible 30th Anniversary Edition includes the WS6 performance package, distinctive blue-tinted wheels, white upholstery with blue trim, a blue convertible top, and special graphics. There were 535 30th Anniversary Trans Am convertibles built in the 1999 model year. ***Below:*** The 1999 Trans Am 30th Anniversary Edition was also available as a hatchback coupe. This coupe had the same unique features as the convertible and was finished in Arctic White (10) with 17-inch blue-tinted wheels and white interior trim with blue accents. There were 1,065 30th Anniversary Trans Am coupes built for the 1999 model year.

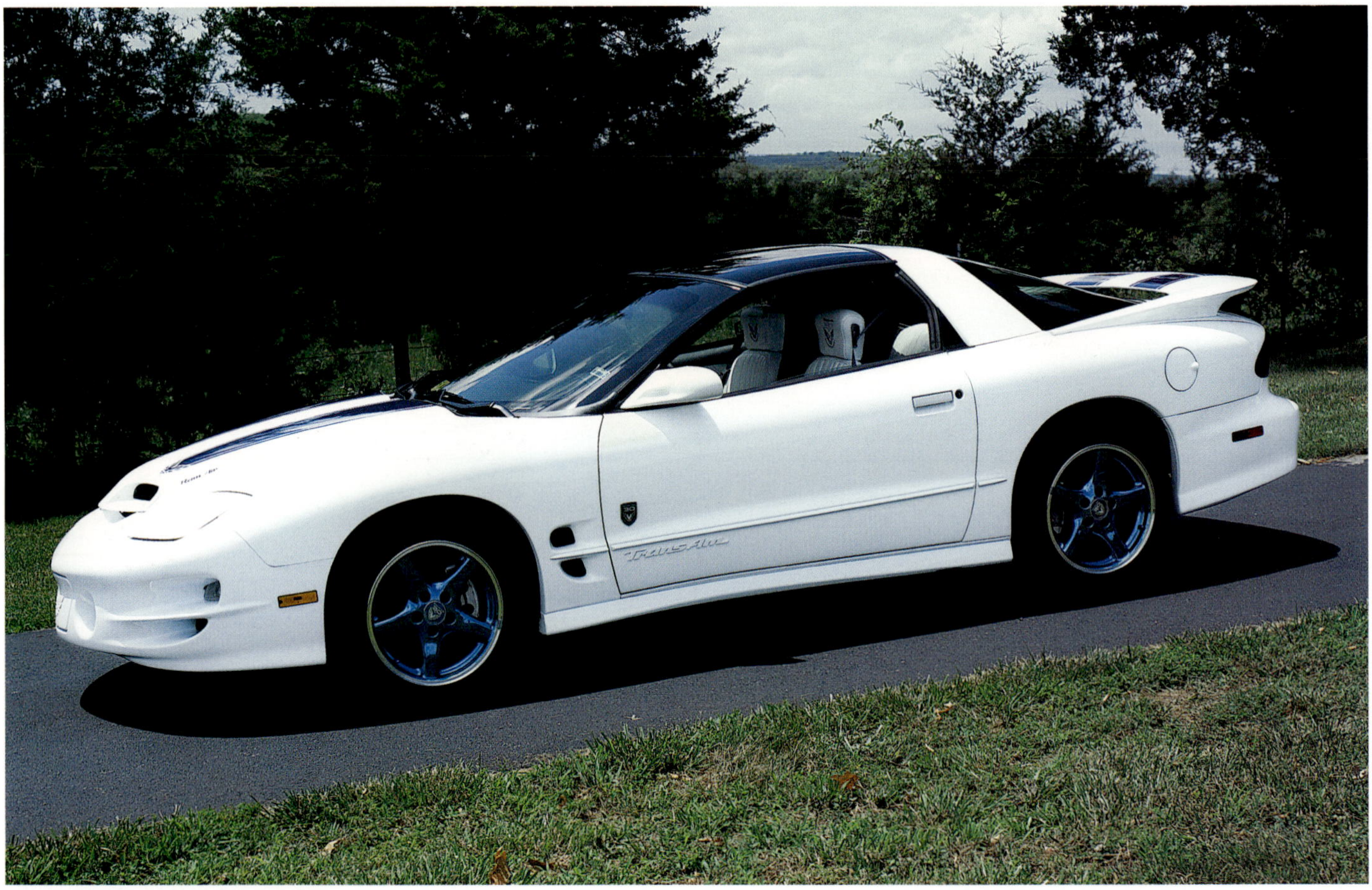

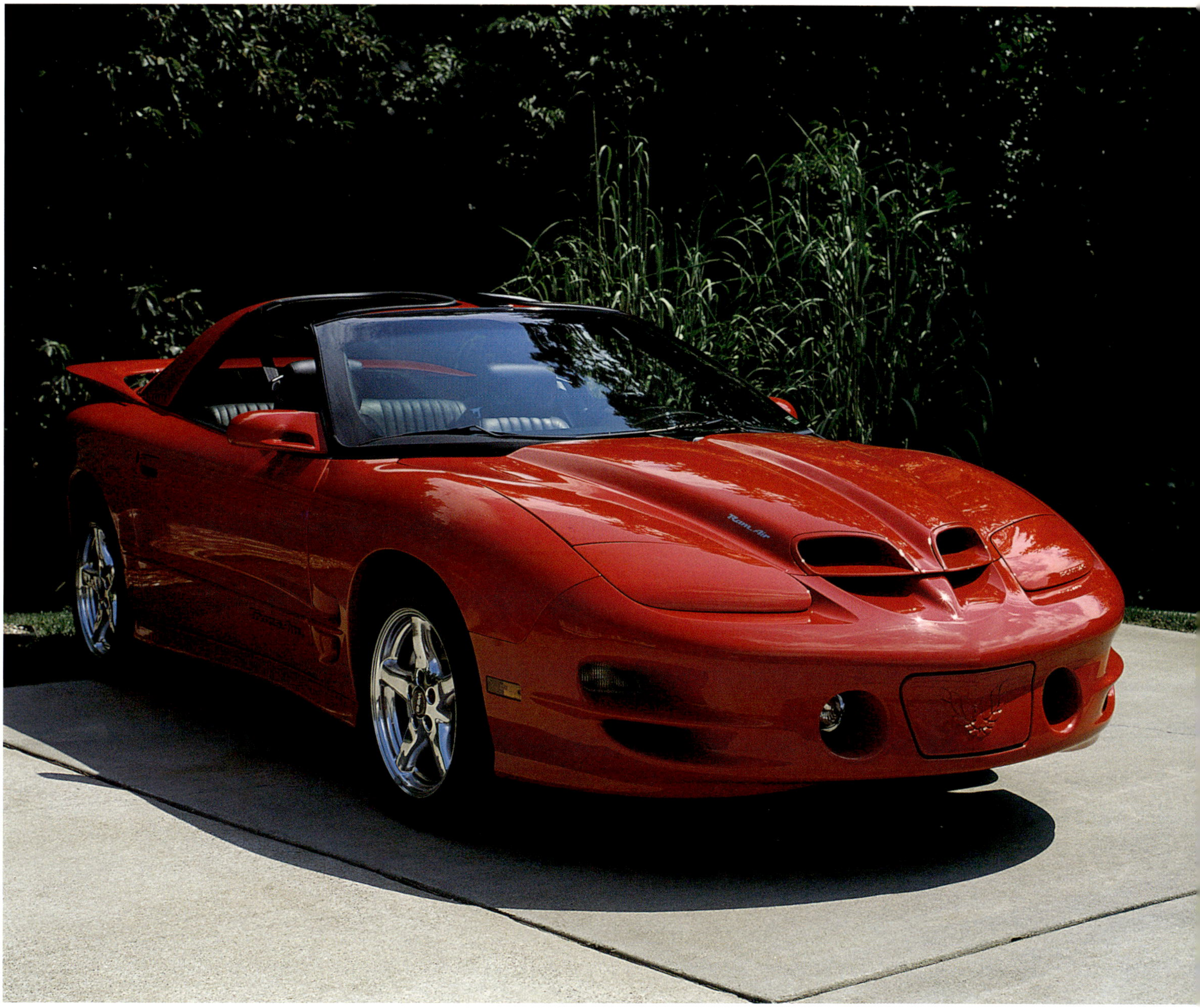

This right front quarter view of a Bright Red 2000 Trans Am Ram Air WS6 hatchback coupe with T-top shows the new front fascia and air intake styling for the 1998–2002 Trans Ams.

The 1993 Firebird was available with eight body-color choices. For 1994–1998, there were 10 exterior colors each year. There were nine exterior colors available in 1999 and eight in each of 2000–2002. There were generally three to five interior trim combinations available in cloth and leather for all years and models. Convertible tops were available in three colors.

Total Firebird production was 14,112 for 1993; 45,922 for 1994; 50,987 in 1995; 30,982 in 1996; 30,756 in 1997; 32,155 for 1998; 36,219 in 1999; 31,826 in 2000; 21,436 in 2001; and 30,690 for 2002 (the final year of production). All Firebird production ended at the St. Therese plant in September 2002.

Body Sheet Metal and Trim

The 1993–2002 Firebird continued the unitized-construction concept of previous Firebirds, but the latest execution included a monocoque construction with overall body rigidity being increased 20 percent. The windshield was angled at 68 degrees, giving a sleeker and more aerodynamic appearance to the design, helping to provide a drag coefficient of 0.32. The new body construction consisted of the steel floorpan with virtually straight frame rails and integral roof and door-opening structures. The only visible outer steel panels were the rear quarters and the hood. The roof panel was shared with the fourth-generation

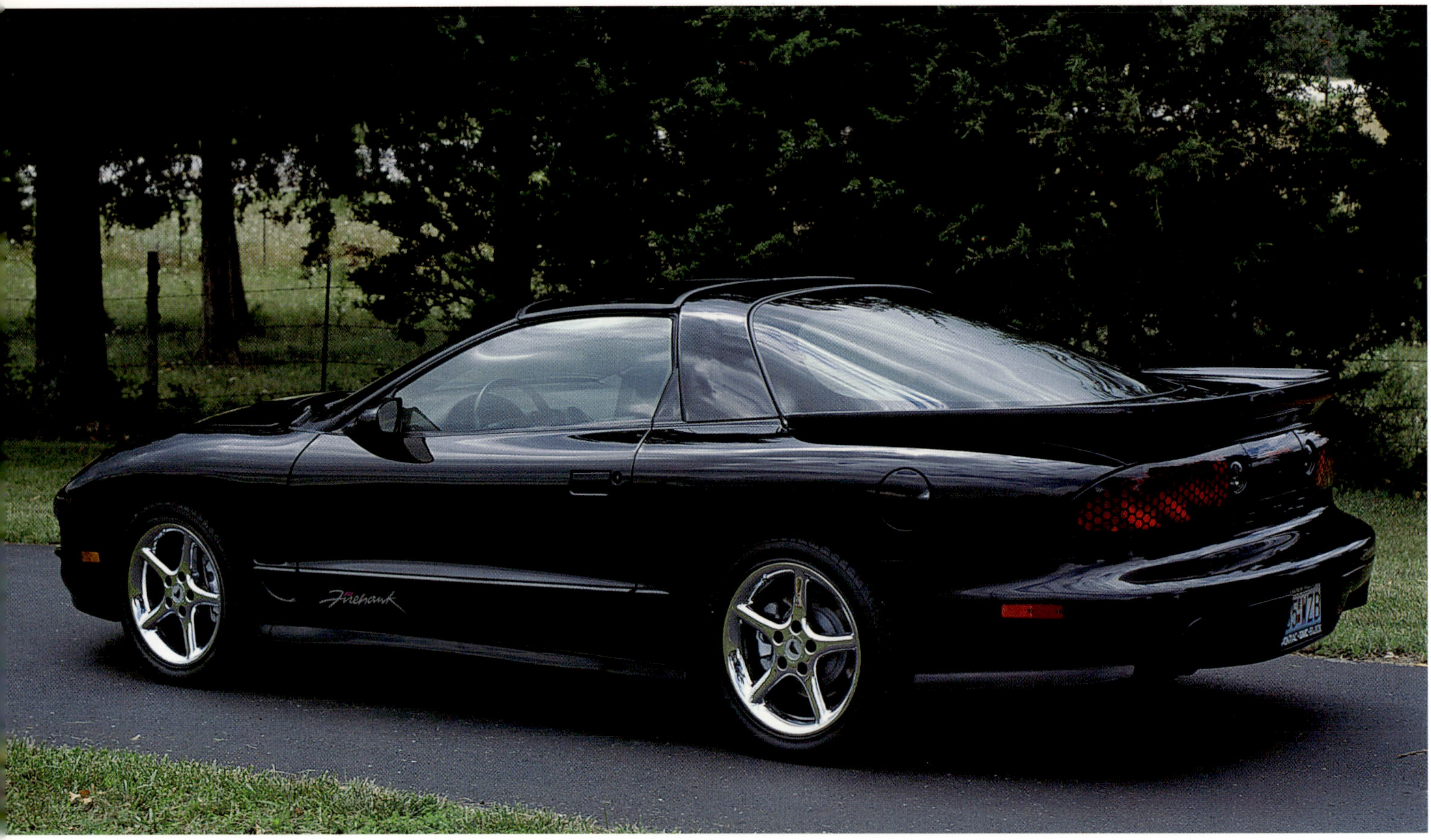

Above: This black 2002 Trans Am Firehawk was specially built by Straight Line Performance (SLP) and had a number of unique features, including a high-performance 335-horsepower LS1 V-8 and Ram Air with a special hood air intake design. Note the 17x9-inch aluminum wheels with black-and-silver center hubs and the silver Firehawk body graphics. ***Below:*** The final special-edition Trans Am was the 2002 Collector Edition hatchback coupe with T-top finished in special Collector Edition Yellow (54). In addition to the distinctive finish, the Collector Edition Trans Ams included special graphics, badges, and black wheels.

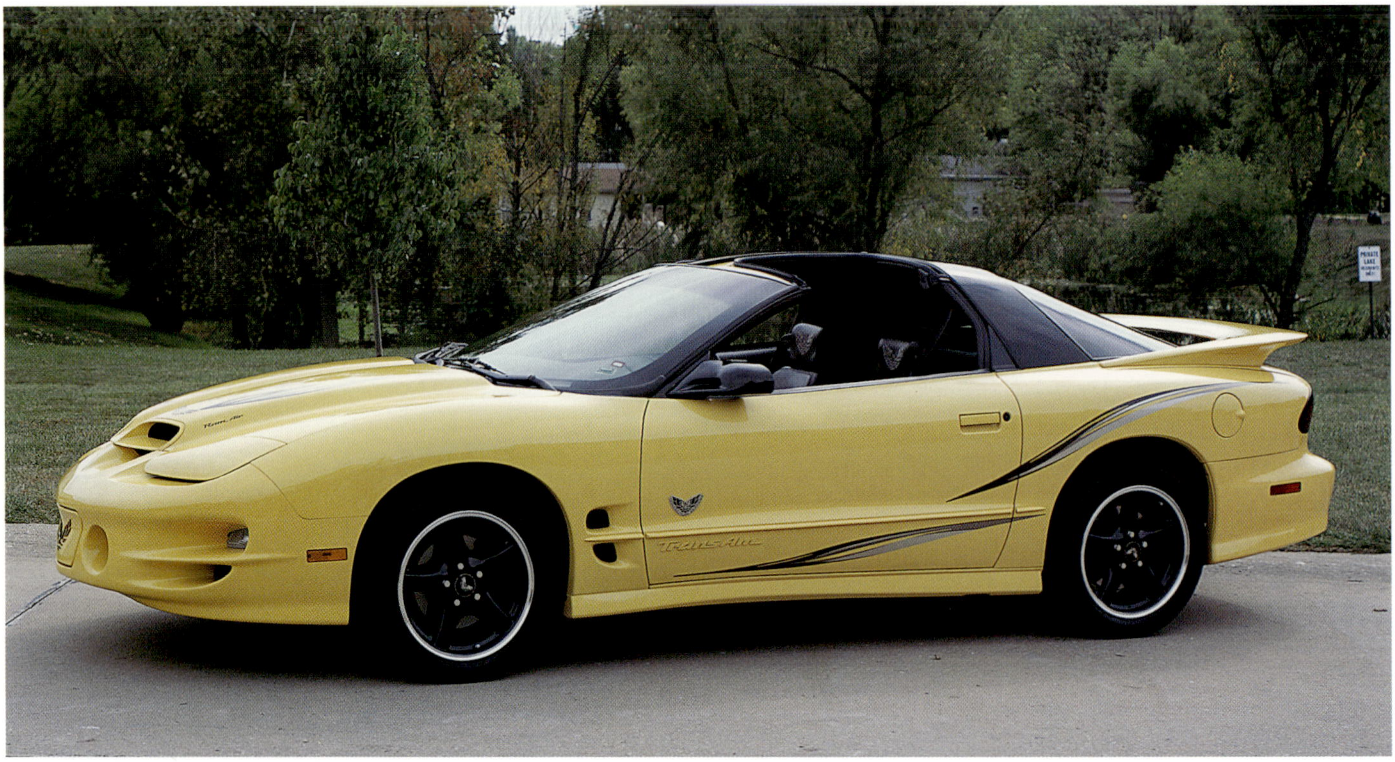

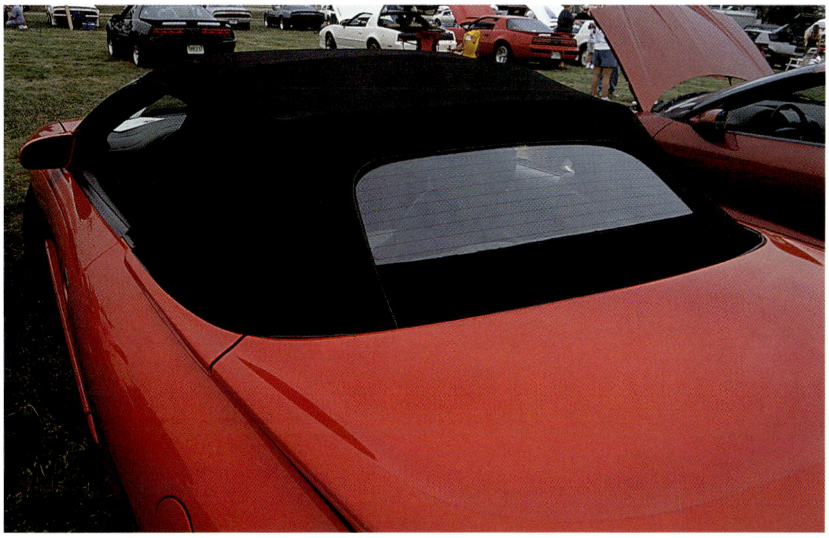

Left: This photo shows the rear of a black convertible top on a red 1995 Firebird Formula. Note the design of the rear deck and spoiler unique to the convertible body.

Below: This right rear view of a Sport Gold Metallic 1998 Firebird convertible with the top lowered shows the design of the rear deck and standard spoiler. This Firebird has a dark gray vinyl interior trim and black convertible top.

Camaro and constructed from composite plastic. Roof panels varied according to whether or not a T-top hatch roof was ordered. The door-opening structure was stamped from a single piece of steel. The body was not a space-frame design like the Fiero, but essentially a steel unitized structure with a number of plastic and composite exterior panels. All 1993–2002 Firebirds had a 15.5-gallon fuel tank mounted at the rear of the body pan. All 1993–2002 Firebirds were based on a two-door sport coupe or two-door convertible configuration on a 100-inch wheelbase.

The front structure of the body shell included the front suspension and engine supports. The inner front-fender support structure was tied to the body firewall and radiator support. The stiffer construction provided better ride and handling properties. The stable platform also allowed the springs and shock absorbers to function more efficiently, as less energy was lost controlling the torsional movements of the body. Because the body shell and support structure were painted as a single unit, all components were finished in body color.

In addition to the standard steel-frame composite roof, all 1993–2002 Firebirds were available with an optional T-top (hatch) roof with two removable dark-tinted glass panels (RPO CC1). When removed, the glass roof panels were stored in slots for that purpose in the rear cargo compartment. The removable T-top hatch roof with

Inset: When the convertible top is lowered, the folded top assembly is hidden with a three-piece snap-on molded hard plastic tonneau cover.

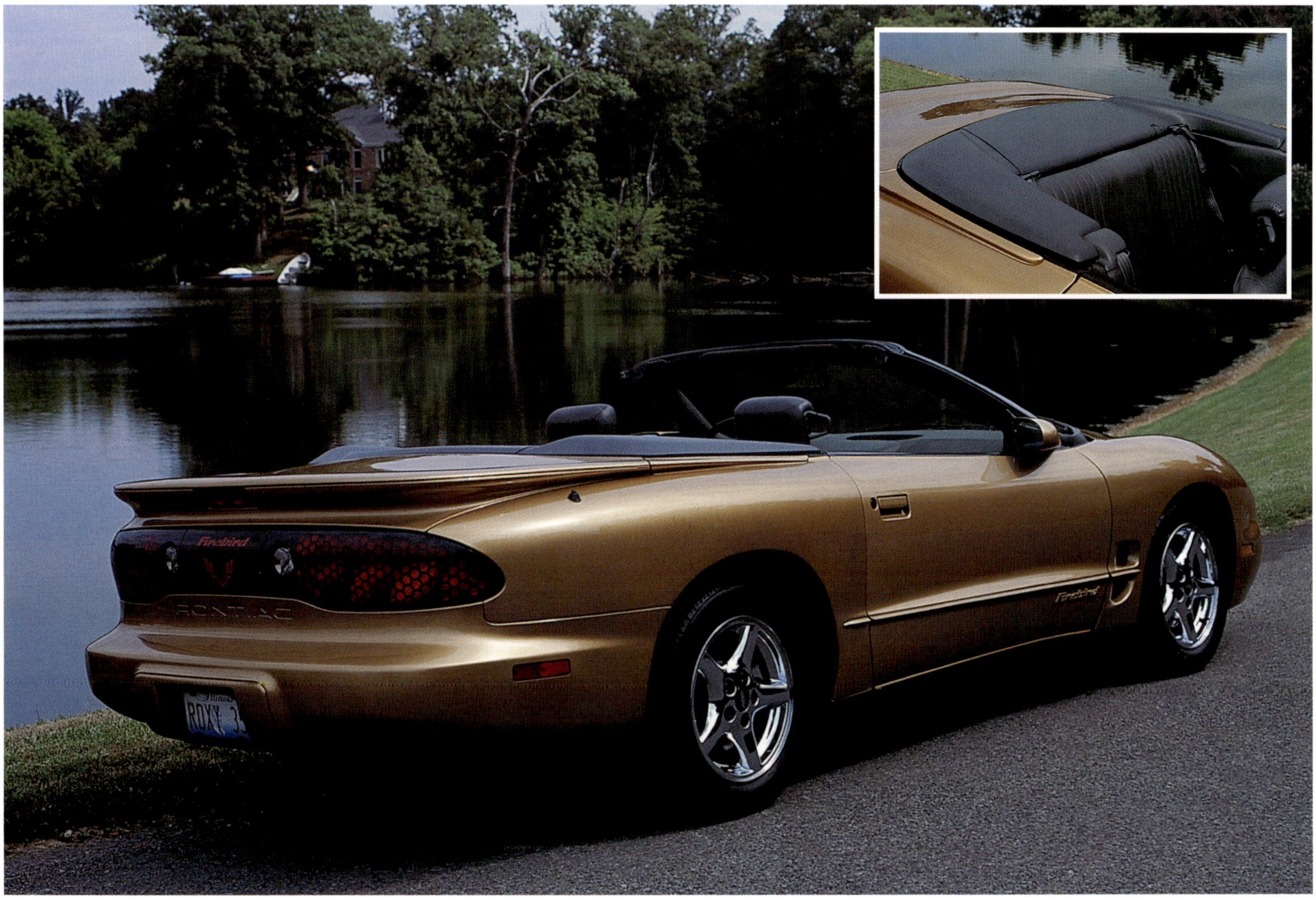

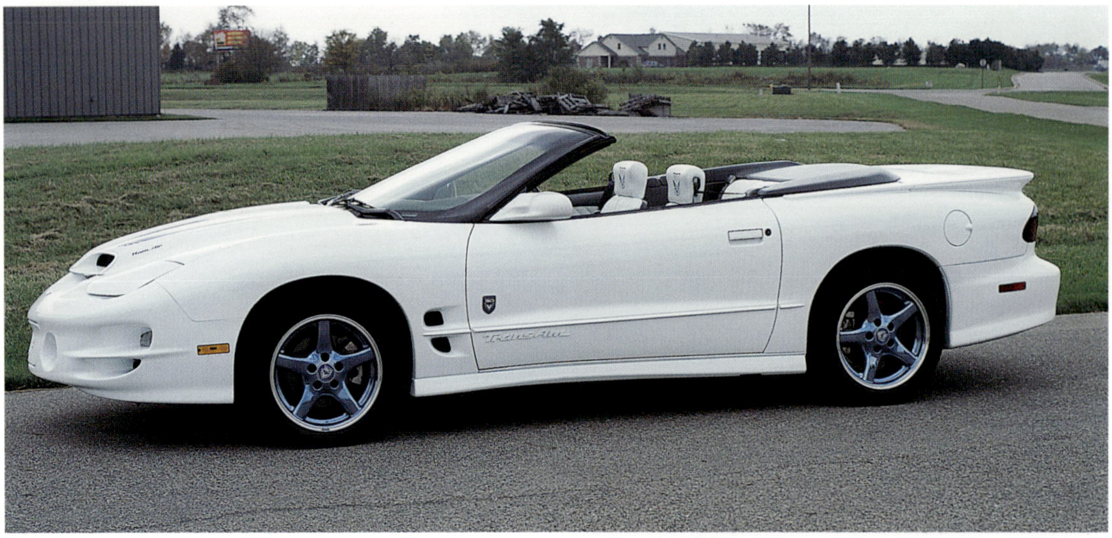

This left side view of an Arctic White (10) 1999 Trans Am 30th Anniversary Edition convertible with the top lowered shows the lower body air dam and special badges. The rear quarter panels are the only steel components on the fourth-generation Firebird and Trans Am body.

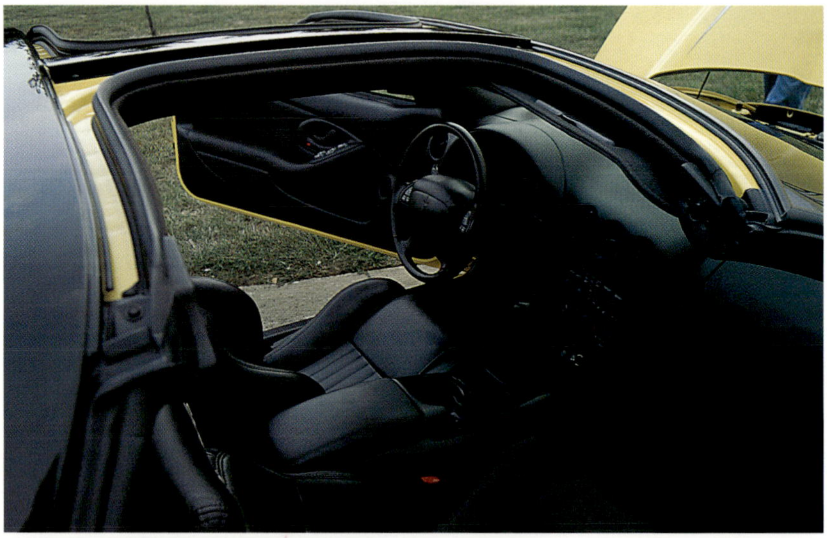

Right: This detail view of the roof on a 2002 Trans Am Ram Air yellow Collector Edition coupe with optional T-top shows the soft black rubber seal surrounding the perimeter of the opening.

sunshade (RPO DE4) was standard with the 1998–2002 Trans Am. No vinyl roof options were available with the 1993–2002 Firebirds.

All 1993–2002 Firebirds used the same left and right door shells. Firebird doors were made from sheet-molded compound (SMC), the same material used to make Corvette body panels. This new construction method allowed the door panels to be formed into more complex sculpted shapes than conventional steel stamping could provide. The SMC doors were also significantly lighter than equivalent steel parts. The doors

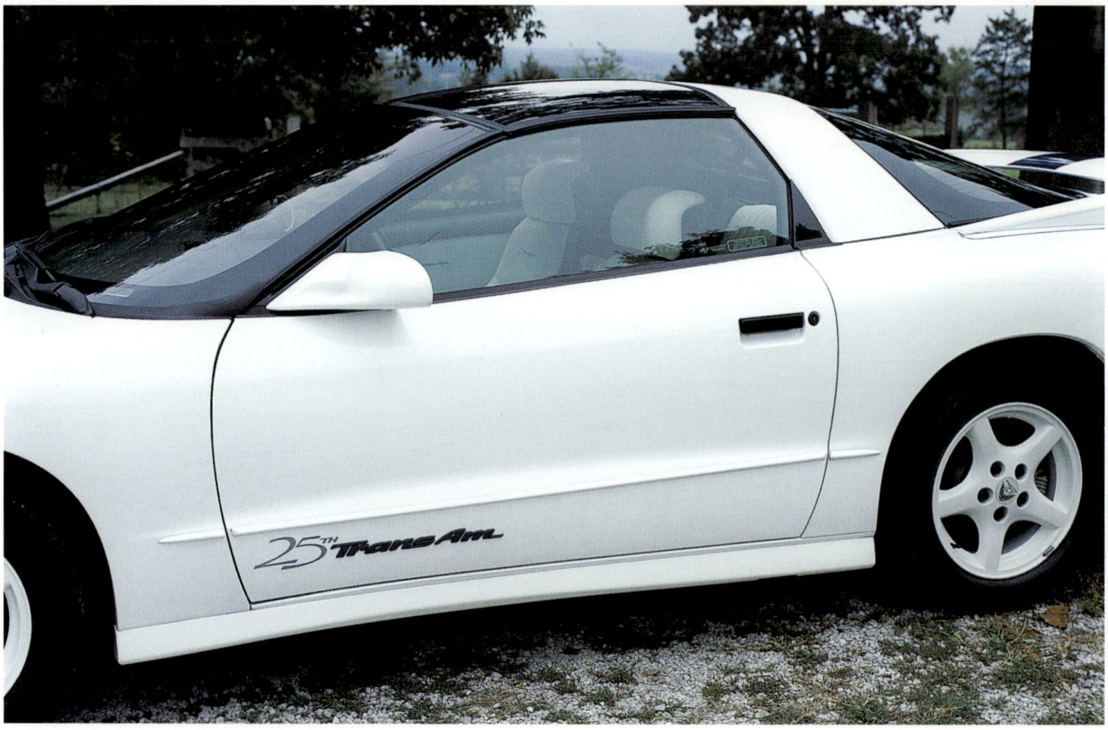

Left: Detail view of the molded composite door on a white 1994 Trans Am 25th Anniversary Edition hatchback coupe with T-top. Note the black door handle, the distinctive 25th Anniversary Trans Am graphics on the lower door panel, and the special white-painted wheels. This is one of 1,412 25th Anniversary coupes with T-tops made for the 1994 model year.

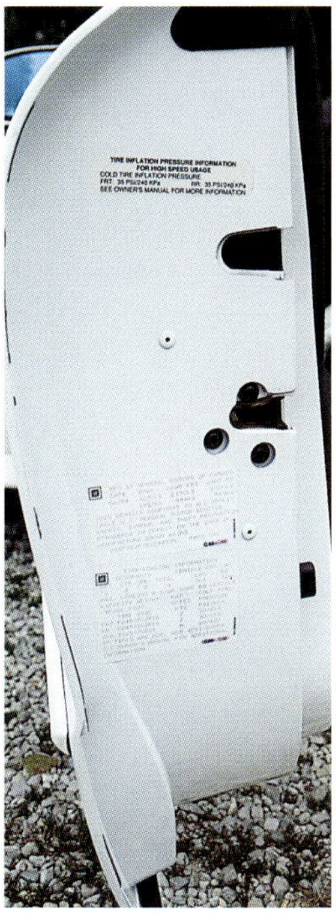

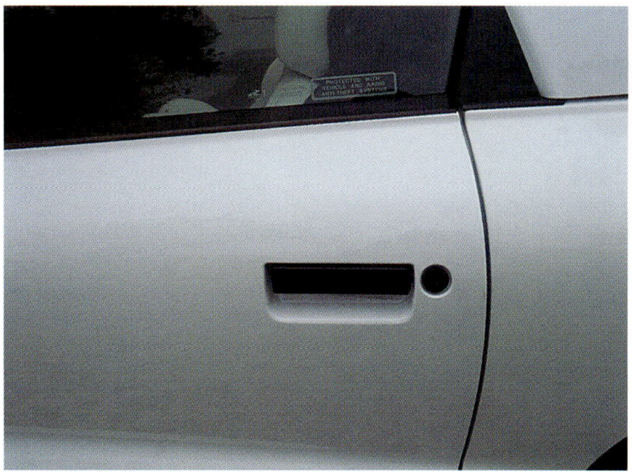

Above: Detail view of the door and door handle on a white 1994 Trans Am GT 25th Anniversary Edition. The door lock is also finished in black. ***Left:*** The outer door panel on the left side door of a white 1994 Trans Am GT 25th Anniversary Edition hatchback coupe diplays the three white decals with information on vehicle weight and tire loading and inflation data.

were operated by rectangular left and right door handles painted to match the body color. The rear of the door had an internal latch attached with three round-head socket-head black phosphate screws. The outer end of the driver's door for the 1998–2002 models also had a white service parts information decal, white build number information decal, and white tire loading information decal. The SLP Firehawk Firebirds had an additional white decal with an alteration notification decal on the driver's-door lock panel.

Left and right outside body-color aerodynamic sport mirrors were standard on all 1993–2002 Firebirds. The RPO D35 package provided a left side remote-control outside mirror with a convex manual passenger-side outside mirror. RPO DD9 brought breakaway-body left and right remote-control outside mirrors. Blue-tinted right convex power and left power mirrors were available with RPO D7.

All 1993–2002 Firebird doors were sealed with black soft sponge rubber weatherstrip that

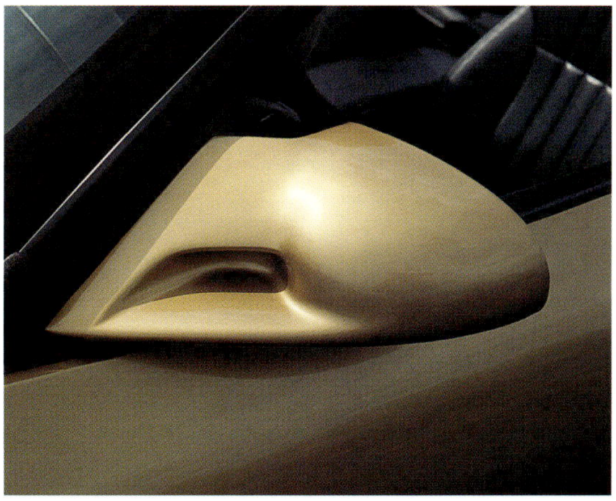

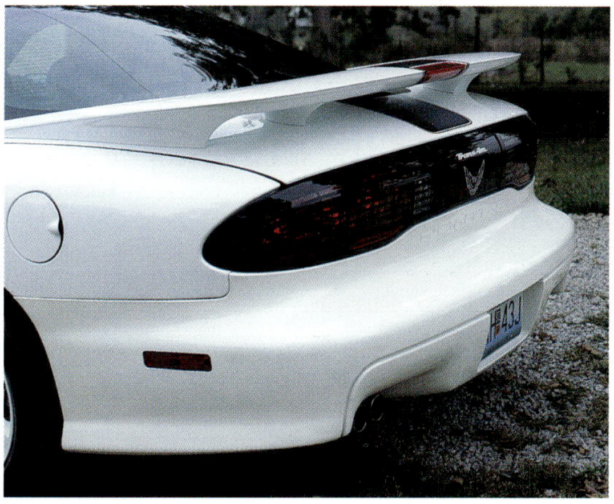

Right: This is a detail view of the left side body-color sport mirror of a Sport Gold Metallic (63) 1998 Firebird convertible and its distinctive aerodynamic mirror. ***Far right:*** This is a detail view of the left rear quarter of a white 1994 Trans Am GT 25th Anniversary Edition showing the rear deck and hatchback liftgate. Note the design of the high-angle spoiler and high-mounted stop light. ***Right:*** This close view of the left side roof and door of a Bright Red 2000 Trans Am Ram Air coupe shows the design of the molded composite door panel. Note the distinctive horizontal character lines of the body side, the iconic engine compartment extractor vents in the rear of the front fender, and the body-color Trans Am nameplate in the lower door panel.

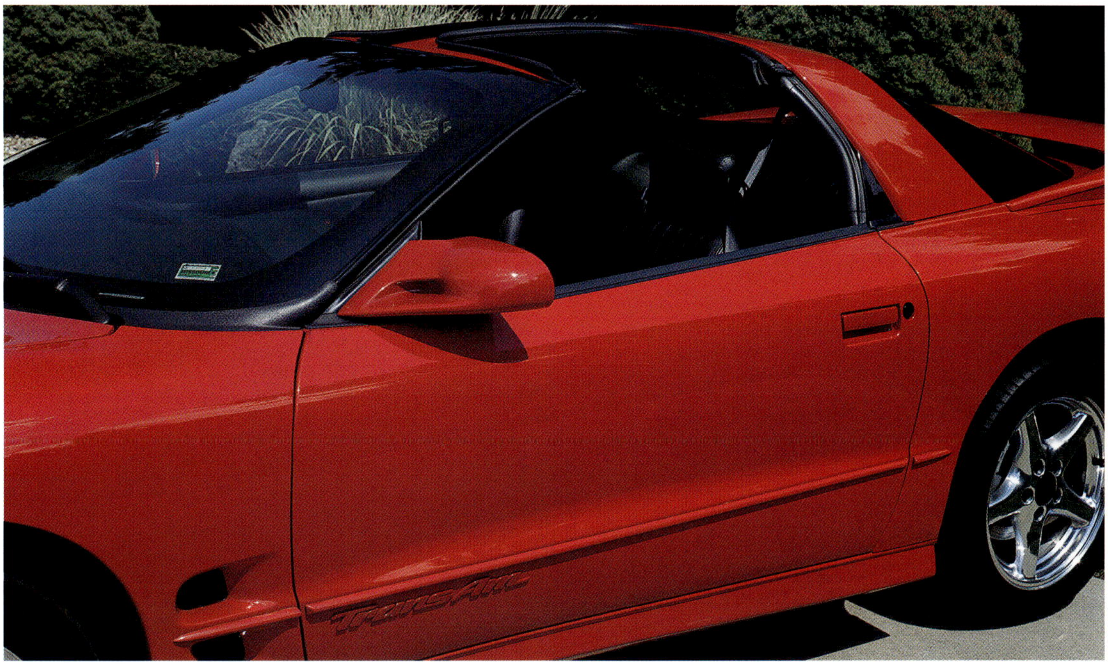

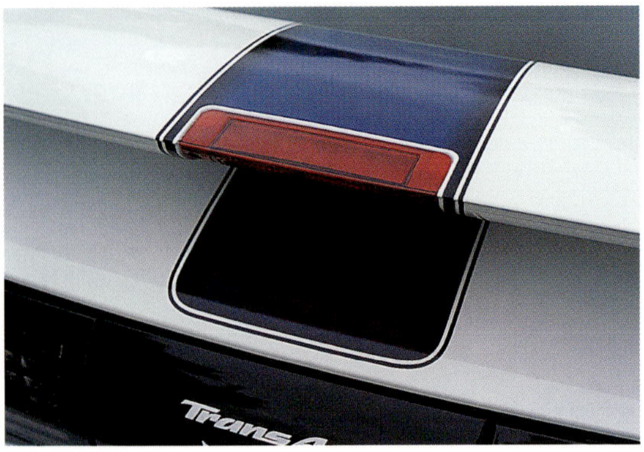

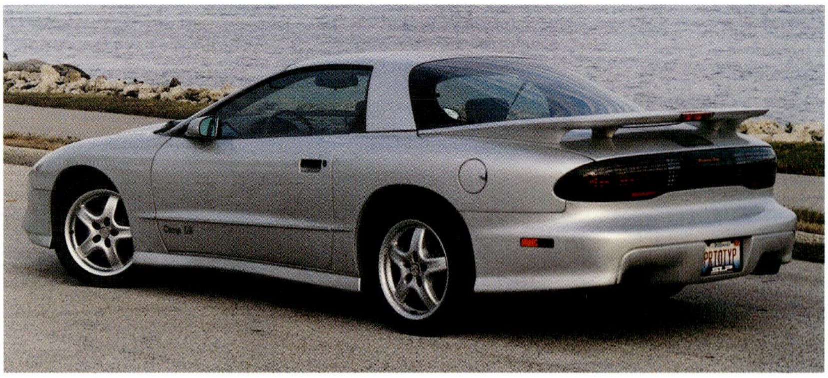

Above left: This is a detail view of the rear spoiler on the liftgate of a white 1994 Trans Am GT 25th Anniversary Edition with the standard center stoplight and distinctive blue stripe. ***Above right:*** This photo shows a left rear quarter view of a Bright Silver Metallic (13) 1995 Comp T/A Trans Am coupe. Note the rear spoiler and body air dam and the Comp T/A decal on the front of the lower door panel. This is one of 164 Comp T/As built in 1995–1997. *Dean Fait*

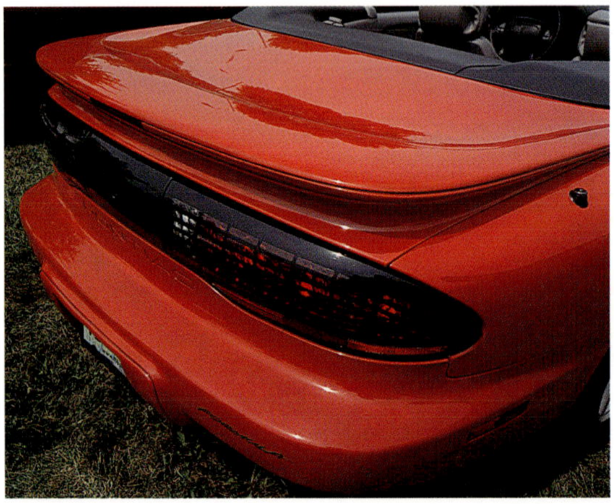

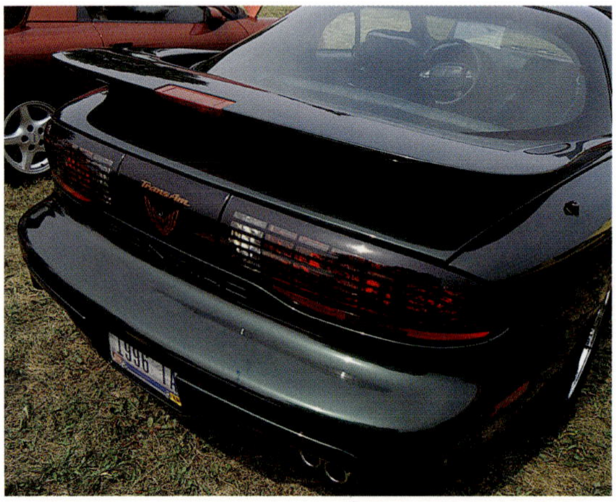

Far left: This photo shows the rear of the hatchback liftgate and spoiler on a Bright Red 1995 Firebird Formula convertible. Note the relatively flat spoiler design with integral center stoplight and the black power radio antenna bezel on the right rear quarter panel. ***Left:*** This photo shows the upward-angled rear spoiler and hatchback liftgate on a Dark Green Metallic (48) 1996 Trans Am coupe with optional T-top roof. The red Trans Am logo and bird are visible in the center of the rear deck lower panel.

surrounded the outer perimeter of the body door opening. The upper door-opening seal was molded to accept the raised side window glass. There was no seal on the door shell except a small molded rubber seal at the upper rear corner. The lower door sill had a black plastic cover with a pattern of two rows of squares. The rear door opening pillar had a black phosphate-finish Torx-head latch striker and a two-post lock catch.

All 1993–2002 Firebird sport coupes used a body-color SMC molded-hatchback-design rear compartment lid with a curved Soft-Ray tinted glass that sealed against the rear of the body roof. The lid was hinged at the top, latched at the rear center, and sealed at the body with a black sponge rubber seal on the body-opening perimeter. A remote-control rear compartment lid lock was available with RPO A90. All hatch lids had a wide integral flat, curved aero-deck spoiler with two support posts and a center-mounted brake light on the trailing edge of the spoiler. The Trans Am spoiler design was unique. A semigloss-black hinge assembly and small-diameter strut on each side supported the raised lid.

In the convertible Firebird models, the rear hatch was replaced with a special SMC molded deck lid without a rear window. The deck lid incorporated a spoiler similar to that used on the standard rear hatch. When the convertible roof was lowered, it folded completely into the body behind the rear seat and was covered with a removable three-piece snap-on hard plastic cover. The cover had a textured finish and was color-coordinated to match the interior trim color.

Like the previous model, the 1993–2002 Firebird sport coupe did not have a conventional trunk. The entire carpeted rear cargo compartment

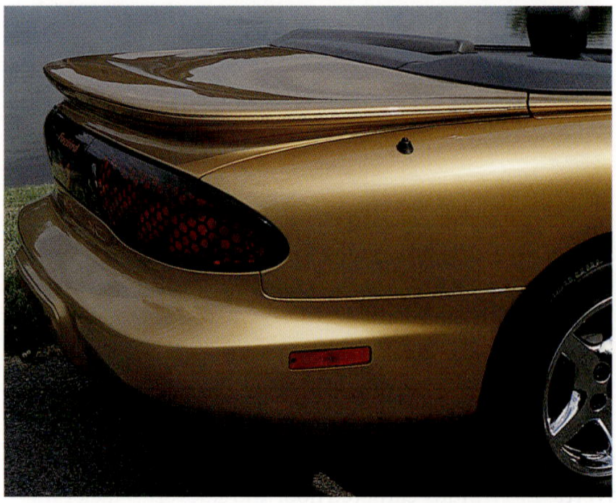

This photo shows the right rear view of a Sport Gold Metallic 1998 Firebird convertible with the top lowered. Note the flat design of the spoiler and rear deck and the red side marker light in the rear fascia.

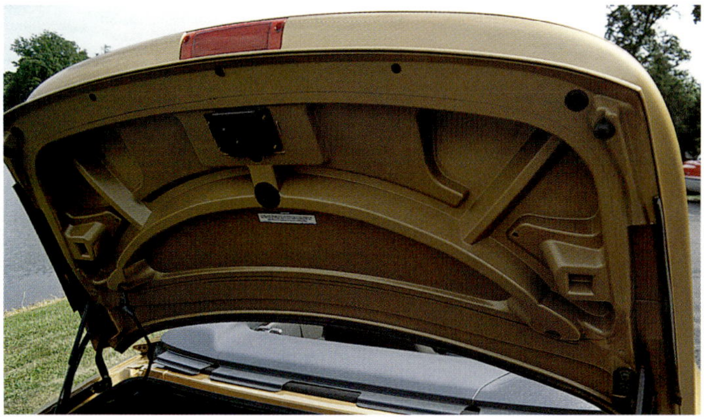

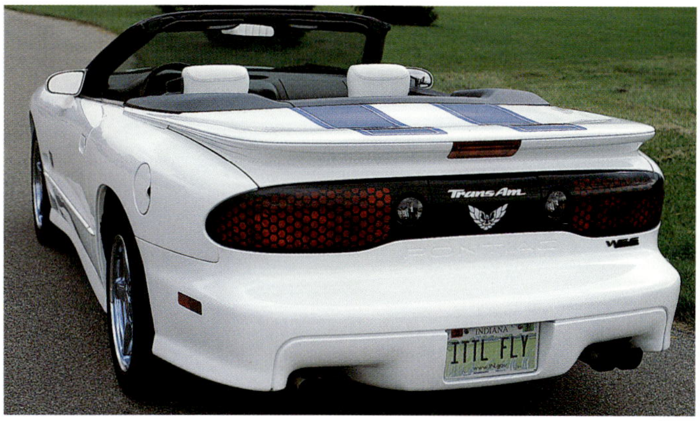

Above left: This is a detail view of the inside of the unique deck lid on a 1998 Firebird convertible shows the small instruction decal in the center of the inner panel. ***Above right:*** This rear view of an Arctic White 1999 Trans Am 30th Anniversary Edition convertible with top lowered includes the unique white Trans Am logo and bird on the rear deck lower panel. Note the design of the convertible rear hatch and spoiler.

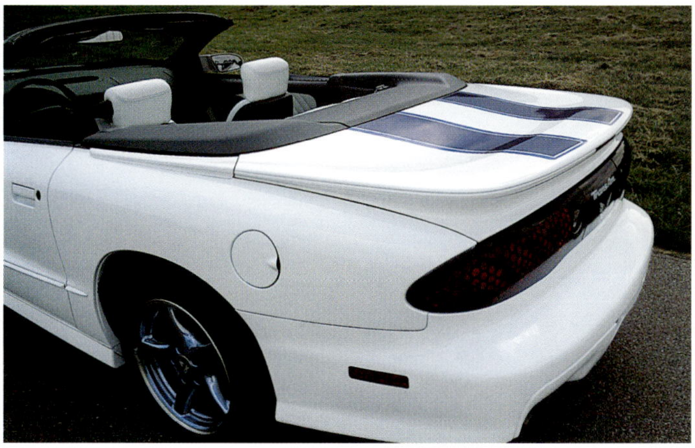

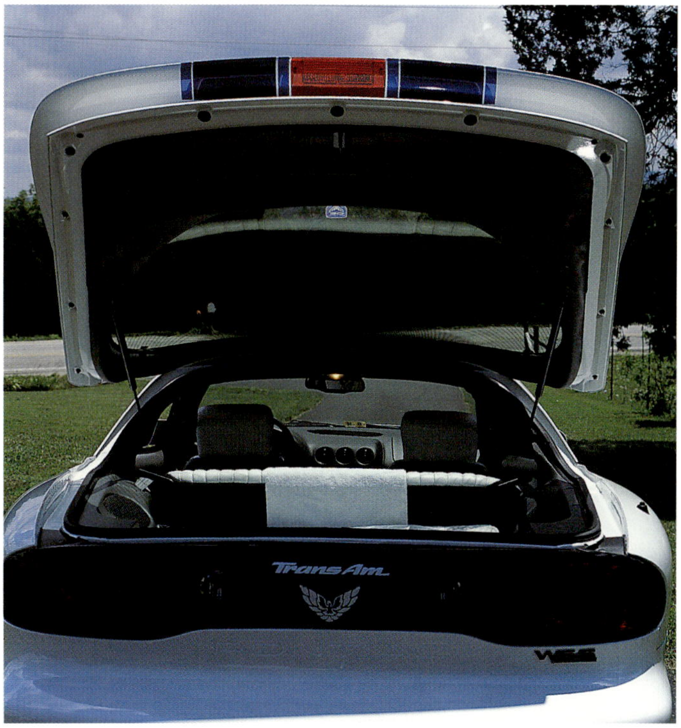

Above: This left rear view of the rear deck and spoiler on a white 1999 Trans Am 30th Anniversary Edition convertible shows the design of the spoiler and dual blue stripes. This Trans Am is one of 35 30th Anniversary convertibles delivered to Canada, and it has a kilometer speedometer. ***Right:*** This is a detail view of the interior of the raised rear liftgate hatchback on a white 1999 Trans Am. Note the hatch support struts on either side and the tinted rear window. The brake light is mounted in the center of the spoiler.

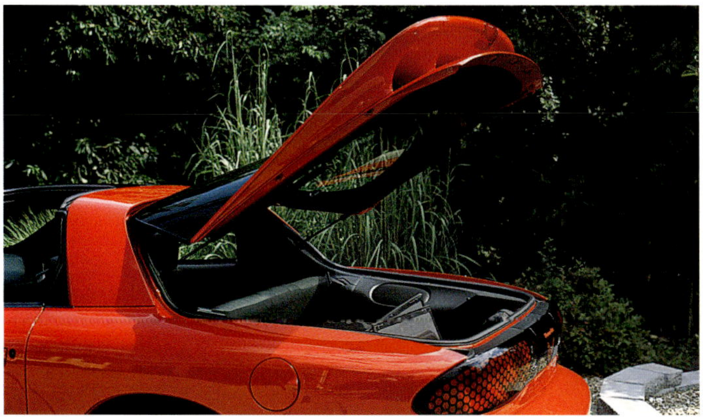

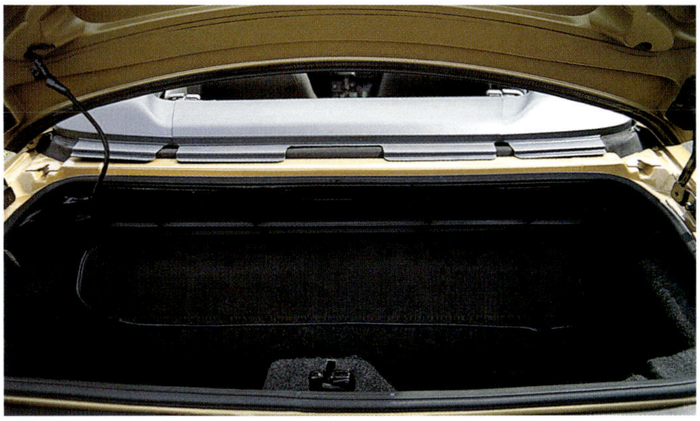

Above left: This photo shows a left side view of the raised rear hatchback liftgate on a Bright Red 2000 Trans Am Ram Air coupe with optional T-top roof. Note the black finish of the inner panel and the twin support struts on either side. ***Above right:*** This is a detail photo of the trunk compartment in a Sport Gold Metallic 1998 Firebird convertible. The fully carpeted floor and sides and black rubber seal around the perimeter of the trunk opening are visible.

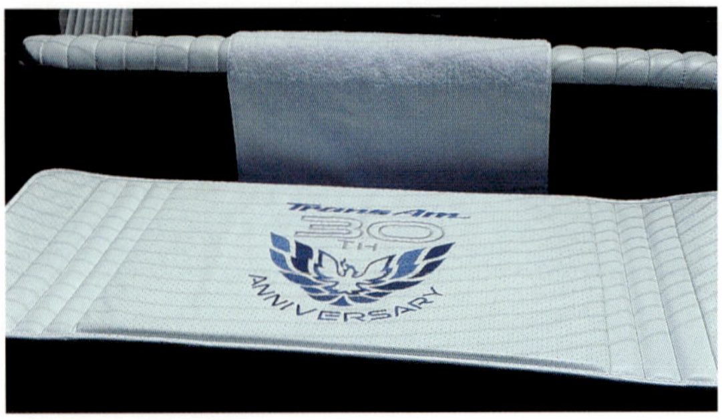

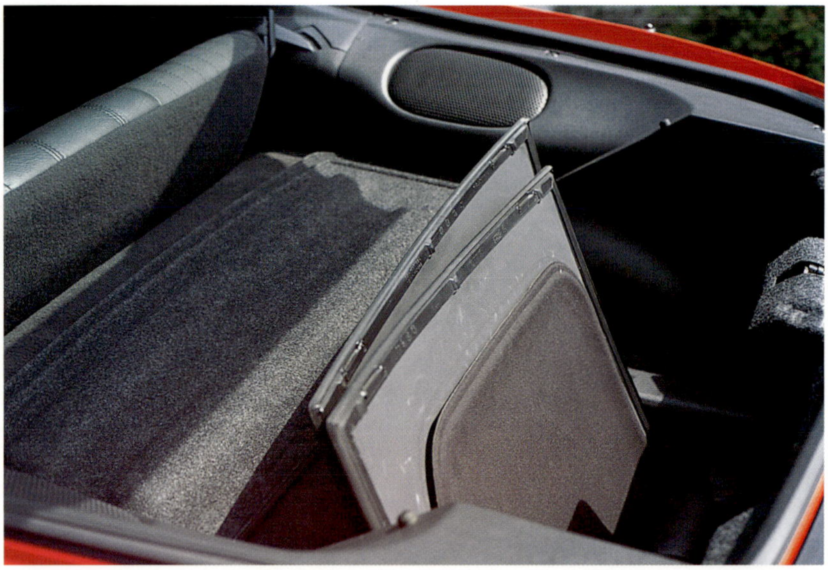

Above: This white cargo compartment pad is provided as part of the special package in the 1999 Trans Am 30th Anniversary Edition. It has a distinctive blue logo and bird that matches the interior trim colors. ***Right:*** The cargo compartment in a Bright Red 2000 Trans Am Ram Air hatchback coupe with optional T-top. The T-top removable roof panels are shown in their storage position. The sound system speaker is visible on the right side of the compartment.

was exposed when the rear lid was opened. There was a deeper well to the rear of the axle hump. The deeper well held the T-top roof panels when they were removed. A wide carpeted cover folded over the deep rear cargo compartment to hide the contents from view. The rear seat also folded, creating more flat carpeted cargo area in the rear compartment. The SLP Firehawk special editions had a custom flat cover carpet available with the name of the owner and the car's number embroidered on the center in color. Since the convertible models did not have the rear hatch compartment lid, they had a more conventional trunk configuration, although deep and limited in space.

In the right side of the rear compartment, a cover (part number 10251237) hid the standard compact spare wheel and tire. The wheel for the 1993–1996 Firebird was a 15x4 with part number 9591849. The wheel for the 1997–2002 models was a 16x4 (part number 9592913). The right compartment also held the standard folding jack and jack-handle/wheel wrench assembly (part number 25606055).

The rear deck lower panel on the 1993–2002 Firebird was smooth and vertical, with a horizontal sculptured design for the taillights and panel. The taillight panel was flat black, and the body-color panel beneath the dark lens taillights flowed smoothly into the bumper and featured large recessed block letters spelling "Pontiac." The energy-absorbing rear fascia was a single piece of reaction-injection-molded (RIM) polyurea composite material. The license plate was mounted in the lower center of the bumper portion of the rear panel.

The 1993–1997 taillights had seven vertical sections on each side with black dividers and a backup lamp on the inside. There were also seven narrow horizontal sections with narrow black dividers in each left and right taillight assembly. A flat black panel between the taillights had a red bird with either "Firebird," "Formula," or "Trans Am" in red script above it. Some special editions had the bird and script in white. The 1998–2002 rear deck panel was similar, but the taillights were redesigned as a flat black honeycomb pattern on

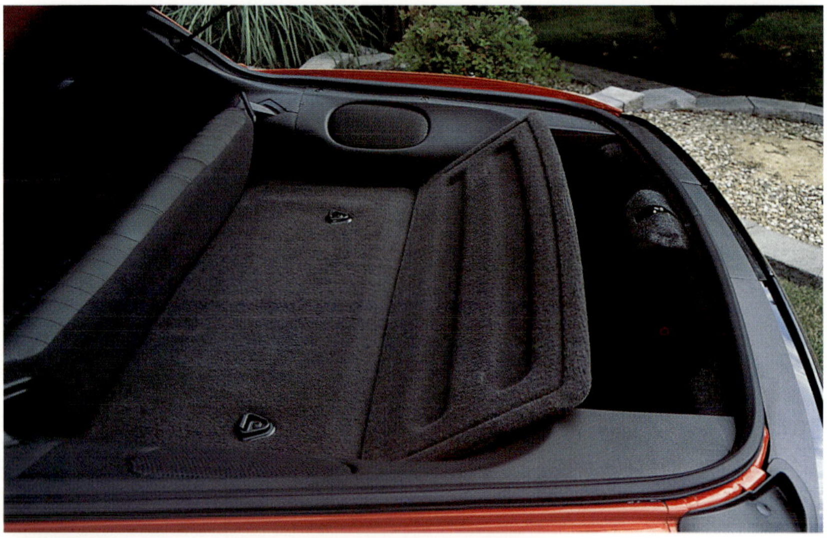

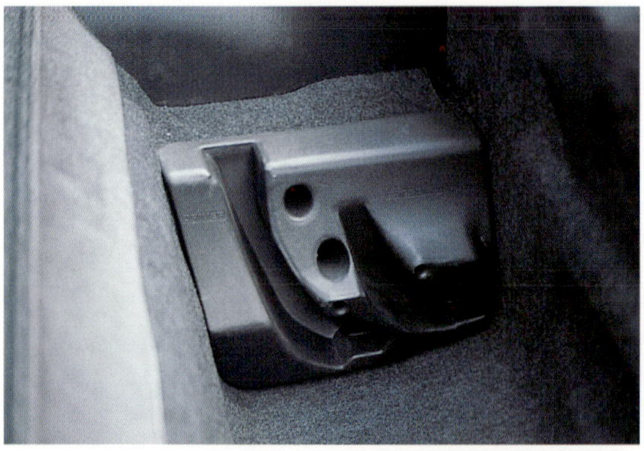

Above: This view shows the folding cargo compartment cover in a Bright Red 2000 Trans Am Ram Air hatchback coupe. The cover is carpet-covered hard plastic. ***Left:*** The removable T-top roof panels fit into these special slots in the cargo compartment of the 2000 Trans Am coupe. The right side bracket is marked "passenger" to indicate its proper installation position.

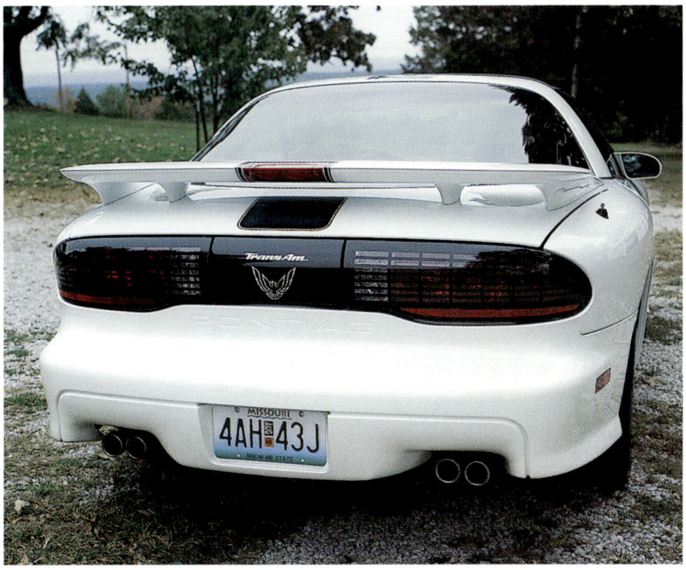

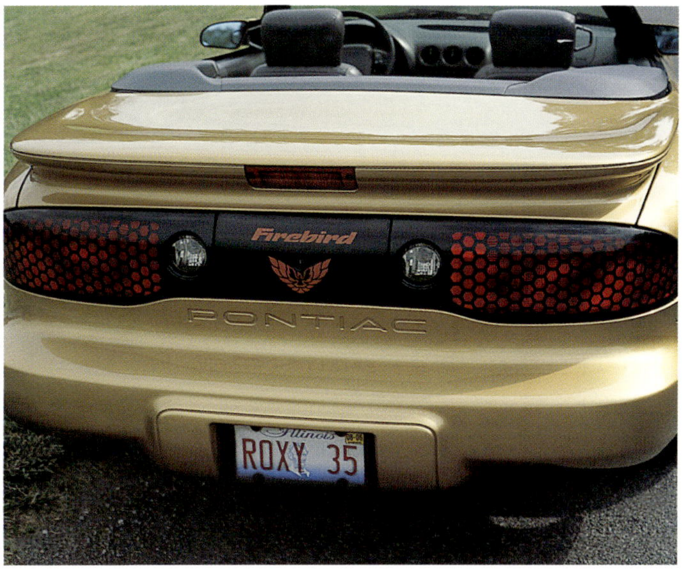

Above left: Detail view of the rear deck lower panel and taillight design on a white 1994 Trans Am GT 25th Anniversary Edition hatchback coupe with the distinctive white Trans Am logo and bird in the center. Note the design and mounting of the spoiler. ***Above right:*** This is the rear deck lower panel of a Sport Gold Metallic Firebird convertible (S67V). Note the octagonal honeycomb design of the taillights and the red Firebird name and bird logo on the center of the panel.

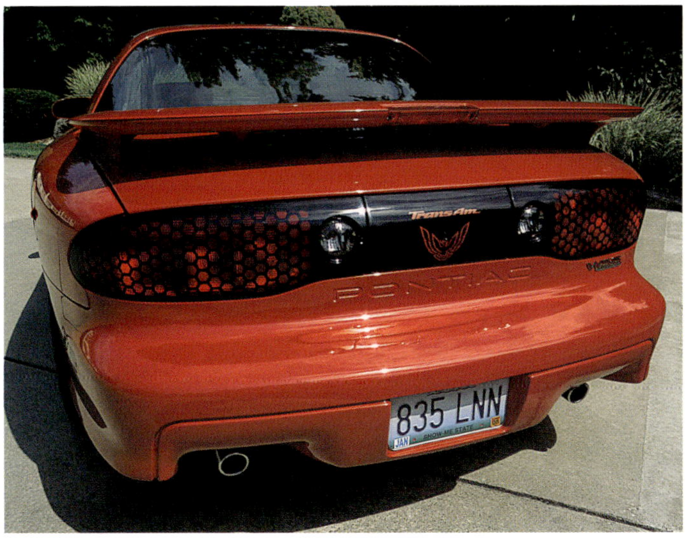

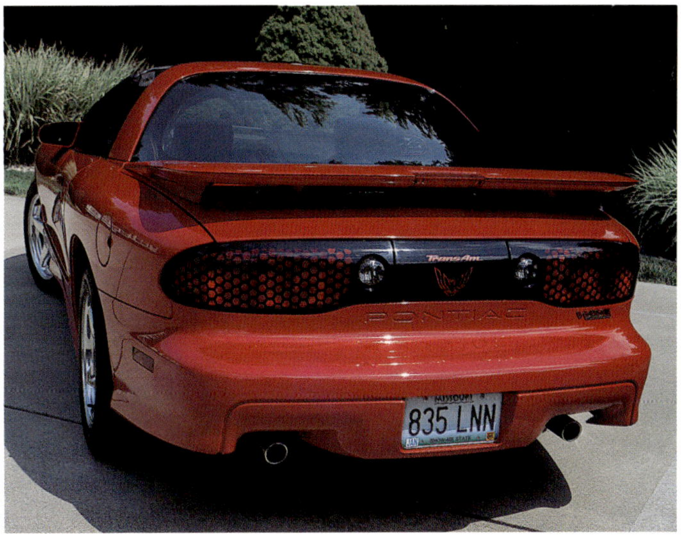

Above left: This view of the rear deck lower panel of a Bright Red 2000 Trans Am Ram Air WS6 hatchback coupe shows the design of the lower panel and air dam. Note the WS6 badge on the right of the panel. ***Above right:*** This is a detail view of the rear deck lower panel on a Bright Red (81) 2000 Trans Am WS6 Ram Air with T-top roof. Note the unique hexagonal honeycomb pattern in the taillight panel, the red Trans Am logo and bird in the center, and the design of the spoiler.

each side with round backup lights on the inside of each taillight assembly. All 1993–2002 taillights wrapped around the sides of the body.

The rear quarter panels of the 1993–2002 Firebird were stamped steel and rounded with a distinct horizontal curve on the sides. The wheel openings were rounded, and the round body-color fuel filler door was mounted on the upper left panel just behind the wheel opening. A small rectangular side marker light was mounted in the outer sides of the wraparound bumper. The radio antenna was mounted in the upper right rear quarter panel. There were no bright wheel opening moldings available on the 1993–2002 Firebirds.

All 1993–1997 Firebirds used the same front fenders (part numbers 10404898 right and 10404899 left) that featured a strong horizontal curve on the top and a sloping front. The fenders were made from resilient, reaction-injection-molded plastic that was imbedded with microscopic pieces of mica to give the panels the same reflective qualities as steel panels. The lower edge of the front of the fenders was attached to the outer ends of the front fascia, leaving a horizontal seam from the rear of the fascia to the front of the wheel openings. The lower side of the rear of the fender panel behind the wheel opening had a horizontal molding crease that followed back to the rear wheel opening. On the Trans Am, the front of the one-piece lower-body side dam was attached to the lower edge of the front fender. For 1998–2002, the front fenders were redesigned and added twin simulated extractor scoops behind the front wheel openings for all models. The 1998–2002 fenders used part numbers 10420065 (right) and 10420066 (left).

There were two hoods for the 1993–1997

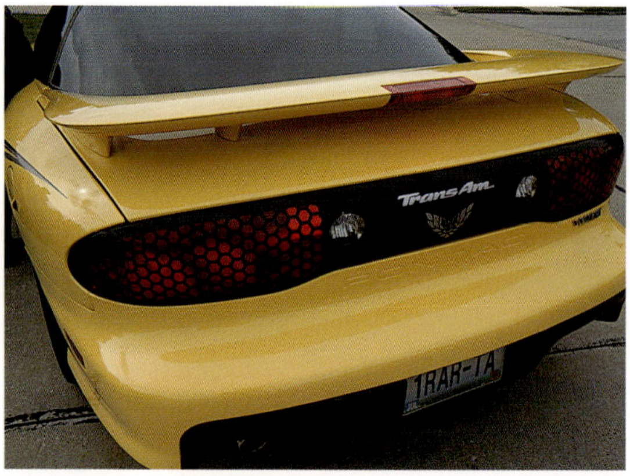

This view of the rear deck lower panel on a 2002 Trans Am WS6 Ram Air Collector Edition Yellow coupe shows the black finish of the lower air dam and silver Trans Am name and bird on the rear panel. Note the WS6 badge on the right of the panel and the difference in the spoiler design from the 2000 Trans Am.

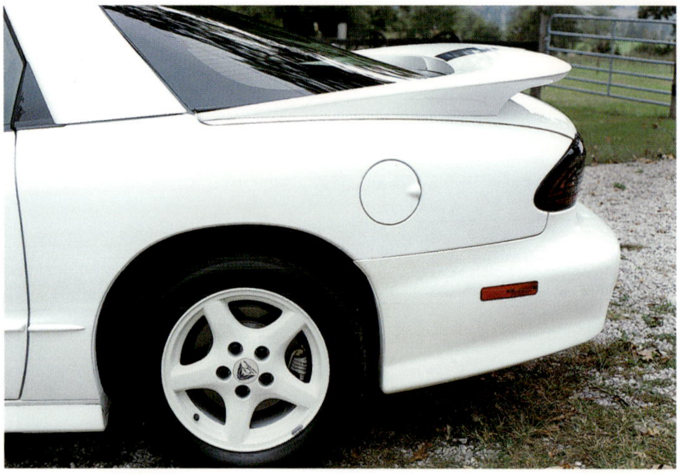

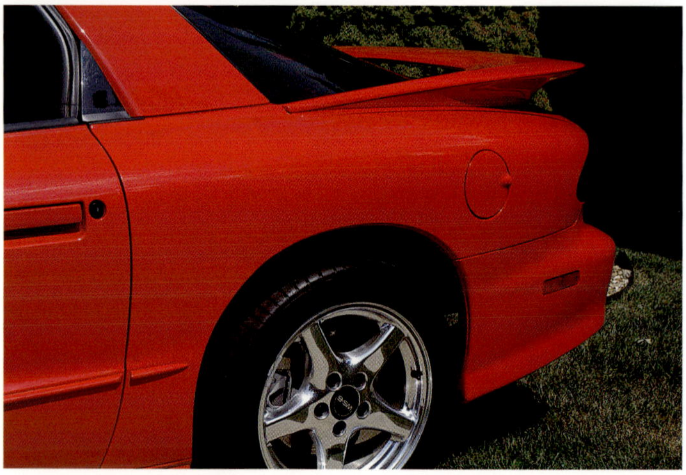

Above left: This detail view of a white 1994 Trans Am GT 25th Anniversary Edition shows the design of the left rear quarter panel, including the round fuel filler door. The rear quarter panels are the only steel body parts on a fourth-generation Firebird or Trans Am. ***Above right:*** This photo shows the left rear quarter panel and rear spoiler on a Bright Red 2000 Trans Am Ram Air hatchback coupe with T-top roof. It has rectangular side marker lights in the rear fascia.

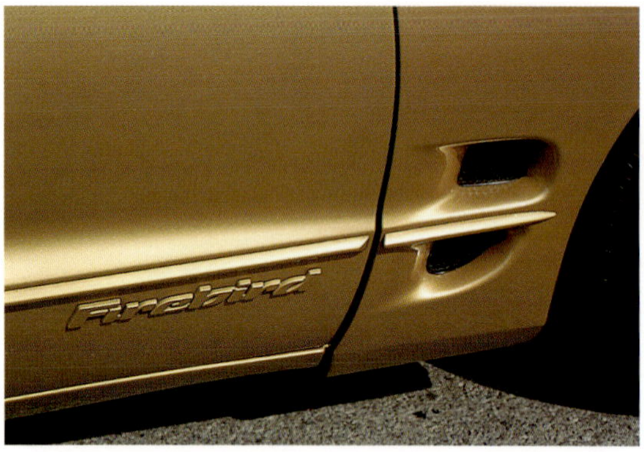

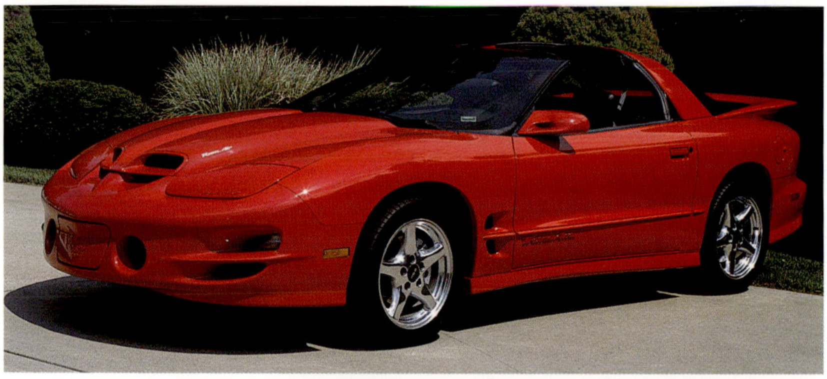

Above left: This is a detail view of the right front fender of a Sport Gold Metallic 1998 Firebird front fender showing the extractor vents and horizontal body character line. A body-color Firebird nameplate appears on the door panel. ***Above:*** This photo of a Bright Red 2000 Trans Am Ram Air hatchback coupe with T-top shows the horizontal character line on the body and fender side and extractor vents on the rear of the fender. ***Right:*** This is a detail view of the left front fender of a Bright Red 2000 Trans Am WS6 Ram Air coupe with the red Trans Am nameplate on the lower door panel. Note the lower body air dam.

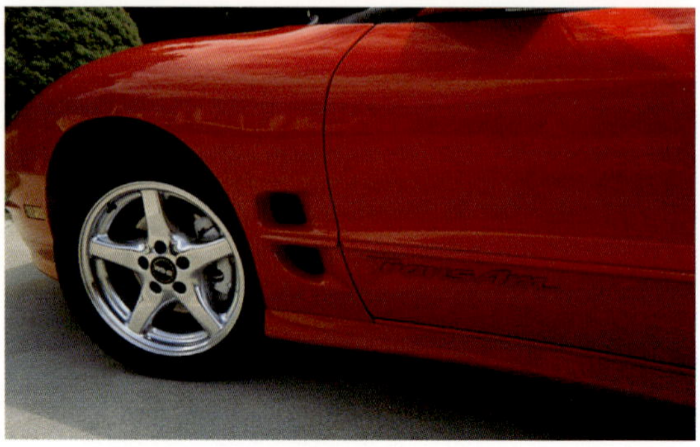

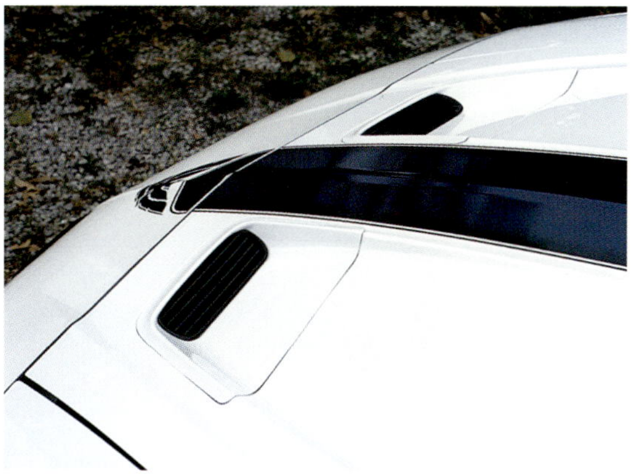

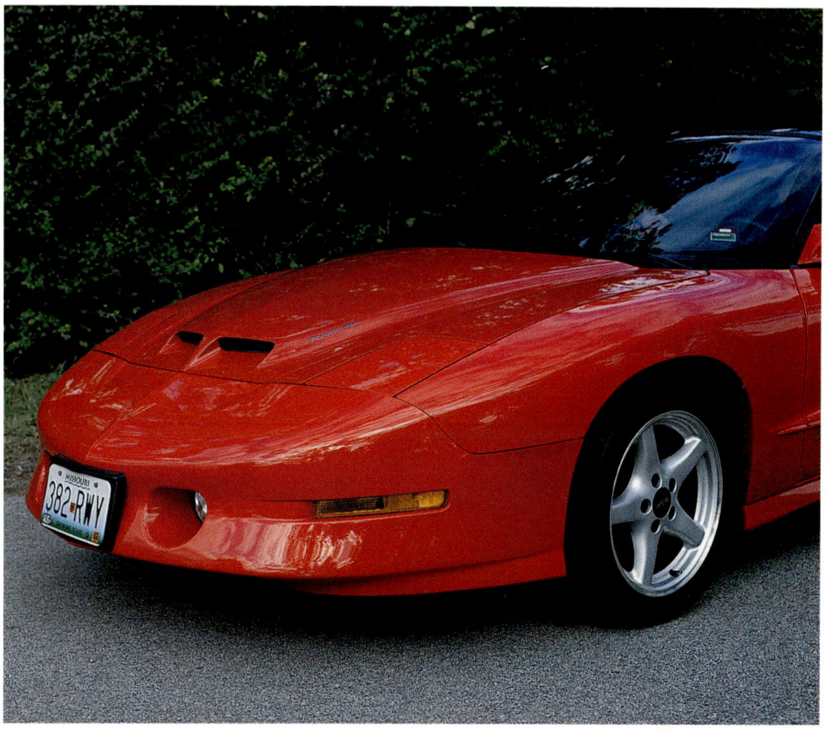

Above: This is a detail view from the rear showing the twin grilles in the hood of a white 1994 Trans Am GT 25th Anniversary Edition coupe. Note the distinctive blue stripe. ***Right:*** This is a left front view of the hood and front fascia of a Bright Red 1996 Trans Am Ram Air hatchback coupe. This was the first year for the new Ram Air hood intake system on the fourth-generation Trans Am, and the special Ram Air components were produced by SLP.

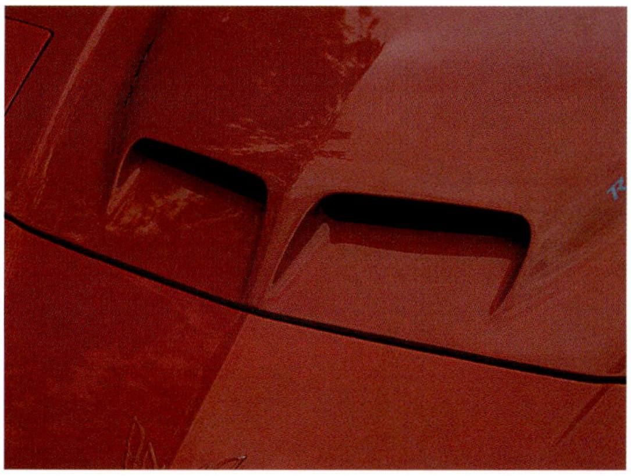

The dual air intake openings on a Bright Red 1996 Trans Am WS6 Ram Air hatchback coupe feature a fine longitudinal crease in the center of the hood and front fascia.

Firebirds. The base Firebird, Formula, and Trans Am without Ram Air had a relatively flat two-sided galvanized-steel hood (part number 10259276) with a fine longitudinal crease in its center and a small reversed indentation with insert on either side. A black transverse louvered grille was mounted in the front of each indentation insert. When the WS6 Ram Air Induction Package was ordered in the 1996 and 1997 Formula and Trans Am, it featured a unique molded-composite hood (part number 12359196) with a wide raised center hump that tapered toward twin functional air intake scoops. A Ram Air decal was mounted on each side of the front of the raised hump. The initial 1996 Ram Air production was done by SLP for Pontiac, so some hoods on these first 499 cars may show a variation in the finish shade or quality.

In 1998–2002, two new hoods were used. The Firebird, Formula, and Trans Am without Ram Air again had a smooth two-sided galvanized-steel hood (part number 10269572), but this new design was rounder and smoother with a slightly raised center and lower sides that flowed to meet the edges of the fenders. Twin air intakes were cut into the top center of the front fascia on all models to give even the standard hood an aggressive appearance.

The 1998–2002 Firebird Formulas and Trans Ams with the 5.7-liter Ram Air V-8 used a

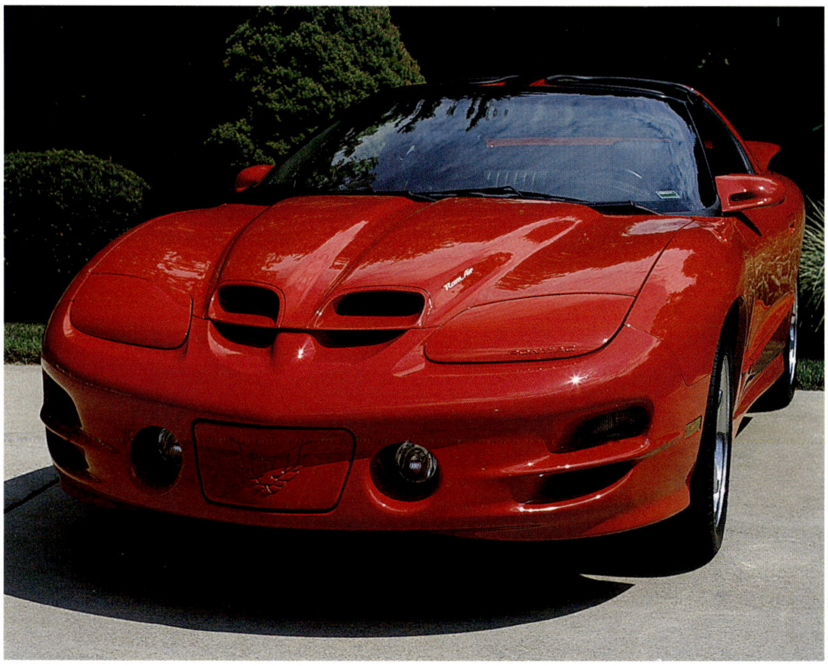

Left: This photo shows the distinctive hood and front fascia of a Bright Red 2000 Trans Am Ram Air coupe with T-top roof with the four distinct openings for the Ram Air induction system. Note the removable body-color license plate cover with embossed bird.

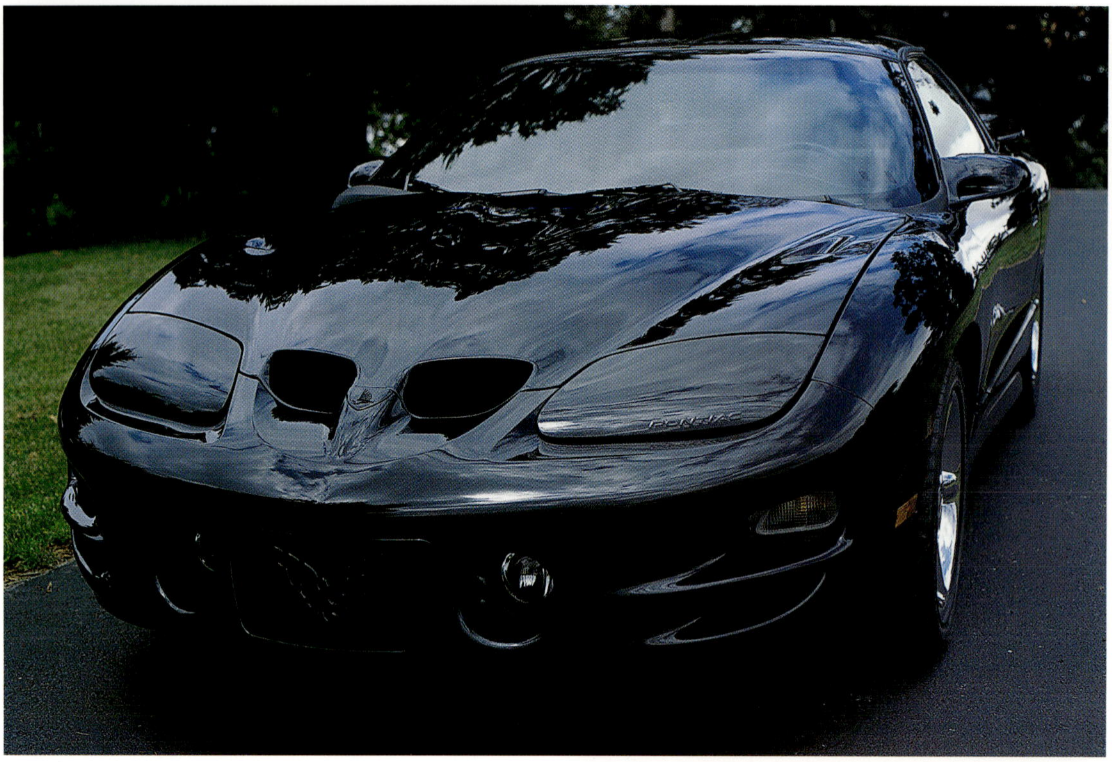

This view of a black (41) 2002 Trans Am Firehawk coupe shows the special Firehawk composite hood and the unique Ram Air intakes that differ from those on the standard Trans Am. The Firehawk logo is visible in the center of the upper fascia.

Below: The Ram Air scoops on the hood and front fascia of a yellow 2002 Trans Am Collector Edition with the distinctive black-and-silver body graphics included on the collector-edition package.

distinctive molded-composite hood (part number 12455210) with a massive dual-hump center scoop with twin openings that matched the already-present vents in the front fascia, giving one of the most impressive front views on any car. Ram Air decals were mounted on each side of the large scoop. The 2002 SLP Firehawk model used a unique composite hood with a different Ram Air intake design and air extractors. All 1993–2002 Firebird hoods had a left and right front corner notch for the standard concealed headlamps, and all hoods opened to 80 degrees for easier engine compartment access.

There were two different body-color reaction-injection-molded front fascias used on the 1993–1997 Firebirds. The base Firebird and Formula used a peaked front fascia that included dual wide openings on either side of a distinctive and

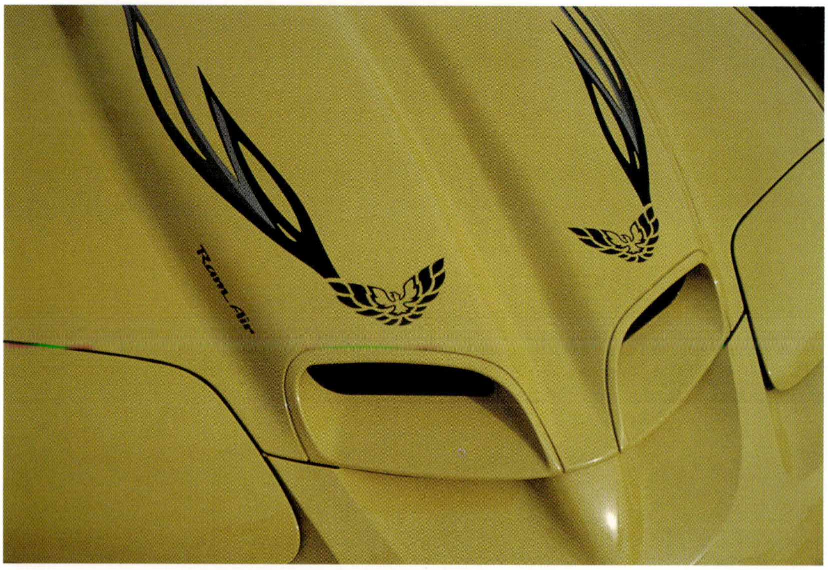

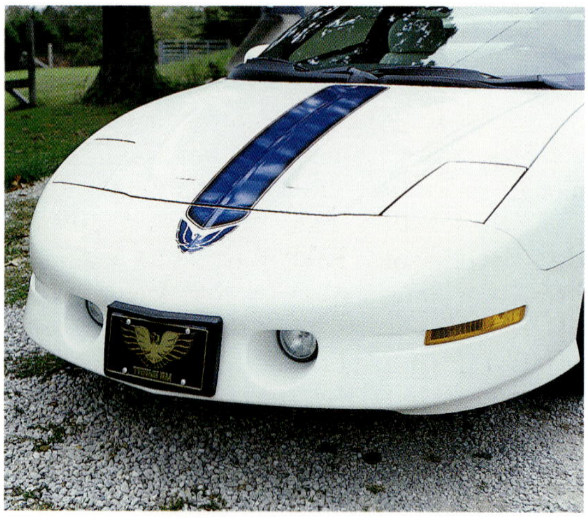

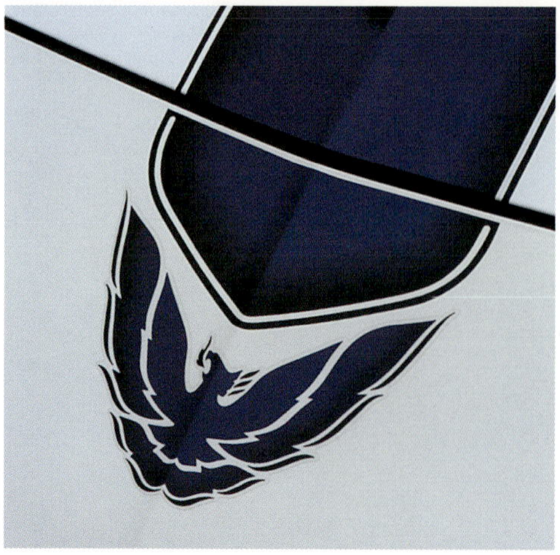

Far left: This view of the front fascia of a white 1994 Trans Am GT 25th Anniversary Edition coupe shows the relatively smooth hood surface with special blue stripe, standard front license plate mounting, and wraparound side marker lights. *Left:* The blue bird on the front fascia of a white 1994 Trans Am GT 25th Anniversary Edition coupe. Note the fine stripe around the border of the main panel.

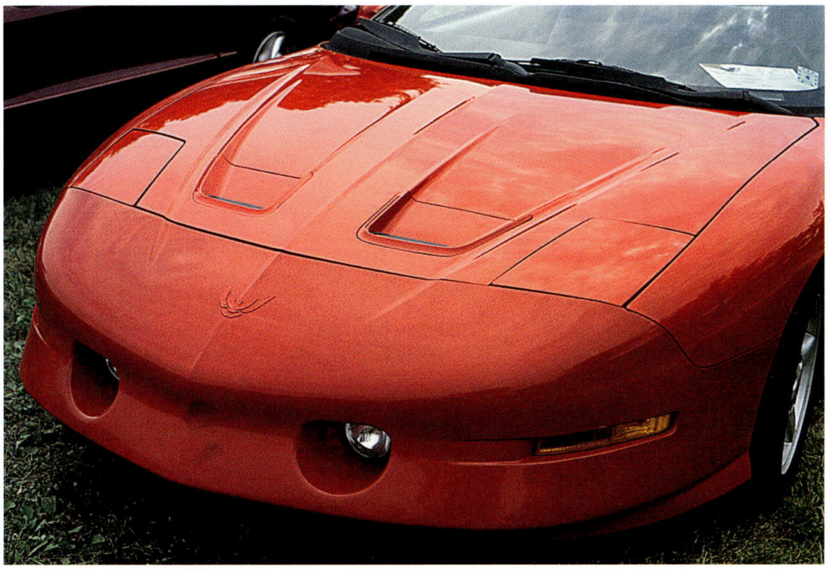

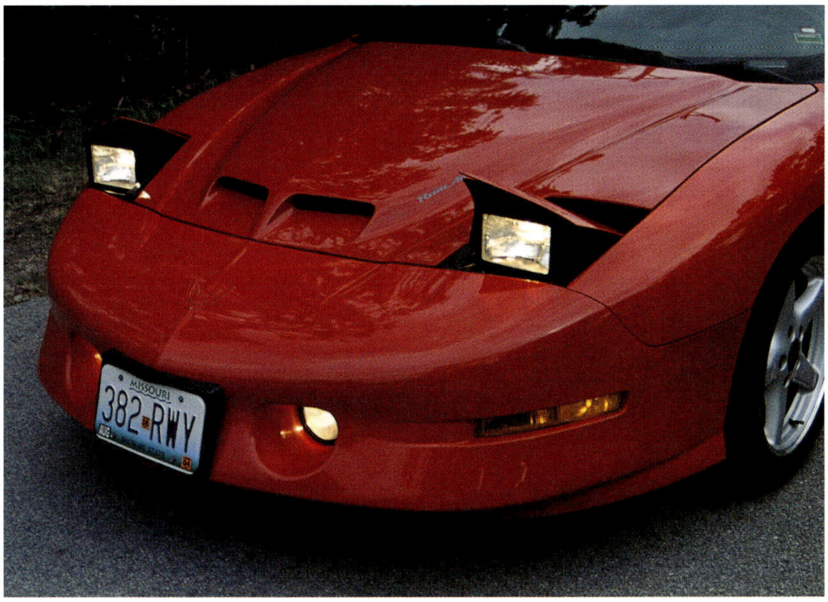

Top: This Bright Red 1995 Trans Am coupe has round driving lights on either side of the front of the panel. ***Above:*** This photo shows the headlights raised and the parking and driving lights turned on in this Bright Red 1996 Trans Am coupe The Ram Air intake openings were new for 1996 in the Trans Am.

Firebird Production

1993

Model	Production
Firebird	5,006
Formula	3,985
Trans Am	5,121

1994

Model	Production
Firebird coupe	25,669
Firebird conv.	174
Formula coupe	9,234
Formula conv.	168
Trans Am coupe	3,852
Trans Am conv.	468
Trans Am GT coupe	6,142
Trans Am GT conv.	215

1995

Model	Production
Firebird coupe	26,230
Firebird conv.	2,926
Formula coupe	7,448
Formula conv.	1,038
Trans Am coupe	10,943
Trans Am conv.	2,402

1996

Model	Production
Firebird coupe	17,773
Firebird conv.	976
Formula coupe	3,033
Formula conv.	302
Trans Am coupe	7,981
Trans Am conv.	917

1997

Model	Production
Firebird coupe	16,394
Firebird conv.	1,226
Formula coupe	2,766
Formula conv.	324
Trans Am coupe	8,656
Trans Am conv.	1,390

1998

Model	Production
Firebird coupe	15,869
Firebird conv.	704
Formula	2,123
Trans Am coupe	12,046
Trans Am conv.	1,413

1999

Model	Production
Firebird coupe	17,170
Firebird conv.	1,245
Formula coupe	1,427
Formula WS6 coupe	175
Trans Am coupe	10,343
Trans Am conv.	1,027
Trans Am WS6 coupe	2,765
Trans Am WS6 Conv.	467
Trans Am 30th Anniv. coupe	1,065
Trans Am 30th Anniv. Conv.	535

2000

Model	Production
Firebird coupe	13,529
Firebird conv.	1,149
Formula	1,302
Formula WS6	233
Trans Am coupe	6,639
Trans Am conv.	783
Trans Am WS6 coupe	7,166
Trans Am WS6 conv.	1,025

2001

Model	Production
Firebird coupe	7,191
Firebird conv.	2,347
Formula	1,037
Trans Am coupe	2,596
Trans Am conv.	396
Trans Am WS6 coupe	7,073
Trans Am WS6 conv.	796

2002

Model	Production
Firebird coupe	8,423
Firebird conv.	1,498
Formula	901
Trans Am coupe	3,962
Trans Am conv.	998
Trans Am WS6 coupe	12,212
Trans Am WS6 conv.	2,696

Right: This photo shows a close-up view of the right side driving and parking lights in a Sport Gold Metallic 1998 Firebird convertible. The shape of the headlight panels also changed.

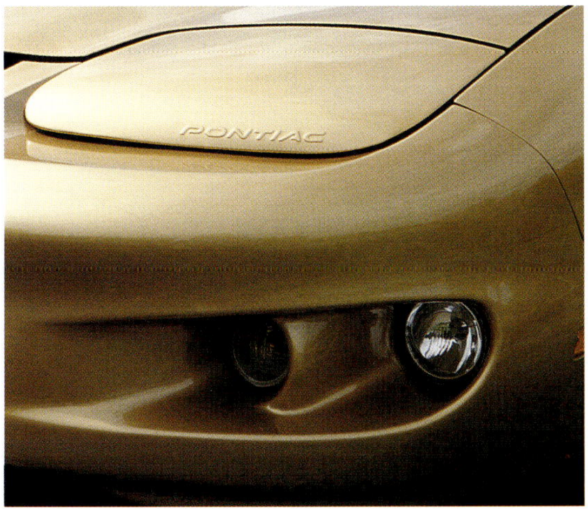

iconic Pontiac split. The openings housed optional driving/fog lights (RPO T96) when ordered. The upper surface of the fascia was relatively smooth, and the lower sides had wraparound wide rectangular amber marker/parking lamps. All standard front fascias had a narrow lower air dam across the entire width and a molded-in bird emblem on the top center.

The 1993–1997 Trans Am had a completely unique body-color RIM front fascia with two round openings and a smooth aerodynamic peaked appearance. The round openings housed standard driving lights. The lower edge of the Trans Am fascia angled forward with a distinctive air dam. The Trans Am front fascia also had wide wraparound side marker/parking lights like the standard front end.

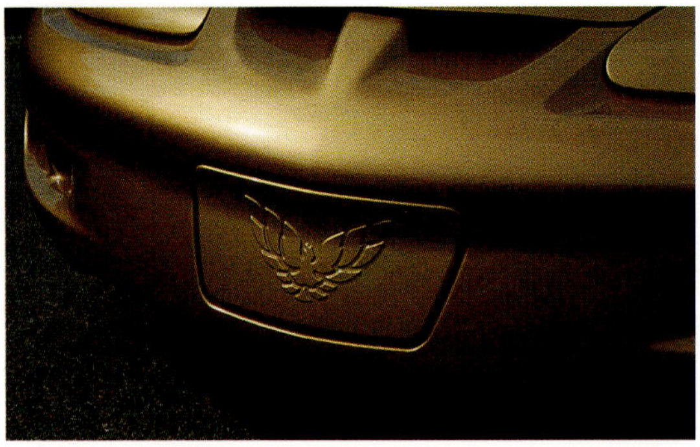

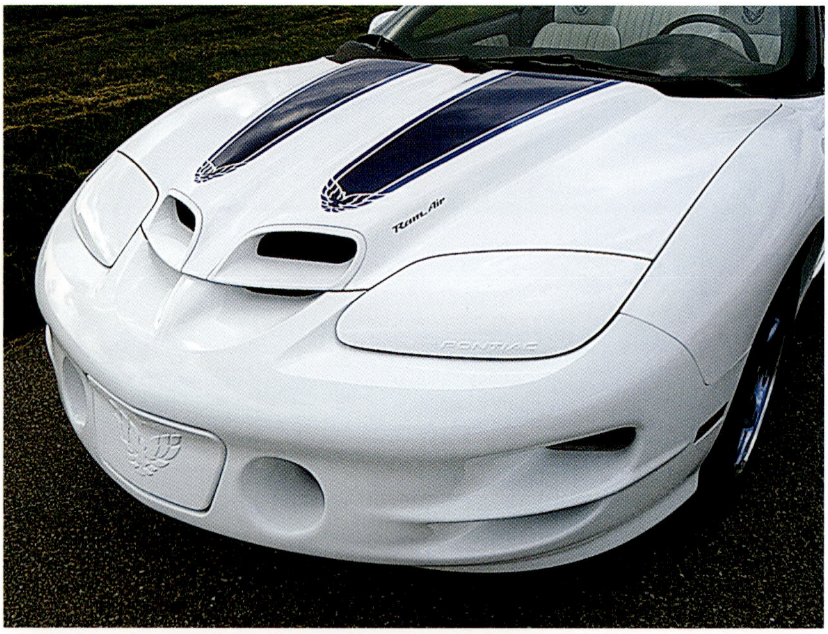

Above: All 1998–2002 Firebirds and Trans Am were equipped with this removable license plate opening cover with bird logo. It was installed to improve the appearance when the front plate was not required by law or when the car was parked. ***Right:*** This is a view of the front fascia of a white 1999 Trans Am 30th Anniversary WS6 Ram Air convertible. Note the hood stripe and Ram Air decal on the side of the scoop.

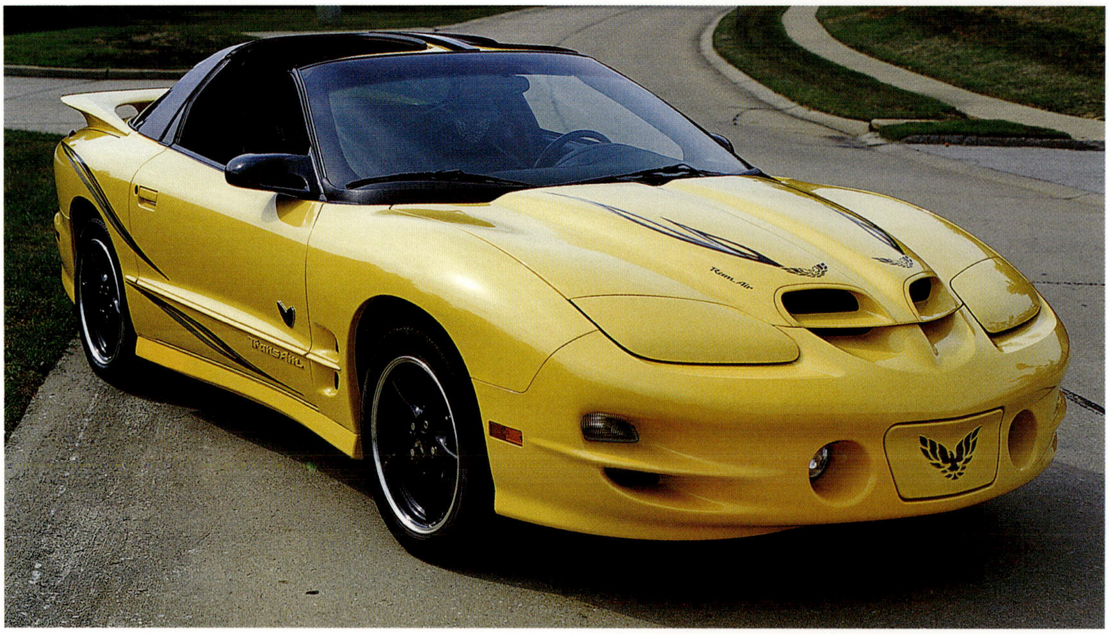

Left: This photo shows the front fascia and hood design on a yellow (54) 2002 Trans Am WS6 Ram Air Collector Edition hatchback coupe with optional T-top roof. The special yellow finish and body graphics were unique to the 2002 Collector Edition.

There were two different body-color RIM front fascias used for the 1998–2002 Firebird. The base Firebird and Formula used a front fascia that was derived from the Trans Am design in the previous model with a smooth front. The upper center of the fascia had two small scoop inlets divided by the iconic Pontiac split. The lower front fascia angled forward and had a center license plate mounting with a removable cover. The cover had a molded-in bird. The outer ends of the fascia had two small round openings in an inline recess for parking lights (inner) or driving lights (outer). There were rectangular amber side-lights just ahead of the wheel opening on each side.

The 1998–2002 Trans Am front fascia was similar to the standard front, but there were large round openings for driving lights on each side of the license plate mounting. There were also two oval, vertically stacked, recessed openings on each end for parking lights on top and an unused opening on the bottom. A horizontal windsplit divided the two openings, and a small rectangular side marker was just behind the rear end of the windsplit.

Interior

The 1993–2002 Firebird was available with a variety of interior trim combinations and materials, all with standard reclining front bucket seats and deep-cushion rear bucket seats with a solid folding rear seatback. A front center floor console was standard equipment on all 1993–2002 Firebirds. A pull-up hand-brake lever with vinyl boot was

Body Colors

1993 Body Colors

Code	Color
10	Bright White
41	Black
45	Dark Green Metallic
54	Yellow
71	Medium Red Metallic
80	Bright Blue Metallic
81	Bright Red
91	Gray Purple Pearl

1994 and 1995 Body Colors

Code	Color
10	Bright White
41	Black
45	Dark Green Metallic
54	Yellow
72	Medium Red Metallic
80	Bright Blue Metallic
81	Bright Red
91	Gray Purple Metallic

1996 Body Colors

Code	Color
05	Medium Dark Purple Metallic
10	Bright White
13	Bright Silver Metallic
37	Dark Aqua Metallic
41	Black
48	Dark Green Metallic
79	Blue-Green Chameleon
80	Bright Blue Metallic
81	Bright Red
96	Red-Orange Metallic

1997 Body Colors

Code	Color
10	Bright White
13	Bright Silver Metallic
31	Bright Green Metallic
41	Black
48	Dark Green Metallic
79	Blue-Green Chameleon
81	Bright Red
88	Bright Purple Metallic
96	Red-Orange Metallic

1998 Body Colors

Code	Color
10	Bright White
13	Bright Silver Metallic
28	Navy Blue Metallic
31	Bright Green Metallic
41	Black
63	Sport Gold Metallic
79	Blue-Green Chameleon
81	Bright Red
88	Bright Purple Metallic
96	Red-Orange Metallic

1999 Body Colors

Code	Color
10	Arctic White
11	Pewter Metallic
13	Silver Metallic
20	Medium Blue Metallic
28	Navy Blue Metallic
31	Bright Green Metallic
41	Black
79	Blue-Green Chameleon
81	Bright Red

2000 Body Colors

Code	Color
10	Arctic White
11	Pewter Metallic
13	Silver Metallic
28	Navy Blue Metallic
41	Black
44	Maple Red Metallic
79	Blue-Green Chameleon
81	Bright Red

2001 and 2002 Body Colors

Code	Color
10	Arctic White
11	Pewter Metallic
28	Navy Blue Metallic
41	Black
44	Maple Red Metallic
71	Sunset Orange Metallic
79	Blue-Green Chameleon
81	Bright Red

The interior in this white 1994 Trans Am GT 25th Anniversary Edition hatchback coupe has a special interior trim scheme with white Prado leather and dark gray contrasting vinyl trim. The seatbacks and door panels also include special embroidered 25th Anniversary logos in blue.

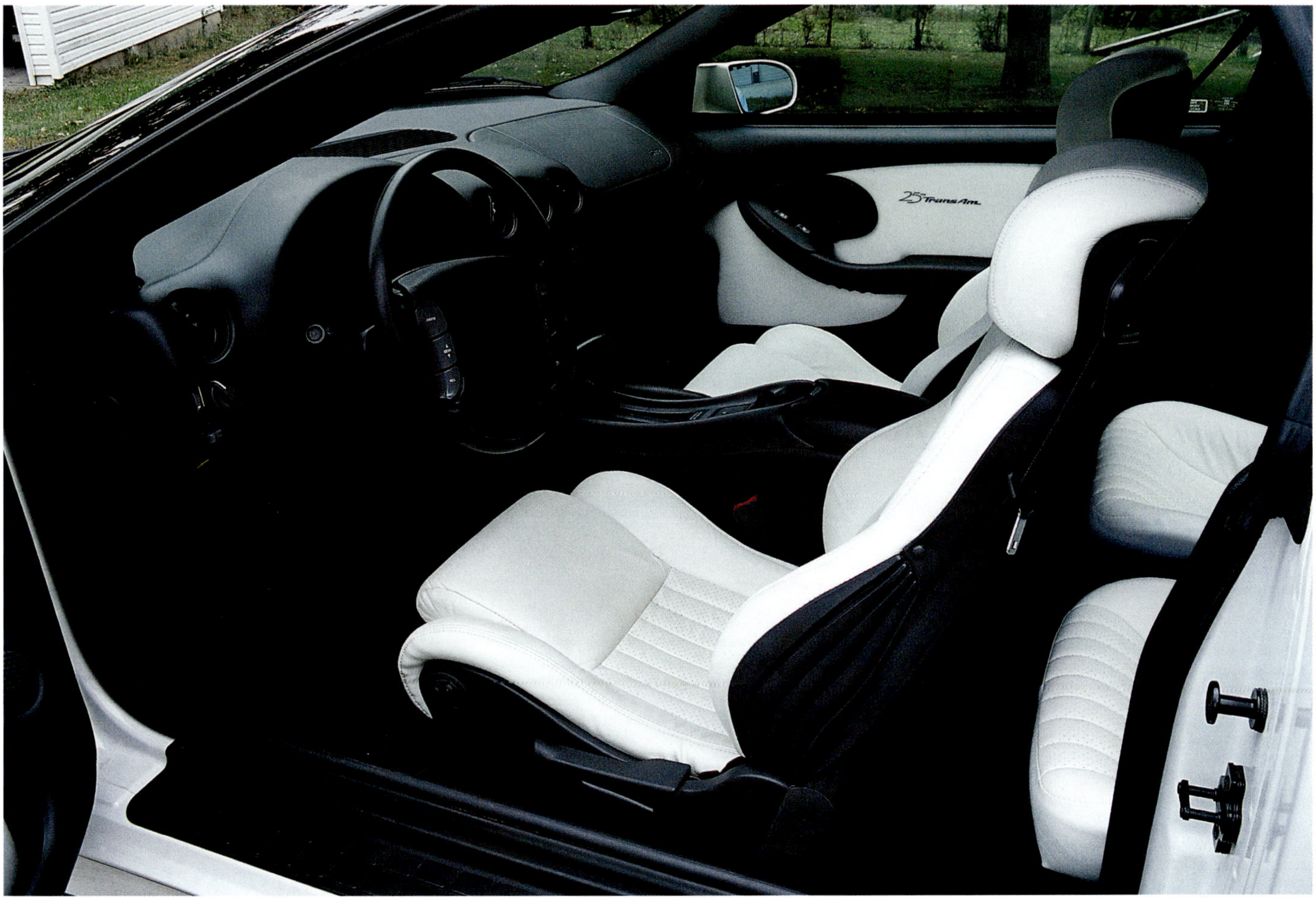

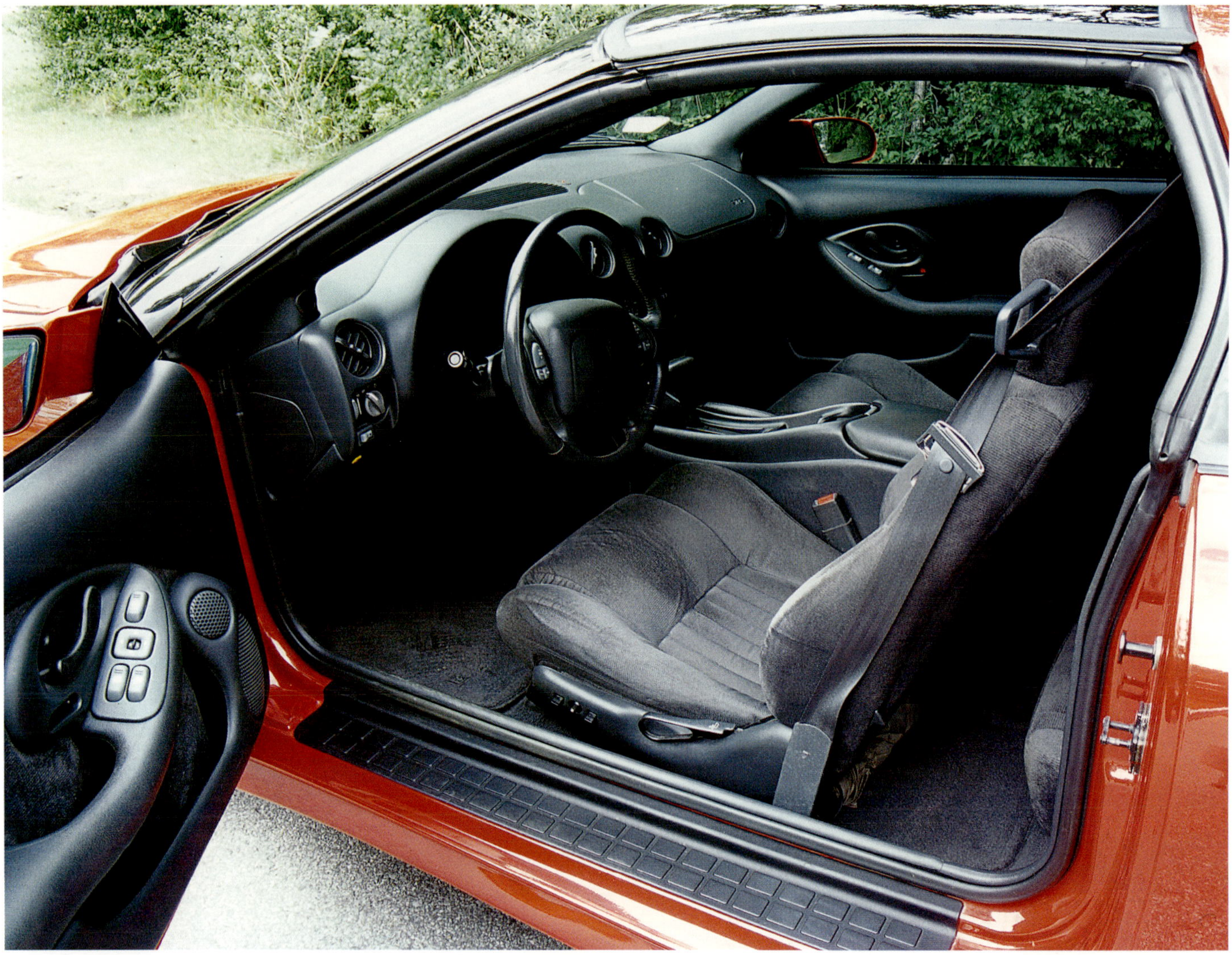

This is the graphite cloth interior in a Bright Red 1996 Trans Am hatchback coupe with optional T-top roof. The air bag panel is visible in the center of the steering wheel.

Interior Trim Combinations

1993–1995

Code	Color
12B, D	Graphite cloth
122	Graphite leather
14B, D	Medium Gray cloth
142	Medium Gray leather
64B, D	Medium Beige cloth
642	Medium Beige leather

1996 and 1997

Code	Color
102	White Prado leather
12B, D	Graphite cloth
122	Graphite leather
52B, D	Neutral cloth
522	Neutral leather
702	Red Prado leather

1998–2002

Color (codes not available)

Taupe Cartegena cloth
Ebony Cartegena cloth
Taupe Prado leather and vinyl
Ebony Prado leather and vinyl
Medium Dark Oak Prado leather and vinyl
Camel Prado leather w/Camel and Ebony accents (2002 only)

mounted on the right side of the console on all models. The new interior design had an integrated cockpit look with the door panels, instrument panel, and console tied together visually.

The standard 1993–2002 seat designs featured well-formed backs and smooth cushion bolsters with inserts of longitudinal sewn pleats forward to about ⅔ of the lower cushion. The front of the seat cushion had a smooth raised front leg bolster. The sides of the seatbacks had very deep, smooth side bolsters to provide excellent lateral support and integral headrests. The new seat designs were similar to that used for the 1985–1992 deluxe interior trim. The interior trim for 1993 was available in Metrix cloth in medium gray (64), graphite (12), and beige (14) shades only.

At the beginning of the 1994 model year, the cloth interior was available in the original shades of medium gray, graphite, and beige, but flame red (70) was added before the end of the model year. Later in the 1994 and into the 1995 model years, Prado leather became available in tan and graphite only. In 1996 and 1997, the Metrix cloth was available in graphite (12) and neutral (52).

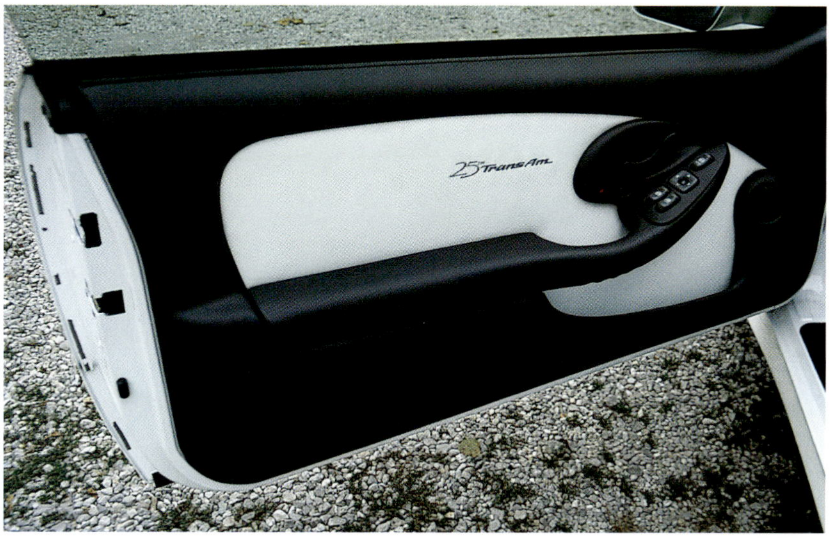

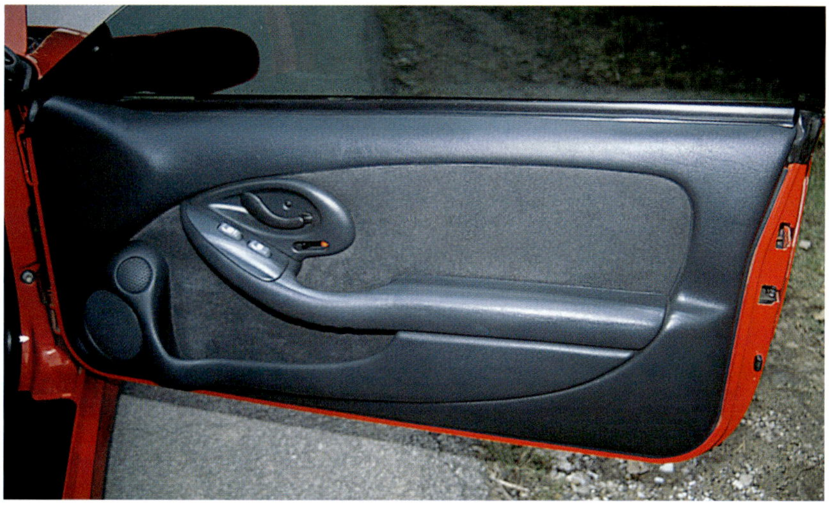

Top: This left door panel trim in a 1994 Trans Am GT 25th Anniversary Edition features the distinctive embroidered 25th Anniversary logo on the white panel. **Above:** This is the right door panel of a Bright Red 1996 Trans Am Ram Air WS6 coupe. Note the gray cloth, graphite vinyl trim scheme, and speakers in the front of the door panel.

For 1996 and 1997, the leather was also available in red (70). Color-coordinated carpet covered the floors, rear seatbacks, and cargo compartment.

The 1998 and 1999 interior trim schemes were available in Cartagena cloth in dark gray and neutral and Prado leather in dark gray, neutral, and red. The leather was standard in the Trans Am coupe and convertible and optional in the Firebird and Formula. The cloth interior was standard in the Firebird and not available in the Trans Am.

The 1999 Trans Am 30th Anniversary Edition had standard arctic white (10) Prado leather seating surfaces with blue embroidery and special 30th Anniversary door panel inserts, leather-and-vinyl headrests with medallion, floor mats, and leather cargo mat. The outer seat frames were graphite plastic. There was also a special numbered 30th Anniversary emblem on the console. The carpets were black.

For 2000 and 2001, interiors were available in Cartagena cloth in taupe and ebony (19) for the base Firebird coupe and convertible, and the Formula coupe. Trans Am coupe and convertible interiors were available in Prado leather seating with perforated inserts. The Prado leather was available in taupe and ebony with all exterior colors and in dark oak (67) with all exterior colors except pewter metallic. The Prado leather interiors were optional in the Firebird and Formula.

In 2002, the Firebird and Formula had standard Cartagena cloth in ebony available with all exterior colors and in taupe with all except bright silver metallic. The 2002 Trans Am had standard Prado leather with perforated inserts in ebony with all exterior colors, in taupe with all but bright silver metallic, and in camel (671) with all but pewter metallic. The Prado leather trim was optional in the Firebird and Formula. The 2002 Trans Am Collector Edition had a unique interior

Selected 1993–2002 Regular Production Options

RPO	Description	RPO	Description	RPO	Description
AC3	Six-way power driver's seat	KC4	Engine oil cooling system	NW9	Traction control system
AR9	Articulating bucket seats, leather trim	K34	Cruise control	PW7	16x8 cast-aluminum wheels
AQ9	Reclining seats	LS1	5.7-liter V-8	QA7	16x7.5 cast-aluminum wheels
AU0	Remote lock control	LT1	5.7-liter V-8	T61	Daytime running lamps
A31	Power windows	L32	3.4-liter V-6	T96	Fog lamps
A90	Rear compartment remote lock	L36	3.8-liter V-6	UQ0	Four-speaker system
B84	Body-color side moldings	MD8	Four-speed automatic	UW2	10-speaker system
CC1	Removable roof hatch panels (T-top)	MM5	Five-speed manual	U18	Kilometer speedometer
C49	Rear window defogger	MN6	Six-speed manual	U73	Fixed antenna
C60	Air conditioning	MX0	Automatic overdrive transmission	U75	Power antenna
DD9	Outside mirrors, remote LH, breakaway	M28	Six-speed, BW, 3.36 low gear	UK3	Steering wheel radio controls
DE4	Removable hatch roof sunshade	M29	Six-speed, BW, 2.97 low gear	WS6	Ram Air performance and handling package
DG7	Dual sport power mirrors	M49	Five-speed, BW, 3.95 low gear	W68	Sport appearance package
J41	Power front disc, rear drum brake system	NC3	Tailpipe modifications	Y87	3800 performance package
J65	Power front and rear disc brake system	NP5	Leather-wrapped steering wheel		
		N36	Four-spoke sport steering wheel		

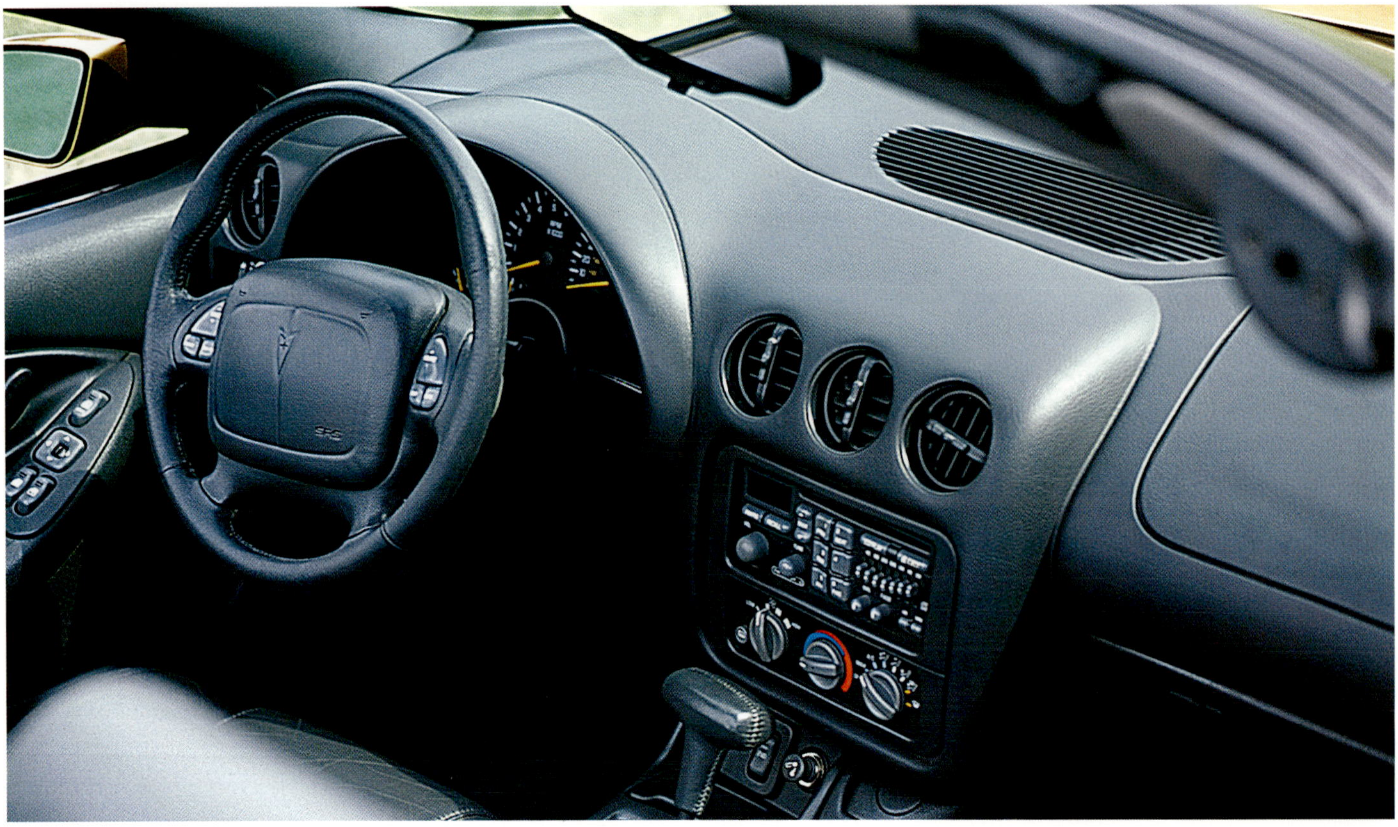

This is a detail view of the instrument panel of a Sport Gold Metallic 1998 Firebird convertible with optional gray leather interior. There are controls on the steering wheel.

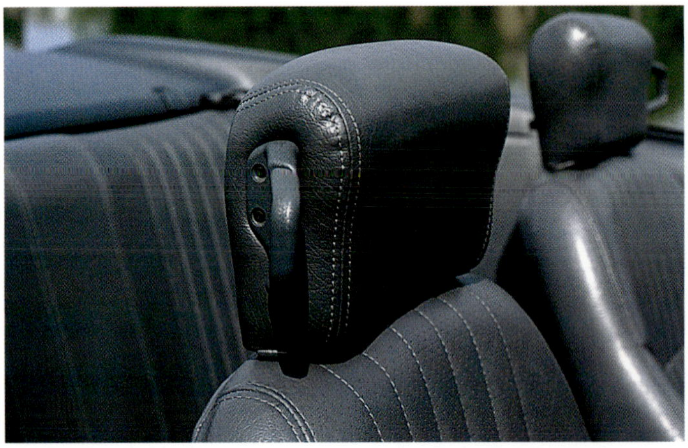

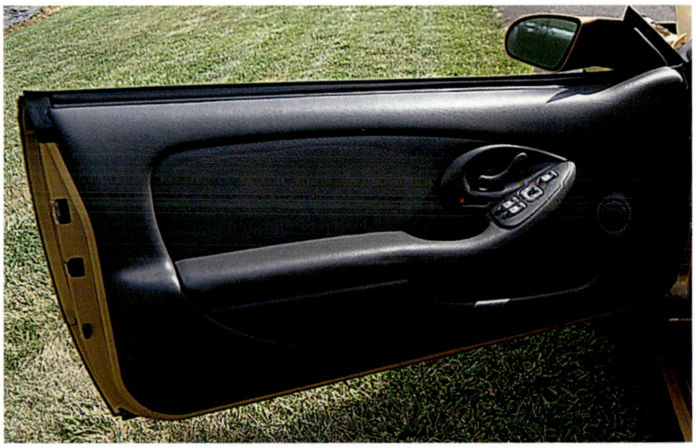

Above left: This is a detail view of the seat headrests in a Sport Gold Metallic Firebird convertible with optional gray leather interior trim. There is light color stitching on the seams. ***Above right:*** This is the left door panel of a 1998 Firebird convertible with optional gray leather interior trim. The window controls on the front of the armrest and the speakers on the front of the panel are visible.

ebony-leather trim scheme that featured silver-embroidered Collector Edition birds on the headrests and the outer rear corners of the standard front floor mats.

The 1993–2002 Firebird instrument panel was completely redesigned from the previous year. All panels were finished in dark gray vinyl with a distinctive dome over the instrument cluster. Inside the large domed cluster area were clear analog gauges in black faces with white indicators. At night, the gauges were illuminated with red backlighting to increase instrument legibility. A single round adjustable air duct was mounted to the upper left of the cluster dome with a backlighted light switch just below the cluster. All 1993–2002 Firebird models had a standard passenger-side air bag installed in the right side of the instrument panel.

Each cluster had two small gauges on each side of two large, partially round gauges in the center. The large gauge on the left was the 7,000-rpm

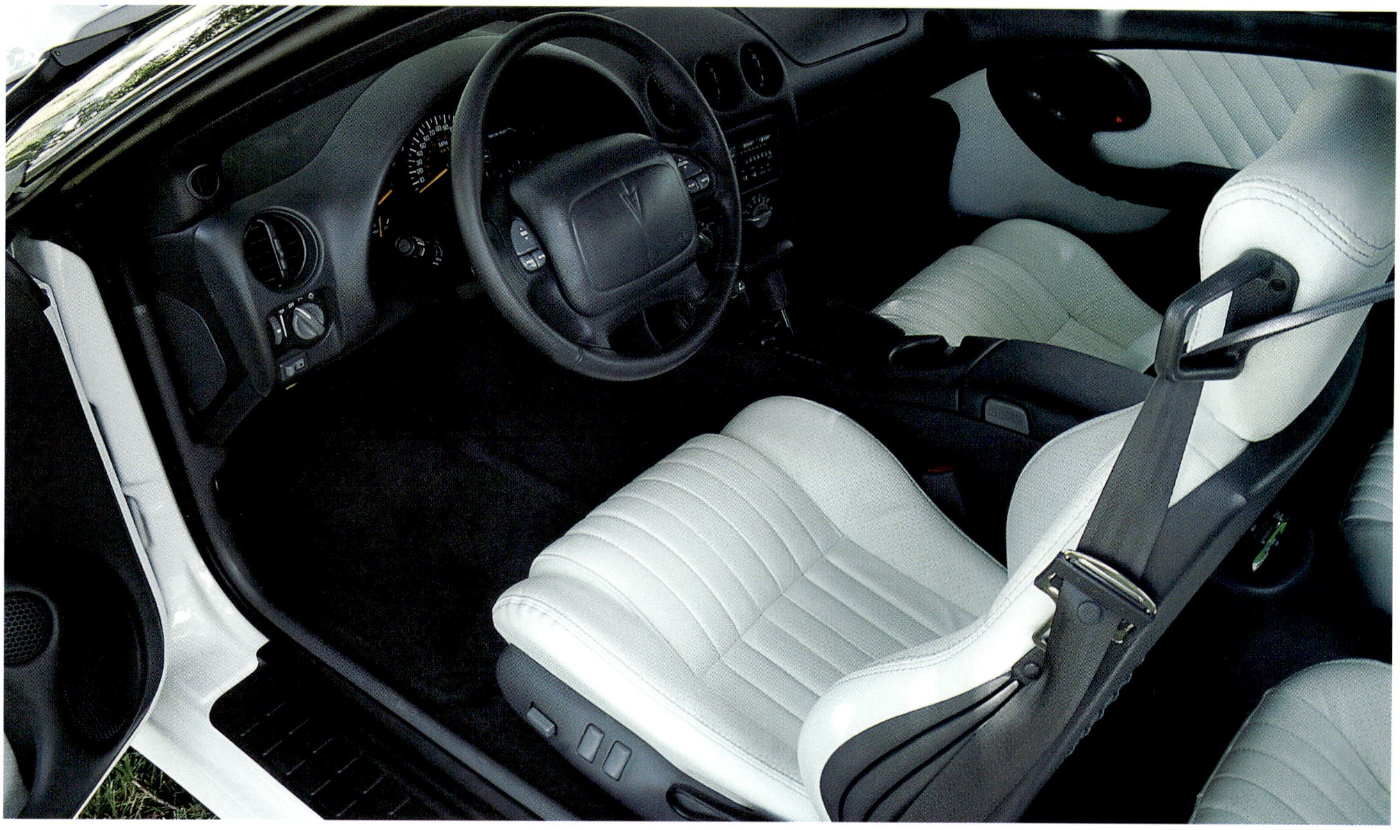

This is the white leather interior in a white 1999 Trans Am 30th Anniversary Edition coupe. The instrument panel, steering wheel, and side panels are graphite vinyl, and the carpet is black.

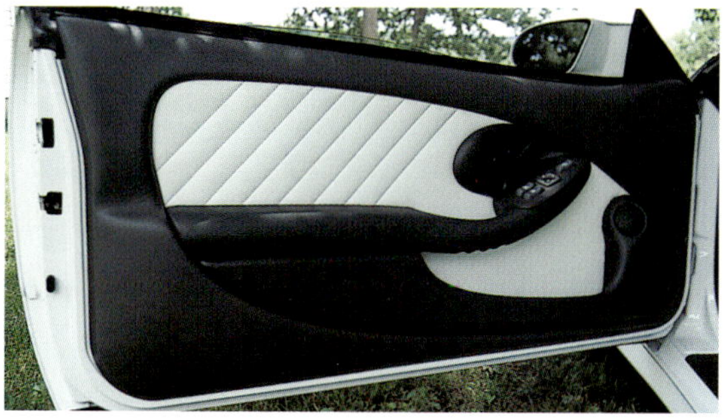

Above: This special door panel on a white 1999 Trans Am 30th Anniversary Edition has distinctive angled pleats in the center panel and the window and lock switches in the front of the armrest.

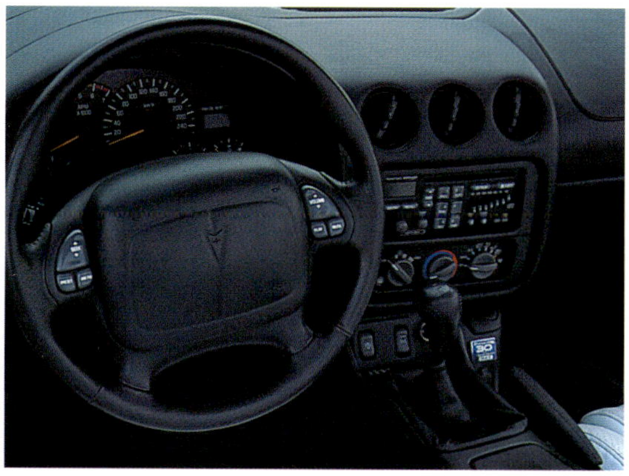

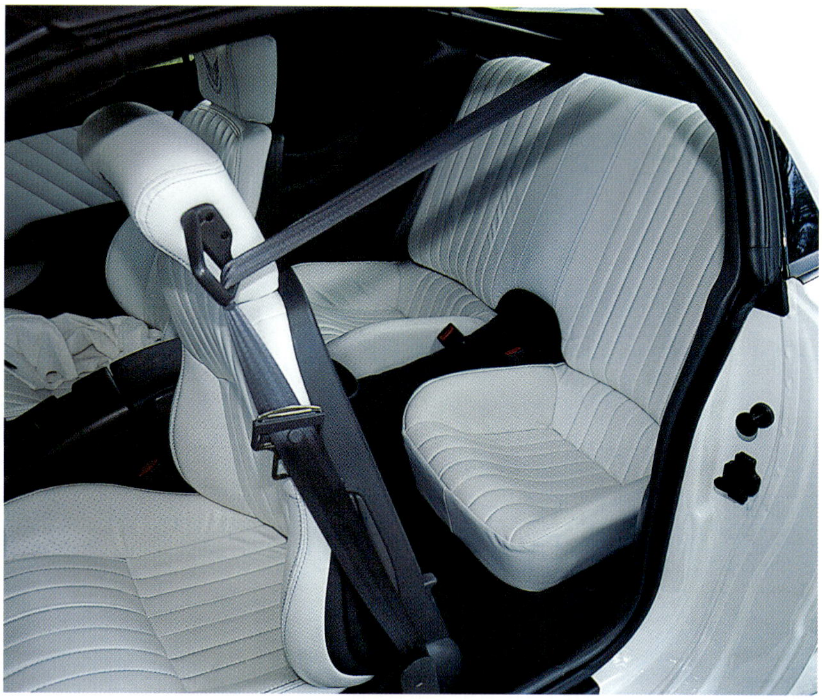

Above: This view of the rear compartment of a white 1999 Trans Am 30th Anniversary Edition coupe shows the distinctive deep-bucket design of the rear seat cushions and the perforated leather in the seat panels. ***Left:*** This is a detail view of the instrument panel of a white 1999 Trans Am 30th Anniversary Edition convertible. Note the radio controls on the steering wheel. This is a Canadian-delivered convertible so the speedometer is calibrated in kilometers.

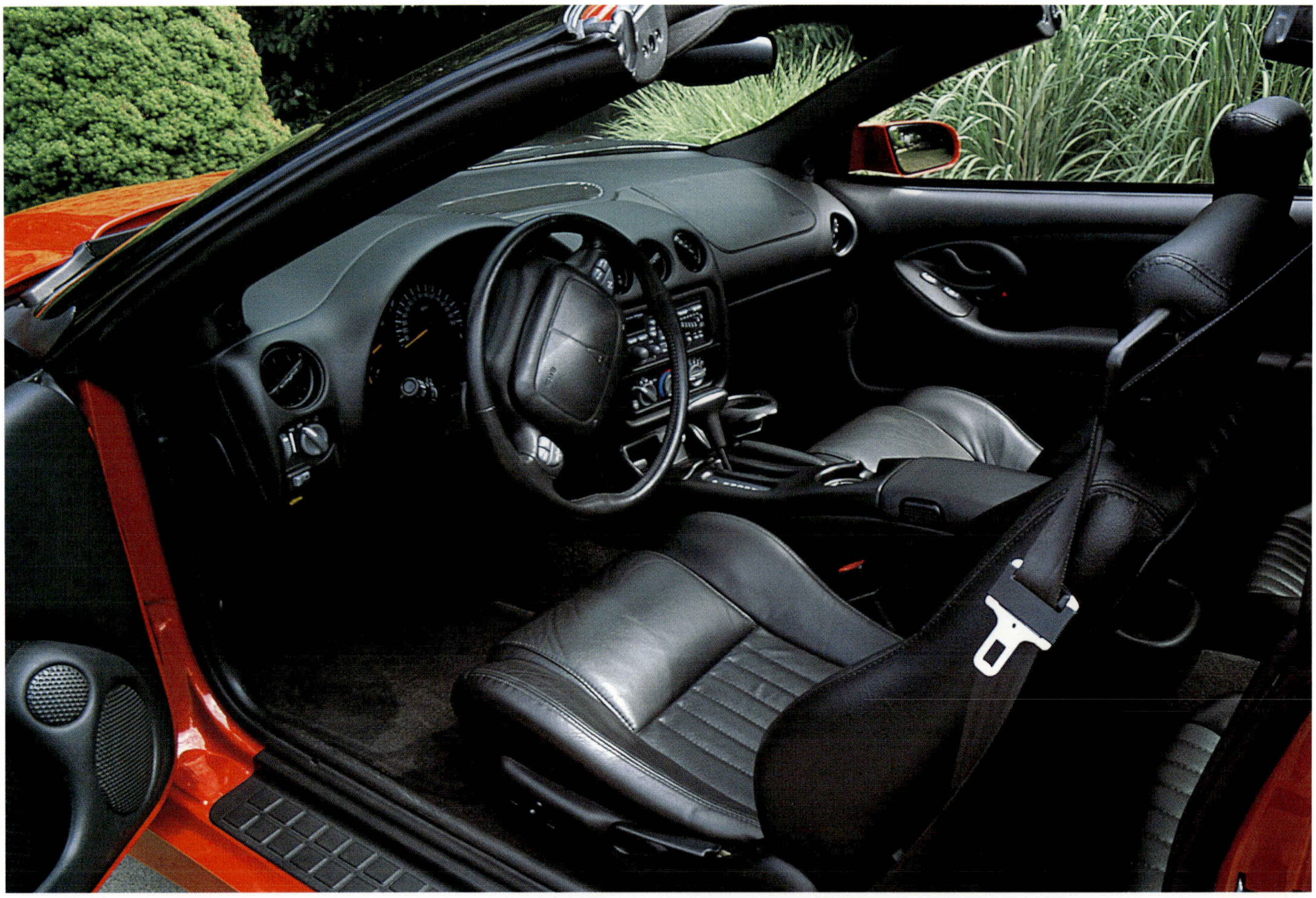

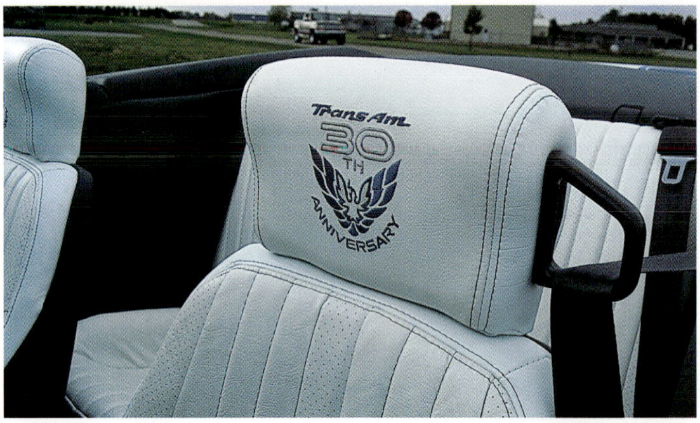

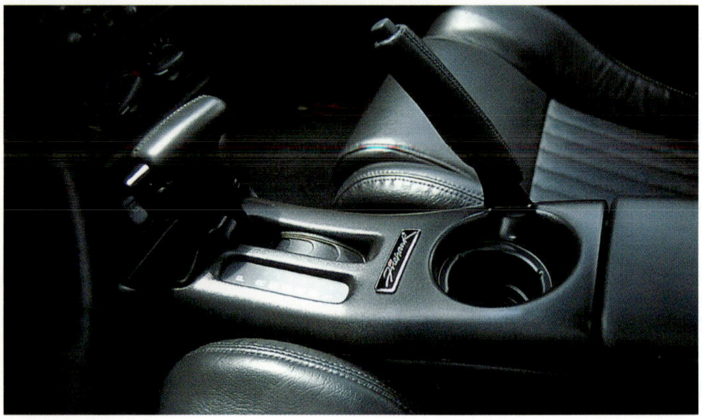

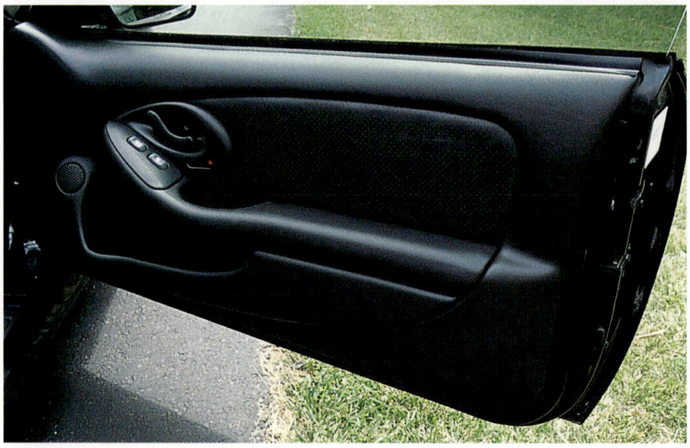

Top: This is the interior of a Bright Red 2000 Trans Am WS6 Ram Air hatchback coupe with ebony leather interior trim. The radio controls and air bag SRS panel in the steering wheel center are visible. ***Above left:*** This is a detail view of the left front headrest in a white 1999 Trans Am 30th Anniversary Edition convertible with the special blue embroidered 30th Anniversary logo. ***Above right:*** This is a detail view of the center floor console in a black 2002 Trans Am Firehawk hatchback coupe equipped with automatic transmission. Note the distinctive Firehawk badge on the top of the console. ***Left:*** This is a view of the right door panel of a 2002 Trans Am Firehawk coupe with ebony leather interior trim. Note the perforated leather in the center panel.

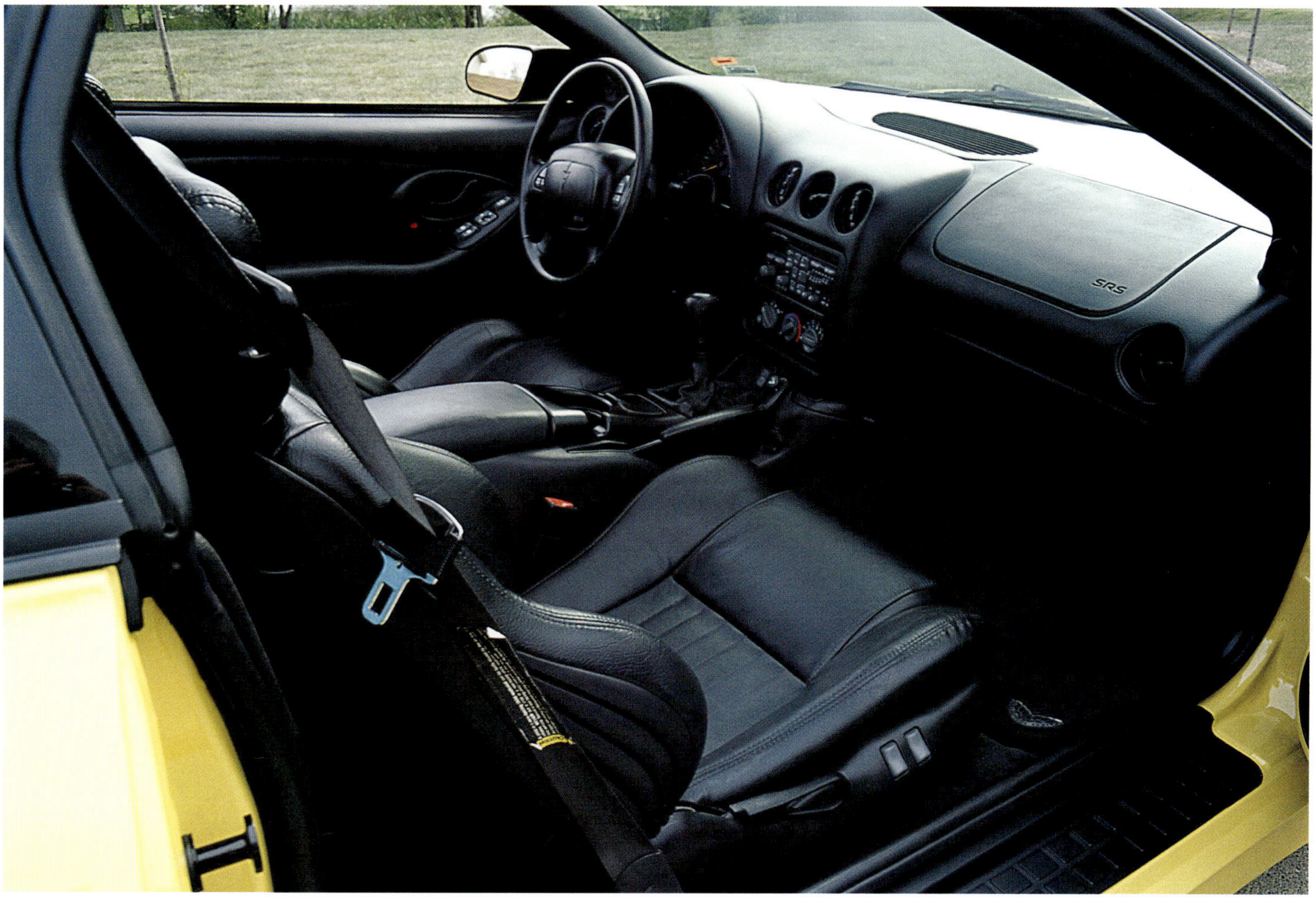

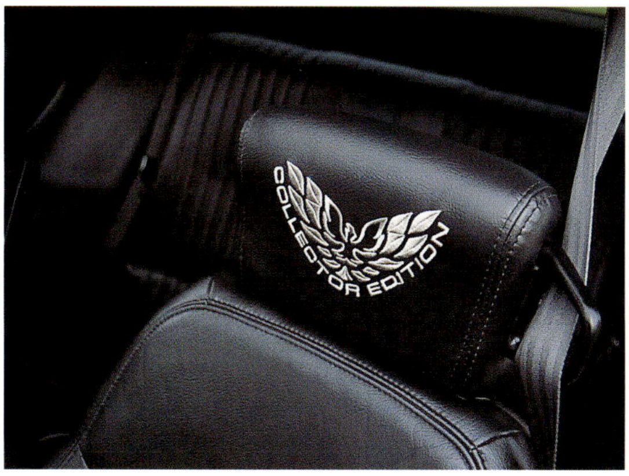

Above: This photo shows the ebony leather interior in a yellow 2002 Trans Am WS6 Collector Edition hatchback coupe with the optional six-speed manual transmission (RPO MN6) and short-throw Hurst Performance shifter (RPO BBS). ***Right:*** Detail view of the headrest with silver embroidered bird logo on a yellow 2002 Trans Am WS6 Collector Edition hatchback coupe. The interior trim is ebony leather.

tachometer. The large gauge on the right overlapped the left gauge and housed the speedometer that displayed both miles per hour and kilometers per hour. The Firebird and Formula speedometer read to 110 miles per hour, and the Trans Am speedo read to 150 miles per hour. The smaller gauges on the lower left displayed the coolant temperature and oil pressure. The voltmeter and fuel gauge were on the lower right.

In the center of the instrument panel was a separate recessed panel insert that held the radio and heater/air-conditioning controls. The radio controls were at the top of the insert and varied according to which optional sound system was ordered. The standard sound system for the 1993–1996 Firebird and Formula was a Delco ETR AM stereo with cassette and clock (RPO UM6). This system was not available in the 1993–1996 Trans Am, which had a standard Delco ETR stereo AM/FM with auto-reverse cassette and five-band equalizer. It included a clock, seek (up and down) and search buttons, and a 10-speaker system, all with steering wheel controls (RPO UX1). This system was optional in the Firebird and Formula. All models were available with a Delco ETR AM stereo with compact disc player, equalizer, and seek/scan system with 10-speakers and steering wheel controls (RPO U1A).

The standard sound system for all 1997 and 1998 Firebird models was the Delco 2001 Series ETR AM/FM stereo with cassette player, seven-band equalizer, clock, touch control, and four speakers (RPO W52). The optional sound system was the Delco 2001 Series with compact disc player, seven-band graphic equalizer, clock, touch control, and four speakers (RPO W73). There was also an optional Delco 2001 Series with AM/FM stereo, auto-reverse cassette, seven-band graphic equalizer, touch control, and Monsoon sound system with 10 speakers (RPO W54). This system was not available in convertibles. A second Monsoon system with compact disc player, four-band graphic equalizer, and 10 speakers was available with RPO W55; it was also not available in convertibles. In 1998, two special sound systems were available only in the convertibles.

In 1999, the standard sound system for the Firebird coupe was a Delco 2001 Series ETR AM/FM stereo with compact disc player, seven-band graphic equalizer, touch control, search and seek, and four speakers (RPO W53). The Firebird and Trans Am convertible had a similar system standard but with eight speakers, 500-watt Monsoon system, and subwoofer amplifier (RPO X20). These systems were not available in the coupes.

The standard sound system for the 1999–2001 Formula and Trans Am coupes and optional in the Firebird coupe was the Monsoon Series ETR AM/FM stereo with compact disc player, seven-band graphic equalizer, 500-watt power, 10 speakers, and touch control (RPO W55). Optional in all models but the convertibles was a Monsoon Series ETR AM/FM stereo with auto-reverse cassette, seven-band graphic equalizer, touch control, 800-watt power, seek up and down, and 10 speakers (RPO W54). A similar system was optional in the convertibles with eight speakers and a subwoofer amplifier (RPO X10).

For 2002, sound system options changed slightly, and the standard system in the Firebird coupe was a Delco 2001 Series ETR AM/FM stereo with CD player, seven-band graphic equalizer, clock, and four speakers (RPO W53). Standard with the Firebird and Trans Am convertible was the Monsoon Series ETR AM/FM stereo with CD player, seven-band graphic equalizer, 500-watt power, and eight speakers. The Formula and Trans Am coupes had a standard Monsoon Series ETR AM/FM stereo with CD player, seven-band graphic equalizer, 500-watt power, and 10 speakers (RPO W55). It was optional in the Firebird coupe. A trunk-mounted 12-disc CD changer was optional in all models.

The standard steering wheel for the 1993–1996 Firebird coupe and Formula coupe was the sport four-spoke wheel in dark gray vinyl with tilt column. The Trans Am had a standard dark gray leather-wrapped four-spoke wheel with radio controls that was optional on the Firebird and Formula with UX1 and U1A radios. The control buttons were mounted on either side of the center hub. Both wheels had a flat center with standard air bag and a Pontiac arrowhead logo in the center. There was a visible vertical seam in the center of the wheel.

For 1997–2002, the standard Trans Am steering wheel was a dark gray leather-wrapped wheel that was not available in the Firebird coupe or Formula coupe. A steering wheel with radio controls was optional with the radio option packages and was also available in the Firebird, Formula, and Trans Am. It was standard in the 1998 Formula and Trans Am and all convertible models. All steering wheels included a standard tilt column.

Engine and Engine Compartment

The 1993–2002 Firebird was available with three basic engine choices. The standard (and only engine available in the base 1993–1995 Firebird) was the 3.4-liter (207-cubic-inch) V-6 with electronic fuel injection available with 160 horsepower. The V-6 displacement was increased to 231 cubic inches (3.8 liters) in 1996–2002 with the horsepower increased to 200. The V-6 was not available in the Formula or Trans Am.

The standard engine for the 1993–1997 Formula and Trans Am was the 5.7-liter (350-cubic-inch) V-8. The 5.7 V-8 was available as the 270–285-horsepower base LT1 version from 1993 to 1997 and Ram Air LT1 in 1996 and 1997. A new 350-cubic-inch (5.7-liter) V-8 was also available in 1998–2002 as the standard LS1 all-aluminum version with 305–310 horsepower and Ram Air LS1 with 320–325 horsepower. The 5.7-liter V-8 was not available in the base Firebird.

Overhead-Valve V-6

The 1993–1995 3.4-liter (207-cubic-inch) overhead-valve V-6 (RPO L32) had a compression ratio of 9.0:1, a bore and stroke of 3.62x3.31 inches, and developed 160 horsepower at 4,600 rpm and 200 foot-pounds of torque at 3,200 rpm. The L32 V-6 used electronic fuel injection and had a VIN engine code of 8.

In 1996, a new larger cast-iron-block overhead-valve V-6 was introduced with 231 cubic inches (3.8 liters) with a 9.0:1 compression ratio. The RPO L36 engine had a bore and stroke of 3.80x3.40 inches and developed 200 horsepower at 5,200 rpm and 225 foot-pounds of torque at 4,000 rpm with electronic fuel injection. The VIN engine code was X in 1996 and K in 1997–2002.

Overhead-Valve V-8

The 1993–1997 Formula and Trans Am had a standard 350-cubic-inch (5.7-liter) overhead-valve V-8 with a cast-iron block and aluminum heads and intake manifold. The 5.7-liter V-8 (RPO LT1) had a bore and stroke of 4.00x3.48 inches, a compression ratio of 10.5:1, and developed 270 horsepower at 4,800 rpm and 325 foot-pounds of torque at 2,400 rpm. In 1994, sequential-port fuel injection was added to the 5.7-liter V-8. The horsepower was increased to 275 in 1995 and 285 at 5,000 rpm in 1996. The 1993–1996 LT1 V-8 had electronic fuel injection. The VIN engine code was P.

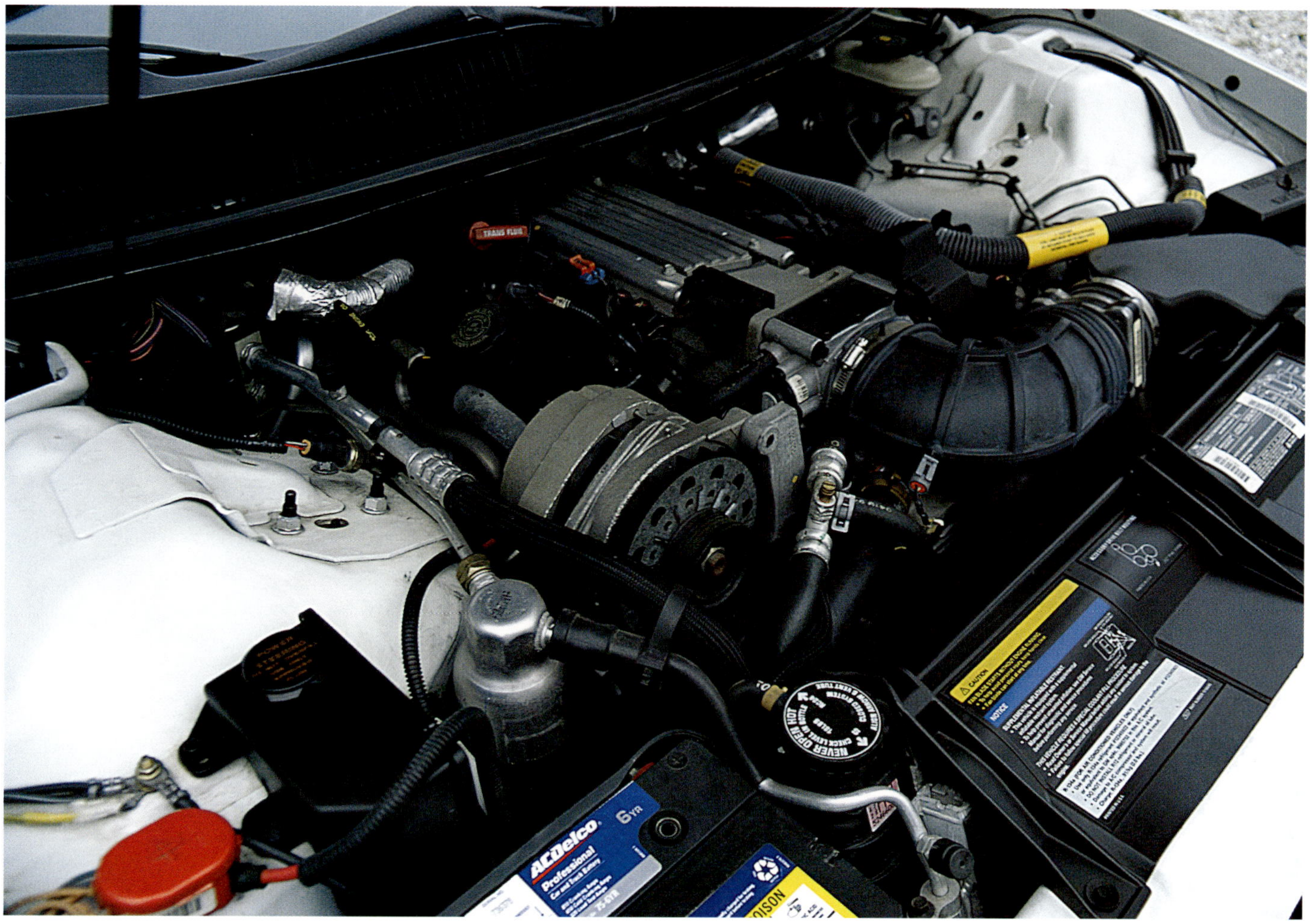

This is the engine compartment of an original white 1994 Trans Am GT 25th Anniversary Edition hatchback coupe. This Trans Am has the standard 5.7-liter (350-cubic-inch) RPO LT1 Chevrolet V-8 engine.

In 1996 and 1997, the 5.7-liter LT1 V-8 became available in a Ram Air version with a compression ratio of 10.5:1. The LT1 Ram Air V-8 was part of the WS6 Ram Air Performance Package and developed 305 horsepower at 5,000 rpm and 325 foot-pounds of torque at 2,400 rpm with electronic sequential-port fuel injection. The VIN engine code was 5.

In 1998–2002, the standard 5.7-liter V-8 was the RPO LS1 with a bore and stroke of 3.90x3.62 inches with a compression ratio of 10.5:1. The completely new LS1 had an aluminum cylinder block, heads, and intake manifold and developed 305 horsepower at 5,200 rpm and 335 foot-pounds of torque at 4,000 rpm with electronic fuel injection. Horsepower was increased to 310 (and torque to 340) for 2001 with the addition of a new intake manifold and camshaft. The standard LS1 had a VIN engine code of G.

The LS1 V-8 was also available in a Ram Air version with the WS6 Ram Air Performance Package for 1998–2002. The LS1 Ram Air engine had a compression ratio of 10.5:1 and developed 320 horsepower at 5,200 rpm and 345 foot-pounds of torque at 4,400 rpm in 1998–2000, and 325 horsepower and 350 foot-pounds of torque for 2001 and 2002 (with electronic fuel injection). The VIN engine code was G.

There were also special versions of the 5.7-liter V-8 that were part of the Street Legal Performance (SLP) Firebird and Formula Firehawks from 1995 through 2002. These engines were modified by SLP to increase performance over the standard configurations. In 1995, the SLP Firehawk package offered the 5.7-liter V-8 in 300- and 315-horsepower versions. In 1999, the modified SLP Trans Am Firehawk developed 327 horsepower and 345 foot-pounds of torque.

The 2000 Trans Am 10th Anniversary SLP Firehawk had a specially tuned 5.7-liter V-8 that developed 335 horsepower and 350 foot-pounds of torque using a specially designed composite hood with smaller air intake openings. The 2001 and 2002 versions of the Firehawk also developed 335 horsepower and 350 foot-pounds of torque with a special high-flow induction system and the Ram Air hood.

Engine Compartment

The firewall, inner fender panels, and radiator support of all 1993–2002 Firebirds were finished in body color, as the entire unitized body was painted as a unit. The inner fenderwells and firewall had a flat finish and did not have a gloss

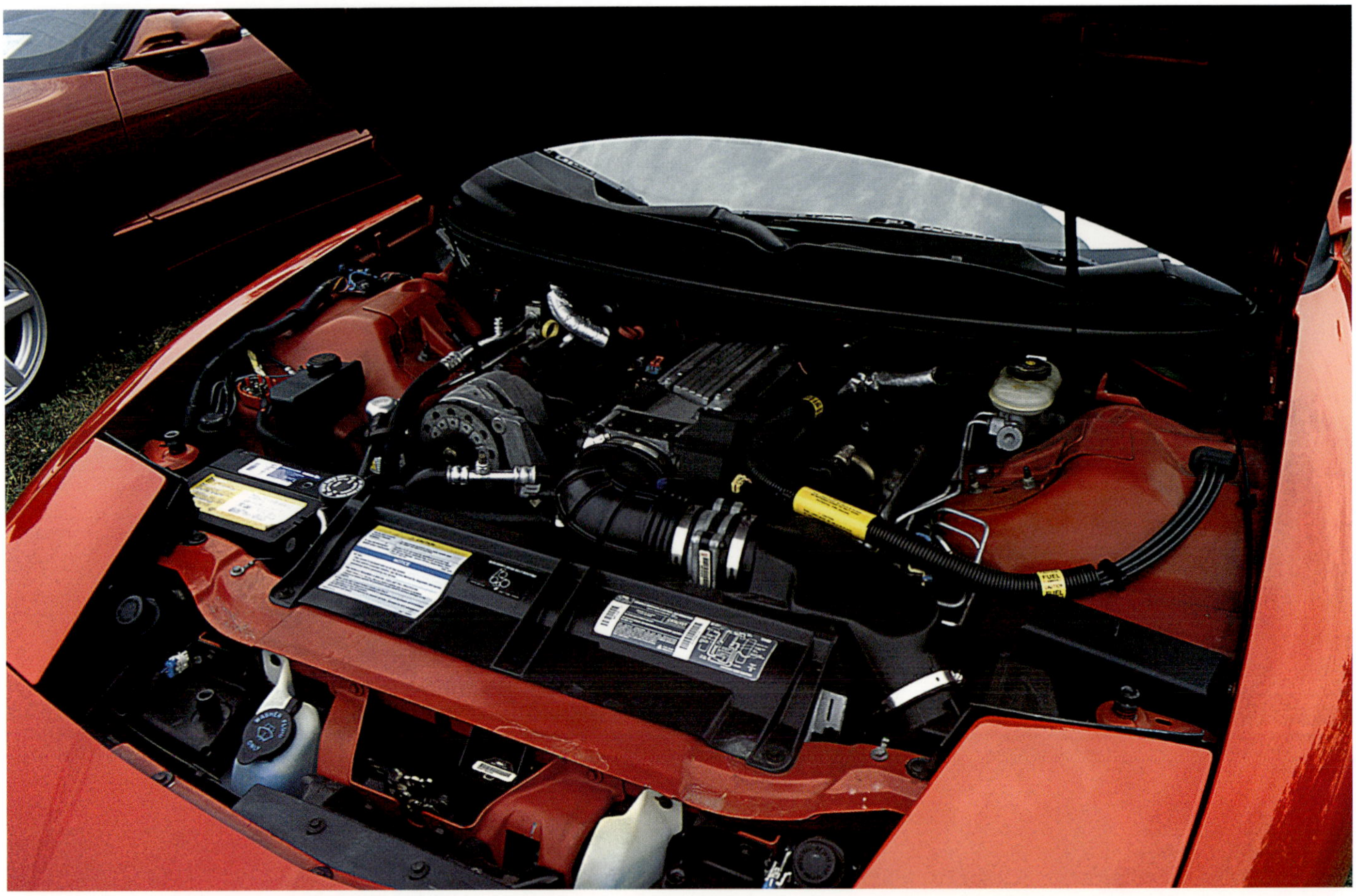

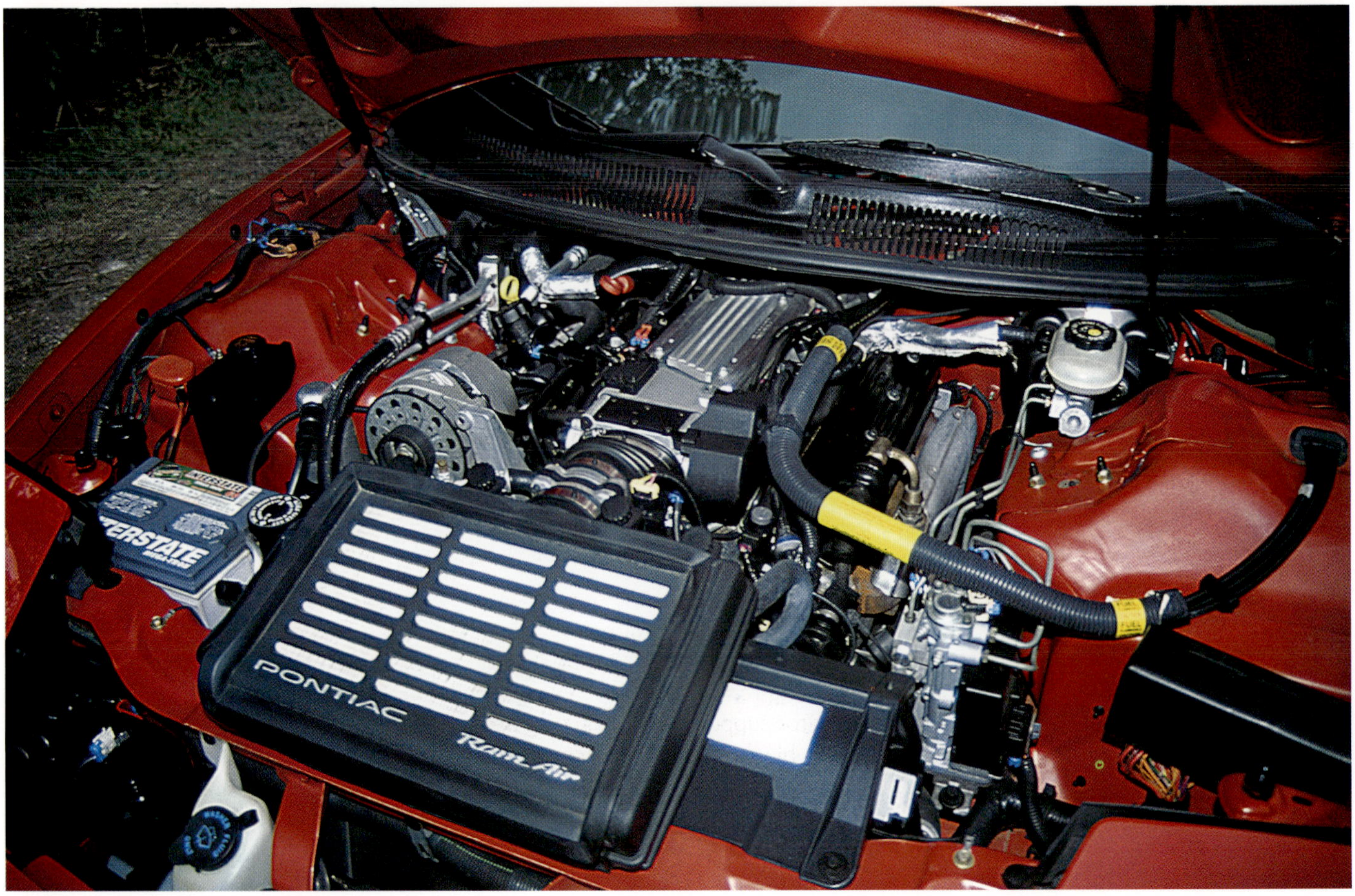
PONTIAC
Ram Air

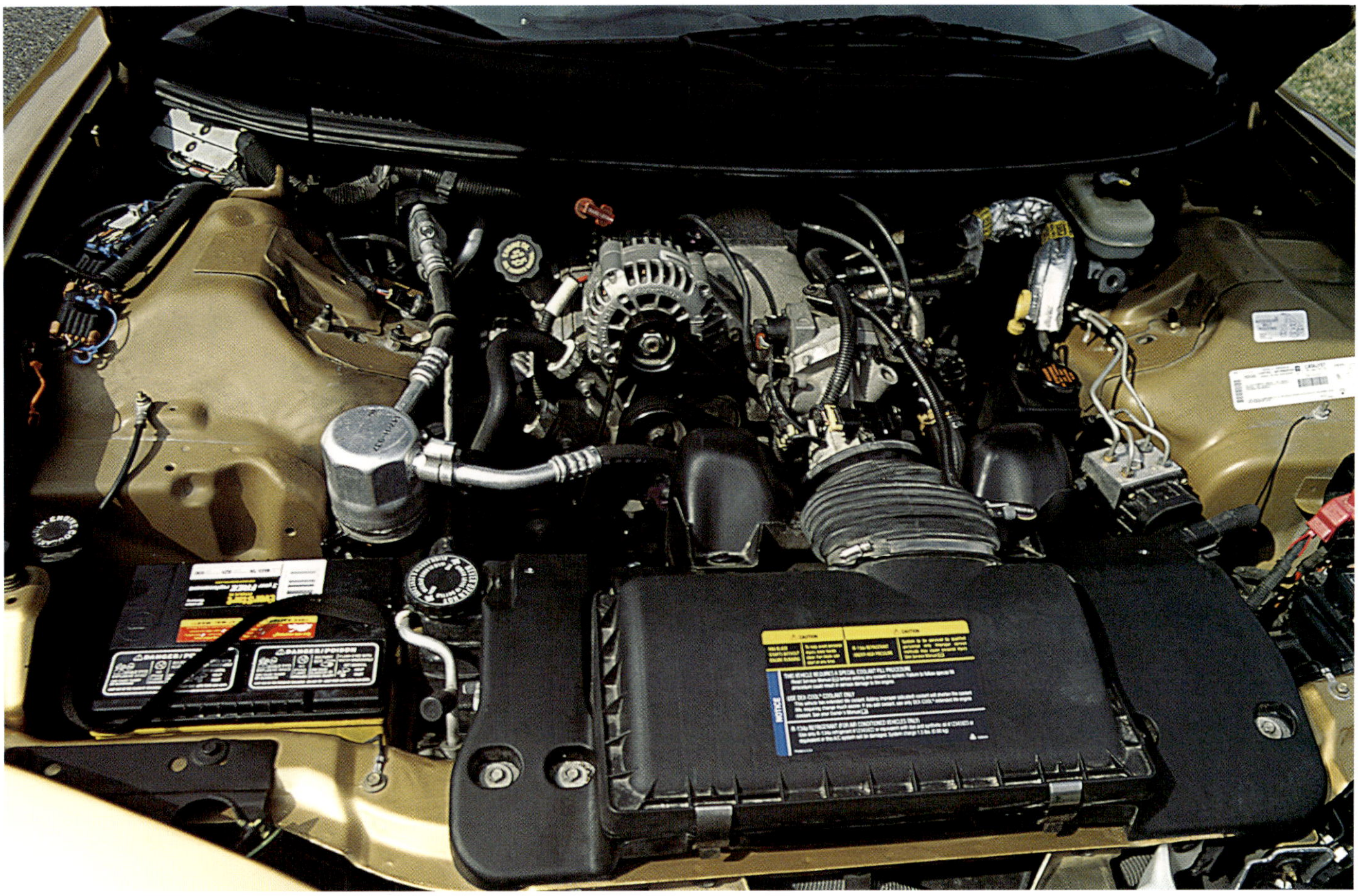

Opposite top: This is a front view of the engine compartment on an original red 1995 Firebird Formula Ram Air hatchback coupe showing the standard LT1 V-8 engine. Note the decals on the black front valance panel. *Opposite bottom:* This view of the engine compartment of an original Bright Red 1996 Trans Am WS6 Ram Air coupe with the LT1 V-8 engine shows the design of the air intake with Pontiac Ram Air logo. *Above:* This is the engine compartment of an original Sport Gold Metallic 1998 Firebird convertible equipped with the standard 231-cubic-inch V-6 (RPO L36). Note the air cleaner housing and decals. This Firebird is equipped with air conditioning.

clear coat like the outside of the body. The fenders were attached to the body with body-color hex-head bolts and washers from the inside of the engine compartment. The most significant item on the driver-side inner fenderwell was the large body-color wheelhouse bulge with the upper strut mounting studs and nuts on its inside edge. There were two white decals on the front top of the wheelhouse. The rear decal was the routing information for the serpentine accessory belt. The front decal was the emission control information decal. A small black ground wire is attached to a brass stud and flat steel hex nut on the front side of the wheelhouse.

Two flat, black-plastic-covered fuse and relay boxes with white printed markings were mounted in front of the wheelhouse. A black positive cable with red connector cover was attached to the right side of the rear box. Small yellow, blue, and orange wires exit from the right side of the front box. A body-color small steel tower holding a rubber hood bumper on a stud was mounted at the left front corner of the compartment.

The body-color radiator support was covered across its center with the black-plastic air intake shroud. The air filter canister attached with two hex-head bolts and washers on each side and its flat black rectangular lid was secured in the front with two small metal clips. An oval flexible hose was attached to the air filter with a metal clamp, exited the rear of the canister, and attached to the front of the throttle body plenum on the engine intake manifold.

A yellow-and-black coolant fill warning decal was mounted on the upper center of the air filter canister on the standard system. On the Ram Air system, the warning decal was mounted on the left side of the air filter, and a large black-and-yellow Ram Air Pontiac decal was in the top center of the filter. A black radiator filler cap was mounted to the right of the air intake housing. A white plastic windshield-washer reservoir with right side filler was mounted in front of the radiator support and surrounded the center hood latch mounting. The black Delco Freedom battery was mounted in the right front corner of the engine compartment behind the radiator support.

When the V-6 engine was ordered, the alternator was mounted on the upper right of the engine. The V-8 alternator was mounted lower on the engine and was not as visible as the V-6 unit. If air conditioning was ordered, the aluminum A/C receiver/dryer was mounted to the rear of the battery in the front right of the engine compartment, and the lines exit from the left and rear of the canister. The body-color right strut tower was to the rear of the A/C receiver/dryer, and the engine oil filler and dipstick handle were

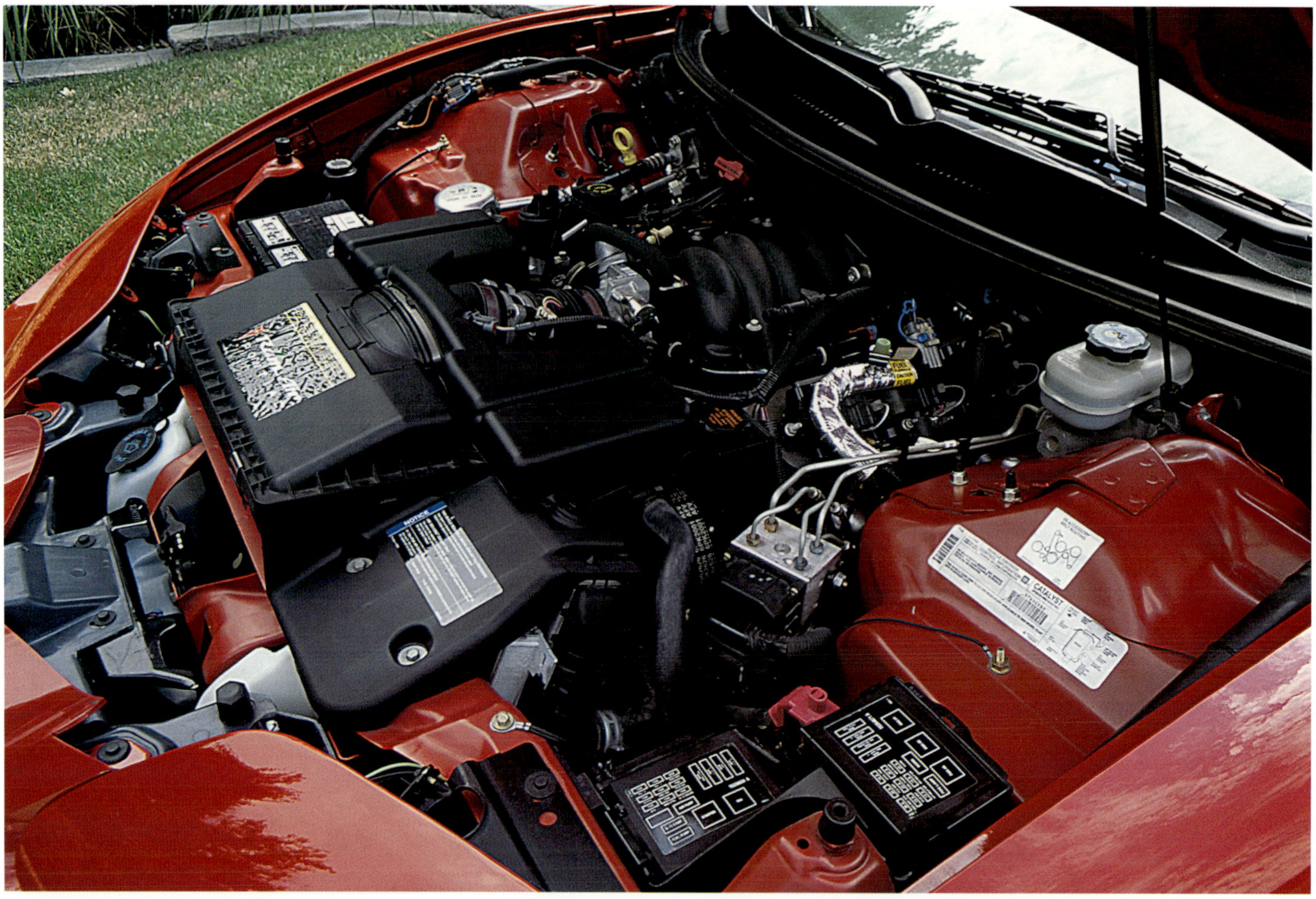

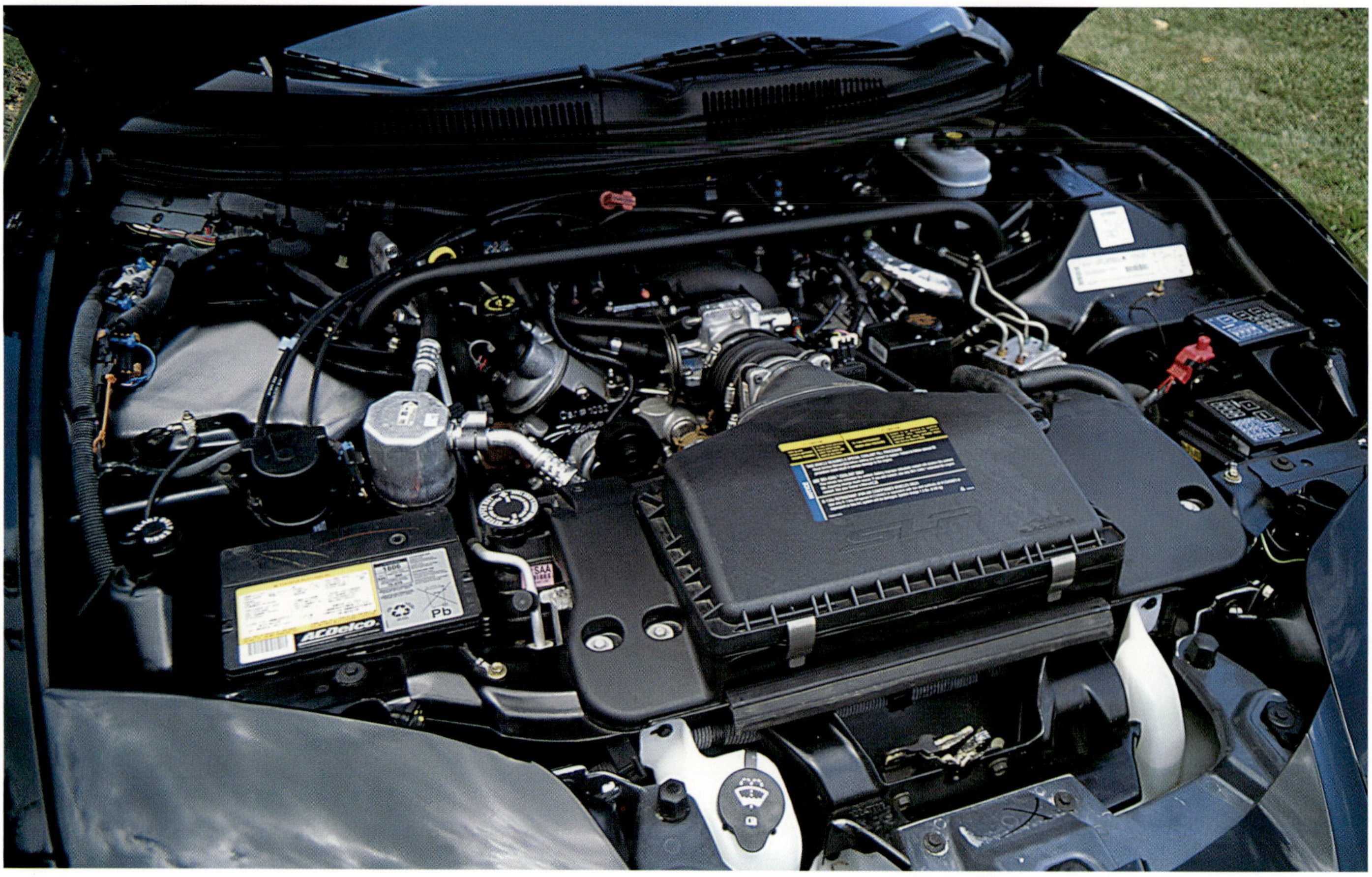

Opposite top: This photo shows the left side of the engine compartment of a Bright Red 2000 Trans Am WS6 Ram Air coupe equipped with the 5.7-liter LS1 aluminum V-8. Note the design of the air intake. *Opposite bottom and below:* This is the engine compartment of a black 2002 Trans Am Firehawk hatchback coupe equipped with a 345-horsepower 5.7-liter LS1 Ram Air V-8. Note the distinctive SLP logo embossed on the top of the intake box. The transverse chassis reinforcement is an add-on accessory. There is a white plastic windshield washer bottle on either side of the hood latch assembly.

on the right side of the engine. The computer control module and related wiring were installed at the right rear corner of the engine compartment next to the passenger side of the firewall under the upper cowl.

The driver side of the firewall held the brake master cylinder and vacuum booster. The dual master cylinder reservoir was white translucent plastic with a black plastic cap with yellow lettering. The single body-color hood hinge was mounted at the rear of the hood at each rear corner, and the hood was held open with a thin black gas strut on each side.

Frame, Transmission, and Driveline

All 1993–2002 Firebirds used welded-steel construction with an integral front subframe to support the engine and front suspension crossmember. There were two different front crossmembers in 1993, two in 1994, five in 1995, four in 1996 and 1997, and four in 1998–2002. Crossmember part numbers varied according to engine options and years. The body structure consisted of a welded-steel floorpan and monocoque body frame structure including the front fender supports, radiator support, and rear quarters. The front body structure, firewall, and rear quarters were finished in body color. The underside of the body had light gray primer with body-color overspray heavier in the center of the pan and lighter at the rear. A thick black undercoat-type material was sprayed from the outside along the outer body frame member with a narrow line of overspray on the floorpan. The purpose of this coating was for appearance only and was used to show black under the outside edge of the body rather than body color.

Front Suspension

The 1993–2002 Firebird suspension used a short/long arm (SLA) front suspension with power rack-and-pinion steering and orange-painted deCarbon tubular shock absorbers with French-language labels. The semigloss-black-painted front coil spring/shock absorber units were attached between the inside end of the long lower control arm and the upper fenderwell in the front body structure. The upper control arm was a wishbone design. The lower control arms were attached to the outer ends of the front crossmember that also supported the engine. The standard Firebird front suspension included a 30-millimeter tubular anti-roll bar with a number of variations each year according to engine options and suspension packages. The new front suspension design provided a smoother ride with better handling and control. Both upper and

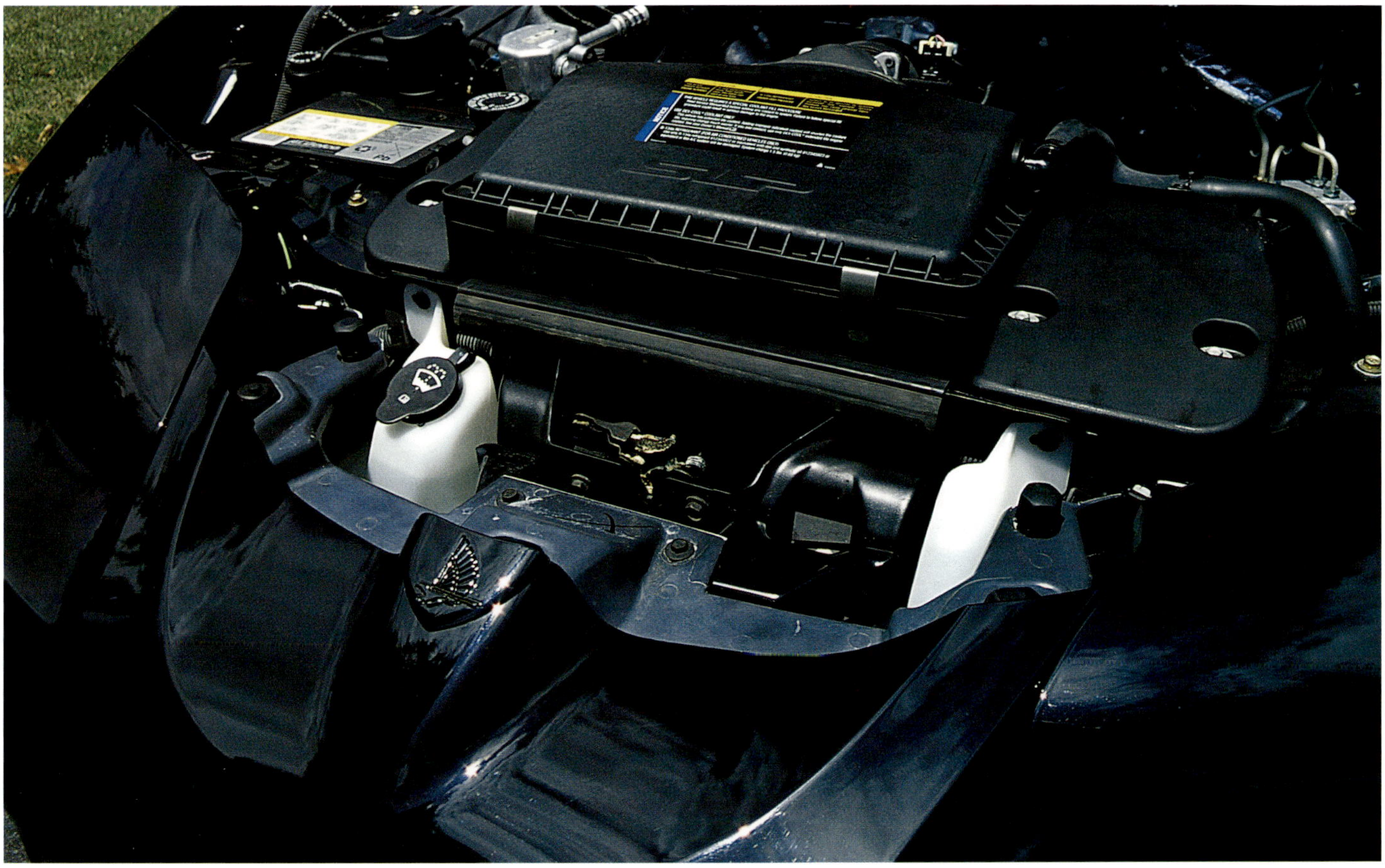

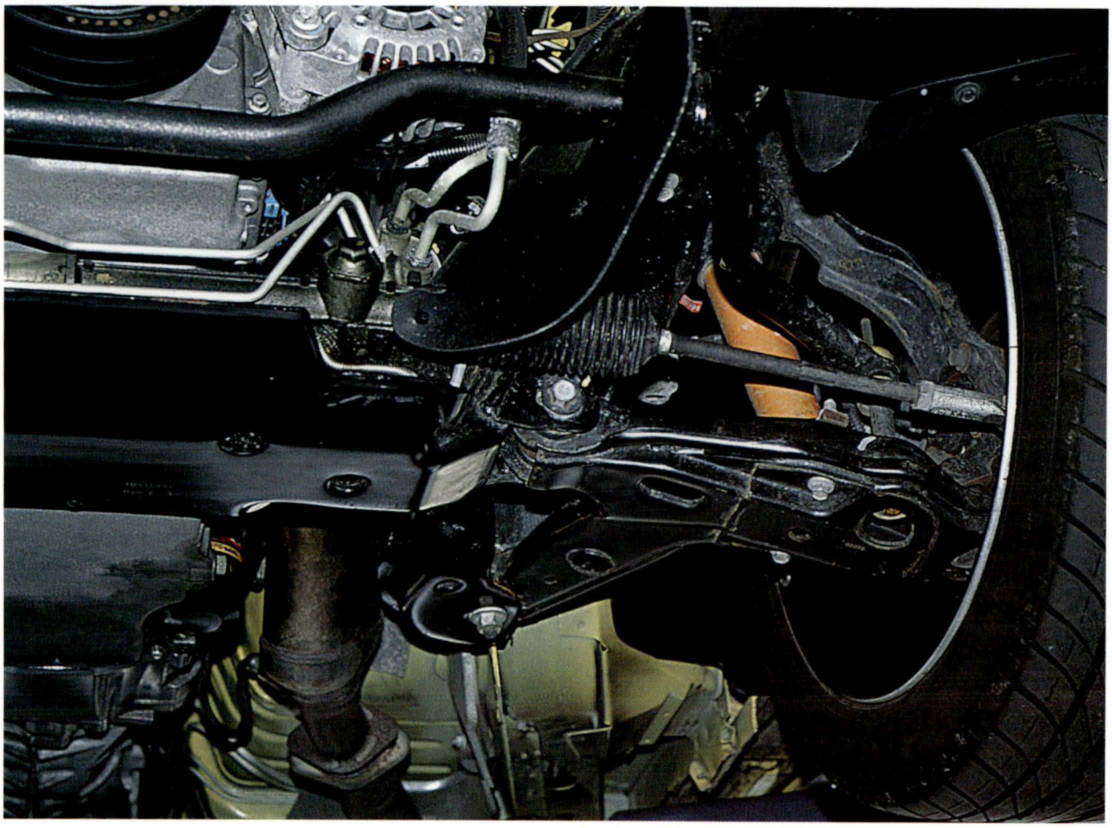

This detail view of the left front suspension on a 2002 Trans Am Collector Edition shows the rubber boot for the rack-and-pinion steering and the orange deCarbon shock absorber.

lower control arms and the anti-roll bar were painted semigloss black on all models.

The standard front brakes for all 1993–1997 Firebirds were 10.9-inch-diameter vented power discs with single-piston cast-iron-finish calipers and standard semimetallic pads. The 1998–2002 front brakes were 11.9-inch discs, and the calipers were dual-piston units. The 1998–2002 pads were organic material. The Firebird front disc/rear drum and four-wheel disc brake systems included a standard Delco Moraine four-wheel ABS VI three-channel four-wheel anti-lock system. In 1998, a new Bosch 5.3 ABS system was adopted along with automatic traction control.

The standard Firebird power rack-and-pinion steering gear had an overall ratio of 16.9:1 and 2.67 turns lock to lock with the F41 suspension package. The Trans Am and Formula equipped with the FE2 Firm Ride and Handling Package had a faster standard 14.4:1 steering ratio with 2.3 turns lock to lock. In each year from 1993 to 2000, there were six different steering gear assemblies according to the model, engine, and suspension package. In 2000–2002, there were only two steering gear assemblies used. All except the 3800 GT with the Y87 package used part number 26077996. Those with the FE2, FE4, F41 suspension packages, and the GT with the Y87 package used part number 28062311. A convoluted black rubber boot was used to cover the rack-and-steering-arm connection.

Rear Suspension

The 1993–2002 Firebird rear axle was a Salisbury-type semifloating design with a 7.5-inch ring gear and 10-bolt cover. The axle was available in 1993 and 1994 with open and Safe-T-Track (RPO G80) differential ratios of 2.73:1 (RPO GU2) and 3.23:1 (RPO GU5). For 1995–2002, the rear axle ratios were available in 2.73:1, 3.08:1 (RPO GU4), and 3.23:1. The 3.23:1 was considered a performance ratio and was only available in the Formula and Trans Am with automatic transmission and QLC or QLK tires.

Axle codes varied for each year, and the gear ratio varied according to the model and engine/transmission configuration. The axle code was stamped on the front passenger side of the axle tube or on an identification tag attached to the carrier cover. The rear axle assembly was lightly painted flat black and had paint codes identifying the various configurations. The 2002 SLP Firehawk was available with a special high-performance Bilstein suspension system that included an Auburn high-torque performance differential with an AAM cast-aluminum cover.

The 1993–2002 Firebird rear suspension design was similar to that used in the third-generation Firebirds and consisted of outboard semitrailing lower control arms with semigloss- black-painted coil springs, tubular shock absorbers, and an aft-mounted transverse track bar. The 1993 rear suspension had softer springs than the previous year and featured long-life deCarbon high-pressure

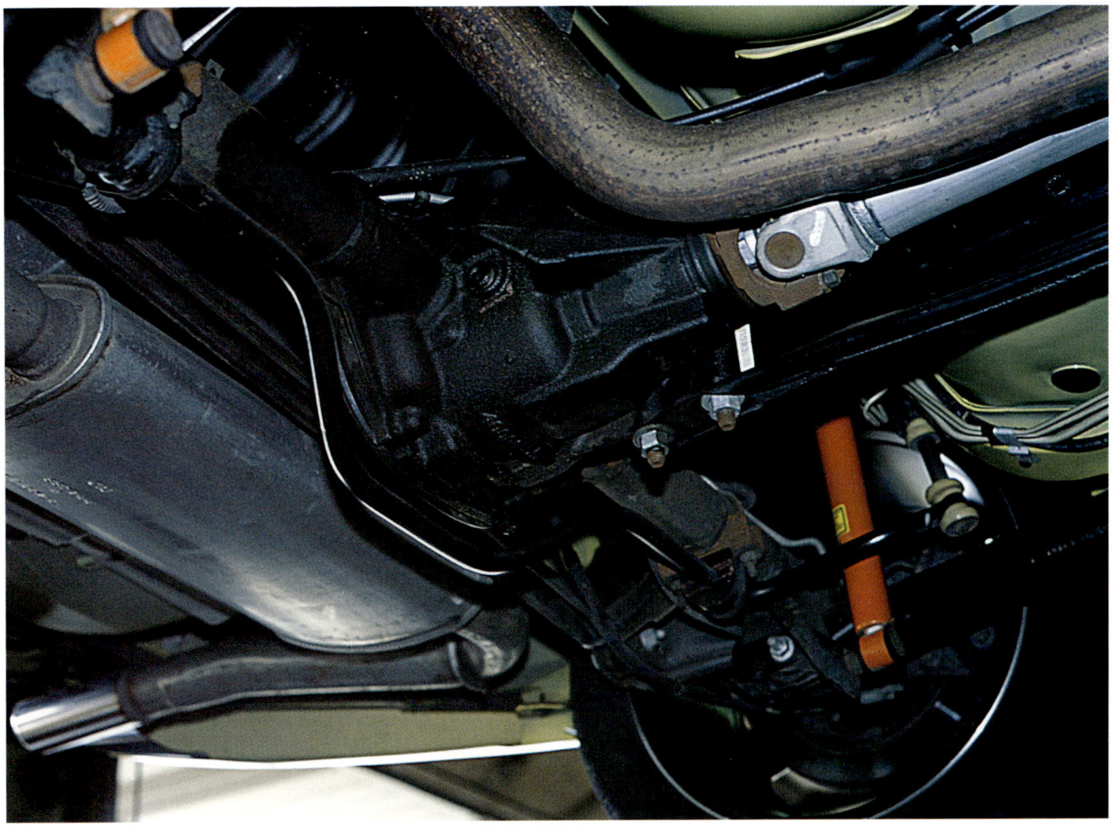

This detail view of the rear axle and rear suspension of a 2002 Trans Am Collector Edition shows the 10-bolt General Motors axle assembly and transverse muffler mounting.

gas-charged shock absorbers. The shock absorbers were painted bright orange and had French-language labels. The 1993–2002 rear suspension also included the previous model's semigloss-black-painted torque arm that extended from the differential housing through the transmission tunnel to the transmission. The Firebird rear suspension included a semigloss-black-painted stabilizer bar for all models with a 17-millimeter bar used for the Firebird and a 19-millimeter bar for the Formula and Trans Am.

The standard rear brakes on all 1993–2002 base Firebirds were drum-type hydraulic with 9.5-inch cast-iron finned drums. Standard asbestos linings were 2 inches wide. Four-wheel disc brakes (RPO J65) were standard on the 1993–2002 Formula and Trans Am. The rear brake calipers were single piston with the first design caliper assembly used in 1993–1997 and another in 1998–2002. The 1993–1997 AC/Delco calipers (18H223 part number 18031697) fit left and right and had a 1⁹⁄₁₆-inch bore diameter and included a parking brake assembly. The 1998–2002 calipers used part number 12455127 (left) and 12455128 (right). The 1993–1997 brake rotors were vented with 11.4-inch diameter, and the 1998–2002 rotors were 12 inches in diameter. The 1998–2002 rotors incorporated a new inner drum for the parking brake shoes. The 1993–1997 brake pads were semi-metallic, but they were changed to organic material in 1998–2002.

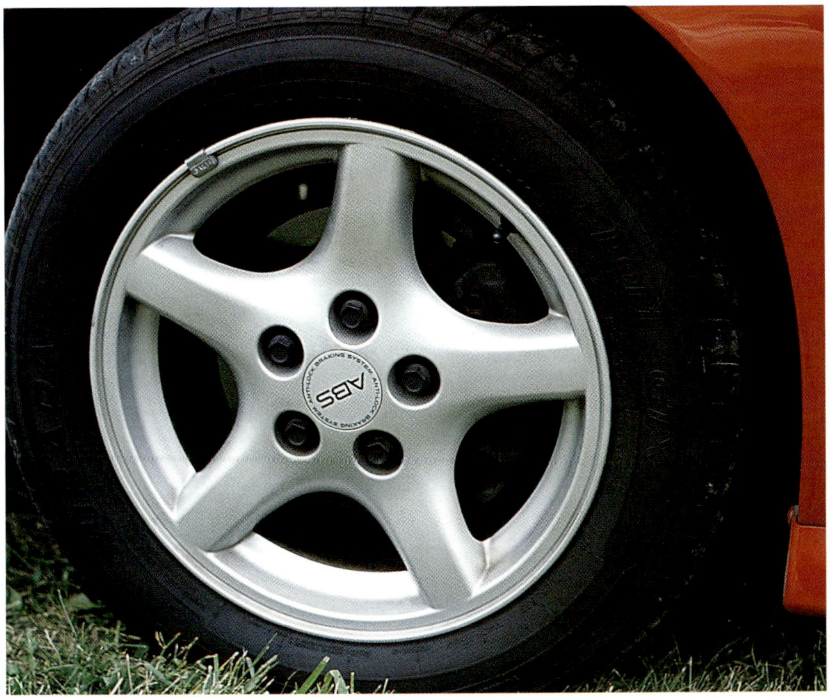

This is the left front wheel of a red 1995 Trans Am coupe equipped with the standard 16x8 five-spoke sparkle silver sport cast-aluminum wheels (RPO N60). Note the anti-lock braking system badge in the center hub.

Tires and Wheels

The standard wheels for the 1993 and 1994 base Firebird were 16x7.5 cast-aluminum (RPO QA7). Firebirds prior to VIN 214500 used a wheel with part number 12525669, and those after that VIN used a Dark Argent wheel with part number 12513701. Standard wheels for the 1993 and 1994 Formula and Trans Am were 16x8

Sport cast-aluminum (RPO PA7) in bright-sparkle silver color with part number 12517528. This same wheel was also available with the Formula and Trans Am in bright white with part number 12513702. The 1994 25th Anniversary Trans Am (RPO B71) used a unique Arctic White five-spoke aluminum wheel with part number 12523763.

The standard wheels for the 1995 base Firebird were the same Dark Argent 16x7.5 wheels used since 1993. Optional with the Firebird and standard with the Formula and Trans Am were five-spoke bright cast-aluminum sparkle silver 16x8 Sport wheels with part number 9592446 (RPO N60). A similar five-spoke Sport wheel in chrome with part number 9592454 was available with RPO P05.

For 1996, the standard wheels for the Firebird, Formula, and Trans Am were cast-aluminum bright-silver five-spoke 16x8 Sport wheels with part number 9592446 (RPO N60). A similar wheel in bright-chrome finish was available with RPO P05. A unique wheel was available only with the WS6 Ram Air Performance and Handling Package. It was a cast-aluminum five-spoke 17x8 wheel (RPO N66) with part number 9592510.

For 1997, the standard wheels for the Firebird, Formula, and Trans Am were 16x8 bright-silver cast-aluminum five-spoke Sport wheels (RPO N60) with part number 9593120 for the first design. A second design was used with part number with RPO P05 and part number 9593122. Optional wheels for all models were a similar 16x8 cast-aluminum five-spoke Sport wheels with chrome finish (RPO P05) and part number 12365482. A 17x8 polished cast-aluminum five-spoke Sport wheel (RPO N66, part number 9593305) was available only with the WS6 Ram Air package in the Formula and Trans Am.

In 1998, wheel selections and options changed for all models. The standard wheels for the Firebird were 16x8 Sport five-spoke bright-silver cast-aluminum wheels (RPO N60, part number 9593301). The standard wheels for the Formula and Trans Am were 16x8 cast-aluminum five-spoke Sport wheels in silver finish (RPO PA6, part number 9592907). The optional wheels for the Firebird, Formula, and Trans Am were 16x8 cast-aluminum chrome-finish five-spoke Sport wheels (RPO P05, part number 9593303). The 17x9 five-spoke cast-aluminum polished Sport wheels (RPO N66, part number 9593305) were available only with the WS6 Performance and Handling Package in the Formula and Trans Am.

In 1999–2002, the standard wheels for the Firebird were the same 16x8 RPO N60 wheels used in 1998. Standard wheels for the 1999–2002 Formula and Trans Am were also the same RPO PA6 wheels used in 1998. The optional RPO P05

Below: This is a standard 16x8 sport five-spoke bright silver cast-aluminum wheel (RPO N60) on a Sport Gold Metallic 1998 Firebird convertible. Note the black-and-silver ABS badge in the center hub. ***Bottom:*** This is the special 17x8 five-spoke cast-aluminum wheel finished in blue tint with special 30th Anniversary center cap medallion. This wheel is standard on the 1999 Trans Am 30th Anniversary Edition coupe and convertible.

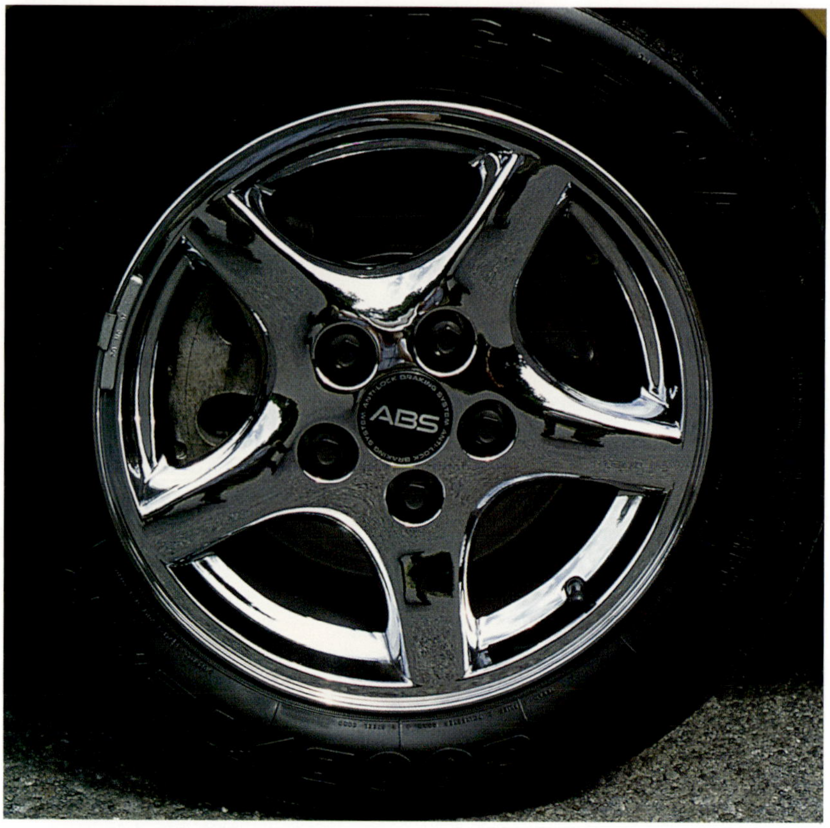

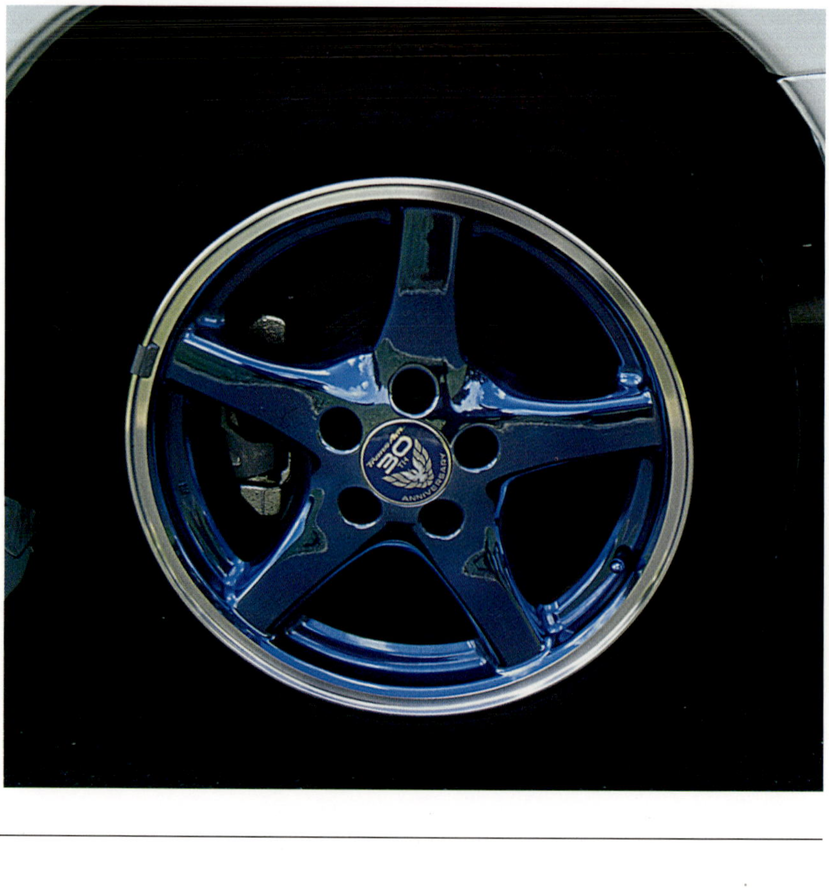

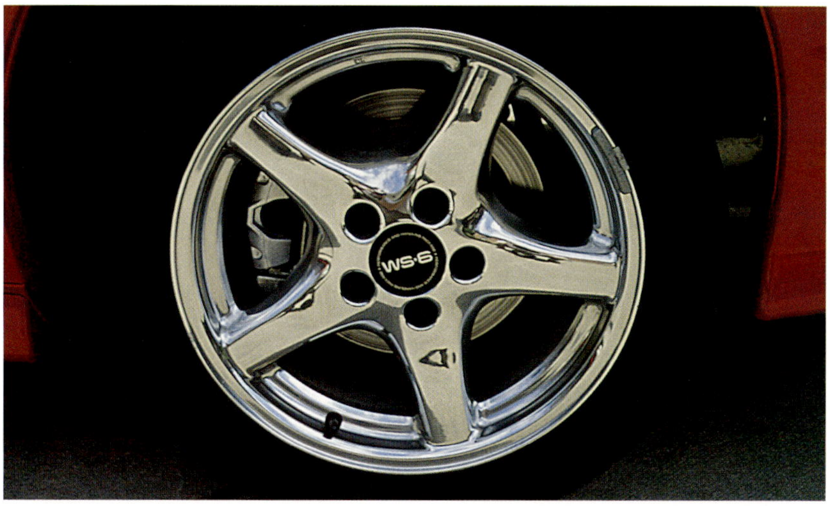

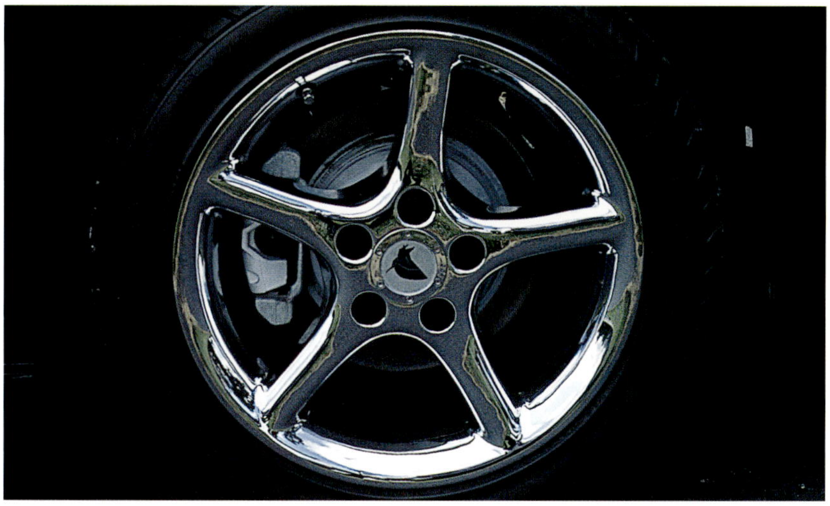

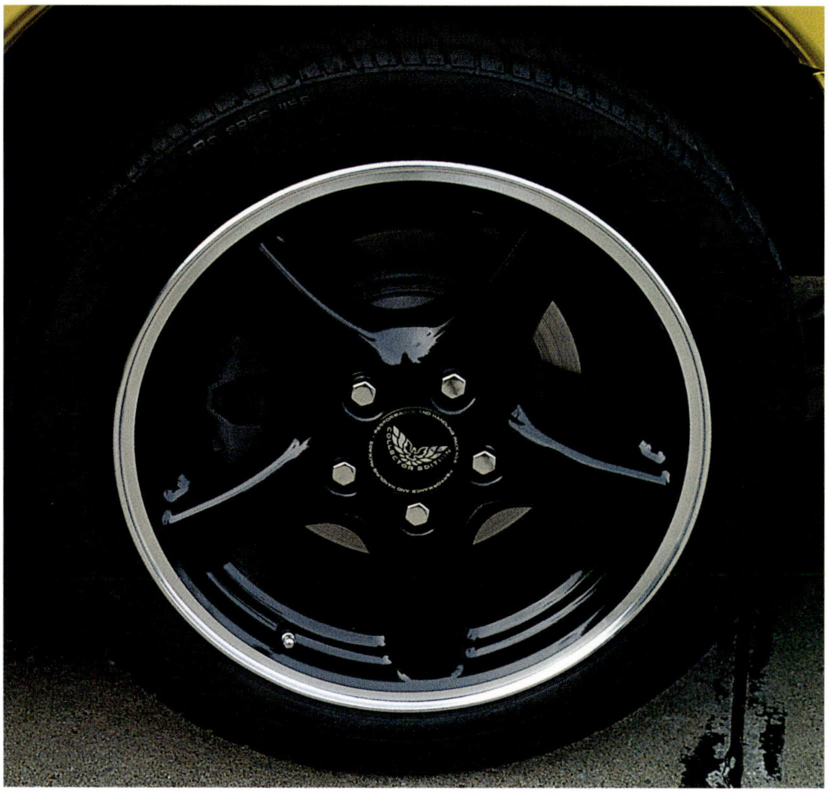

Top: This is the left rear wheel on a Bright Red 2000 Trans Am WS6 Ram Air coupe with T-top. The standard wheel was a bright-finish 17x9 sport spoke cast-aluminum (RPO QF6). Note the WS6 Performance and Handling Package badge in the center hub. ***Middle:*** The standard wheel on a black 2002 Trans Am Firehawk coupe. This 17x9 bright highly polished cast-aluminum sport five-spoke wheel (RPO QB6) has a special Firehawk center hub medallion. The standard tires were 275/40ZR17 black-sidewall Firehawk radials. ***Bottom:*** This is a black painted version of the 17x9 cast-aluminum five-spoke sport wheel on a 2002 yellow Collector Edition Trans Am. Note the bright outer rim and special silver bird in the center hub.

wheels for 1999 were the same part number (9593303) used in 1998. The optional RPO N66 17x9 spoke Sport wheels used since 1997 were continued for 1999 with the WS6 package. In 1999, the 30th Anniversary Appearance Package (RPO Z4C) on the Trans Am had standard 17x8 five-spoke highly polished cast-aluminum wheels finished in medium-blue tint with a special blue-and-silver 30th Anniversary hubcap (part number 9593526).

For 2000, a standard wheel came with the WS6 Performance and Handling Package with a new dished, slotted design with RPO N66 and part number 9583474. Optional for 2000 and standard with the 2001 WS6 package was a 17x9 Sport five-spoke cast-aluminum wheel with RPO QF6 and part number 9593305. In 2002, a new 17x9 highly polished cast-aluminum Sport-spoke wheel became optional with the WS6 package with RPO QB6 and part number 9594403. The 2002 Collector Edition package included gloss-black-painted 17x9 aluminum wheels with a distinctive center medallion. The SLP Firehawk package included special Firehawk hubcaps with a black bird in the center.

The standard tires for the 1993–1995 base Firebird were black sidewall 215/60R16 Goodyear Eagle GA steel-belted touring (RPO QPE). Standard tires for the Formula and optional for the Firebird were 235/55R16 Goodyear Eagle GA steel-belted touring (RPO QMT). Standard for the Trans Am and optional for the Formula were 245/50ZR16 Goodyear Eagle GSC steel-belted high-performance tires (RPO QLC). In 1995, the 245/50ZR16 black-sidewall tires were also available in all-weather tread (RPO QFZ) in the Trans Am convertible only.

In 1996 and 1997, the standard Firebird tires were 215/60R16 steel-belted touring tires. The standard tires for the 1996 Formula and optional with the Firebird were 235/55R16 steel-belted touring tires (RPO QCB). The standard tires for the Trans Am and optional for the Formula were

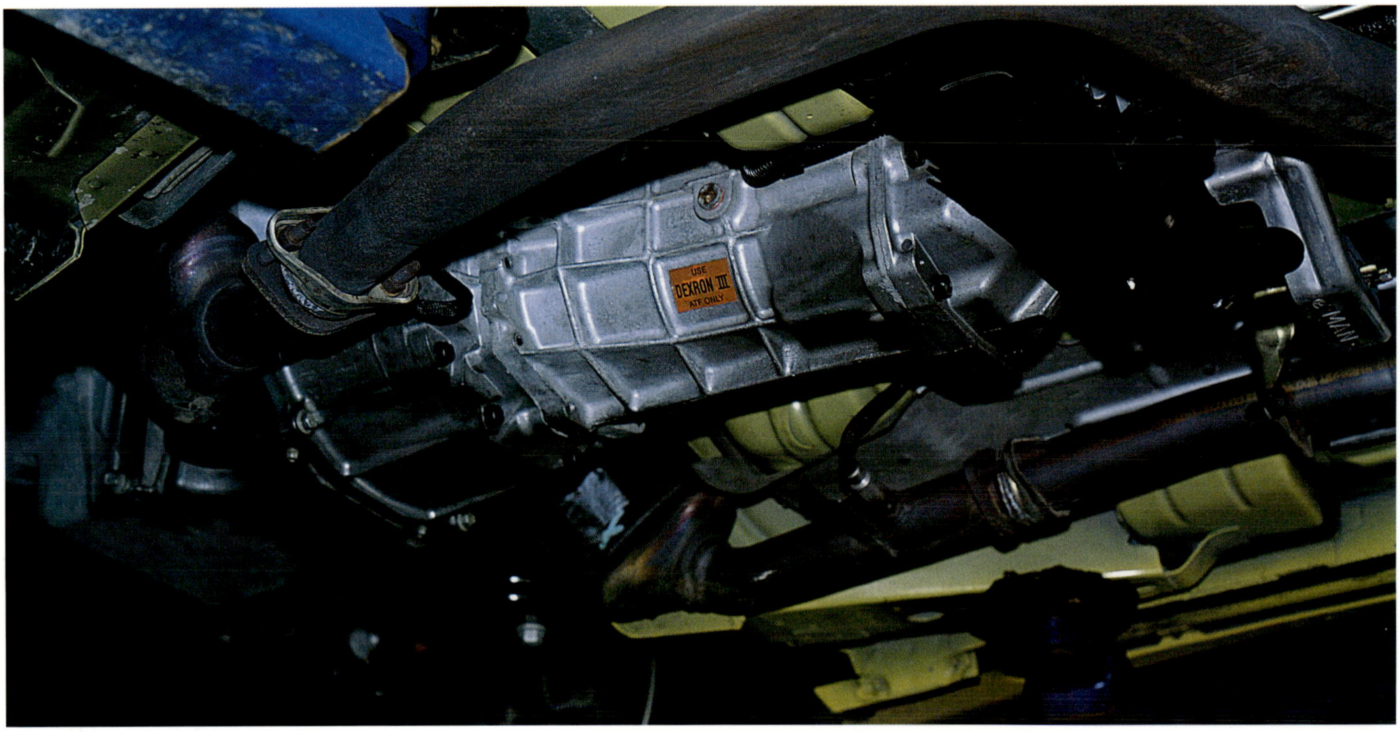

This is a detail of the underside of a 2002 yellow Collector Edition Trans Am equipped with the optional six-speed Warner T56 manual transmission and optional Hurst short-throw shifter. Note the natural-aluminum finish of the ribbed transmission case and the catalytic converter mounted at the front of the body.

245/50ZR16 black-sidewall radials. In 1996 and 1997, the WS6 Performance and Handling Package was available with optional 275/40ZR17 black-sidewall Goodyear tires (RPO QLC).

The standard Firebird tires for 1998–2002 were 215/60R16 Goodyear touring (RPO QEA). The base Firebird was available with optional (RPO QCB) 235/55R16 black-sidewall touring tires that were also part of the 3800 V-6 Performance Package (with automatic transmission only). Neither of these tires was available with the Formula or Trans Am. The standard tires with the 1998–2002 Formula and Trans Am were 245/50ZR16 all-weather black-sidewall radials (RPO QFZ). The Formula and Trans Am were available with optional 245/50ZR16 high-performance black-sidewall tires (RPO QLC). Speed-rated 275/40ZR17 black-sidewall radials were available only with the WS6 package in the Formula and Trans Am. A space-saver spare was standard on all models with a 15x4-inch wheel used in 1993–1996 and a 16x4-inch wheel used in 1997–2002.

Transmissions

The 1993–2002 Firebirds were equipped with a choice of three transmissions depending on the engine and model. The standard transmission in the Firebird with V-6 engine was a Warner T5 five-speed manual with console-mounted floor shift (RPO MM5). The 1993 and 1994 Formula and Trans Am had a standard Warner T56 six-speed manual with floor shift (RPO MN6) that was not available with the base Firebird. The ribbed cast-aluminum case T56 was developed from the T5 basic design in 1988 but entirely different, weighing 125 pounds with dual-cone synchronizers for all gears, including reverse. The T56 used in the Formula was the M28 wide-ratio version with a 3.36:1 low gear. The Trans Am used the M29 close-ratio version with a 2.97:1 low gear. All T56 transmissions had a direct fourth gear with overdrive fifth and sixth gears. The six-speed manual transmission was optional in the 1995–2002 Formula and Trans Am. In 2000–2002, an optional short-throw Hurst Performance shifter (RPO BBS) was available only with the six-speed manual transmission.

All 1993–2002 Firebirds and 1993 and 1994 Formula and Trans Am were available with an optional 4L60 four-speed overdrive automatic transmission (RPO MX0) until 1994, when the transmission was updated to a computer-controlled 4L60-E. The new computer control improved shifting performance. For the 1999 model year, a second-gear start system (SGS), optional in the earlier models, became standard. The four-speed automatic transmission was standard with the 1995–2002 Formula and Trans Am.

All 1993–2002 transmissions were connected to the rear axle by a natural-finish one-piece welded-steel driveshaft when used with the 5.7-liter V-8 engine. The V-6 engine used a two-piece natural-steel-finish driveshaft with a center support until the 1999 model year, when a new one-piece driveshaft was adopted. The driveshafts varied according to the engine and transmission applications and were marked with a black or brown stripe for identification.

Index